PERIOPERATIVE CARE

Anesthesia, Medicine, and Surgery

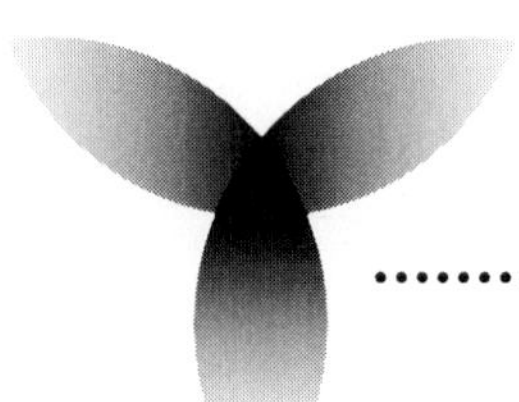

PERIOPERATIVE CARE

Anesthesia, Medicine, and Surgery

David J. Stone, M.D.
Associate Professor of Anesthesiology
Board Certified in Anesthesiology, Internal Medicine and Critical Care Medicine
University of Virginia Health Sciences Center
Charlottesville, Virginia

David L. Bogdonoff, M.D.
Associate Professor of Anesthesiology and Surgery
Board Certified in Anesthesiology and Surgery
University of Virginia Health Sciences Center
Charlottesville, Virginia

George S. Leisure, M.D.
Assistant Professor of Anesthesiology
Board Certified in Anesthesiology and Internal Medicine
University of Virginia Health Sciences Center
Charlottesville, Virginia

Burkhard F. Spiekermann, M.D.
Assistant Professor of Anesthesiology
Board Certified in Anesthesiology
University of Virginia Health Sciences Center
Charlottesville, Virginia

Donald D. Mathes, M.D.
Assistant Professor of Anesthesia
Board Certified in Anesthesia and Internal Medicine
The Bowman Gray School of Medicine of Wake Forest University
Winston-Salem, North Carolina

with 39 contributors

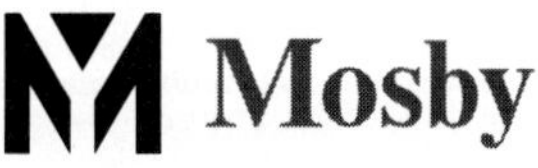

St. Louis Baltimore Boston Carlsbad Chicago Minneapolis New York Philadelphia Portland
London Milan Sydney Tokyo Toronto

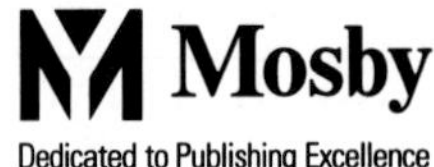

A Times Mirror Company

Senior Editor: Laurel Craven
Developmental Editor: Kimberley J. Cox
Project Manager: Chris Baumle
Production Editor: Eric Van Gorden
Manufacturing Supervisor: William A. Winneberger, Jr.
Designer: Carolyn O'Brien

First Edition

Printed in the United States of America

Mosby–Year Book, Inc.
11830 Westline Industrial Drive
St. Louis, Missouri 63146

Printed in the United States of America

Library of Congress Cataloging-in-Publication Data

Perioperative care: anesthesia, medicine, and surgery / David J. Stone . . . [et al.].
p. cm.
Includes bibliographical references and index.
ISBN 0-8151-4639-6
1. Therapeutics, Surgical. I. Stone, David J.
[DNLM: 1. Preoperative Care—methods. 2. Intraoperative Care—methods. 3. Postoperative Care—methods. WO 179 P445 1997]
RD49.P45 1997
617'.91—dc21
DNLM/DLC
for Library of Congress 97-16896
CIP

---

97 98 99 00 01 / 9 8 7 6 5 4 3 2 1

Contributors

Victor C. Baum, M.D.
Associate Professor of Anesthesiology and Pediatrics
Attending Physician, Departments of Anesthesiology and Pediatrics
University of Virginia Health Sciences Center
Charlottesville, Virginia

Daniel M. Becker, M.D., M.P.H.
Professor and Chief, Division of General Medicine
Department of Internal Medicine
University of Virginia Health Sciences Center
Charlottesville, Virginia

Frederic A. Berry, M.D.
Professor of Anesthesiology and Pediatrics
University of Virginia Health Sciences Center
Charlottesville, Virginia

David L. Bogdonoff, M.D.
Associate Professor of Anesthesiology and Surgery
University of Virginia Health Sciences Center
Charlottesville, Virginia

Stephen H. Caldwell, M.D.
Assistant Professor of Internal Medicine
Director, Clinical Hepatology
University of Virginia Health Sciences Center
Charlottesville, Virginia

Alison S. Carr, M.B., B.S. (Lond.), F.R.C.A.
Assistant Professor in Clinical Anesthesiology
Department of Anesthesiology
University of Virginia Health Sciences Center
Charlottesville, Virginia

John M. Dent, M.D.
Assistant Professor of Medicine, Cardiovascular Division
Director of Echocardiography
University of Virginia Health Sciences Center
Charlottesville, Virginia

David J. Di Benedetto, M.D.
Resident, Department of Anesthesiology
University of Virginia Health Sciences Center
Charlottesville, Virginia

Cosmo A. DiFazio, Ph.D., M.D.
Professor of Anesthesiology
University of Virginia Health Sciences Center
Charlottesville, Virginia

Carolyn J. Driscoll, R.N., M.S.N.
Hepatology Nurse Coordinator
University of Virginia Health Sciences Center
Charlottesville, Virginia

Charles G. Durbin, Jr., M.D., F.C.C.M.
Professor of Anesthesiology and Surgery
Medical Director, SICU
University of Virginia Health Sciences Center
Charlottesville, Virginia

Nicholas C. Gagliano, M.D.
Resident, Department of Anesthesiology
University of Virginia Health Sciences Center
Charlottesville, Virginia

Thomas J. Gal, M.D.
Professor of Anesthesiology
Attending Anesthesiologist
University of Virginia Health Sciences Center
Charlottesville, Virginia

A. Sinan Gursoy, M.D.
Assistant Professor of Medicine
Division of Cardiology
University of South Florida
Director, Interventional Electrophysiology and
Cardiac Arrhythmia Services
Tampa, Florida

Jerry A. Hall, M.D.
Senior Associate Consultant
Mayo Clinic Jacksonville
Jacksonville, Florida

Timothy N. Harwood, M.D.
Assistant Professor of Anesthesiology
Bowman Gray School of Medicine
Wake Forest University
Attending Anesthesiologist
North Carolina Baptist Hospital
Winston-Salem, North Carolina

Cassandra A. Kennedy, M.D.
Chief Surgical Resident, General Surgery
Kern Medical Center
Bakersfield, California

Daniel J. Kennedy, M.D.
Assistant Professor of Cardiac Anesthesia/Critical Care Medicine
Department of Anesthesia
Bowman Gray School of Medicine
Winston-Salem, North Carolina

John A. Kern, M.D.
Resident, Division of Thoracic and Cardiovascular Surgery
University of Virginia Health Sciences Center
Charlottesville, Virginia

Alan T. Lefor, M.A., M.D.
Professor of Clinical Surgery
University of California, San Diego School of Medicine
San Diego, California
Program Director in General Surgery
Kern Medical Center
Bakersfield, California

George S. Leisure, M.D.
Assistant Professor of Anesthesiology
University of Virginia Health Sciences Center
Charlottesville, Virginia

Neil P. Lewis, M.B., B.S., M.D., M.R.C.P.
Assistant Professor of Internal Medicine (Cardiology)
University of Virginia Health Sciences Center
Charlottesville, Virginia

Robert C. Li, M.D.
Chief Resident, Department of Anesthesiology
University of Virginia Health Sciences Center
Charlottesville, Virginia

Jonathan R. Lindner, M.D.
Assistant Professor, Cardiovascular Division
University of Virginia Health Sciences Center
Charlottesville, Virginia

Mark E. Lovelock, M.B., B.S., F.R.A.C.S.
Vascular Surgeon
St. Vincent's Hospital, Fitzroy
Angliss Hospital, Ferntree Gully
Victoria, Australia

Stuart M. Lowson, M.B., B.S., M.R.C.P., F.R.C.A.
Assistant Professor
Department of Anesthesiology
University of Virginia Health Sciences Center
Charlottesville, Virginia

Donald D. Mathes, M.D.
Assistant Professor of Anesthesia
The Bowman Gray School of Medicine
Wake Forest University
Winston-Salem, North Carolina

George Monir, M.D.
Fellow in Cardiovascular Medicine
University of South Florida
Tampa, Florida

Jennifer E. O'Flaherty, M.D., M.P.H.
Assistant Professor of Anesthesiology
University of Virginia Health Sciences Center
Charlottesville, Virginia

Lawrence H. Phillips, II, M.D.
Professor and Vice-Chairman of Neurology
University of Virginia
Charlottesville, Virginia

Timothy L. Pruett, M.D.
Professor of Surgery
Chief, Transplantation Surgery
University of Virginia Health Sciences Center
Charlottesville, Virginia

William T. Ross, Jr., M.D., M.B.A.
Professor of Anesthesiology
University of Virginia Health Sciences Center
Medical Director
Virginia Ambulatory Surgery Center
Charlottesville, Virginia

Marc A. Rozner, Ph.D., M.D.
Assistant Professor of Anesthesiology
Assistant Professor of Pharmacology and Therapeutics
Medical Director, Perioperative Assessment Center
Medical Director, Post Anesthesia Care Unit
University of South Florida College of Medicine
Staff Anesthesiologist, Tampa General Hospital
Staff Anesthesiologist, H. Lee Moffitt Cancer Center
Staff Anesthesiologist, James A. Haley Veterans Hospital
Tampa, Florida

Bruce David Schirmer, M.D.
Stephen H. Watts Professor of Surgery
University of Virginia Health Sciences Center
Director, Laparoscopy Institute of Virginia
University of Virginia Health Sciences Center
Charlottesville, Virginia

David M. Sibell, M.D.
Assistant Professor
Department of Anesthesiology
Oregon Health Sciences University
Portland, Oregon

Burkhard F. Spiekermann, M.D.
Assistant Professor of Anesthesiology
University of Virginia Health Sciences Center
Charlottesville, Virginia

David J. Stone, M.D.
Associate Professor of Anesthesiology
University of Virginia Health Sciences Center
Charlottesville, Virginia

Curtis G. Tribble, M.D.
Professor of Surgery
University of Virginia Health Sciences Center
Charlottesville, Virginia

Mary Lee Vance, M.D.
Professor of Medicine and Neurosurgery
University of Virginia Health Sciences Center
Charlottesville, Virginia

Guy L. Weinberg, M.D.
Assistant Professor
University of Illinois College of Medicine
Staff Anesthesiologist
V.A. West Side Medical Center
Chicago, Illinois

Rebecca W. West, J.D.
Assistant Professor of General Medicine
University of Virginia Health Sciences Center
Managing Director
Piedmont Liability Trust
Charlottesville, Virginia

Brian Wispelway, M.S., M.D.
Associate Professor of Medicine
Director, Infectious Diseases Clinic
University of Virginia Health Sciences Center
Charlottesville, Virginia

Terrance A. Yemen, M.D.
Associate Professor
Anesthesia Department
McGill University
Anesthetist-in-Chief
Montreal Children's Hospital
Anesthetist-in-Chief, Shriners Hospital for Children
Montreal, Quebec

Jeffrey S. Young, M.D.
Assistant Professor of Surgery and Emergency Medicine
Director, Trauma Center
University of Virginia Health Sciences Center
Charlottesville, Virginia

Foreword

The physiologic state of the anesthetized patient differs significantly from the physiologic state of the unanesthetized preoperative patient and the patient receiving postoperative analgesia. The postoperative patient takes several days to weeks after his surgery to return to his preoperative physiologic state. Thus, each patient with a medical illness who undergoes an elective surgical procedure is actually three distinctly different patients physiologically whose common medical illness is addressed by three physicians with distinctly different approaches to patient care—the primary care physician preoperatively, the anesthesiologist intraoperatively, and the surgeon postoperatively. Perioperative medicine melds these three specialties. An important component of perioperative medicine is practicing at the two interfaces between medicine and anesthesia preoperatively and between anesthesia and surgery postoperatively. The perioperative physician does not need to know everything that the primary care physician, the anesthesiologist, and the surgeon need to know. But he, or she, needs (1) to possess a body of knowledge that must be common to internists, anesthesiologists, and surgeons, (2) to appreciate the physiologic response to surgery as modified by anesthesia and by medical illness, and (3) to emphasize the importance of effective and timely communication between internists, anesthesiologists, and surgeons regarding this three-in-one patient. The authors of this book make a strong first attempt to define that common body of knowledge and to tie it together with basic physiologic principles.

The new economics of medicine is creating a vacuum which physicians who practice perioperative medicine must abhor and fill. Primary care physicians are being asked to focus so much of their effort on preventive and ambulatory medicine that they are losing their edge when it comes to caring for patients who are entering a hospital setting. Similarly, incentives in managed care systems are designed to encourage surgeons to concentrate their activity in the operating room and busy surgical clinics and away from the ambulatory preparation of the patients they have scheduled for surgery. Finally, anesthesiologists are being pressured to develop a "red line" approach to the administering of anesthesia. The red line is the line on the floor in an operating room suite that you can only cross if you are garbed in operating room attire. They feel pressured to concentrate their attention on the technical task of administering or supervising anesthesia and to delegate all tasks on the other side of the red line to other health care providers. In this health care delivery system the stage is set for these three groups of physicians to define sharply the interfaces between them rather than to blur them.

Quality of care requires the smooth passage of the elective surgical patient from his preoperative physiologic state through his intraoperative and postoperative physiologic states if he is to return successfully to his preoperative physiologic state. The editors and authors of this book understand this. They are not red line anesthesiologists. They all take seriously their responsibilities as perioperative physicians. I would feel comfortable knowing that any one of them was responsible for directing my care should I require surgery. They want you to know the breadth and depth of what is important to them in their daily practice of medicine at the two interfaces.

Raymond C. Roy, Ph.D., M.D.
Distinguished Professor and Chair
Department of Anesthesiology
University of Virginia Health Sciences Center

Preface

In this book, we attempt to provide our definition of a relatively new specialty, perioperative medicine, the non-surgical care of the adult patient in the pre- and postoperative periods. The introductory chapter, "Issues and Philosophy" defines some of the past and present problems in this area and states one opinion as to what comprises this area. The next section of the book covers the preoperative evaluation of the patient who is scheduled for or being considered for surgery. It is organized in a traditional way along system areas but it also attempts to be driven primarily by physiology rather than by the "differential diagnosis" approach most frequently practiced in medical education. While drugs and medical procedures change continuously, human physiology remains relatively constant. We also hope to present at least as great an emphasis on treatment as on diagnosis. The next section includes two views on the art and science of perioperative consultation and ends with a chapter on the relatively new concept of the preoperative evaluation clinic.

The book's fourth section considers selected relevant surgical concerns, we continue to try to present a viewpoint that includes input from more than one specialty for each topic. For this reason, most chapters will have more than one author, usually of different specialties. The surgical sections cover some newer procedures but also several older, but still complicated, areas of surgery. We believe that further knowledge of the concerns of the surgeons will benefit other involved physicians whether they be primary doctors, medical subspecialists, or anesthesiologists.

The block of chapters on anesthesiology cannot provide an entire summary of the specialty, but in it, we hope to provide the non-anesthesiologist (or the future or novice anesthesiologist) with some important concepts so that they learn something about what actually occurs in the operating room. Our goal is to stimulate more informed and effective communication, commentary, and consultation among the involved physicians. The chapters on postoperative care have a similar function. A significant percentage of perioperative problems will occur, or at least will first be detected in the recovery room. Pain management is a burgeoning specialty that has exploded with new concepts and knowledge: It contributes greatly to patient comfort and possibly, to improved outcome in the surgical patient. The chapter on critical care is not a treatise on management of the intensive care unit patient so much as a discussion about who belongs in the unit (and for how long) in the postoperative period.

The final section of the book considers some non-medical areas that are important to the current practice of perioperative medicine. The medicolegal chapter is groundbreaking in considering the legal implications of consultation: Physicians' concerns have always included a fear of not asking for a consult when it is indicated, and possible liability for not following the precise recommendations of the consultant (e.g., "insert pulmonary artery catheter"). The consultant's concerns include her/his liability for recommendations that are followed but somehow resulted in a bad outcome. We also wished to cover the issues of cost, outcome, and the application of modern management principles to medical practice.

Under today's systems of managed care, physician gatekeepers have increased control over who gets expensive surgical procedures. They must ensure that optimal yet cost-effective care is provided for these patients. It is important that patients not be operated on unnecessarily but even more important to ensure that patients are not denied essential procedures for economically driven reasons. Surgeons are likewise increasingly responsible for cost-effectiveness and efficiency in their area of care. Anesthesiologists in many institutions are applying and extending their knowledge of perioperative medicine to the time periods before and after surgery. Undergraduate medical education appears to suffer from time restraints that limit the ability of medical schools to teach perioperative medicine. Residencies may overlook this area of medical overlap as what is perceived as more essential, core information in the specialty is imparted. This book hopes to provide a heretofore unavailable source of information that all these doctors need to take optimal care of their patients. It is neither a manual nor a definitive textbook as we do not pretend that the data available indicates the 'right' way to deal with a particular problem in perioperative medicine. Rather, this book is intended as a basis for thinking about the perioperative period so that each patient can be approached in a collaborative fashion with subsequent care based on knowledge of the patient and the procedure, and attention paid to the special concerns generated by this interaction. The intended result is better and more efficient patient care practiced in a collegial environment in which the concerns of patients and colleagues are understood and taken into consideration when formulating and carrying out the process of perioperative medicine.

David J. Stone, M.D.
David L. Bogdonoff, M.D.
George S. Leisure, M.D.
Burkhard F. Spiekermann, M.D.
Donald D. Mathes, M.D.

How to use this book

This is an unusual medical book in that it is intended to cross the usual denominational boundaries of the traditional specialties. Therefore, some of the material will be new for readers of one specialty but "old hat" for readers of another. Medical students and novice trainees in any specialty should find all the material to be useful, or at least new. This may also apply to those training in the primary care specialties and those who are practicing primary care but received little or no experience in perioperative care. Medical subspecialists may not gain much new knowledge from the chapters in their areas but may gain a new perspective on the particular problems of the perioperative period that will aid them in providing perioperative consultations. Surgeons may choose to skim or skip the section on special surgical considerations and anesthesiologists beyond the earliest stages of training are unlikely to gain much from the anesthesia section. On the other hand, anesthesiologists trained before acute pain services became the norm may be interested in this chapter and surgeons may learn something new in the areas of transplants, laparoscopy, or new developments in thoracic surgery.

We have chosen to include the material selected in order to cover the field of perioperative medicine in a fairly comprehensive fashion. We realize that this means that the material in selected chapters will be very basic to some experienced readers. However, it will be the very unusual clinician who can not gain some insights into perioperative medicine from some parts of this book. We also hope that reviewers will take these comments into consideration when they question in print the goals and audience of the book. This book is just a beginning intended to stimulate further thoughts, reading, and research into a very special kind of patient care.

Table of Contents

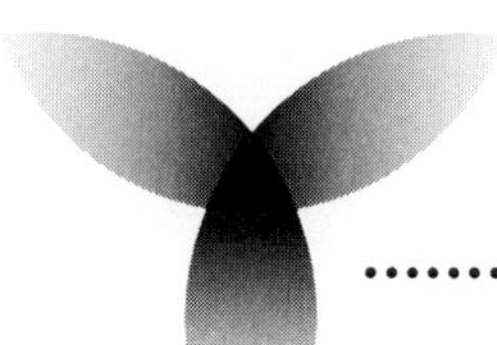

Section I

INTRODUCTION
Philosophy and Issues in Perioperative Medicine

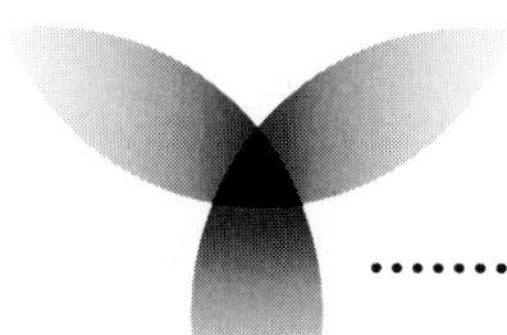

Chapter 1

Issues and Philosophy

David J. Stone, MD

A classic dictum of military strategy is that one of the most vulnerable points of a defensive alignment is at the junction of two armies under separate commands. This is especially so if the allied armies speak different languages and are somewhat suspicious of the capabilities of their comrades on the flanks. While perioperative medicine is not quite war, it has suffered in both an academic and practical sense from the historical alignment of family practice (FP), internal medicine (IM), anesthesiology, and surgery in which the individual parts do not always add up to an optimal whole. Each specialty has its own body of knowledge, its own language ("dialects" of the mother language we all struggle to acquire in medical school), its own unfounded assumptions, and, oftentimes, the prejudice that one's own specialty is the most difficult (or hard-working, intellectual, useful, etc.) of all. This chapter will attempt to state some of the problems of the perioperative care of the adult patient in the more general sense. The rest of the book will then go on to speak to some of these problems in a more specific fashion.

As implied above, many of the problems that arise in the interaction of the varying specialties in the perioperative period are those of communication, language, and respect. In addition, there is a tendency on the part of many doctors, regardless of specialty, to provide an opinion in spite of inadequate knowledge in or experience with some aspect of perioperative care. For example, my training in internal medicine at the University of Virginia was superb in many regards but simply did not touch on the care of the perioperative patient in more than the most superficial manner. Subsequently, in the private practice of general internal medicine, I was called on to "clear" patients for anesthesia, usually at the end of a long, hard day of seeing patients in the office and hospital. In fact, I had no basis for "clearing" patients for anesthesia and usually went on to describe the patient's current condition and make a few recommendations on improving his or her condition in the next 12 or so hours before surgery. I really didn't understand the problems and special requirements of the perioperative period and felt rather frustrated and inadequate in this function; not only was I uncertain of what was being asked of me, I had inadequate knowledge of and experience with perioperative medicine to make a truly useful contribution.

The first step in learning medicine may lie in learning to say "I don't know" (I think the second step is learning to say "I'm sorry, I was wrong") and then proceeding to find out if the knowledge is available or if this area has simply never been adequately addressed. In the busy practice of clinical medicine, it may be difficult to ascertain what knowledge is available with the resources at one's disposal. Perhaps the advent of electronic communications through the World Wide Web and electronic mail will facilitate searches for information as it has already done for those who have access to MEDLINE library searches. This book is, at least, a start in the search for information on clinical perioperative issues and one that may be accessed easily and quickly. The practice of perioperative medicine is a blend of internal medicine, surgery, and anesthesiology in proportions that may fluctuate on the basis of the nature and acuity of the patient's problem, the surgical procedure and its postoperative implications, and the particular point in time in the patient's course (i.e., pre-, intra-, early postoperative, later postoperative). A relatively small amount of awareness concerning what the "other guy" knows and is capable of, goes a long way in carrying out this mission.

THE MECHANICS OF PERIOPERATIVE MEDICINE

The precise way in which perioperative medicine functions depends on how the patient enters the surgical system. If a patient is well-known to a primary care physician at a community hospital and is referred to a local surgeon for a procedure of low or moderate risk at that institution, it is likely that the patient's personality and medical problems will be well-understood and the lines of medical communication will be clear. In general, the physician will choose a surgeon with whom he or she works well and has trust. However, the patient may still have complex problems that require special knowledge of perioperative concerns that can be communicated through the mini-Internet of patient-surgeon-physician-anesthesiologist. The major advantage to this setting is that the patient has a physician who knows him or her well and for whom the physician can go to bat, both medically and emotionally. Both the institution and removal of therapies can occur without the painful gaps in communication that may occur in the academic medical center. Medical egos generally do not come into the picture in a negative way as they seem to do in the academic setting: the goal is to take care of the patient well and efficiently, rather than show the other guy how smart you are. In addition, nursing services may be more available in a well-run community hospital. Possible disadvantages include an absence of relevant medical subspecialty consultants, relative unfamiliarity with an unusual medical or anesthetic problem due to the primary care nature of the setting, relative lack of experience with the technical aspects of an infrequently performed procedure, and absence of some potentially beneficial support systems such as a full-service intensive care unit with 24-hour physician staffing and an acute postoperative pain consultative service.

Patients may be referred to larger tertiary care centers, which may or may not be academic medical centers. This referral may be because of patient request even if the procedure can be done at the community hospital, because the procedure cannot be performed at the community hospital, or because the patient's medical problems or potential problems justify referral to a center where specialized medical and anesthetic care is available. In any case, the patient has lost an important advocate and source of wisdom as the primary care physician is no longer at the bedside. It is evidently critical that the patient be accompanied by whatever relevant information can be provided by the referring physician. An echocardiogram report or thyroid function tests can prevent a lot of wasted time, frustration, and anguish on the part of both patient and physicians on the referral end. This applies even more so in the current era of "same-day" surgery where patients are not routinely admitted the night before. On the other hand, it is also the physician's duty to independently review the case and not assume that all previous findings are necessarily valid.

Patients are often screened by physicians or nonphysician health personnel in a preadmission assessment center well before the day of surgery. This is an excellent time to make certain that all the necessary test results and radiographs are available and appropriate consultations obtained. Dr. Donald D. Mathes addresses this concept in detail in a later chapter. In fact, this type of area represents the primary care aspect of perioperative medicine as it has a screening function and sees many people who are well, except for their need for a particular operation or procedure. If patients are being referred for a radiological procedure alone, it is important to establish who will assume the patient's care in case complications arise that necessitate admission. In some cases, the cost of supporting this kind of unit can be defrayed by billing for a preoperative consultation if sufficient time elapses between consultation and procedure.

For patients referred to a larger center, the primary care physician role is developed in several ways. For those surgical specialties, such as general and cardiovascular surgery that assume responsibility and take pride in their patient care abilities, the surgeon may provide this role. For other surgical specialties, it may be best to obtain a consultation in general internal medicine if the patient has numerous and/or significant medical problems, especially if these require pre- and/or postoperative intervention and follow-up. For same-day surgery and for patients who have not been seen by a general internist, the anesthesiologist may assume the functional role of primary care physician. At times, the anesthesiologist will be the first physician to carry out a careful history in the referring institution and be aware of significant medical problems that require further attention in the perioperative period.

COLLEAGUES AND OTHER MISUNDERSTANDINGS

One of the obstacles in perioperative medicine is the nonanesthesiologist's perception of the anesthesiologist's role, knowledge, and abilities, particularly by nonsurgical medical practitioners. The practice of anesthesia does not merely involve the administration of anesthetic gases during an operation. In the operating room, the anesthesiologist must have an awareness and understanding of the patient's medical status that will allow for the administration of an anesthetic, but more importantly, must provide for the patient's safety and total medical care through this period, as well as the immediate postoperative period. In specific instances, this may extend into care in an intensive care unit and specialized pain management. The preoperative medical evaluation of the patient is critical in that it sets the stage for planning a safe and practical anesthetic that considers the patient's special needs and problems. The result of this is that the practicing anesthesiologist is quite knowledgeable about medical problems as they present throughout the perioperative period. This knowledge should not be underestimated or dismissed by consulting physicians who may be unaware of the extensive role that anesthesiologists now play in helping surgeons to perform more and more complex operations on sicker and sicker patients. In addition, there is a remarkable degree of overlap between the problems that an anesthesiologist or primary care physician will treat on a daily basis such as hypertension, angina, diabetes, congestive heart failure (CHF), anemia, and chronic obstructive pulmonary disease (COPD)/asthma. This overlap is more impressive if one considers and eliminates the amount of time the primary care physician treats functional problems caused by anxiety and depression, and the time that the anesthesiologist is monitoring a stable patient. The degree to which the perioperative medical role of the anesthesiologist will expand is not currently clear but it is likely that in selected institutions, the anesthesiologist will become the dominant physician in the overall provision of perioperative medical care. One problem is that while the anesthesiologist may coordinate medical care, the patient may miss the personal touch of someone accustomed to primary care. This may be solved by the evolution of anesthesiology into a true perioperative specialty, special devotion of part of the general medical consultation service to this function, or to an expanded role for nonphysician practitioners such as nurses and physicians' assistants.

PUTTING IT ALL TOGETHER

In any case, the preoperative period involves screening for and evaluation and treatment of medical problems that are important enough to potentially impact on the patient's intra- and postoperative course. Questions inevitably arise about the need for further data (e.g., an echocardiogram) and the need for formal consultation by a medical specialist, most often, a cardiologist. If possible, it is optimal to consult an attending cardiologist who has developed an interest in, knowledge of, and an intuitive feel for this aspect of patient care. In the academic center, the rotating attendings on the consult service may provide an unfortunate roller coaster of attending quality and interest. The main question is often whether the particular problem that has been noted requires the postponement of surgery or whether modifications in anesthetic, surgical, and postoperative care can justify going ahead as planned. Early evaluation by knowledgable individuals of whatever specialty can avoid this kind of delay and anguish on the day of the planned operation. They can facilitate optimal care, probably reduce "near-miss" kinds of anesthetic complications, and possibly even contribute to improved outcome. They can clearly contribute to patient satisfaction and a feeling that first-rate care is being provided.

The next preoperative step is communication between physician, surgeon, and anesthesiologist, which is the "Mount Everest" of all steps in actual practice. This issue is further discussed in the chapter on perioperative consultation. Finally, a plan is conceived that may involve further testing, simple postponement, or a modification of anesthetic and/or surgical care. Another important goal in this period is the prevention of infection and pulmonary thromboembolism. These are discussed in later chapters in the context of overall perioperative pharmacology.

The move into the intraoperative period generally leaves the physician at the operating room door; but the events of this period are important so far as they impact on overall care. For this reason, we have included a section on selected surgical procedures and the specific problems they entail, as well as a section that very briefly summarizes the nature of intraoperative anesthetic care, with a particular emphasis on the physiological consequences of anesthesia and surgery. It is the anesthesiologist's job to utilize the available monitors and techniques to safely shepherd the patient through the controlled trauma of surgery. It is also the anesthesiologist's job to determine which of these techniques and monitors should be employed in a given case. It is our feeling that some knowledge of intraoperative events will help physicians to provide effective perioperative consultation and to do so in a more intellectually satisfying manner than simply "clearing" patients for surgery. This knowledge will unquestionably improve communications as the knowledge gained involves some element of new language acquisition as well as that most important element: a demonstration of interest in what someone else is doing and spending some effort, no matter how small, to learn something about it. Furthermore, this kind of knowledge can only increase respect among the specialties for what the others are doing. Intellectually, it is a requirement for the development of an efficient, collegial, and effective perioperative medical team.

The postoperative period presents a whole new set of difficulties and, again, represents a body of knowledge that should be acquired by those who are to participate in perioperative care. Recovery room care is generally provided by anesthesiologists but problems may require medical and surgical involvement, as well. Practitioners should be aware of the kinds of problems that arise in the recovery room, particularly as they relate to preoperative evaluation (e.g., myocardial ischemia, respiratory failure in COPD). Furthermore, it is important to be aware of the modalities currently available for pain management. This awareness may even extend into patient care outside the perioperative period as surgeons and primary care physicians learn about potential pain clinic care for chronic pain if such a facility is available for their referral. While the medical details of intensive care are now covered in a slew of texts, handbooks, and pamphlets, the issues of who needs intensive care and for how long are not frequently addressed. What happens to patients after discharge from an intensive care unit? Who, perhaps, should have been in the unit but was not? These kinds of questions are relevant to the practitioner even if he or she does not actually provide care in the intensive care unit.

Finally, in the current era of great changes in the delivery of health care, issues of economics, efficiency, quality improvement, and medicolegal issues cannot be ignored. What has already been learned about efficient perioperative medical care and what can be improved? What costs are involved and what can be trimmed without undue risk? What special medicolegal issues arise in this period when consultation or lack of it may play such an important role in patient care? Perioperative medicine involves all these concerns, as well. They are to be ignored at one's peril.

CODA

So what is perioperative medicine? When you fly in an airplane, what is important? Building the plane? Maintaining the plane? Piloting the plane? Making sure you have a ticket and a seat and the plane actually takes off sometime near the scheduled time and you make your connections? Making certain there is something to eat and drink on a 10-hour flight? Obviously, all these things are important although some may be more important for convenience, comfort, and cost than for actual safety. The provision of first-rate perioperative care is similarly a team effort. The actual coordination of this effort may come from a general surgeon, an anesthesiologist, or a primary care physician, but the important point is that they are all aware of the patient's problems and the concerns of the other involved team members. Only in the case of a minor procedure taking place under local anesthesia can a surgeon assume all the responsibility. Perioperative medicine involves filling in the cracks between the formal specialties so that care is not fragmented. The ultimate perioperative medicine improves communication between the formal specialties to take advantage of what is already known so that first-rate care can be given. It provides a forum for improved care in both the medical and administrative senses.

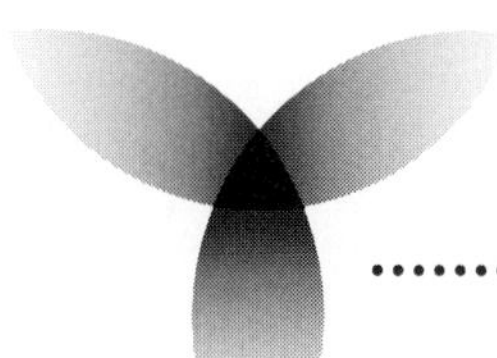

Section II

PREOPERATIVE MEDICAL ASSESSMENT AND TREATMENT

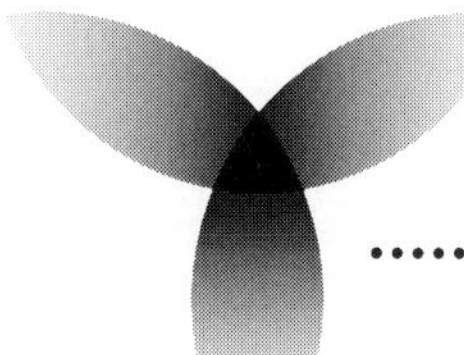

Chapter 2

Hypertensive and Ischemic Heart Disease

Definitions, Statistics, and Current Cardiology

David J. Stone, MD, John M. Dent, MD

DEFINITION OF THE CLINICAL PROBLEM

This chapter considers the problems of the patient with coronary artery disease (CAD) and hypertension in tandem because they are often inseparable in clinical practice. Certainly, many patients do have hypertension without CAD but the treatment of these patients is carried out to prevent congestive heart failure (CHF) and CAD, among other long-term complications of hypertension. Many patients with CAD have hypertension or were hypertensive before a failing left ventricle ceased to pump forcefully enough to raise the blood pressure to unacceptable levels. Drugs such as angiotensin-converting enzyme (ACE) inhibitors, calcium-channel blockers (CCBs), vasodilators and beta-blockers are used to treat both processes. Certainly, blood pressure control is probably one factor in the onset of perioperative ischemia. Finally, ischemia and hypertension separately and in combination form the most common etiology(ies) of CHF.

Hypertension

The perioperative problem of hypertension per se has not been clearly shown to affect outcome. However, an inquiry into most anesthesia texts reveals a statement to the effect that elective surgery should not be performed in patients with diastolic pressures at or above 110 mmHg. The choice of this particular number is not unreasonable but may be as much a matter of faith as of science. Perioperative problems in the poorly controlled hypertensive patient include hemodynamic instability, with consequent predisposition to both cardiovascular and cerebrovascular sequelae. Experienced clinicians realize that patients with relatively poorly controlled blood pressure will tend to experience more of an "Alpine anesthetic," but when questioned about their own practice, they are likely to admit to a clinical course of action other than case cancellation. The patient receiving first-rate medical care is rarely a problem in this regard, but the problem may lie in the fact that the patient has never previously entered the medical system, is a true therapeutic dilemma, or is noncompliant. The perioperative period, thus, represents a great screening and educational opportunity in the care of hypertensive patients. The clinician must decide, on a case-by-case basis, the appropriate course of action in proceeding with surgery and anesthesia in the patient whose hypertension is not well-controlled. Issues to be considered include the urgency of surgery, the social situation, the possibility of truly improving the situation by delay, and the response to a trial of therapy, as well as the absolute values of the systolic and diastolic integers.

Coronary Artery Disease

Patients with CAD represent a vast spectrum of disease ranging from minimal occlusion of one vessel to severe, multivessel disease that may produce myocardial infarction (MI), unstable angina, CHF, or dysrhythmias. Historically, perioperative MI was first identified as a clinical problem almost 50 years ago and it was subsequently learned that a history of (especially recent) MI or CHF appeared to be important perioperative risk factors. This was followed in the 1970s by the advent of the cardiac risk index (a.k.a. the Goldman study), which is still commonly referred to in consultations. Improvements in operative and postoperative anesthetic care since that time have had substantial impact in making this period safer, even for high-risk patients. Many of these improvements lie in the spectrum of overall anesthetic care. Credit should be given to this specialty for these improvements.

Over the past 10 to 15 years, cardiologists have developed a number of screening tests, most of which have been subsequently applied to the perioperative period.

The use of these tests seems to be undergoing a healthy, revisionist reevaluation. The recent joint publication of a short review article by the leading cardiologist and anesthesiologist in this area is a good prognostic sign, at least in the sense of communication and collaboration.[1] In fact, after all the diagnostic tests are in, no one is quite sure what is the best course to take therapeutically.

The development and application of more sophisticated diagnostic and treatment methods has altered the characteristics of the patient population undergoing evaluation for surgery. Because inducible myocardial ischemia and extensive CAD are now frequently detected and often corrected through revascularization, patients who may have been judged "high risk" by previous criteria, may in fact be low risk after revascularization. The fact that the characteristics of the patients being studied are a moving target further complicates the application of older, accepted risk assessment criteria to our current patients.

Congestive Heart Failure

This and the following chapter are specifically concerned with the patient who has myocardial dysfunction on the basis of hypertension, CAD, or both. The problems of valvular, congenital, and other cardiomyopathic heart diseases are addressed in separate chapters. Although diastolic dysfunction commonly accompanies significant systolic dysfunction, it is convenient to classify myocardial dysfunction as either predominantly diastolic or systolic. The syndrome of diastolic left ventricular dysfunction is characterized by reduced left ventricular compliance, but not necessarily a reduction in ejection fraction. This is commonly observed with hypertensive heart disease, acute ischemia, and more rarely, with infiltrative disease leading to restrictive cardiomyopathy. Systolic dysfunction, then, is defined by a reduced ability of the heart to eject a normal fraction as is seen with dilated ischemic cardiomyopathy, when acute ischemia is extensive enough to reduce ejection fraction, in the more advanced stages of hypertensive cardiomyopathy, and in dilated or idiopathic cardiomyopathy. Both types of dysfunction are likely to result in dyspnea when the system is stressed, pulmonary vasculature pressures increase, and vascular, interstitial, and even alveolar fluid congestion ensue. Systolic dysfunction is more likely to produce symptoms of generalized reduced perfusion.

Perioperative Cardiology

In short, the role of the perioperative physician is to ensure that a reasonable level of cardiological care has been provided. That is to say, a quality and quantity of medical input has been provided that should have been provided whether surgery was scheduled or not! For those patients under the care of cognizant physicians, perioperative management should be greatly simplified as myocardial function and risk for ischemia have already been thoughtfully analyzed. Unfortunately, a large number of patients who enter the perioperative screening process have not received cardiac care at this level and represent unsolved diagnostic and therapeutic conundrums. This also represents an opportunity to have an impact on patient care in a fashion that spreads beyond the perioperative period. For example, some diagnostic or therapeutic options have implications for long-term and not just perioperative outcome.

More simply, it allows an entry into the medical care system for those patients who have avoided it but who actually need it.

In these chapters, we attempt to make some clinical sense out of our experience and the extensive literature that is now available on perioperative ischemic risk and to discuss clinically practical options rather than textbook platitudes. There are many approaches to these patients, ranging from the minimalist history and physical to catheterization of nearly all patients. Some options depend on the expertise and skills available at local institutions and in no sense has a standard of care been established. More does not equal better in the realm of perioperative testing for ischemic risk. All this must now be interpreted in a managed care, cost-conscious environment in which thallium does not flow like water. In addition, cardiac care has a special emotional overlay for patients that may be inexplicable but is definitely real. This must also be kept in mind when discussing the risks and options with individual patients.

Adverse Cardiovascular Events

One basic problem with the study of cardiac risk is the definition of an adverse event. These events may include cardiac death, nonfatal MI, angina (generally unstable, by definition), cardiogenic pulmonary edema, and severe ventricular dysrhythmias. One can see potential problems here immediately. When is a death clearly cardiac? Resolving this question is especially difficult in the setting of the operating or recovery rooms where concurrent misadventures are not uncommon. The diagnosis of MI is particularly difficult in the perioperative period because it may be confounded by nonspecific electrocardiogram (ECG) changes and muscle enzyme changes as a result of surgical trauma. The presence of a small amount of MB fraction in skeletal muscle creatinine phosphokinase (CPK) may make certainty elusive.[2] The use of cardiac troponin I measurements may prove useful in this regard. Yet, how important is the diagnosis of MI, per se? Sometimes, physicians become so focused on determining the presence or absence of infarction that they fail to heed ongoing issues such as left ventricular dysfunction, ongoing ischemia, and risk of further ischemia. The frequency of worrisome but nonspecific changes in the ECG and the low frequency of chest pain in this setting make angina a difficult perioperative diagnosis. Some studies have required chest pain to be present before angina is diagnosed, but in these patients classic chest pain is uncommon. When is pulmonary edema clearly due to CHF vs. fluid overload or noncardiogenic sources of infiltrates such as aspiration or atelectasis? Some studies include dysrhythmias as adverse events while others do not. Obviously, the former studies will have a higher incidence of adverse events and probably a better success rate at treating them, as many perioperative dysrhythmias are not ischemic in origin. These points are made to demonstrate how muddy the waters of perioperative cardiac care may be, whether the care is given by anesthesiologist, primary care physician, surgeon, or cardiologist.

Planned Surgical Procedure

As for the respiratory system, perioperative cardiac care must consider the nature of the planned surgical procedure in conjunction with the patient's medical problems.

Studies of cardiac risk have often targeted the vascular surgery population as a high-risk group based on both patient pathology and surgical stress. In fact, infrainguinal vascular procedures that do not involve cross-clamping of the aorta appear to manifest as high a cardiac risk as aortic aneurysm repair or aortobifemoral bypass. Minor risk procedures would include opthalmological surgery, especially under local anesthesia, and minor patient procedures such as knee arthroscopy and inguinal hernia repair. Intermediate risk procedures would include major abdominal, thoracic, and orthopedic surgeries, but these may turn into high risk if marked blood loss, large fluid shifts, coagulopathy, and so on ensue. The baseline cardiac risk of a high-risk procedure appears to be on the order of 10%.

• DAMN LIES AND STATISTICS

Perhaps more than for any other clinical area, a critical appreciation of the clinical research literature on cardiac ischemic risk requires some understanding of statistics. In many cases, the level of statistical analysis far exceeds the sort of introductory understanding that many of us possess. While we do not claim to be statisticians, we believe it would be useful to define some of the terms encountered in this literature. For those interested, the suggested reading at the end of the chapter has several references in this area. Feel free to skip this section but it may be a useful reference when encountering some of the terms in the literature.

Sensitivity

This is the likelihood that the test in question will be positive if the patient has the "disease." This is in contrast to the **positive predictive value**, which refers to the probability of having the disease if the test is positive. Sensitivity may also be referred to as true positive rate or power. If the sensitivity is high, the incidence of false-negative tests (1-sensitivity) will be low. The latter is also referred to as **Type II** or **β error**. Both sensitivity and specificity (viz infra) must be applied and interpreted in terms of the prior or pretest probability (or the prevalence) of the disease in the population under consideration (Bayesian analysis).

Specificity

This is the likelihood that the test will be negative if the patient does *not* have the "disease." Again, this in contrast to the **negative predictive value**, which is the probability of not having the disease if the test is negative. Note that unless a disease has a very high prevalence in a population, a test is more likely to have a high negative than positive predictive value. If the specificity is high, the incidence of false-positive tests (1-specificity) is low. The latter is referred to as **Type I** or **α error** or that holy grail of statistics, the **P value**. Note that as a test is made more specific, it becomes less sensitive or, in other terms, if Type I error is decreased, Type II error will increase. Therefore, to keep the P value in the arbitrarily accepted range of less than .05, the sensitivity of the test may have to be decreased so the incidence of false positives is reduced.

Likelihood Ratio

This expression is commonly noted in the literature and is the ratio of the true positive rate (sensitivity) to the false-positive rate, i.e., the "likelihood" that a positive test represents a true rather than false positive. In conjunction with information on the prior probability of disease, the likelihood ratio can be employed to calculate the predictive value of the test result. To calculate this value, known as posterior odds, the likelihood ratio is multiplied by the prior odds. For a disease with a 10% prior probability, the prior odds would be 1 to 9.

A **receiver operating characteristic** (ROC) curve may be generated by plotting true-positive and false-positive rates on the y and x axes, respectively. An ROC curve that is steep in the upper left quadrant, therefore, represents a "better" test, i.e., one with a high true-positive rate and low false-positive rate. ROC analysis offers a comprehensive method for comparing and selecting appropriate tests for particular patient populations. It assesses diagnostic test performance about all possible pairs of sensitivity and specificity values.

95% Confidence Interval

Range of values within which test results would fall 95 times if the test were repeated 100 times. As confidence interval increases in percentage (i.e., to 99%), the range itself must necessarily increase to include 99% of possible outcomes. In other words, confidence intervals represent the limits between which an observation falls, with a given probability.

Univariate vs. Multivariate Analysis

The commonly used statistical tools such as the T-test are known as univariate methods because they analyze the influence of a treatment on a single variable, one variable at a time. Multivariate analysis considers the effects of several variables at once, as in the original Goldman cardiac risk index, for example. These methods are based on multiple linear regression, which is the equivalent generalization of the simple linear regression technique used to draw a best straight line through a data plot. While the mathematics is beyond the scope of this discussion (and the authors), multivariate analysis is a powerful way of looking at complex and poorly controlled studies. In addition, parameters may enter in a nonlinear fashion requiring even more complex analyses of nonlinear regression.

• CURRENT CARDIOLOGY AND PERIOPERATIVE MEDICINE

This section is intended to present some of the tools cardiovascular medicine currently possesses in the diagnosis of cardiac disease. The next chapter will present several approaches to the patient who has symptomatic CAD or a recent MI.

New Concepts in Myocardial Ischemia

These are not truly new to the physiologist but may be unfamiliar to the clinician. **Hibernating myocardium** refers to areas of myocardium that are dysfunctional as a result of a reduced blood flow. The reduced level of blood flow is too low to provide for normal muscle function but is sufficient to preserve the viability of the myocardial cells. It is analogous to the ischemic penumbra in the brain when the electroencephalogram (EEG) is flat because of reduced blood flow, but the neurons remain viable. This dysfunction may also be remediable by revascularization, either coronary artery bypass surgery (CABG) or percutaneous transluminal coronary angioplasty (PTCA). In contrast, **stunned myocardium** refers to muscle that has suffered a significant but not irreversible ischemic insult. While blood flow has been restored, the functional state of the myocardium has not yet returned to normal. Repeated episodes of stunning, although reversible as individual events, may lead to infarction. While, in general, hibernating myocardium is found distal to a fixed stenosis, and stunned myocardium is subtended by a transiently occluded coronary artery, recent evidence from the animal laboratory suggests that there may be considerable overlap between these two causes of left ventricular dysfunction.

Exercise Electrocardiography/Exercise Tolerance

The standard, now rather old-fashioned ECG stress test (ST) may be useful if results are extremely positive, particularly if performed in a population with a high prior probability of disease. These results would include marked ST depression (downsloping >4 mm), severe dysrhythmias, or evidence of ischemic myocardial dysfunction, e.g., hypotension. In clinical practice, the test is more likely to produce ambiguous results with borderline ST-T wave changes at less than desired heart rates. Predicted maximal heart rate is 220 minus age and the goal is to get the patient's heart rate as close to that number as possible and within reason.

There are a number of factors that may limit the utility of the exercise ECG in detecting ischemia with both a high sensitivity and specificity. First, the use of β-blocking drugs and CCB with a negative chronotropic effect may prevent patients from reaching a diagnostic heart rate. Also, patients with baseline ST-segment changes are essentially ineligible for analysis due to the poor positive predictive value of additional ECG changes. Finally, false-positive tests are common if upsloping ST depression is interpreted as positive, particularly in young women.

The real utility of the exercise ECG test may lie in the exercise rather than in the ECG. Clinicians have long employed some less than strictly quantitative measures of exercise tolerance as an indicator of overall cardiovascular-pulmonary function. These may include the ability to walk up a flight of steps without stopping (some add a second flight or a bag of groceries to the equation), or the ability to walk a fairly long distance on the flat without angina or dyspnea. This may also be referred to in terms of metabolic equivalents (METS) with one MET representing oxygen consumption at rest, approximately 250 ml per minute for the 70-kg adult. Walking up two flights of steps requires about 4 METS for a brief time. These abilities probably correlate with an ejection fraction of at least 35% to 40%, although, occasionally, patients with severely reduced left ventricular systolic function will have a satisfactory exercise tolerance. This evaluation can also be formalized by having the patient bicycle in an upright or supine position to determine if heart rate can be raised to 100 bpm without undue disaster. Upper extremity exercise can be employed if the lower extremities are dysfunctional because of vascular or rheumatologic disease. The importance of exercise tolerance was demonstrated in a study in which patients who could raise their heart rates to 85% of predicted maximum, even with ST changes, appeared to be at less perioperative risk than patients who could not exercise to these levels.[3] Unfortunately, only approximately 30% of the vascular surgery population, a high-risk group for perioperative cardiac problems, can reach this level of exercise by any form of work. In addition to the aforementioned vascular and rheumatological limitations common to these patients, there is an important incidence of limiting neurological and especially pulmonary disease, as well.

The "catch-22" of the situation is that the patient who can exercise does not need an exercise tolerance test (± ECG) and the patient who cannot exercise will not generate meaningful results. Therefore, there is not really much role for the application of these particular tests in perioperative medicine. In essence, if we had one question to ask a patient it would be that of exercise tolerance. The ability to walk up a flight of stairs does seem to *work* as an indicator that the stresses of an operation can be weathered. Unfortunately, this still leaves a large segment of the at-risk population with undefined status concerning myocardial function and risk for ischemia.

Ambulatory Electrocardiography (Holter Monitoring)

Long-term monitoring of patients for evidence of dysrhythmia or heart block is quite familiar to clinicians. Recently, this technology has been applied to patients in terms of analyzing at least two ECG leads for evidence of myocardial ischemia either in the hospital or during normal activity at home. Computer analysis is employed with ischemia defined as a certain degree of ST depression lasting a defined period of time. An example of a definition of ischemia would be at least a 1-mm planar or down-sloping ST depression persisting in consecutive beats for longer than a minute. Baseline ECG abnormalities such as bundle branch block, pacemaker-dependent tracing, left ventricular hypertrophy (LVH) ± strain, or pronounced baseline ST-T wave changes preclude the use of this test in at least 10% of a moderate-to-high-risk population. The test is relatively inexpensive ($300–$500) compared to nuclear studies, but it has not gained widespread acceptance because of disagreement about the significance of ST-segment changes.

One notable finding of these Holter studies has been that the majority of apparent ischemic ECG changes have not been accompanied by symptoms, i.e., they represent so-called "silent ischemia." Initial studies reported a very high (≈99%) negative predictive value if preoperative ischemia was absent. However, the majority of even high-risk patients with preoperative ischemia on testing do not suffer an adverse postoperative cardiac event (positive predictive value ≈20%). Furthermore, additional work did not reproduce the extremely high negative predictive value for the absence of preoperative ischemia and claimed rather, that postoperative ischemia was the most important predictor of adverse cardiac events. However, the latter information is obviously unavailable to the physician attempting to care for the patient preoperatively.

The ambulatory ECG approach to evaluating the perioperative patient is not employed extensively at the current time, but analysis of this data has taught us that the immediate postoperative period may be a time to continue or step-up close monitoring for and treatment of myocardial ischemia. Prolonged postoperative ischemia caused by tachycardia and other factors may result in myocardial stunning or infarction with resultant ischemic left ventricular dysfunction and dysrhythmias, as well.

Echocardiography

The rest two-dimensional (2-D) echocardiogram is a measure of ventricular function rather than myocardial ischemia per se. Changes in segmental wall motion during the perioperative course may represent areas of new ischemia or infarction and have been monitored for this purpose during high-risk procedures. However, even at rest, areas of wall motion abnormalities (hypo-, a-, or dyskinesia) indicating decreased function from infarction or hibernating myocardium may be markers for patients with coronary disease who would benefit from CABG. Rest echocardiography may be indicated if severe myocardial dysfunction is suspected on the basis of poor exercise tolerance or inability to exercise at all. Several findings on echocardiography may be helpful in determining the severity of diastolic dysfunction. Patients with significant LVH and left atrial enlargement (without a history of sustained atrial fibrillation to account for the atrial enlargement) probably have diastolic dysfunction and will require especially careful fluid management. A more precise quantitation of function may lead to changes in anesthetic technique, intraoperative monitoring, and intensity of postoperative care. Echocardiography can be performed at bedside after hours, without requiring scheduling in the radiology department. This is particularly useful in perioperative medicine where the evaluation may be taking place on the night before surgery but after regular radiology hours. Echocardiography also provides the advantage of evaluation of other structures, including heart valves and pericardium.

STRESS ECHOCARDIOGRAPHY

The cardiovascular system may be stressed by exercise, dipyridamole (see under Thallium for mechanism), or dobutamine ± atropine to produce abnormalities in segmental wall motion that are presumably caused by ischemia. After division of the left ventricular wall into a number of segments, a positive test may be defined as changes in two or more segments. Potentially serious side effects of the dobutamine/atropine test include dysrhythmias, hypo- or hypertension, and uncontrollable shaking. Fortunately these side effects are rare and generally resolve with discontinuation of the medication. The test is fairly new but appears to have a positive predictive value for adverse perioperative cardiac events, roughly similar to dipyridamole/thallium (viz infra); however, nuclear scintigraphy may be superior to dobutamine echocardiography for the detection of multivessel CAD, and for patients with baseline wall motion abnormalities. The test may also be informative in giving some rough idea of how well the heart will *function* when stressed. These tests are slightly less expensive than nuclear tests (≈$1000 vs. $1500).

Nuclear Cardiology

This technology is based on radioactive-labelled agents that can be used to trace the distribution of coronary blood flow or the volume of the left ventricular chamber.

In the latter case, **gated blood pool scanning** is employed to calculate ejection fraction. This test is infrequently used today because echocardiography can yield this data as well as other information (viz supra) in a more convenient, repeatable, and inexpensive manner.

Thallium (^{201}TL) Scanning

The distribution of thallium correlates with perfusion so that areas of old myocardial infarction will manifest themselves as defects in thallium distribution. Areas of hibernating myocardium may be represented by absent or reduced thallium penetration. Defects on the rest scan presumably should represent one of these two pathophysiologic entities with an increased number and size of defects representing more severe disease. In addition, defects may fall into a grey zone of less than complete perfusion or lack of perfusion. Increased lung uptake of thallium has a particularly poor prognosis, because it indicates that the ischemic heart has become dysfunctional, producing increased pulmonary venous pressures. Left ventricular dilation in the immediate poststress image also bodes a worse prognosis. Until recently, thallium scans have been 2-D or *planar*. Cardiologists can now also employ single photon-emission computed tomography (SPECT) scans that allow a 3-D evaluation of more segments. In clinical practice, this may actually lead to a higher number of false-positive scans (more sensitive, less specific tests). Thallium studies are subject to variability in interpretation and highly dependent upon the available local talent, which affects their utility as a clinical tool.

Stress Thallium

The increased demand for coronary blood flow (CBF) generated by exercise is satisfied by dilation of small coronary vessels that is, at least in part, mediated by the production of adenosine. The ability of these vessels to dilate is referred to as "coronary reserve." When coronary stenoses are severe enough (≈70% ⇓ diameter) to result in significant reductions in blood flow, poststenotic dilatation begins to compensate. Flow is improved until all coronary reserve is exhausted and no further dilation is possible. In this latter case, if demand is increased by exercise, flow will be diverted to areas perfused by normal or lesser stenosed vessels, resulting in critically low flows to poststenotic areas. Stress thallium takes advantage of this physiology to detect areas of absent or reduced thallium uptake during exercise. However, the presence of reduced thallium uptake during exercise does not distinguish between ischemia, infarction, and hibernation.

Redistribution refers to refilling of these defects by thallium on a second scan after some defined period of time, usually about 4 hours. Redistribution will not occur if the area represents infarction and may not occur if the areas represent hibernation, depending on the level of blood flow at that time. Some centers reinject thallium for this redistribution scan to improve scan quality, but reinjection may alter clinical interpretation. Defects that do not refill at this time are referred to as "fixed defects."

The dipyridamole (Persantin) scan was developed to obtain this kind of information in patients who cannot exercise. Dipyridamole produces a vasodilatory state by inhibiting adenosine reuptake that is analogous to that produced by exercise. If bronchospasm or unacceptable ischemia is produced, intravenous theophylline is used for reversal. Adenosine itself has been employed with thallium, but in clinical practice it often produces chest pain and nausea so that its use for this purpose is minimized. In patients with significant bronchospasm, dobutamine infusions can be used to increase heart rate with secondary changes in coronary blood flow. However, this mode of producing ischemia is not identical to the administration of dipyridamole. In any case, it is not clear that any of these "stress" tests truly reproduce the actual stresses of the perioperative period, which are not only hemodynamic, but may be metabolic, vascular, and hypercoagulopathic as well.

The early reports on thallium testing presented a picture of a test that was an excellent screening device with virtually no false negatives. For example, in the original report by Boucher et al.[4] in 1985, no patient without redistribution suffered an adverse cardiac event. In an effort to better define the population who might be best served by thallium screening, Eagle et al.[5] attempted to define groups at such low and high risk that scanning was not useful. They found that patients with none or >2 of the following risk factors (Q waves, age >70, angina, diabetes, ventricular ectopy) seemed to fit this definition. Eagle's concept of an intermediate risk group is one that begins to solve the fundamental dilemma of preoperative testing; after patients who clearly need and do not need further cardiologic workup have been eliminated, a group of patients remains whose proper care is unclear in the area of diagnostic screening.

As is often the case, further studies have removed the blush somewhat from the stress thallium scan and problems have been noted with false-negative scans. These include problems with the interpretation of fixed defects (i.e., old MI vs. hibernating myocardium), diffuse coronary disease causing global but, generally, equal flow reductions, and technical problems with the interpretation of results when they are not clear-cut. Quality of technique and interpretation is, indeed, an issue. A truly normal (no fixed defects, no globally reduced flow, no zones of questionably reduced uptake) scan does seem to be a marker for substantially reduced cardiac risk. However, thallium results do not specifically mark which of the patients with abnormal scans are candidates for CABG or angioplasty on the basis of their anatomy and physiology.

More recent studies have begun to question the role of stress thallium studies in preoperative testing. Mangano's group reported no association between redistribution or fixed defects and perioperative ischemia/adverse cardiac outcomes in vascular surgery patients.[6] In addition, they did not find the high negative predictive value originally noted by Boucher's group. Mangano et al. suggested the following reasons for this discrepancy: differences in scan interpretation, differences in patient enrollment methods, blinding of involved clinicians, and tight control of intraoperative hemodynamics. They postulate that thallium studies may not be predictive of cardiac events due to thrombosis or increased demand for CBF. Seeger et al. reported that stress thallium was not more helpful than clinical evaluation and a knowledge of EF in stratifying risk in an aortic surgery population.[7] Thallium testing did not contribute to improved 36-month outcome in that study. Costs reported in the Seeger study included angiography ($3295), angioplasty ($14,765), and CABG ($64,420). Baron et al.[8] reported that SPECT dipyridamole-thallium scans performed before aortic surgery were not useful predictors of outcome. Note that none of these studies has specified standards for monitors, anesthetic and surgical technique and quality, and hemodynamic interventions. A recent study by Fleisher's group[9] reported that quantitation of thallium results did have some long-term predictive ability. In conclusion, results of preoperative thallium testing probably need to be taken with a bit more of a grain of salt than we have done over the past 10 years.

TECHNETIUM SESTAMIBI

This is a relatively new nuclear agent that produces a better, brighter image in patients over 200 lb, an important advantage in our obesity-ridden population. This agent does not redistribute like thallium. In order to obtain information analogous to a thallium redistribution scan, sestamibi testing is performed in the opposite fashion by first obtaining a scan at rest and then reinjecting the patient just before exercise or dipyridamole administration. At present, it is not certain that this information is the precise equivalent of that gained with thallium. However, many clinical cardiologists are proceeding with this not unreasonable assumption, which is supported by data from the canine model of reversible ischemia. The ability to observe increased lung uptake of a nuclear agent as a prognostic marker is not observed. However, the sestamibi scan has the added advantage that an ejection fraction, as well as segmental wall abnormalities, can be measured by "gating" the scan, i.e., monitoring the images at many parts of the cardiac cycle. Such monitoring may also be helpful for distinguishing artifacts from true perfusion defects.

SUMMARY

Since stress echocardiography and stress nuclear techniques are roughly equivalent techniques for the detection of CAD, the choice of imaging technique, either nuclear or echocardiography, must be informed by the strength of the available laboratories. Detection of wall motion abnormalities by echocardiography is inherently subjective, and is one of the more difficult aspects of echocardiography to master. While the newer SPECT nuclear techniques are highly sensitive, there is a significant potential for false-positive tests in experienced hands, due to the potential for artifacts that simulate perfusion defects. The advent of certification examinations for echocardiography and nuclear cardiology may improve the consistency of these tests.

REFERENCES

1. Goldman L and Mangano DT: Preoperative assessment of patients with known or suspected coronary disease, *N Engl J Med* 333:1750, 1995.
2. Adams JE, et al: Diagnosis of perioperative myocardial infarction with measurement of cardiac troponin I, *N Engl J Med* 330:670, 1994.
3. McPhail L, et al: The use of preoperative testing to predict cardiac complications after arterial reconstruction, *J Vasc Surg* 7:60, 1988.
4. Boucher CA, et al: Determination of cardiac risk by dipyridamole-thallium imaging before peripheral vascular surgery, *N Engl J Med* 312:389, 1985.

5. Eagle KA, et al: Combining clinical and thallium data optimizes preoperative assessment of cardiac risk before major vascular surgery, *Ann Intern Med* 110:859, 1989.
6. Mangano DT, et al: Dipyridamole thallium-201 scintigraphy as a preoperative screening test: A reexamination of its predictive potential, *Circulation* 84:493, 1991.
7. Seeger JM, et al: Does routine stress-thallium cardiac scanning reduce postoperative cardiac complications? *Ann Surg* 219:654, 1994.
8. Baron JF, et al: Dipyridamole-thallium scintigraphy and gated radio nuclide angiography to access cardiac risk before abdominal aortic surgery, *N Engl J Med* 330:663, 1994.
9. Fleisher LA, et al: Preoperative dipyridamole thallium imaging and ambulatory electrocardiographic monitoring as a predictor of perioperative cardiac events and long-term outcome, *Anesthesiology* 83:906, 1995.

BIBLIOGRAPHY

Baron JF, et al: Dipyridamole-thallium scintigraphy and gated radionuclide angiography to assess cardiac risk before abdominal aortic surgery, *N Engl J Med* 330:663, 1994.

Eagle KA, et al: Guidelines for perioperative cardiovascular evaluation for noncardiac surgery, *Circulation* 93:1278, 1996.

Eichelberger JP, et al: Predictive value of dobutamine echocardiography just before noncardiac vascular surgery, *Am J Cardiol* 72:602, 1993.

Fleisher LA, Barash PG: Preoperative cardiac evaluation for noncardiac surgery: A functional approach, *Anesth Analg* 74:586, 1992.

Glantz SA, Slinker BK: *Primer of Applied Regression and Analysis of Variance,* New York, 1990, McGraw-Hill.

Glantz SA: *Primer of Biostatistics,* 3rd ed, New York, 1992, McGraw-Hill.

Mangano DT: Perioperative cardiac morbidity, *Anesthesiology* 72:153, 1990.

Mangano DT: Preoperative risk assessment: many studies, few solutions, *Anesthesiology* 83:897, 1995.

Mangano DT, et al: Association of perioperative myocardial ischemia with cardiac morbidity and mortality in men undergoing noncardiac surgery, *N Engl J Med* 323:1781, 1990.

Mangano DT, Goldman L: Preoperative assessment of patients with known or suspected coronary disease, *N Engl J Med* 333:1750, 1995.

Mantha S, et al: Relative effectiveness of four preoperative tests for predicting adverse cardiac outcomes after vascular surgery: a meta-analysis, *Anesth Analg* 79:422, 1994.

Poldermans D, et al: Dobutamine stress echocardiography for assessment of perioperative cardiac risk in patients undergoing major vascular surgery, *Circulation* 87:1506, 1993.

Raby KE, et al: Correlation between preoperative ischemia and major cardiac events after peripheral cardiac surgery, *N Engl J Med* 321:1296, 1989.

Rosner B: *Fundamentals of Biostatistics,* 2nd ed, Boston, 1986, Duxbury Press.

Wong T, Detsky AS: Preoperative cardiac risk assessment for patients having peripheral vascular surgery, *Ann Intern Med* 116:743, 1992.

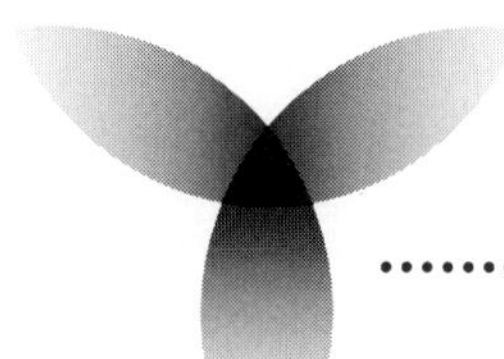

Chapter 3

Hypertensive and Ischemic Heart Disease

Evaluation and Intervention

David J. Stone, MD, John M. Dent, MD

• PREOPERATIVE EVALUATION

Clinical Risk Indices

The granddaddy of all these indices is of course, the Goldman Cardiac Risk Index, which is known far and wide and oft quoted on preoperative cardiology consultations. It was a new concept, performed at Massachusetts General Hospital, and published in the *New England Journal of Medicine.*[1] Basically, the index weighs a number of preoperative risk factors to produce a number that presumably represents perioperative cardiac risk. There are still some questions remaining as to the statistical validity of the original study done more than 20 years ago. For example, the data was gathered prospectively but analyzed retrospectively to pick out significant items. Furthermore, one analysis of the data noted that the P value of the study was .092, "a value usually considered unacceptable."[2]

More importantly, we have not found application of the index to be clinically useful. While the magnitude of the risk predicted by the index is roughly accurate, it is not clearly superior to that of a clinician with a moderate degree of experience and judgment. Most importantly, we have noted that consultants may begin and end a consult with a so-called "Goldman number" representing perioperative risk. This does not constitute a useful consultation. While it is the responsibility of the clinician requesting the consultation to pose the questions "What is wrong with the patient and what should be done about it?" the perioperative consultation in this situation should resolve these questions. The production of a Goldman number on a consult form does not answer these questions. If the consultant is so unfamiliar with perioperative cardiac care that the Goldman number is the only contribution he/she can make to the case, there is a need for a different consultant more cognizant of the medical requirements of perioperative care. A cardiac risk calculation, whether by the Goldman or another index, does not inform the involved physicians as to what actually needs to be done in any particular case. Notably, recent studies of cardiac risk have found that the Goldman index is not predictive, while other studies simply ignore it.[3]

The Problems of Ischemic, Hypertensive, and Congestive Heart Failure Risk

The basic questions can be formulated in several different ways. For example, is there myocardium at risk for ischemia and how well does the heart work? Alternatively, can the heart achieve the work levels demanded during the perioperative period and what is the ischemic cost (ST depression, angina, infarction) of this work? Finally, are coronary artery and/or myocardial pathologies present that demand changes from the norm of perioperative care? If Jane Austen were to write a novel based on perioperative cardiac care, she might entitle it *Tolerance and Reserve*.

The questions of ischemia and myocardial function (MI) are invariably intertwined. Ischemia may produce dysfunction, and dysfunction may predispose to or produce ischemia. The former is graphically demonstrated during intraoperative echocardiography when wall motion deteriorates in the face of acute ischemia. Increased wedge pressures in conjunction with decreased stroke volumes can also be demonstrated during acute ischemia if a pulmonary artery catheter is employed.

Heart failure may contribute to ischemia when associated left ventricular hypertrophy (LVH) reduces subendocardial perfusion. Ischemia can actually be produced by LVH even in the absence of severe coronary occlusions. Electrocardiographic and echocardiographic evidence of LVH increases perioperative ischemic risk as well as that of congestive heart failure (CHF).

The failing heart has a decreased ability to augment cardiac output when there is an increased demand for coronary blood flow (CBF). This inability to increase coronary flows will predispose to ischemia. In this sense, there is a reduced reserve so far as cardiac output is concerned. Furthermore, the dilated heart has a higher myocardial oxygen consumption (M_VO_2) due to increased LV end-diastolic volume (preload). In addition, coronary perfusion pressure may be reduced by increases in LV end-diastolic pressure. A heart with reduced EF and stroke volumes will also require higher heart rates to provide a given cardiac output, thereby setting the stage for a vicious cycle of ischemia and worsening dysfunction.

Hypertension may be a factor in both acute and chronic presentations. Severe acute uncontrolled hypertension enters the picture if afterload is increased to the extent that myocardial ejection is impaired in a failing heart. Ischemia may ensure if the increase in M_VO_2 and reduction in supply are beyond the capacity of a challenged coronary vasculature. The chronic effects of hypertension include contributions to the occurrence of CHF and coronary artery disease (CAD). Even in the absence of CAD or full-blown CHF, hypertension tends to result in a perioperative patient with decreased LV compliance, vasoconstriction, hypovolemia, and hemodynamic instability. In addition to the obvious problem of severe hypotension that may ensue due to all of these factors, decreased LV compliance (a.k.a. diastolic dysfunction) represents a particular intraoperative challenge, because a balance must be maintained between adequate cardiac filling and ejection versus pulmonary edema.

Directed Clinical Examination

The patient's history and physical are directed at detecting the presence and severity of coronary disease and myocardial dysfunction. In the case of patients with known CAD, it is important to establish whether the anginal pattern is stable, the magnitude of exertion required to produce angina (part of the exercise tolerance issue), and if there is a history of MI. A history of coronary artery bypass surgery (CABG) or angioplasty, along with response to these interventions, is obviously important. For other patients, it is important to screen for the possible presence of CAD manifested by typical or atypical patterns of chest pain. Other important factors include age (>70 is probably a risk factor), diabetes, hypertension, dysrhythmias, and other coronary risk factors. A history of CHF is solicited and questioning of its severity completes the exercise tolerance inquiry. Current medications are noted, with special attention to an increased requirement for antianginals. Physical examination is directed towards evidence of CHF, including the more subtle findings such as gallops; however, it is important to remember that even experienced clinicians may underestimate the degree of left ventricular dysfunction on physical examination, particularly when a gallop is absent. Other factors that should be especially considered are overall medical condition and the possible presence of aortic stenosis. The resting electrocardiogram (ECG) is reviewed with particular attention to evidence of CAD, LVH ± strain, and significant dysrhythmias. Important basic laboratories include hematocrit, as anemia may lower the threshold for myocardial ischemia, and glucose, especially if diabetes was not previously diagnosed. The basic findings on history, physical, and routine lab studies (including ECG) should give the clinician a fairly good idea of the patient's cardiac status and the need or lack of need for further testing.

Recent Myocardial Infarction

The patient who has suffered an MI in the previous 6 months has been especially worrisome ever since the original reports of increased perioperative risk appeared.

While perioperative morbidity appeared to level off after a 6-month post-MI interval, perioperative MI incidence was reported to range from 16% (3–6 months) to 37% (<3 months) after recent MI, with overall mortality of about 50% if an infarction occurred. Since that time, the situation appears to be somewhat ameliorated by improvements in drug therapy, anesthesia, and monitoring. Even so, the combination of surgery and recent MI has continued to be worrisome on both medical and medicolegal grounds.

Recent changes in cardiovascular knowledge and practice have definitely changed the picture, although these changes have been slow to enter the arena of perioperative medicine. For example, there are differences between Q wave and non-Q wave infarctions, in that the non-Q wave patients appear to be at somewhat increased risk for postinfarct ischemia. Non-Q wave MIs are now considered similar to unstable angina. This instability may occur because the territory supplied by the partially occluded vessel has not been completely infarcted as in the case of Q wave infarction. More important are advances in therapy for MI that include thrombolytic therapy and balloon angioplasty. Thrombolytic treatment is so effective that these patients are likely to be at much lower subsequent perioperative risk than MI patients who have not received such therapy. Also, patients who receive thrombolytic therapy appear to have a lower prevalence of multivessel CAD than infarction patients who don't receive thrombolytic therapy. However, data are not yet available to confirm this supposition.

From a diagnostic standpoint, cardiologists are much more aggressive about catheterization in the early post-MI period. Some cardiologists will catheterize virtually all their patients on day 3 to 4 postinfarction and claim that this actually represents a cost-effective approach, since appropriate risk stratification and therapy gets selected patients out of the hospital earlier. Other cardiologists are more selective and will only catheterize patients with continued angina or CHF at this time. There is general agreement concerning the need for some kind of reduced level stress testing of patients post-MI. One approach is to perform a low-level stress test (up to 70% maximal heart rate) with thallium or echo about day 6 after MI. This data is then used to decide whether there appears to be myocardium at risk for ischemia that may benefit from angioplasty or CABG. Operations other than the most urgent are best delayed for some period (≈10–14 days?) after these cardiotherapeutic procedures. In any case, the postinfarction patient who has received modern, high-quality cardiology care will already have answers in hand regarding the questions of ischemic risk and myocardial function. If the patient is able to perform low-level exercise without symptoms or worrisome changes in thallium redistribution or wall motion, it is reasonable to go ahead with surgery that is best not delayed (e.g., for cancer). The exact time of delay is a matter of judgment that depends on the magnitude of the planned procedure and the patient's response to therapeutic interventions and recovery from the MI. Should litigation arise, there is always the potential for a plaintiff's expert witness to claim that all surgery must wait until 6 months after an MI. This is simply no longer the standard of care. However, the exact details of the changes in care are in the process of being worked out and are best managed in a collaborative manner between surgeon, anesthesiologist, and cardiologist.

The patient who has had a possible or definite recent MI and has not had this kind of work-up will require some evaluation of myocardial function and risk for ischemia. Further work-up is clearly indicated if the patient manifests symptoms of CHF or angina. However, this may constitute quite a difficult judgment call if the patient had an MI 5 months ago, has been reasonably active and asymptomatic since, and requires surgery fairly urgently. Even in this situation, it is probably reasonable to obtain cardiologic consultation for several reasons. These include acute and long-term postoperative follow-up for appropriate cardiac care and to determine the need for a test such as echocardiography that will define functional state and extent of old infarction. The echocardiogram can usually be obtained quickly and conveniently. Finally, the patient and family are, thereby, notified that while the perioperative team is aware of some increase in risk, it has taken appropriate measures to evaluate the problem in more detail before proceeding with surgery. One of the keys to effective perioperative medicine is to prevent such patients from "showing up on the doorstep" on the day of surgery with a history of recent MI. In short, effective preoperative screening is necessary and should not be too difficult in this situation.

Known and Uncertain Coronary Artery Disease/Congestive Heart Failure

Patients with well-controlled, stable angina who have received adequate medical care and have reasonably good exercise tolerance (no symptoms of CHF) can certainly undergo low or intermediate-risk procedures without further work-up. The decision to pursue further work-up for high-risk procedures may involve the precise level of exercise tolerance and the nature of the work-up to date. Similarly, patients who have undergone coronary angioplasty or CABG with good results (asymptomatic or mild, controlled symptoms, good exercise tolerance) can proceed, even with high-risk surgery.

The patient with angina that appears to be unstable or has LV dysfunction on an ischemic basis deserves further work-up whether surgery is planned or not. Until recently, unstable angina has been an indication for urgent coronary catheterization. Unstable angina presents a very high perioperative cardiac risk with a reported incidence of adverse events of nearly 30%.[4] While angina of increasing severity or at rest may be evident, the clinician must be alert to more subtle signs, such as increased drug use or decreased activity. Previously undiagnosed classic angina may fit the definition of unstable angina and is an indication for further medical care before all but the most urgent operations. Ischemic myocardial dysfunction is not only important per se, but is generally an indicator of severe coronary disease. Patients with CHF (EF <45%) and triple vessel disease (or left main disease alone) demonstrate improved outcome from CABG and should be worked-up appropriately whether surgery is planned or not. Unfortunately, the extent of CAD cannot be determined by clinical means alone.

The aforementioned represents the relatively clear-cut cases of how to proceed, but many patients' risks fall into more nebulous categories. These may include patients with possible CAD/atypical chest pain, patients with remote histories of MI, patients who have received a less than complete cardiac work-up but are reasonably stable, and patients who simply present an enigmatic clinical picture on the basis of poor or unclear histories and inadequate medical records. Another group of patients consists of those who cannot exercise on the basis of disease in other systems (respiratory, neurological, vascular, etc.), or simply on the basis of old age or marked debilitation. The real question is how much good do we actually do these patients by delaying surgery and causing inconvenience, expense, discomfort, and worry with further medical testing? Currently, the answer to this question is that this is a matter of clinical judgment and it is up to the physicians involved to optimize patient care on a case-by-case basis. This may involve further testing or deciding that further testing is not indicated, especially if surgical risk is low or intermediate and patient benefit seems unlikely. Note that the entire team, including the anesthesiologist, should be involved in this decision, as well as a patient/family conference, if necessary.

Testing—1,2,3

The presently available noninvasive options have been discussed in the preceeding chapter and include ambulatory electrocardiography, echocardiography (± stress), and nuclear studies, generally with an element of stress. These tests should be approached with several goals/questions in mind. Most importantly, will the results change patient care in that cardiac catheterization followed by possible CABG or angioplasty will take place, if judged necessary? What do the physicians actually hope to learn from the test that will change perioperative management? Are the tests indicated for general medical reasons whether surgery is planned or not? The perioperative period may simply speed up a process of patient evaluation which should take place in any case. Is the test being done only because a physician feels *something* must be done or because something truly useful may ensue?

Ambulatory ECG is not commonly employed as a screen for ischemic heart disease and is not a measure of myocardial function. If a perioperative patient is undergoing 24-hour ECG monitoring for other purposes, the trace should certainly be evaluated for evidence of ischemia. The role of preoperative ECG monitoring is especially unclear because recent studies have indicated that postoperative changes are what count, i.e., correlate with adverse cardiac events. It is likely that the ambulatory ECG will serve as an intense and continuous monitor of postoperative ischemia in the future, rather than as a preoperative screening test.

The most commonly employed test for ischemia is the stress thallium, whether accomplished via exercise or dipyridamole. Unfortunately, the perioperative stress thallium may have begun to replace the Goldman number as a "requirement" for perioperative cardiac consultation by some clinicians. The stress thallium, performed and interpreted by experts, may provide evidence for the exclusion or presence of CAD if the diagnosis cannot be made clinically. This would fall under a general medical indication that may be useful perioperatively, as well. In fact, most of the indications for preoperative thallium probably fit in this category, i.e., the test would be indicated whether surgery was planned or not. Useful findings include ischemic LV dysfunction and extensive ischemia that may represent indications for catheterization. Specific preoperative indications for testing are harder to come by. In an attempt to specify a population that might benefit from the test, Eagle and coworkers noted that patients with one or two of the following factors (Q waves, age >70, diabetes, angina, ventricular ectopy) can be successfully stratified into risk groups by the test. They noted that patients with none of the factors were at extremely low risk and that patients with three or more factors possessed an increased risk that did not require thallium for identification. Clinicians may or may not be comfortable conducting their own practice on these findings alone.

Patients who cannot exercise or have reduced exercise tolerance may possibly be candidates for a dipyridamole thallium study if there is some question about the extent of myocardium at risk for ischemia and high or high-intermediate risk surgery is planned. The need for thallium studies is questionable if CABG or angioplasty are not considerations, e.g., refused by the patient or surgeon. The question remains: how will scan results alter management, especially when false-negatives are not unheard of and the positive predictive ability of the test is approximately 20%? The next section on intervention addresses this issue in more detail.

These conclusions basically apply to the stress echocardiogram, as well, except that the echocardiogram invariably provides some information on myocardial function. The choice of thallium or echo concerning the detection of ischemic risk may depend on local expertise, economics, and politics, but we may find the echo supplanting the nuclear studies in view of the increased information on LV function the stress echocardiogram provides. Advocates of nuclear imaging may counter this with increased use of the sestamibi scan which, as noted, does provide an estimate of ejection fraction. Unfortunately, a test that truly duplicated all the stresses of the perioperative period would represent a real risk in itself! Ultimately, the perioperative period may represent its own kind of stress test, one that screens for patients who require further cardiologic evaluation and treatment.

The resting two-dimensional (2-D) transthoracic echocardiogram is an undervalued screening test that is less expensive and more readily available than stress echocardiographic or nuclear studies. In the patient with newly diagnosed angina, the absence of wall motion abnormalities at rest reduces the potential benefit of revascularization and supports a medical approach with aspirin, β-blockers, and modification of lipid profile. If wall motion abnormalities are present, the results of a stress test with thallium or echo may provide further clinical impetus for cardiac catheterization vs. medical therapy. The rest echo is extremely useful for the perioperative patient who has reduced exercise tolerance or cannot exercise at all, since it can point to the presence or absence of systolic myocardial dysfunction, LVH, valvular heart disease, and even less common problems such as myxomas and pericardial constriction/tamponade.

The need for cardiac catheterization is determined by the consultant cardiologist and clearly falls into the category of a test that is done because it is indicated, regardless of planned surgery. It is reasonable to catheterize patients with unstable angina, angina after recent MI, ischemic myocardial dysfunction, and suspected left main or triple vessel coronary disease, particularly in the setting of reduced LV function. There is accumulating evidence that patients with hibernating myocardium or double vessel CAD and LV dysfunction receive more than symptomatic benefit from CABG.

Catheterization is expensive, uncomfortable, and does have a small risk of its own; so it should be applied selectively and thoughtfully.

• PREOPERATIVE INTERVENTIONS

Except for emergency procedures, patients with significant ischemic or CHF risk should not pose a "surprise" on the day of surgery. Such a discovery almost invariably results in surgical delay or cancellation, so that medical therapy can be instituted, intensified, or revascularization can be performed. Unfortunately, surprises do occur for a number of reasons, both avoidable and unavoidable, and it is incumbent upon the physicians involved to do the right thing regardless of patient or physician convenience. In the ideal perioperative situation, the patient has come to medical attention some time, preferably at least a week, before the scheduled surgery so that the "state of the heart" can be determined. Patients who have received thorough care will generally require no further intervention preoperatively, since both pharmacological and other measures have already been considered or instituted. Patients who have received less than optimal or no care, benefit most from this early cardiac preoperative evaluation. The first part of preoperative intervention is evaluation.

Invasive Interventions

After the results of evaluation are in, an important issue arises: the possible need for cardiac catheterization. The real question is whether perioperative CABG or angioplasty is indicated specifically as a perioperative adjunct. In general, the answer to this question is no. Patients who have received previous successful (improved re angina ± CHF) CABG surgery are clearly at reduced risk for subsequent surgery. However, applying this knowledge to the perioperative period must account for the added risk of the catheterization and CABG themselves. It appears that subsequent risk is mainly reduced by transferring risk to the peri-CABG period, rather than by eliminating risk entirely. Revascularization is appropriate if CABG is indicated, surgery or not, but may not be so if CABG is planned solely because of anticipated surgery. There is also a small, but real, risk in delaying procedures such as aortic aneurysm repairs and carotid endarterectomies. An aggressive approach to catheterization and CABG for high-risk vascular surgery patients has been taken in the past and probably does benefit some individual patients at the cost of hurting others. It is also extremely expensive.

The role of coronary angioplasty in the perioperative period is just beginning to be worked out with some initial reports of mixed success. It is important to schedule subsequent surgery in the window between the acute complications of the procedure and the onset of restenosis (2–4 weeks postangioplasty). The decision to proceed with angioplasty vs. CABG is a cardiologic one and involves the extent and location of the coronary occlusions, ejection fraction, and available expertise. As for CABG, it is likely that angioplasty should be reserved for patients for whom it is indicated, surgery or not. However, it is possible that for carefully selected patients undergoing high-risk procedures, angioplasty provides an option for reduction of perioperative cardiac risk that should be undertaken for this reason alone. However, all the data is not in on this issue.

Noninvasive Interventions

After the need for invasive interventions has been excluded, the main job is to optimize medical therapy for hypertension, angina, and CHF. This should be done thoughtfully, as overaggressive treatments may lead to increased intraoperative instability and, possibly, increased morbidity. There is otherwise no special magic to medical care at this time and internists/cardiologists should not decide to become especially aggressive in their recommendations. It is easier for the anesthesiologist to add a necessary drug later than to remove one that is causing difficulties. For instance, patients should not be overdiuresed just before anticipated surgery because anesthetics tend to cause vasodilation and reduced inotropy. In patients with reasonable renal function, it may be best to hold diuretics on the day of surgery if they are only part of an antihypertensive regime. On the other hand, if diuretics are required to control CHF, they should be administered on the morning of surgery. The decision to continue digoxin for CHF on the morning of surgery should be individualized, but digoxin should be continued for control of heart rate in atrial fibrillation. Beta-blockers are extremely useful and may turn out to play an increased perioperative role if postoperative tachycardia is established as a key determinant of outcome. There has long been a temptation on the part of consultants to recommend an intravenous nitroglycerin infusion for patients at ischemic risk. Recent work indicates that nitroglycerin infusion is not an effective maneuver, possibly because of differing mechanisms of ischemia in surgical patients.

It cannot be overemphasized that anesthesiologists are well-versed in the cardiovascular care of patients with these problems and are well aware of the perioperative implications of antihypertensives, antianginals, and drugs for CHF. Most anesthesiologists care for patients with CHF, hypertension, and angina on a near-daily basis. There is no substitute for a team approach at this time when members learn about the strengths of the other players. Furthermore, while thoughtful suggestions are welcome, the provision of intraoperative care, including monitoring, is the province of the anesthesiologist. Recommendations for specific monitors or cardiovascularly active drugs should be phrased carefully. For example, write "consider placement of PA catheter" rather than "place PA catheter." There is no need to make statements such as "careful fluid management" or "monitor ECG." The competent, well-trained anesthesiologist has already considered the need for particular monitors and drugs. If possible and reasonable, state why you think the particular monitor or agent is recommended. Recommendations for specific kinds of anesthesia are best not part of the written consultation but may justify verbal inquiry on the part of the consultant or primary care physician. For example, does a recommendation for "cardiac anesthesia" imply a need for a specific drug on drugs, a specific individual, or for the use of cardiopulmonary bypass? It is not a meaningful or appropriate recommendation. Take advantage of this interaction to learn from each other!

The goal of medical care at this time is similar to that in any setting: the optimization of patient care within the bounds of "*non nocere*." The anticipation of surgery may speed the clock up a bit, but there is no need to try to prepare a "superpatient" who can leap all operations at a single bound. Sometimes, physicians try to invent new medicine at this juncture, rather than apply the principles of care that serve them well on a daily, nonperioperative basis.

INTRAOPERATIVE PHYSIOLOGY

While intraoperative hemodynamic stability is still the major goal of patient care recent work has demonstrated that intraoperative blood pressure and heart rate control is only part of the picture. For example, work done by Slogoff and Keats[5] in the mid 1980s revealed that only approximately half the episodes of intraoperative ischemia they detected were associated with a hemodynamic change previously defined as significant. More recent studies of Mangano et al. have found that the incidence of intraoperative ischemia is less than during the postoperative period and not much different from the preoperative period. Their work has pointed to postoperative ischemia as being most important in determining adverse cardiac outcome. These findings do not relegate the intraoperative period to the realm of the unimportant, but certainly move it out of the primary suspect position when a source for a bad outcome is investigated.

Monitoring

In general, the patient with mild disease, whether it be hypertension, coronary disease, or CHF can be monitored with "routine" methods. The word "routine" is somewhat deceptive, as routine measures are fairly intensive. In most cases, these would include continuous monitoring of two ECG leads, including a limb lead and V_4 or V_5. The addition of the frontal lead has been shown to boost test sensitivity for ischemia to the 80% to 90% range. The range can be further increased with the addition of a second frontal lead but this is not usually available. Some clinicians will have computerized analysis of ST segments available to them, whereby the ECG tracing is continuously analyzed by an inmonitor computer that reports potentially significant changes. Blood pressure is measured with an automatic oscillometer that is usually cycled every 2 to 3 minutes but can cycle every minute or even more often when employed for short periods in a so-called "stat" mode. The oscillometer provides an extremely accurate mean pressure measured by the cuff but provides somewhat less accurate systolic and diastolic measurements, which are calculated. The capnometer that measures expired carbon dioxide requires pulmonary blood flow and, hence, cardiac output, to provide carbon dioxide for measurement. However, it is not a useful monitor of cardiac output within the normally acceptable range because expired carbon dioxide does not drop off significantly until cardiac output has fallen to unacceptable levels, i.e., approximately half of normal. At that point, a more linear relationship is established between cardiac output and expired carbon dioxide so that the monitor has been shown to be useful during cardiac arrest/CPR situations.

As the magnitude of surgery increases and as patient disease state worsens, monitoring is intensified. The intraarterial cannula, or "A-line" in medical jargon, is an extremely useful monitor that provides continuous monitoring of blood pressure at relatively little cost, discomfort, and risk. A variety of engineering factors in the fluid-filled tubing can lead to some overestimation of systolic pressures, but the mean pressure is extremely accurate. The precise systolic and diastolic pressures recorded will also depend on the location of the catheter, as more distal locations (e.g., dorsal pedis) will result in higher systolic and lower diastolic pressures. This is mainly due to reflection and amplification of pressure waves in smaller vessels. Mean pressures remain reliable and decrease slightly with distance from the heart because this is the direction of blood flow. As discussed in the monitoring chapter, analysis of the pressure pulse waveform can give quite an accurate picture of volume status. This analysis rests on the interaction of mechanical ventilation with cardiac preload and afterload, as well as direct mechanical factors, and is ideal in the anesthetized, paralyzed patient.

It is reasonable to place an arterial cannula in patients with moderate to severe CHF (EF <40% to 45%), patients with poorly controlled hypertension, and patients with a significant amount of myocardium at ischemic risk. The latter would include urgent or emergent surgery in the patient with unstable angina or recent MI, the patient with severe CAD that is not amenable to intervention, or the patient presenting a truly unclear, but worrisome, clinical picture. While the patient with stable angina may not require intraarterial monitoring for every procedure, one's threshold for intraarterial monitoring should be somewhat reduced so that it may be employed for procedures perceived to be moderately stressful but in which the "A-line" would not be inserted in a healthy patient. These procedures *might* include laparoscopic intraabdominal procedures, hip surgery or replacement, and prolonged procedures of any sort. The presence of LVH on ECG or echocardiography might also lower the threshold for intravascular blood pressure monitoring, since these patients are quite sensitive to alterations in preload. Placement before the induction of anesthesia allows continuous monitoring during this stressful period and is generally recommended.

The central venous pressure (CVP) catheter is not a particularly useful intraoperative monitor in these patients. Analysis of the cycling of the arterial waveform is a more accurate monitor of volume status. The CVP may be useful postoperatively when spontaneous ventilation makes arterial waveform analysis difficult to impossible. The pulmonary artery (PA) catheter is a good monitor of cardiac function, especially when stroke volume is analyzed in tandem with filling pressures. It might be employed in the patient with severe CHF for procedures of even moderate stress but only for more stressful procedures in the case of lesser degrees of myocardial dysfunction. However, the relationship between pulmonary capillary wedge pressure and LV end-diastolic pressures may be muddled by a number of factors so that the recorded wedge pressure does not accurately track preload. For example, wedge pressures may be normal in the face of hypovolemia if the left atrium and/or ventricle is noncompliant or there is pulmonary venoconstriction. The absolute wedge pressure remains a good indicator of the propensity for cardiogenic pulmonary edema. The PA catheter is not a particularly good monitor for myocardial ischemia because changes in waveform morphology or filling pressures that are due to ischemia will not occur until sufficient myocardium is ischemic so that the change occurs. In other words, there must be substantial myocardial dysfunction before stroke volume falls and filling pressures rise as evidence of ischemia. The PA catheter may be placed before or after the induction of anesthesia. Some practitioners find placement facilitated by patient cooperation (head elevation and turning), while others feel the discomfort is not justified by any utility during induction.

Intraoperative transesophageal echocardiography (TEE) appears to be an excellent way to monitor both ischemia and function but requires availability of expensive equipment and significant skill in technique and interpretation. The relatively noninvasive nature of the monitor makes it especially implementable in cases when it is not clear that a PA catheter is indicated or when insertion presents extreme risk or difficulty. There is little question that the TEE is a better monitor of preload as the LV chamber can be visualized. In addition, EF can be estimated and, if a PA catheter is in place, LV end diastolic volume (LVEDV) can actually be calculated: LVEDV = stroke volume ÷ EF. The echocardiogram is clearly a better monitor for ischemia than the PA catheter. Ischemia is detected by noting new abnormalities in segmental wall motion, which may manifest as a-, hypo-, or dyskinesis, depending on the severity of the ischemia. These changes should occur earlier and be more accurate than ST changes in ischemia. However, interpretation is highly operator-dependent and may be muddled by the concomitant changes in preload, inotropy, and afterload that occur during anesthesia and surgery. Care must be taken to not overinterpret and overtreat changes thought to represent ischemia. With these caveats in minds, TEE represents an impressive modality of monitoring for ischemia and is a reasonable monitor during general anesthesia for any procedure when there is a significant risk of myocardial ischemia. The question still remains as to whether the TEE is a more useful monitor of intraoperative ischemia than a two-lead ECG, since there is no gold standard for ischemia. Caution should be employed in neurosurgical procedures requiring extreme neck flexion in which the area of the oropharynx may already be compromised by positioning and in whom severe swelling of upper airway and oral structures may ensue if lymphatic and vascular drainage is further limited.

Anesthesia

Anesthetic care is planned and carried out with an aim to minimization of hemodynamic aberration while maintaining an adequate cardiac output. At times, consultants request a "cardiac anesthesiologist" and/or "cardiac anesthesia" for a particular case. Cardiac anesthesiologists are specialists within anesthesiology who anesthetize patients for procedures requiring cardiopulmonary bypass. The techniques involved often include high doses of narcotics, which maintain hemodynamic stability and baseline inotropy at the cost of a prolonged requirement for mechanical ventilation. What the consultants mean to say is that they have specific concerns regarding the potential for ischemia or heart failure that require attention from a clinician cognizant of these issues. This clinician may or may not be one who also covers bypass cases and, in many instances, the clinicians who ordinarily cover major noncardiac cases are at least as qualified.

For the patient with myocardium at risk for ischemia, the simultaneous occurrence of tachycardia and hypotension is the worst possible combination so far as supply and demand are concerned. Severe bradycardia and hypertension may also be deleterious by reducing supply and increasing demand, respectively. Care is taken to blunt the tachycardic/hypertensive response to painful stimuli such as laryngoscopy, intubation, and surgical incision, but this must be done without overcorrection that results in hypotension and/or marked bradycardia (with β-blockers, for example). A variety of methods are available to carry out this mission including application of local anesthesia to the airway, inhaled and intravenous anesthetics, β-blockers, narcotics, and vasodilators. Care must be taken to avoid hypotension subsequent to the use of longer-acting agents followed by the withdrawal of a severe, acute stimulus. While techniques such as high-dose narcotics may be employed, as for cardiac cases, they are generally avoided for shorter and less extensive cases, because they will result in prolonged recovery times that are generally unnecessary. The anesthesiologist is best qualified to decide whether a regional anesthetic technique, whether alone or in combination with general anesthesia, is an appropriate and reasonable option in any particular combination of surgeon, procedure, and patient. For coronary disease without underlying CHF, spinal or epidural anesthesia may offer no particular benefit. However, these techniques, as well as upper extremity blocks, may be quite effective and applicable as an option. It must be realized that regional anesthesia is no panacea and that spinal or epidural anesthesia can lead to severe hemodynamic aberration, patient anxiety with $\Uparrow M_VO_2$, and, possibly, adverse intramyocardial hemodynamics if the level of anesthesia does not include the upper thoracic segments.

Care of the hypertensive patient involves many of the previous concerns in conjunction with awareness of the patient's current antihypertensive regimen and an awareness that the patient may be functionally hypovolemic and possess a particularly reactive peripheral vasculature. In addition to concern about severe elevations in blood pressure, attention must be paid to decreases that may be even more concerning if the cerebral blood flow autoregulatory curve is shifted to the right by an uncorrected chronic hypertensive state. Interventions to blunt increases in blood pressure should be conceived so as to avoid the creation of a new problem with prolonged, significant hypotension. This is carried out with small doses of short-acting drugs given to mildly undercorrect the problem, rather than to severely overcorrect it. If appropriate, regional anesthesia is a fine option once intravascular hypovolemia has been corrected before spinal or epidural anesthesia.

The patient with moderate-to-severe CHF must be anesthetized without causing significantly reduced inotropy or changes in preload or afterload that severely affect cardiac output. The actual physiology involved may depend on the pathophysiology of the patient's CHF. This is why preoperative echocardiography may be particularly useful in planning an anesthetic. For example, the patient with long-standing hypertension may have severe LVH without major coronary occlusions. Such a patient may be quite preload dependent and sensitive to changes in volume status. However, this patient may be relatively well adapted to tolerate some decline in inotropic state and increase in afterload. This patient may tolerate anesthesia well with a potent inhaled agent as long as normovolemia is maintained. On the other hand, the patient with a dilated ischemic cardiomyopathy may tolerate or even mildly benefit from some decrease in preload, yet be very sensitive to increases in afterload or decreases in inotropy. Anesthesia can be planned to avoid negative inotropes as far as possible, and might involve a basic nitrous oxide-narcotic technique. The introduction of etomidate has provided practitioners with an intravenous induction agent that is less cardiovascularly depressant than previously available nonnarcotic agents. Note that circulation time is slowed in these patients so that particular patience must be employed in the administration of intravenous drugs. In addition, drug metabolism may be slowed due to reductions in hepatic and renal perfusion.

Regional anesthesia is a reasonable alternative in these patients especially since neither spinal nor epidural anesthesia causes a decrease in inotropy. The decrease in afterload may also be beneficial in cases of dilated cardiomyopathy. Care must be taken to maintain preload when these techniques cause vasodilation, as higher segmental dermatomes supplying sympathetic vasoinnervation are blocked. Dramatic falls in cardiac output can also occur when cardioaccelerator fibers are blocked by a high level of spinal or epidural anesthesia. The combination of regional with general anesthesia may improve outcome in selected patients with CHF. At the least, a successful combined technique will improve pain management during the immediate and early postoperative period. Care must be taken to avoid hypotension when these techniques are combined intraoperatively. One way to accomplish this is to markedly limit the administration of vasodilating local anesthetics intraoperatively until near the end of the case when an infusion of dilute local anesthesia with a narcotic is begun through an epidural catheter.

• POSTOPERATIVE INTERVENTIONS

As the effects of anesthesia wear off and the metabolic and vascular effects of surgical stress and pain take full effect, the patient enters a most dangerous period as far as hypertension, myocardia ischemia, and heart failure are concerned. After the last stitch is in, the surgeon will often call the family and tell them that everything has gone well. However, the potential for problems is not over for any patient at that time, and especially, not for this population. The postoperative care of hypertension is discussed in the recovery room chapter. In brief, hypertension is quite common in the recovery period and, in addition to antihypertensive treatment, remediable etiologies such as pain, hypoxemia, hypercarbia, and bladder or gastric distention must be considered.

The diagnosis of myocardial ischemia in this time period is particularly difficult and often involves cardiologic consultation. The ECG may have nonspecific changes due to stress, hypothermia, surgery, electrolyte shifts, and drugs that suggest the possibility of ischemia. Breslow and coworkers reported that mild T-wave changes without ST changes are unlikely to represent ischemia.[6] Most of the diagnostic problems involve some degree of ST-segment depression with ST-elevation and Q waves much less common than in an emergency room setting, for example. Neurovascular procedures, especially if preceded by subarachnoid hemorrhage, may result in impressive ECG changes (especially deep inverted T waves) that may or may not represent some element of microscopic cardiomyopathy. In addition, most of the ischemia that does occur is silent, because of a variety of factors including altered consciousness, predominant incisional pain, analgesics, and, possibly, endogenous endorphins. The baseline ECG is very useful at this time to draw comparisons with the postoperative 12-lead ECG. Interpretation of the ECG is extremely difficult during this period and is best tempered with some element of judgment and experience. The transthoracic echocardiogram has not been used much to date in identifying postoperative segmental wall abnormalities that might tend to substantiate the importance of nebulous ST-T wave changes. If a baseline echocardiogram is not available, it might be difficult to sort out the significance of observed wall motion abnormalities. Although there is little-to-no data on this, postoperative echocardiography might be useful in guiding the next stage of care. For example, the patient with totally normal wall motion is unlikely to have significant ischemia, and triage to an unmonitored floor bed may be more reasonable than for one with suspicious wall motion abnormalities.

It is critical to carry out presumptive therapy while the diagnosis is under serious consideration. This might involve rate control with β-blockers and the administration of nitroglycerin in some form (transdermal, intravenous [IV], sublingual, or nebulized if the patient is intubated). Basic care of pain, electrolyte disturbances, and respiratory status should not be forgotten. One frequent conclusion of clinicians/consultants is that MI must be "ruled-out." Unfortunately, such a conclusion seems to preclude further care in some cases, as if "ruling out MI" by drawing cardiac enzymes was sufficient therapy in itself and the patient can be sent to a general surgery bed on the floor. Relevant issues include: (1) Where should MI be "ruled-out?" Is anywhere other than the critical care unit (CCU) or a carefully monitored bed appropriate if the diagnosis is being seriously considered? (2) How are enzymes interpreted in the perioperative period? Does a borderline test have no significance if slightly low, yet tremendous significance if slightly high? and (3) Does a negative workup for MI signify that a patient has no further risk for ischemia? The last may, in fact, be just as important as the actual occurrence of MI per se. It is essential to ensure that basic therapeutics are continued during the "rule-out" stage including treatment of ischemia, CHF, and dysrhythmias. This may be difficult to accomplish for a patient in an unmonitored bed on a surgical floor and may be the best reason for transfer to a location and/or service where these factors will be addressed. If MI is an obvious consideration, urgent cardiologic consultation and transfer to a CCU should be arranged. In any case, the family should be informed of the problem, particularly since it is likely that they just received a call from the surgeon telling them that everything went perfectly.

The patient with CHF is at increased risk for postoperative fluid overload acutely as the intravascular volume space is decreased due to cold, vasoconstriction from stress and pain, and the wearing off of vasodilating anesthetics. Care must be taken not to overdiurese acutely, because these patients will tend to vasodilate as they rewarm and pain is better controlled, particularly if epidural local anesthetics are being used. Many consultants are flabbergasted by the volumes of crystalloid that have been administered in the operating room and are quick to blame the anesthesiologist for fluid overload, even when what are appropriate volumes have been administered. The amount of crystalloid may seem quite large since it is given in a 3:1 or 5:1 ratio to replace blood loss and must replace normal fluid requirements as well as third space and evaporative losses. Third spacing represents displacement of fluid to a nonfunctional extravascular space and may involve liters of fluid. Evaporative losses can be 500 ml an hour for major abdominal cases. In general, the anesthesiologist is coming from a viewpoint in which the administration of a little extra fluid may be an inconvenience, but a hypovolemic cardiac arrest is a disaster. However, fluid overload does occur, especially if myocardial function is compromised and accounts for a substantial proportion of those patients who require continued intubation/ventilation or reintubation with ventilation in the University of Virginia recovery room. (Terrance Yemen, MD, personal communication.)

Postoperatively the clinical diagnosis is made more difficult by the fact that bibasilar crackles may represent atelectasis rather than left-sided CHF. Furthermore, it is difficult to sit up most surgical patients for a good physical examination. A good PA chest radiograph is difficult to obtain and even a technically adequate portable film may be difficult to interpret, due to artifactual cardiac enlargement, atelectasis, and postsurgical changes. Other postoperative etiologies for infiltrates include aspiration, drug or blood transfusion related noncardiogenic pulmonary edema, and negative pressure pulmonary edema that can follow episodes of upper airway obstruction. These are reasons that surgeons pay such careful attention to "Is and Os" on their postoperative rounds (along with WBC count as an indicator of wound infection). In the first few postoperative days, fluid is mobilized from extravascular spaces into the vasculature so that vigilance must be maintained for fluid overload during this time as well. Other elements that may predispose to postoperative myocardial decompensation include tachydysrhythmias, myocardial ischemia/infarction, and poorly controlled hypertension.

REFERENCES

1. Goldman L, et al: Multifactorial index of cardiac risk in nonardiac surgical procedures, *N Engl J Med* 297:845, 1977.
2. Teplick R: American Society of Anesthesiologists Refresher Course Lectures 113, 1988.
3. Younis, et al: Preoperative clinical assessment and dipyrydamole thallium-201 scintigraphy for prediction and prevention of cardiac events in patients having major noncardiovascular surgery and known or suspected coronary artery disease, *Am J Cardiol* 74:311, 1994.
4. Shah KB, et al: Angina and other risk factors in patients with cardiac diseases undergoing noncardiac operations, *Anesth Analg* 70:240m 1990.
5. Slogoff S, Keats AS, et al: Further observations on perioperative myocardial ischemia, *Anesthesiology* 65:539, 1986.
6. Breslow MJ, et al: Changes in T-wave morphology following anesthesia and surgery: A common recovery room phenomenon, *Anesthesiology* 64:398, 1986.

BIBLIOGRAPHY

Elmore JR, et al: Myocardial revascularization before abdominal aortic aneurysmorrhaphy: effect of coronary angioplasty, *Mayo Clin Proc* 68:637, 1993.

Fleisher LA: Perioperative assessment of the patient with cardiovascular disease undergoing noncardiac surgery, *Curr Opin Anesth* 6:24, 1993.

Gersh BJ, et al: Evaluation and management of patients with both peripheral vascular and coronary artery disease, *J Am Coll Cardiol* 18:203, 1991.

Goldman L: Cardiac risk in noncardiac surgery: an update, *Anesth Analg* 80:810, 1995.

Goldman L: Multifactorial index of cardiac risk in noncardiac surgery: ten-year status report, *J Cardiothorac Anesth* 1:237, 1987.

Goldman L, et al: Multifactorial index of cardiac risk in noncardiac surgical procedures, *N Engl J Med* 297:845, 1977.

Hollenberg M, et al: Therapeutic approaches to postoperative ischemia, *Am J Cardiol* 73:30B, 1994.

Mangano DT, et al: Dipyridamole thallium-201 scintigraphy as a preoperative screening test—A reexamination of its predictive potential, *Circulation* 84:493, 1991.

Massie BM, Mangano DT: Risk stratification for noncardiac surgery—How and why? *Circulation* 87:1752, 1993.

Seeger JM, et al: Does routine stress thallium cardiac scanning reduce postoperative cardiac complications? *Ann Surg* 219:654, 1994.

Shah KB, et al: Reevaluation of perioperative myocardial infarction in patients with prior myocardial infarction undergoing noncardiac operations, *Anesth Analg* 71:231, 1990.

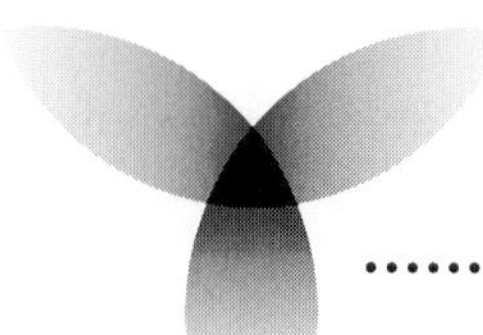

Chapter 4

Management of Valvular Heart Disease

George S. Leisure, MD, John M. Dent, MD

Valvular heart disease comprises a variety of disorders, each of which requires a different approach. Perioperative management demands a thorough understanding of the physiologic derangement imposed on the cardiovascular system by the specific valvular lesion. In order to manage the hemodynamic status of these patients appropriately, the severity and chronicity of the valvular lesion must be considered, as well as the state of left ventricular contractile function. The presence of significant coronary artery disease must also be considered. Depending on the lesion involved, specific attention must be paid to the patient's preload (intravascular volume), afterload (systemic vascular resistance), and cardiac rhythm. In general, stenotic lesions are more difficult to manage than regurgitant lesions because stenotic lesions cause the systemic cardiac output to be relatively fixed within a narrow range.

The risk of noncardiac surgery for a given valve defect is difficult to quantify. In the case of aortic stenosis, Goldman in 1977 identified this lesion as an independent risk factor for postoperative cardiac death, citing a 13% mortality rate. However, O'Keefe reported in 1989 no perioperative deaths in a series of 48 patients with severe aortic stenosis undergoing noncardiac surgery. Although large scale studies are lacking, it is possible that current diagnostic and therapeutic options may decrease the risk of noncardiac surgery in this population. In some cases, the best preparation of the patient with valvular heart disease for noncardiac surgery may be surgical repair or replacement of the valve. Balloon valvuloplasty as a nonoperative alternative in valvular stenosis may also be considered, although the long-term results of this procedure have been disappointing.

In this chapter, we will focus primarily on defects of the mitral and aortic valves as they usually have the most significant hemodynamic consequences. The etiology, pathophysiology, and perioperative concerns for each lesion will be described. Finally, indications for valve surgery will be briefly outlined.

MITRAL STENOSIS

Etiology

Stenosis of the mitral valve occurs when either scarring or some other pathologic process causes obstruction of blood flow through the mitral valve, leading to left atrial enlargement, pulmonary edema, pulmonary hypertension, and right heart failure. The primary cause of mitral stenosis (MS) is rheumatic heart disease (RHD). Rheumatic fever is caused by Group A, β-hemolytic streptococcal infection usually acquired between the ages of 5 and 15 years. It is an insidiously progressive disease and patients often become symptomatic between the third and fifth decades of life. As a result of the rheumatic fever, the mitral valve apparatus becomes inflamed which ultimately leads to leaflet thickening and calcification, commissural fusion, and chordal fusion. This process leads to a funnel-shaped mitral valve with decreased orifice size, and obstruction to blood flow. Thrombus formation in the left atrial appendage and other areas of the atrium is a common occurrence, and systemic embolization can result.

More rare causes of mitral stenosis include atrial myxoma, thrombus, vegetations, the parachute mitral valve deformity, and calcification of the mitral leaflets and annulus. Calcification occurs most commonly in the elderly and in those with chronic renal failure but only rarely produces significant stenosis.

Pathophysiology

The normal mitral valve area is about 4 to 6 cm^2, and patients become symptomatic when the orifice area is decreased by more than half. As the resistance to flow increases, the left atrial pressure increases to maintain normal left ventricular filling. Left atrial hypertrophy and dilation result. For a period of time, the augmented left atrial pressure maintains reasonable diastolic flow. However, the dilated and scarred left atrium often develops paroxysmal and then chronic atrial fibrillation, and the loss of atrial systole may severely impair ventricular filling. Forward flow now becomes increasingly dependent on the diastolic filling period, and the increased heart rate will further raise the left atrial pressure. In addition, dynamic exercise can cause an elevation in the left atrial pressure by increasing the transvalvular flow and reducing the diastolic filling time.

Left atrial hypertension leads to pulmonary venous congestion and subsequent pulmonary venous hypertension. Pulmonary arterial constriction ensues as the intima and media of the pulmonary arterial walls undergo hyperplasia in an effort to protect the capillaries from fluid transudation. Finally, irreversible pulmonary hypertension develops with right ventricular hypertrophy, tricuspid regurgitation, severe venous congestion, and edema. Left ventricular function usually remains essentially normal. However, left ventricular function can be affected by an overloaded right ventricle. Patients develop dyspnea on exertion, paroxysmal nocturnal dyspnea, and may develop hemoptysis due to bronchial vein rupture. These symptoms may be exacerbated by other stresses such as pregnancy or infection. The clinician must be aware that the symptoms of pulmonary hypertension and right ventricular failure may be mistaken for those of chronic obstructive pulmonary disease.

Perioperative Concerns

Significant mitral stenosis (MS) is rarely overlooked on the preoperative evaluation because the symptoms usually correlate with the severity of the hydraulic defect. However, some patients may remain minimally symptomatic despite significant stenosis by progressively reducing their activity level. The murmur on physical examination may correlate poorly with the degree of obstruction, and even the classic findings of MS may be missed on casual auscultation. The chest radiograph reveals a characteristic distortion of the cardiac silhouette with enlargement of the left atrium, right ventricle, and pulmonary artery. The findings on electrocardiography include left atrial enlargement, right ventricular enlargement, and the presence of atrial fibrillation. Doppler echocardiography can be used to assess the severity of the lesion by estimating the gradient across the valve and by determining the valve area, using the pressure half-time method.

As a result of the obstruction of flow from the left atrium to the left ventricle, the left ventricle has inadequate preload, and an abnormally elevated left atrial pressure is needed to maintain acceptable left ventricular diastolic pressures. Clearly, inadequate volume may lead to a drop in cardiac output and overzealous fluid administration may lead to pulmonary edema. Consequently, the clinician should have a low threshold for placing a flow-directed pulmonary artery catheter to help guide the fluid replacement. Interpretation of this data must be with caution. The pulmonary capillary wedge pressure will be greater than the left ventricular end-diastolic pressure because of the obstruction to flow. In addition, the clinician should beware of catheter balloon inflation in the presence of pulmonary hypertension, advanced age, and anticoagulant use. The presence of these factors has been associated with an increased risk of pulmonary artery rupture during balloon inflation.

Tachycardia can be deleterious in this population because it reduces the time for blood to flow from the left atrium to the left ventricle, and, thus, can lead to the sudden development of pulmonary edema. Heart rate must be controlled aggressively. If the patient is in sinus rhythm, β-adrenergic receptor blockers may blunt rises in heart rate. If atrial fibrillation is present, the ventricular response must be well-controlled before the surgical procedure. Medications that may cause tachycardia such as atropine, glycopyrrolate, ketamine, pancuronium, and Demerol should be avoided. If the patient is on anticoagulant treatment preoperatively, this should be taken into consideration. Prophylactic antibiotics should be administered if indicated for the procedure. Both general or regional anesthesia can be employed safely if the physiologic consequences of this lesion are fully understood.

If the patient is symptomatic from the mitral stenosis in the perioperative period, further cardiac evaluation should be strongly considered because mitral valve surgery or percutaneous mitral balloon valvotomy may be indicated prior to an elective surgical procedure. Balloon valvotomy offers an effective nonsurgical alternative that has provided excellent long-term relief in patients whose valve anatomy is suitable for this procedure. Fortunately, sudden death in asymptomatic patients with mitral stenosis is rare. Consequently, if the patient is asymptomatic in the perioperative period, there is no justification for prophylactic mitral valve surgery or balloon valvotomy.

AORTIC STENOSIS

Etiology

Aortic stenosis (AS) can be divided into four categories: congenital, calcific bicuspid, rheumatic, and calcific senile. Congenital AS may result from a unicuspid valve, hypoplasia of the annulus, or congenital fusion of the commissures. In the case of calcific bicuspid AS, the patient is born with a nonstenotic bicuspid aortic valve, a common congenital defect affecting approximately 1% of the population. As a result of the altered mobility of the valvular cusps, chronic trauma results in progressive fibrosis, calcification, and, ultimately, valvular stenosis. Rheumatic aortic stenosis results from acquired thickening of cusps and fusion of commissures. However, this rarely results in isolated AS. Most patients will have associated mitral valve disease that is clinically apparent. Aortic incompetence is frequently present. Calcific senile AS is caused by sclerosis which results in calcification of the valve over a long period of time. The obstruction to flow is generally mild, but can progress to the point of requiring surgical intervention. Concomitant mitral annular calcification is frequently present in these patients.

In general, the etiology of AS in a patient under the age of 30 years is a congenitally stenotic aortic valve. In patients presenting with AS between the ages of 30 to 70 years, the stenosis is likely caused by rheumatic disease or calcification of a congenital bicuspid valve. Beyond the age of 70 years, the most common cause of AS is senile or degenerative calcification of the aortic valve.

Pathophysiology

The normal aortic valve area is 3 to 4 cm^2. Patients do not generally become symptomatic until the valve area falls below 1 cm^2, presenting with symptoms of angina pectoris, exertional syncope, and exertional dyspnea. Severe AS is present when the valve area is less than 0.7 to 0.8 cm^2. A peak instantaneous gradient across the valve of greater than 70 mm Hg or a mean gradient greater than 50 mm Hg obtained from echocardiogram are also indicative of significant AS.

Obstruction to blood flow leads to a pressure-overloaded left ventricle which, initially, results in left ventricular hypertrophy. This hypertrophied ventricle increases cardiac work and oxygen consumption which, ultimately, can lead to left ventricular failure. Poststenotic dilation of the ascending aorta also can occur. Symptoms are more likely to be precipitated by exercise because stroke volume and heart rate are increased during exercise which further increases oxygen consumption. The development of angina reflects the imbalance of the oxygen supply/demand relationship and can occur even in the absence of significant coronary artery disease. Angina pectoris occurs in approximately 60% of symptomatic patients.

Exertional dyspnea occurs in approximately 90% of symptomatic patients. It may herald the onset of left ventricular failure because it is caused by pulmonary venous hypertension. Exertional syncope or dizziness results from decreased cerebral perfusion due to an inability to increase further the cardiac output and to peripheral vasodilation. Exertional syncope or dizziness occurs in approximately 35% of symptomatic patients. As left ventricular failure progresses, orthopnea and dyspnea at rest ensue. Right ventricular failure due to pulmonary hypertension is rare, however, because patients usually die before reaching this stage. Other more rare consequences of AS include dissecting aneurysm, infective endocarditis, and systemic embolism.

Atrial fibrillation is a serious complication of aortic stenosis. It occurs in nearly 10% of patients with isolated AS in the absence of associated mitral valve disease. The hypertrophied left ventricle becomes less compliant. As a result, it is quite dependent on atrial contraction for diastolic filling. Consequently, the loss of atrial contraction, coupled with a rapid heart rate which decreases diastolic filling time, may lead to a progression in the symptoms of left ventricular failure. Other serious arrhythmias can also occur in the face of AS. Sudden death can occur because of ventricular fibrillation or complete heart block caused by extension of the calcification of the aortic valve into the conducting system.

Perioperative Concerns

Aortic stenosis is a progressive disease. The valvular obstruction increases over time as fibrosis and calcification of the valve lead to valve immobility and decreased valve orifice area. However, the rate of this progression varies greatly. Patients who have symptomatic AS are at increased risk for sudden death. If they present in the perioperative period, immediate medical evaluation is warranted. Aortic valve replacement may be indicated prior to elective noncardiac surgery. Asymptomatic patients with AS, however, are at extremely low risk for sudden death. The risk of prophylactic aortic valve replacement in this population is not justified. Although severe aortic stenosis was originally identified as a major risk factor for patients undergoing general anesthesia for noncardiac operations, more recent studies suggest that selected patients with severe AS can undergo noncardiac procedures at a reasonably low risk with careful monitoring.

Because the degree of aortic stenosis is commonly quantitated by either echocardiography or catheterization, it is important for anesthesiologists to have a basic understanding of how these measurements are made. Transthoracic echocardiography provides a measurement of left ventricular function, determines the mechanism of stenosis and presence or absence of other valve lesions, and can quantitate the degree of stenosis by either the pressure gradient across the valve or valve area. Continuous wave Doppler imaging is used to measure the peak instantaneous transvalvular gradient, which is the maximal pressure gradient, and the mean pressure gradient. Using Doppler-determined pressure gradients and measurement of the left ventricular outflow tract, the valve area can be accurately determined using the continuity principle. Both the technical quality of the study and the experience of the sonographer and echocardiographer must be considered when applying the results of the study to patient management, since small errors in technique can lead to significant underestimation or overestimation of the severity of stenosis.

There are important differences between the echocardiographic and catheter-derived measurements of aortic stenosis. For traditional reasons, the most commonly used pressure gradient in the catheterization laboratory is the "peak-to-peak" gradient, measured between the left ventricular and aortic pressure tracings; these two peaks are nonsimultaneous. While the peak-to-peak gradient is always less than the peak instantaneous gradient obtained from echocardiography, the mean gradient measured in the catheterization laboratory usually agrees with the mean gradient from Doppler echocardiography. Using the Gorlin equation, aortic valve area is measured after determination of the mean gradient and cardiac output. There are a number of reasons that the measurements made by catheterization and echocardiography may differ significantly, and in these not infrequent cases it can be difficult to decide which measurements should be used. Finally, since all of these measurements are flow-dependent, they can change with changes in left ventricular function or volume status. Patients with reduced left ventricular function, for example, can have critical aortic stenosis with low peak or mean pressure gradients because of reduced cardiac output.

Adequate hydration is essential in the patient with AS since these patients have a limited ability to increase stroke volume. Consequently, an adequate heart rate is essential to maintain cardiac output. However, tachycardia must be avoided as it increases myocardial oxygen demand and decreases supply by decreasing left ventricular diastolic filling time and decreasing the diastolic perfusion time of the hypertrophied left ventricle. In addition, atrial fibrillation may not be well tolerated. It must be promptly recognized and treated aggressively. The ventricular rate should be controlled and normal sinus rhythm restored, if possible, by cardioversion.

These patients may not tolerate a reduction in systemic vascular resistance (SVR). Coronary blood flow is dependent upon diastolic arterial pressure to maintain adequate coronary perfusion. A decrease in the SVR may lead to a decrease in the diastolic perfusion pressure, leading to irreversible myocardial ischemia and cardiovascular collapse. Serious consideration should be given to placing a pulmonary artery catheter and arterial pressure catheter preoperatively in those with tight AS to aid in judicious fluid administration and rapid correction of hemodynamic instability. Myocardial depressants and hypotension must, therefore, be avoided. Spinal anesthesia may be hazardous because of the unpredictable vasodilation. Epidural anesthesia has been used safely but must be used with extreme caution. Local anesthetics containing epinephrine should be avoided due to the possibility of accompanying tachycardia.

MITRAL REGURGITATION

Etiology

The causes of mitral regurgitation (MR) are diverse. The most common causes of MR in the United States are myxomatous degeneration and coronary heart disease. Myocardial infarction caused by coronary artery disease may result in MR caused by left ventricular systolic dysfunction, which alters the geometry and function of the mitral apparatus, or rupture of a papillary muscle. Rheumatic fever is also an important cause of MR. Less common causes of MR include bacterial endocarditis, calcification of the mitral annulus, inherited connective tissue disorders such as Marfan's syndrome, congenital heart disease, and systemic lupus erythematosus.

Pathophysiology

There is a profound difference between the manifestations of acute and chronic mitral regurgitation. The major sequelae of acute MR involve the pulmonary venous circulation and the lungs. In acute MR, the left atrial pressure tracing reveals a large regurgitant wave, that reflects a systolic pressure wave transmitted to the pulmonary veins, capillaries, and, occasionally, the pulmonary arteries. This acute pressure and volume overload of the pulmonary vasculature can result in pulmonary edema. In chronic MR, however, the burden is carried more by the left ventricle.

In acute MR the normal left ventricle exhibits an increase in ejection fraction due to an increased preload and a decreased afterload. The major transition from acute to chronic MR involves enlargement of the left ventricle. Myocardial changes characteristic of chronic MR include myocardial hypertrophy with left ventricular chamber dilation, normal end-diastolic pressure, and normal contractility. In addition, the left atrium enlarges and becomes more compliant and able to accommodate a large atrial volume with minimal changes in pulmonary venous pressures. The development of atrial fibrillation is better tolerated than in MS because there is no obstruction to diastolic blood flow. Patients with compensated MR may remain asymptomatic for years.

The pathophysiology of the transition from compensated to decompensated MR is poorly understood. Unfortunately, an insidious deterioration of left ventricular function can occur without major clinical manifestations before the patient presents with congestive symptoms such as fatigue, dyspnea, orthopnea, paroxysmal nocturnal dyspnea, and peripheral edema. Myocardial changes characteristic of decompensated MR include substantial left ventricular enlargement with inadequate hypertrophy, increased end-diastolic pressure, increased wall stress, and depressed contractility.

Perioperative Concerns

Patients with acute MR should not present for elective noncardiac surgery because this is a medical emergency requiring treatment with vasodilators, diuretics, and inotropes as needed, as well as consideration of urgent valve replacement or repair. Patients with chronic, compensated MR who present for elective noncardiac surgery should be able to tolerate the physiologic demands of anesthesia and surgery. It is a difficult decision when to send the patient with compensated chronic MR for mitral valve replacement or repair because there is no evidence that mitral valve replacement prolongs life in chronic MR. In the asymptomatic patient, it is difficult to distinguish between compensated and uncompensated MR. Echocardiography can be useful in these patients, by providing a measure of left ventricular systolic function, determining the mechanism of regurgitation, and by detecting and measuring chamber enlargement that occurs as a consequence of the regurgitation. For example, patients with mitral regurgitation, marked left atrial enlargement (in the absence of chronic atrial fibrillation to account for this enlargement), and increased left ventricular dimensions often have severe regurgitation, while the presence of normal atrial and ventricular dimensions argues against significant chronic mitral regurgitation.

In the perioperative period, prophylactic antibiotics should be administered if indicated. The patient may be systemically anticoagulated if there has been a history of systemic embolism or chronic atrial fibrillation. Systemic anticoagulation may preclude the use of neuraxial blockade, but this risk must be considered for each individual patient. Patients with chronic MR usually withstand vasodilation well. Consequently, general anesthesia, as well as regional anesthesia including epidural and spinal anesthesia, are well-tolerated. Hypovolemia should be avoided to maintain an adequate cardiac output. Normal sinus rhythm should be maintained and adequate rate control should be achieved in those with preexisting atrial fibrillation. Profound depression of the myocardium should be avoided. As a result, β-blockers should be used judiciously. Right-heart pressure monitoring may be indicated in patients with severely depressed ventricular function.

AORTIC REGURGITATION

Etiology

Syphilis and rheumatic fever were previously the major causes of aortic regurgitation (AR). However, due to the diminished frequency of these clinical entities, anatomic abnormalities of the aortic valve and ascending aorta have become more prominent causes of AR. Ankylosing spondylitis, Marfan's syndrome, systemic lupus erythematosus, osteogenesis imperfecta, rheumatoid arthritis, and Reiter's syndrome are all examples of connective tissue diseases that can be associated with AR. In the case of Marfan's syndrome, however, the regurgitation may be caused by both aortic dilation and prolapse of the aortic cusps as a result of myxomatous changes. Annuloaortic ectasia and aortic dissection can both lead to dilation of the aortic root with subsequent AR. Valvular abnormalities such as rheumatic fever, infective endocarditis, myxomatous degeneration, congenital bicuspid valve, and previous aortic valve surgery can all lead to MR. Any process that leads to aortic stenosis likely will lead to incomplete valve closure with resultant AR. Finally, long-standing hypertension and atherosclerosis can lead to AR through aortic dilation.

Pathophysiology

As with mitral regurgitation, a distinction must be made between acute and chronic AR because the hemodynamic changes are different. In the case of acute AR, a volume overload is suddenly imposed on the left ventricle which is unable to adapt by dilating and increasing its compliance. Consequently, diastolic filling is impaired and left ventricular end-diastolic pressure may rise dramatically, leading to pulmonary venous hypertension and acute pulmonary edema. In chronic AR, however, the volume overload applied to the left ventricle allows for physiologic adaptation. Left ventricular end-diastolic volume gradually increases since the left ventricle receives blood from both the left atrium and the systemic circulation. The left ventricle dilates and the diastolic compliance is increased without an associated appreciable rise in end-diastolic pressure. These adaptations permit an increase in total left ventricular stroke volume so that an adequate effective stroke volume to the systemic circulation can be maintained.

At some point, chronic compensated AR turns to decompensated AR as myocardial fibrosis and fiber slippage develop. The left ventricle becomes less compliant and the left ventricular-end diastolic pressure rises. Severe bradycardia may exacerbate the regurgitant volume as a result of the increased diastolic duration. Initially, the mitral valve is competent, which protects the pulmonary circuit from the rise in left ventricular end-diastolic pressures. However, as myocardial contractility declines, mitral regurgitation increases, exposing the left atrium and pulmonary system to these rising pressures, resulting in pulmonary venous hypertension. Finally, the massive chamber enlargement that can occur in chronic AR, as well as the compensatory hypertrophy, will increase the pressure-volume work on the left ventricle so that myocardial oxygen consumption will be significantly elevated.

Perioperative Concerns

The distinction must once again be made between the treatment of acute and chronic AR in the perioperative period. Acute AR is often a surgical emergency. These patients may present with cardiovascular collapse and acute pulmonary edema. They should be monitored in an intensive care setting with both intraarterial and Swan-Ganz catheters. If the systemic pressure is adequate to maintain reasonable perfusion pressures, sodium nitroprusside can be started to lower the pulmonary artery wedge pressure. In the presence of wide open AR, an intraaortic balloon pump is contraindicated. These measures are, obviously, of only temporary benefit while emergency surgical intervention is being arranged. If the acute AR is caused by bacterial endocarditis and the patient is stable, antibiotics can be instituted to control the infection. Most of these patients will need valve replacement within a matter of days to weeks. Left ventricular dysfunction can occur in the setting of acute AR, but it often reverses after valve replacement.

Chronic AR, however, may be well-tolerated for years before left ventricular dysfunction and the onset of symptoms occur. In fact, significant impairment of left ventricular function may develop without symptoms. It is important to identify and closely follow these patients because left ventricular dysfunction because of AR may be irreversible and may compromise results of valve replacement. Consequently, if these patients are identified in the perioperative period, consultation with a cardiologist for appropriate follow-up is essential.

The timing of aortic valve replacement (AVR) is difficult and requires serial measurements of left ventricular function and dimensions. The patient must not be exposed prematurely to the risk of aortic valve replacement, but the valve should be replaced before irreversible left ventricular dysfunction occurs. The symptomatic patient with AR should be considered strongly for AVR. Asymptomatic patients with normal left ventricular dimensions at rest are not considered for surgery. However, patients with significantly decreased left ventricular function or an end-systolic left ventricular diameter greater than 55 mm by echocardiography, should be considered for exercise testing to measure exercise tolerance. If this is significantly reduced, then AVR may be appropriate.

Asymptomatic patients with AR should tolerate anesthesia and surgery well, but with some precautions. If indicated by the proposed surgical procedure, antibiotics should be administered to prevent bacterial endocarditis. A reasonable heart rate and preload should be maintained and large increases in systemic vascular resistance (SVR) should be avoided to provide adequate cardiac output. Profound myocardial depressants should be avoided. Regional anesthesia is well-tolerated as long as sudden and profound drops in SVR, which can cause a precipitous fall in coronary perfusion pressure, are avoided.

BIBLIOGRAPHY

Carabello BA: Indications for valve surgery in asymptomatic patients with aortic and mitral stenosis, *Chest* 108:1678–1682, 1995.

Goldman L, et al: Multifactorial index of cardiac risk in noncardiac surgical procedures, *N Engl J Med* 297:845–850, 1977.

O'Keefe JH, Shub C, Rettke SR: Risk of noncardiac surgical procedures in patients with aortic stenosis, *Mayo Clin Proc* 64:400–405, 1989.

Rozich JD, et al: Mitral valve replacement with and without chordal preservation in patients with chronic mitral regurgitation, *Circulation* 86:1718–1726, 1992.

Schlant RC, Alexander RW, editors: *Hurst's the heart*, ed. 8, New York, 1994, McGraw-Hill.

Wagner HR, et al: Clinical course in aortic stenosis, *Circulation* 56(suppl 1):47–56, 1977.

initial introduction. The NASPE/BPEG pacemaker code now contains five positions describing: (1) chamber(s) paced; (2) chamber(s) sensed; (3) the generator's response to a sensed signal; (4) programmability and rate modulation; and (5) antitachyarrhythmia function(s). Table 5-1 shows the current generic pacemaker code. (A similar code system has been defined for ICDs. The next chapter describes these devices.)

In general, each of these five positions is independent of any other position (except that a pacemaker without a sensing function will have no sensing response), and older pacemakers that were implanted when the pacemaker code had only three positions have "OO" appended to their designations; that is, they are not programmable nor do they have antitachyarrhythmia function. Programmable pacemakers have a "default" mode, and they operate in this mode at start-up, prior to programming. Internal circuitry can switch the pacemaker back to the default mode after an unexpected internal reset or electrical fault, which can be caused by internal generator failure or direct electrical activity applied to the generator (such as electrocautery or defibrillation).

In the older programmable devices (simple programmable), only the pulse rate and/or stimulating current was programmable. In the newer devices, available since the late 1980s, programmable features include:

Mode—current devices have considerable microcomputing ability and nearly every newer device is capable of operating in multiple modes. The two–chamber devices (DDxxx) can be programmed to operate in single chamber mode (either Axxxx or Vxxxx) and the sensing function(s) can be enabled or disabled.

Upper Rate Limit—newer generators programmed to DDDxx include an upper rate limit (also called the maximum atrial tracking rate) for ventricular pacing in case a patient develops an atrial tachyarrhythmia. In older devices, such an event could cause the pacemaker to pace the ventricles at a rapid rate. Thus, DDDxx devices will: (1) pace the atria (as well as the ventricles when A-V conduction is absent) when the patient's rate falls below the generator's lower (or programmed) rate; (2) track the atrial rate, with ventricular pacing as needed, when the atrial rate is between the lower rate and the upper rate limit; and (3) alter the ventricular pacing rate when the atrial rate exceeds the upper rate limit.

When a dual-chamber device is placed in a patient with a history of atrial fibrillation or flutter, the generator must be programmed to DDIxx* mode or it must be programmed to respond appropriately to the atrial tachycardia. Depending upon the manufacturer and/or programming, when the sensed atrial rate exceeds the upper rate limit, generators can either: (1) introduce

** DDIxx generators provide A-V synchrony ONLY when the generator issues an atrial pulse; i.e., the patient's underlying atrial and ventricular rates are lower than the programmed lower rate for the generator. DDDxx generators provide A-V synchrony (tracking) as long as the atrial rate (either intrinsic or paced) is below the upper rate limit. In both DDIxx and DDDxx modes, the atrial "timer" is reset by either an atrial or ventricular depolarization.*

Table 5-1. NASPE/BPEG Generic Pacemaker Code

POSITION I	POSITION II	POSITION III	POSITION IV	POSITION V
Pacing Chamber(s)	Sensing Chamber(s)	Response(s) to Sensing	Programmability, Rate Modulation	Antitachyarrhythmia Function(s)
O = None	O = None	O = None	O = None	O = None
A = Atrium	A = Atrium	I = Inhibited	P = <simple> Programmable	P = Pacing
V = Ventricle	V = Ventricle	T = Triggered	M = <multi> Programmable	S = Shock
D = Dual	D = Dual	D = Dual (T + I)	C = Communicating	D = Dual (Pace + Shock)
			R = Rate Modulation	

Source: *Handbook of pulse generators and leads*. Reproduced with permission by Cardiac Pacemakers. St. Paul, MN, 1994, Publication 8-488-1194.
* The designation of Rate Modulation takes precedence over the other Position IV modes.

Wenkebach A-V block; (2) introduce 2:1 type II second-degree block; (3) switch to DDIxx mode; or (4) switch to VVIxx mode.

Hysteresis—generators with hysteresis have two "pacing rates." The lower of these rates represents the threshold for initiation of pacing. The higher rate is the true pacing rate, and the generator accelerates to this rate over a prescribed number of beats (programmable). The purpose of hysteresis is to prevent pacemaker firing when the intrinsic heart rate is only slightly below the set rate of the generator or an R-R interval is lengthened by an inspiration. Hysteresis prevents competition for control of chamber activation and reduces energy consumption of the pacemaker. It is not needed in the patient who has no underlying cardiac rhythm.

Some newer pacemakers can be programmed to decrease the pacing rate at regular intervals (also programmed), in order to search for resumption of intrinsic activity. If none is found, the pacemaker resumes pacing at the programmed pacing rate.

R-Wave (or P-Wave) Sensitivity—adjustment of the sensitivity of the sensing function(s) can eliminate noise or artifact that then inhibits (or triggers) the output of the generator. In the default mode, electrical sensitivity is set low, and it is adjusted upward during programming to a threshold that is just below the point at which the pacemaker fails to detect the patient's intrinsic electrical activity. For dual-chamber, dual-sensing devices, the sensitivity for both chambers can be programmed, but care must be taken so that signals from one chamber do not affect pacemaker sensing for the other chamber (termed "crosstalk"). New onset crosstalk is theoretically possible, but no such reports can be found in the literature.

Atrioventricular Delay—the dual-chamber generators permit adjustable "P-R" intervals, allowing the cardiologist to program the pacemaker for optimal filling time of the ventricles. In some pacemakers, the generator can be programmed to alter this time, based upon the heart rate. This feature is called "dynamic AV delay" or "rate adaptive AV delay."

Rate Modulation—current "rate adaptive" generators determine the need to increase the heart rate via one of three mechanisms: (1) a mechanical sensor can be contained within the generator and it can detect motion or vibration; (2) the transthoracic impedance can be measured to detect changes in respiration; or (3) metabolic parameters such as central venous blood temperature or saturation can be monitored. Typically, a device with rate modulation is placed in a patient who lacks the ability to increase his/her heartrate to appropriate stimuli (termed "chronotropic incompetence").

Generators with mechanical sensors are the most common. However, mechanical sensors can be affected by vibration, motion, or pressure that is not due to patient activity. For example, patients with mechanical sensors should expect an increase in heartrate when subjected to strong vibration, such as during helicopter transport (French and Tillman 1989), and care must be exercised when placing patients into hyperbaric chambers exceeding 1.5 to 2 atm pressure.

Upper Sensor Rate—rate adaptive generators will not increase the pacing rate above some programmed value, called the "upper pacing limit" or "upper activity rate." This term (and function) should not be confused with the "upper rate limit," which is programmed independently in DDDRx generators.

Most pacemakers (although not all of them) respond to magnet placement by converting to an "asynchronous" mode (designated "DOOxx," "VOOxx," or "AOOxx") in which all sensing functions are disabled and the generator fires at a predetermined rate, regardless of underlying atrial or ventricular activity. However, the "magnet mode" of some generators can be reprogrammed, which can make the magnet response unpredictable. The generator manufacturers strongly recommend against alteration of the magnet mode, but some patients who work in areas of strong magnetic or electric fields might require deactivation of the magnet mode. In some generators, an "event sequence monitoring mode" can be activated by magnet placement, so these generators also will behave as though they have a disabled magnet mode.

The placing of the magnet triggers a reed switch within the generator, alerting the device that an operator is present. For many generators, the magnet must be held tightly against the skin over the generator pocket, and the thickness of wrapping paper (often found around the "sterilized" magnet in the operating room) can be sufficient to prevent activation of the reed switch. For most generators, the pacing rate in the asynchronous magnet mode can be used to predict remaining battery life or battery status. In order to interpret this data, though, one must have information supplied by the pacemaker manufacturer. Pacemaker data is available from the manufacturer, and the patient should have been given a card with the manufacturer name, phone number, model and serial number of the device, and the date of implantation. The manufacturer and a device identification code can also be obtained (in many cases) from a radiograph of the device. At least two World Wide Web sites now provide considerable information about generators. At:

www.webaxis.com/heartweb/pulsegen.htm

one can enter either the pacemaker model or the radiograph code. (This site also contains an on-line journal for those interested in cardiac electrophysiology.) At:

www2.interpath.net/devcomp/guide.htm

nearly every device ever made can be found by manufacturer and/or model number. Neither site provides information about ICDs. All of the companies have 24-hour technical assistance available by telephone, although some of the telephones are answered by voice-mail devices, which page a technician who returns a call. Toll-free telephone numbers for many companies are found in Box 5-1, and many of the companies publish handbooks that contain information about all pacemakers.

• PACEMAKER INDICATIONS

Permanent pacemaker placement is indicated for patients with a deficit in cardiac impulse formation or conduction that is uncorrectable by other means. These deficits typically include: (1) sick sinus syndrome; (2) chronic sinus node dysrhythmias that produce unwanted clinical symptoms (sinus bradycardia, sinus arrest, sinoatrial exit block); (3) atrioventricular block (third degree, second-degree type II, symptomatic

Box 5-1 Toll-Free Phone Numbers

American Pacemaker Corporation (Intermedics, Inc)	800-231-2330
ARCO Medical Products (Intermedics, Inc)	800-231-2330
Biotronik, Inc	800-547-0394
Cardiac Control Systems	800-227-7223
Cardiac Pacemakers, Inc	800-227-3422
Cook Pacemaker Corporation	800-245-4715
Coratomic (Biocontrol Technology)	800-245-6886
Cordis Corporation (Telectronics Pacing Systems)	800-525-7042
Diag/Medcor	800-328-3873
Edwards Pacemaker Systems (Medtronic, Inc)	800-328-2518
ELA Medical	800-352-6466
Intermedics, Inc	800-321-2330
Medtronic, Inc	800-328-2518
Pacesetter, Inc	800-722-3774
Siemans-Elema	800-722-3774
Telectronics Pacing Systems	800-525-7042
Ventritex	800-733-3455
Viatron (Medtronic, Inc)	800-888-5252

second-degree type I); (4) tachycardia-bradycardia syndrome; and (5) symptomatic carotid sinus syndrome. Indications for temporary pacing include: (1) fixed stroke volume necessitating rate augmentation to enhance cardiac output (e.g., postcardiopulmonary bypass pump); (2) temporary conduction abnormalities secondary to electrolyte or drug disturbances; and (3) temporary bradycardia with hemodynamic compromise unresponsive to pharmacologic therapy (e.g., high subarachnoid block).

A patient who has no underlying rhythm without a generated systole is considered "pacemaker dependent," and his/her cardiac output can be limited by a fixed rate generator. The determination of pacemaker type, lead type, and site of implantation is usually made by a cardiologist who specializes in electrophysiology. A patient with a pacemaker should have regular follow-up with his/her cardiologist.

The placement of a sophisticated, multichamber generator is reserved for those patients who have atria that will respond to pacing. Generators that have atrial functions are contraindicated in patients with: (1) chronic refractory atrial tachyarrhythmias (such as atrial fibrillation or flutter) or (2) retrograde pathways likely to induce pacemaker-generated tachycardias. Furthermore, pulse generators employing only unipolar leads are contraindicated in a patient with an ICD, since the activation pulse from the pacemaker might also activate or inhibit the ICD therapy.

PREANESTHETIC EVALUATION

The initial evaluation of the patient with a pacemaker should be no different from the evaluation of any other patient scheduled for a procedure with anesthesia. The majority of patients with permanent pacemakers have ischemic cardiomyopathy, and many, if not most, of these patients have a high incidence of concomitant diseases (hypertension, pulmonary dysfunction, diabetes) that have the potential to exacerbate their preexisting heart disease. For elective procedures, these diseases should be optimized (as with any patient), and for urgent or emergent interventions, therapies should be instituted to minimize untoward outcomes from these coexisting diseases. Thus, the history and physical exam of the patient should be directed toward eliciting signs and symptoms of: (1) worsening congestive failure; (2) increasing exercise intolerance; (3) new or unstable angina; or (4) intercurrent infection or illness.

A patients with a pacemaker should be questioned about the initial indication for pacemaker placement, and his/her history should be examined for a return of these symptoms. Such symptoms could indicate pacemaker dysfunction. Since pacemaker batteries have expected lives of 4 to 10 years, the date of placement or last testing can be important. Pacemaker battery function can be interrogated with a pacemaker programmer or predicted from the asynchronous rate when in the magnet mode. A patient with a pacemaker exhibiting "end of life" behavior (which is defined by the manufacturer) should not undergo elective surgery until the pacemaker has been changed. A discussion with the cardiologist who last evaluated both the patient and his/her pacemaker parameters can be useful and should be attempted. Finally, many of newer generators maintain a history of abnormal cardiac events, which can be obtained by pacemaker interrogation.

The patient should also be questioned about palpitations (which might suggest competition in the patient with an asynchronous pacemaker or sensing failure in a newer device). Furthermore, all patients should be questioned about the signs and symptoms of "pacemaker syndrome." Pacemaker syndrome results from retrograde ventriculoatrial conduction, causing atrial contraction against closed atrioventricular valves. It produces elevated venous pressures, causing symptoms of dyspnea, fatigue, head and neck pulsation, right upper quadrant tenderness due to hepatic congestion, and peripheral edema. It can lead to peripheral vasodilation via stimulation of atrial vagal receptors, causing significant reduction in blood pressure if it occurs acutely.[1] The onset of pacemaker syndrome in a patient with a dual chamber, multiple-mode pacemaker represents dysfunction in the detection of atrial systole or in the sequencing of the pacer spikes.

The physical exam must include determination of the pacemaker site, since this site must be protected from electrocautery. As part of the exam, the patient's cardiac rhythm should be palpated while observing the ECG to insure that pacer discharges are captured (i.e., become p waves or QRS complexes) and that QRS complexes become mechanical systoles. Patients with native heart rates exceeding the programmed (or hysteresis) rate should have no pacemaker discharges. Evidence of generator dysfunction includes: (1) noncaptured generator "spikes"; (2) atrial or ventricular rate slower than the programmed (or hysteresis) rate without generator spikes; and (3) defects suggestive of improper sensing (i.e., atrial or ventricular pacing "spikes" that occur without appropriate delay from the patient's own chamber depolarization).

Some authors state that a chest (or generator site) radiograph is mandatory; however, in a patient with a functioning pacemaker of known manufacturer and model type, radiographs should be obtained only for appropriately indicated reasons. When question(s) about the generator site or model remain, a radiograph might provide the "x-ray code," but not all generators contain such codes. Some authors recommend a radiograph to ensure lead integrity, but radiographs will fail to detect insulation breakdown, and they have insufficient sensitivity to detect small lead fractures.

Selection of laboratory tests should be based upon the expected procedure, the patient's medication(s), and the patient's prior medical problem(s). Some authors suggest the need for a preoperative potassium level, since hypo- or hyperkalemia can affect myocardial sensitivity to pacemaker operation. If any preanesthetic labs are ordered because "the patient has a pacemaker," care should be taken to ensure that the tests are performed in a timely manner with respect to the procedure. Most of the patient's ambulatory drug therapy should be continued throughout the perioperative period; and drug levels (e.g., antiarrhythmics, theophylline) should be obtained only when necessary.

Pacemaker evaluation should include a recent interrogation of the generator to determine programmed mode and rate, lead integrity, and battery performance. Other data, such as hysteresis rate, upper rate limit (for generators in DDDxx mode), or upper sensor rate (for rate responsive generators) might also be obtained. Considerable effort must be made to determine the generator's response to magnet placement, since the response to magnet placement on some generators is programmable.

A magnet can be placed over the pacemaker (while the patient's vital signs, including ECG display, are monitored) to help determine the magnet response. The pacemaker magnet rate should be determined, because it might be greater than the programmed lower rate. This magnet rate should be kept in mind while caring for the patient with a pacemaker, because a patient with significant blood loss, fluid shifts, or need to increase tissue oxygen delivery might benefit from the temporary rate increase that can be obtained with magnet placement. In general, magnet mode should be enabled for all procedures except MRI.

The reprogramming of pacemaker mode remains controversial. In general, conversion of a demand generator to asynchronous mode (AOOxx, VOOxx, or DOOxx) eliminates the possibility of any interference with generator behavior during a procedure. Competition between the patient's native rhythm (if any) and generator spikes can be prevented by setting the programmed rate to exceed the patient's native rate or by pharmacologic therapy designed to lower the patient's native heart rate. Such mode and rate reprogramming should be strongly considered in any patient undergoing major surgery or in situations likely to require monopolar cautery.

• INTRAOPERATIVE (AND OTHER PROCEDURE) MANAGEMENT

The presence of a pacemaker does not necessitate any special monitoring that exceeds the standard monitors usually applied. The use of invasive arterial or pulmonary arterial monitoring should be based upon the severity of preexisting disease and the planned intervention. Pulmonary artery catheters seem to be considered "safe" and unlikely to dislodge a transvenous pacemaker electrode if the electrode has been in place for more than 4 to 6 weeks. If electrocautery use is planned, a method to evaluate cardiac rhythm that will not be affected by electrocautery is required. Such methodology includes auscultation, palpation, or pulse oximetry plethysmography.

No special anesthetic technique is required for patients with pacing devices, and the induction, maintenance, and emergence technique often require no modification for patients with pacemakers. However, higher levels of central neuraxial block (from an epidural or subarachnoid anesthetic) could reduce intrinsic heart rate below the generator's lower pacing rate, which would result in the initiation of pacing. Also, the paced heart might be unable to compensate for any hypotension produced by the block, and the combination of pacing with symptoms of hypotension might provoke anxiety in the awake patient.

Some authors raise the issue of muscle fasciculation with succinylcholine or myoclonus with etomidate as reasons to avoid these drugs in patients with "sensing" pacemaker devices. Using a MEDLINE search, one article was found suggesting that fasciculations during succinylcholine use resulted in a shutdown of a VVIRO pacemaker. However, this elderly patient promptly developed ventricular fibrillation and was defibrillated.[2] Because of lead failure after the defibrillation, no conclusive data was published in this report. Some authors have suggested the use of a "defasciculating" dose of nondepolarizing muscle relaxant. As always, the use of succinylcholine and adjuncts should be guided by the clinical situation. No data was found regarding etomidate use and pacemakers.

Nearly all authors and generator manufacturers agree that electrocautery remains the principal intraoperative issue. Electromagnetic interference (EMI) can confuse a sensing pacemaker, which might cause excessive firing or inhibit the pacemaker output. Microprocessor current consumption can be affected by "signals" from monopolar electrocautery, which could result in premature discharge of the generator battery. A direct strike of electrocautery current onto the pacemaker or unintended conduction via the pacemaker leads can cause pacemaker failure, pacemaker reset, or myocardial microshock.

Pacemakers have been known to become reprogrammed during electrocautery use, and Domino and Smith (1983) report one instance of rate change in a VVIOO device while operating with a magnet. They correctly state that magnet placement on some devices conditions them to receive new programming instructions, which apparently took place in their patient. However, the programming sequence in newer devices is embedded with "network communication data," which should prevent incidental reprogramming from stray electromagnetic interference. Still, some manufacturers recommend against magnet placement during electrocautery. Most manuals state that a pacemaker-dependent patient should have his/her generator reprogrammed to asynchronous mode (rather than temporary magnet placement) if interference from electrocautery is expected.

Generally accepted guidelines for electrocautery use include:

1. The ECG must be monitored when using cautery of any kind.
2. Avoid monopolar cautery when possible (use bipolar cautery).
3. Always position the grounding pad so that the generator is not in the path of cautery current flow. When possible, the expected current path for monopolar cautery should be perpendicular to a line drawn from the patient's ventricle to the generator, to reduce the possibility of induced current on the pacemaker leads.
4. Request that the surgical personnel not activate the cautery device until it is actually needed, and then use the cautery only in short bursts.
5. Request that the smallest possible current be used.
6. Never use cautery over the generator or along the lead path to the heart.
7. If a magnet is placed over the generator, the patient must be monitored during magnet removal to ensure the integrity of the generator function. If any doubt remains, the generator should be interrogated with a pacemaker programmer.

Other equipment and procedures that might require special attention in pacemaker patients include lithotripsy, transurethral resection of the prostate, hysteroscopic resection of the uterus, magnetic resonance imaging (MRI), electroconvulsive therapy, or nerve stimulator therapy (see following).

Lithotripsy

The manufacturers of generators state that "lithotripsy may damage the pulse generator." However, in their review of the literature, Celentano et al. (1992) cite numerous studies that show no damage to single-chamber pacemakers when exposed to lithotripsy *in vitro*. In addition, a few studies have been published suggesting that lithotripsy is safe in patients with pacemakers. In the largest of these studies, Drach et al. surveyed urologists in the United States and Europe. They reported learning of 142 treatments in 131 patients without any major pacemaker problems (i.e., lethal arrhythmia, need for pacemaker replacement), and only 4 minor problems arose, which were easily corrected. No study to date was found that suggested patients with pacemakers should be denied lithotripsy treatment.

Transurethral Resection of the Prostate (TURP) and Hysteroscopic Uterine Resection

The primary risk from transurethral prostate resection (TURP) comes from the use of monopolar electrocautery. A few case reports of pacemaker problems during this procedure appear in distant literature. In hysteroscopic uterine resection, a monopolar resectoscope (similar to the TURP resectoscope) is used, with similar potential risk of pacemaker interference. Both TURP and hysteroscopy can be associated with significant changes in sodium concentration, but seizure activity from hyponatremia represents greater risk to the patient than does the small change in myocardial resting potential. In addition, seizure activity might be misinterpreted by a sensing pacemaker as intrinsic myocardial activity, with resultant inhibition of generator output. In hysteroscopy, 32% dextran-70 (Hyskon) is infused into the uterus to maintain the visual field and irrigate away the bleeding; Hyskon infusion has been associated with anaphylaxis, anaphylactoid reactions, and severe decreases in sodium concentration (Manger, 1992). For patients with a vasodilating reaction, cardiac output might become limited due to a fixed pacemaker rate.

Magnetic Resonance Imaging (MRI)

The manufacturers of implantable generators recommend against subjecting patients with pacemakers to MRI for a variety of reasons: (1) the strong magnetic field of the MRI scanner can alter the operation of the pacemaker; (2) the pacemaker can be damaged directly by either magnetic interference or electromagnetic interference (EMI); and (3) MRI can cause movement of the pacemaker within the pectoral pocket, resulting in lead breakage or pain to the patient. However, a recent report by Lauck et al. (1995) suggests that pacemakers are not damaged by MRI, and a report of an uncomplicated head MRI in a patient with a pacemaker has appeared (Inbar et al., 1993).

The pacemaker manufacturers state that other forms of radiologic imaging are unlikely to damage a generator or lead system. Some do warn, though, that radiation therapy (such as cobalt-60) can produce generator malfunction or failure. Thus, generators should have lead shielding placed prior to irradiation of the patient.

Electroconvulsive Therapy (ECT)

The presence of a pacemaker has been considered a relative contraindication for ECT, but uncomplicated ECT has been reported in patients with pacemakers.[3] Many authors believe that the presence of a pacemaker will protect a patient from the initial bradyarrhythmia caused by vagal discharge. ECT produces profound hemodynamic changes, and patients with pacemakers often have an ischemic cardiomyopathy. Thus, as with all interventions, one must carefully weigh the risks and benefits of a procedure, and the patient scheduled for ECT should be carefully examined. The possibility exists for seizure activity to be interpreted by a sensing pacemaker as intrinsic myocardial activity. Thus, patients who are pacemaker-dependent, with sensing pacemakers, should have the mode changed to asynchronous pacing prior to ECT.

Nerve Stimulator Therapy

Placement of a transcutaneous electrical nerve stimulator (TENS) unit, neuromuscular stimulator, or spinal cord stimulator must be carried out while carefully monitoring the patient. The manufacturers of pacemaking devices suggest caution be employed when using nerve stimulators. Like electrocautery, currents from these devices should not cross the path from the generator to the heart, and patients with stimulators that have surface electrodes should be cautioned so that they do not "explore" unusual electrode positioning.

Miscellaneous

Two other reports of unusual pacemaker problems have been published. Lamas et al. (1985) reported the failure (presumed to be from nitrous oxide) of a VVIOO pacemaker with a unipolar ventricular lead (i.e., the case was used for the grounding electrode) during hip replacement surgery. They stated that air entrapped in the recently placed generator pocket expanded during nitrous oxide use, disrupting the circuit continuity and resulting in apparent pacemaker failure. Placement of a magnet and manual expression of the gas resulted in return of pacing capture. Purday and Towey reported a case in which the placement of a magnetic instrument mat over a generator initiated a ventricular threshold test, (this generator's appropriate response to magnet placement), which resulted in cessation of pacing. These problems, again, alert anesthesiologists that vigilance to all activity in the operating room remains paramount.

PACEMAKER FAILURE

Pacemaker failure has three etiologies: (1) generator failure; (2) lead failure; and (3) failure of capture. In patients with intrinsic, perfusing rhythms, who have a sensing, inhibiting pacemaker device, failure of the pacemaker will be difficult to detect.

Lead failure can cause: (1) undersensing of intrinsic activity, which will result in excessive and undesired pacemaker activity; (2) oversensing of intrinsic activity, which will result in inappropriate generator pauses; (3) lack of pacemaker spikes if the lead is completely fractured, which will result in; (4) loss of pacemaker capture if sufficient energy cannot reach the myocardium to produce a depolarization (Note: a defect in the inner insulation of a pacemaker lead can also prevent sufficient energy from reaching the myocardium).

Failure of capture, owing to a defect at the level of the myocardium (i.e., the generator continues to fire but no myocardial depolarization takes place), remains the most difficult problem to treat. Myocardial changes that lengthen the refractory period, or increase the energy requirement for depolarization, can result from myocardial ischemia, MI, acid-base disturbance, electrolyte abnormalities, or abnormal levels of antiarrhythmic drug(s).

In the pacemaker-dependent patient, any pacemaker system failure represents a "code" situation. The initial evaluation of presumed pacemaker failure rests with the accurate determination that no ventricular activity is present (i.e., the patient is pulseless). At that time, all personnel attending to the patient must be informed, the procedure must be stopped, any drapes should be removed, a call for help must be issued, and attention must be given to the basics: Airway, Breathing, and Circulation. Some patients might develop an escape rhythm. The adequacy of this rhythm to produce sufficient cardiac output must be determined.

The next response depends upon the clinical situation; patients with perfusing rhythms and relatively stable vital signs can be observed while personnel are mobilized to attempt "repair" of the pacemaker. For the patient with inadequate perfusion, the following steps can be tried (while cardiopulmonary resuscitation [CPR] is in progress if appropriate):

1. A magnet can be applied to the pacemaker known to revert to asynchronous mode. Such application will inhibit sensing and, in many pacemakers, maximizes the current available for pacing. If myocardial ischemia resulted in increased threshold for pacing, placement of a magnet might temporarily restore capture.
2. Chronotropes can be administered in an attempt to increase the rate of a bradycardic heart. Isoproterenol (0.5μg/min) is often recommended, but its administration can be accompanied by hypotension. Epinephrine (0.5–1 μg/min) can also be infused. Antimuscarinic drugs (atropine, glycopyrrolate) might be useful for the patient with atrial activity but conduction system disease, since release of vagal tone might have some benefit. In patients who depend upon ventricular escape, vagolytic drugs will fail to produce any increase in heart rate, and these drugs rarely work in a denervated (transplanted) heart.
3. External pacing can be initiated, and it can be transthoracic, transvenous, or transesophageal. Transesophageal (atrial) pacing requires a functional atrium and sinoatrial (SA) node for ventricular activation.
4. Electrolyte, antiarrhythmic, and acid-base disturbances should be corrected. Potassium, calcium, and magnesium all affect myocardial thresholds for depolarization. Hypokalemia, hypercalcemia, hypomagnesemia, and severe acidosis or alkalosis can inhibit myocardial capture. Remember that potassium flux, as well as acid-base equilibrium, can be affected by hyper- or hypoventilation.
5. If all else fails, consideration should be given to sternotomy or thoracotomy by the surgical staff to permit application of epicardial leads.

Tachyarrhythmias

Unstable tachyarrhythmias must be treated appropriately; often, these problems require cardioversion. Cardioversion can damage the pacemaker, and an attempt should be made to place the paddles away from the generator (consider transthoracic placement). Any patient who undergoes cardioversion or defibrillation must have his or her pacemaker system interrogated shortly afterwards.

As previously stated, in patients with dual chamber pacemakers set to DDDxx mode and without an appropriate upper-rate limit setting, the onset of atrial fibrillation can produce a rapid, hemodynamically unstable ventricular response as the generator attempts to drive the ventricles at the sensed atrial rate. Placement of a magnet over the generator, changing the generator to DOOxx mode, should terminate this problem (assuming that the magnet mode is not disabled). Reprogramming the generator to DDIxx mode will prevent this problem (see "upper rate limit" described earlier in this chapter).

Postoperative (or Postprocedure) Management

A patient with a pacemaker who undergoes a procedure uncomplicated by pacemaker problems should be monitored according to the needs of the procedure. A patient who maintains a native rhythm that inhibits pacemaker firing might need to have his/her pacemaker interrogated to ensure that no damage has occurred. Shivering and/or seizure activity in the postprocedure period can inhibit a sensing generator or increase the rate of an adaptive pacemaker, and attention should be given to prevention of these untoward activities. Finally, a patient who has undergone a significant procedure can develop a catabolic state and might need to have his/her heart rate increased to meet their new, postprocedure oxygen delivery need. Box 5-2 summarizes the care for the patient with a cardiac pacemaker.

Box 5-2 Management of the Patient with a Pacemaker

1. Identify pacemaker manufacturer, date of placement, indication(s) for placement, and current operational mode. Verify pacemaker function to the extent possible from patient history. Time permitting, obtain report of pacemaker settings and magnet response from the patient's cardiologist. Also, time permitting, the procedure and pacemaker management (i.e., the need for reprogramming) should be discussed with the patient's cardiologist. At some time prior to the procedure, the magnet mode and rate should be checked.
2. Optimize medical therapy for coexisting diseases.
3. Continue all antiarrhythmic drug therapy.
4. Obtain labs and radiographs as needed.
5. Perform the surgery or procedure while maintaining continuous cardiac rhythm monitoring. If electrocautery is required, see the text for precautions. Also see the text for information regarding treatment of pacemaker failure and tacharrhythmias.
6. Some patients might need to have their pacemakers interrogated and/or reprogrammed after completion of the surgery or procedure. Such patients include those who underwent pacemaker reprogramming prior to the procedure, those who were exposed to significant monopolar cautery, and any patient with a significant untoward (pacemaker) event during the procedure.

• SUMMARY

The miniaturization of computing equipment has permitted the design and use of sophisticated electronics in patients who have need for external pacing of their hearts. Both the aging of the population and our ability to care for patients with increasingly complex disease, suggest that we will be caring for patients with these devices, and we must be prepared. Safe and efficient clinical management of these patients depends upon our understanding of pacemaker systems, indications for their use, and the perioperative needs they create.

Acknowledgments

Although many of the pacemaker manufacturers provided information helpful in the preparation of this document, special thanks must be accorded to Mr. Ken Kinser and Mr. Scott Andre of the Medtronic Corporation.

REFERENCES

1. Forand JM, Schweiss JF: Pacemaker syndrome during anesthesia, *Anesthesiology* 60(6):588–589, 1984.
2. Finfer SR: Pacemaker failure on induction of anaesthesia, *Br J Anaesth* 66:509–512, 1991.
3. Alexopoulos GS, Frances RJ: ECT and cardiac patients with pacemakers, *Am J Psychiatry* 137:(9)1111–1112, 1980.

BIBLIOGRAPHY

Celentano WJ, Jahr JS, Nossaman BD: Extracorporeal shock wave lithotripsy in a patient with a pacemaker, *Anesth Analg* 74:770–772, 1992.

Domino KB, Smith TC: Electrocautery-induced reprogramming of a pacemaker using a precordial magnet, *Anesth Analg* 62:609–612, 1983.

Drach GW, Weber C, Donovan JM: Treatment of pacemaker patients with extracorporeal shock wave lithotripsy, *J Urol* 143:895–896, 1990.

French RS, Tillman JG: Pacemaker function during helicopter transport, *Ann Emerg Med* 18:305–307, 1980.

Handbook of pulse generators and leads, St Paul, Mn, 1994, Cardiac Pacemakers Publication 8–488–1194.

Inbar S, et al: Case report: nuclear magnetic resonance imaging in a patient with a pacemaker, *Am J Med Sci* 305(3):174–175, 1993.

Jauhar P, et al: Electroconvulsive therapy for patients with cardiac pacemakers, *BMJ* 1:90–91, 1979.

Lagergren H: 25 years of implanted intracardiac pacers, *Lancet* 1 (8586):636–638, 1988.

Lamas GA, et al: Pacemaker malfunction after nitrous oxide anesthesia, *Am J Cardiol* 56:995–996, 1985.

Lauck G, et al: Effects of nuclear magnetic resonance imaging on cardiac pacemakers, *PACE* 18(8):1549–1555, 1995.

Manger D: Anaesthetic implications of 32% dextran-70 (Hyskon) during hysteroscopy: hysteroscopy syndrome, *Can J Anaesth* 39:975–979, 1992.

Purday JP, Towey RM: Apparent pacemaker failure caused by activation of ventricular threshold test by a magnetic instrument mat during general anaesthesia, *Br J Anaesth* 69:645–646, 1992.

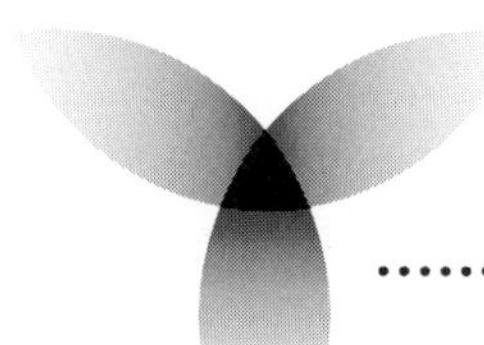

Chapter 6

Care of the Patient with an Implantable Cardioverter Defibrillator

Marc A Rozner, PhD, MD, Sinan Gursoy, MD, FACC

This chapter is designed to educate the perioperative physician about the function and behavior of implantable cardioverter defibrillators (ICDs).* Two underlying assumptions have guided the writing of this chapter. First, understanding the behavior of ICDs will lead to better perioperative care of a patient with such a device. Second, the previous chapter "Care of the Patient with a Pacemaker" should have been read and understood, since much of ICD technology has been built around pacemaker technology.

** Although many authors and references refer to these devices as "automatic implantable cardioverter defibrillators or AICDs," the term* AICD *is a brand name and belongs to CPI Cardiac Pacemakers Incorporated, St Paul, MN. The term* PCD *(for "programmable cardioverter defibrillator") belongs to Medtronic Corporation, Minneapolis, MN.*

GENERAL OVERVIEW

In 1980, the report of an implantable, battery-powered device able to deliver sufficient energy to terminate a lethal ventricular tachyarrhythmia represented a major medical breakthrough for patients with a history of sudden death or ventricular tachycardia that could not be controlled by pharmacologic means. The Federal Food and Drug Administration (FDA) first approved ICDs for implantation into patients in 1985. By 1989, approximately 5000 devices had been inserted into patients. From 1989 to 1994, more than 25,000 additional devices had been implanted. Numerous reports from uncontrolled studies have suggested that ICD placement is associated with significant reduction in death from ventricular tachyarrhythmias. The first randomized, prospective study comparing ICD placement to pharmacologic therapy for life-threatening arrhythmias was published in 1996; the presented data suggest that mortality from lethal ventricular tachyarrhythmias could be reduced by more than 50% with ICD implantation.

Initially, one major difficulty with ICD placement rested upon the need for thoracotomy to attach epicardial leads, which precluded insertion into many patients believed to be poor candidates for major thoracic surgery. The subsequent development and FDA approval (12/93) of transvenous lead systems, that could be placed without thoracotomy, significantly reduced the morbidity and mortality associated with ICD insertion. Next, refinements in generator technology that have taken place since introduction of ICDs have resulted in further miniaturization of these devices, and they now contain electronics able to detect and treat multiple tachyarrhythmias. These electronic advances, when coupled with new, transvenous lead systems, have significantly expanded the number of patients who could (or will) undergo placement of an ICD device.

ICD DESIGNATION

Like pacemakers, ICDs incorporate a generator, which contains a power source and electronic components needed for sensing, pacing, and shocking the patient's heart. The shock produced by an ICD is direct current, and it can be mono- or biphasic (biphasic shocks seem to be more effective than monophasic shocks when using transvenous lead systems). The shock is created by electronic circuitry designed to change the battery voltage (typically 3–6 volts) into approximately 660 to 750 volts needed to produce a maximum energy shock (approximately 30 J). The lead systems for ICDs are considerably more complex than those for pacemakers, and each lead must contain multiple electrodes for sensing, pacing, and shocking the myocardium.

Currently, only four companies (CPI, Intermedics, Medtronic, and Ventritex) manufacture and market FDA-approved ICD devices. Pacesetter[†] has a device in clinical

[†] *Pacesetter is a wholly owned subsidiary of St Jude Medical, Minneapolis, MN. Pacesetter recently acquired Ventritex. Prior to the acquisition, Pacesetter was in clinical trials with an Angeion device, which will likely be marketed under the Ventritex name.*

testing expected to enter the ICD marketplace sometime in 1997. Most of the ICD generators are large when compared to pacemaker generators, and ICDs typically have been placed in the abdomen. In 1995 Medtronic introduced the first ICD small enough for implantation in a pectoral pocket. With dimensions of approximately 7x7cm, these devices are only slightly larger than typical pacing generators. Other companies also have reduced the size of their generators, so one can no longer assume that a device in a pectoral pocket is a pacemaker.

Most of the ICDs marketed since February 1993 also provide some type of antibradycardia pacing therapy. Since this pacing function was designed to provide only emergency antibradycardia therapy, patients who need an ICD and have indication for a permanent pacemaker usually require two separate devices. Currently, only VVIOO mode pacing is available from ICD generators.

Another feature found in newer ICDs includes the ability to perform overdrive pacing to treat tachyarrhythmias. This feature requires less energy than a countershock, but it requires additional computational ability.

In a similar style to pacemakers, the North American Society of Pacing and Electrophysiology (NASPE) and the British Pacing and Electrophysiology Group (BPEG) have produced a four-position code to designate ICD lead placement and function. The NASPE/BPEG defibrillator code contains four positions describing: (1) chamber(s) shocked; (2) chamber(s) paced for antitachycardia therapy; (3) tachycardia detection algorithm; and (4) chamber(s) paced for antibradycardia therapy. Table 6-1 shows these codes. In this current scheme, older devices that had detected and treated only ventricular fibrillation, as well as devices that detect abnormal rhythms and provide only shock therapy to the ventricle, are designated VOEO.

At present, only the ventricles are shocked, paced, or sensed, and the only tachycardia detection scheme involves analysis of the electrical rhythm of the ventricle (electrogram detection). Each manufacturer has developed its own tachycardia detection algorithm, which can be found in the physician's manual for the ICD. Generator manufacturers are developing hemodynamic tachyarrhythmia algorithms, and the NASPE/BPEG code has been designed with these future improvements in mind.

ICDs have a large number of programmable features, most of which are beyond the scope of this chapter. Briefly, these features are divided into: (1) tachyarrhythmia detection; (2) tachyarrhythmia therapy; and (3) bradycardia pacing therapy. ICDs continuously monitor ventricular rhythm; any abnormality (termed an "event" or "episode") initiates either a pacing sequence (in devices with antitachycardia-pacing capability) or a shocking sequence. ICDs typically operate under the following set of rules for antitachycardia therapy: (1) within an event, each therapy delivered must be greater or equal to the strength of the previous therapy, even if the current presentation would have required a lower energy; (2) shock therapy is considered stronger than overdrive pace therapy, so once a shock has been delivered, no further antitachycardia pacing will be attempted; (3) overdrive pacing therapy is limited and the ICD will convert to shock therapy should it detect an event that is not corrected by pacing within a specified time or pacing sequence; and (4) each event can have no more than a limited number of shocks (typically 4 to 6, although some of the more advanced ICDs subclassify events and will deliver as many as 18 shocks

Table 6-1. NASPE/BPEG Defibrillator Code

POSITION I	POSITION II	POSITION III	POSITION IV
Shock Chamber(s)	Antitachycardia Pacing Chamber(s)	Tachycardia Detection	Antibradycardia Pacing Chamber(s)
O = None	O = None	E = Electrogram	O = None
A = Atrium	A = Atrium	H = Hemodynamic	A = Atrium
V = Ventricle	V = Ventricle		V = Ventricle
D = Dual (A + V)	D = Dual (A + V)		D = Dual (A + V)

in 1 event). Thus, a patient who develops ventricular fibrillation and is defibrillated (by the ICD) into ventricular tachycardia will continue to receive shock therapy, even if the ICD has antitachycardia-pacing function.

Once the decision is made to deliver a shock, the ICD must charge its capacitor with sufficient energy to produce the shock. Charging time is dependent upon the desired output, and it can be 6 to 15 seconds for a maximum shock (typically in the 30-J range). In an ICD programmed to detect an event in only 6 to 8 beats and deliver a low energy shock (2–4 J), time from event start to shock can be as little as 4 seconds. Charging time is lengthened by lower battery voltage, longer time from last charge[‡] and lower temperature (i.e., significant hypothermia). Additional time can pass after charging while the device attempts synchronization with the ventricular depolarizations. Some ICDs recheck the rhythm just prior to a shock and "cancel" (also called "abort") or alter the therapy if the rhythm has changed. All ICDs store information about events that can be downloaded into an ICD programmer.

The effect of magnet placement on an ICD depends on the manufacturer, model, and ICD programming. Calling the manufacturer represents the most reliable method for the determination of magnet response. Although most ICDs will disable antitachycardia (i.e., shock) therapy when a magnet is placed over the generator, the "magnet mode" can be disabled by programming. At present, no ICD disables the antibradycardia therapy or switches to asynchronous pacing when in the magnet mode. Ventritex warns that effectiveness of the magnet placement varies and is not a reliable means of disabling antitachycardia therapy. Ventritex states that magnet placement is indicated only for temporary inhibition of the antitachyarrhythmia therapy. CPI devices can be programmed to emit tones when the magnet is detected, which can be used to identify and change the current antitachycardic mode. Applying the magnet will produce an audible "beep" tone, which is synchronous

[‡] *The internal capacitor in an ICD "deforms" during periods of inactivity. Capacitor deformation decreases capacitor performance, which increases the time needed to charge the capacitor to a desired level. To mitigate the effects of deformation, all ICDs perform a nontherapeutic charging of their capacitors (called "reforming") at periodic intervals from 1 to 6 months.*

with the R waves if antitachycardia therapy is enabled, and a continuous tone if not. Applying the magnet for 30 or more seconds can change the mode (and the tone) in a CPI device only if the ICD is programmed to permit mode change with magnet placement. Intermedics has a device that responds to magnet placement by changing the VVI pacing rate to 100 beats per minute for the next 13 cardiac cycles (then returning to the programmed rate), provided that the battery-sensing circuit finds the battery at its "beginning of life" voltage.

Like patients with pacemakers, patients with ICDs should have been given a card with the manufacturer name, phone number, ICD identification, and date of implantation. Often, the manufacturer code can be obtained from a radiograph of the device. Current manufacturers' phone numbers can be obtained from Box 5-1 in Chapter 5 ("Care of the Patient with a Pacemaker").

● ICD INDICATIONS

ICDs are designed for use in patients who have a history of ventricular tachyarrhythmias (ventricular fibrillation or tachycardia) with hemodynamic compromise. Patients who have experienced hemodynamically significant ventricular tachycardia and who have responded to overdrive pacing are candidates for the ICDs with this function. Before placement of a device, a patient should have undergone electrophysiology testing to determine rates of inducible and spontaneous ventricular arrhythmias, as well as maximum sinus rate and the rate of any inducible supraventricular tachycardia. This testing should have been performed after stabilization of the patient's underlying medical problems and pharmacologic antiarrhythmic therapy. The data obtained from electrophysiologic testing serves as a guide to the selection of the device, as well as its programming. Depending upon the ICD manufacturer and model, the expected battery life of an ICD is 5 to 7 years.

Relative contraindications to placement of an ICD include: the presence of a pacemaker with unipolar leads (they generate large pacer spikes than "bipolar pacemakers" and can confuse the sensors in an ICD, which might prevent detection of a tachyarrhythmia), tachyarrhythmias resulting from transient or correctable factors (e.g., drug toxicity, electrolyte imbalance, acute myocardial infarction, drowning, electrocution, or sepsis); or history of nonsupressible supraventricular tachycardia with a rate above the tachyarrhythmia detection range (although some manufacturers now claim that their ICD can differentiate supraventricular from ventricular tachycardia). The expected need for frequent shocks or pacing represents an additional relative contraindication to placement, because battery life can be reduced by more than 50% in the presence of repeated need for shock or pace therapy.

● PREANESTHETIC EVALUATION

The patient with an ICD is likely to have severely depressed left ventricular function, most commonly from ischemic cardiomyopathy. The patient should also have a history of sudden death or hemodynamically significant ventricular tachyarrhythmia(s), and this patient frequently takes many medications. Like a patient with a pacemaker, a patient with an ICD has a high likelihood of concomitant disease, and considerable effort should be expended in the optimization of treatment within the preoperative time frame.

A patient with an ICD should be questioned about the indication for device placement. The site of the ICD placement should be determined, and a radiograph might provide information about lead placement or device code. The patient should be asked about any untoward events with the ICD and how any problem was corrected. Time permitting, ALL patients with ICDs should undergo device interrogation, which can be performed by a cardiologist or an ICD technician. The interrogation report will provide information about the frequency of ICD activation, the therapies delivered by the ICD, and the responses exhibited by the patient. For example, knowledge that the patient requires two or three shocks at the high output of the ICD suggests that low energy shocks during the perioperative period will be ineffective. Symptoms of improper ICD sensing function(s) include inappropriate delivery of shock therapy or inappropriate ventricular pacing. Furthermore, a patient with an ICD capable of antibradycardia therapy should be questioned about palpitations or pacemaker syndrome (see Preanesthetic Evaluation in Chapter 5, "Care of the Patient with a Pacemaker").

• INTRAOPERATIVE (AND OTHER PROCEDURE) MANAGEMENT

The manufacturers of ICDs recommend that the ICD be disabled during any procedure likely to "confuse" the ICD. Such procedures include surgery (with electrocautery or use of a nerve stimulator), therapeutic radiation, lithotripsy, and the placement of temporary pacing. At least one report of inappropriate shock therapy has appeared after electrocautery was used, and Stamato et al. (1996) report a case of inappropriate heart rate sensing by an ICD during train-of-four stimulation.[§] Reprogramming the ICD represents the best method to disable the ICD, since both the antitachycardia (overdrive pace or shock) and antibradycardia (pace) therapies can be inhibited. In an emergency, placement of a magnet might disable the antitachycardia therapy, but it will not disable nor alter any possible antibradycardia therapy. Most manufacturers believe that magnetic resonance imaging (MRI) and diathermy should be prohibited in patients with ICDs (see following).

Intraoperative monitor selection depends on the patient and proposed surgery. Electrocardiogram monitoring and the ability to deliver manual antitachycardia therapy must be present from the time that the ICD is disabled until the ICD is reenabled and tested. If electrocautery is planned, then a method to evaluate cardiac rhythm that is not affected by electrocautery is required.

....

§ *Stamato NJ et al (1996): Sensing of a transcutaneous nerve stimulator by an ICD device.* **www.webaxis.com/heartweb/1096/stamato.htm** *(an electronic journal on the World Wide Web).*

No special anesthetic technique appears necessary for the patient with an ICD, and most authors believe that an anesthetic technique should be the same that normally would be used for the scheduled procedure and the pathophysiological state of the patient. One must be prepared for the onset of ICD antibradycardia pacing should the heart rate fall below the programmed lower pacing rate while the ICD is "disabled" by magnet placement. Since only VVI mode pacing is available in current ICDs, cardiac output might be insufficient without an atrial contraction. Also, no method (except generator interrogation) is available to determine the bradytherapy pacing rate.

As with pacemakers, the manufacturers of ICDs believe that electrocautery remains a principal intraoperative issue. Although no report of damage to an ICD generator or lead system has been published, ICD manufacturers believe that appropriate cautions with electrocautery should be observed. These guidelines include the following:

1. Electrocautery can confuse the generator's sensing algorithms, which could lead to application of therapy (either shock or pace). All ICD functions should be disabled with the programmer, if time permits. Magnet placement might temporarily inhibit antitachycardia function. If magnet placement is to be used, the manufacturer should be contacted to determine appropriate magnet type, size, and placement instructions (directly over the ICD generator or off to one side). Remember that the patient with a disabled ICD MUST HAVE HIS/HER ELECTROCARDIOGRAM CONTINUOUSLY MONITORED until such time as the ICD function is restored and tested.
2. Avoid monopolar cautery when possible (use bipolar cautery).
3. If monopolar cautery cannot be avoided, then position the grounding pad so that the generator is not in the path of cautery current flow. When possible, the expected current path for any monopolar cautery should be perpendicular to a line drawn from the patient's ventricles to the generator, to reduce the possibility of induced current on the ICD leads.
4. Never use cautery over the generator or along the lead path to the heart.
5. Request that the smallest possible electrocautery current be used, that it be used only in short bursts, and that cautery not be activated until actually needed. Short bursts with resting periods (one manufacturer recommends 10-second resting periods between electrocautery bursts) will permit the sensing function to "clear" false senses, since most algorithms for detection of tachyarrhythmias search for periods of continuous, or near continuous, high ventricular rates.
6. Any patient who has undergone a procedure with electrocautery, external pacing, external defibrillation, or ICD reprogramming must have his/her ICD function(s) reenabled and tested after completion of the procedure, but before external monitoring is discontinued.

Specific Procedure Management

At this time, no reports have been published with specific information about equipment or procedures that might require special attention to patients with ICDs. ICD manufacturers state that MRI be absolutely contraindicated in patients with ICDs, since the behavior of the ICD and its leads in such a strong, alternating electromagnetic field is unknown. Possible effects of exposure to MRI could include: pain at the implanted site (from heating or movement); inhibition of ICD therapy; inappropriate delivery of therapy; reprogramming of the generator; damage to the ICD; damage to the patient's heart; or patient death if induced current on the ICD lead(s) produces a malignant cardiac rhythm.

According to the manufacturers, lithotripsy is permitted if the intended therapy site is not near the ICD generator or leads. Like the patient with a pacemaker, electroconvulsive therapy, nerve stimulator therapy, or procedures requiring monopolar cautery (i.e., transurethral resection of the prostate, hysteroscopic resection of the uterus) might be contraindicated or require special planning. If these procedures are contemplated, consultation with a cardiologist and the ICD manufacturer should be sought.

TREATMENT OF PERIOPERATIVE TACHYARRHYTHMIAS

A patient with an ICD has had previous episode(s) of hemodynamically significant tachyarrhythmias that has responded to defibrillation or cardioversion. Thus, when caring for a patient with an ICD, one should be prepared to treat such a problem. Treatment options for a tachyarrhythmia include the use of the ICD programmer to attempt overdrive pacing or internal shock therapy, or the use of other internal or external defibrillators. Should a patient develop a nonperfusing rhythm, the procedure must be stopped, cardiopulmonary resuscitation (CPR) should be started, and appropriate therapy should be instituted. Some sources recommend gloves be used when providing the CPR, since a discharge from an ICD might be perceived as a shock by the CPR personnel. At least one manufacturer cautions that sufficient energy might be present at the patient's skin to initiate an abnormal cardiac rhythm in the caregiver.

If the ICD programmer is to be used to deliver therapy, note that the charging or other operation of a nearby external defibrillation device can interfere with communication between the implanted ICD and the programmer. Guidelines for (non-ICD) defibrillation include:

1. If internal defibrillator paddles are used, the ICD leads must be disconnected to prevent damage to the generator.
2. Position external defibrillator paddles as far from the pulse generator as clinically possible.
3. Attempt to minimize induced current on the implanted leads by placing the external paddles in such a way that current flow between the external paddles is perpendicular to the path of the implanted leads.
4. Set the energy output of the external device as low as clinically possible.
5. Always have the ICD generator function retested after any external defibrillation.
6. Remember that the treatment of the patient takes precedence over worry about the ICD.

Box 6-1 Management of the Patient with an ICD

1. Identify ICD manufacturer, date and indication(s) for placement, and operational mode. Verify ICD function to the extent possible from patient history and the patient's cardiologist. Use the ICD programmer to obtain ICD treatment history (time permitting). Call the ICD manufacturer to determine magnet type and placement if ICD function cannot be disabled for the procedure.
2. Optimize medical therapy for coexisting diseases.
3. Continue all antiarrhythmic drug therapy.
4. Just prior to procedure, apply external cardiac rhythm monitor(s) and disable all ICD functions. Defibrillator equipment and pads should be immediately available.
5. Perform the surgery or procedure while maintaining continuous cardiac rhythm monitoring. If electrocautery is required, see the text for precautions. Also see the text for information regarding treatment of tachyarrhythmias.
6. Reenable ICD functions and verify performance of the ICD.
7. Discontinue external cardiac rhythm monitoring.

POSTOPERATIVE (OR POSTPROCEDURE) MANAGEMENT

A patient with an ICD MUST have his/her cardiac rhythm monitored continuously until the ICD operation is restored to its previous parameters. The ICD should be interrogated and tested to ensure appropriate function if the procedure involved the use of electrocautery, nerve stimulators, or the need for external pacing or defibrillation. No information is available about the possible misinterpretation of seizure or shivering activity, which might interfere with ICD sensing function. Box 6-1 presents a summary of management for the patient with an ICD.

SUMMARY

Implantable cardioverter defibrillators (ICDs) have been designed to provide continuous monitoring and treatment for lethal tachyarrhythmias. Recent literature suggests that placement of ICDs in selected patients has the potential to significantly reduce mortality from sudden death and other ventricular tachyarrhythmias. Since their approval by the FDA in 1985, ICD generators and lead systems have undergone a number of important improvements that will increase the number of patients who could (or will) undergo placement. As the number of patients with these devices increases, so does the probability that these patients will need perioperative care. Our ability to provide this care in a safe and efficient manner rests upon our understanding of these devices and the patients who have them.

Acknowledgement

Special thanks for assistance with this manuscript must be given to Mr. Jay Wilcox, Senior Technical Consultant, and Mr. Ken Kinser of the Medtronic Corporation.

BIBLIOGRAPHY

Deutsch N, et al: Perioperative management of the patient undergoing automatic internal cardioverter defibrillator implantation, *J Cardiothorac Vasc Anesth* 4(2):236–244, 1990.

Gaba DM, et al: Anesthesia and the automatic implantable cardioverter defibrillator. *Anesthesiology* 62:786–792, 1985.

Handbook of pulse generators and leads, St Paul, Mn, 1994, Cardiac Pacemakers. Publication 8–488–1194.

Moss AJ, et al: Improved survival with an implanted defibrillator in patients with coronary disease at high risk for ventricular arrhythmia, *N Engl J Med* 335(26):1933–1940, 1996.

Naccarelli GV, et al: Advances in implantable cardioverter/defibrillators. In Lynch, Carl III editor: *Clinical cardiac electrophysiology,* Philadelphia, 1994, Lippincott.

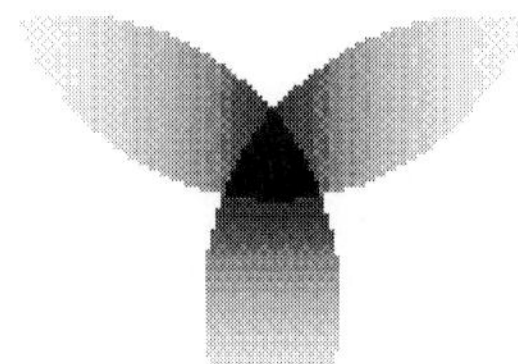

Chapter 7

The Adult with Congenital Heart Disease

Victor C. Baum, MD

Although management of patients with congenital heart disease has long been the purview of anesthesiologists specializing in the care of children with congenital heart disease, the marked success of pediatric cardiologists, cardiac surgeons, and pediatric cardiac anesthesiologists over the past several decades has resulted in more and more of these children surviving. As they survive and age, they will be seen for a host of noncardiac problems, not in specialized pediatric cardiac care centers, but increasingly in general referral and community hospitals, as well as ambulatory facilities.

Currently, an estimated 500,000 to 600,000 adults in the United States suffer from structural congenital heart disease, and each year 20,000 patients undergo intracardiac procedures for it. Over 80% of children currently born with congenital heart disease can expect to grow into adulthood. Approximately 6% to 8% of the adult congenital heart population requires hospitalization annually. The number of young adults who have undergone cardiac surgery in the first year of life has expanded to nearly 12,000 per year. As this patient population ages, it will bring with it to the operating room concerns of postoperative residua and sequelae, the acquired cardiovascular and noncardiovascular diseases of adulthood and old age, and increasingly complex intracardiac repairs, all superimposed on underlying physiology.

Cardiac surgery is considered *curative* if no residua, sequelae, or complications of the heart and circulation are present after surgery. In fact, very few congenital cardiac malformations are completely amenable to cure in the literal sense, with cure requiring that normal cardiovascular function is achieved and maintained, life expectancy is normal, and further medical or surgical treatment of the congenital heart disease is unnecessary. These few examples include uncomplicated closure of a nonpulmonary hypertensive patent ductus arteriosus, often, but not necessarily in childhood, and closure of an uncomplicated ostium secundum atrial septal defect in childhood. With few exceptions, however, cardiac surgery is followed by residua and sequelae, and curative heart surgery does not preclude noncardiac residua. Cardiac residua and sequelae include electrophysiologic, valvular (native or prosthetic), ventricular and vascular disorders, and infective endocarditis substrate.

Space limitations do not allow for a discussion of all of the various congenital heart defects and their natural histories and perioperative management. Instead, this chapter will concentrate on general principles of the perioperative care of the adult with congenital heart disease. First will be a discussion of the noncardiac manifestations of chronic cyanotic and acyanotic congenital heart disease, followed by a discussion of the perioperative considerations. Descriptions of the anatomy and physiology of lesions and their surgical repair is available in any number of texts, and complete discussions of the medical and surgical issues involved in caring for adults with congenital heart disease are also available (see Bibliography). Long-term ventricular function of a number of defects has been reviewed by Graham, and Hickey has reviewed the anesthetic management of patients following cardiac surgery (see Bibliography).

One factor which tends to make caring for patients with congenital heart disease intimidating to those not accustomed to it, is that most, if not all, patients will have had a surgical procedure that is identified eponymously. A list of pediatric cardiac surgical eponyms is given in Table 7-1.

PULMONARY ISSUES

Increased pulmonary blood flow from left-to-right shunting causes decreased pulmonary compliance, which, in turn, increases the work of breathing. Increased interstitial lung fluid may impinge upon small airways, increasing airway resistance and resulting in "cardiac asthma." Patients with chronic hypoxemia tend to have increased ventilation with normal arterial pCO_2. The ventilatory response to hypercarbia has not been extensively studied in cyanotic patients, though it has been evaluated in the related physiology of high altitude. Cyanotic patients appear to have normal ventilatory responses to hypercarbia but have blunted responses to hypoxemia, which resolve following surgical correction. End-tidal pCO_2 correlates well with arterial pCO_2 in acyanotic patients with normal or increased pulmonary blood

Table 7-1. Congenital Heart Disease Surgical Eponyms

NAME	DESCRIPTION	COMMENT
Blalock-Hanlon	closed atrial septectomy	a palliative procedure to increase shunting in TGA
Blalock-Park	end-to-side LSCA to descending aorta	an early repair of coarctation
Blalock-Taussig	subclavian to pulmonary artery shunt	see Figure 7-1
Damus-Kaye-Stansel	ligate MPA distally, anastomose proximal ascending aorta and proximal MPA; RV-distal PA valved conduit	for single ventricle with subaortic stenosis
Fontan	connection of right atrium or both venae cavae to right pulmonary artery	for tricuspid atresia or defects with only a single functional ventricle—(Figure 7-2)
Glenn	anastomose superior vena cava to right pulmonary artery; classic Glenn divides RPA with end-to-end anastomosis; "bidirectional Glenn" is end-to-side anastomosis	palliation for same indications as Fontan with decreased pulmonary blood flow; now done as palliation prior to completing Fontan
Jatene	arterial switch	for TGA
Konno	AVR with patch enlargement of RVOT	for AVR with small aortic annulus
Mustard	redirects atrial blood to opposite ventricle using an intraatrial baffle of pericardium	atrial repair of TGA; high incidence of atrial tachyarrhythmias or RV failure long-term, also SVC obstruction; (Figure 7-3)
Norwood	enlarge ascending aorta and anastomosis with MPA, atrial septectomy, ligate PA, aortopulmonary shunt; later Glenn, then Fontan	for hypoplastic left heart; done in 2-3 stages
Potts	descending aorta to left pulmonary artery anastomosis	see Figure 7-1
Rashkind	balloon atrial septostomy	a palliative procedure to increase shunting for TGA; done in cath. lab
Rastelli	conduit from LV through VSD to RVOT with external valved-conduit from RV to PA	for TGA with VSD
Ross	resect and transfer native pulmonary valve to aortic position and place homograft in pulmonary position	for AVR; prosthetic valve longer-lived on right side

(continued)

Table 7-1. Congenital Heart Disease Surgical Eponyms *(Continued)*

NAME	DESCRIPTION	COMMENT
Senning	functionally the same as Mustard, but uses atrial septum and free wall to redirect blood	see Figure 7-3
Waldhausen	ligate and divide LSCA, open proximal segment as a patch to relieve coarctation	subclavian flap repair of aortic coarctation
Waterston	ascending aorta to right pulmonary artery anastomosis	also known as Waterston-Cooley; modified shunt uses Gore-Tex rather than native artery; see Figure 7-1

Abbreviations: AVR, aortic valve replacement; LSCA, left subclavian artery; LV, left ventricle; MPA, main pulmonary artery; PA, pulmonary artery; RPA, right pulmonary artery; RV, right ventricle; RVOT, right ventricular outflow tract; SVC, superior vena cava; TGA, d-transposition of the great arteries; VSD, ventricular septal defect

flow; however, it underestimates arterial pCO_2 in cyanotic patients with decreased, normal, or increased pulmonary blood flow.

A Waterston aortopulmonary shunt (Fig. 7-1) may have resulted in asymmetric pulmonary blood flow, with increased flow to the ipsilateral lung and an oligemic contralateral lung. With time the flow may have been so excessive to the overperfused lung that it may develop the changes of pulmonary vascular disease. A pulmonary arterial band may, in time, migrate distally, also causing asymmetric pulmonary blood flow.

In adults, enlarged pulmonary arteries only rarely result in chronic compression of bronchi, causing recurrent or chronic atelectasis, pneumonia, or localized emphysema. At risk for compression are the left mainstem and upper lobe bronchi, which can be compressed by a large, hypertensive left pulmonary artery and the right middle lobe bronchus, which may be compressed by a large, hypertensive right lower lobe pulmonary artery. The right middle lobe syndrome is chronic right middle lobe pneumonia/atelectasis from bronchial compression. The left mainstem and upper lobe bronchi can also be compressed between the left upper lobe pulmonary artery and an enlarged left atrium. An enlarged hypertensive pulmonary trunk can compress the recurrent laryngeal nerve. Hemoptysis is a complication of Eisenmenger physiology. Previous surgery may have resulted in diaphragmatic paresis or paralysis from phrenic nerve injury.

Although not directly related to structural heart disease, there may be involvement of the airways relating to an underlying dysmorphic syndrome, which was responsible for the cardiac defect. A variety of dysmorphic syndromes are not only associated with congenital heart disease but also with difficult intubations. Aboussouan, for example, surveyed a group of adult patients with Down syndrome, both with and without cardiac disease. Aboussouan found decreased tracheal diameters in these adult patients (which had previously been described in pediatric patients with Down syndrome) unrelated to body habitus or the presence of cardiac disease.

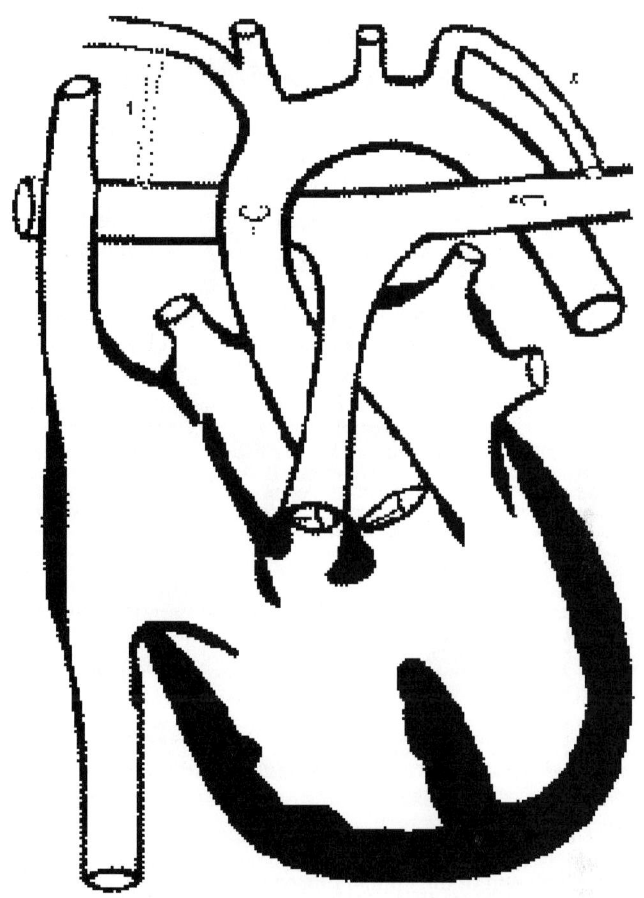

Figure 7-1

Palliative aortopulmonary anastomoses. The anastomoses superimposed on a heart with tetralogy of Fallot represent: 1, modified Blalock-Taussig; 2, classic Blalock-Taussig; 3, Waterston; 4, Potts. (Reprinted from Baum VC: The adult with congenital heart disease. *J Cardiothorac Vasc Anesth* 10:261–282, 1996, with permission of the publisher. Original modified with permission from Dr. Allen Everett, Department of Pediatrics, University of Virginia.)

Patients with congenital heart disease have an increased incidence of scoliosis, reported to be up to 19%, although the degree is rarely sufficient to impair pulmonary function. Scoliosis is more common in patients with cyanotic disease and may develop in adolescence, even though cyanosis had been relieved by corrective surgery years earlier during early childhood.

Pulmonary vascular disease, or an abnormal increase in pulmonary vascular resistance, is one of the most serious consequences of structural cardiac defects, cyanotic or acyanotic, causing increased pulmonary blood flow. This increase in pulmonary

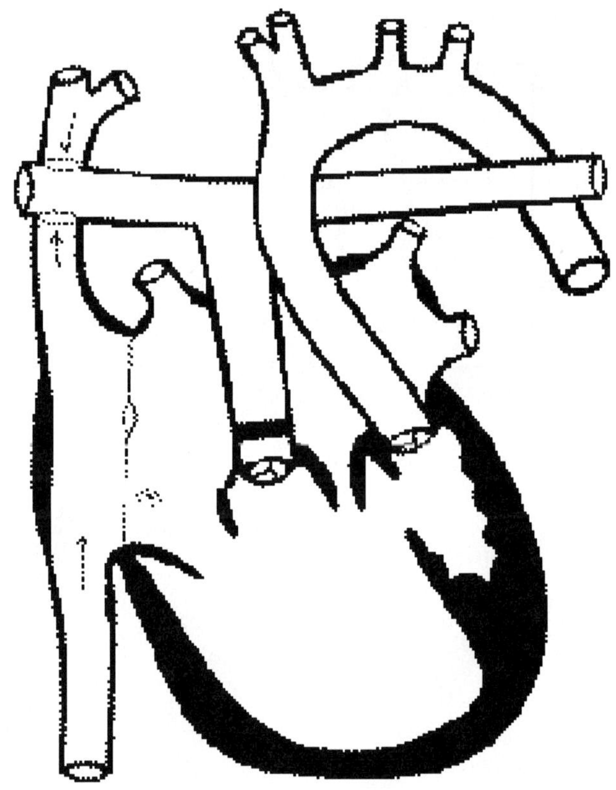

Figure 7-2
Lateral tunnel modification of the Fontan procedure in a patient with single ventricle. A fenestration has been placed in the atrial baffle to allow decompression of the right atrium, if necessary. The pulmonary artery has been ligated proximally. The coronary sinus (*CS*) has been incorporated into the low pressure neoleft atrium, which results in minor arterial desaturation. It can be appreciated that the superior limb of the cavopulmonary anastomosis represents a bidirectional Glenn shunt. (Reprinted from Baum VC: The adult with congenital heart disease. *J Cardiothorac Vasc Anesth* 10:261–282, 1996, with permission of the publisher. Original modified with permission from Dr. Allen Everett, Department of Pediatrics, University of Virginia.)

vascular resistance is the hemodynamic manifestation of physiologic and anatomic changes in the pulmonary arterial vasculature. During gestation, the pulmonary arteries and arterioles become heavily muscularized in a centrifugal manner, so that by term, vessels as small as 180 μm are muscularized. In the normal newborn this heavy muscularization regresses, accounting in large measure, for the decrease in pulmonary vascular resistance manifested over the first few months of life. Lesions that result in increased shear forces on the pulmonary arterial system will cause delayed regression of the pulmonary arterial musculature. Early on, these changes are solely manifested by increased tone of the musculature and are reversible, either

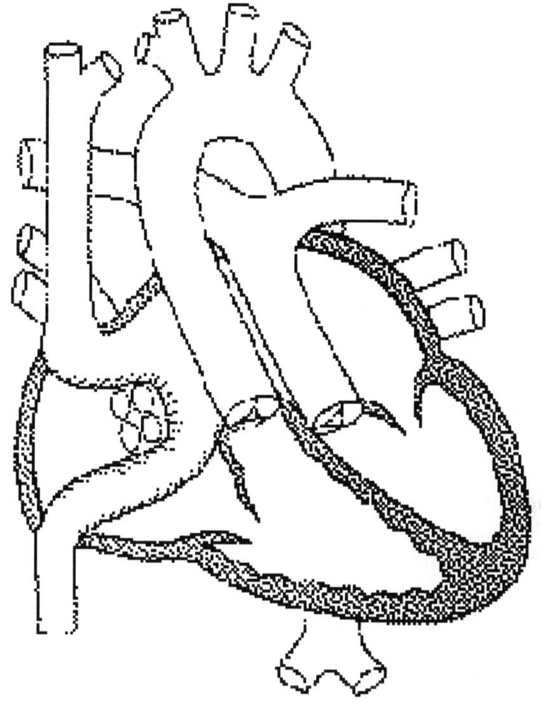

Figure 7-3
The Mustard operation for d-transposition of the great vessels. An intraatrial pericardial baffle directs vena caval return posterior to the baffle to the left ventricle. Pulmonary venous return flows anterior to the baffle across the tricuspid valve to the right ventricle. A Senning operation utilizes native atrial tissue to accomplish the same physiologic result. (Reprinted from Mullins C, Mayer D: *Congenital heart disease: a diagrammatic atlas,* New York, 1988, Alan R. Liss with permission of Wiley-Liss, Inc., a subsidiary of John Wiley & Sons, Inc.)

acutely with pharmacologic manipulation or permanently following surgical intervention. With time, anatomic changes develop and the elevations in pulmonary vascular changes are fixed and nonreversible. Surgical correction at this time is not only useless but may be fatal. The time course for the development of anatomic changes in the pulmonary vasculature is related to shear force. Ventricular or great vessel level shunts, such as a large ventricular septal defect or patent ductus arteriosus, may develop changes in childhood, while patients with a large atrial septal defect may not develop major increases in pulmonary vascular resistance until latter middle age.

Perioperative modification of pulmonary vascular resistance by relative hyperventilation or hypoventilation is one of the major therapeutic tools of pediatric cardiac anesthesia. These maneuvers are likely to be less useful in the adult population with congenital heart disease. In lesions with diminished pulmonary blood flow, pulmonary vascular resistance will already be low, and pulmonary blood flow will not increase in response to efforts at further lowering by hypocarbia. The main obstruction to pulmonary blood flow is the proximal one, typically pulmonary stenosis. Adult patients with left-to-right shunts will tend to segregate themselves into two groups. In one group the shunt is relatively small and will be of no clinical significance. The other group will have had a large left-to-right shunt and will have developed fixed pulmonary hypertension by adulthood. The one exception might be adults with atrial level left-to-right shunts who have not yet developed fixed pulmonary vascular disease. However, the effects of acute ventilatory changes to modify pulmonary blood flow is unclear, because the most important determinant of shunting in these patients is the relative diastolic compliance of the two ventricles, rather than the ratio of pulmonary to systemic vascular resistance as in ventricular or great vessel levels shunts. That being said, it would certainly seem prudent to avoid factors which will increase pulmonary vascular resistance in patients with preexisting pulmonary vascular disease.

Eisenmenger Physiology

Although Eisenmenger originally described a patient with a nonrestrictive ventricular septal defect, pulmonary vascular disease and reversed shunt, the term "Eisenmenger Syndrome" has come to be used in the wider context of patients with pulmonary vascular disease secondary to left-to-right shunting, regardless of the level of the shunt. Eisenmenger physiology is consistent with patient survival into adulthood. The presence of pulmonary arterial hypertension and elevated pulmonary vascular resistance can be inferred from the physical examination (loud pulmonic component of the second heart sound, single or narrowly split second sound, Graham-Steell murmur of pulmonary insufficiency, pulmonary ejection sound "click"), or can be documented by cardiac catheterization or echo-Doppler examination. Pulmonary arterial hypertension may also be suggested by findings on the electrocardiogram (right ventricular and, possibly, right atrial hypertrophy) and the chest radiograph (prominent main pulmonary artery and branches with "pruning," or a rapid decrease in size, of the distal intrapulmonary branches).

Patients with Eisenmenger physiology constitute a fair percentage of adult patients referred for preoperative anesthesia consultation for noncardiac surgery. They are, as a group, at particularly high perioperative risk. Fixed pulmonary vascular resistance precludes rapid adaptation to intraoperative hemodynamic changes. Given the widely patent connection(s) between the pulmonary and systemic circulations, hypovolemia and changes in systemic vascular resistance will be manifested by changes in the degree of right-to-left shunting. Particularly close monitoring of intravascular volume and extremely cautious use of systemic vasodilators, including regional anesthesia, are mandatory. Despite real concerns, epidural anesthesia has been used successfully in patients with Eisenmenger physiology, but the local anesthetic must be given slowly and in carefully titrated increments. Postoperative postural hypotension can also increase the degree of right-to-left shunting and postoperative patients should be cautioned to change position slowly.

Placement of a pulmonary arterial catheter in patients with congenital heart disease and Eisenmenger physiology, with or without a coagulopathy, is problematic and not without risk. Pulmonary hypertension is a risk factor for pulmonary artery perforation by a catheter. Both the abnormal intracardiac anatomy, and the right-to-left flow of blood may make successful placement of the catheter into the pulmonary artery difficult, if not impossible without the aid of fluoroscopy. Although seemingly useful in patients with pulmonary hypertension, thermodilution pulmonary arterial catheters are much less useful than what might be presumed. The relative resistances of the systemic and pulmonary arterial circulations are usually reflected rather well by changes in systemic arterial oxygen saturation, readily measured by pulse oximetry. Systemic cardiac output as estimated by thermodilution right ventricular output is erroneous, due to the right-to-left shunt. Acute intraoperative right ventricular failure is almost never a problem, because the large ventricular or great vessel level communication allows decompression of the right ventricle and maintenance of systemic output (albeit at a somewhat lower systemic oxygen saturation due to the increased right-to-left shunt). Potential exceptions to this are patients with single ventricle physiology and diminished ventricular function, and patients with atrial septal defects and pulmonary vascular disease, who may develop right ventricular failure secondary to suprasystemic pulmonary arterial pressure.

Long-standing pulmonary vascular disease becomes fixed in nature and unresponsive to pulmonary vasodilators including nitric oxide. Nevertheless, prudence would seem to dictate that in caring for patients with pulmonary vascular disease, factors known to elevate pulmonary vascular tone be avoided to minimize vasoconstriction in any segments of the pulmonary vasculature still dynamic. These include hypothermia, acidosis, hypercarbia, hypoxia (as opposed to the preexistent hypoxemia), and endogenous or exogenous catecholamines with α-adrenergic activity. Although this last comment, that α-adrenergic agents be avoided, is often seen, it is clear in clinical practice that their effects on the systemic circulation are more pronounced. In patients with ventricular or great vessel level shunts, use of α-adrenergic agents such as phenylephrine routinely and uniformly increase pulmonary blood flow and systemic oxygen saturation. The increase in pulmonary vascular resistance is more than compensated for by an increase in systemic vascular resistance.

Appropriate nerve blocks offer an appropriate alternative to general anesthesia of neuraxial blockade in patients with Eisenmenger physiology. If major surgery requires general endotracheal anesthesia, consideration should be given to plans for gradual recovery from anesthesia and extubation of the trachea in several hours. Because of the high risk, patients with Eisenmenger physiology should probably be observed in a monitored unit overnight after major surgery. After an appropriate period of observation in the postanesthesia care unit, same-day discharge is a reasonable option for these patients, however, following uncomplicated minor surgical procedures.

HEMATOLOGIC ISSUES

Congenital heart disease is associated with abnormalities of red cell regulation as well as hemostatic defects. Chronic hypoxemia results in increased production of renal erythropoietin and increased red blood cell production (erythrocytosis). The relationship among red blood cell mass, oxygen saturation and 2,3-diphosphoglycerate (2,3-DPG) is relatively poor in patients with cyanotic congenital heart disease. The oxygen-hemoglobin dissociation curve is usually normal or slightly right-shifted with chronic cyanosis. Although the majority develop a new, stable, higher equilibrium point for hematocrit, allowing for stable and adequate oxygen delivery, compensating for decreased arterial oxygen saturation, some patients will not develop and equilibrium and will have excessive hematocrit levels. These patients are often iron-deficient.

The major sequelae of high hematocrit levels are related to associated hyperviscosity. Symptoms of hyperviscosity include headache, faintness or dizziness, diplopia or blurred vision, myalgias, weakness, paresthesias, or depressed mentation and a feeling of dissociation. Hyperviscosity symptoms are rare at hematocrits less than 65% in the iron-replete patient. Iron-deficient red cells are less deformable than iron-replete cells, and iron-deficient blood will have a higher viscosity than iron-replete blood at any hematocrit. Iron deficiency is usually due to excessive inappropriate phlebotomies and is reflected by hypochromic microcytic indices, despite an apparent erythrocytosis. Treatment with oral iron is occasionally required, but patients need to be observed closely because this may result in an acute significant increase in hematocrit.

In young children erythrocytosis and hyperviscosity are associated with cerebral venous thrombosis. However adults with cyanotic congenital heart disease are not at risk for cerebral thrombosis, either arterial or venous, regardless of the hematocrit. Thrombosis may occur, however, in the upper lobes of the lungs in patients with Eisenmenger physiology.

Temporary relief of major hyperviscosity symptoms is afforded by isovolemic phlebotomy, assuming the hematocrit is greater than 65% and not the result of dehydration. Phlebotomy is recommended based on the presence of symptoms and not on a predetermined hematocrit level. Reductions in hematocrit by phlebotomy have been shown to improve, but only transiently, systemic blood flow, stroke volume, and oxygen transport. Five hundred milliliters of blood are withdrawn and replaced by an equal volume of crystalloid or colloid. Improvement in symptoms usually occurs within 24 hours. It is unusual for any patient to require removal of more than one unit of blood. It is appropriate to coordinate this with the blood bank in patients scheduled for major surgery to allow this blood to be used for autologous transfusion perioperatively.

Because dehydration can cause an increase in hematocrit to worrisome levels in some patients with already elevated hematocrits, prolonged preoperative fasting should be avoided. Newer recommendations for fasting, allowing a more limited preoperative fast, should make this issue less problematic.

Erythrocytosis results in plasma trapping and falsely elevated hematocrits if the hematocrit is measured with microhematocrit tubes. If possible, hematocrit levels should be measured by automated techniques. Because there is less plasma for each volume of erythrocytotic blood compared to normal blood, clinical laboratories may require larger samples of whole blood to obtain adequate volumes of plasma or serum for analysis.

Hemostatic defects occur widely in cyanotic, erythrocytotic patients but are poorly understood. If the hematocrit is less than 65%, bleeding diatheses are usually mild or absent, although excessive bleeding can occur with surgery or trauma. In general, the extent of the bleeding diathesis mirrors the degree of erythrocytosis.

Although platelet counts are typically reported in the low to low-normal range in erythrocytotic patients, bleeding is unrelated to thrombocytopenia. In fact, the platelet count is normal in almost all patients. When the diminished plasma volume in the laboratory samples from these patients is accounted for, the total platelet count is closer to normal (Fig. 7-4). Abnormalities in platelet function have, however, been reported in patients with chronic cyanosis. In addition, there may be iatrogenic reasons for abnormal platelet function. Patients with indwelling synthetic vascular grafts or atrial fibrillation may be maintained on a platelet inhibitor (aspirin or dipyridamole), which may increase the degree of perioperative bleeding.

Abnormalities of both the intrinsic and extrinsic coagulation systems, as well as deficiencies in specific factors, have been reported in some cyanotic patients; but, these are not uniformly present, and the etiology remains unclear. The fibrinolytic pathways are normal. Some patients with both cyanotic and acyanotic lesions have been described with deficiencies of the largest von Willebrand factor multimers which normalize after corrective surgery.

The increased hematocrit in erythrocytotic patients may result in spuriously elevated values of prothrombin and partial thromboplastin times (PT and PTT). The reason for this is that the tubes for the determination of PT and PTT contain a fixed amount of citrate as anticoagulant. This volume of citrate assumes a normal hematocrit. However, because erythrocytotic blood contains less plasma per unit volume of blood, this amount of citrate will be excessive (see Fig. 7-4). If the laboratory is informed of the patient's hematocrit in advance, it can prepare a blood tube containing the appropriate amount of citrate specifically for that patient. This correction is indicated for hematocrits over 55%. Correcting to an idealized hematocrit of 45% (plasma volume 55%), the amount of citrate to be added to the tube can be calculated as follows:

ml of citrate = (0.1 x blood volume collected) x (100 – patient's hematocrit)/55

In severely erythrocytotic patients isovolumic phlebotomy should be used to improve preoperative hemostasis. A 500 ml isovolemic phlebotomy is repeated every 24 hours to obtain a hematocrit of just under 65%. Again, the phlebotomized blood can be banked for autologous transfusion if needed perioperatively.

In addition to the intrinsic defects in coagulation previously described, there are other factors that may increase perioperative bleeding in patients with congenital heart disease. These include (for cyanotic patients) increased tissue vascularity and aortopulmonary collateral vessels, which increase blood loss when surgically interrupted. Elevated central venous pressure may also increase perioperative bleeding. Furthermore, many, if not most, of these patients will have had some type of intrathoracic surgical procedure in the past. Fibrosis increases the risk of bleeding with subsequent intrathoracic procedures.

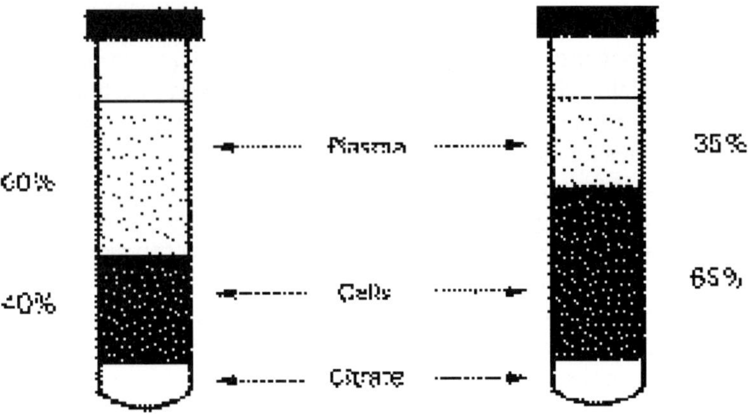

Figure 7-4
Basis for artifactual thrombocytopenia and elevated PT and PTT in the erythrocytotic patient. The fixed anticoagulant volume and decreased plasma volume in the erythrocytotic sample result in artifactual elevations in the PT and PTT. Similarly, although the platelet concentration is identical in both samples of plasma, the platelet count per ml of whole blood will be lower in erythrocytotic blood. (Reprinted from Baum VC: The adult with congenital heart disease. *J Cardiothorac Vasc Anesth* 10:261–282, 1996, with permission of the publisher).

• RENAL FUNCTION

Adult patients with chronic cyanosis have distinctive renal histopathology with hypercellular glomeruli, basement membrane thickening, focal interstitial fibrosis, tubular atrophy, and hyalinization of both afferent and efferent arterioles. High plasma–uric acid levels may be present; they are not the result of urate overproduction but inappropriately low levels of fractional uric-acid excretion. Enhanced urate reabsorption is thought to be caused by renal hypoperfusion superimposed on a high filtration fraction. Despite elevated levels of plasma uric acid, urate nephropathy and urate stones are rare. Arthralgias are common, but acute gouty arthritis is less frequent than what would be expected from the levels of plasma uric acid.

• NEUROLOGIC CONSIDERATIONS

Two major concerns in any patient with a real or potential intracardiac communication are brain abscess and paradoxical cerebral embolization. Adult patients remain at risk for the development of cerebral abscess, which may require surgical drainage, and a healed childhood abscess may present in the adult as a seizure disorder. Paradoxical emboli originating as lower extremity thrombi are of particular concern in the postoperative adult with congenital heart disease. Patients are at risk of paradoxical emboli from lower extremity thrombophlebitis, even in the face of the predominant left-to-right shunt such as atrial septal defect (ASD). Scrupulous attention must be paid to intravenous lines to avoid the introduction of intravascular air. Embolism of intravenous air into the left atrium has been reported with increases in intrathoracic pressure, such as high levels of positive end-expiratory pressure (PEEP) or a Valsalva's maneuver. Unlike children with cyanotic congenital heart disease, adults do not appear to be at risk for the development of either arterial or venous cerebral thrombosis, independent of hematocrit or the presence of hyperviscosity symptoms.

Prior surgery may have resulted in iatrogenic peripheral nerve injury. Surgery at the apices of the lung may have resulted in injury to the recurrent laryngeal nerve with hoarseness, to the phrenic nerve with diaphragmatic paresis or palsy, or to the sympathetic chain with the development of an ipsilateral Horner's syndrome. The presence of any of these should be documented preoperatively to clarify the possible development of new findings.

GASTROINTESTINAL FUNCTION

Because of increased hemoglobin turnover with erythrocytotic cyanotic heart disease, these adults have an increased incidence of calcium bilirubinate gallstones, which may present as acute cholecystitis. Biliary colic may develop years after reparative cardiac surgery and resolution of the cyanosis. Patients with right-sided failure and elevated systemic venous pressure may develop a protein losing enteropathy. Patients with profound ventricular failure may have passive hepatic congestion with mild-to-moderate elevation of the PT.

PREOPERATIVE CARE

Most adults with congenital heart disease lead normal and completely functional lives. One issue that these patients will face as they reach the age of majority is that they will no longer be able to obtain medical insurance coverage through their parents or through crippled children's services. Presently in the United States, over half are denied health insurance coverage entirely or in part because of preexisting conditions.

Vascular Access

Individual patients may have abnormalities that restrict placement of venous or arterial vascular access. Access to the right atrium from the femoral approach may be impossible because of thrombosis of one or both femoral veins from earlier catheterizations. Routine cardiac catheterization in children has been done for approximately 25 years percutaneously, even in neonates. However, adult patients may have had catheterization by means of femoral venous cutdown. The cardiologist may have either repaired or ligated the vein. More recently, some children still require a venous cutdown for technical reasons. This is typically by means of the saphenous vein in the groin, leaving the femoral vein patent. It will not be in any way apparent which of these approaches was used without reviewing the original catheterization report. Patients with visceral heterotaxy and polysplenia (these patients are bilaterally left-sided) will have interruption of the inferior vena cava with return of lower extremity blood to the heart through the hemiazygous vein, which makes passage of a catheter from the groin to the right atrium in the operating room difficult, requiring fluoroscopy. However, short intravenous catheters can be placed into the femoral veins in these patients without difficulty. Many practitioners prefer not to catheterize the superior vena cava in patients who have had either a Glenn shunt or a lateral tunnel modification of the Fontan procedure (both of which involve a superior vena cava to pulmonary artery anastomosis). Catheter-related thrombosis of the superior vena cava, although rare, can be catastrophic in these patients.

Because of the risk of intravenous air passing right-to-left, all intravascular lines must be maintained scrupulously free of bubbles. This is not only true in patients with right-to-left shunts, but also in those with predominant and even pure left-to-right shunts. The risk of paradoxical embolization in patients with ostium secundum atrial septal defects, for example, has been shown to increase with elevations in intrathoracic pressure. Although air and particle filters for intravenous lines are available, they tend to be inadequate for the administration of large amounts of fluids to adults.

Arterial access may also be compromised. If a residual aortic coarctation is present, there will be a disparity between blood pressures obtained proximally, (right arm and variably left arm) and from the legs. Patients with classic Blalock-Taussig shunts have discontinuity of the subclavian artery. The ipsilateral brachial and radial pulses are most often absent, but occasional patients have adequate collaterals to reconstitute a palpable pulse, albeit with questionable reliability of the blood pressure measured in that extremity. Blood pressure should be measured in the contralateral arm. Patients who have had bilateral Blalock-Taussig anastomoses require blood pressure monitoring in a lower extremity. Although the use of a synthetic aortopulmonary shunt (the modified Blalock-Taussig anastomosis) maintains the continuity of the subclavian artery, there may be partial obstruction at the site of the anastomosis. Blood pressure should only be obtained from the operative side when it has been confirmed that it correlates with blood pressure in the other arm or the legs. The left subclavian artery may have been utilized in repairing an aortic coarctation. Patients with supravalvar aortic stenosis have artifactually elevated systolic blood pressure in the right arm—the Coanda effect.

Infective Endocarditis Prophylaxis

The advent of surgical repairs has altered the natural history of endocarditis. Some operations eliminate the risk (e.g., ligation of patent ductus arteriosus), whereas others (prosthetic valves or shunts) increase the risk. There are two major predisposing factors for the development of infective endocarditis, namely a susceptible cardiac or vascular lesion and a source of bacteremia. The lesions at risk are characterized by high velocity flow, jet impact, and local increases in shear rate. Among the congenital lesions, those at greatest risk for the development of endocarditis are bicuspid aortic valve, restrictive ventricular septal defect, tetralogy of Fallot, high pressure atrioventricular valve insufficiency, and aortic insufficiency. A rationale for the current approach to antibiotic prophylaxis of infective endocarditis is offered by Durack.[1]

A list of conditions for which endocarditis prophylaxis is or is not warranted is given in Box 7-1. Because not all surgical or invasive procedures require endocarditis prophylaxis, a partial list of procedures not requiring prophylaxis is given in Box 7-2. Appropriate regimens are given in Box 7-3. It is notable that orotracheal intubation is not associated with bacteremia, unlike passage of catheters through the nose.

PREOPERATIVE MEDICATIONS

There is no contraindication to appropriate preoperative sedation in patients with cyanotic or acyanotic defects. In fact, patients with unpalliated tetralogy of Fallot or pulmonary vascular disease specifically benefit from good preoperative anxiolysis. Some patients will be receiving chronic digoxin or diuretic therapy. If digoxin is being given as an inotrope, and the surgical procedure will involve manipulation of the heart either by the surgeon or by the placement of intracardiac catheters, it is not unreasonable to withhold digoxin on the morning of surgery. Patients taking digitalis preparations have an increased incidence of arrhythmias with mechanical cardiac stimulation. Digoxin has a long half-life, and should the patient require additional inotropy perioperatively, numerous more potent inotropic agents are available. Patients who are receiving digoxin as an antiarrhythmic should receive their usual dosage. In general, it is better to withhold diuretics on the day of surgery to assure optimal intravascular volume prior to induction of anesthesia. Other cardiac medications are routinely continued up to the time of surgery.

Induction and Maintenance of Anesthesia

The presence of congenital heart disease, with or without cyanosis, is not in and of itself an indication for more than routine monitoring intraoperatively. A wide variety

Box 7-1 Conditions Requiring Antibiotic Endocarditis Prophylaxis

PROPHYLAXIS RECOMMENDED
- Prosthetic valves (bioprosthetic and homograft)
- Previous endocarditis
- Systemic-pulmonary shunts (e.g., Blalock-Taussig)
- Most cardiac structural abnormalities

PROPHYLAXIS NOT REQUIRED
- Isolated secundum atrial septal defect
- Surgical repair of secundum atrial septal defect, ventricular septal defect, or patent ductus arteriosus without residua beyond 6 months of repair

Box 7-2 Procedures Not Requiring Antibiotic Endocarditis Prophylaxis

Injection of intraoral anesthetics
Tympanostomy tube placement
Orotracheal intubation
Flexible bronchoscopy with or without biopsy
Cardiac catheterization
Endoscopy with or without biopsy (includes transesophageal echocardiography)
Cesarean section
In the absence of infection: urethral catheterization, dilatation and curettage, uncomplicated vaginal delivery, therapeutic abortion, sterilization procedures, insertion or removal of intrauterine devices

of anesthetic agents has been used to induce and maintain anesthesia in patients with congenital heart disease. An awareness of the varied hemodynamic effects of the various anesthetic agents is assumed. Space does not permit a discussion of appropriate anesthetic regimens for all of the possible congenital cardiac defects. Anesthesia for each of these is detailed in texts such as that by Lake (see Bibliography). The appropriate regimen is dictated by the specific pathophysiology, by appropriate preoperative evaluation of the history, physical examination, and relevant laboratory data.

The effects of anesthetic agents can be additive or opposite in action. For example, systemic arterial oxygen saturation routinely increases following the induction of anesthesia in cyanotic patients, despite the fact that the vasodilatory property of most of these drugs would be expected to decrease pulmonary blood flow (and, therefore, systemic saturation) in patients with right-to-left shunts. Presumably, the effect of the anesthetics to decrease oxygen consumption, thereby increasing mixed venous saturation, more than offsets the effect on pulmonary blood flow. Another example would be the negative inotropic effects of many anesthetics, which would be expected to be of benefit in lesions where dynamic obstruction inhibits emptying of one of the ventricles.

Although one often encounters discussions of the relative rapidity with onset of anesthesia in the patient with right-to-left or left-to-right shunts, the clinical implications with modern anesthetics is minimal.

In adults, nitrous oxide decreases cardiac output and systemic arterial blood pressure and increases pulmonary vascular resistance, particularly in patients in whom pulmonary vascular resistance is already elevated. An iatrogenic increase in pulmonary vascular resistance would be problematic in patients with pulmonary vascular disease or in those who depend on low pulmonary vascular resistance, such as patients who have had the Fontan procedure. However, in children with congenital heart disease, no increase in pulmonary vascular resistance has been observed with the use of 50% N_2O, regardless of the pulmonary vascular resistance. Nitrous oxide and halothane have long been used to induce anesthesia in cyanotic pediatric patients. Oxygen saturation routinely increases, also suggesting nitrous oxide has minimal, if any, significant effect on pulmonary vascular resistance in these patients.

Box 7-3 Regimens for Infective Endocarditis Antibiotic Prophylaxis

I. STANDARD PROPHYLAXIS FOR DENTAL, ORAL, OR UPPER RESPIRATORY PROCEDURES
   - A) Routine oral: amoxicillin 3.0 g 1 hour before procedure, then 1.5 g in 6 hours
   - B) Oral, penicillin allergic: erythromycin ethylsuccinate 800 mg (or 1.0 g erythromycin stearate) 2 hours before procedure, then 1/2 dose 6 hours later

     -or-

     Clindamycin 300 mg 1 hour before procedure, then 150 mg 6 hours later
   - C) Routine parenteral: Ampicillin 2.0 g IM or IV 30 minutes before procedure, then 1.0 g IM or IV, or 1.5 g orally, 6 hours later
   - D) Parenteral, penicillin allergic: clindamycin 300 mg IV 30 minutes before procedure, then 150 mg 6 hours later

     -or-

     Vancomycin 1.0 g slowly before surgery. No repeat dose necessary

II. STANDARD PROPHYLAXIS FOR GASTROINTESTINAL OR GENITOURINARY PROCEDURES
   - A) Standard parenteral: ampicillin 2.0 g IM or IV + gentamicin 1.5 mg/kg (not to exceed 80 mg) 30 minutes before procedure, then either 1.5 g amoxicillin orally in 6 hours or repeat parenteral regimen in 6 hours
   - B) Low risk oral (no prosthetic valve or prior bacterial endocarditis): amoxicillin 3 g orally 1 hour before procedure then 1.5 g orally 6 hours later
   - C) Parenteral, penicillin allergic: vancomycin 1.0 g + gentamicin 1.5 mg/kg (not to exceed 80 mg) 1 hour before procedure, then repeat in 8 hours

Although nitrous oxide precludes the use of 100% oxygen, even 30% oxygen is significantly greater than the 21% oxygen these patients normally breathe. Also, increments or decrements in F_1O_2 have only minimal effects on systemic saturation in patients whose cyanosis is due to right-to-left shunts. One precautionary note is due regarding the use of nitrous oxide in patients with shunt lesions. Nitrous oxide should probably be used cautiously in patients at risk for paradoxical emboli who are having surgical procedures, which may introduce air emboli, since nitrous oxide would enlarge such emboli.

For patients with large left-to-right shunts, efforts at increasing pulmonary vascular resistance by means of moderate hypercarbia and minimizing F_1O_2 as much as possible will decrease the degree of the shunt, decreasing left ventricular diastolic volume and improving the left ventricular oxygen supply-demand relationship. However, it is expected that most patients with large left-to-right shunts will have developed adequate pulmonary vascular disease by adulthood to have limited excessive flows on their own.

Intravascular volume replacement is of course guided by the operation. As a generalization, patients with good ventricular function and decreased pulmonary blood flow will not be hurt by slight overhydration but may have increased cyanosis with decreased intravascular volume.

POSTOPERATIVE MANAGEMENT

Patients with congenital heart disease clearly warrant close observation in the postanesthesia care unit. The specific duration of observation cannot be generalized, being dependent on both underlying physiology and the type of surgery. Patients with good cardiac function following successful surgical repair or palliation, who undergo minor noncardiac surgical procedures, can be treated as any other patient, and are in no way excluded from ambulatory surgery. Patients with cyanosis from right-to-left shunting will have only minimal increases in systemic oxygenation with supplemental oxygen, which should be made known to those caring for the patient to avoid needlessly prolonged courses of high inspiratory oxygen concentrations and delayed discharge from the postanesthesia care unit. Hypovolemia, a frequent consequence of surgery, will result in many cyanotic patients, in increased right-to-left shunting and should be corrected rapidly. Cyanotic patients, who require increased hematocrits, should have hematocrits evaluated serially, especially when significant blood loss has occurred. Patients should be encouraged to ambulate slowly to avoid hemodynamic changes from postural hypotension.

If patients with Glenn or Fontan procedures require protracted postoperative positive pressure ventilation, efforts should be made to minimize pulmonary artery pressure by limiting inspiratory pressure as much as is practical and by using low, physiologic levels of PEEP to optimize functional residual capacity.

The presence of congenital heart disease is in no way a contraindication to appropriate postoperative pain relief. These patients have a normal carbon dioxide response curve and may be given appropriate doses of parenteral, subarachnoid, or epidural opiates.

REFERENCES

1. Durack DT: Prevention of infective endocarditis, *N Engl J Med* 332:38–44, 1995.

BIBLIOGRAPHY

Aboussouan LS, et al: Hypoplastic trachea in Down's Syndrome, *Am Rev Resp Dis* 147:72–75, 1993.

Baum VC: The adult with congenital heart disease,. *J Cardiothorac Vasc Anesth* 10:261–282, 1996.

Dajani AS, et al: Prevention of bacterial endocarditis. Recommendations by the American Heart Association, *JAMA* 264:2919–2922, 1990.

Elkayam U, Gleicher N: Cardiac problems in pregnancy: diagnosis and management of maternal and fetal disease, New York, 1990, Alan R. Liss.

Emmanouilides GC, et al, editors: *Moss' heart disease in infants, children, and adolescents*, Baltimore, 1995, Williams and Wilkins.

Graham TP Jr, Cordell GD, Bender HW: Ventricular function following surgery. In Kidd BS, Rowe RD editors: *The child with congenital heart disease after surgery*, Mt. Kisco, 1995, Futura Publishing Co.

Hickey PR: Anesthetic evaluation for the reconstructed heart, *Adv Anesthesia* 8:91–113, 1991.

Lake CA, editor: *Pediatric cardiac anesthesia*, Norwalk, Ct, 1993, Appleton and Lange.

Perloff JK, Child JS editors: *Congenital heart disease in adults*, Philadelphia, 1991, WB Saunders.

Rudolph AM: *Congenital diseases of the heart*, Chicago, 1974, Yearbook Medical Publishers.

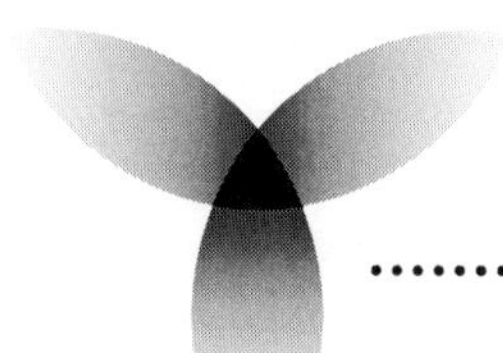

Chapter 8

The Cardiomyopathies

Stuart M. Lowson, MB.Bs, FRCA, MRCP
Neil P. Lewis, MB.Bs, MD, MRCP

The World Health Organization (WHO) defines a cardiomyopathy (CM) as a heart muscle disease of unknown cause and divides it into three types: dilated (DCM), hypertrophic (HCM), and restrictive (RCM). DCM accounts for 90% of cases with RCM being the least common of the three.

• DILATED CARDIOMYOPATHY (DCM)

According to the WHO definition, DCM should be idiopathic. However, a dilated cardiomyopathy may be secondary to a number of underlying conditions, the most important of which are ischemic, valvular heart disease, and alcoholism. It is estimated that idiopathic DCM is approximately one tenth to one fourth as common as ischemic left ventricular dysfunction. Epidemiologic studies in a defined Swedish population demonstrate an annual incidence of DCM in 5.3 cases per 100,000 population. Approximately 20,000 new cases are diagnosed each year in the United States.

The Pathophysiology

DCM is characterized by markedly decreased ventricular contractility and enlargement of both the right and left ventricles. The increase in end-diastolic volume (EDV) serves as a compensatory mechanism to preserve stroke volume (SV) in the face of a decreased ejection fraction (EF). In fact, resting SV may be almost normal despite a significantly reduced EF and a "latent stage." That stage, in which cardiomegaly precedes symptoms, is well documented and may exist for many years. With time, however, this compensatory mechanism fails to keep pace with the disease process, resulting in overt congestive heart failure (CHF).

Ventricular dilation may produce both mitral and tricuspid regurgitation, which will further compromise forward flow and exacerbate congestive symptoms. There is a high incidence of mural thrombi with the attendant risk of embolic events.

The Natural History of DCM

Mortality in DCM is closely related to LV function and the patient's functional status, which represent the best prognostic indicators. The 1-year mortality of CHF in patients with New York Heart Association (NYHA) classification IV is quoted as more than 50%. However, different studies have reported a highly variable outcome. While much of the data demonstrating a poor prognosis comes from tertiary referral centers, studies performed on population-based cohorts have demonstrated a significantly better survival. Furthermore, there is a strong suggestion that survival has improved as a result of improvements in treatment, namely the use of angiotensin convertase enzyme inhibitors (ACEIs) and perhaps β-blockers.

The Symptoms

The symptoms of DCM may vary from mild to severe, depending upon disease severity, the efficiency of the compensatory mechanisms, and the efficacy of treatment. The majority of patients with severe DCM will already be known to the medical profession, and it is unlikely that such a patient will turn up unannounced in the surgical admission suite on the morning of the operation; however, we do live in uncertain times. The onset of symptoms may be gradual or dramatic. Common symptoms include fatigue, weakness, exertional dyspnea, orthopnea, and paroxysmal nocturnal dyspnea. Chest pain, typical of angina, occurs in 10% of patients, while 3% of patients experience thromboembolic events. Arrhythmias, particularly ventricular tachycardia and atrial fibrillation, are an early manifestation of DCM in 50% of patients.

The patient's level of activity is a significant factor in outcome and can be defined according to the NYHA Functional Classification:

Class I—patients have no limitation of ordinary activity.
Class II—patients have some limitation of physical activity, experience symptoms with ordinary activity, but are comfortable at rest.
Class III—patients are comfortable at rest but less than ordinary physical activity causes fatigue, palpitations, dyspnea, or anginal pain.
Class IV—any physical activity causes discomfort and patients may be symptomatic at rest.

Goldman and others have demonstrated that the incidence of perioperative cardiac events correlates with the NYHA class. More recently, the ability to increase oxygen consumption (baseline oxygen consumption is expressed as 1 metabolic equivalent—1 MET) has been used as a measure for risk stratification. It has been demonstrated that patients who are unable to increase their oxygen consumption by at least 4 times have a significant increase in perioperative cardiac events. Levels of activity that exceed 4 METs include climbing a flight of stairs, walking uphill, walking on the level at a normal pace, and running a short distance.

The Physical Examination

Physical signs of DCM will vary with the severity of the disease and the response to treatment. They include a displaced and diffuse precordial impulse, low volume arterial pulse, jugular venous distension, hepatomegaly, peripheral edema, pulmonary rales and/or dullness, signifying pulmonary edema and/or effusion, murmurs of mitral and/or tricuspid regurgitation, gallop heart sounds, and pulsus alternans (usually an indicator of advanced left ventricular failure [LVF]). The presence of jugular venous distension, a third heart sound, and pulmonary congestion has been classically associated with increased perioperative risk. Importantly, the physical signs (and symptoms) may not accurately reflect the degree of physiologic impairment, and the absence of cardiomegaly, edema, and pulmonary rales does not exclude the diagnosis of CHF. In the early stages, a patient may be asymptomatic with relatively normal hemodynamic parameters at rest but will not have a normal response to stressful stimuli, which includes surgery. This behooves us to request more detailed patient evaluation.

The Laboratory Findings

When ordering any laboratory test we should always ask ourselves what we are looking for and how the result will influence patient management. Blood chemistry is routinely ordered for patients with cardiac disease. Hyponatremia (defined as a plasma sodium less than 135 mEq/l) is a frequent finding in patients with poorly controlled CHF, tends to correlate with the degree of fluid overload, but may be due to saline depletion secondary to overdiuresis. While acute hyponatremia is associated with central nervous system (CNS) disturbances and an enhanced response to CNS depressant drugs (in animals), there is no evidence of an interaction between chronic hyponatremia (to the level commonly encountered in patients with CHF) and anesthetic agents. Hypokalemia is also a feature of diuretic treatment. While the relationship between hypokalemia and perioperative arrhythmias is controversial, it would appear prudent to attempt to correct a potassium deficit in patients receiving digoxin, patients who have frequent preoperative arrhythmias, and perhaps those likely to require perioperative inotropic support (β-agonists will produce increased intracellular potassium movement and worsen the extracellular hypokalemia) or require hyperventilation as part of the anesthetic technique (hypokalemia induced by the respiratory alkalosis). Acute attempts to correct the potassium deficit are unlikely to be successful and may be hazardous. If hypokalemia is to be corrected, potassium should be infused over at least 24 hours, with the understanding that this is also unlikely to replace the total deficit, particularly if hypomagnesemia is also present. The amount of potassium infused per hour will depend on how aggressive replacement therapy is to be and the clinical setting. Many textbooks recommend adding no more than 20 mM of potassium per litre of infusion fluid, which will result in a very conservative rate of replacement if the patient is not to be volume-overloaded. In the intensive care unit, however, where cardiac monitoring facilities are available and most patients will have central venous access, it is not unknown to infuse potassium at rates of 20 mM per hour. Hypomagnesemia commonly results from prolonged use of diuretics and, unless treated, most of the administered potassium will simply be lost in the urine. Elevated blood urea and creatinine may also be seen. This may be secondary to either a low cardiac output and/or volume depletion, producing a corresponding low renal blood flow and glomerular filtration ratio.

Patients with CHF cannot respond to anemia with the normal increase in cardiac output, so it is important to aim for an "optimum hematocrit" in the perioperative period. What constitutes an "optimum hematocrit" is still debated and probably varies between individuals and disease states, but a hemoglobin concentration of at least 10 g/dl is probably appropriate. Coagulation studies are clearly required for any patient receiving anticoagulants, particularly if regional anesthesia is contemplated. Coagulation may also be deranged in a patient with cardiac-induced hepatic dysfunction.

Chest radiography may demonstrate cardiomegaly with or without pulmonary congestion and effusions. The electrocardiogram (ECG) is nonspecifically abnormal in the majority of symptomatic patients. ECG abnormalities include left axis deviation, low QRS voltage, evidence of left ventricular hypertrophy and atrial enlargement, nonspecific ST-segment changes, and Q waves (associated with patchy myocardial fibrosis). Almost any arrhythmia may be found. Continuous ambulatory monitoring shows atrial fibrillation and ventricular tachycardia in 20% and 50% of patients, respectively. Conduction defects, both atrioventricular and intraventricular (particularly left bundle branch block), are common.

Two-dimensional echocardiography is valuable in both the diagnosis and assessment of DCM. Echocardiography will show enlargement of the cardiac chambers, the decreased cardiac contractility, and may reveal mural thrombi and AV valve regurgitation, as well (Fig. 8-1). In addition to the patient's functional status, an accurate assessment of the EF is one of the most useful pieces of information the

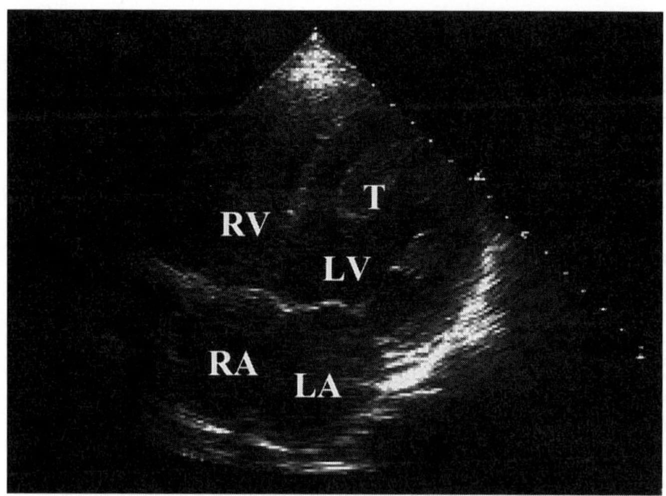

Figure 8-1
Two-dimensional echocardiogram in a patient with dilated cardiomyopathy secondary to a prior anterior (septal) myocardial infarction. This apical four-chamber view shows four-chamber dilatation, septal thinning, and a mobile thrombus (*T*) attached to the apex of the left ventricle (*LV*).

anesthesiologist can receive. Although the EF is usually obtained with the patient at rest, it does provide a measure of baseline cardiac function, and, therefore, an estimate of the likely response to anesthetic agents and hemodynamic pertubations. Furthermore, a reduced LVEF (less than 40%) has been shown to be significantly associated with increased perioperative cardiac events. Echocardiography will also differentiate DCM from other possible diagnosis such as HCM, RCM, and long-standing valvular disease.

Cardiac catheterization provides a measure of left- and right-sided heart pressures, and cardiac output. If the diagnosis of either DCM or ischemic left ventricular dysfunction is in doubt, then either radionuclide imaging and/or coronary angiography should be performed. These two conditions cannot be reliably differentiated by history alone, as myocardial ischemia may be silent and chest pain may be a feature of DCM. The importance of diagnosing ischemia lies in its potential for reversibility.

Electrophysiologic testing may be performed to determine whether ventricular arrythmias are inducible and whether they can be effectively suppressed by antiarrhythmic drugs.

Endomyocardial biopsy may be needed to rule out certain diseases such as sarcoidosis, hemochromatosis, and myocarditis.

The Treatment

Over the last decade there have been a number of changes in the treatment of CHF based on the results of large multicenter studies. These changes and the studies that conceived them are described in detail in this section. Most patients with severe DCM are placed under the care of a cardiologist. Perioperative management of such patients involves a joint consultation between specialities who should be familiar with modern treatment modalities.

General measures include weight reduction, salt restriction, and abstinence from alcohol and tobacco. If the patient has symptoms or signs of congestion then diuretics, usually loop diuretics, are given with the addition of a thiazide (metolazone) if the dose of the loop diuretic is increasing and the response diminishing.

Vasodilators have become the mainstay of treatment. In the first Veterans heart failure trial (V-HEFT I), survival was improved by the combination of hydralazine and isosorbide dinitrate compared to prazosin or placebo. In the second Veterans trial (V-HEFT II) mortality was lower in those patients treated with enalapril compared to the hydralazine/isosorbide combination. The efficacy of angiotensin converting enzyme inhibitors (ACEI) was also demonstrated in the 1987 Cooperative North Scandinavian Enalapril Survival Study (CONSENSUS) and the 1992 Studies of Left Ventricular Dysfunction (SOLVD). ACEIs may not be tolerated in all patients because of renal dysfunction, hypotension, hyperkalemia, or cough. In these patients, the combination of hydralazine and isosorbide dinitrate provides a useful alternative.

Digitalis glycosides have been the cornerstone of treatment for CHF since Withering first brewed his tea with foxglove in 1785. Over the last decade, treatment of CHF with digoxin was considered routine, then not indicated in patients in sinus rhythm, and is now back in favor. The 1993 Randomized Assessment of Digoxin on Inhibitors of the Angiotensin Converting Enzyme (RADIANCE) demonstrated clinical deterioration in patients with CHF already receiving ACEIs, when digoxin was randomly withdrawn. While digoxin may improve symptoms and decrease hospitalization rate, it does not appear to confer any survival advantage as shown by the results of the Digitalis Investigators Group study presented in 1997. The possible beneficial effects of digoxin are now thought to be due to its sympatholytic properties, rather than any positive inotropic ones. In fact, positive inotropes in general have fallen into disfavor for the chronic management of CHF. Attempts to develop oral β-adrenergic agonists have been frustrated by the rapid development of tolerance. Trials with the phosphodiesterase inhibitors were suspended as a result of the 1991 Prospective Randomized Milrinone Survival Evaluation (PROMISE) study which showed that cardiovascular mortality was 34% higher in those patients on long-term oral milrinone. While long-term treatment with positive inotropes is in disfavor, these agents may be beneficial in the acute setting, such as the perioperative period.

A new agent that has appeared on the scene is oral vesnarinone. Vesnarinone is a weak phosphodiesterase III inhibitor, delays inward and outward potassium currents, and opens sodium channels. It prolongs the action potential, slows the heart rate, and may also have an anticytokine action. In a randomized study of 500 patients with symptomatic CHF (EF <30%) an intermediate dose of vesnarinone (60 mg/day) reduced all causes of mortality and morbidity by more than 50%. Interestingly, the high-dose arm (120 mg/day) increased mortality.

It is generally thought that β-blockers should be avoided in CHF. However, recent trials have shown that treatment with β-blockers may decrease morbidity, the frequency of hospitalizations, and mortality. The 1992 Metoprolol in Dilated Cardiomyopathy and the 1994 Cardiac Insufficiency with Bisprolol Study both demonstrated a nonstatistically significant survival benefit with β-blockers in CHF. Treatment with β-blockers is, therefore, still viewed as experimental, must be introduced gradually, and may not be tolerated by all patients. Newer agents such as bucindol and carvedilol have additional vasodilating properties and both agents have been shown to produce a sustained increase in left ventricular EF. Bucindolol is currently being evaluated in the on-going β-blocker Evaluation Survival Trial. The mechanism of action in β-blockers is unknown. It may be due to upregulation of the β-adrenergic receptor or, as is now considered more likely, to a reduction of the adverse effects of sustained catecholamine release on the failing heart.

The probability of mural thrombi and thromboembolic phenomena increase when the EF is less than 30%. Therefore, it is logical (but still controversial) to consider long-term oral anticoagulation in these patients. This is particularly true if additional risk factors, such as age over 60 years, previous embolism, and/or atrial fibrillation are also present. The value of anticoagulation in mild DCM (EF > 40%) and sinus rhythm is not known.

Arrhythmias are common in patients with DCM. Over 50% of patients have nonsustained ventricular tachycardia (VT) during ambulatory monitoring. Neither class I antiarrhythmics nor amiodarone have been shown to improve prognosis, and may be proarrhythmogenic in patients with nonsustained VT. CHF is exacerbated in 4% to 25% of patients, especially when class I drugs are used. Patients with sustained VT or out of hospital ventricular fibrillation are at high risk of recurrent life-threatening tachyarrhythmias and sudden death. Prevention of these arrhythmias can be difficult and drug selection may be aided by electrophysiologic and electropharmacologic testing. Studies from Europe have shown that, in approximately 30% to 50% of patients with DCM, the ventricular arrhythmia can be reproducibly induced and responds favorably to antiarrhythmic therapy. Amiodarone is the preferred agent because its negative inotropic effect is less than other antiarrhythmics and rarely clinically apparent. If the ventricular arrhythmia cannot be reliably induced and/or no pharmacologic agent appears effective, then the high-risk patient should be offered an automated cardioverter-defibrillator (AICD). Recent studies (albeit involving small numbers) have shown that an AICD may considerably improve outcome in patients with DCM and sustained ventricular arrhythmias. Atrial arrhythmias, particularly AF, are common. Efforts should be made to restore sinus rhythm to maintain cardiac output and decrease the risk of embolic events. Inadequately controlled AF may also contribute to the ongoing deterioration in ventricular function.

In patients with DCM unresponsive to pharmacologic therapy, recent studies have shown that dual-chamber pacing, with a short atrioventricular interval, may improve hemodynamics and symptoms. Increased left ventricular filling, reduced mitral regurgitation, and decreased ventricular wall stress are thought to account for this improvement.

Dilated cardiomyopathy remains the most common indication for cardiac transplantation and the outcome of transplanted patients with severe DCM (NYHA class IV) is better than with medical therapy. The 1- and 5-year survival after transplantation is 85% and 70%, respectively. Unfortunately, the shortage of donor hearts means that there are twice as many patients added to the waiting list in the United States each month than patients who actually undergo cardiac transplantation. Only the most severe case receives a new heart. The shortage provides the impetus for improvements in medical therapy and novel surgical techniques such as cardiomyoplasty (wrapping the heart in the latissimus dorsi muscle). Mechanical circulatory-assist devices may be used short-term as a bridge to transplantation.

Surgery in Patients with DCM

Patients with DCM may undergo cardiac or noncardiac surgery. Common cardiac procedures include placement of an AICD, mechanical-assist device, electrophysiologic testing, and cardiac transplantation. Operative correction of mitral regurgitation is associated with a high mortality and is thought by some to be inadvisable.

It is important to establish the cause of the CHF before surgery; perioperative management will differ if the patient's CHF is secondary to DCM, ischemic or valvular heart disease. Studies from the 1970s and 1980s showed that patients with a current or past history of CHF were at an increased perioperative risk. Additional risk factors were found to be age over 60 years, an abnormal ECG, and major surgery (particularly emergency surgery) associated with large fluid shifts and/or blood loss. The degree of risk associated with each NYHA class has probably improved over the last 2 decades because of improvements in both medical therapy and anesthetic management. Although it has never been conclusively shown that preoperative optimization of the patient's cardiac status affects outcome, this deduction makes intuitive sense. It is indeed, the very foundation upon which the subspeciality of perioperative medicine is built. Ideally, patients should arrive in the operating room free of congestive signs and symptoms and with maximized tissue perfusion (see following text).

The aims of intraoperative management are to avoid myocardial depression and increases in afterload, and to maintain preload. These patients are extremely sensitive to myocardial depressant drugs, which favor a narcotic-based anesthetic technique. As previously stated, inotropic support may be required to sustain the patient over the perioperative period. The degree of monitoring employed depends on the patient's condition and the nature of the procedure. Patients in NYHA class I and II will generally tolerate minor noncardiac surgery well and do not require invasive monitoring. In contrast, the peri- and postoperative management of patients in NYHA class III or IV undergoing major surgery will be facilitated by the use of invasive monitoring (arterial line, pulmonary artery catheter, and/or transesophageal echocardiography). In between these two poles lies the ever present "grey area" in which management is determined by clinical judgment. In theory, regional anesthesia by decreasing afterload may be of benefit. However, no study has conclusively demonstrated that the outcome of patients with CHF is influenced by anesthetic technique. An expertly conducted procedure is likely to be associated with a better outcome than an "anesthetic thrash," irrespective of the particular method chosen. Therefore, the old axiom of "when in doubt, stick to what you are familiar and comfortable with" is never more appropriate than with the high-risk patient.

The treatment, as well as the disease, may influence the patient's response to anesthesia. Patients with DCM will commonly be receiving several vasoactive agents, may be anticoagulated, and perhaps have a cardiac pacer. Diuretics will result in fluid and electrolyte disturbances. Most anesthetic agents are vasodilators (either directly or indirectly) and will produce hypotension in a patient who has been excessively diuresed. Angiotensin-convertase enzyme inhibitors have been associated with a greater sensitivity to the cardiovascular depressent effects of anesthetics and a decreased response to vasopressors. Amiodarone has been associated with isolated reports of perioperative atropine-resistant bradycardia, slow nodal rhythm, complete heart block, myocardial depression, increased requirements for perioperative circulatory support, and the acute respiratory distress syndrome. However, two recent studies found no difference in the rate of perioperative complications between patients treated with amiodarone and control patients.

In recent years it has been realized that it is the postoperative, rather than the intraoperative period that represents the most hazardous time for the high-risk patient. Major surgery imposes a greater sustained physiologic stress on patients than any aspect of their normal daily activity. Patients with poor physiologic reserve are unlikely to cope with this stress and are unlikely to have a rapid and event-free recovery. It is in the postoperative period that the team approach to maximize perfusion, support respiration and decrease respiratory work, and minimize further stressful stimuli, such as pain, is particularly important.

• HYPERTROPHIC CARDIOMYOPATHY (HCM)

Hypertrophic cardiomyopathy (HCM) is now the accepted term for, what in the past has been called, "hypertrophic obstructive cardiomyopathy," "asymmetric septal hypertrophy," and "muscular subaortic stenosis." There are no clear diagnostic criteria for HCM, which is believed by many to represent a spectrum of disease rather than a single entity. The diagnosis is commonly based on finding significant myocardial hypertrophy in the absence of an underlying cause, in the presence or absence of an outflow tract gradient. The prevalence of HCM is 19.7 cases per 100,000 population.

HCM is inherited as an autosomal-dominant condition with a high degree of penetrance. There is an association between HCM and pheochromocytoma and neurofibromatosis.

The Pathophysiology

In the past, pathological descriptions of HCM were dominated by the dynamics of the left ventricular outflow tract (LVOT) gradient. It is now understood that severe symptoms and sudden death may occur in the presence of a severe, mild, or absent LVOT gradient, and attention has focused upon the diastolic dysfunction present in HCM. Impaired diastolic filling is one of the paramount features of HCM and results from a combination of abnormal diastolic relaxation and increased chamber stiffness. Diastolic filling is especially dependent upon maintaining a normal sinus rhythm, and atrial contraction contributes up to 75% of LV filling in patients with

HCM. Diastolic dysfunction leads to increased diastolic pressures, pulmonary congestion, and dyspnea. Systolic function is usually normal or increased. Most patients have a normal-to-supernormal EF, with a pronounced increase in the speed and extent of ventricular emptying.

An LVOT gradient was emphasized in the original description of HCM by Brock in 1957. Although the occurrence of a true LVOT gradient in HCM has been questioned, Doppler studies have demonstrated that such a gradient does exist. What is clear, is that the severity of the LVOT obstruction is highly variable, not only between individuals but also in the same individual when examined at different times. This may explain why the LVOT gradient measured on a single occasion does not correlate with symptoms or prognosis.

Mitral regurgitation (MR) is common in patients with an LVOT gradient and correlates with the degree of obstruction. In HCM, unlike other situations, vasodilators will increase while vasoconstrictors decrease the severity of MR. Relief of the LVOT gradient by myomectomy usually cures the MR, and the need for mitral valve replacement is rare.

Thallium scintigraphy has demonstrated regional myocardial ischemia in the majority of patients with HCM. Coronary blood flow may be decreased by increased compressive forces from the hypertrophied myocardium, decreased coronary perfusion pressure secondary to the elevated LV end-diastolic pressure, and a decrease in aortic pressures secondary to LVOT obstruction. The coronary vasculature has also been found to be abnormal in HCM. Myocardial hypertrophy further increases the mismatch between oxygen supply and demand.

Arrhythmias are common in HCM. Ambulatory monitoring detects ventricular arrhythmias in up to 75% of patients with HCM: supraventricular arrhythmias in 25%, and atrial fibrillation (AF) in 10% of patients. Atrial fibrillation often produces clinical deterioration because of the dependence of diastolic filling on atrial systole. Rapid atrial tachycardias are seen in 50% of cases, often due to the presence of accessory conduction pathways, which are associated with HCM. Arrhythmias may be asymptomatic but can also result in syncope and are probably the main cause of sudden death.

The Natural History of HCM

This is highly variable. Annual mortality is 3% to 4% in patients younger than age 65. Very young children have a very poor prognosis; 30% experienced clinical deterioration and 30% died suddenly over a 7-year follow-up in one series. Young adults usually have severe hypertrophy and tend to follow a stable course but are prone to sudden death, particularly if there is a strong family history of an abrupt demise. Sudden death may occur after severe exertion but may also occur at rest. Arrhythmias, particularly ventricular, are believed to be the primary cause of sudden death. Elderly patients usually have mild or no symptoms until the sixth to seventh decade when they develop CHF and angina. In this age group, there appears to be a functional overlap between HCM and hypertensive hypertrophic cardiomyopathy. In both groups, symptoms develop secondary to diastolic dysfunction and/or outflow obstruction. They are exacerbated by afterload reduction and diuretics. The survival rate of patients in whom the diagnosis of HCM is made after age 65 is similar to that of an age- and sex-matched control group.

Other complications of HCM include infective endocarditis (5% of patients), embolic events (10% of patients), and CHF (10% of patients).

The Symptoms

These are typically nonspecific and include dyspnea, chest pain, and syncope. Symptoms usually appear in the second or third decade and increase with age. As stated previously, symptoms do not correlate with the LVOT gradient. Dyspnea occurs in up to 90% of patients and is believed to arise from the diastolic dysfunction. Angina is present in 75% of patients and evidence of a past MI is found in 15% of individuals at autopsy. Syncope occurs in 20%, but presyncopal symptoms are experienced in 50% of patients. Cardiac arrhythmias are the most likely cause of syncopal symptoms. Deterioration to CHF is uncommon and occurs in less than 7% of patients. A form of HCM has recently been described in elderly patients, usually in the sixth decade, in which CHF appears to be a prominent feature.

Given the vague, nonspecific nature of the symptoms, it is possible that patients previously undiagnosed with HCM may present for surgery.

The Physical Signs

The classic pulse waveform is a bisferiens pulse characterized by a rapid upstroke followed by a midsystolic drop, and, finally, a delayed slower wave. The pulse waveform distinguishes HCM from aortic valve stenosis (AS), in which there is a decrease in both the rate of rise and the amplitude of the pulse. The apical impulse is forceful, may be bifid (palpable S4), and is associated with a thrill in 40% of patients. Auscultation reveals a normal S1, usually preceeded by a loud S4, and a split S2. The outflow murmer is systolic, crescendo-decrescendo in nature, heard best at the left sternal border, and, in contrast to the murmur of AS, seldom radiates to the carotid. The murmur can be increased by factors that decrease LV volume and increase the outflow gradient, such as a Valsalva maneuver, amyl nitrate, and the upright position. The murmur is decreased by factors that increase LV volume such as squatting, leg raising in the supine position, or phenylephrine. An apical pansystolic murmur of MR is present in most patients.

The Laboratory Studies

The ECG is abnormal in the majority of cases of HCM. A normal axis is present in 60% of patients and a left axis in 30%. ECG findings of left ventricular hypertrophy are found in up to 80% of patients. Abnormal Q waves are common (25%), may appear in any lead system, and are believed to be caused by abnormal activation of the interventricular septum. Patients are usually in sinus rhythm but, as stated previously, continuous ECG monitoring reveals a high incidence of supraventricular and ventricular arrhythmias, which have prognostic implications. Twenty-five percent of patients with nonsustained VT die suddenly within 3 years. Conversely, the incidence of symptomatic arrhythmias is low in patients without VT on Holter monitoring. Annual Holter monitoring is recommended for all patients with HCM. Electrophysiologic testing has been used to stimulate arrhythmias in selected patients with HCM (previous cardiac arrest or syncope) but remains an investigational tool at present.

There is usually mild-to-moderate cardiomegaly on the chest x-ray (CXR) with signs of left atrial enlargement. The presence of aortic valve calcification or a dilated ascending aorta should raise the suspicion of aortic valve disease.

Echocardiography has now largely replaced cardiac catheterization in the diagnosis and pathophysiologic delineation of HCM. The classic echocardiographic features of HCM are asymmetric septal hypertrophy, decreased rate of septal thickening, systolic anterior motion of the mitral valve, and early systolic closure of the aortic valve (Fig. 8-2). However, the hypertrophy may involve the septum to a variable extent and may, in some cases, be concentric. Furthermore, asymmetric hypertrophy may occur in conditions other than HCM. Hypertrophy is most severe in the young patient and may progress in children up to puberty but does not appear to progress in adults. The degree of hypertrophy appears to correlate with the diastolic dysfunction, the presence of nonsustained ventricular tachycardia on Holter monitoring, and the risk of sudden death. An unusual ground-glass texture of the involved myocardium has been described but is not specific for HCM (it may be seen in cardiac amyloid and chronic renal failure).

Doppler echocardiography can provide valuable hemodynamic information as to the presence and severity of an LVOT gradient or mitral regurgitation. Pulsed-wave Doppler of the mitral flow velocities has been used to assess diastolic filling. Abnormal relaxation is reflected in a lower, initial velocity of the E wave, prolongation of the deceleration time, and a lower E:A ratio.

The echocardiographic features of HCM may be seen in severe left ventricular hypertrophy secondary to long-standing hypertension, infiltrative diseases such as cardiac amyloid and hemochromatosis, chronic renal failure requiring hemodialysis, and Friedreich's ataxia. HCM should be diagnosed with caution in patients with these conditions.

The Treatment of HCM

This is mainly medical and includes β-blockers, calcium channel blockers, and antiarrhythmics. β-blockers, usually in large doses (320 mg of propranolol per day), relieve symptoms in most cases but have not been shown to improve diastolic function. They have no proved benefit in decreasing the risk of sudden death and have not been shown to improve survival. Calcium channel blockers, of which verapamil has been the most studied, improve exercise tolerance and angina, improve diastolic function, and have been shown to decrease myocardial hypertrophy. The initial dose of verapamil is 80 mg 3 times per day, increasing to 240 mg 3 times per day as tolerated, until symptoms are relieved. Calcium channel blockers may produce a hemodynamic deterioration in some patients, particularly in those with a large, resting LVOT gradient, as a result of their vasodilating properties. It is for this reason that some cardiologists prefer β-blockers rather than calcium channel blockers as the treatment of choice in HCM.

No drug has been shown to be effective in the prevention of sudden death. Of the antiarrhythmics available, amiodarone has shown the greatest promise in the

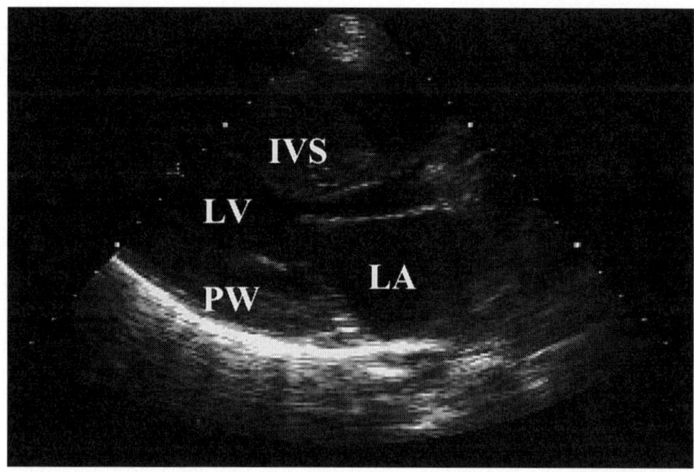

Figure 8-2
Two-dimensional echocardiogram in a patient with hypertrophic cardiomyopathy. This parasternal long-axis view shows concentric left ventricular hypertrophy, which is more marked in the interventricular septum (*IVS*) than the posterior left ventricular wall (*PW*), and slight left atrial (*LA*) enlargement.

abolition of both supraventricular and ventricular arrhythmias on Holter monitoring. In selected cases, electrophysiologic testing may be warranted. If the patient is found to be at high risk of arrhythmias, an automatic implantable defibrillator may be indicated.

In patients refractory to medical therapy, dual-chamber pacing has recently been shown to improve symptoms and hemodynamic function, decrease LVOT gradients, and cause regression of myocardial hypertrophy. The reduced gradient is thought to be caused by the abnormal septal motion induced by the right ventricular pacing.

Transaortic septal myectomy is the operation of choice in patients who have failed medical therapy. It has a mortality of 1.2% in patients younger than age 65. Myectomy relieves the outflow obstruction, improves diastolic function, significantly decreases MR, and usually produces a dramatic improvement in symptoms. Complications of myectomy include immediate or delayed complete heart block, left bundle branch branch block, ventricular septal defect, and septal aneurysms. Retrospective studies have shown an improved survival in surgically treated patients as compared to those who are medically treated. However, no randomized, prospective study has been performed to support this claim. Although mitral valve replacement has been proposed as an alternative to septal myectomy, current opinion is that this should only be performed if primary mitral valve disease and significant MR is present or if the septum is not thought to be sufficiently thickened to undergo myectomy.

Surgery in Patients with HCM

Patients with HCM may present for electrophysiologic testing, placement of an automatic implantable defibrillator, transaortic septal myectomy, as well as noncardiac surgery.

The aims of anesthetic management are to avoid exacerbating the outflow obstruction and maintain diastolic filling. The LVOT gradient is increased by both decreases in afterload and preload and by increases in myocardial contractility. Maintaining an adequate filling pressure is important and is best guided by monitoring of the CVP, pulmonary artery occlusion pressures (PAOP), or by TEE. Isolated measurements of CVP or PAOP will not provide an accurate guide to LV filling because of the abnormal LV compliance; however, repeat measurements will provide a useful trend. While some monitoring of preload appears ideal, in a recent series of patients with HCM undergoing surgery, 51% had no intravascular monitoring and pulmonary artery catheters were inserted in only 18% of patients. However, perioperative CHF occurred in 16% of patients, which underscores the importance of diastolic dysfunction in this disease. Focusing on the LVOT gradient and aggressively providing fluid support to avoid hypotension may well precipitate CHF if preload is not carefully monitored. Hypotension should be treated with Trendelenburg position, fluids, and vasopressors rather than inotropes. Atrial arrhythmias requiring treatment were the most common perioperative complication in one study. They are poorly tolerated in HCM and should be treated promptly with cardioversion.

Halothane has become the agent of choice for anesthetic maintenance. Animal studies have suggested that halothane should be used with caution in patients receiving verapamil, as the combination may produce conduction disturbances and markedly depressed cardiac function.

Regional techniques have been described in HCM. Providing hypotension is avoided by the judicious use of vasopressors and fluids, such techniques are not contraindicated if the patient may otherwise benefit from avoiding a general anesthetic.

• RESTRICTIVE CARDIOMYOPATHY (RCM)

This is the rarest and the least well defined of the cardiomyopathies. The recognition of RCM as a distinct disease category arose from the identification of certain patients with the clinical and hemodynamic abnormalities of constrictive pericarditis (CP) but without pericardial disease. In 1980, the WHO defined primary RCM to include only the eosinophilic endomyocardial diseases (EED), all other cases being secondary to a separate disease process. Currently, it is understood that a separate idiopathic form of RCM does exist, and EED now falls into the specific heart muscle disease category, which also includes amyloid, hemochromatosis, carcinoid syndrome, progressive systemic sclerosis, postradiation, doxorubicin and daunorubicin cardiotoxicity, and post–heart transplantation.

The Pathophysiology

The primary abnormality in RCM is abnormal diastolic ventricular filling. Early diastolic filling is rapid but abruptly ceases, resulting in a fixed limitation to end-diastolic volumes, identical to that which occurs with CP. Systolic function is preserved, but cardiac output is limited by the fixed stroke volume and is dependent upon an adequate heart rate and preload (to maintain diastolic filling). Coronary artery disease is usually absent in RCM. Mural thrombi and embolic events are uncommon in RCM but are prominent features of EED. Atrial fibrillation has been noted in 50% of patients and is presumably a consequence of the atrial enlargement produced by the chronically elevated filling pressures and/or AV valve incompetence.

It is now realized that the diastolic filling abnormality does not always correspond to such a strict description. As a consequence, many workers now use a broader definition of RCM to include a spectrum of conditions with decreased diastolic compliance of unknown cause, that is, in the absence of such known causes such as severe ventricular hypertrophy, systolic dysfunction, or pericardial disease. RCM is, therefore, a diagnosis of exclusion.

The Natural History of RCM

The progress of EED is usually one of progressive cardiac dysfunction with a 10-year survival of 25%. However, the clinical course is variable, with some patients manifesting minimal symptoms for many years while others undergo a relentless downhill course secondary to increasing diastolic dysfunction, obliteration of the ventricular cavities, and AV valve insufficiency. The prognosis appears to be worse in children than in adults.

The Symptoms

Fatigue and dyspnea are symptoms of both RCM and CP. However, chest pain tends to be a feature of RCM. Patients may have the history, symptoms, or stigmata of the specific heart muscle diseases (as previously mentioned), or a history of pericarditis, which would obviously favor a diagnosis of CP.

The Signs

These are nearly identical to those of CP, namely, jugular venous distension with a prominent Y descent, peripheral edema, and ascites in the absence of cardiomegaly. Pulmonary congestion, a third heart sound, and murmurs of AV valve incompetence favor a diagnosis of RCM.

The Laboratory Studies

Most of these are directed towards excluding CP. Electrocardiogram findings are usually nonspecific but may include conduction abnormalities, ST-T wave abnormalities, and AF. The chest radiograph may show pulmonary congestion while heart size is normal or mildly increased. Pericardial calcification suggests a diagnosis of CP. Certain echocardiography features may allow RCM and CP to be distinguished. Pericardial thickening (hard to appreciate with echocardiography), a pericardial effusion, and increased variation of flow across the mitral valve with respiration are associated with CP but not RCM. Computed tomography and magnetic resonance imaging are both accurate in identifying pericardial thickness and calcification. Cardiac catheterization reveals elevated right heart pressures with the prominent Y descent and the classical dip-plateau waveform of ventricular diastolic pressures in both CP and RCM. The dip is caused by the rapid, early diastolic relaxation and is associated with the rapid, early diastolic filling, whereas the plateau results from the abrupt cessation of diastolic filling.

Surgery in Patients with RCM

Endocardiectomy and valve replacement has produced symptomatic improvement with an 80% survival at 4 years. However, cardiac transplantation is frequently the only option, particularly for young patients.

As in HCM, cardiac output is dependent upon adequate preload and heart rate. Agents or techniques that decrease these two factors should be avoided and monitoring of PAOP is recommended, particularly if the surgery is associated with hemodynamic fluctuations and fluid shifts. Unlike HCM, cardiac output is also dependent upon cardiac contractility, cardiac depressent agents should be avoided and inotropes may be needed to support the patient through the perioperative period.

BIBLIOGRAPHY

Goldman L: Multifactorial index of cardiac risk in non-cardiac surgery: ten-year status report, *J Cardiothorac Vasc Anesth* 1(3):237–244, 1987.

Guidelines for peri-operative cardiovascular evaluation for non-cardiac surgery. Report of the American College of Cardiology/American Heart Association Task Force on Practice Guidelines, *Circulation* 93:1278–1317, 1996.

Kaplan JA: Cardiac anesthesia, ed 3, Philadelphia, 1993, WB Saunders.

Licker M, et al: Long-term angiotensin-convertase enzyme inhibitor treatment attenuates adrenergic responsiveness without altering hemodynamic control in patients undergoing cardiac surgery, *Anesthesiology* 84(4):789–800, 1996.

Ramahi TM, Forrester AL: Medical therapy and prognosis in chronic heart failure: lessons from clinical trials, *Cardiol Clin* 13(1):5–26, Feb. 1995.

Wigle ED, et al: Hypertrophic cardiomyopathy: clinical spectrum and treatment, *Circulation* 92:1680–1692, 1995.

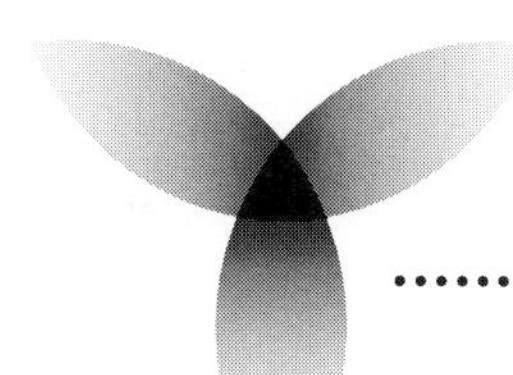

Chapter 9

Arrhythmias and Disturbances of Conduction

Stuart M. Lowson, MBBS, FRCA, MRCP, Jonathan R. Lindner, MD

Arrhythmias are the most commonly reported perioperative complication, occurring in 60% to 80% of surgical patients monitored with continuous electrocardiographic recordings. Fortunately, most of these are not clinically significant, the incidence of clinically significant arrhythmias being approximately 1%. Disturbances of heart rhythm or conduction may manifest in different ways. Patients may present with a preoperative history of arrhythmias, which may be either permanent or paroxysmal. Alternatively, arrhythmias and conduction disturbances may present for the first time in the perioperative period. Whether the arrhythmia is supraventricular or ventricular in origin, the operative team needs to be aware of the likely cause of the arrhythmia, especially the presence of underlying heart disease, precipitating factors, the history of the arrhythmia (its frequency and hemodynamic consequences), and measures used to treat both acute episodes and prevent recurrence. The chapter begins with a general overview of the perioperative considerations that apply to any patient with a history of arrhythmias. The nature and prevalence of any underlying heart disease and the possible treatment(s) patients may be receiving varies and is addressed in the sections describing the specific arrhythmias. Also included in the specific sections are the recommended treatments should the arrhythmia occur in the perioperative period.

General Perioperative Considerations

Planning the perioperative management for any patient with a history of arrhythmias requires the patient's past cardiac history. The following questions must be asked: If the arrhythmia is paroxysmal how frequently does it recur and what are the hemodynamic consequences? How has the arrhythmia been treated? Has treatment been accomplished with one drug or has it required multiple attempts and combination therapy? Questions concerning the patient's drug history are essential. What antiarrhythmic drugs is the patient presently receiving and what are their side effects and drug interactions (see Box 9-1)? Which drugs have proved to be effective or ineffective? If the arrhythmia recurs during surgery how should this be treated?

Preoperative drug levels may be useful but should be viewed in the context of the patient's clinical status. This applies particularly to digoxin levels. A high digoxin level supports a diagnosis of toxicity, whereas a low level may indicate inadequate dosing. Intermediate digoxin levels, however, have a poor correlation with clinical effect and cannot be used to "fine tune" therapy. In addition to the prescribed medications, the patient should be questioned as to the use of "social drugs," particularly tobacco, alcohol, caffeine, and both illegal and "over the counter" substances, all of which are either associated with an increased risk of heart disease or are directly arrhythmogenic.

It is the foundation of perioperative care that patients should present for surgery in the best possible medical condition. Therefore, medical problems that may precipitate or exacerbate an arrhythmia should be addressed. The significance of any preexisting coronary artery or valvular heart disease should be assessed and managed in an appropriate manner (see the chapters describing these conditions). The patient's volume status should be optimized, respiratory disorders and blood gases treated, and endocrine (thyroid status), electrolyte abnormalities (particularly hypokalemia and hypomagnesemia), and drug effects (digitalis toxicity, alcohol, sympathomimetic stimulants) corrected.

All patients with a history of arrhythmias, palpitations, syncope, chest pain, or congestive heart failure (CHF) should have a preoperative electrocardiogram (ECG), which may reveal underlying heart disease (coronary or congenital heart disease), proarrhythmic conditions (long QT interval, Wolff-Parkinson-White syndrome), electrolyte disorders, and drug effects (digitalis toxicity). Occasionally, prolonged rhythm strips or 24-hour Holter monitoring may be used to document the arrhythmia or conduction disturbance. More sophisticated methods to determine arrhythmic risk may be used in patients with recurrent ventricular tachycardia, particularly post–myocardial infarction.

The sympathetic nervous system plays an important role in the induction and exacerbation of the "tachycardias." The perioperative period is associated with heightened sympathetic activity and it is, therefore, not surprising that arrhythmias are a frequent complication of surgery and anesthesia, in particular the more "stressful" procedures, e.g., cardiothoracic surgery. It is logical to select an anesthetic technique that avoids further stimulation of the sympathetic nervous system, and reduces the sympathetic response to known stimulating procedures (intubation, skin incision, sternotomy). This is sound anesthetic practice with any patient, but is particularly appropriate if there is a risk of precipitating a clinically significant arrhythmia. The anesthetic plan should include a suitable calming premedicant individualized to the patient's age, size, anxiety level, and medical condition. While no one anesthetic technique has been clearly shown to be superior, certain anesthetics may be better than others in a patient with arrhythmias. The volatile anesthetics, and halothane in particular, reduce the amount of epinephrine required to produce ventricular arrhythmias, depress the sinoatrial (SA) node and prolong atrioventricular (AV) conduction. AV dissociation with a junctional pacemaker is frequently seen with halothane. Opiates are noted for their hemodynamic stability and have been shown to increase the threshold for ventricular fibrillation. Bradycardia is a common finding when high doses of opiates are given, but is rarely a problem and may be beneficial.

The postoperative period is associated with the highest frequency of cardiac complications and "at risk" patients require constant care and vigilance during this time. Good quality pain control and attention to the patient's cardiorespiratory and electrolyte status is vital. The level of postoperative monitoring is determined by the perceived level of risk and may vary from an intensive-care-unit bed to continuous, bedside ECG monitoring on the floor, to discharge home, depending upon the patient's medical condition and the type of surgery performed.

The management of individual arrhythmias and conduction disturbances are described in more detail in the following.

THE SUPRAVENTRICULAR TACHYCARDIAS

General Considerations

In recent years there has been a rapid growth in our understanding of the origin and the mechanisms underlying the supraventricular tachycardias (SVTs). Electrophysiologic mapping of the cardiac conduction system has provided greater insight into the way the electrical impulse is generated and conducted through the heart, in both normal and diseased states. This has further provided the impetus to develop new

Box 9-1 Side Effects of Antiarrhythmic Agents

CLASS 1A

Quinidine.

Cardiac: Vagolytic effect, which may increase the baseline heart rate and the ventricular rate in the presence of AF or A-flutter (pretreat with AV blockers), QT prolongation (above). Quinidine may also cause hypotension.

Noncardiac: Gastrointestinal (nausea, vomiting, and diarrhea producing dehydration), central nervous system (tinnitus, hearing loss, visual disturbances, delerium, and psychosis), thrombocytopenia.

Procainamide.

Cardiac: Vagolytic effect that can increase the ventricular rate in the presence of AF or A-flutter, QT prolongation (above).

Noncardiac: Lupuslike syndrome (arthralgia, fever, pleuropericarditis, pericardial effusions, vasculitis, and Raynaud's phenomenon but brain and kidney spared), agranulocytosis, central nervous system (giddiness, psychosis, and hallucinations).

Disopyramide.

Cardiac: Myocardial depression (particularly in the presence of preexisting LV dysfunction), QT prolongation.

Noncardiac: Urinary retention, blurred vision, and dry mouth due to its anticholinergic effects.

CLASS 1B

Lidocaine.

Cardiac: May enhance conduction over an accessory pathway in a small percentage (<5%) of patients with preexcitation.

Noncardiac: Central nervous system (dizziness, paresthesias, confusion, seizures, coma).

Mexiletine.

Cardiac: Hypotension, bradycardia (both usually after IV dosing).

Noncardiac: Central nervous system effects (tremor, dysarthria, diplopia, anxiety, confusion, and nausea), nausea and vomiting common.

Tocainide.

Cardiac: As for lidocaine.

Noncardiac: Central nervous system (as for lidocaine), nausea and vomiting common, pulmonary fibrosis, hematologic disorders (agranulocytosis, anemia, thrombocytopenia).

CLASS 1C

Flecainide.

Cardiac: May increase the ventricular rate in the presence of AF, marked slowing of cardiac conduction, proarrhythmic effects, myocardial depression, increased mortality when given to patients after myocardial infarction.

Noncardiac: Frequent central nervous system effects (dizziness, visual disturbances).

Propafenone.

Cardiac: Conduction abnormalities (AV block, sinus node depression), myocardial depression.

Noncardiac: Central nervous system (dizziness, headache), exacerbation of bronchospasm (due to its β-blocking activity), cholestatic jaundice (rare).

Box 9-1 *Continued*

CLASS II (β-ADRENERGIC BLOCKERS)
Cardiac: Interact with anesthetic agents to produce hypotension and bradycardia, blocks sympathetic response to hypovolemia, myocardial depression, AV block, withdrawal syndrome if suddenly stopped (angina, arrhythmias), exacerbation of peripheral vascular disease.
Noncardiac: Exacerbation of bronchospasm, increased risk of hypoglycemia in diabetics, insomnia, fatigue.

CLASS III
Amiodarone.
Cardiac: Hypotension and bradycardia (particularly after IV administration), myocardial depression (mild compared to other agents), QT prolongation (this does not appear to be a significant problem with amiodarone).
Noncardiac: Pulmonary toxicity (pulmonary alveolitis [fever, dyspnea, cough]), one report of postoperative acute respiratory distress syndrome, hypo- and hyperthyroidism, elevated liver enzymes, neuropathy, corneal deposits, drug interactions (increases digoxin levels).
Sotalol.
Cardiac: Proarrhythmias, QT prolongation (precipitation of torsades de pointes), side effects of β-blockers (sotalol has β-blocking activity).
Noncardiac: As for β-blockers.

CLASS IV (VERAPAMIL AND DILTIAZEM)
Cardiac: Hypotension, bradycardia, AV block (particularly if the patient is already receiving β-blockers), myocardial depression, enhances conduction over accessory pathways (may increase the ventricular rate in patients with the Wolf-Parkinson-White syndrome and AF), hemodynamic collapse when given to patients with the common form of VT, increased digoxin levels.
Digoxin.
Cardiac: Disturbances of impulse formation and conduction (in decreasing order of frequency these are VPCs, second- and third-degree heart block, AV junctional tachycardia, atrial tachycardia with block [Fig. 9-1], VT, and sinoatrial block), accelerated conduction over accessory pathways.
Noncardiac: Multiple drug interactions (digoxin levels increased with amiodarone, quinidine, propafenone, verapamil, erythromycin, teracycline, omeprazole, cyclosporine, levels decreased with antacids, cholestyramine, bran, albuterol), gastrointestinal (nausea, vomiting), central nervous system (lethargy, agitation, visual disturbances), thrombocytopenia (rare).

therapeutic techniques to treat the SVTs, a field that truly represents one of the fastest growing areas of cardiology today. It is clear that our ability to provide appropriate therapy for an arrhythmia is determined by our ability to make the correct diagnosis. A general overview of the SVTs is, therefore, first provided to aid in the differentiation of the individual arrhythmias.

The SVTs can be divided into those tachycardias originating above the AV node (sinus tachycardia, unifocal and multifocal atrial tachycardia, atrial fibrillation [AF], and atrial flutter) and those in which the AV node comprises an integral part of the abnormal circuitry (AV nodal reentry and AV reciprocating tachycardia). All arrhythmias can be further divided according to their mechanism of origin: automatic, reentry, or triggered. Briefly, an automatic focus is an area of excitable myocardium capable of spontaneous depolarizations at a rate faster than the normal sinus rate. Reentry refers to the mechanism whereby a circular circuit is generated as a result of conduction down more than one pathway possessing different conduction velocities and refractory periods. Triggered activity is caused by membrane depolarizations that occur during or following an action potential (afterdepolarizations). Most SVTs arise from automatic foci or reentrant circuits. These classifications into the mechanism and site of origin may provide important clues to the diagnosis of the individual SVTs.

Key factors in the diagnosis of an SVT are the age of the patient, the medical history (particularly cardiac disorders), the characteristics of the SVT (onset and offset), the duration of the tachycardia and, importantly, certain ECG features. Misdiagnosis of the individual SVTs are common. Features that may help to diagnose a specific SVT are listed in Box 9-2. Distinguishing between an SVT or a ventricular tachycardia (VT) may be difficult. VT is, by far, the most common cause of a wide QRS complex tachycardia, particularly if the patient has had a previous myocardial infarction. Thus, if in doubt, think and treat VT. Electrocardiographic features that may help distinguish an SVT from VT are listed in Box 9-3.

• INDIVIDUAL SUPRAVENTRICULAR ARRHYTHMIAS

Premature Atrial Contractions (PAC)

Premature atrial contractions may originate from any of the supraventricular structures (sinus node or atrial tissue). A PAC is diagnosed on the ECG by the presence of a premature P wave, whose configuration is usually different from the sinus beat, with a PR interval exceeding 120 msec (Fig. 9-1). The P wave is usually best seen in leads V_1 or II, but may be difficult to visualize if buried in the preceeding T wave. The QRS complex is usually identical to the sinus beat but may be different due to aberrant conduction. Unlike ventricular premature complexes, there is no compensatory pause after a PAC as the atrial reset to the baseline sinus rate.

PERIOPERATIVE CONSIDERATIONS

Premature atrial complexes can be triggered by a number of disorders including myocardial ischemia, valvular heart disease, systemic or local infections and inflammation, electrolyte and acid-base abnormalities, anxiety, "social" drugs (tobacco, alcohol, caffeine), surgical manipulation, and central line insertion.

Although Goldman identified PACs on the preoperative ECG as an indicator of perioperative cardiac events, PACs usually do not require treatment unless they serve as the trigger for an SVT. The significance of PACs is that frequently they mark

Box 9-2 Features that Help to Identify a Specific SVT

1. Is a P wave or F (flutter) wave visible? If not, this suggests AF, with an irregular RR interval, or AVNRT, with a regular RR interval. In the most common form of AVNRT an inverted P wave occurs in leads II, III, and AVF, but this is usually buried in the QRS complex. If the P wave morphology and PR interval during the tachycardia is different from that in sinus rhythm, this suggests atrial tachycardia. If a P wave is not visible on the surface ECG, then it may be detected by esophageal leads, using the "saline bridge" of a central venous catheter (or the right atrial port of a pulmonary artery catheter), or by using epicardial electrodes. Epicardial recordings are obtained by connecting the atrial wire of the temporary pacing electrode (commonly placed after cardiac surgery) to a standard ECG. Leads II or III will provide a unipolar atrial electrogram of both atrial and ventricular activity.
2. Are the RR intervals irregular? Irregularity suggests AF, multifocal atrial tachycardia, or atrial flutter with variable AV nodal block. A regular RR interval suggests sinus tachycardia, atrial flutter, AV nodal reentrant tachycardia (AVNRT), or AV reciprocating tachycardia (AVRT).
3. Ventricular rate; a rate of approximately 150 beats per minute suggests atrial flutter with 2:1 AV block. A rate greater than 200 beats per minute in an adult suggests an accessory pathway.
4. The presence of AV block excludes the participation of the AV node in the abnormal circuit and, therefore, excludes AVNRT and AVRT.
5. Examination of the ECG in sinus rhythm may demonstrate preexcitation (see below).
6. Rhythms that abruptly start and stop with premature beats suggest reentry (AVNRT, AVRT, AF, atrial flutter), whereas a gradual change in rate suggests sinus tachycardia.
7. Is electrical alternans present? This refers to sustained differences in the amplitudes of the QRS complex (>1mm). This is said to be diagnostic of a concealed accessory pathway; however, some authors feel it is simply a rapid rate-related phenomenon.
8. Do vagal maneuvers (carotid sinus massage or Valsalva) slow or terminate the tachycardia? If the answer is yes, then this suggests that the AV node participates in the abnormal circuit, i.e., AVNRT or AVRT. If vagal maneuvers produce AV block but do not terminate the tachycardia, then this points to an origin above the AV node, i.e., sinus tachycardia, AF, atrial flutter, or atrial tachycardia. Vagal maneuvers may, however, slow the ventricular response to atrial flutter and allow the flutter waves to be identified. Unfortunately, many patients who experience these tachycardias in the acute setting are stressed, in a parasympatholytic state, and are unresponsive to vagal maneuvers.
9. What is the response to adenosine? If adenosine abruptly stops the tachycardia then it originated from a reentrant circuit involving the sinoatrial (SA) or AV node. Adenosine will convert over 95% of such tachycardias, i.e., AVNRT, and sinus node reentrant tachycardia. If the adenosine-induced AV block slows but does not terminate the tachycardia, this suggests that it originates from a site of automacity, i.e., atrial tachycardia, or from a reentrant circuit that does not involve the SA or AV node, i.e., AF or atrial flutter.

Box 9-3 Features that Help Distinguish an SVT from VT

FAVORS AN SVT:

1. Narrow QRS complex (<140 msec).
2. Slowing or termination by vagal maneuvers.
3. Onset with a premature P wave.
4. Linkage of the P wave and QRS suggest that the ventricle is being discharged by a supraventricular source.
5. Initial vector of the QRS similar to that of a sinus beat.
6. RP interval <100 msec.

FAVORS VT:

1. Fusion beats and capture beats indicate that the ventricle has been activated by two different foci which implies that one of the foci was from the ventricle.
2. AV dissociation is strong evidence of a VT. However, retrograde VA conduction may occur with VT, in which case atrial and ventricular activity will be associated.
3. Left axis deviation (–60° to –120°) or superior axis.
4. QRS duration >140 msec, with a QRS of normal duration during sinus rhythm.

an underlying disorder, which should be the focus of therapeutic measures, i.e., myocardial ischemia, electrolyte disorders, or hypoxia.

Sinus-Node Reentrant Tachycardia

This uncommon SVT (less than 10% of SVTs) originates from a reentrant circuit incorporating the sinus node. The P wave is identical to that of the sinus beat but, unlike sinus tachycardia, sinus-node reentry begins and ends abruptly, a feature common to all reentrant tachycardias. The tachycardia is often precipitated by a PAC. The rate is usually 130 beats per minute (range 100 to 160 beats per minute).

PERIOPERATIVE CONSIDERATIONS

Patients with previous surgical trauma to the right atrium (prior atrial cannulaton or repair of congenital heart disease) seem to be predisposed to this arrhythmia. If the arrhythmia occurs perioperatively and does not cause any hemodynamic problems, then the patient may simply be observed as the arrhythmia often terminates spontaneously. If treatment is considered necessary then vagal maneuvers, adenosine, β-blockers or a calcium channel blocker (CCB) should be tried in that order.

Atrial Tachycardia (AT)

Atrial tachycardia (AT) may arise from an automatic focus, reentry, or triggered activity. Opinions differ as to the relative importance of each of these three mechanisms. Unifocal AT is present in fewer than 15% of patients with symptomatic SVTs. The atrial rate is usually 150 to 200 beats per minute (which helps distinguish AT from atrial flutter). The P wave usually preceeds the QRS and has a different morphology from that of the sinus P wave (Fig. 9-2). The atrial rate may be regular or

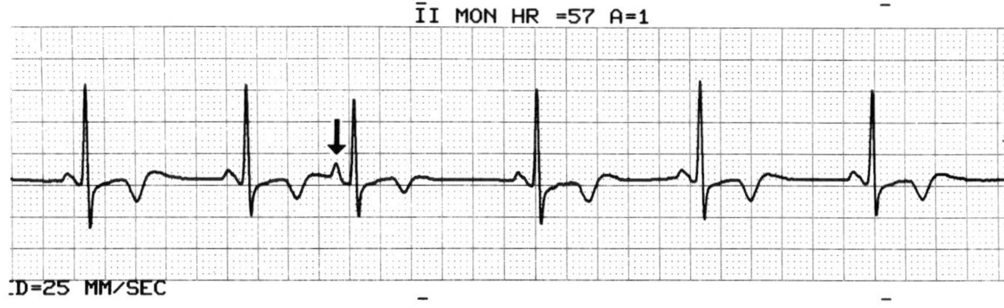

Figure 9-1
Premature atrial complex (PAC). The third complex in the recording occurs early and is identified as a PAC by the presence of a narrow QRS complex preceded by a P wave morphology (**arrow**) and PR interval that is different from that found during normal sinus rhythm.

irregular (particularly during the onset of the tachycardia). Vagal maneuvers and adenosine may produce AV block but do not usually stop AT.

PERIOPERATIVE CONSIDERATIONS

Atrial tachycardia occurs most commonly in patients with ischemic or structural heart disease, chronic lung disease, hypoxia, after acute alcohol intoxication, and, importantly, with digitalis intoxication. Atrial tachycardia, with either Mobitz type 1 or type 2 AV block, is frequently seen with digitalis toxicity (usually, premature ventricular complexes are also present).

The first goal of the management of AT is the correction of precipitating factors (above). If digitalis toxicity is present, hypokalemia and hypomagnasemia should be treated. Frequently, the ventricular rate is not excessive and AT will respond to simply withholding the cardiac glycoside. In a patient not receiving digitalis, the ventricular rate may be slowed with digoxin, CCBs, or β-blockers. Cardioversion (begin at a 100 J) may also be used if the patient is hemodynamically compromised and should be successful if the AT arises from a reentrant circuit. If AT persists, procainamide (15 mg/kg IV at a rate not greater than 20 mg/min) is the recommended treatment although other class IA, IC, and III agents have also been tried. Atrial tachycardia may be difficult to abolish with antiarrhythmic drugs and, often, control of the ventricular response must be accepted as the best possible treatment option.

Multifocal Atrial Tachycardia (MAT)

The origin of this tachycardia (also called chaotic atrial rhythm) is from multiple automatic sites within the atria. The diagnosis of MAT is based on the presence of three or more different morphologic patterns of P waves on the ECG, an isoelectric baseline between the P waves, and an irregular atrial rate of 100 beats per minute or greater. Because of the irregular ventricular response, MAT is frequently misdiagnosed as atrial fibrillation (Fig. 9-3). It has a reported incidence of 0.3% in hospitalized patients and predominantly occurs in the acutely ill.

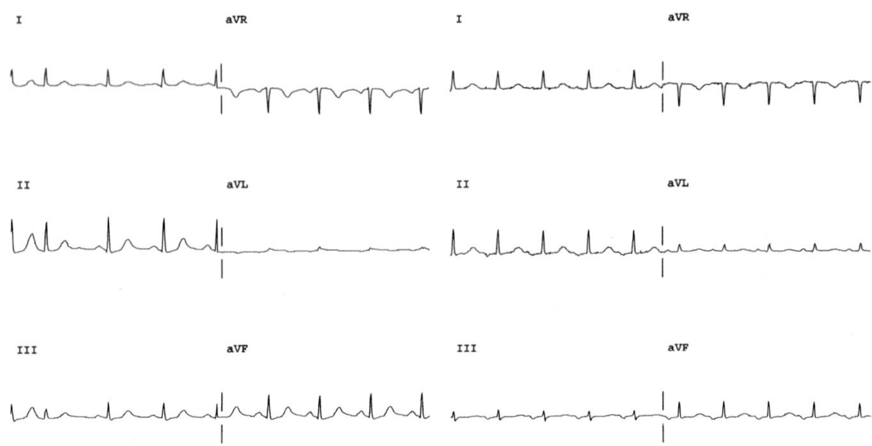

Figure 9-2

Atrial tachycardia. Limb lead recordings from a single patient during sinus rhythm (**left panel**) and after paroxysmal initiation of an atrial tachycardia (**right panel**). The patient's heart rate abruptly increased and, during the tachycardia, a different P wave morphology and PR interval are found, indicating an atrial focus other than the sinoatrial node.

PERIOPERATIVE CONSIDERATIONS

Multifocal atrial tachycardia is classically encountered in patients with severe chronic lung disease (60% of patients with MAT) or congestive heart failure who are hypoxic, hypercarbic, acidotic, and have increased levels of endogenous catecholamines. Hypoxia is the most common cause of MAT and should be immediately corrected.

The primary goal of the management of MAT is the correction of the underlying disease and its complications. Hypoxia, hypercarbia, hypokalemia, and hypomagnesemia should be identified and corrected. If the MAT requires treatment, β-blockers or CCBs are the first line of therapy but are often ineffective. β-blockers (metoprolol) have been used to treat patients with chronic obstructive pulmonary disease (COPD) and MAT without compromising the patient's respiratory status. Verapamil may slow ventricular rate but may worsen the hypoxia in patients with COPD by inhibiting hypoxic pulmonary vasoconstriction. Cardioversion is seldom effective in MAT.

Atrioventricular Nodal Reentrant Tachycardia (AVNRT)

This is the second most common cause of an SVT after atrial fibrillation, and is the most common cause of a paroxysmal **regular** SVT. Atrioventricular nodal tachycardia is usually a narrow complex regular tachycardia, with a sudden onset and termination, and a rate of between 130 and 250 beats per minute (commonly 180 to 200 beats per minute in adults). However, aberrant conduction may occur, particularly in the elderly, and be difficult to distinguish from VT.

Electrophysiologic studies have demonstrated two functionally distinct pathways in the AV node in patients with AVNRT: a slow pathway (slow conduction, short

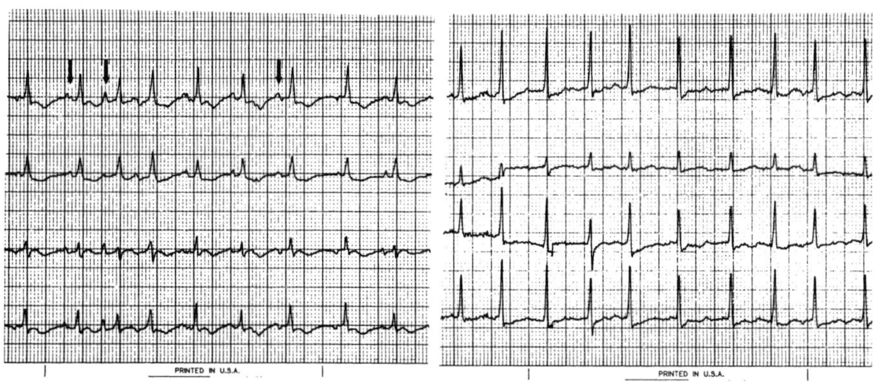

Figure 9-3
Although both recordings represent narrow complex tachycardias, multifocal atrial tachycardia (**left panel**) can be distinguished from atrial fibrillation (**right panel**) by the presence of at least three different P wave morphologies (**arrows**). During atrial fibrillation, distinct P waves are absent and a fine, undulating baseline is observed.

refractory period) and a fast pathway (fast conduction, long refractory period). In sinus rhythm the impulse is conducted down the fast pathway and usually produces a normal PR interval in the baseline ECG. Commonly, the tachycardia is precipitated by a PAC that is blocked in the fast pathway and conducts anterograde in the slow pathway (Fig. 9-4). If conduction in the slow pathway is slow enough that the fast pathway has time to recover, then the impulse is conducted retrograde up this latter route, thereby completing the reentrant circuit. Since retrograde conduction to the atria is rapid, the P waves are usually obscured by the QRS on the ECG. If visible, the P waves are negative in leads II, III, and aVf. In approximately 10% of cases of AVNRT the reentrant circuit is reversed with anterograde conduction down the fast pathway and retrograde conduction back up the slow pathway. In this form of AVNRT, imaginatively referred to as "uncommon AVNRT," the P waves still appear negative in leads II, III, and aVf but are delayed, with a long PR interval, and appear just before the next QRS complex.

PERIOPERATIVE CONSIDERATIONS

Atrioventricular nodal reentrant tachycardia is seldom associated with underlying heart disease and may occur at any age, most commonly in the fourth or fifth decade of life. Seventy percent of patients with AVNRT are women. Symptoms are common and range from the sensation of palpitations and nervousness to angina, CHF, syncope, or shock depending upon the ventricular rate and the presence of underlying heart disease. The prognosis for patients without heart disease is good.

Patients with recurrent AVNRT may or may not be receiving antiarrhythmic drugs. Treatment may not be needed if the episodes are infrequent, of short duration, and cause minimal symptoms. If treatment is required, CCBs are the most popular agents

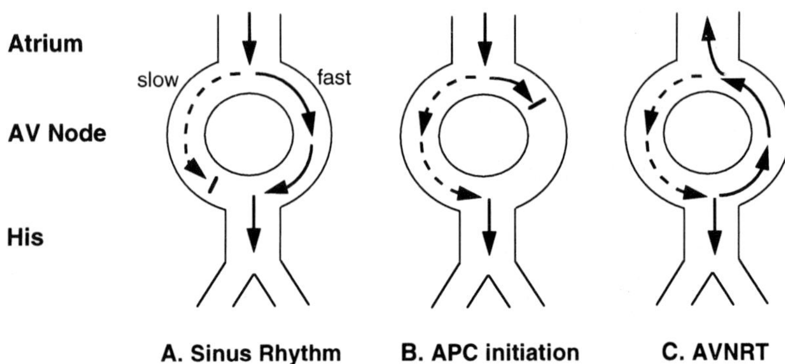

Figure 9-4
Schematic representation of the generation of atrioventricular nodal reentrant tachycardia (AVNRT). **A.** During normal sinus rhythm, although dual AV nodal pathways are present, conduction to the His bundle occurs primarily via the fast pathway. **B.** Because of variable refractoriness of the two AV nodal pathways, a premature atrial complex may be blocked in the fast pathway, yet conducted down the slow pathway. **C.** Recovery of the fast pathway during impulse propagation down the slow pathway, allows retrograde conduction and a reentrant circuit is formed.

although their superiority over digoxin or β-blockers has not been demonstrated. In patients who do not respond to or do not tolerate AV blockers, the choice is between a class IA (procainamide), IC (flecainide, propafenone), or III (amiodarone, sotalol) agent. Radiofrequency (RF) catheter ablation can cure patients of their AVNRT and may offer the best option for long-term control of AVNRT. Either the fast or slow pathway can be ablated with success rates of 90%. In 5% to 10% of cases, AVNRT recurs, requiring a second ablation. The incidence of complete heart block after RF ablation has been recently reported as 1.2%.

If AVNRT occurs perioperatively then vagal maneuvers are the first line of therapy and frequently terminate the tachycardia. Adenosine (6–12 mg given rapidly IV) is the initial drug of choice and is effective in over 90% of cases of AVNRT. Adenosine's effects are apparent within 15–30 seconds. Transient side effects such as facial flushing, chest pain, and dyspnea are common. Adenosine-induced bronchospasm in patients with reactive airways remains a theoretical, but undocumented, problem. Although adenosine is effective in terminating AVNRT, it does not prevent recurrence of the arrhythmia. Verapamil (75 μg/kg, 5–15 mg IV in an adult) or diltiazem (0.25–0.35 mg/kg IV) terminates AVNRT in approximately 2 minutes in 90% of cases, and are given if vagal maneuvers and adenosine fail. An IV bolus of a CCB may produce hypotension, which can be treated with an IV bolus of calcium; this does not affect the drug's electrophysiologic effects. A β-blocker may also be given, either esmolol (slow IV bolus of 0.5 mg/kg followed, if necessary, by an IV infusion of up to 250 μg/kg/min, titrating to ventricular rate), metoprolol (5–15 mg IV), or propanolol (0.25–0.5 mg IV titrated to effect or until a total dose of 0.2 mg/kg is given).

Patients with Accessory AV Pathways

An accessory pathway is an abnormal band of conducting tissue connecting the atria and ventricles that is separate from the AV node. Most accessory pathways are capable of conducting in both an anterograde and retrograde direction. Anterograde conduction of the sinus impulse down the accessory pathway, results in preexcitation of the ventricle and the combination of a short PR interval (<120 msec) and delta wave, the ECG signature of the Wolff-Parkinson-White (WPW) syndrome (Fig. 9-5).

The most common arrhythmia in patients with an accessory pathway are orthodromic atrioventricular reciprocating tachycardia (AVRT) (80%), followed by AF (15% to 30%), and atrial flutter (5%). Because the impulse travels anterograde down the AV node and retrograde up the bypass tract, no delta wave is seen during orthodromic AVRT. The ECG appearance of AVRT is similar to that of AVNRT, except that it is frequently associated with a retrograde P wave visible in the ST segment. In 10% of patients with WPW and AVRT the impulse is conducted anterogradely down the bypass tract, producing a wide QRS complex with a delta wave. Approximately 25% of accessory pathways are only capable of retrograde conduction. They are still capable of contributing to an orthodromic reentrant circuit but show no evidence of their presence on the ECG: so called "concealed bypass tracts." Orthodromic AVRT caused by a concealed accessory pathway is the third most common SVT after AF and AVNRT. Approximately 30% of patients referred for electrophysiologic studies

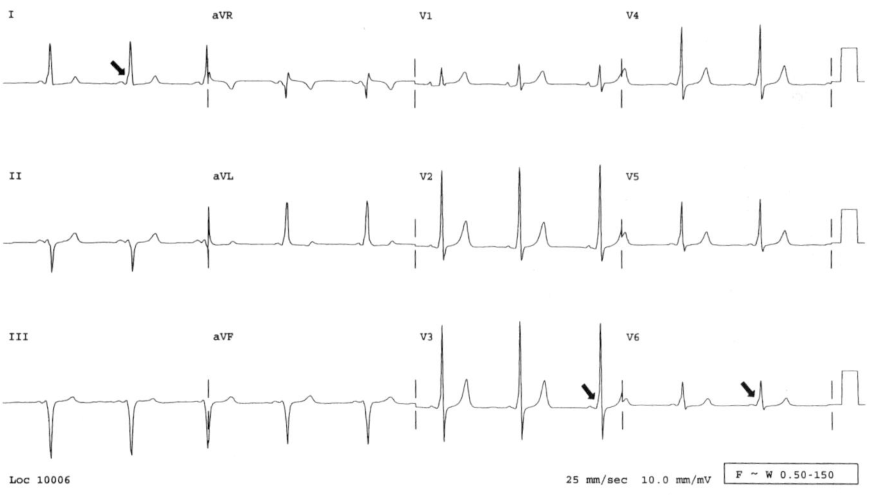

Figure 9-5

Wolff-Parkinson-White syndrome (WPW). Twelve-lead ECG obtained from a patient with WPW. Conduction down an accessory AV pathway results in a short PR interval (≈80 msec) and delta waves, which are observed as an initial slurring of the QRS complex (*arrows*).

with no prior evidence of an accessory pathway prove to have orthodromic AVRT. As mentioned previously, if a tachycardia is associated with electrical alternans this is believed to be highly suggestive of a bypass tract with retrograde VA conduction. During AF the impulse conducts anerogradely down the accessory pathway so that the delta wave is visible, distorting the QRS complex.

PERIOPERATIVE CONSIDERATIONS

The preexcitation syndrome has an average incidence of 0.5 to 2 per 1000 in a healthy population. Arrhythmias are most problematic in the first year of life, in the teens and 20s, and then in the 50s and 60s. The disorder appears to be familial and relatives of a patient with WPW have an increased incidence of preexcitation. Therefore, a preoperative ECG should be ordered for the patient with a positive family history of a relative with recurrent arrhythmias, particularly at an early age. If preexcitation is discovered on the preoperative ECG, this does not automatically mean that the patient is at high risk for arrhythmias or underlying heart disease. The majority of patients with preexcitation never experience an SVT and the prognosis of the syndrome in the absence of SVTs or cardiac disease, such as Ebstein's anomaly, mitral valve prolapse and cardiomyopathies, is excellent. The prognosis is also good for most patients with SVT although sudden death occurs rarely (less than 0.1%).

Until recently most patients requiring chronic prophylaxis for AVRT would be receiving either class IA or IC agents. However, the usefulness of these drugs is limited by their side effects (see Box 9-1), particularly, their proarrhythmic properties. Class III agents (amiodarone, sotalol) have also been shown to be effective in controlling tachycardias because of an accessory pathway. The pharmacologic approach to chronic management is falling in disfavor with the demonstrated efficacy of RF ablation. This approach is curative, has low risk, and is now considered early for symptomatic patients.

If an arrhythmia occurs in the perioperative period and produces hemodynamic compromize then electrical cardioversion is the initial treatment. If the AVRT is tolerated, vagal maneuvers should be tried first and will either terminate or slow the tachycardia. If this fails, adenosine will be effective in over 90% of cases. In patients with preexcitation, adenosine may precipitate AF with a fast ventricular rate so an external cardioverter-defibrillator should be available. If vagal maneuvers and adenosine fail, CCBs, β-blockers are alternative treatments.

Atrial fibrillation or flutter may be associated with a rapid ventricular rate which progresses to ventricular fibrillation. Electrical cardioversion is the treatment of choice. In patients with a known preexcitation syndrome procainamide (combined with a β-blocker), sotalol, or amiodarone are the treatments of choice, as these agents slow conduction over the accessory pathway. Digoxin and CCB do not block accessory pathway conduction and may produce a rapid ventricular rate if used alone for the treatment of AF. Lidocaine rarely terminates AF and may also enhance conduction over the accessory pathway.

Anesthesia should be conducted with the goal of reducing any stimuli, particularly sympathetic stimulation, that may precipitate arrhythmias. No particular anesthetic agent or technique is either prohibited or recommended.

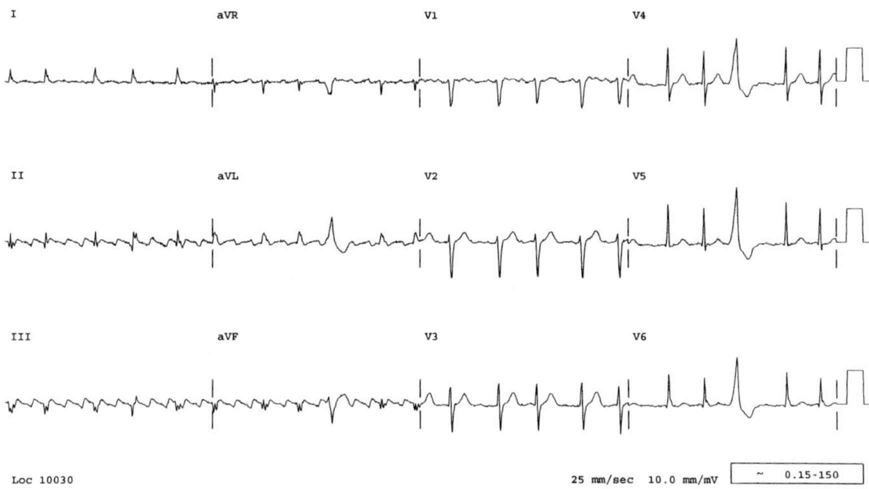

Figure 9-6
Twelve-lead ECG demonstrating atrial flutter. The classic "sawtooth" flutter (F) waves are often seen best in the inferior leads (II, III, aVF). Both 2:1 and 3:1 AV conduction are observed, as well as occasional wide-complex ventricular premature complexes.

Atrial Flutter (A-Flutter)

The atrial rate in A-flutter is 250 to 350 beats per minute. The tachycardia is commonly associated with a 2:1 block, resulting in a ventricular rate of approximately 150 beats per minute. In children, and patients with thyrotoxicosis or preexcitation, 1:1 AV conduction may occur producing a ventricular rate of 300 beats per minute. The ECG displays regular sawtooth flutter waves, often best seen in leads II, III, aVf, or V_1. The rate is usually regular although varying degrees of AV block can produce an irregular ventricular response (Fig. 9-6).

PERIOPERATIVE CONSIDERATIONS

While paroxysmal A-flutter may occur in healthy individuals, persistant A-flutter is usually associated with heart disease, as well as metabolic abnormalities (hypokalemia, hypomagnesemia, thyrotoxicosis, acute alcohol intoxication), inflammation (pericarditis), or postcardiothoracic surgery. Chronic A-flutter is uncommon, as this is an unstable tachycardia that tends to convert to either sinus rhythm or AF. Its prevalence increases with age. Patients with chronic A-flutter may be receiving AV blockers to control the ventricular response, or class IA, IC, or III agents in the hope of restoring sinus rhythm and preventing recurrence.

If A-flutter occurs in the perioperative period, vagal maneuvers and adenosine may initially be tried. These rarely terminate the tachycardia but may slow the ventricular rate and reveal flutter waves if the diagnosis is in doubt. Synchronous DC cardioversion, using low energy levels (50 J), is effective and is the initial treatment of choice. The cardioversion will either restore the A-flutter to sinus rhythm or convert it to AF, in which case, either the cardioversion should be repeated with a higher energy level, or the AF can be left untreated. If cardioversion fails, then CCBs, β-blockers, or digoxin may be given to control the ventricular response. The class 1A drugs (quinidine, procainamide, and disopyramide) possess vagolytic properties which may slow the atrial rate and facilitate AV conduction, resulting in 1:1 conduction. If a class 1A agent is given to a patient with A-flutter it should be preceded by an AV blocker (CCB or β-blocker). Atrial flutter may also respond to overdrive pacing through pacing leads or an esophageal catheter.

It is a widely held belief that the risk of a thromboembolic event is far less common in patients with A-flutter than in those with AF. However, in one study of hospitalized patients with A-flutter, atrial thrombus was detected by echocardiography in 21% of cases and thromboembolism has been reported after cardioversion of A-flutter. This is an area of controversy with many cardiologists adopting the same approach to the cardioversion of A-flutter as they do to AF, i.e., give anticoagulants if the duration of the arrhythmia is greater than 48 hours (see following).

Atrial Fibrillation (AF)

Atrial fibrillation is the most common sustained arrhythmia encountered in clinical practice. The prevalence of AF increases with age: 0.05% in the 25- to 35-year age group, 0.5% from 50 to 59 years of age, and increasing to over 5% in individuals over 65. In the past, AF was commonly a consequence of rheumatic heart disease (particularly mitral stenosis), however, CHF and hypertension are now the two disorders most commonly associated with AF. Atrial fibrillation is also seen in ischemic heart disease, dilated and hyperthrophic cardiomyopathy, mitral valve disease, alcohol ingestion, thyrotoxicosis, diabetes, pulmonary embolism, and chronic lung disease. Approximately 10% of cases of AF are not associated with any underlying disease, so called "lone AF." In the presence of heart disease, AF may be paroxysmal at first but tends to become chronic with the progression of the underlying disease. In contrast, AF is usually self-limited after acute myocardial infarction (5% to 18% of cases) and surgery, particularly cardiothoracic surgery.

Most patients with AF are symptomatic. Palpitations are common, while fatigue, dizziness, presyncope, and dyspnea are also frequent complaints. The loss of effective atrial contraction may decrease cardiac output. This decrease will be greatest in patients with impaired diastolic ventricular filling (mitral stenosis, ventricular hypertrophy, poor LV contractile function, and pericardial disease). The increased heart rate will also increase myocardial oxygen demand and may precipitate angina in susceptible individuals.

There are three clinical goals in the treatment of AF: relief of symptoms, improved cardiac performance, and decreasing the risk of thromboembolism (Fig. 9-7). The first two goals may be achieved by either control of the ventricular rate or pharmacologic restoration of sinus rhythm. The right option is currently a source of debate in the cardiac literature and the subject of an ongoing trial, the Atrial Fibrillation Follow-up and Antiarrythmic Management (AFFIRM) study. Patients with recurrent paroxysmal or chronic AF may, therefore, present to surgery receiving either AV blocking drugs (digoxin, CCBs, or β-blockers) or class IA, IC, or III agents.

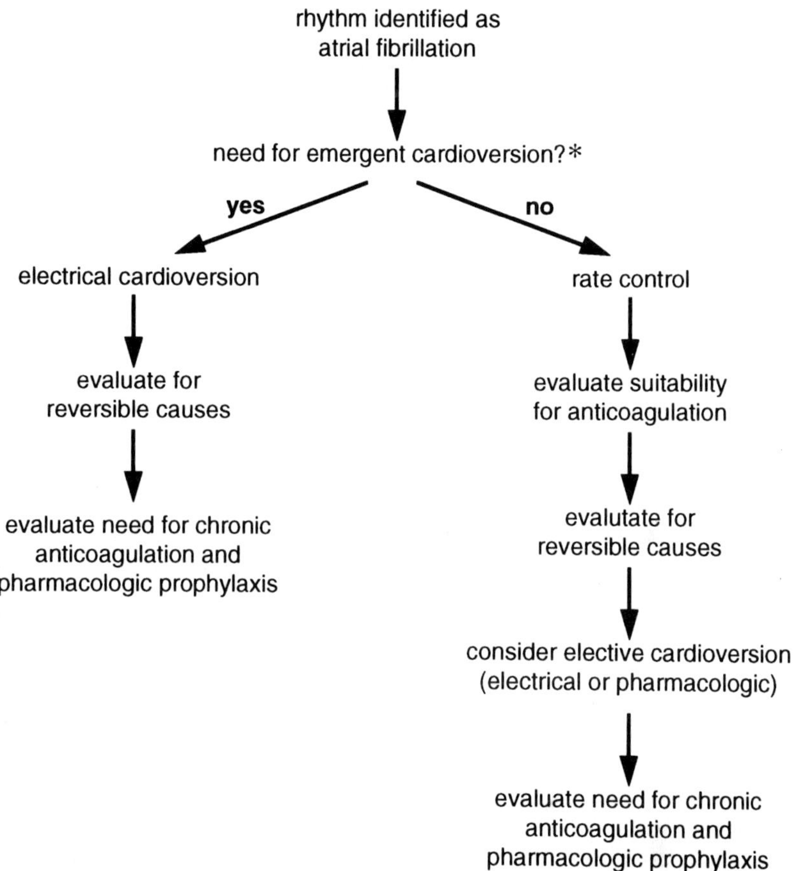

Figure 9-7

Conventional paradigm for the management of recent-onset atrial fibrillation. *Emergent cardioversion should be performed in any individual with hypotension, congestive heart failure, chest pain, or mental status changes. Electrical direct-current countershocks should always be synchronized to the QRS complex.

While any arrhythmia may occur during or after surgery, AF is by far the most common tachycardia and has been reported in 5% to 40% of patients after coronary artery bypass grafting (CABG). It most commonly occurs on the second to third day post-CABG. Reported risk factors for post-CABG atrial fibrillation include patient's age (the most significant factor), male sex, preoperative use of digoxin, preoperative withdrawal of β-blockers, COPD, valvular heart disease, LV dysfunction, pericarditis, increasing aortic cross-clamp time, and the presence of persistant atrial activity during cardioplegic arrest. Post-CABG atrial fibrillation has been associated with an increased incidence of postoperative stroke (3-fold increase), ventricular tachycardia or fibrillation, a need for permanent pacemaker placement, and increased hospitalization.

If AF occurs in the perioperative period the treatment options are either to control the ventricular response, or to attempt pharmacologic or electrical conversion to sinus rhythm. The management plan should be determined by the hemodynamic effects of the arrhythmia, the patient's preexisting cardiac status, the understanding that the patient will best be able to tolerate the stresses of the perioperative period if cardiac function is optimized, and the fact that perioperative AF is usually transient.

If control of the ventricular response is the chosen management plan, then the physician is confronted with the questions of which agent(s) should be given and what the target ventricular rate should be. Digoxin was traditionally the agent of choice for rate control, but its role has become more limited. There is a delay in the therapeutic effect of digoxin of at least 60 minutes after IV administration, and the full effect is not seen for 6 hours. Furthermore, digoxin is no more successful than placebo in converting patients back into sinus rhythm. It may prolong the duration of episodes of paroxysmal AF and does not successfully control ventricular rate during exercise or in the presence of increased sympathetic drive (commonly seen in the perioperative period). Digoxin is still considered to have a role in the chronic management of patients with AF and LV dysfunction. If acute rate control is the goal then the choice is between a CCB or β-blocker alone or in combination with digoxin. Verapamil (IV bolus of 5–15 mg followed by an infusion of 0.05–0.2 mg/min) or diltiazem (IV bolus of 15–25 mg followed by an infusion of 10–15 mg/hour), are both 95% successful in slowing ventricular rate within 5 minutes, the most common reported side effect being hypotension (8% of cases). Esmolol, metoprolol (5–15 mg IV over 5–15 minutes), or propranolol are also effective, particularly in the presence of thyrotoxicosis or increased sympathetic tone, and are potentially the agents of choice in the management of perioperative AF. Esmolol, because of its short half-life of 9 minutes, may be particularly useful in this setting. Neither digoxin nor the AV blockers appear to influence the conversion rate of AF to sinus rhythm. It should be reemphasized that patients with preexcitation and AF should not be given CCBs, digoxin, and probably β-blockers; the options instead are electrical cardioversion and procainamide. Adenosine has no role in the management of AF.

The question of what is meant by a "controlled ventricular rate" is a source of debate in the cardiology literature. Reducing the rapid ventricular rate in AF increases diastolic filling time and left ventricular stroke volume, but this is offset by a decreased contractility and stroke rate. In one study of patients with chronic AF a "controlled" rate was defined as that rate above which increases in heart rate were associated with an increased cardiac output. If an increase in heart rate was associated with a decreased cardiac output, this was considered a poorly "controlled" rate. It was determined that a target rate of 90 beats per minute was the ideal ventricular response, which resulted in the least compromise of cardiac output. This would, therefore, appear to be a reasonable goal for rate control of perioperative AF.

If the decision is made to pharmacologically convert the patient with perioperative AF, then the class IA, IC, or III antiarrhythmics may be used. Both amiodarone and propafenone have β-blocking properties and will slow the ventricular rate, even if pharmacologic cardioversion is not achieved. The ability of these agents to maintain sinus rhythm decreases with the duration of AF, large left atrial size (although this has been disputed in recent studies investigating pharmacologic conversion of AF), and multiple previous pharmacologic failures. A new class III agent, ibutalide fumarate, has recently been evaluated for the chemical cardioversion of AF. It appears to be effective in up to 50% of cases of recent onset AF (less than 30 days), and produces its effect within 30 minutes in most patients. It is only available in a parenteral formulation and is given as a 1 to 2 mg slow IV injection over 10 minutes. Giving these agents is not without risk. The class 1A and 1C (flecainide, propafenone) agents may facilitate AV conduction, resulting in an increased ventricular rate. It is recommended that an AV blocker should be given before these agents are administered. Drugs that prolong the QT interval, (particularly quinidine, but also other class 1A and III agents), may precipitate *torsades de pointes*, a rapid polymorphic ventricular tachycardia. Patients most at risk are those with CHF, hypokalemia, and baseline prolonged QT interval.

Electrical cardioversion is the correct therapy if the AF is associated with hemodynamic compromise, myocardial ischemia, or CHF. Treatment should begin with 200 J, but higher energy levels may be required in the patient who has recently undergone cardiothoracic surgery. After a median sternotomy, it is recommended that the anterior paddle be placed to the right of the sternum between the third and sixth intercostal spaces, and the other paddle should be positioned in the fourth to sixth intercostal space as far left in the axilla as possible, or in a posterior location under the tip of the left axilla. While the role of electrical cardioversion in the patient with hemodynamic compromise is not questioned, does it have a role in the management of perioperative AF that is hemodynamically tolerated? If the AF occurs intraoperatively or in the intensive-care unit, then the patient will already be anesthetized or sedated and have the airway protected. Electrical cardioversion has a reported success rate of approximately 85% in patients with AF of short duration (less than 1 year), although anecdotal reports suggest a lower success rate in the treatment of perioperative AF. Electrical cardioversion is certainly less likely to be successful if the precipitating cause of the AF is still present. Therefore, blood gases, electrolyte disorders, inadequate anesthesia, or pain relief should be corrected, if possible, before attempting cardioversion. Arguments in favor of electrical cardioversion include the restoration of the atrial contribution to the cardiac output, which should improve the patient's ability to tolerate the recognized stresses of the perioperative period. It also spares the patient from receiving antiarrhythmic drugs, which may have negative inotropic or proarrythmic properties. Furthermore, echocardiographic studies have demonstrated a thrombogenic environment in the atria of patients with recent onset AF (less than 48 hours' duration). Allowing the patient to remain in AF may, therefore, expose him or her to an increased risk of thromboemboli.

Against the argument in favor of electrical cardioversion of perioperative AF, are the reports of arrhythmias induced by cardioversion. All of these reports are from the cardiology literature and do not address the question of acute onset of perioperative AF. Asystole, AV block, and significant bradycardia can be precipitated by cardioversion, are more common in patients treated with antiarrythmic drugs, or with preexisting sinus node dysfunction or AV block, and are usually transient. Ventricular arrhythmias are usually the result of the shock not being correctly synchronized with the QRS complex, or cardioversion of patients with digitalis toxicity. Electrical conversion of a patient with a pacemaker can damage the pulse generator, the lead system, and/or the myocardium if certain precautions are not taken. The paddle should be at least 12 cm from the pacemaker battery (the anteroposterior paddle position is recommended), and the lowest effective energy settings should be used. The final decision of whether to attempt to rapidly restore sinus rhythm in a patient who appears to be hemodynamically tolerating a perioperative episode of AF will doubtlessly depend upon the experience and bias of the physician managing the patient. One of the present authors clearly remembers the maxim of an experienced cardiologist in the United Kingdom—"if your hospital's pharmacy bill is larger than its electricity bill, then you are not managing arrhythmias correctly." That teaching has influenced this author's bias.

Several studies have evaluated the efficacy of prophylactic therapy to prevent AF after cardiac surgery. Prophylactic β-blockers alone, or in combination with digoxin, were the most effective. Procainamide has demonstrated efficacy in one report, whereas prophylactic digoxin, verapamil, amiodarone, or sotalol failed to reduce the frequency of SVTs after cardiac surgery.

The final goal in the management of AF is the prevention of thromboembolism. Most thromboembolic events originate from thrombus formed in the atria, in particularly, the left atrial appendage. Emboli may be shed into either the systemic (commonly to the brain) or pulmonary circulation. The incidence of stroke is, on average, 6 times greater in patients with AF than those without AF. The risk is even higher in patients with AF and mitral stenosis. Other risk factors for stroke in patients with AF include:

1. Age—the risk of stroke increases with age. Patients younger than 60 years of age with no cardiovascular disease have a low risk of stroke. In the Framingham study, AF was the only cardiovascular condition associated with an increased risk of stroke in individuals over 80 years of age.
2. Coexistant diseases—mitral stenosis, prosthetic heart valves, valvular disease, previous stroke or transient ischemic attack (TIA), diabetes mellitus, hypertension, ventricular dysfunction, ischemic heart disease, and thyrotoxicosis.
3. Certain echocardiographic findings—large left atrium, LV dysfunction, and mitral annular calcification.

Patients over 75 years of age with at least one risk factor (hypertension, diabetes mellitus, or previous stroke/TIA) have a stroke rate of 8.1% per annum. Five recent randomized controlled trials have demonstrated a 70% reduction in the incidence of ischemic stroke with the use of long-term oral anticoagulants. This therapy is now recommended by the American College of Chest Physicians (ACCP) in all patients with AF older than 65 years of age and for younger patients with any of the risk factors listed previously. If oral anticoagulants are contraindicated, aspirin 325 mg/day should be given (aspirin demonstrated a 36% risk reduction of stroke). Aspirin may also be used in low-risk patients younger than 65 years with "lone AF." Patients with AF older than 75 years have the highest stroke rate but also have the greatest risk of bleeding complications with anticoagulant therapy. It is recommended that anticoagulation should be maintained in the lower end of the therapeutic range (international normalized ratio ([INR] 2.0 to 3.0) in these patients.

The perioperative physician may now be faced with the problem of the patient with AF on anticoagulants scheduled for surgery. Management options include:

1. Stopping the oral anticoagulation 3 to 5 days prior to surgery and restarting treatment as soon as possible postoperatively.
2. Reducing the dose of oral anticoagulation prior to surgery and considering giving fresh frozen plasma or a small dose of vitamin K preoperatively; (0.5–1 mg IV of vitamin K will significantly reduce the INR in 12–24 hours without producing a state of relative resistance to oral anticoagulants when they are restarted).
3. Stopping oral anticoagulation 3 to 5 days before surgery; giving heparin (to maintain a blood heparin level of 0.2–0.4 U/ml), up until 4 hours before surgery and restarting heparin postoperatively.

There are no studies to guide the management of such patients. Instead, the physician must balance the risks of reducing the anticoagulation and exposing the patient to the risk of a stroke versus continuing the anticoagulation and risking perioperative bleeding. Some guidance can be obtained from the recommendations for the perioperative management of patients with bileaflet prosthetic heart valves in the aortic position (who have a similar risk of thromboembolism compared to the elderly patient with AF and at least one risk factor). Studies have shown that it is safe to stop the oral anticoagulants 3 to 5 days prior to surgery in such patients (see option 1, previously).

If the decision is made to cardiovert a patient with postoperative AF, should anticoagulants be given? The ACCP currently recommends that oral anticoagulants be given for 3 weeks prior to either electrical or chemical cardioversion of patients who have been in AF for more than 2 days, and be continued until normal SR has been maintained for at least 4 weeks. Recent studies have examined the role of transesophageal echocardiography (TEE) prior to cardioversion. If no thrombus is detected by TEE, then a shortened course of oral anticoagulants may be given prior to cardioversion but a 4-week course postcardioversion is still recommended.

VENTRICULAR ARRHYTHMIAS

Ventricular Premature Complexes

A ventricular premature complex (VPC) is characterized as a premature QRS complex differing in morphology and duration (usually greater than 120 msec) from the dominant rhythm, and associated with a large T wave that has a direction opposite to the major deflection of the QRS. A P wave does not proceed the QRS. The atria may be activated retrograde, but the P wave is usually buried in the QRS and is rarely seen. A fully compensatory pause usually follows the VPC, i.e., the RR interval of the sinus beat on either side of the VPC equals twice the normally conducted RR interval (Fig. 9-8).

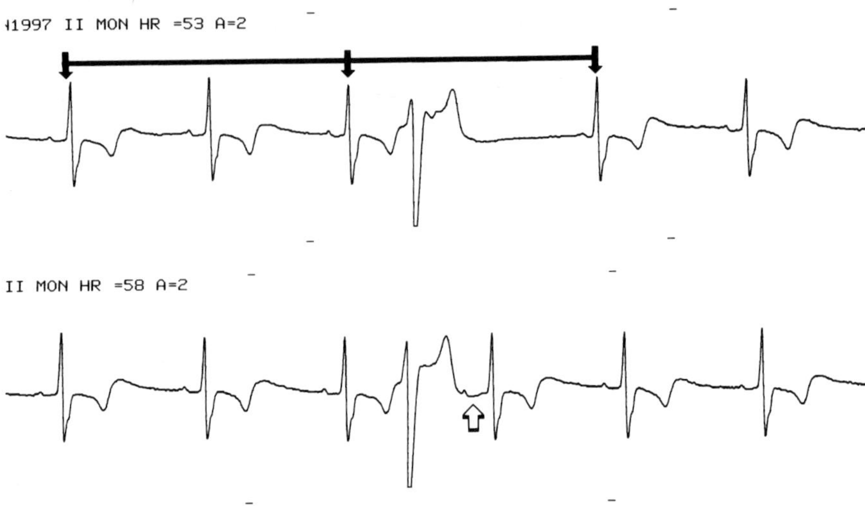

Figure 9-8
Ventricular premature complexes (VPCs). These are characterized as early, wide QRS complexes without preceding P waves. Most commonly, a VPC is followed by a compensatory pause **(top panel)** because the VPC does not reset the intrinsic sinus rate, but does produce AV refractoriness. When the VPC occurs earlier or the sinus rate is slower, a compensatory pause may not be present **(bottom)** due to partial recovery of the AV node. As illustrated in this example, when a compensatory pause is absent after a VPC, a prolonged PR interval often follows the next sinus beat ***(empty arrow)*** since the AV node has not completely recovered.

Ventricular premature complexes may have similar (unifocal, uniform, monomorphic) or differing morphology (multifocal, multiform, polymorphic). The rhythm can be described as bigeminy when the VPC occurs regularly after each normal complex, and trigeminy when the VPC occurs after two normal complexes. Two successive VPCs are referred to as a pair or couplet. Three or more VPCs are arbitrarily referred to as VT which is called nonsustained if it lasts less than 30 seconds, or sustained if lasting longer than 30 seconds or associated with hemodynamic collapse.

PERIOPERATIVE CONSIDERATIONS

Ventricular premature complexes are common in healthy individuals and increase in frequency with age. They are associated with a wide range of pathologies including electrolyte and respiratory disorders, infection, inflammation, structural heart disease (most importantly, coronary artery disease), and the intake of alcohol, tobacco, caffeine, or any other synaptomimetic drug. Ventricular premature complexes may be asymptomatic or associated with palpitations. They may precipitate angina or hypotension in patients with heart disease if they are frequent and significantly increase the heart rate. Asymptomatic individuals with VPCs, but no underlying heart disease, do not appear to be at risk of cardiac events and are usually offered reassurance rather than antiarrhythmic agents. Ventricular premature complexes occur in the majority of patients after CABG surgery but have not been found to be a risk factor for VT, a finding born out by several other studies. The chief significance of VPCs is that they appear to be a marker of underlying heart disease rather than the cause of subsequent problems. This is supported by Goldman's assertion that frequent preoperative VPCs (>5 VPCs per minute) represent a significant risk factor for postoperative cardiac events only in patients with underlying heart disease and not in healthy individuals.

After myocardial infarction (MI) (including a perioperative MI) VPCs are common. Certain VPCs (those occurring close to the preceding T wave, in salvos of three or more, more than five per minute, bigeminal or multiform) have been considered to presage the onset of ventricular fibrillation (VF). However, approximately 50% of patients with these "high-risk" VPCs do not develop VF. While frequent VPCs can identify postMI patients at increased risk of VT or sudden death, the Cardiac Arrhythmia Suppression Trial has cast doubt on the wisdom of antiarrhythmic therapy in this setting, because of the higher mortality in those patients whose VPCs were pharmacologically suppressed.

If frequent VPCs are observed perioperatively a search should be made for precipitating factors, especially myocardial ischemia. Myocardial ischemia should be treated by correcting acute adverse hemodynamic events (hypotension and tachycardia), nitroglycerin, and β-blockers. Hypoxia and hypercarbia are potent triggers of VPCs and should be treated. Electrolyte abnormalities, e.g., hypokalemia and hypomagnesemia, should also be corrected, particularly in patients receiving digoxin in whom frequent VPCs should alert the clinician to possible toxicity. Frequently, the VPCs will respond to these measures. If no precipitating cause can be found or corrected and frequent VPCs are considered to be a problem, then the pharmacologic agent of choice is either a β-blocker or lidocaine IV, followed by procainamide. The sympathetic nervous system is an important trigger of ventricular arrhythmias, so β-blockers may be particularly useful in the perioperative setting. While lidocaine is effective in suppressing VPCs, the use of prophylactic lidocaine to prevent sustained VT or VF after cardiac surgery does not appear to be so. Simple VPCs can often be suppressed by increasing the atrial rate if a pacing wire is in place.

Ventricular Tachycardia (VT)

The diagnosis of VT is suggested by the finding of three or more abnormal QRS complexes with a duration greater than 120 msec and an ST-T vector pointing in the opposite direction to that of the QRS complex. The distinction between VT and an SVT with aberrant conduction may be difficult (Box 9-3). The ventricular rate is highly variable (usually between 70–250 beats per minute). As with VPCs, the VT may be labelled monomorphic or polymorphic, depending upon whether the QRS complexes have a uniform or variable morphology, respectively.

PERIOPERATIVE CONSIDERATIONS

The predominant etiology of VT is ischemic heart disease (over 50% of patients with symptomatic VT), followed by the cardiomyopathies (both dilated and hypertrophic) and an assortment of cardiac disorders, which include valvular and congenital heart disease. After MI the risk of VT increases with decreasing ejection fraction, previous VT, and persistent occlusion of the infarct-related artery. Nonsustained VT is common after CABG surgery occurring in up to 58% of patients. However, sustained VT and VF are rare (0.41%–1.4%). Valve surgery has been associated with an increased incidence of VT occurring late after surgery. Sustained VT or VF, within the first postoperative year, accounts for 24% of the annual deaths after aortic valve replacement.

Patients who have experienced an episode of VT may or may not be on antiarrhythmic therapy. There is a growing awareness that all of the current antiarrhythmic drugs are themselves proarrhythmic, and this risk increases in those patients with the most marked ventricular dysfunction who are the very patients at most risk of VT. Treating patients with asymptomatic episodes of nonsustained VT does not decrease mortality, and there is a general consensus that such patients should not be prescribed antiarrythmic agents (except, perhaps, β-blockers). Treatment is reserved for patients who have had a symptomatic (hemodynamic compromise, cardiac arrest) episode of VT, and can be divided into measures to terminate the arrhythmia and measures to prevent it from recurring. Prevention of VT is more difficult than cure of the acute event. While there appears to be no "right" agent at present, recent clinical trials favor the use of amiodarone, particularly in patients with coronary artery disease. When single agents fail, drug combinations may then be used, or placement of an automatic implantable cardioverter-defibrillator (AICD) be considered. Studies have demonstrated a high mortality (about 30%) and a high incidence of sustained VT after CABG surgery in patients with an ejection fraction of less than 35%. The ongoing CABG Patch Trial is addressing this issue and evaluating the benefits of prophylactic AICD placement in this patient population.

If VT occurs in the perioperative period and produces hemodynamic collapse then synchronized electrical cardioversion is the first line of therapy, starting with energy levels of 200 J. If VT does not compromise the patient (hypotension, angina, CHF, symptoms of cerebral hypoperfusion), then it may initially be managed pharmacologically. Intravenous lidocaine is usually the first line of therapy, followed by procainamide; procainamide actually appears to be superior to lidocaine in converting VT. After conversion of the VT to sinus rhythm it is essential to institute measures to prevent its recurrence. This includes correction of precipitating factors such as myocardial ischemia, respiratory and electrolyte disorders (hypoxia, hypercarbia, acidosis, hypokalemia, hypomagnesemia), and CHF.

Specific Types of VT

Three particular varieties of VT deserve mention: accelerated idioventricular rhythm, monomorphic VT in structurally normal hearts, and *torsade de pointes*. Accelerated idioventricular rhythm (AIVR) is uncommon but seen in perioperative patients and patients in the intensive care unit. It usually occurs in patients with underlying heart disease. The firing rate of the ectopic ventricular focus is slow (60–110 beats per minute) and competes with the sinus node for the dominant control of the ventricle. The onset of the arrhythmia is slow and occurs when the rate of the ectopic rate exceeds the sinus rate. The arrhythmia is usually transient and rarely produces hemodynamic compromise, except in patients who depend on their atrial contraction to maintain ventricular preload. The rhythm rarely needs treatment but can be blocked by simply increasing the sinus rate with atropine, or by cardiac pacing.

Monomorphic VT is rare in patients with structurally normal hearts but may arise, often in young healthy individuals, from a focus in the right ventricular, and, less commonly, the left ventricular outflow tract. Those VTs arising from the right side of the heart have a left bundle branch block configuration with an inferior axis on the ECG. The VT is often triggered by exertion, sympathetic stimulation, or administration of β-adrenergic agonists and can be treated or prevented with β-blockers. Some variants also respond to adenosine or verapamil, wrongly suggesting that the arrhythmia is an SVT. This form of VT is rarely associated with ventricular fibrillation or sudden death. Endocardial catheter ablation of the ectopic focus is curative.

Torsade de pointes is a polymorphic VT, which often arises in the setting of a prolonged QTc interval (often >50 seconds) (Fig. 9-9). There are two clinical forms of prolonged QT interval: the acquired and the congenital form. The acquired form is the most common. The QT interval may be prolonged by antiarrhythmic agents, (quinidine, sotalol, procainamide, and its metabolite, N-acetylprocainamide, disopyramide and amiodarone), electrolyte abnormalities, (hypokalemia, hypocalcemia, hypomagnesemia), severe bradycardia, subarachnoid hemorrhage, myocardial ischemia,

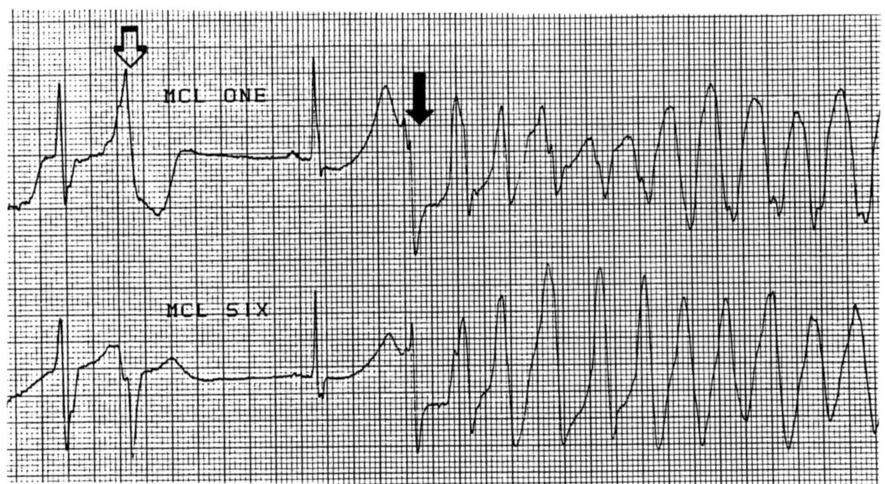

Figure 9-9
Torsade de pointes (TdP). Recording from a patient admitted with syncope and hypokalemia, demonstrating initiation of TdP. The third complex of the recording has a prolonged QT interval (580 msec). A ventricular premature complex (VPC) occurs during the T wave (***solid arrow***), resulting in a polymorphic ventricular tachycardia with an axis that resolves around the baseline. The third complex in the recording is also preceded by a long pause caused by a VPC (***empty arrow***), resulting in the classic "long-short" initiation sequence.

and an assortment of drugs (phenothiazines, tricyclic and tetracyclic antidepressants, erythromycin, pentamidine, nonsedating antihistamines, (terfenadine, astemizole), and probucol. The arrhythmia typically occurs after a prolonged RR interval (a pause), followed by a prolonged QT interval in which the T wave is interrupted by a VPC, which is the first beat of the arrhythmia. The VT may spontaneously terminate or degenerate into VF, which requires immediate electrical cardioversion. Magnesium (bolus of 1–2 grams IV over 1–2 minutes followed, if needed, by an infusion of 3–20 mg per minute with monitoring of neuromuscular blockade) should be given to prevent recurrences. Magnesium is often effective even if serum magnesium levels are normal. If magnesium is ineffective, the RR interval may be shortened by β-adrenergic agonists such as isoproterenol titrated to a dose that suppresses ventricular ectopy. Alternatively, overdrive atrial or ventricular pacing may be added at a rate that suppresses ventricular ectopy (usually at a rate of 100–120 beats per minute). In the acquired form of QT interval prolongation, adrenergic stimulation (see isoproterenol previously) shortens the QT interval and may be beneficial. Virtually every anesthetic agent has been associated with QT prolongation and precipitating VT in vulnerable patients. Whether this is caused by some intrinsic effect of slowing ventricular conduction, or is simply because of the sympatholytic effect of anesthesia per se, is not known. Droperidol has been shown to produce a dose-related QT prolongation but has not been definitely shown to increase the risk of VT.

The congenital form of prolonged QT interval is rare. It may have an autosomal-recessive pattern of inheritance and be associated with congenital deafness (the Jervell and Lange-Nielson syndrome), or have autosomal-dominant inheritance (Romano Ward syndrome). Typically, patients experience episodes of VT and have syncope or cardiac arrest before the third decade. Unlike the acquired form, sympathetic stimulation may precipitate the arrhythmia in the congenital form, and β-blockers represent the first line of treatment and prevention.

• DISTURBANCES OF CONDUCTION

Left Bundle Branch Block (LBBB)

The diagnostic criteria for LBBB (Fig. 9-10) are:

1. QRS duration is longer than 0.12 seconds.
2. Broad monophasic R wave in leads I, V_5 and V_6 without Q waves.
3. A QS or RS complex in lead V_1.
4. Displacement of the ST segment and T wave in an opposite direction to that of the major vector of the QRS complex.

Left bundle branch is also frequently associated with poor R wave progression in right and midprecordial leads and left axis deviation.

PERIOPERATIVE CONSIDERATIONS

The incidence of LBBB increases with age. Most cases of LBBB are the result of underlying heart disease such as coronary artery disease, hypertension, dilated cardiomy-

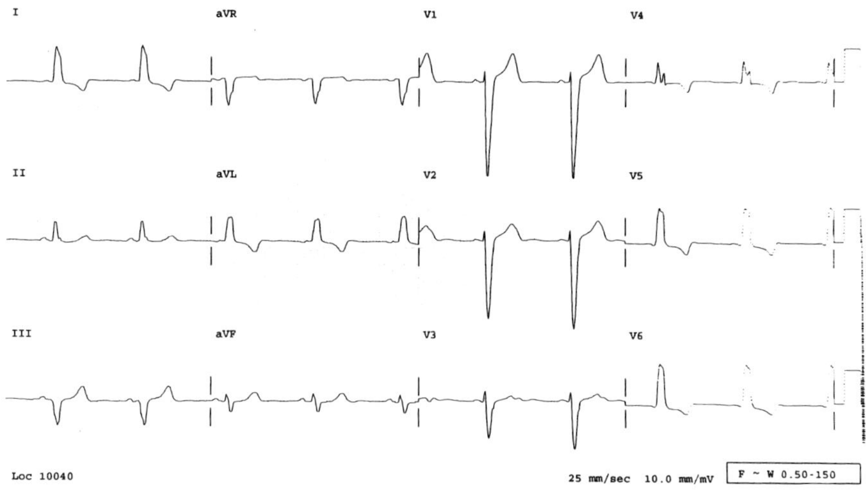

Figure 9-10
Twelve-lead ECG demonstrating a left bundle branch block. The QRS duration is 136 msec. There is a broad RS complex in leads V_1 and V_2 and a broad monomorphic R wave in leads I, V_5, and V_6.

opathy, valvular heart disease (14% of patients with aortic stenosis), and primary degenerative disease of the conducting system. It may also be present without overt heart disease.

The diagnosis of LBBB is clinically significant and should prompt a detailed cardiac evaluation of the patient. In the population-based Framingham study, clinically apparent cardiovascular disease was detected in 89% of individuals who developed LBBB. Fifty percent of these individuals died from cardiovascular-related causes within 10 years of the onset of LBBB. In hospital-based studies, patients with coronary artery disease and LBBB survive an average of 3 years. In the Coronary Artery Surgery Study, LBBB was a marker for more extensive coronary artery disease, worse left ventricular function, and increased mortality. Complete AV block is an infrequent cause of death.

The perioperative management of a patient with LBBB depends on the underlying cause of the block. There has been concern that insertion of a pulmonary artery catheter may precipitate complete heart block in patients with LBBB. While several studies have not found this to be a problem, the anecdotal evidence (as well as the author's own experience) indicates that this may occur.

Left Anterior Hemiblock (LAH)

The diagnostic criteria for LAH are a normal QRS complex duration with a leftward QRS axis, usually 60° or greater. It is found in 2% to 5% of adults and increases with age. Approximately 60% of individuals with LAH have evidence of heart disease, usually coronary artery disease or hypertension. Left anterior hemiblock, by itself, should not alter perioperative management.

Left Posterior Hemiblock (LPH)

The diagnostic criteria for LPH are a normal QRS duration with a rightward QRS axis of +90° to +180° and an S_1Q_3 pattern. Isolated LPH is rare, is usually associated with coronary artery disease or hypertension, but does not by itself, affect perioperative management.

Right Bundle Branch Block (RBBB)

The diagnostic criteria for RBBB are:

1. QRS duration is longer than 0.12 seconds.
2. An RSR' configuration in V_1 with the secondary R wave (R') having a greater amplitude than the initial R wave.
3. A wide S wave in leads I, V_5, and V_6.

The axis of the initial portion of the QRS is normal. There is no displacement of the ST segment and the T wave is in the opposite direction to the vector of the final portion of the QRS complex. Right bundle branch block is best diagnosed in lead V_1.

Right bundle branch block is present in 1% of hospitalized patients and has been found to be the most common perioperative conduction defect after CABG surgery. The frequency of RBBB increases with age. The majority of individuals with RBBB have no apparent cardiovascular disease and their prognosis is similar to that of the general population. Finding an RBBB in the preoperative ECG does not appear to influence patient management. However, RBBB may be a sign of underlying heart disease (most commonly, coronary artery disease) and was associated with an increased number of cardiovascular-related deaths in the population-based Framingham study.

Bifascicular Block

Bifascicular block refers to RBBB plus blockade of one of the fascicles of the left bundle (Fig. 9-11). The combination of RBBB and left anterior hemiblock (LAH: frontal plane axis of –30° to –90°) is the most common variety and has been detected in 1% of hospitalized patients. Coronary artery disease is the most common etiology, (40%–60% of cases), followed by hypertension (20% of cases), aortic valve disease, cardiomyopathies, and degenerative changes in the conduction system. Bifascicular block with intermittent type II AV block, irrespective of symptoms, is a definite indication for pacing, as is symptomatic bifascicular block with intermittent complete heart block. The combination of RBBB and left posterior hemiblock is uncommon, but more of these patients progress to complete heart block (60% in one series).

The risk of perioperative complete heart block developing in a patient with bifascicular block is low and, in the absence of the specific conditions listed previously, prophylactic pacing is not required.

First-Degree Atrioventricular Block

The diagnostic criteria for first-degree AV block are a PR interval of more than 0.2 seconds. This is found in 0.5% of apparently healthy males and does not affect prognosis. First-degree AV block is usually caused by a degenerative disease of the

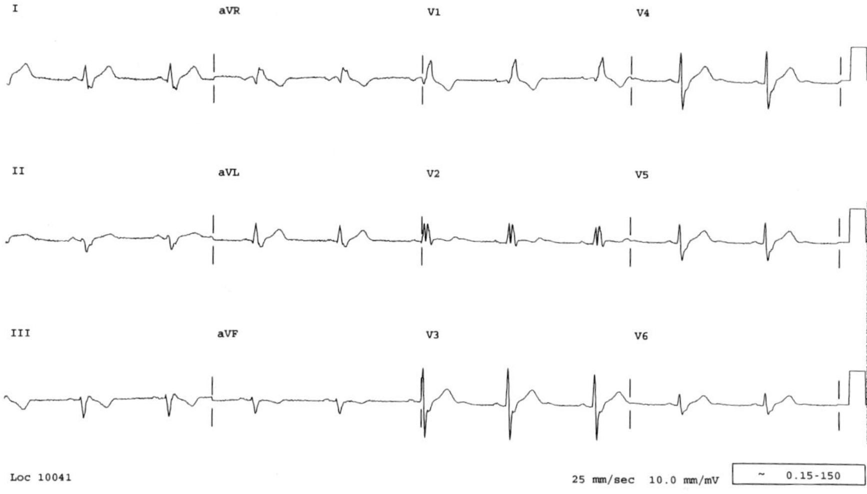

Figure 9-11
Twelve-lead ECG demonstrating bifascicular block. A right bundle branch block is present with a prolonged QRS duration (130 msec), and an RSR' best seen in leads V_2, as well as a broad S wave in leads I and V_6. A left anterior hemiblock is also present, denoted by a leftward deviation of the QRS axis further than –60°.

conducting system, but may also result from coronary artery disease, infiltrative myocardial disease, drugs (digoxin), enhanced vagal tone, and congenital heart disease. First-degree block does not usually require pacing, however, some patients develop symptoms as a consequence of the loss of physiologic AV synchrony. Pacing may correct the abnormal AV interval and restore cardiac function. Patients with first-degree AV block generally have an excellent prognosis and require no specific changes in perioperative management. The only exception is the patient who develops first-degree heart block and LBBB in the setting of an MI. These patients require temporary and possibly permanent pacing.

Second-Degree Atrioventricular Block

In second-degree AV block there is an intermittent failure of the P wave to conduct to the ventricles. There are two types of second degree AV block: type I and type II. The ECG findings in type I are a progressive lengthening of the PR interval and shortening of the RR interval until a P wave is blocked (Fig. 9-12); the RR interval containing the blocked P wave is shorter than the sum of two PP intervals. When type I block is associated with QRS of normal duration, the site of the conduction block is in the AV node. If the QRS is prolonged, the block may be in the AV node, within the His bundle or more distal. The ECG findings in type II AV block are intermittent, blocked P waves with a normal PR interval. Type II block is almost always associated with a bundle branch block, and the site of the block is within or below the His bundle. The causes of second-degree AV block are similar to that of first-degree block, although myocardial ischemia plays a more prominent role.

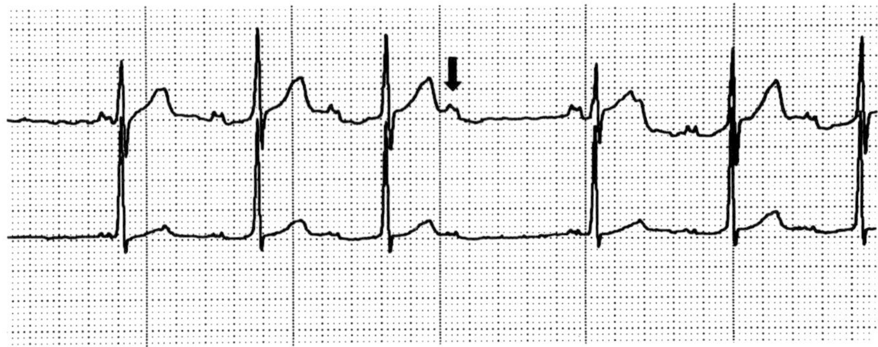

Figure 9-12

Type I, second-degree atrioventricular block or "Wenckebach" block. The PP interval is constant, whereas a gradual prolongation of the PR interval occurs until conduction through the AV node is blocked and a QRS complex fails to follow a P wave (*arrow*).

PERIOPERATIVE CONSIDERATIONS

Type I block occurs in some healthy individuals during sleep (and perhaps anesthesia), and in highly trained athletes. In the absence of associated heart disease, type I block has a good prognosis and rarely progresses to more advanced AV block. When it is associated with heart disease, such as coronary artery disease or aortic stenosis, the prognosis is usually determined by the nature of the underlying disease and not the conduction abnormality. Pacing is not recommended unless patients are symptomatic. This is also applicable to the management of the patient during surgery.

Unlike type I, type II block frequently progresses to complete AV block, producing Adams-Stokes syncopal attacks. The American College of Cardiology—American Heart Association guidelines recommend permanent pacemaker insertion in all symptomatic patients with type II block and asymptomatic patients with heart rates less than 40 beats per minute. Perioperative patients should also be managed according to these guidelines. Some practitioners feel that all patients with type II block should be offered a pacemaker, irrespective of symptoms, and temporary transvenous pacing may be prudent in the patient who is unlikely to tolerate an episode of intraoperative bradycardia. Certainly, mechanisms to treat a bradycardia (atropine, isoproterenol, transcutaneous and/or transvenous pacing facilities) should be readily available.

Third-Degree Atrioventricular Block

Third-degree AV block is characterized by a complete failure of the atrial impulse to excite the ventricles (Fig. 9-13). The ventricular rate is normally 40 to 60 per minute with a junctional pacemaker, and 20 to 40 per minute with a ventricular pacemaker.

PERIOPERATIVE CONSIDERATIONS

Third-degree AV block may be either acquired or congenital. The most common causes of the acquired form are fibrous degeneration of the conducting system,

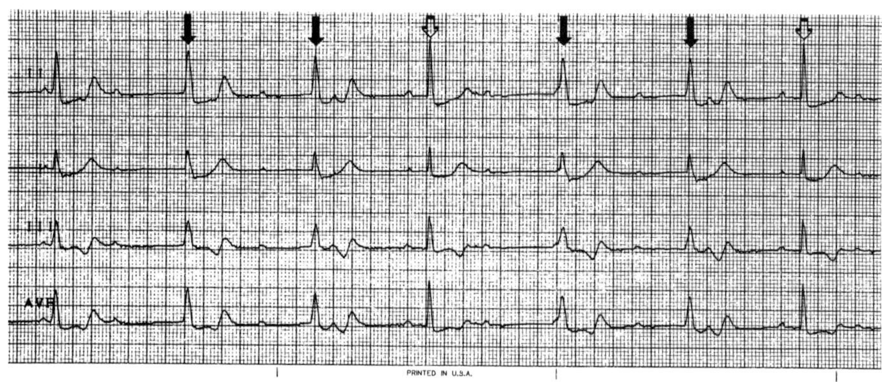

Figure 9-13
Recording demonstrating complete heart block. P waves are seen marching through the tracing at a sinus rate of approximately 75 beats per minute and are dissociated from the wide-complex ventricular escape beat (***solid arrows***). Occasional AV nodal conduction of sinus beats occurs, resulting in intermittent, narrow complexes (***empty arrows***) with similar PR intervals.

coronary artery disease, and drug toxicity (digoxin, β-blockers). Permanent cardiac pacing is recommended, particularly if the bradycardia is symptomatic (syncope, presyncope, worsening of CHF), if pauses in the QRS exceed 3 seconds in duration, and/or the escape rate is less than 40 beats per minute. Even if the patient is asymptomatic at presentation, the natural history of the disease is for symptoms to occur with time; so a pacemaker is often recommended. If third-degree AV block occurs unexpectedly during surgery, then either atropine, an isoproterenol infusion (1–5 μg per minute), or transcutaneous pacing may maintain a sufficient rate until a transvenous pacemaker can be inserted.

Sinus Node Dysfunction

The sick sinus syndrome is caused by a failure of the SA node to either generate an impulse or transmit it to the atria. It may present as severe sinus bradycardia, sinus arrest, sinoatrial block and/or the tachycardia-bradycardia syndrome. Many patients with this disorder also have other conduction defects such as AV block and bundle branch block. The sick sinus syndrome most commonly presents in elderly individuals and can result from a number of different disorders. A sclerodegenerative process involving the SA node is the most common etiology but other causes include coronary artery disease, primary and secondary (amyloid, sarcoid, scleroderma) cardiomyopathies, hypertensive, rheumatic and congenital heart disease, mitral valve prolapse, familial form, and drugs (β-blockers, digoxin, quinidine, CCBs, lithium, amitryptyline, cimetidine, and the phenothiazines). Sinus node dysfunction is the primary indication for a permanent pacemaker in the United States. Before recommending permanent pacing, an attempt should be made to correlate the sinus node dysfunction with the patient's symptoms. Documented symptomatic bradycardia is a definite indication for permanent pacing. While opinions differ on the need for pacing in a patient with no definite correlation between symptoms and sinus function, it would appear prudent to insert a temporary transvenous pacemaker in any patient with this disorder, and a history of syncope, who present for all but the most minor surgery. The individual aspects of the sick sinus syndrome are described in the following:

Sinus Pause or Arrest and Exit Block

Sinus pause or arrest is a transient failure of the SA node to generate an impulse. It can occasionally occur in healthy young individuals and trained athletes. Sinus exit block is a failure of the sinus impulse to exit the SA node and excite the atrium. As with AV block it can be categorized as first degree (conduction time prolonged, but normal 1:1 response), second-degree (some of the impulses fail to capture the atrium), or third degree (complete failure of sinoatrial conduction). Only second-degree exit block can be diagnosed by the surface ECG.

Tachycardia-Bradycardia Syndrome

This syndrome is characterized by spontaneous periods of bradycardia, not caused by drugs and innapropriate for the physiologic circumstance, interrupted by episodes of tachycardia which may be AF or A-flutter (40% of cases), atrial tachycardia, AVNRT, ventricular tachycardia, or fibrillation. The disease frequently follows an intermittent and unpredictable course. Pharmacologic treatment of the tachycardia can exacerbate the bradycardia. Pacing is indicated if the bradycardia produces symptoms (syncope, worsening CHF) and indicated in patients who require chronic antiarrhythmic therapy to treat the tachycardia. There is evidence that dual-chamber pacing can significantly reduce or prevent episodes of recurrent AF and improve survival. Thromboembolism has been reported in up to 20% of patients with this disorder, (particularly in association with AF), and anticoagulation should be considered.

BIBLIOGRAPHY

Braunwald E, editor: Heart disease, ed 5, Philadelphia, 1997, WB Saunders Company.

Ganz LI, Friedman PL: Supraventricular tachycardias, *N Engl J Med* 332(5):162–173, 1995.

Goldman L: Cardiac risks and complications of noncardiac surgery, *Ann Intern Med* 98:504–513, 1983.

Kusumoto FM, Goldschlager N: Cardiac pacing, *N Engl J Med* 334(2):89–98, 1996.

Lynch C, editor: *Clinical cardiac electrophysiology: perioperative considerations*, Philadelphia, 1994, JB Lippincott.

Pires LA, et al: Arrhythmias and conduction disturbances after coronary artery bypass graft surgery: epidemiology, management and prognosis, *Am Heart J* 129:799–808, 1995.

Prystowsky EN, et al: Management of patients with atrial fibrillation, *Circulation* 93(6):1262–1277, 1996.

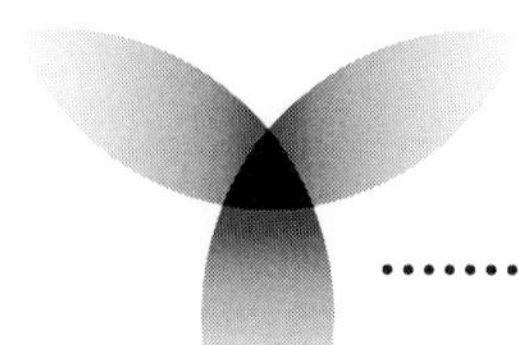
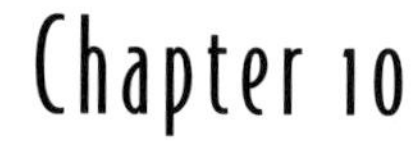

Chapter 10

Pericardial Disease

Alison S. Carr, MB BS, FRCA

Pericardial disease covers a spectrum of pathology from acute pericarditis, with or without pericardial effusion, to cardiac tamponade and chronic constrictive pericarditis. Pericardial disease may present insidiously with minimal symptoms or may present abruptly with severely disabling symptoms, leading rapidly to death, unless appropriate intervention occurs.

There are several reasons why the perioperative physician is increasingly likely to encounter patients with pericardial disease. Patients with malignant neoplasms, end-stage renal disease, and connective tissue disease are living longer and may well require surgery for other manifestations of their disease process. Pericardial disease may arise from complications of modern therapy, such as postcardiac surgery, and secondary to invasive diagnostic procedures. Drug therapy, such as the use of procainamide, phenytoin, hydralazine, and anticoagulants, is another source of pericardial disease. More cases of pericarditis and pericardial effusion are being diagnosed since the widespread introduction of echocardiography. In spite of this, surgery for pericardial disease, per se, is required in only a minority of these patients who have severe hemodynamic impairment or chronic pain.

The perioperative physician may encounter patients whose primary disease may be pericardial. More commonly, the disease of the pericardium represents the local manifestation of a systemic disease or distant malignancy. In treating these critically ill patients perioperatively, a knowledge of the pathophysiology of pericardial disease and its modification by anesthetics and other pharmacologic agents is required. In addition, when the pericardial disease is part of a systemic disease process, it is important to consider how other manifestations of the underlying disease may be important perioperatively.

THE PERICARDIUM

The pericardium is a fibroserous structure with external fibrous and internal serous components. The serous portion is composed of two layers, visceral and parietal. A small amount, (approximately 50 mls) of pericardial fluid, an ultrafiltrate of plasma, is housed in the pericardial space. The visceral pericardium, which is also called the epicardium, covers the heart and the first 3 cm of the great vessels. It is then reflected to form the outer parietal layer. Parietal pericardium lines the inner surface of the fibrous pericardium. The anterior and lateral parts of the fibrous/parietal layer contact the mediastinal pleurae and the inferior part is attached to the diaphragm. Reflections of the serous pericardium give rise to the pericardial sinuses. The pericardium overlying the left atrium is functionally isolated from the rest of the pericardium and is infrequently involved in pericardial effusions, generally being included only in large ones. Intrapericardial pressure is approximately 0 mm Hg or slightly subatmospheric, decreasing on inspiration and increasing on expiration, similar to intrapleural pressure.

Although not an essential structure, the pericardium has several physiologic functions. It separates the heart from other structures and prevents adhesions. It permits smooth cardiac contraction due to the smooth surface in contact with the myocardium. It may prevent the heart from acute dilatation and helps maintain normal ventricular compliance. It also provides the lymphatic drainage of the myocardium. It may retard the spread of infection and inflammatory disease between the intrapericardial contents and the mediastinum. Patients with congenital absence of the pericardium or pericardiectomy, however, do not suffer from an increased incidence of cardiac or mediastinal disease. Thus, the true role of the pericardium is unknown.

ACUTE PERICARDITIS

Etiology

Acute pericarditis is an inflammatory process of the pericardium, which can result from a variety of causes, the most common of which are idiopathic (acute benign pericarditis), infectious (bacterial, tuberculous, viral, fungal, amebic), postmyocardial infarction (MI) (rapid-onset or delayed-onset Dressler's syndrome), postcardiotomy, neoplastic (primary or metastatic), systemic diseases (rheumatoid arthritis, systemic lupus erythematosus, scleroderma, mixed connective tissue disease, polymyositis, dermatomyositis), thyroid disease, posttraumatic, uremic, postradiation, and drug-induced (procainamide, hydralazine, anticoagulants, penicillin). Acute, benign pericarditis is the most common cause and is thought to be caused by viral infection.

Viral pericarditis is treated symptomatically with salicylates, nonsteroidal antiinflammatory drugs, and short courses of corticosteroids. The response to treatment is usually fairly rapid. Recurrent (relapsing) pericarditis is poorly understood and may result from any of the causes of acute pericarditis. It may be idiopathic or may follow cardiac surgery, cardiac trauma, MI, or intrapericardial bleeding. Management with salicylates, nonsteroidal antiinflammatory drugs, and then steroids, usually leads to clinical improvement.

Anesthesiologists are most likely to encounter patients with acute pericarditis caused by MI, the postcardiotomy syndrome, or uremia. Acute pericarditis complicates 15% to 20% cases of acute MI and can be detected by the appearance of a pericardial friction rub. Acute pericarditis may develop during the first week after MI or may develop 2 to 3 months later (Dressler's syndrome).

In the postcardiotomy syndrome, acute pericarditis develops between 10 days and 2 to 3 months after cardiac surgery or cardiac trauma, and is probably immune-mediated. Its prevalence varies from 5% to 30% in reported series. A pericardial friction rub is frequently heard and many cases are complicated by the development of a pericardial effusion. The characteristic electrocardiogram (ECG) findings (described further on) are present in less than 50% of cases. Cardiac tamponade is more likely to develop if the patient is taking anticoagulants. Both Dressler's syndrome and the postcardiotomy syndrome tend to be relapsing: chest pain, pericardial rub, pyrexia, frequently, the development of a pericardial effusion mark relapses.

Uremic pericarditis is present in up to 20% of patients with end-stage renal failure treated with hemodialysis or peritoneal dialysis. Classical pleuritic chest pain is less commonly present in uremic pericarditis than in idiopathic pericarditis. Pericardial effusion is a common complication of uremic pericarditis: approximately two thirds of patients with chronic renal failure have a pericardial effusion detected by echocardiography, although only one third of these are symptomatic.

Preoperative Evaluation

The most common symptom of acute pericarditis is chest pain. The patient will complain of severe, sharp, chest pain of sudden onset, centrally located, radiating to the back and to the scapulae. The pain is frequently accentuated by respiration, exacerbated by lying supine, and relieved by sitting up and leaning forward. When evaluating a patient with acute pericarditis perioperatively, the most important objective is to distinguish the chest pain from that of myocardial ischemia. A number of important differentiating factors should be sought from the history, examination, and investigations (Table 10-1).

On auscultating the chest, a pericardial friction rub may be heard over the precordium, usually best heard in the third and fourth intercostal spaces adjacent to the

Table 10-1. The Differences Between Ischemic and Pericardial Pain

CHARACTERISTIC	ISCHEMIC (MYOCARDIAL)	PERICARDIAL
Nature	Constrictive, crushing	Sharp, often pleuritic, varying in intensity
Site	Central	Precordial but less precisely retrosternal
Radiation	Classically to left arm, neck, jaw, or tongue	To trapezius ridge
Duration	Less than 30 mins and usually intermittent if angina. May last hours if MI.	Persistent, often lasting for several days
Severity	Severe and crushing in MI	Varies: may be very severe and crushing as in MI
Pericardial rub	Present only when complicated by pericarditis	Almost always present
Effect of respiration	No effect	Exacerbated by inspiration
Effect of posture	No effect	Exacerbated by lying supine and relieved by sitting up and leaning forward
Effect of coughing	No effect	Exacerbated
Effect of swallowing	No effect	Exacerbated
Effect of body movement	No effect	Tends to be exacerbated
Effect of nitroglycerin	Often relieved	No effect
Heart rhythm	Frequent conduction disturbances and arrhythmias	Sinus rhythm in 90% cases, arrhythmias rare if no associated ischemic heart disease
ECG changes	Localized ST segment elevation in MI with reciprocal depression. Q waves and T wave inversion associated with ST segment elevation in MI.	Widespread concordant concave ST-segment elevation without reciprocal depression; return of ST-segment to baseline with later T-wave change, T-wave negativity and then return to normal. Absent Q waves and T-wave inversion associated with ST-segment elevation.
Associated symptoms	Dyspnea, diaphoresis, nausea and vomiting	Fever, dyspnea
Cardiac enzymes	Elevated in MI	Unchanged

MI = myocardial infarction

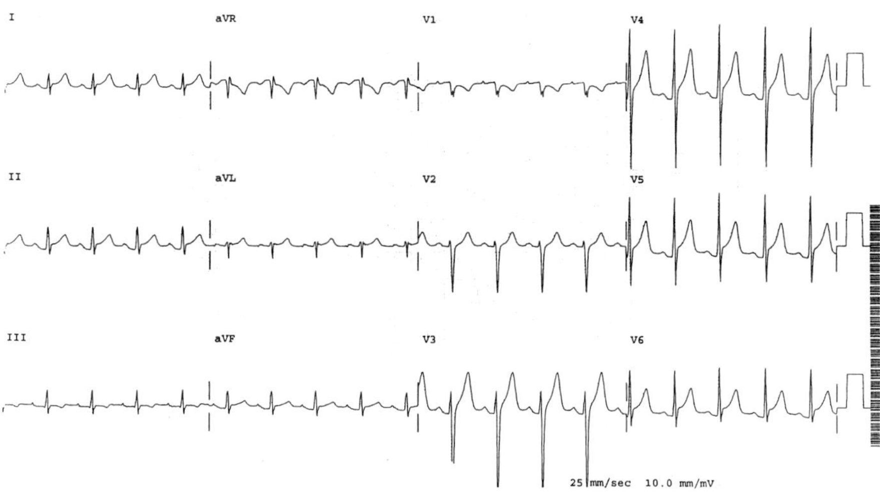

Figure 10-1
An ECG in a patient with acute pericarditis. ST-segment elevation is present in most ECG leads, particularly those derived from the epicardium of the left ventricle—mainly I, II, aVL, aVF, and V_3–V_6. Lead aVR and lead V_1 show ST-segment depression.

sternum. The rub has three classic components: atrial systole, ventricular systole, and ventricular diastole. It is best heard by asking the patient to lean forward. The rub may be transient, lasting a few hours or may be present for days.

Typical ECG findings are virtually diagnostic. There is ST segment elevation in most ECG leads, particularly those derived from the epicardium of the left ventricle—mainly I, II, aVL, aVF, and V_3–V_6. Lead aVR, consistently, and lead V_1, usually, show ST segment depression. Most patients with pericarditis are in sinus rhythm. However, a few may have rhythm disturbances such as sinus tachycardia, atrial fibrillation, and atrial flutter. An ECG from a patient with acute pericarditis is shown in Figure 10-1.

Acute pericarditis may be complicated by the development of a pericardial effusion. A pericardial effusion can result from most causes of pericardial disease: for example, idiopathic, trauma, malignancy, infection, inflammation, and uremia. Pericardial fluid accumulates when fluid is produced by the pericardium at a faster rate than it is reabsorbed. The pericardial fluid may be serous, purulent, or hemorrhagic, or a combination of these. In assessment of the pericardial effusion, a preliminary simple investigation is a chest radiogram. Cardiac size will be normal, however, if the pericardial effusion is less than a few hundred milliliters. Larger effusions produce cardiomegaly on chest radiogram and the heart may adopt a water-bottle shape. Two-dimensional and time-motion echocardiography are sensitive and specific in the detection of pericardial effusions. They are widely available and can be performed at bedside. Pericardial effusions are also readily diagnosed by computerized tomography (CT) and by magnetic resonance imaging (MRI). Magnetic resonance imaging

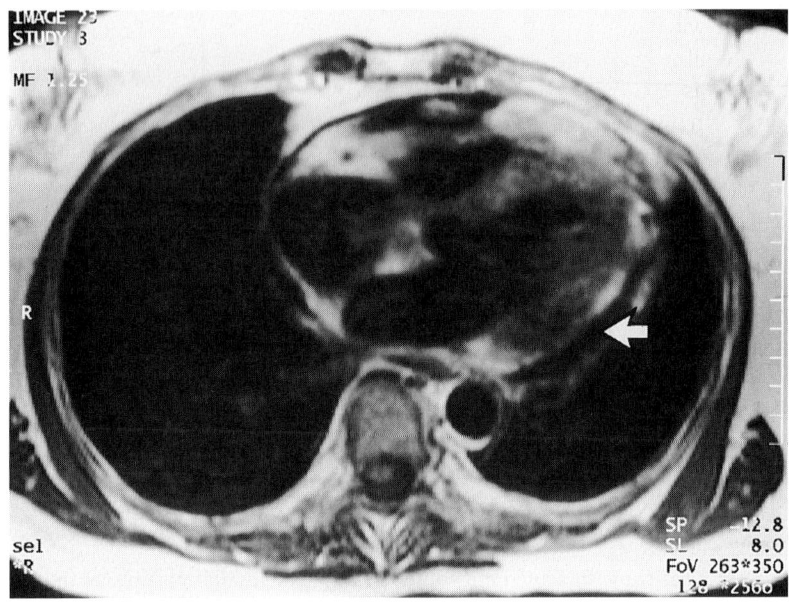

Figure 10-2
Magnetic resonance image in a patient with a pericardial effusion. Kindly provided by Dr Jayashree Parekh.

is highly sensitive in the detection of small pericardial effusions, even when no effusion is evident on echocardiography. Magnetic resonance imaging outlines the distribution of the pericardial effusion well and provides an estimate of pericardial fluid volume comparable with an echocardiographic estimate. Figure 10-2 shows an MR image, which clearly illustrates the presence of a pericardial effusion. Magnetic resonance imaging has an advantage over CT in that images of the pericardium can be taken in more planes. Newer diagnostic approaches include pericardioscopy and thoracoscopy, followed by pericardial and epicardial biopsy.

Perioperative Management

There are several indications for surgery in acute pericarditis. Purulent pericarditis requires antibiotic therapy and pericardiocentesis. If acute pericarditis is complicated by a pericardial effusion, it may require surgical drainage for diagnostic purposes or to relieve symptoms. In patients with acute pericarditis who do not respond to medical therapy, or who are unable to discontinue adrenal steroids after 6 months to 1 year, or who cannot tolerate the side effects of the adrenal steroids, pericardiectomy is the treatment of choice. If pericardiectomy is performed, it should be complete or further relapses may follow. Complete pericardiectomy provides tissue for diagnosis and avoids the possibility of cardiac tamponade or constrictive pericarditis complicating the disease.

Patients with acute pericarditis usually tolerate anesthesia and surgery well. Cardiac function will be unaffected in acute pericarditis per se, unless there is associated myocardial ischemia, or if a pericardial effusion causes hemodynamic compromise. Patients with acute pericarditis may require surgery for complications such as cardiac tamponade and constrictive pericarditis. These conditions pose great challenges to the perioperative physician and are described below.

CARDIAC TAMPONADE

Pathophysiology

Cardiac tamponade is defined as the cardiovascular syndrome caused by impairment of diastolic filling of the heart, caused by an unchecked rise in intrapericardial pressure. Elevated intrapericardial pressures result from the accumulation of fluid in the intrapericardial space.

In the absence of a pericardial effusion, the parietal pericardium is in direct contact with the heart and is able to restrain the heart chambers from undergoing acute enlargement. In the presence of a pericardial effusion, the parietal pericardium loses contact with the heart chambers and a uniform pressure in the pericardial space is transmitted equally to all heart chambers. When this pressure is small (less than 5 mm Hg), the heart is able to fill normally because diastolic pressure exceeds intrapericardial pressure. When the intrapericardial pressure approaches or equals the diastolic pressure in the heart, diastolic expansion of the heart chambers becomes limited. Consequently, chamber size is reduced and stroke volume and cardiac output fall. The effects of tamponade are first seen when the intrapericardial pressure briefly exceeds the pressure in a cardiac chamber. This is manifest by transient inward motion of the wall of the chamber, which is termed "collapse." Cardiac chamber size becomes more limited as the intrapericardial pressure continues to rise until severe tamponade; then, the heart chamber sizes, the stroke volume, and the cardiac output are reduced to approximately 50% of their normal values. Intrapericardial pressures of 15 to 20 mm Hg are associated with severe hemodynamic disturbances.

As tamponade increases, the ventricles fill only during atrial systole, particularly, at rapid heart rates. The right-atrial-pressure waveform becomes elevated with amputation of the Y descent and preservation of the X descent, consistent with the inflow into the right atrium, occurring mainly in systole. In cardiac tamponade, there is equalization of the right atrial, pulmonary artery end-diastolic, and pulmonary capillary wedge pressures (right and left ventricular end-diastolic pressures). Figure 10-3 illustrates the equalization of right and left ventricular pressure along with intrapericardial pressure in a patient with cardiac tamponade. At each site, diastolic pressure is elevated (to 17 mm Hg) and all three pressures are equal. In the ventricular pressure tracing, an early diastolic dip is absent.

Compensatory mechanisms are activated by stimulation of the sympathetic nervous system in an attempt to maintain cardiac output and blood pressure by peripheral vasoconstriction and tachycardia. While pressures in the central veins exceed right ventricular end-diastolic pressures, cardiac output and blood pressure are

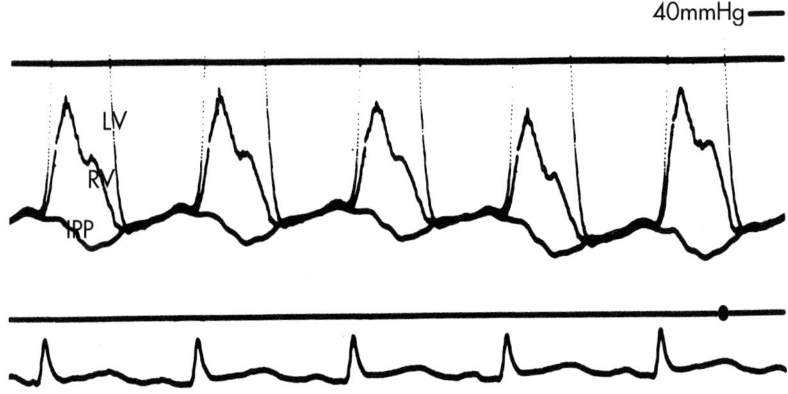

Figure 10-3
Simultaneous recordings of right (RV) and left (LV) ventricular pressure along with intrapericardial pressure (IPP) in a patient with cardiac tamponade. (From Reddy PS, et al. Cardiac tamponade: hemodynamic observations in man, *Circulation*; 58:265, 1978. Reproduced with permission from the authors and from the American Heart Association.)

preserved. As intrapericardial pressure rises further, the compensatory mechanisms fail to compensate, and cardiovascular collapse ensues. Hemodynamic changes in cardiac tamponade depend on the rapidity and the amount of accumulation of pericardial fluid. Cardiac tamponade can result from the rapid accumulation of a small volume of fluid in the pericardium (for example, 200 ml) or from the gradual accumulation of a large volume of pericardial fluid (for example, 700 ml). In either case, the intrapericardial pressure rises when the elastic limit of the pericardium is overcome. Figure 10-4 shows the pericardial pressure–volume relationship. The steepness of the pericardial pressure–volume relationship after the inflection point, shows that even small increases or decreases in pericardial fluid volume near this point have enormous effects on the intrapericardial pressure.

Etiology

The perioperative physician may encounter patients with cardiac tamponade arising from a variety of clinical conditions. Trauma to the heart or proximal aorta, either blunt or penetrating, can result in intrapericardial bleeding, producing hemopericardium. Intrapericardial bleeding can occur in the immediate postoperative period following cardiac surgery or later, in association with postoperative pericarditis. A postcardiotomy syndrome can occur many months after cardiac surgery. Common causes of cardiac tamponade in medical patients are metastatic malignant tumor, idiopathic pericarditis, renal failure, infections (bacterial and tuberculous), connective tissue disease, anticoagulants, and complications of diagnostic procedures. Spread of metastatic cancer to the pericardium is the most common cause of cardiac tamponade in medical inpatients. Lung cancer, breast cancer, and the hematologic

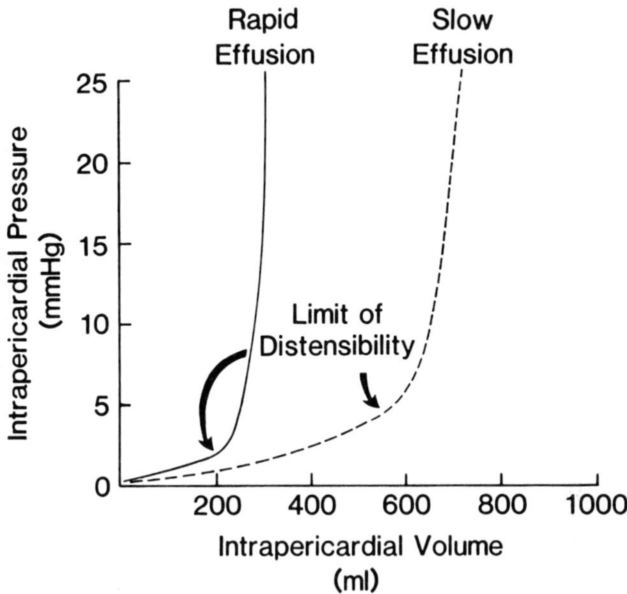

Figure 10-4

Pericardial pressure–volume relationship. (From Ameli S, Shah PK: Cardiac tamponade—pathophysiology, diagnosis and management, *Cardiol Clin* November; 9(4):666, 1991, with permission from the authors and from WB Saunders Company.)

malignancies account for approximately three quarters of the cases. Cardiac tamponade can result as a complication of invasive procedures in the cardiac catheterization laboratory, for example, from perforation of the heart during balloon valvuloplasty, endomyocardial biopsy, temporary ventricular pacing, coronary angioplasty, and from high-pressure angiographic injections as well.

Preoperative Evaluation

What signs and symptoms should be looked for in a patient suspected of developing cardiac tamponade? In 1935, Beck described two triads for cardiac compression caused by tamponade. The acute tamponade triad consisted of decreasing arterial pressure, increasing venous pressure, and a small, quiet heart. The chronic tamponade triad consisted of high-venous pressure, ascites, and a small, quiet heart. Beck's triad for acute cardiac tamponade was based largely on the effects of intrapericardial bleeding from cardiac trauma or aortic or cardiac rupture. Patients with more gradual onset of symptoms (most medical patients) develop the pleural effusion slowly. Effusion may be extensive before cardiac tamponade develops. Often, these patients lack one or more of the signs in Beck's triad; they frequently have a large cardiac silhouette on chest radiogram and may not be hypotensive.

More recently, a clinical definition of tamponade was proposed consisting of moderate or extensive pericardial effusion, elevated systemic venous pressure, dyspnea and tachycardia, relief of venous hypertension, pulsus paradoxus and dyspnea, and tachycardia by pericardial fluid drainage. These changes are more frequently present in patients with cardiac tamponade than the symptoms or signs in Beck's triad. The diagnosis of cardiac tamponade can be made when a patient with a large or moderately large pericardial effusion has elevated systemic venous pressure, dyspnea, tachypnea, orthopnea, diaphoresis, and tachycardia with a paradoxical arterial pulse. In evaluating a patient with cardiac tamponade, these symptoms should be sought.

Paradoxic pulse is the most specific physical sign of cardiac tamponade. The paradoxic arterial pulse may be defined as an inspiratory decline of systolic arterial pressure exceeding 10 mm Hg. It is present in nearly every case of cardiac tamponade. Pulsus paradoxus can be diagnosed easily from the waveform of an indwelling arterial catheter, as shown in Figure 10-5. It may also be diagnosed by auscultation of Korotkoff's sounds while a blood pressure cuff is slowly deflated. Two blood pressures are recorded: the blood pressure at which Korotkoff's sounds are first present (occurring during expiration), and the first blood pressure at which Korotkoff's sounds are present throughout the respiratory cycle. The difference between the blood pressures recorded provides the measure of paradox. Pulsus paradoxus may be absent in cardiac tamponade if there is an atrial septal defect, obstruction to the pulmonary artery, left ventricular dysfunction (when left ventricular end-diastolic pressure exceeds intrapericardial pressure), or severe aortic regurgitation. Positive-pressure ventilation may mask the signs of pulsus paradoxus. When the cardiac tamponade is distributed over the right atrium only, there may be no pulsus paradoxus. Regional cardiac tamponade is most common after cardiac surgery. Several other signs are suggestive of cardiac tamponade: visibly distended neck veins, an absent Kussmaul's sign (a rise in venous pressure with inspiration), and faint heart sounds (although they may be normal). The cardiac apical pulse is usually not palpable, and cardiac murmurs and gallop rhythm are usually absent. Removal of the pericardial collection relieves symptoms by reducing intrapericardial pressure below the right atrial pressure and facilitating venous return. Once pericardial pressure falls below the right atrial pressure, no further hemodynamic improvement results from withdrawal of further fluid.

The most common heart rhythm seen in cardiac tamponade is sinus rhythm. The ECG may show a low-voltage QRS complex, although this is not a consistent finding, electrical alternans, and total alternans. In electrical alternans, there is a beat-to-beat alternation of QRS voltage caused by an abnormal mobility of the heart within the pericardial space. The heart swings on alternate beats between two positions, producing beat-to-beat change in the QRS axis and in the QRS voltage in a given lead. The above ECG findings have, however, recently been shown to be neither specific nor sensitive enough to diagnose pericardial effusion or cardiac tamponade on their own.

Cardiac catheterization and echocardiographic criteria remain the gold standards for diagnosing pericardial effusion and cardiac tamponade. Cardiac catheterization allows documentation of a significant improvement in hemodynamic parameters upon drainage of a cardiac tamponade. Echocardiography, being less invasive, is

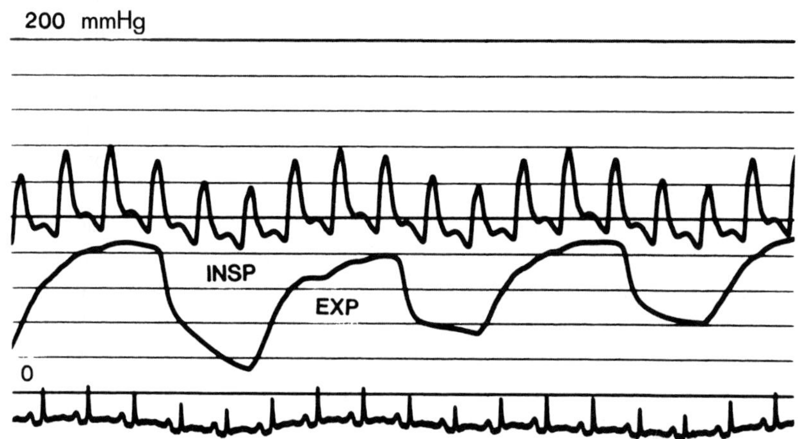

Figure 10-5
Pulsus paradoxus. During inspiration, arterial systolic pressure falls by more than 12 mm Hg. Vertical axis represents systemic arterial pressure. INSP, inspiration; EXP, expiration. (From Reddy PS, Curtiss EI: Cardiac tamponade, *Cardiol Clin* November; 8(4):628, 1990, with permission from the authors and from WB Saunders Company.)

usually the test of choice in making these diagnoses. Echocardiographic features of cardiac tamponade include:

- right atrial compression and right atrial diastolic collapse
- right ventricular diastolic collapse
- abnormal inspiratory increase of right ventricular dimensions and abnormal inspiratory decrease of left ventricular dimensions
- exaggerated inspiratory increase of blood flow velocity through the tricuspid valve, and exaggerated inspiratory decrease of mitral-valve-flow-velocity
- dilated inferior vena cava with lack of inspiratory collapse and
- a swinging heart.

Right-atrial and right-ventricular diastolic collapse are perhaps the most commonly used echocardiographic evidence of cardiac tamponade. Figure 10-6 illustrates right ventricular diastolic collapse in cardiac tamponade by M-mode echocardiography and by two-dimensional echocardiography in the short-axis view. A large pericardial effusion surrounds the anterior and lateral aspects of the heart.

Preanesthetic Preparation

Definitive management of cardiac tamponade is by drainage of the pericardial fluid. The decision to proceed with pericardial drainage will depend on the clinical status of the patient and the etiology of the effusion. If hemodynamic compromise is marked

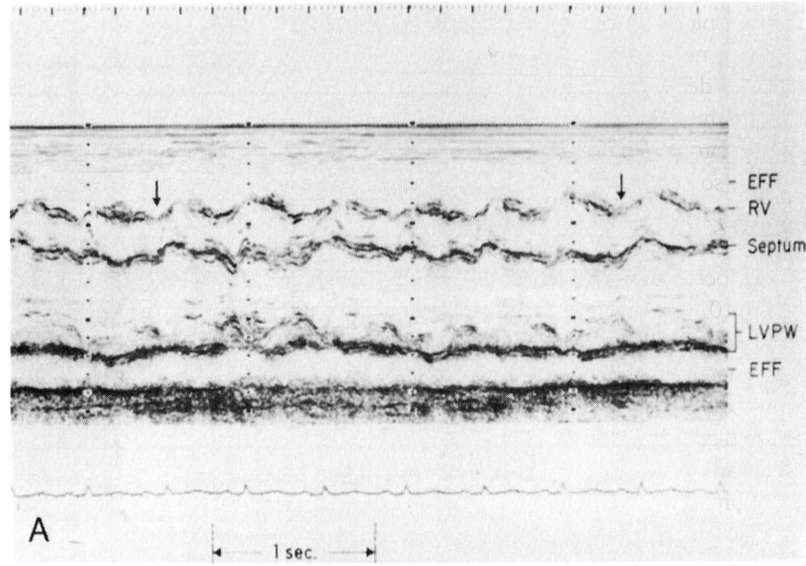

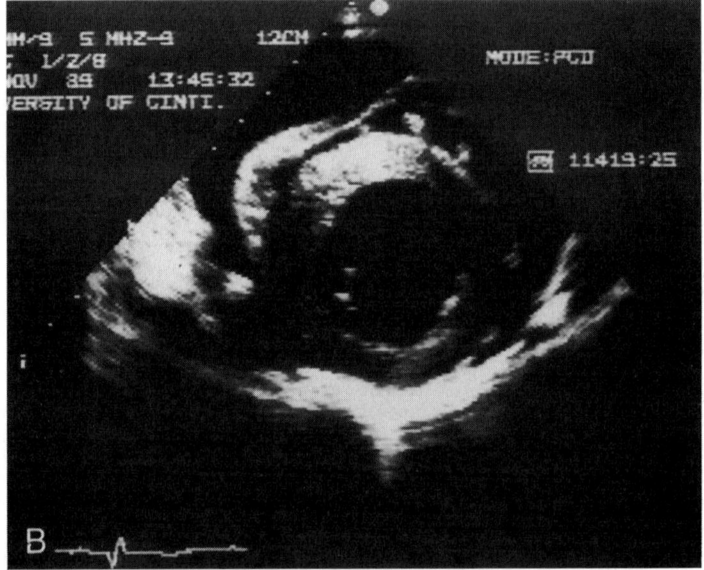

Figure 10-6

Right ventricular diastolic collapse in cardiac tamponade. **A.** M-mode echocardiogram. Note posterior motion of right ventricle (*RV*) free wall during diastole (*arrow*) and the abnormal septal motion. EFF, effusion; LVPW, left ventricular posterior wall. **B.** Two-dimensional echocardiogram in the short-axis view showing early diastolic collapse of right ventricle. A large pericardial effusion surrounds anterior and lateral aspects. (From Hoit BD: Imaging the pericardium, *Cardiol Clin* November 8(4):592, 1990 with permission from the author and from WB Saunders Company.)

with falling blood pressure and impaired consciousness or severe dyspnea, pericardial drainage by needle pericardiocentesis should be performed emergently, regardless of etiology, or death will follow. Intrapericardial drainage should be done under local anesthetic through a percutaneous pericardiocentesis, through a subcostal or subxiphoid approach. Pericardiocentesis is best performed in the cardiac catheterization laboratory so that the diagnosis can be established, and improvements in hemodynamic parameters can be documented on drainage of the pericardial effusion. If required emergently, however, pericardiocentesis should be performed at bedside under echocardiographic guidance. Removal of only a small amount of pericardial fluid (50–100 ml) results in marked clinical improvement and restores hemodynamic stability; after removal, a more definitive drainage procedure may be undertaken under general anesthesia. Figure 10-7 illustrates the hemodynamic improvements which accompanied aspiration of pericardial fluid in a patient with cardiac tamponade resulting from uremia. Marked hemodynamic improvements occurred until intrapericardial pressure fell below right atrial pressure, at which point, ventricular diastolic pressures and the inspiratory fall in arterial systolic pressure did not change.

Cardiac tamponade may now be diagnosed well before hemodynamic compromise requiring emergent pericardial drainage is necessary. By definition, cardiac tamponade causes impairment of diastolic filling of the heart. This can be seen on echocardiography at an earlier stage than diagnosis of cardiac tamponade can be made from clinical symptoms and signs. This poses a dilemma over when to drain a pericardial effusion. Echocardiographic Doppler criteria for cardiac tamponade should probably not be used on their own to decide when to perform pericardial drainage, because they may be too sensitive. The benefit of early diagnosis of tamponade by echocardiography is that, in combination with the clinical picture and known etiology of the pericardial effusion, a decision can be made to drain or to treat medically, and observe the tamponade closely with echocardiography.

Profound hypotension and death have been reported following general anesthesia, intermittent positive-pressure ventilation of the lungs in patients with severe hemodynamic compromise from cardiac tamponade. Anesthesia in these cases can produce myocardial depression, peripheral vasodilatation, and reduced venous return. Myocardial ischemia can result from reduced coronary blood flow because of elevated transmural pressures in the heart, confounded by reduced coronary filling due to hypotension and tachycardia.

How should the perioperative physician improve the patient's clinical condition in preparation for surgical intervention? If the hemodynamic consequences of the tamponade are not severe, time taken to resuscitate the patient preoperatively will optimize the clinical condition of the patient for general anesthesia. Invasive cardiovascular monitoring should be started as soon as possible. An arterial line, a central venous line, and a pulmonary artery catheter (if necessary), should be inserted and baseline measurements obtained. A pulmonary artery catheter is not usually required. However, it can show equalization of diastolic pressures when the diagnosis of tamponade is uncertain.

Several physiologic manipulations may improve the clinical condition. Blood volume expansion is of key importance to maintain the venoatrial gradients and cardiac

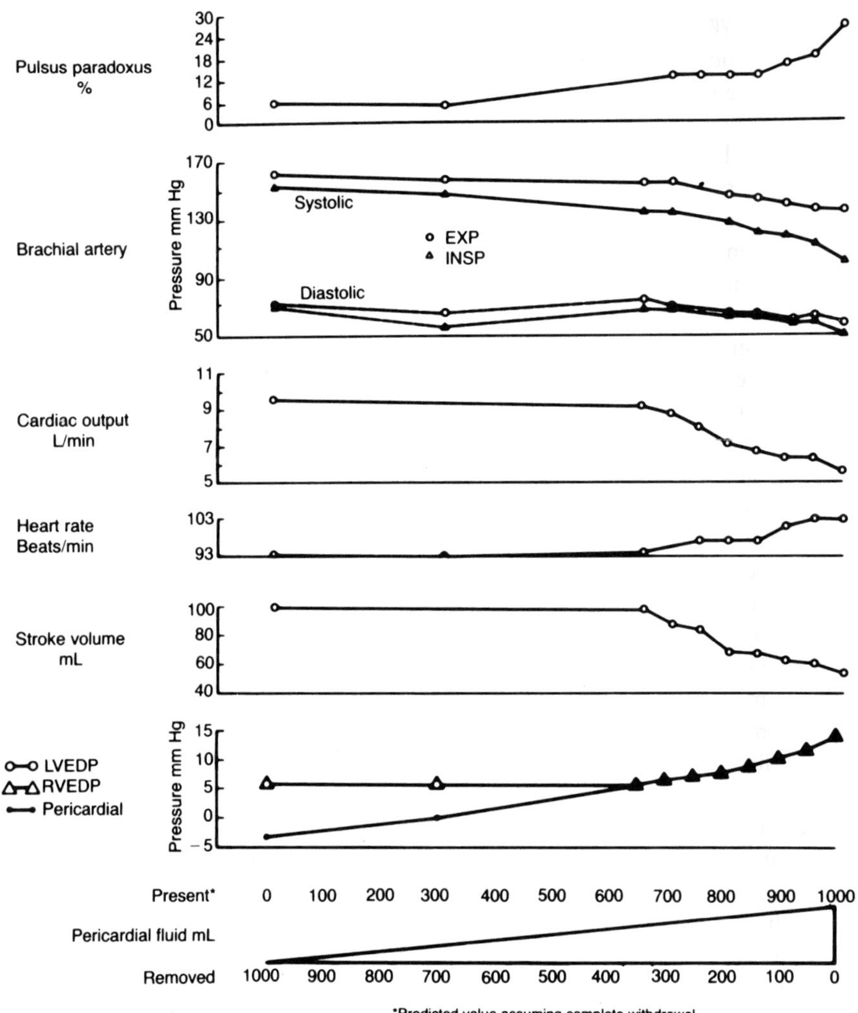

Figure 10-7
Hemodynamic changes during pericardial fluid aspiration in a patient with pericarditis due to uremia. (From Reddy PS: Hemodynamics of cardiac tamponade in man. In Reddy PS, Leon DF, Shaver JA, editors: *Pericardial disease*. New York, 1982, Raven Press, p. 177, with permission.)

output. Inotropes will increase stroke volume and/or support systemic vascular resistance by systemic vasoconstriction. Agents to reduce afterload may improve cardiac output in patients who have adequate intravascular volume replacement. Atropine may be required to offset vagal reflexes provoked by stretching of the pericardium by the effusion. Metabolic acidosis caused by low cardiac output, should be treated by intravenous sodium bicarbonate to improve cardiac contractility. Frequent blood gas analyses should be measured during correction.

Intraoperative Management

These manipulations are also important if general anesthesia has to be induced in the presence of hemodynamic compromise, where temporary drainage of the cardiac tamponade has not been successful. Continuous monitoring of intraarterial pressure and central venous pressure should be instituted before induction of general anesthesia. Cardiovascular stability at induction may be maintained by the use of anesthetic agents such as ketamine and etomidate. These drugs do not greatly decrease venous return or cause myocardial depression. Ketamine may be the drug of choice, although it will depress the myocardium and impair hemodynamics if used in the presence of maximal sympathetic outflow and hypovolemia. Positive-pressure ventilation should be avoided, if possible, until pericardial drainage has relieved the tamponade. Otherwise, it will increase the intrathoracic pressure and further reduce venous return and cardiac filling. If artificial ventilation of the lungs is required, small tidal volumes and a fast respiratory rate should be used. Positive end-expiratory pressure (PEEP) is preferably not used, although if vital to maintain oxygenation in the presence of coexistent pulmonary pathology, PEEP with a fast respiratory rate is favored. Coughing or straining during induction should also be avoided because this will also reduce venous return. If hemodynamic improvement has been obtained by a small pericardiocentesis under local anesthesia, high-dose opioids, midazolam, and pancuronium could be used to induce anesthesia for more definitive surgical drainage. Other muscle relaxants with minimal effects on the circulation may be used, such as *cis*-atracurium besylate, vecuronium, or rocuronium. Filling pressures should be maintained and bradycardia avoided. Transesophageal echocardiography can provide useful intraoperative information on the adequacy of venous return, the volume status of the heart, and the contractility of the ventricles to guide the anesthesiologist in the intraoperative management. Some patients with malignant tamponade will have received chemotherapy (i.e., doxorubicin) and may have an element of cardiomyopathy, which can confound the hemodynamic instability on induction of anesthesia. A surgeon must be present with the necessary equipment to perform emergency pericardiocentesis or sternotomy, in the event of hemodynamic collapse after induction of general anesthesia. If ventricular fibrillation occurs, a higher voltage may be required to defibrillate because of the presence of the pericardial fluid.

Subxiphoid pericardiostomy is commonly performed as a primary approach to intrapericardial drainage. An incision is made into the inferoanterior parietal pericardium and a tube inserted to allow drainage to the outside, initially. Drainage continues into the anterior mediastinum when the tube is removed. When cardiac tamponade results from trauma or postcardiac surgery, a pericardiotomy is usually performed under local or general anesthesia. Surgical drainage or pericardial biopsy may also be done for diagnostic purposes if the etiology is uncertain and the clinical condition is stable. If the tamponade recurs, it will usually indicate the need for pericardiectomy or a pericardial window under general anesthesia. To remove large amounts of pericardial fluid, a drainage procedure into the right or left pleura can be performed by thoracotomy or by median sternotomy. Recently, video-assisted thoracoscopy under general anesthetic, and tracheal intubation with a double-lumen endotracheal tube, has been used safely and effectively to visualize the whole pericardial and pleural cavity. The procedure is especially useful in patients with combined pericardial and pleural/lung diseases, to obtain pericardial fluid for diagnosis, to form an adequate pericardiopleural window in patients with massive pericardial effusion, and to perform pericardiectomy.

Postoperative Considerations

Significant hemodynamic improvement follows relief of pericardial tamponade; the postoperative course should be uneventful. It is important, however, to look for signs of recollection of the pericardial effusion in case the route of pericardial drainage becomes obstructed. Myocardial ischemia should be considered as a cause in a patient who fails to improve hemodynamically following drainage of the tamponade. Occasionally, pulmonary edema may occur after relief of cardiac tamponade. This arises because as the filling pressure of the right ventricle returns to normal, the systemic vascular resistance remains elevated. Improvement may occur after treatment with systemic vasodilators such as sodium nitroprusside.

CONSTRICTIVE PERICARDITIS

Pathophysiology

Constrictive pericarditis results from chronic fibrous thickening of the pericardial membrane, which is so contracted that it prevents the normal diastolic filling of the heart. The fibrotic process typically involves both the parietal and visceral pericardium, and the space between the two layers usually becomes obliterated. Rarely, an effusion may collect between the fibrotic layers of pericardium. Normally the disease progresses slowly over years. It has been known, however, to develop over as short a period as a few months. Most causes of acute pericarditis can also cause chronic pericarditis, although the most common cause is idiopathic. Patients having surgery for constrictive pericarditis often suffer from idiopathic, malignant, or uremic pericarditis.

Restriction of diastolic filling causes elevation and equilibration of pressures in the atria and ventricles. Ventricular filling is severely limited by pericardial constriction. Equalization of filling pressures of right and left sides of the heart result. Unlike cardiac tamponade, the heart is not compressed in early diastole and tends to relax quickly. This permits ventricular filling until the pericardial constricting limit is reached. The jugular venous pressure rises and pulse volume and cardiac output are reduced. Constrictive pericarditis affects filling of both sides of the heart. However, the predominant clinical picture resembles that of right heart failure.

Preoperative Evaluation

In evaluating a patient with constrictive pericarditis, the following symptoms should be sought: dyspnea on exertion, cough, orthopnea, fatigue and exhaustion, abdominal swelling, and discomfort. Chest pain is characteristically absent. Before operative treatment was available, patients with end-stage constrictive pericarditis invariably had significant ascites and peripheral edema. On examination, the neck veins are distended and Kussmaul's sign is present. The jugular venous-pressure waveform shows prominent X and Y descents. Pulsus paradoxus may be present. On examination of the precordium, there may be decreased activity, no murmurs, or a pericardial knock may be heard. There is hepatomegaly, ascites, and peripheral edema. There may also be pleural effusions as well. Unlike a patient with congestive heart failure, these latter-mentioned signs do not regress after diuretic therapy and a low-sodium diet. There may also be a history of previous pericarditis. The heart size is usually normal on chest radiogram and calcification of the cardiac outline may be present as illustrated in Figure 10-8. The ECG often shows a rather low-voltage QRS with an intraatrial conduction defect. T waves show nonspecific changes. Atrial arrhythmias are common in constrictive pericarditis because of involvement of the sinoatrial node. One quarter of patients have atrial fibrillation and 5% have atrial flutter.

The pressure waveform tracing, typical of constrictive pericarditis, shows the following abnormalities: an elevated, right atrial pressure; an early diastolic dip in right ventricular pressure, followed by a rapid rise to a plateau (the square-root pattern); elevated end-diastolic pressures in both ventricles; and equalization of mean right atrial pressure, right ventricular end-diastolic pressure, and pulmonary artery diastolic pressure. Echocardiography commonly shows pericardial thickening, a significant increase in left-ventricular-isovolumetric relaxation time, and an abrupt end to left ventricular filling. Figure 10-9 shows an M-mode echocardiographic tracing from a patient with constrictive pericarditis. In the absence of pericardial fluid, pericardial thickening may be difficult to define by echocardiography. In such a case, conventional CT can show pericardial thickening easily and can visualize calcification of the pericardium. Magnetic resonance imaging can also provide excellent visualization of thickened pericardium in constrictive pericarditis.

Constrictive pericarditis must be differentiated from restrictive cardiomyopathy before treatment by pericardiectomy. Both diseases have similar clinical presentations, overlapping hemodynamic profiles at cardiac catheterization, and are difficult to distinguish. Restrictive cardiomyopathy results from endomyocardial fibrosis or myocardial involvement by sarcoidosis, amyloidosis, or tumor, and is not amenable to treatment by pericardiectomy. Computerized tomography or MRI are useful in this respect by showing pericardial thickening (greater than 4 mm) in constrictive pericarditis, which excludes a diagnosis of restrictive cardiomyopathy.

Intraoperative Management

Surgical treatment of constrictive pericarditis is by pericardiectomy. Pericardiectomy for chronic constrictive pericarditis was first performed in 1928 in the United States by Churchill. It was the first cardiac operation to be widely practiced many years before extracorporeal circulation became available. In his account of the operation, Churchill reports that while he was freeing adhesions around the vena cava, he had to press on the right side of the heart and, at that time, the anesthetist reported that he could not obtain the blood pressure. Surgery may be complicated and associated with hemodynamic disturbances. Often, the pericardium is very scarred and adherent to the myocardium. The surgeon may need to manipulate the heart to a great

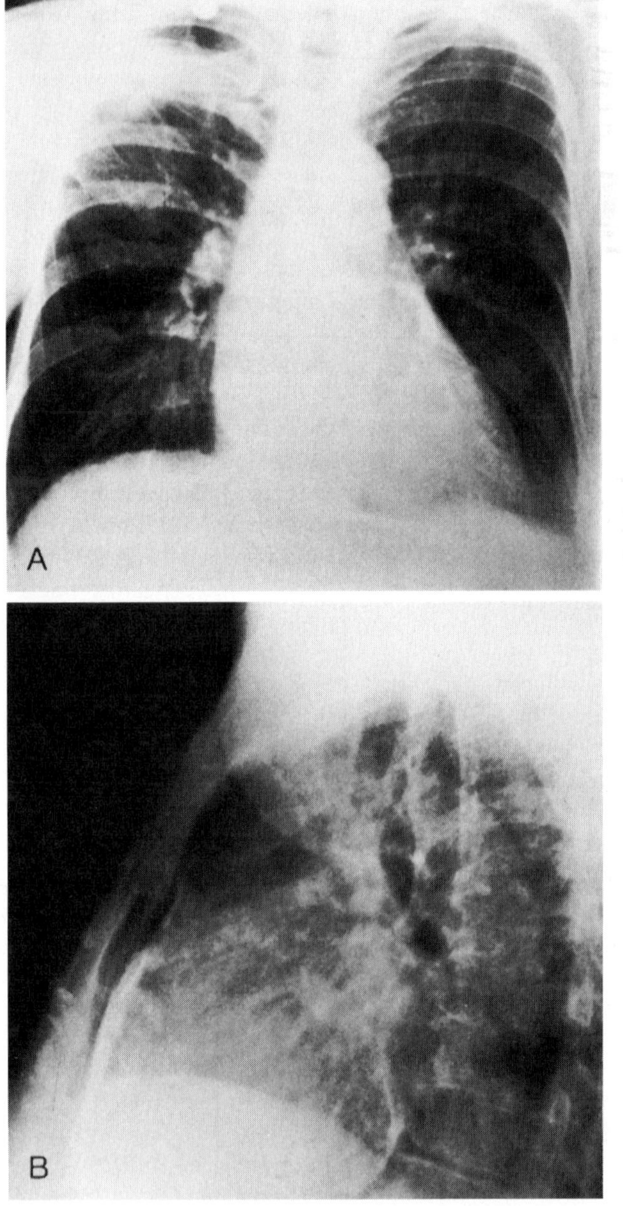

Figure 10-8
Posteroanterior (A) and lateral (B) chest radiograms demonstrating extensive calcification of the pericardium in a patient with idiopathic constrictive pericarditis. (From Tuna IC, Danielson GK: Surgical management of pericardial disease, *Cardiol Clin* November; 8(4):685, 1990 with permission from the author and WB Saunders Company.)

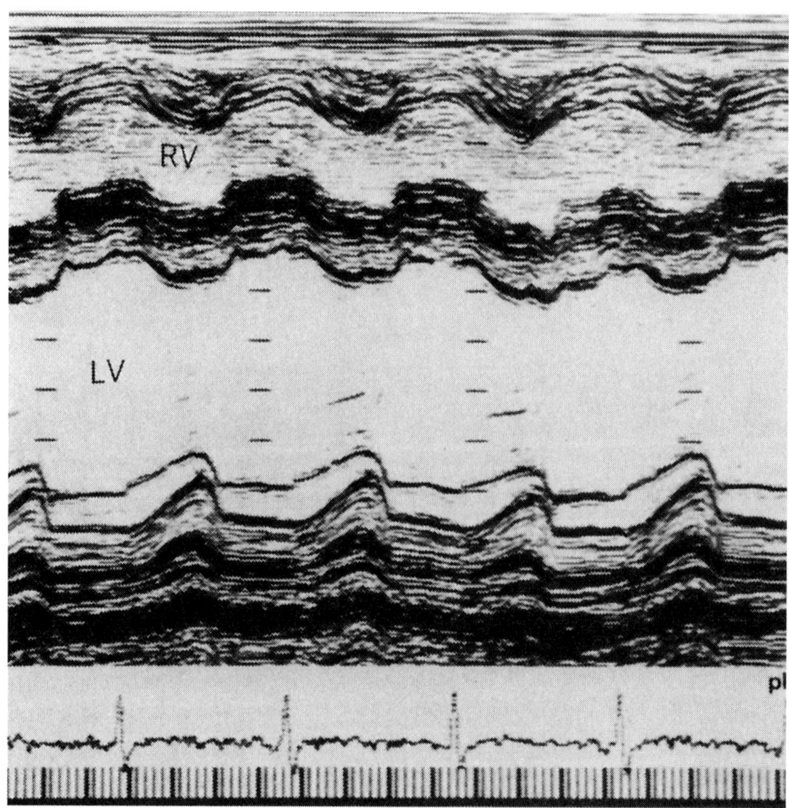

Figure 10-9
M-mode echocardiographic tracing from a patient with constrictive pericarditis. The thickened pericardium appears as multiple dense lines moving in concert (*arrow*). The posterior left ventricular (*LV*) wall shows a brisk early diastolic expansion followed by abrupt flattening. RV, right ventricle. (From Brockington GM, et al: Constrictive pericarditis, *Cardiol Clin* November; 8(4):652, 1990 with permission from the author and WB Saunders Company.)

extent. This may affect myocardial filling, leading to loss of cardiac output, and may provoke cardiac arrhythmias. Bleeding may be a problem, especially if the myocardium is penetrated. The coronary blood flow may be impaired by damage to the coronary arteries during pericardial dissection.

Before surgery, it is important to secure good intravascular access. Large-bore peripheral intravenous cannulae should be sited or a pulmonary artery catheter-introducer sheath may be used if peripheral venous access is poor. An arterial line and central venous catheter should be sited to allow continuous monitoring of hemodynamics. A pulmonary artery catheter may be useful in the intraoperative management of a patient with constrictive pericarditis, but it is not essential. Bleeding can be profuse, and blood products should be immediately at hand. A cell saver should be used if there are no contraindications. Cardiopulmonary bypass should be available in case there is massive hemorrhage or cardiovascular instability is produced during surgical dissection. In some hospitals, femoral-femoral bypass is occasionally used to allow more rapid surgical exposure and permit blood salvage.

For induction of anesthesia, cardiovascular stability may be maintained by the use of anesthetic agents such as ketamine and etomidate. Opioids, midazolam, and nitrous oxide could also be used as anesthetic techniques. These drugs do not greatly decrease venous return or cause myocardial depression. Muscle relaxants with minimal effects on the circulation such as *cis*-atracurium, vecuronium, or rocuronium are favored. They may be preferable to the use of pancuronium because it may induce tachycardia. Positive-pressure ventilation should be avoided, if possible, until surgery for pericardiectomy is underway, because it will increase the intrathoracic pressure and further compromise venous return and cardiac filling. Coughing or straining during induction will also reduce venous return and should be prevented.

The principles of intraoperative management aim to maintain hemodynamic stability. They are maintain preload, avoid bradycardia, avoid myocardial depression, and maintain afterload. Ventricular diastolic filling is limited, resulting in cardiac output being rate dependent. The development of atrial fibrillation may be catastrophic because of the rapid ventricular rate and the loss of the atrial component of ventricular filling. As with any other arrhythmia causing reduction in cardiac output, treatment should be started at once. A defibrillator and antiarrhythmic drugs should be immediately available. Hemodynamic stability may be maintained by blood volume expansion to maintain filling pressures and maximize cardiac output. Inotropes may be required to maintain cardiac contractility and/or support systemic vascular resistance. Agents to reduce afterload may improve cardiac output in patients with adequate intravascular volume replacement.

Pericardiectomy may be performed through a median sternotomy or through a left anterior thoracotomy. The pericardium may be removed completely, or some surgeons remove only that part overlaying the ventricles. Rarely, the epicardium may cause constriction and may also require removal.

Postoperative Considerations

Patients should be transferred postpericardiectomy to an intensive care unit where continuous, invasive hemodynamic monitoring should be continued. Postoperative mechanical ventilation of the lungs may also be required because of respiratory insufficiency. In contrast to the dramatic improvement in right atrial pressure following surgery for cardiac tamponade, right atrial pressures may take several days to return to normal after pericardiectomy for constrictive pericarditis. Improvement in cardiac function may not be maximal for many weeks. The immediate postoperative course may be stormy, and the perioperative physician must monitor the hemodynamic status closely.

The most important cause of morbidity and mortality after pericardiectomy in these patients is a persistently low cardiac output state. Failure to improve after pericardiectomy is usually caused by inadequate resection of the visceral and parietal pericardium, although a number of other factors may be responsible. Sclerotic epicardium may be providing constriction. The myocardium may have been damaged during the dissection; this may be permanent or temporary. There may be myocardial involvement in the disease process. This can occur in viral, infectious, amyloid, sarcoid- or radiation-induced myocarditis, and pericarditis. Myocardial atrophy can accompany constrictive pericarditis of long or even short duration. When the disuse atrophy is advanced, the heart may continue to dilate as it fails in "the exploding heart syndrome." Fortunately, in some patients the atrophy reverses over a few days if adequate hemodynamic support is provided during this time. Cardiac output should be optimized by the use of volume expansion, inotropes, and vasodilator drugs as guided by the hemodynamic data obtained at regular intervals from the pulmonary artery catheter. Success has also been reported with the use of intraaortic balloon counter-pulsation.

Cardiac arrhythmias may occur in the immediate postoperative period and treatment should be immediately available.

The most significant factor in outcome after pericardiectomy is the preoperative clinical condition of the patient. If pericardiectomy is performed before myocardial damage has occurred because of the constriction, mortality is significantly reduced. Patients presenting in New York Heart Association (NYHA) classes I and II have better survival postpericardiectomy than those presenting in NYHA classes III and IV. High, right-sided pressures postpericardiectomy are also associated with raised mortality. Other causes of mortality are infection, hemorrhage, and cardiac arrhythmias.

SUMMARY

Pericardial disease, although not commonly encountered perioperatively, provides great challenges in management for the perioperative physician. A sound knowledge of the pathophysiology associated with conditions, such as cardiac tamponade and constrictive pericarditis, and appropriate manipulation of the hemodynamics will allow the clinician to optimally manage patients with pericardial disease in the perioperative period. Modern imaging techniques, such as echocardiography and nuclear MRI, greatly aid the perioperative physician in the diagnosis and management of pericardial disease.

BIBLIOGRAPHY

Ameli SA, Shah PK: Cardiac tamponade: pathophysiology, diagnosis, and management, *Cardiol Clin* 9(4):665–674, 1991.

Brockington GM, Zebede J, Pandian NG: Constrictive pericarditis, *Cardiol Clin*, 8(4):645–661, 1990.

Fowler NO: Cardiac tamponade: a clinical or an echocardiographic diagnosis? *Circulation* 87(5):1738–1741, 1993, (review).

Fowler NO: Pericardial disease: heart disease and stroke 1(2):85–94, 1992, (review).

Hoit BD: Imaging the pericardium, *Cardiol Clin*; 8(4):587–600, 1990.

Lake CL: Anesthesia and pericardial disease. *Anesth Analg* 62:431–443, 1983, (review).

Oliver WC, DeCastro MA, Strickland RA: Uncommon diseases and cardiac anesthesia. In Kaplan JA, editor: *Cardiac anesthesia*, ed 3, Philadelphia, 1993, WB Saunders Ltd.

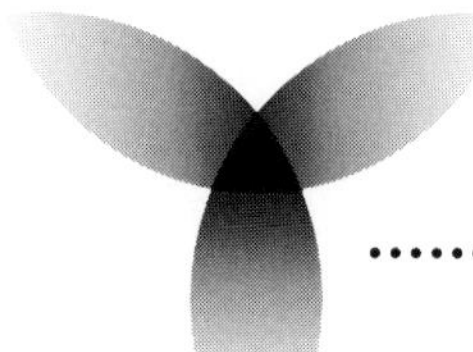

Chapter 11

A Physiologic Approach to Perioperative Respiratory Care

David J. Stone, MD, Thomas J. Gal, MD

This chapter, as well as the subsequent two on bronchial hyperresponsiveness and perioperative respiratory failure, address the issue of nonthoracic surgery. The special considerations of thoracic surgery will be covered separately. The respiratory risk of nonthoracic surgery arises from the interaction between the underlying physiology of the patient and the site of the operation, and its appreciation requires a physiological, yet practical approach. The recent proliferation of laparoscopically aided intraabdominal surgery has added a new array of potential perioperative problems and has shifted some of the peril from the postoperative to the intraoperative stage of patient care. These problems are also addressed in a separate chapter.

In brief, respiratory impairment as a result of general anesthesia arises from reduced lung volumes and respiratory system compliance, increased pulmonary resistance, impaired oxygenation, and depressed respiratory drive. These changes are most important intraoperatively and for several hours after surgery ends. The respiratory consequences of surgery relate strongly to the incision site so that thoracic or abdominal procedures result in the most impairment. The effects of such operations on respiratory mechanics are obviously important during the course of the surgery, but residual effects, such as reduced lung volumes, may last for a week or more. The severity of fluid shifts from bleeding, subsequent volume replacement, loss of fluid into a nonfunctional extravascular space, as well as positioning, postoperative pain, and length of the procedure are other important factors. Thus, major head and neck or orthopedic procedures, which do not invade the thorax or peritoneum, may still cause major respiratory problems. It is also unfortunate that the operations most likely to cause significant problems are unlikely to be those that can be approached with regional or local anesthetic techniques alone.

While many patients with some degree of pulmonary impairment undergo surgery, relatively few have devastating or irreversible pulmonary complications. The ability to limit complications requires input from primary and specialty physicians to define the nature and extent of the patient's problems and provide optimal prior medical therapy. In preparing the respiratory section of this book, we became keenly aware that other than aggressive treatment, prevention of bronchospasm, and reduction of secretions, there are few specific preoperative measures that are likely to be of real benefit for the patient with pulmonary disease. Unlike the area of cardiac risk in which a patient can receive surgical correction of the problem through angioplasty or coronary bypass grafting (CABG), there is no quick fix for patients with respiratory disease. Care of such patients requires thoughtful application of clinical skills and judgment. The following constitutes an approach to these problems in the preoperative period. Rather than define the clinical problem through the usual means of differential diagnosis or disease categorization, we have adopted a physiologically based approach, which tends to direct therapy in a logical way. In fact, many patients will have overlapping symptoms and problems, regardless of the precise diagnoses that has been applied to their conditions. Table 11-1 lists perioperative respiratory concerns that may well overlap in any given patient. For example, a patient labelled as having chronic obstructive pulmonary disease (COPD) may present with all of the table's listed elements. Nevertheless, these divisions should form a useful mental construct in the approach to evaluating and treating all patients.

Just what are the complications we are trying to prevent? These have been fairly well defined for the postoperative period and include bronchospasm, atelectasis, pneumonia, and pulmonary edema; all of which can alone or in combination lead to respiratory failure and, on occasion, death. For the intraoperative period, the onset of respiratory failure, per se, is not an issue because the patient is usually ventilated with supplemental oxygen through an artificial airway; but even so, there may be difficulties with adequate oxygenation or ventilation, as well as with bronchospasm and secretions. It is generally in the postoperative period that actual respiratory failure becomes a problem.

Clearly, our division of this clinical problem is as artificial as one based on disease entity. However, we hope that a different and more physiological approach to perioperative pulmonary care can stimulate thought about problems as they exist in clinical reality. Bronchial hyperresponsiveness, smoking, inadequate lung volumes with ventilation/perfusion (V/Q) mismatch, hypercapnia, muscle weakness, and excessive secretions contribute in varying degrees to produce pulmonary dysfunction. Each individual patient should be analyzed in terms of the relative contribution of each of these pathologic elements, so that appropriate preventions and interventions can be instituted.

Table 11-1. Perioperative Respiratory Concerns

I. Bronchial Hyperresponsiveness/Smoking and Secretions
II. Low Lung Volumes/Atelectasis
III. Neuromuscular Disease/Chest Wall and Spinal Deformity
IV. Ventilatory Failure

DEFINITIONS OF THE CLINICAL CONCERNS

Bronchial Hyperresponsiveness/Smoking and Secretions

Patients may be labelled as having asthma, COPD, chronic bronchitis, or emphysema with clinical evidence of wheezing. However, heavy smokers or patients who seldom report such symptoms may develop bronchial hyperreactivity in association with respiratory infections, intraoperative aspiration, and, especially, with the mechanical instrumentation of the airway necessary during anesthesia. Other patients who develop wheezing on exposure to cold or with exercise, may also be prone to perioperative bronchospasm. Finally, patients with allergies to drugs or substances such as latex or preparation solutions used during this time period can develop severe degrees of airway reactivity.

The bronchoconstrictive response may be partly caused by reduced, resting airway caliber, but also results from changes in airway smooth muscle, damage to airway epithelium, mucosal edema and inflammation, and airway secretions. The parasympathetic nervous system plays a key role as well, with both afferent and efferent components contributing. At selected times, pulmonary function tests (PFTs) may be used to evaluate severity and response to therapy in these patients. However, evaluation of symptoms and response to therapy represent the cornerstones of clinical management. It is not always evident that PFTs alter the approach to therapy, even in patients with severe COPD. Furthermore, actual values are not established in terms of indicating a need for postoperative ventilation or avoiding surgery entirely.

Patients who appear to have bronchospasm (i.e., obstruction to airflow at the bronchial level) may actually have obstruction to airflow more proximally in the airway. This can occur at the level of the trachea or larger bronchi from tumor or foreign bodies. It is especially more likely to occur, and be more difficult to diagnose, at the level of the trachea or larynx. Patients with a history of prolonged intubation or tracheostomy (look for scar) are especially at risk, but other otolaryngologic disorders (e.g., tumor, vocal cord paralysis) can result in a patient with laryngeal or tracheal obstruction, which mimics wheezing and will not respond to bronchodilators.

The patient who is a heavy smoker is likely to have a stormier perioperative course whether or not any significant postoperative complications actually occur. The smoker often has copious secretions and may be particularly prone to bronchospasm with initial airway instrumentation (laryngoscopy/intubation) as well as positioning, and during emergence from anesthesia. Beneficial clearing of airways takes approximately 1 month to develop after cessation of smoking. In the initial 48 to 72 hours after cessation, the situation may actually be worse because cilia become active and provoke coughing and secretions. While the majority of patients with excessive secretions are smokers, other groups include those with active or recent respiratory infections and, more notably, patients with cystic fibrosis. Patients who have significant neuromuscular weakness, especially bulbar, will have difficulty with secretions, which is worsened by reduced vital capacity, increased pulmonary resistance, and other perioperative factors. Secretions lead to an increased likelihood of bronchospasm and can contribute to the development of atelectasis if they are not adequately cleared from the airway. They may also cause significant obstruction of the endotracheal tube. Obstruction can be a particular problem in operations that limit access to the airway or those done in unusual positions (e.g., prone).

Low Lung Volumes/Atelectasis

Patients may have reduced lung volumes because of restrictive lung disease, previous resectional surgery, or COPD that has gone on to produce large areas of "lung" that do not effectively participate in gas exchange. Other causes include significant pleural effusions, obesity, and pregnancy, all of which impair lung expansion. The patient with small lung volumes may not be able to produce an effective cough with the added limitations imposed during the perioperative period. Attempts at coughing from a low lung volume are less effective because of decreased volume and forcefulness. The patient is, thus, unable to adequately clear secretions or aid in the reexpansion of areas of lung that have developed atelectasis. These areas can range from those too small to be seen on chest radiograph to "white-out" of an entire lung field when endobronchial intubation occurs and is not detected and remedied. The vicious cycle of low lung volumes and atelectasis can produce clinically important hypoxemia, predispose to pneumonia, and, eventually, cause respiratory failure. Of course, an effective cough also requires adequate airflow rates and, consequently, will be limited by the presence of airway obstruction and other factors, such as muscle weakness and overwhelming amounts of secretions.

Neuromuscular Disease/Chest Wall and Spinal Deformity

The patient with neuromuscular disease may have respiratory difficulties that relate to the central and peripheral nervous system, neuromuscular junction, and skeletal muscle. Central nervous system pathology sufficient to affect respiration is likely to be severe in such disorders as brainstem hemorrhage or high spinal cord injuries. The patient with obstructive sleep apnea may also have a central component as the basis for the clinical problem. Peripheral neuropathies and myopathies, conversely, are not likely to affect respiration except in special cases such as severe Guillain-Barré syndrome or congenital myopathy. The patient with myasthenia gravis is a special case, warranting separate discussion in the neurologic disorders chapter.

Patients with spinal and chest wall abnormalities are likely to present for corrective spinal surgery but may require surgery for other reasons, as well. In general, such patients are likely to develop atelectasis, ventilatory failure, and difficulty dealing with secretions in the perioperative period. This is largely because of the impaired chest wall mechanics, which accompany the deformities.

Ventilatory Failure

Ventilatory failure occurs when metabolically produced carbon dioxide cannot be adequately removed by the respiratory apparatus. Inadequate oxygenation will occur as well, unless the inspired oxygen fraction is increased. Ventilatory failure can take place when the pump mechanism is simply impaired, as in neuromuscular or chest wall disorders. This results in a reduction of the volume of gas that actually moves in and out of the lung. In the perioperative period, pharmacologic respiratory depression that decreases total minute ventilation may also result in ventilatory failure. Failure is even more likely if upper airway patency is impaired by residual neuromuscular blockade, glottic or subglottic edema, or surgical factors.

Inefficiency of the respiratory pump will also occur when so-called "dead space" or wasted ventilation is increased. In this case, ventilatory gas is delivered to many areas of lung that are poorly perfused. Normally, such dead space is approximately 2 ml/kg or one third of tidal volume. In normal patients, this is almost entirely caused by the non–gas exchanging areas of the upper airway (i.e., anatomic dead space). In patients with pulmonary disease, further increases in dead space are the result of an increase in alveolar dead space, in which ventilation persists in relatively underperfused areas of lung. Total dead space (anatomic + alveolar) may be precisely measured, but requires a measure of mixed expiratory carbon dioxide; it is not commonly performed in this setting. If mixed expiratory carbon dioxide can be measured total dead space fraction is calculated using the Bohr equation: $(P_aCO_2 - P_ECO_2) \div P_aCO_2$ where P_ECO_2 is mixed expired carbon dioxide pressure. Note that for an arterial carbon dioxide of 40 mm Hg and dead space of 30%, mixed expired carbon dioxide will be approximately 28 mm Hg.

Dead space may be almost doubled in patients with severe lung disease because of severe maldistribution of ventilation, relative to perfusion. Unless minute ventilation or, more specifically, alveolar ventilation can be doubled as well, carbon dioxide tensions in blood will increase proportionately. This increase stems from the fact that arterial carbon dioxide tension is inversely proportional to alveolar ventilation, which is total minute ventilation minus dead space ventilation. Dead space is increased slightly by general anesthesia. However, this increase is offset by endotracheal intubation, which reduces the volume of the upper airway.

Currently, anesthesiologists monitor end-tidal carbon dioxide concentrations as indicators of endotracheal intubation, ongoing ventilation, and pulmonary perfusion. The gradient between the arterial and end-tidal carbon dioxide concentrations reflects the degree of alveolar dead space which is generally small (gradient <5 mm Hg) in normal patients during general endotracheal anesthesia. However, patients with pulmonary disease, pulmonary vascular occlusion, or diminished cardiac output may exhibit much larger arterial to end-tidal gradients. For these reasons, end-tidal CO_2 may not reliably track arterial carbon dioxide, and evaluations of arterial blood gases may be required to prove adequacy of ventilation.

Increases in arterial carbon dioxide tensions may also result from increases in carbon dioxide production. Normal carbon dioxide production is approximately 2.5 to 3 ml per kilogram per minute, so that a 70-kg person produces nearly 160 to 200 ml per minute. This figure is decreased by anesthesia and hypothermia and increased by fever, sepsis, and in malignant hyperthermia. Clinicians may, at times, refer to the respiratory quotient (RQ); that is the carbon production divided by oxygen consumption. With a normal diet, the ratio is approximately 0.8, but a pure carbohydrate diet (without excess carbohydrates converted to fat) yields an RQ of 1.0. In the patient who has minimal reserve in ventilatory capacity, the increased carbon dioxide load in the normal course of perioperative demands, may be excessive and result in significant hypercapnia, and even ventilatory failure.

• PULMONARY FUNCTION TESTING

Understanding, interpreting, and using the results of clinical spirometry or PFTs have proven difficult for generations of physicians. The importance of PFTs in the perioperative period has been variously described as "essential" to "nearly unnecessary." In any case, the information should be applied with the anticipation that specific findings will determine specific clinical actions. Most often, PFTs are done because the patient has lung disease or is having an operation and, therefore, "requires" this test on the chart as an indicator of clinical "completeness." There is a perceived need to apply some quantitation to the defect. It is difficult to characterize the patient who "needs" PFTs. Usually, that patient is the one whose care will benefit in some way from the acquisition of quantitative information. That patient typically has a suspected impairment of respiratory function. Also, that patient is one who is to be subjected to a surgical procedure likely to have a major impact on the respiratory system.

In the majority of cases in which perioperative PFTs are done, a simple forced expiratory spirogram is all that is required (Figure 11-1). Furthermore, of all the information that can be extracted from the spirogram, the most useful items consist of the forced expiratory volume (FEV_1), the forced vital capacity (FVC), and the ratio of the two generally reported as a percentage (FEV_1/FVC%). These forced expiratory indices are determined by the elastic recoil of the lung, the flow-resistive properties of intrathoracic airways, and respiratory muscle strength. The forced midexpiratory flow ($FEF_{25\%-75\%}$) was conceived to avoid considering the initial effort-dependent portion of forced expiration; but, in actual practice it does not add useful information to the FEV_1/FVC ratio.

The term "maximal expiratory flow" has been used in the past for the average flow during the liter of gas exhaled after the initial 200 ml of an FVC maneuver ($FEF_{200-1200}$); but, it is slightly lower than the true peak flow rate. The true peak expiratory flow rate (PEFR) can be measured with a hand-held flowmeter. The meter is particularly useful when repeated measurements are needed, such as after the administration of bronchodilators (Figure 11-2). Furthermore, this test does not require a pulmonary function lab and can be repeated frequently. Values of less than 200 l/min are markers for impaired cough efficiency and an increased likelihood of postoperative complications.

Expected values for PFT results are generally printed out alongside the patient's results so that the two can be compared. Expected vital capacity is predicted mainly

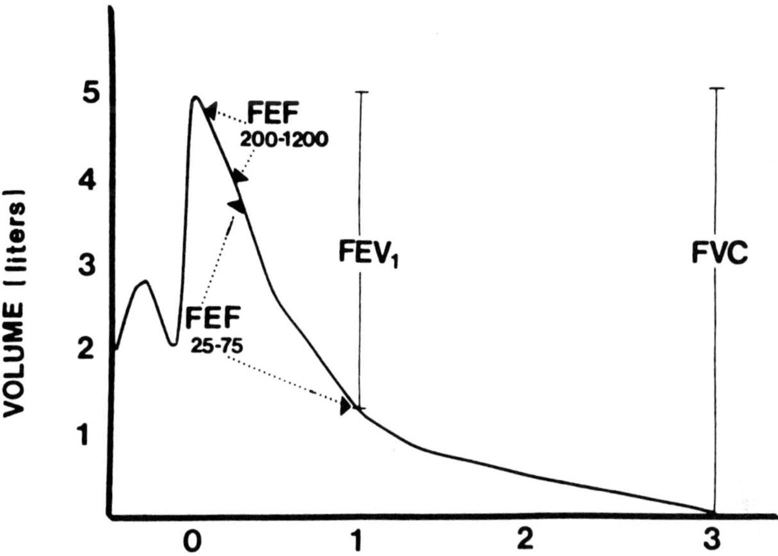

Figure 11-1
Forced vital capacity (*FVC*) maneuver in a normal subject. Exhaled volume is plotted against time as the patient expires forcefully, rapidly, and completely to residual volume (RV), following a maximal deep inspiration. FEV_1, forced expired volume in 1 second; $FEF_{200-1200}$, forced expiratory flow between 200 and 1200 ml of expired volume; $FEF_{25\%-75\%}$, forced expiratory flow over the midportion of vital capacity: that is, from 25% to 75% of expired volume. (From Gal TJ: *Respiratory physiology in anesthetic practice*, Baltimore, 1991, Williams & Wilkins.)

from height and age and is considered abnormal when it falls clearly below 80% of the expected value. The FEV_1 is normally 75% to 80% of the predicted vital capacity. Lower FEV_1/FVC ratios designate mild (<70%), moderate (<60%), or severe (<50%) degrees of airway obstruction. The absolute size of the FEV_1, which essentially tracks FVC, is important to consider as well, because the patient with an FEV_1 of 1000 ml and an FEV_1/FVC ratio of 50% is not as impaired as one with an FEV_1 of 500 ml and the same FEV_1/FVC ratio. This is because the patient with the lower absolute number has far less pulmonary reserve caused by the smaller FVC. Thus, the ability to cough effectively and ventilate adequately in the postoperative period are more impaired. Table 11-2 summarizes the basic PFT results in varying disease states.

As can be seen in Table 11-2, the patient with reduced lung volumes, but normal flow ratios, may have restrictive lung disease ("stiff lungs") or respiratory muscle weakness. Respiratory muscle strength can be evaluated by measuring pressure generated against an occluded airway during a maximal forced inspiratory (PImax, from residual volume) or expiratory (PEmax, from total lung capacity) effort. For extreme accuracy in measurement that is not required for clinical purposes, these pressures can be measured at functional residual capacity (FRC, the "resting"

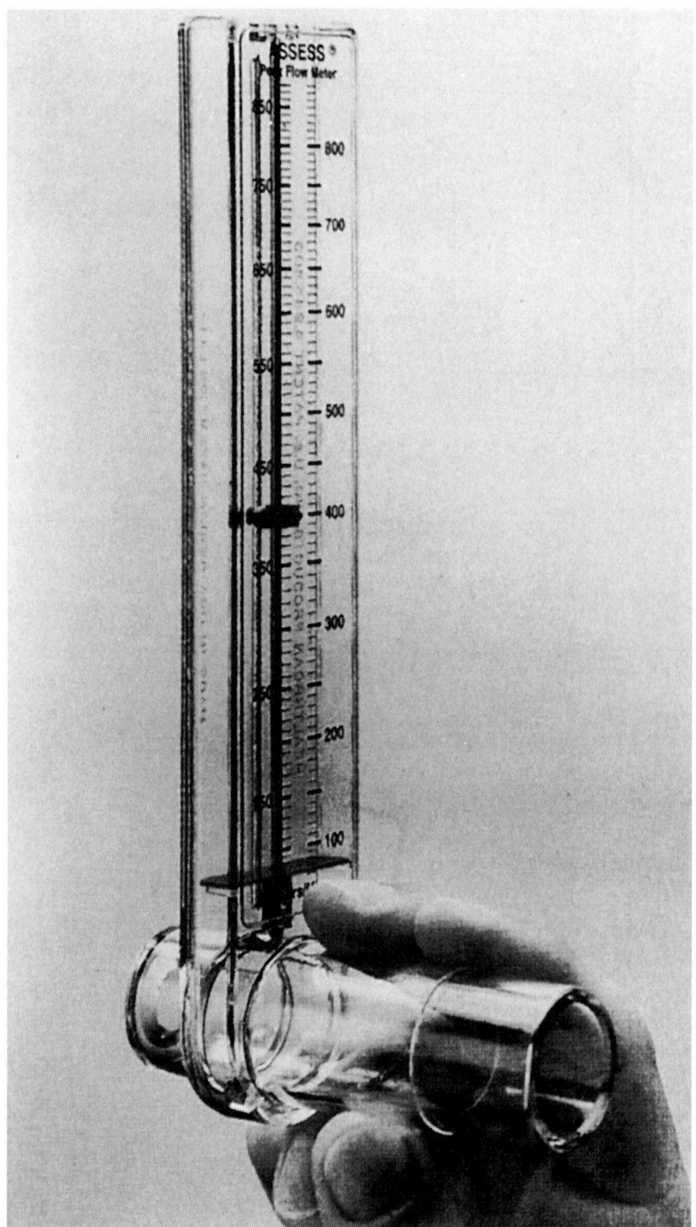

Figure 11-2
The Assess full range (60–880 l/min) peak flow meter. Asthma management zone clips and safety one-way valve disposable mouthpieces are available separately from the manufacturer (with permission from Healthscan Products Inc, Cedar Grove, NJ).

Table 11-2. Airflow and Volumes in Basic Disease States

	AIRWAY OBSTRUCTION	RESTRICTIVE LUNG DISEASE	NEUROMUSCULAR WEAKNESS
FEV_1	⇓	⇓	⇓
FVC	Normal	⇓	⇓
FEV_1/FVC	⇓	Normal	Normal

volume of the lung after a normal breath is exhaled) to eliminate the impact of respiratory system elastic recoil on the total measurement. Healthy, young male patients can generate impressive pressures: PImax of –125 cm H_2O and PEmax of +200 cm H_2O. Trumpet players have been noted to be capable of a PEmax of 235 cm H_2O! Patients with a PImax less than –25 cm H_2O or a PEmax less than +40 cm H_2O have significant weakness and will have problems with deep breathing and coughing. Note that while maximal inspiratory pressures are used at times in the intensive care unit (ICU) setting to evaluate patients for weaning, these tests are not similarly used in the operating room for this purpose. Muscle strength in the anesthetized intubated patient is evaluated by clinical means, including mild electrical stimuli delivered to a peripheral nerve to test the efficacy of neuromuscular transmission and physical examination (after responsiveness to verbal stimuli is restored). The evaluation includes head lift, grip strength, and the ability to protrude the tongue out of the mouth for several seconds. In the ICU, the clinician is testing for muscle weakness, which may be a long-standing problem involving peripheral nerve and muscle. In the operating room, the clinician is primarily testing for neuromuscular weakness produced by the administration of muscle relaxants and reversed by the administration of anticholinesterases and the elimination of volatile anesthetics.

An arterial blood gas analysis provides a useful assessment of overall respiratory function. While significant hypoxemia is an important factor to consider, the level of resting hypercarbia is a more reliable perioperative prognostic marker. It is not possible to correlate the degree of preoperative hypoxemia with respiratory risk; but, in general, hypoxemia caused by V/Q mismatch can be overcome by increasing inspired concentrations of oxygen during and after surgery. Resting hypercarbia is a strong indicator of both potential intraoperative respiratory acidosis (if breathing is spontaneous) and postoperative ventilatory failure. Respiratory depressants, increased carbon dioxide production, and incisional pain all contribute to worsening ventilation.

BIBLIOGRAPHY

Bendixen HH, et al: *Respiratory care*, St. Louis, 1965, Mosby.

Admittedly an old reference that may be hard to find but a real classic with many points still valid in clinical respiratory physiology.

Erice F, et al: Diaphragmatic function before and after laparoscopic cholecystectomy, *Anesthesiology* 79:966–975, 1993.

Ford GT, et al: Respiratory physiology in upper abdominal surgery, *Clin Chest Med* 14:237–252, 1993.

Gal TJ: Pulmonary function testing. In Miller RD, editor: *Anesthesia*, New York, 1994, Churchill Livingstone.

Gal TJ: *Respiratory physiology in anesthetic practice*, Baltimore, 1991, Williams & Wilkins.

Gass GD, Olsen GN: Preoperative pulmonary function testing to predict postoperative morbidity and mortality, *Chest* 89:127–135, 1986.

Jayr C, et al: Preoperative and intraoperative factors associated with prolonged mechanical ventilation: a study of patients following major abdominal vascular surgery, *Chest* 103:1231–1232, 1993.

Stein M, Cassara EL: Preoperative pulmonary evaluation and therapy for surgical patients, *JAMA* 211:787–790, 1970.

Tisi GM: Preoperative evaluation of pulmonary function, *Am Rev Respir Dis* 119:293–310, 1979.

Zibrak JD, O'Donnell CR, Marton K: Indications for pulmonary function testing, *Ann Intern Med* 112:763–771, 1990.

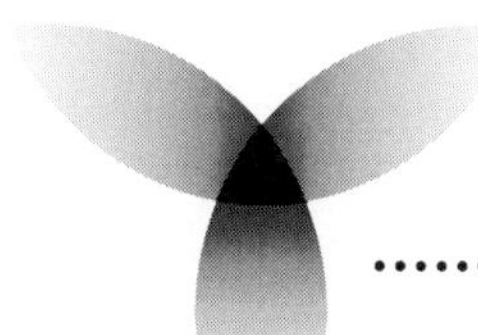

Chapter 12

Bronchial Hyperresponsiveness, Smoking, and Secretions

David J. Stone, MD, Thomas J. Gal, MD

• PREOPERATIVE CLINICAL EVALUATION

The clinical history remains a key part of preoperative evaluation of the patient with bronchospasm. Important questions include: "What symptoms do you have?" "What brings them on?" "What is your exercise tolerance?" These questions provide an overall perspective of the nature of the patient's problem. They should be asked of any patient with respiratory disease including those with problems other than airway obstruction. For exercise tolerance, we frequently ask if the patient can walk up a flight of steps without stopping. This last question appears to be a fairly reliable indicator of the ability of the patient's cardiovascular and respiratory systems to withstand the stress involved in most operations. It correlates surprisingly well with measures of oxygen consumption. Notably, many older patients with chronic obstructive pulmonary disease (COPD) will suffer from other medical problems that also limit exercise tolerance such as heart failure, stroke, arthritis, and vascular insufficiency. More subtle symptoms may include nocturnal dyspnea, morning chest tightness, and cough. These symptoms may be found in patients who respond to noxious stimuli such as cold air, fumes, with bronchospasm.

"What medications at what doses do you normally take?" This also gives some idea as to the severity of the underlying disease (i.e., the quantity and quality of drugs needed to keep symptoms under control). The basic idea is to separate minimal, mild, moderate, and severe degrees of clinical problems.

"Have you recently had to go to the emergency room for bronchospasm, wheezing, or asthma? Have you recently or ever been hospitalized for bronchospasm, wheezing, or asthma? If so, how recently and for how long?" If the answers are positive, the course of the admission should be characterized (e.g., was intubation and ventilation required?). Old records are very helpful, of course.

"Have you had a recent (or current) upper respiratory infection (URI)? Did it exacerbate your bronchospasm?" For 4 to 5 weeks after a URI, patients appear to have particularly reactive airways and elective surgery should be avoided, if this is judged to be medically reasonable.

"Do you feel your bronchospasm is currently well-controlled?" The answer to this question will indicate if anything else should be done to improve the patient's status before surgery, such as increased doses of medication, addition of new medication, or a short course of a corticosteroid.

Physical examination includes simply observing and listening to the patient breathe. The patient who is in distress is not a candidate for elective surgery at that moment. It is helpful to listen to the chest preoperatively or just before the induction of anesthesia to distinguish newly provoked bronchospasm from a baseline condition of chronic wheezing. Some patients with COPD have severely reduced breath sounds. This is important to know before searching for them to verify tracheal intubation. We have never found the traditional "pink-puffer" and "blue-bloater" classifications to be clinically useful.

The chest radiograph can indicate lung hyperexpansion and will occasionally show a previously undiagnosed element of lung or pleural pathology, particularly primary or metastatic malignancies. This discovery may be important since the performance of certain operations may be reevaluated in the face of possible malignancy. The chest radiograph provides baseline information, much like the electrocardiogram, for the perioperative period. If hyperinflation is present on the chest film, there is about a 30% likelihood of respiratory complications. If a respiratory infection is suspected, a chest radiograph is indicated if it will change the clinical plan, especially whether surgery will proceed at all. In other cases, the decision to obtain a chest radiograph remains a clinical one; but all patients with significant disease, or patients with moderate disease undergoing major procedures, should have one. If a chest radiograph has been obtained recently, there is no need to thoughtlessly repeat it, unless there has been a clinical change or the time period since the radiograph is judged to be too long. Younger patients with mild or inactive disease are unlikely to benefit from a preoperative chest radiograph.

Pulmonary function tests (PFTs) are not routinely necessary in the preoperative evaluation of patients with bronchial hyperresponsiveness. This especially applies to the young patient whose problem is limited to intermittent airway hyperreactivity. The standard forced expired volume in the first second (FEV_1) is an indicator of obstruction to airflow when it is reduced, compared to forced vital capacity (FVC). However, in the majority of cases this only reinforces clinical impressions apparent from the patient's history and physical examination. It is in no way a screening test for asymptomatic or stable, mildly symptomatic perioperative patients. Furthermore, while reversibility in response to a bronchodilator may be a specific indication for treatment, most clinicians will empirically treat the wheezing patient with a bronchodilator in any case.

Formal pulmonary function testing may be indicated in the patient who is judged to have clinically moderate-to-severe disease and scheduled to undergo a procedure that will have a major impact on the respiratory system. This testing is especially reasonable if the concurrent complicating factors previously mentioned (i.e., muscle weakness, reduced lung volumes, etc.) are thought to be present. Even in these cases, formal PFTs are often not particularly useful in influencing the pre- and intraoperative management of airway obstruction, per se. Rather, they may help to predict which patients are most likely to suffer postoperative problems with respiratory function because of an extremely limited pulmonary reserve, to which airway obstruction is one contributing factor. The use of the hand-held spirometer to measure peak expiratory flow rate (PEFR) is a cheaper and more convenient way to obtain a repeated measure of airway obstruction if one is deemed necessary. Often, the effect of a therapeutic maneuver can be judged by the clinical observation of the patient's subjective response, including direct questioning and the application of a stethoscope to the chest.

Smoking/Secretions

Obviously, a medical history that identifies significant cigarette smoking should be taken. We have found that patients will sometimes respond negatively to an inquiry about smoking by saying that they have quit, while further questioning reveals that they quit just that morning or the previous day. While a greater number of "pack" years may make COPD more likely, even a novice smoker may present a perioperative problem. Cigarette smoking is likely to make any general anesthetic stormy by producing a patient with copious secretions, significant cough, and an irritable airway prone to laryngospasm (reflex closure of the larynx in response to irritants such as secretions or instrumentation in the setting of deepening or lightening anesthesia) and bronchospasm. A videotape of a smoker emerging from general anesthesia would probably be an effective deterrent to smoking.

The severity of cough and the quantity and nature of secretions will give some idea of the difficulties ahead. Changes may indicate the onset of a respiratory infection, in which case, elective surgery may be deferred. The precise impact of an upper respiratory infection or bronchitis on the course of an anesthetic is difficult to quantitate. Either will tend to make all the elements of a difficult situation (cough, laryngospasm, bronchospasm) worse and, at times, lead to a number of critical "near-miss" events. That is when laryngospasm and/or bronchospasm are so severe that oxygenation is critically impaired, even when the usual countermeasures have been instituted. The significance of minor changes in cough and secretions requires subtle clinical judgment. Certainly, these call for a more careful physical examination and a lower threshold for obtaining a chest radiograph. If significant respiratory infection is present, anesthesia is best delayed for approximately one month after the infection has resolved, unless surgical urgency dictates otherwise. If an infiltrate is present, it is important to establish that it has resolved, especially if the patient has a significant smoking history. This is because the long-term smoker is more likely to have an underlying carcinoma that is obstructing a bronchus or simply hidden behind an acute infiltrate. Often, the decision to cancel or proceed includes the factor of patient convenience ("I took a day off from work and drove 6 hours to get here"). This dilemma is further complicated by our current practices in a competitive and managed medical environment. For example, if the socioeconomics of the situation are such that a patient with a mild cold is unlikely to ever again reenter the medical system for a necessary procedure, it may be best to proceed with all possible medical and anesthetic cautions applied. All of these comments apply to patients with excessive secretions from etiologies other than cigarette smoking, such as cystic fibrosis or environmental chronic bonchitis.

• PREOPERATIVE INTERVENTION

Once the clinician can establish that the patient's wheezing is not caused by mechanical upper airway obstruction or left-sided heart failure, bronchodilator therapy can be undertaken. We do not believe that theophylline preparations have an important role in the perioperative management of these patients, and take no pains to establish or document therapeutic drug levels. Rather, we believe that the toxicity of these agents (particularly dysrhythmias) vastly outweighs their perioperative usefulness. If the patient is taking a theophylline derivative, we would encourage nonadministration on the day of surgery to decrease the likelihood of toxicity.

In contrast, the anticholinergics are critically useful drugs in these patients. Inhaled anticholinergics should be continued up to the time of surgery. These agents, administered intravenously 10 to 20 minutes before and, topically, at the time of airway manipulation are particularly effective at blunting the reflex bronchospasm that may result from necessary instrumentation of the airway (e.g., laryngoscopy, intubation) during an anesthetic. In our practice, we employ glycopyrrolate (Robinul, 0.2 mg/ml) in both inhaled and intravenous administration modes because it causes less tachycardia than atropine and does not cross the blood-brain barrier. To prevent bronchospasm, intravenous doses of 0.4 to 1.0 mg can be given, preferably at least 10 minutes before the induction of anesthesia. Alternatively, a smaller dose (0.2–0.4 mg) can be given intravenously and an additional dose (0.4–1.0 mg) sprayed directly into the trachea during laryngoscopy before the endotracheal tube is inserted. The use of topical administration avoids systemic effects such as tachycardia and prolonged mouth dryness. The agents decrease secretion volume but do *not* increase viscosity and do *not* cause inspissation.

Patients receiving oral and inhaled β-2 agents should continue these on schedule, up to the time of surgery. We encourage patients to take a final inhaler dose in the preoperative waiting area, and even to take an extra puff or two at this time. Patients who do not regularly use an inhaler can receive a dose of a β-2 agent such as albuterol through a nebulizer in the preoperative holding area because they may be unable to master the art of effectively using a hand-held, pressurized inhaler at this time. Albuterol is, in fact, the most favored agent. It appears to be the most β-2 selective agent available when inhaled.

Inhaled steroids should be similarly continued, although not generally begun at this time. If the patient is already taking oral corticosteroids, the dosage can be increased and may be supplemented by an additional dose at bedtime on the evening before surgery. This bedtime dose is suggested to ensure the desired effect occurs before surgery. For example, the patient who normally takes 20 mg a day of prednisone might receive 60 mg the evening before and the morning (with a sip of water) of surgery. If more rapid action is required, and the patient has not taken an increased oral dose, the corticosteroid can be given intravenously before anesthesia. We usually use hydrocortisone (100–200 mg) or dexamethasone (4–10 mg) because we have convenient access to these preparations. Dexamethasone may theoretically have a longer onset time (we have not noticed this to be a problem), but it has the advantage of lasting for the duration of any surgical procedure and well into the early, postoperative period. In contrast, intravenous hydrocortisone must be readministered every 4 to 6 hours. Oral prednisone dosages (in the range of 20–80 mg, generally) may be used for the patient who is not a chronic steroid user. Again, it can be given orally at bedtime and the morning of surgery or through a single, intravenous (IV) dose on the day of surgery. Unless the patient is a very brittle diabetic, the use of one or two doses of steroid does not cause any clinical difficulties and appears to be effective at reducing the maximum bronchoconstrictive response.

An inhaled enzyme preparation (Pulmozyme) should be considered for patients with cystic fibrosis. The usual dose of 2.5 mg can be given via nebulizer or through the endotracheal tube after intubation.

Smoking/Secretions

While our obvious tendency is to advise patients to stop smoking before surgery, unless smoking has ceased 4 weeks before the operation, the benefits are unclear. Clearly, any cessation of smoking will help in reducing carboxyhemoglobin levels. However, we have noticed that smokers who just refrain from smoking just a few days or the day before surgery, lack their normal stimulation to a good, clearing cough and, in fact, may have more difficulty with secretions than those who stop just before the time of surgery. In any case, it is reasonable to encourage the patient to take some good, forceful coughs in the preoperative area and clear up secretions to the extent possible. This applies to any group that has difficulty with secretions such as patients with cystic fibrosis or chronic bronchitis unrelated to smoking. We strongly recommend the administration of glycopyrrolate, 0.2 mg IV, in the preoperative area, to patients who do have a history of copious secretions, which includes most smokers. The anesthesiologist may also choose to administer an antisialagogue for other reasons, such as potential difficult airway, planned, conscious intubation (especially if fiberoptic), or for patients being operated on in positions in which slippage of tape for securing the endotracheal tube would be a disaster (prone neurosurgical patients). While a low dose of antisialagogue may not prevent bronchospasm per se, a reduction in secretions tends to produce a less irritable airway that is not as prone to bronchospasm, laryngospasm, and coughing. The anticholinergic effects do not appear to have an effect on bowel or bladder function that significantly affect surgery. In general, these drugs should not be administered systemically to patients with closed-angle glaucoma. They should be used with caution in those with severe coronary disease in whom an increase in heart rate may produce myocardial ischemia.

• INTRAOPERATIVE PHYSIOLOGY AND INTERVENTION

If regional or local anesthesia is a possibility, it should be strongly considered so that instrumentation of the airway will be avoided. Furthermore, the systemic absorption of lidocaine may produce a mild attenuation of airway reactivity. However, regional techniques are not entirely benign. As higher segmental muscle levels are paralyzed in the normal course of a spinal or epidural anesthetic, the patient progressively loses the ability to exhale forcefully. This may produce difficulty in some patients with airway obstruction who depend on active exhalation for acceptable gas exchange. The need for sedation in combination with this expiratory muscle weakness may further impair the ability to remove secretions. It may then cause atelectasis, V/Q matching problems, and hypoxemia.

If endotracheal intubation is not required with general anesthesia, anesthesia by face mask may require placement of a potentially irritating oral airway or a laryngeal mask airway, which still causes a considerable degree of upper airway stimulation. Intubation is essential for all of the major thoracic and abdominal procedures but may also be indicated for airway maintenance in difficult surgical positions (e.g., prone) and airways judged or known to be difficult to manage. Endotracheal intubation is indicated if access to the airway is problematic, if there is a requirement for muscle relaxants and mechanical ventilation, for the provision of high inspired fractions of oxygen, and to aid removal of secretions. In contrast to the conventional wisdom that slow inspiratory flow rates be used in patients with airway obstruction, we use rapid inspiratory flow rates that allow adequate ventilation and time for exhalation through obstructed airways. This is achieved by the appropriate adjustment of respiratory rate (generally ≈8), tidal volume (≈10 ml/kg), and inspiratory-expiratory times (maintenance at 1:2 allows for short, beneficial end-inspiratory pause); and it still allows adequate time for complete exhalation.

An adequate depth of anesthesia should be achieved before the airway is instrumented. This can be accomplished with intravenous anesthetics, lidocaine, narcotics, and inhaled anesthetics. Endotracheal intubation causes some degree of reflex bronchoconstriction, which should be anticipated. Excess stimulation of the carina or endobronchial intubation should be assiduously avoided. When wheezing occurs in the intubated patient, causes other than bronchoconstriction should be considered. They include mechanical obstruction of the endotracheal tube (secretions, blood, patient biting the tube), aspiration, endobronchial intubation and carinal stimulation, pulmonary edema, tension pneumothorax, and pulmonary embolism.

Once the diagnosis of bronchoconstriction is established, therapy includes the agents discussed in the preoperative section, as well as a variety of other anesthetic drugs. Additional glycopyrrolate and β-2 agonist agents are first-line treatments that can be administered directly into the endotracheal tube, or through a number of available adapting devices that may enhance aerosol delivery. Inhaled agents may not be effective if bronchospasm is especially severe, and may even initially cause mechanical irritation of the airway and worsen the problem. Deepening an inhalational anesthetic is also beneficial because the potent anesthetic gases used in today's practice all produce some degree of bronchodilation. The arrhythmogenic interraction of theophylline and halothane is well known. However, even these potent bronchodilators will not be effective if severe bronchospasm prevents their delivery to airway sites and their use is limited by the hypotension they produce.

Intravenous therapy includes glycopyrrolate as well as anesthetic adjuncts, such as lidocaine (1–1.5 mg/kg), ketamine, propofol, or thiopental sodium in small doses. A drug with β-2 adrenergic properties such as ephedrine (5–20 mg) can be given intravenously. This is an agent commonly used to treat mild-to-moderate hypotension. In fact, airway obstruction and hyperinflation will tend to impair venous return and cardiac output, so that one is often confronted with a patient who is both bronchospastic and hypotensive. Paralysis with an appropriate agent eliminates the contribution of straining and coughing to increased airway pressures, and may be required to ventilate patients who are wheezing, coughing, and hypotensive. In spite of all these measures and the administration of 100% oxygen, severe hypoxemia may occur. Additional measures occasionally necessary include the cautious use of intravenous epinephrine or isoproterenol as small boluses (5–20 μg), followed by an intravenous infusion (start at 1 μg/min and titrate up), and the use of small amounts of positive end-expiratory pressure (PEEP). While using PEEP is generally regarded as undesirable in the patient with airway obstruction and hyperinflated lungs, it may be helpful in maintaining marginal oxygenation when bronchospasm is severe and the usual measures are not working.

Extubation while the patient is still deeply anesthetized has been suggested, at times, as a way to avoid reflex stimulation from the endotracheal tube. However, this may leave the patient without a secure airway while coughing, laryngospasm, and bronchospasm occur and ventilation by face mask is difficult because of the high airway resistance. In general, it is best to leave the patient intubated until awake enough to protect and maintain the airway, and until any bronchospasm is adequately treated. The patient may cough violently on the endotracheal tube, but this can be attenuated somewhat with IV lidocaine with few serious sequelae. Bucking with a tube in place is essentially analogous to laryngospasm without a tube. The decision on when to extubate relies heavily on clinical judgment and experience. It involves consideration of the difficulty of airway management, danger of aspiration, ability to replace the endotracheal tube quickly, adequacy of oxygen saturation, and patient state of consciousness. When in doubt, it is often best to leave the tube in place and wait a few more minutes, even if the patient has to be manually restrained from removing it.

Smoking/Secretions

As noted previously, the use of regional anesthesia with motor blockade above the 10th thoracic level will impair forceful exhalation, cough, and the ability to clear secretions. Conscious or deep sedation as a supplementation to local or regional anesthesia, may further add to the retention of secretions as the patient's awareness of secretions is likely to be reduced. Anesthesia by face mask or with a laryngeal mask airway may be complicated by secretions, especially if an antisialagogue has not been used. Laryngoscopy may also be more difficult in the presence of copious secretions, and mechanical instrumentation of the airway more likely to provoke laryngospasm and bronchospasm. Smokers fall into this category by virtue of the copious secretions most have and by the residual airway hyperirritability that often develops in the airway subjected to smoke inhalation on a daily basis. During anesthesia, secretions may cause obstruction of the endotracheal tube, contribute to difficulties in oxygenation and ventilation, loosen tape that is securing the endotracheal tube, and help create an environment conducive to atelectasis and pneumonia. Patients in surgical positions providing easy airway access can have secretions carefully suctioned, but for those in less accessible positions, such as prone, posterior fossa craniotomy in head pins, secretions and their removal pose a serious threat. In either case, suctioning removes only the most central secretions and cannot reach more peripheral accumulations. As is often the case in medicine, the best cure lies in prevention, with the preoperative or intraoperative administration of glycopyrrolate.

POSTOPERATIVE INTERVENTIONS

Postoperative management continues with the use of the same principles and agents used in the pre- and intraoperative period. Inhaled and intravenous β-2 agonists and anticholinergics, as well as parenteral steroids, should be continued and/or begun as required. Once again, other causes for wheezing must be considered; at this time, heart failure and aspiration are possible etiologies of wheezing that is not primarily bronchospasm. Most importantly, upper airway obstruction becomes a serious consideration and may be caused by glottic or subglottic edema, mild-to-moderate laryngospasm, or more rare injuries to the upper airway, such as vocal cord paralysis. If severe, there will be little or no air movement and, consequently, no wheezing. Upper airway obstruction is manifest by stridor that is clinically detected by noting audible inspiratory noises when a stethoscope is gently placed over the upper trachea. Inspiratory stridor occurs because the relatively high negative-pressure gradient required to move gas, causes dynamic collapse of upper airway structures. The precise diagnosis of upper airway obstruction involves direct visualization; but treatment, in any case, will usually include warmed, humidified gases, with or without nebulized racemic epinephrine (1 ml in 5 ml saline), and intravenous dexamethasone (≈10 mg IV). Careful sedation with an opioid to decrease inspiratory effort and gas flow rates can improve the situation, contrary to popular wisdom which focuses on dangers of depressing respiration. At times, reintubation will be required and should be carried out before the clinical situation becomes critical.

Smoking/Secretions

There are no specific measures for the postoperative care of these patients but, of course, smokers have placed themselves in a physiologic condition in which they are more prone to bronchospasm, atelectasis, and pneumonia than the nonsmoker. Once the endotracheal tube is removed, it is not prudent to thread catheters through the glottis for suctioning. Rather, voluntary coughing and deep breathing, supplemented by some degree of chest physical therapy, is the best technique because secretions are removed from peripheral airways and not just the trachea. If the patient cannot cooperate in these measures and secretions are judged to be a real clinical unacceptable levels of hypoxemia, then the patient may require reintubation for so-called "pulmonary toilet." Mask continuous positive airway pressure (CPAP) may help clear secretions on these occasions by reexpanding areas of lungs behind occluding secretions. These distal areas are accessed by collateral channels for gas flow. This situation is best prevented by avoiding premature extubation in a patient with copious secretions and decreased consciousness, significant muscle weakness, and/or difficulty with airway protection (e.g., postcervical esophagectomy).

BIBLIOGRAPHY

Badgett RG, et al: Can moderate chronic obstructive pulmonary disease be diagnosed by historical and physical findings alone? *Am J Med* 94:188–196, 1993.

Gal TJ: Bronchial hyperresponsiveness and anesthesia: physiologic and therapeutic perspectives, *Anesth Analg* 78:559–573, 1994.

Kroenke K, et al: Postoperative complications after thoracic and major abdominal surgery in patients with and without obstructive lung disease, *Chest* 104:1445–1451, 1993.

Lamberty JM, Rubin BK: The management of anaesthesia for patients with cystic fibrosis, *Anaesthesia* 40:448–459, 1985.

Nunn JF, et al: Respiratory criteria of fitness for surgery and anesthesia, *Anaesthesia* 43:543–551, 1988.

Pizov R, et al: Wheezing during induction of general anesthesia in patients with and without asthma: a randomized, blinded trial, *Anesthesiology* 82:1111–1116, 1995.

Ravin MB: Comparison of spinal and general anesthesia for lower abdominal surgery in patients with chronic obstructive pulmonary disease, *Anesthesiology* 35:319–322, 1971.

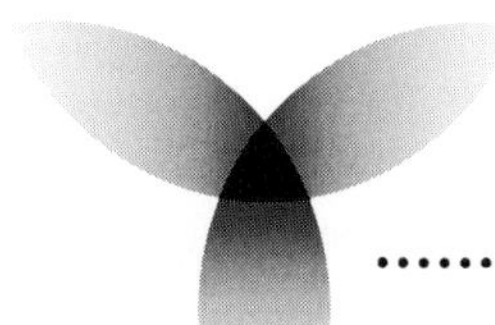

Chapter 13

Respiratory Failure: Predisposing Elements

David J. Stone, MD, Thomas J. Gal, MD

• PREOPERATIVE CLINICAL EVALUATION

Low Lung Volumes/Atelectasis

In addition to questions regarding baseline dyspnea, the patient should be asked about any history of perioperative problems, particularly concerning lung collapse (atelectasis) and pneumonia. It is important to consider potential extrapulmonary manifestations of systemic problems (e.g., rheumatoid arthritis, sarcoid, etc.). Once again, a patient's exercise tolerance is an important indicator of the ability to tolerate perioperative stresses.

Physical examination focuses on the detection of basilar crackles, which could be confused with left-sided heart failure in the perioperative period. Areas of reduced breath sounds are notable and may signify infiltrate, pleural effusion, or previous resection. A chest radiograph can be useful to delineate areas of density caused by fibrosis, which can be confused with congestive heart failure perioperatively, as well as delineate the nature of areas with reduced, or otherwise altered, breath sounds. The radiograph also serves as a valuable baseline with regard to the development of new perioperative problems.

The patient with a reduced lung volume may have difficulty in generating a clinically effective cough. In general, an effective cough requires an expired volume of at least 1 liter, a doubling of the normal tidal volume (≈4–500 ml). This may be verified preoperatively by a vital capacity (VC) of at least 1.6 to 2.0 liters because the VC will be reduced by 50% to 60% in the immediate postoperative period, and persist for as long as a week after upper-abdominal surgery. In addition, the small functional lung volumes that may be present postoperatively will tend to be associated with low ventilation/perfusion (V/Q) areas. This mismatch may be worsened as cardiac output (i.e., perfusion or Q) increases in the postoperative period from pain, tachycardia, fever, and hormonal stress response. Therefore, some estimate of preoperative VC may be useful in patients with symptomatic restrictive lung disease undergoing intraabdominal or thoracic procedures. If the preoperative VC is less than 1.6 to 2.0 liters (depending on the height/age of the patient, postoperative problems with adequate cough and oxygenation should be anticipated.

The severity of disease can also be estimated by the degree of chronic hypoxemia present. The alveolar air equation can be used to quantitate the relationship between inspired oxygen concentrations, arterial carbon dioxide levels, and the respiratory quotient (Box 13-1). The difference between the calculated alveolar and arterial oxygen partial pressures is referred to as the A-a gradient and describes the degree to which oxygenation is impaired. A previously documented need for home oxygen is an obvious marker of significant hypoxemia. While arterial blood gases provide a mildly invasive measure of chronic hypoxemia, the level of oxygen partial pressure in the blood can also be noninvasively estimated by determining hemoglobin saturation with a pulse oximeter. While many factors impact on the hemoglobin-oxygen dissociation curve (temperature, acid-base status, level of 2,3-DPG, P_aCO_2), oxygen saturations of 90%, 80%, and 75% represent P_aO_2s of approximately 60, 50, and 40, respectively.

Neuromuscular Disease/Chest Wall and Spinal Deformity

As usual, the history is the most important element in patient assessment, but the exercise tolerance of these patients may be limited by factors outside the respiratory system, such as lower extremity weakness. Chest radiographs are indicated if there is a significant degree of chest wall deformity and measures of the angles formed by the deformed spine have been used to "quantitate" the likelihood of respiratory dysfunction. Aspiration may also be a problem in patients too weak to protect the airway or in those who have esophageal reflux that may be, at least partly, the result of mechanical deformation of the gastroesophageal junction imposed by a significantly distorted spine. Patients with clinically significant myopathy and/or degrees of thoracic cage abnormalities should probably receive a measure of VC before surgery

Box 13-1 Alveolar Air Equation and A-a Gradient

In equation 1, P_AO_2 is the alveolar partial pressure of oxygen, F_IO_2 is the fractional inspired oxygen concentration, 760 mm Hg is atmospheric pressure, 47 mm Hg is water vapor pressure, and the respiratory quotient (CO_2 production ÷ O_2 production) is assumed to be 0.8.

1. Alveolar air equation: $P_AO_2 = F_IO_2\ (760 - 47 \text{ mm Hg}) - (P_aCO_2 \div 0.8)$.
2. To calculate alveolar-arterial gradient: For F_IO_2 of .21 and P_aCO_2 of 40, $P_AO_2 = .21(713) - (40 \div 0.8) = 150 - 50 = 100$
3. For P_aO_2 of 80, alveolar to arterial or A-a gradient = 20 mm Hg when $P_AO_2 = 100$

involving the thorax or abdomen. It is a matter of clinical judgment as to whether further tests are indicated. This decision considers the patient's symptoms, degree of muscle wasting and weakness on physical examination, as well as the nature of the intended procedure. In patients with muscle weakness, tests of inspiratory and expiratory pressures will provide some quantitation of the respiratory muscular dysfunction. Finally, the measurement of P_aCO_2 may give an integrated result as to the overall capability of the respiratory pump mechanism, even in the presence of normal lung tissue, per se. Patients with the peripheral neuropathies that are commonly seen (i.e., diabetic, uremic) are not particularly prone to respiratory failure on this basis. However, patients with severe, especially acute neuropathy, such as Guillain-Barré syndrome, require some measure of respiratory function such as a VC. Many of these patients will have their VCs monitored serially by their physicians, to identify worsening respiratory function and the need for endotracheal intubation to protect the airway, clear secretions, and provide adequate ventilation.

Severe obesity poses a significant respiratory problem and is partly the equivalent of chest wall deformity, imposed by the massive abdomens of these patients. Further preoperative testing is not likely to be useful unless an additional process is suspected to be present (e.g., chronic obstructive pulmonary disease [COPD] or myopathy), or there is strong suspicion of significant sleep apnea and its attendant problems. A physical examination gives some idea as to how severely breath sounds have been diminished by interceding tissue. A chest radiograph may show basal lung compression that can be confused with atelectasis perioperatively.

Ventilatory Failure

The principal basis is to identify ventilatory failure by assessment of arterial blood gases (ABGs). Arterial partial pressures of carbon dioxide (P_aCO_2) greater than 46 mm Hg are definitely abnormal in the absence of drugs such as opioids, while levels greater than 40 mm Hg are suspicious because patients tend to hyperventilate a bit from the discomfort and anxiety of the blood gas sampling. Hypercapnia may occur with normal lung function if carbon dioxide production is greatly increased, as with fever and thyrotoxicosis. Carbohydrate overfeeding in intensive care unit (ICU) patients may also result in elevated carbon dioxide production and hypercapnia. If respiratory drive is depressed, hypercapnia may occur, even in the presence of normal lung function. For this reason, the patient should not receive respiratory depressants to alleviate the discomfort of arterial puncture. In addition, a baseline P_aCO_2 should not be drawn after depressant premedication has been administered in the preoperative or operative areas.

Clinically, hypercapnia is most often observed in patients with COPD. It also is commonly present in patients with severe cystic fibrosis. In COPD patients, hypercapnia results primarily from ventilation-perfusion mismatch, resulting in a decreased alveolar ventilation (increased dead space), rather than from decreased levels of actual minute ventilation. On occasion, an obese patient will present with hypercapnia as a result of depressed central ventilatory drive ("pickwickian syndrome"), but upper airway obstruction and the increased mechanical load, both of which diminish alveolar ventilation, are important contributors to hypercapnia. Even so, hypercapnia is uncommon in obese patients unless this coexistent pathology is present. It would be unusual to observe hypercapnia in an ambulatory patient with asthma or restrictive lung disease. For this reason, preoperative examination of ABGs as part of a pulmonary function test (PFT) workup would be useful in a moderately symptomatic patient with COPD but probably not indicated with stable asthma. The presence of significant elevation of total carbon dioxide levels on routine chemistry testing (e.g., SMA-6 or -12) may be a clue that chronic hypercapnia may be present and partially compensated by a metabolic alkalosis.

The predicted impact of the operation on the respiratory system, most especially thoracic and upper-abdominal procedures, is an important factor in deciding the need for a preoperative measure of P_aCO_2. There are several practical reasons for evaluating the patient for the presence of chronic ventilatory insufficiency. For one, resting hypercapnia is a marker for advanced disease. Furthermore, these patients are at more risk for excessive respiratory depression, especially if a relatively potent premedication is administered to a patient who is subsequently unsupervised for a period of time. The anesthetic technique and monitoring may be altered by the detection of resting hypercapnia. If allowed to breathe spontaneously during an anesthetic, these patients are likely to develop unacceptably high levels of hypercapnia. In the early postoperative period when the respiratory system is stressed by pain, depressant pain medications, elevated carbon dioxide production, and the residual effects of anesthesia and surgery, marked hypercapnia is likely to persist and require intervention, at times.

PREOPERATIVE INTERVENTIONS

Low Lung Volume/Atelectasis

Since clearance of secretions may be an intra- and postoperative factor that contributes to atelectasis, a reduction in the production of secretions is important. An intravenous dose of 0.2 mg of glycopyrrolate will significantly reduce secretions, although it is not totally effective in the prevention of bronchospasm. Contrary to popular belief, this will not cause inspissation (drying and thickening) of secretions but may cause the patient to complain of a dry mouth for 8 to 12 hours.

Any reversible factors should be adequately investigated and remedied, if possible. If the disease process is one that is responsive to pharmacotherapy, drug dosages should be administered aggressively (for example, steroids in sarcoidosis or collagen-vascular disease). New, preoperative radiograph findings should be appropriately investigated before elective surgery if they are judged to be significant. If emergency surgery is required, the possibility of a pulmonary infiltrate representing a contagious process, such as tuberculosis, should be considered and appropriate measures used to protect personnel and equipment. Large pleural effusions may require drainage to improve lung expansion and gas exchange, but this must be weighed against concerns of postexpansion pulmonary edema.

The patient should receive some instruction about the importance of deep breathing and coughing postoperatively, to enhance lung expansion and secretion clearance, respectively. The likelihood of pain and the measures that will be used to reduce the pain should be mentioned. Epidural anesthesia may be an excellent modality for pain relief following thoracic and abdominal procedures. The catheter is generally inserted at a vertebral level that will afford segmental pain relief through local anesthetic infusion, hopefully without causing undue lower extremity weakness or sympathetic blockade. (The use of epidural anesthesia is discussed in more detail in the pain management and regional anesthesia chapters.) In high-risk patients undergoing major procedures, epidural anesthesia may be used in conjunction with general anesthesia for both intra- and postoperative analgesia. It is important to assure the patient that effective modalities are available to prevent or reduce pain magnitude to a tolerable level, and to emphasize that adequate, deep breaths and forceful coughs are necessary at times, in spite of some pain that these may cause.

If chest physical therapy is to be implemented, it should be shown preoperatively to the patient so that postoperatively, the vigorous stirup and chest pounding is not a source of anxiety. If inspiratory spirometers are to be used, the patient should be instructed in their principles and use preoperatively, to establish incentive for their use as well as some skill. In contrast to maximal inspiratory maneuvers, expiratory maneuvers, such as blow bottles, are counterproductive because forceful expiratory maneuvers actually compress airways and promote collapse of lung tissue. If there is a high likelihood of an uncommonly used item such as mask continuous positive airway pressure (CPAP), it may be a good idea to inform the respiratory therapists of this need to allow preparation of equipment and demonstration of the necessary tight-fitting mask to the patient.

Neuromuscular Disease/Chest Wall and Spinal Deformity

The patient with neuromuscular disease should have proper nutritional and electrolyte (potassium, magnesium, calcium, phosphorus) balance. If there is a predisposition to aspiration, administration of a clear antacid like Bicitra, or an agent to reduce acid production (ranitidine or omeprazole) should be considered. It is reasonable to administer an antisialagogue such as glycopyrrolate because patients with both muscle weakness and deformities are likely to have difficulty with removal of secretions. Preoperative emphasis on lung expansion maneuvers and insight concerning the possibility of postoperative ventilation is also important.

Ventilatory Failure

There are no specific measures to improve the patient with ventilatory failure and COPD, but attention should be paid to the small details of care. For example, the patient should be infection-free. Other contributing factors, such as heart failure, should be optimally treated. The appraisal of the patient's primary care physician is important as to whether the patient appears to be in the best possible state, or has problems that might benefit from further attention. If thoracic or major abdominal surgery is to be undertaken, combined epidural with general anesthesia should be discussed with the patient. The use of epidural anesthesia will allow adequate pain control without large amounts of systemic drugs that can depress ventilation further. It is impossible to quantify the risk of prolonged postoperative ventilation and even a potential inability to be unable to wean the patient from mechanical ventilation. However, these issues should be raised in some form with the patient and family, as well as all the physicians involved. The patient and family should also be educated to the nature of postoperative ventilation and what to expect if continued mechanical ventilation is necessary, i.e., inability to speak, dependence on a machine, and so forth.

• INTRAOPERATIVE PHYSIOLOGY AND INTERVENTIONS

Low Lung Volumes/Atelectasis

As in the case of obstructive disease, the possibility of local or regional anesthesia should be considered with the caveat that higher segmental block levels (i.e., above approximately the 10th thoracic segmental level) may impair respiratory function. However, patients do not usually have the problem of reflex bronchoconstriction and, in fact, may benefit from the large tidal volumes that can be provided through an endotracheal tube. Because of the reduced pulmonary compliance of many of these patients, a lower proportion of applied airway pressure will be transmitted to the pleural space and, hence, effects on venous return and cardiac output are lessened. In this population, tidal volumes slightly higher than usual (i.e., 12–15 ml/kg) may be useful in minimizing the low V/Q areas, which result when functional residual capacity (FRC) decreases with the induction of general anesthesia. This decrease in FRC occurs whether muscle relaxants are used or not, and is the most important intraoperative physiologic change so far as this patient population is concerned. If hypoxemia persists, in spite of the use of reasonably large tidal volumes and 100% oxygen, positive end-expiratory pressure (PEEP) can be used through a number of devices that can be introduced into the anesthesia circuit. Actually, a requirement for PEEP is unusual unless the patient has come from an ICU where PEEP had already been required. Oxygen toxicity from the use of 100% O_2 is not really an issue during the course of most anesthetics, but we would consider attempting to reduce the F_IO_2 after approximately 6 hours by adding air to the inhaled gases. Adding air produces an inhaled gas mixture with a lower F_IO_2 while monitoring for an acceptable P_aO_2 or oxygen saturation.

A long-standing attempt to improve oxygenation in the face of atelectasis/reduced lung volumes is the sigh breath, in which a tidal volume twice normal is administered to more fully expand the lungs. In the past, the use of sigh volumes was virtually standard when mechanical ventilation was used during an anesthetic and a separate control of sigh volume was present on the anesthesia ventilator. In today's practice, the routine use of fairly high tidal volumes (≥10 ml/kg) has eliminated the routine implementation of the sigh volume. The newer anesthesia ventilators may not provide this automatically, but a sigh breath can be given with the breathing bag, with attention to airway pressures and the cardiovascular effects of the maneuver. In fact, there is now evidence from computerized tomographic studies that a breath with inflation to 40 cm H_2O held for 10 seconds will abolish atelectasis.

Neuromuscular Disease/Chest Wall and Spinal Deformity

Unless there is coexisting disease, neuromuscular weakness should not present an insurmountable intraoperative problem. Anesthetic concerns include possible contraindications to the use of succinylcholine and extreme sensitivity to nondepolarizing muscle relaxants. The possibility of concomitant cardiomyopathy or autonomic neuropathy should be considered when planning and managing the anesthetic. It is critically important to be certain that the patient has sufficient strength to protect and maintain upper-airway integrity before extubation. Even if ventilation through the endotracheal tube appears to be reasonable, the patient may still not be strong enough to protect and maintain the airway patency because these functions require a greater return of neuromuscular function than ventilation does per se.

Patients with chest wall and spinal deformity are likely to have the problems of the patient with reduced lung volumes and should respond well to mechanical ventilation, with tidal volumes large enough to provide acceptable oxygenation and ventilation, without impairing cardiac output. These patients will often be operated on in the prone position. Thus, it is important to avoid pressure on sensitive structures (especially eyes and genitals) and to prevent excessive compression of abdominal contents. Abdominal compression can decrease FRC and impair ventilation, usually worsening oxygenation. Compression also can limit venous outflow from the surgical field and contribute to excessive blood loss.

Ventilatory Failure

The principal concern with anesthesia for the patient with chronic hypercapnia is the significant respiratory depression produced by the potent, inhaled anesthetic agents. These drugs produce a spontaneous respiratory pattern of rapid, small, shallow breaths that can result in severe hypercarbia in the patient with COPD who must cope with the mechanical load of airway obstruction. Other respiratory depressants used during the course of anesthetics include narcotics, intravenous induction agents such as thiopental and propofol, and benzodiazepines. In contrast, adjuncts such as nitrous oxide, lidocaine, droperidol, and ketamine are much less depressant.

An additional concern is that the ventilatory response to hypoxia is significantly diminished by the potent agents, even at low, subanesthetic concentrations. The effect will persist into the recovery-room period. Again, this may have the most impact on a chronically hypercapnic patient with reduced arterial oxygen levels who already exhibits both depressed hypoxic and hypercapnic drives. Oxygen should not be withheld from these patients for fear of eliminating the hypoxic drive to breathe. In fact, the hypercarbia that may result from high-inspired fractions of oxygen in these patients is minimal because of an actual decrease in minute ventilation. Rather, the major (80%–90%) component of the observed hypercarbia is caused by increased dead space generated by changes in blood flow distribution that occur when hypoxic pulmonary vasoconstriction is released. It is also a result of the Haldane effect, which refers to the increased ability of deoxygenated blood to carry carbon dioxide. Anesthesiologists are accustomed to coping with patients with diminished ventilatory responses to hypercarbia and hypoxia because they do so on a daily basis in the anesthetized patient.

The overall result is a patient who may become severely hypercarbic if allowed to breathe spontaneously during an anesthetic. Even the respiratory stimulus of surgical pain may not overcome this tendency toward excessive elevations of P_aCO_2. Monitoring end-tidal carbon dioxide with a capnometer may not give an accurate assessment of arterial values. That is because a large dead space may produce a greater than usual arterial to end-tidal carbon dioxide gradient, and falsely underestimate arterial carbon dioxide. Although mild degrees of hypercapnia and respiratory acidosis are acceptable, at some level, elevated levels may produce adverse cardiovascular effects, such as dysrhythmias, and direct cardiovascular depression if the sympathetic response to hypercapnia is insufficient.

For this reason, most anesthetized patients receive mechanical ventilation. The pattern of ventilation must allow sufficient time for complete exhalation. This can be achieved through relatively rapid inspiratory flows, which enable shorter inspiratory times and generous expiratory times. Notably, the overall effect of anesthesia on respiratory dead space in the intubated patient is generally minimal. This is because the increase in dead space that may be generated by anesthesia-induced changes in pulmonary blood flow distribution is offset by the reduction in upper airway anatomic dead space, afforded by an endotracheal tube. Upper-airway anatomic dead space is roughly 2 ml/kg, although it may be somewhat higher in COPD patients who tend to have dilated upper or conducting airways. Thus, the 75 ml extrathoracic anatomic dead space of a 75-kg patient would be replaced by the lesser dead space of an endotracheal tube. For an 8.0 mm internal diameter (ID) tube, this is 12 to 15 ml, depending on length. Note that while a smaller-diameter tube will result in less dead space, it will, to some degree, increase the resistive work of breathing once spontaneous respirations are resumed before extubation. The presence of any size endotracheal tube may provoke reflex distal airway constriction and impair gas exchange.

While most patients can be adequately ventilated, special situations such as laparoscopic surgery and one-lung ventilation (discussed in other chapters) may produce difficulties in ventilation. In addition, some patients may have very compliant lungs, which allow transmission of applied airway pressures, more completely than normal, to the pleural space. This transmission may result in a diminution in venous return and cardiac output that may require volume augmentation and inotropic or pressor support. In most cases, the ability to ventilate the patient adequately is facilitated by the decrease in carbon dioxide production that occurs as a result of general anesthesia (≈15%–20%⇓) and the mild hypothermia (≈7%⇓/°C) that inevitably occurs during surgery. The latter results from a cold operating environment and anesthetic effects on temperature control and compensatory mechanisms. Temperature may drop to some extent, even when warming measures are instituted.

Intraoperative management should consider the residual effect of anesthetic techniques on the postoperative course. Most importantly, the patient should not be left with a large residual of fixed intravenous agents whose elimination cannot be expedited. This procedure is in contrast to the inhalational anesthetics whose elimination can be accelerated by augmenting ventilation while the latter is still controlled. Relief of the pain that is likely to present immediately upon awakening can be approached in several ways, including a regional technique with local anesthetics and narcotics, pre-emergence injection of local anesthetics into the site of the incision or nerves supplying that area, and the use of nondepressant agents, such as nonsteroidal analgesics (e.g., ketorolac tromethamine). The agents may be contraindicated by their mild, anticoagulant effect, particularly in ophthalmologic or neurologic surgery. Parenteral narcotics can certainly be used cautiously, with a smaller dose designed to give some degree of analgesia without excessive respiratory depression on emergence. This dosage can then be carefully and slowly increased as required, according to clinical indicators such as respiratory rate and depth, autonomic responses, and patient demand, once awake. In spite of their theoretical advantages with the so-called "limited" or "ceiling effect," we have not found the use of narcotic agonist/antagonist agents to be useful.

• POSTOPERATIVE INTERVENTIONS

Low Lung Volume/Atelectasis

It is important to maintain adequate lung volumes once the mechanical advantage of positive-pressure ventilation is lost. In general, adequate oxygenation should be demonstrated in the spontaneously ventilating patient before the patient is extubated. If adequate oxygenation cannot be maintained, CPAP can be added to the breathing circuit while a reversible cause for the relative hypoxemia is investigated. The chest radiograph can reveal endobronchial intubation or large areas of collapse that call for vigorous chest physical therapy and CPAP. It can also show unsuspected pneumothoraces or pleural effusions. Adequate reversal of neuromuscular blockade should be evidenced by nerve stimulator or physical examination with additional reversal agent administered, if judged necessary, and a full, reversal dose has not already been given. A cooperative patient can be asked to take some deep breaths through the endotracheal tube; but, often the patient is sufficiently sleepy that a few large "sigh" breaths can be delivered with a breathing bag. Excess secretions should be suctioned, abdominal distention identified, and a sufficient F_1O_2 assured. If severe hypercapnia from a relative excess of narcotics is suspected, small incremental doses of naloxone (40 µg) can be given intravenously, in hopes of gradually increasing tidal volume and minute ventilation. This must be done slowly so that pain relief is not simultaneously eliminated in an abrupt fashion. Some patients may simply need a longer period of mechanical ventilation to allow elimination of inhaled anesthetics, intravenous anesthetics, and muscle relaxants.

Once oxygenation and ventilation, as well as airway patency, are judged to be adequate, the patient is extubated under conditions of careful clinical observation. We often encourage the patient to take a few good deep breaths and vigorous coughs, right after the endotracheal tube is removed. Deep breathing and coughing can be encouraged throughout the time the patient is under the intense nursing care of the recovery room. The nurses can also apply chest physical therapy to help loosen secretions which are causing difficulty. The patient must have sufficient analgesia to tolerate these maneuvers, but not so much that she/he is uncooperative or unarousable. If oxygenation is unacceptably poor, even on maximal oxygen therapy (high F_IO_2 by face mask), a trial of CPAP (or PEEP with spontaneous ventilation) by tight-fitting mask can be applied before reintubation is necessary. Usually, approximately 10 cm H_2O CPAP is applied for 10 to 15 minutes every hour because the apparatus is uncomfortable. However, it may effectively reverse micro- or macroatelectasis in the nonintubated patient and eliminate the need for reintubation. It should not be applied to the patient who is sleepy because it may predispose to aspiration. We rarely administer intermittent positive-pressure breathing (IPPB) to the extubated patient. While others have had some success with IPPB in the past, it is more technically difficult to perform than mask CPAP and not clearly more beneficial. It may, however, be beneficial in the setting of severe neuromuscular weakness or chest deformity.

After the initial recovery period, lung expansion and toilet can be achieved with the aforementioned deep breathing and coughing. These can be supplemented by incentive spirometry, in which the patient has an inexpensive feedback for the magnitude of the inspiratory effort, and chest physical therapy, which may loosen secretions and reexpand collapsed lung areas. Pulse oximetry may be a useful monitor to continue in the patients judged to be at highest risk, but is not of much use if no one is watching the monitor. The key clinical principal here is to intervene with the aforementioned measures before atelectasis is so severe that hypoxemia, pneumonia, and respiratory failure ensue. Good care can only be accomplished by the frequent patient observations of the clinician at bedside. If pain seems to be an important limiting factor and conventional management is not successful, consultation of an acute pain management service, if available, may be helpful in providing excellent pain relief that does not depress respiration. The question of reintubation is always a difficult one, and it is probably better to consult too early than too late. It is best to request the presence of the anesthesiologist as a consultant rather than simply ordering reintubation of the patient, and it is best to be physically present at bedside to discuss the problem. For example, the anesthesiologist may be more sensitive to the possibility that upper-airway obstruction, (rather than atelectasis), is the problem, or be able to suggest a change in respiratory care that avoids reintubation. The patient may well need to be moved to a patient-care area where closer monitoring is possible.

Neuromuscular Weakness/Chest Wall and Spinal Deformity

The postoperative problems of the patient with neuromuscular weakness include sensitivity to muscle relaxants with subsequent inadequate airway patency and protection. In addition, hypoventilation may be caused by upper airway obstruction, sensitivity to central respiratory depressants, or, simply, respiratory muscle weakness.

Difficulty clearing secretions is common because of weakness which limits the ability to take deep breaths and cough forcefully. Relaxants should be used with care and only as necessary surgery in these patients as the requirements for neuromuscular blockade are reduced in already weakened muscle. Adequate reversal, with particular attention to upper airway integrity, must be shown without question before extubation. This is a population in which conventional ICU criteria for weaning/extubation, such as inspiratory pressures more negative than –25 cm H_2O and VC, can be usefully applied in the recovery room.

After extubation, deep breathing and coughing may be inadequate in these patients with chest wall and spinal deformities; it may need to be supplemented with active maneuvers such as chest physical therapy. This may be the one group of patients who potentially benefit from IPPB. IPPB provides a degree of pulmonary inflation that they can't accomplish on their own. Patients with severe myasthenia gravis (see neurologic chapter) or extreme thoracic deformities, may receive continued periods of mechanical ventilation on the basis of preoperative findings such as angle of deformity, VC, and the location of surgery. Certainly, weaning from mechanical ventilation and extubation must be done more cautiously than usual while realizing the possibility that prolonged postoperative ventilation will be required at times.

Ventilatory Failure

For the patient with reduced volumes or with neuromuscular weakness, the immediate postoperative period is critical to good outcome. Before extubation, care is taken that muscle relaxants are adequately reversed and pain is under reasonable control without excessive sedation. If an epidural catheter is in place, adequate analgesia, primarily with local anesthetic infusion, should be established. On occasion, the endotracheal tube may represent an important obstacle to ventilation in these patients; so extubation actually improves ventilation. However, the lumens of the standard endotracheal tubes (7-mm ID in women, 8-mm ID in men) do not disproportionately increase the work of breathing. A small amount of pressure support ventilation, (8–10 cm H_2O), can be added to the circuit to eliminate the work of breathing represented by the endotracheal tube, if this is deemed necessary. The early postoperative period is stressful because patients' already inadequate ventilatory ability is further compromised by many factors. Factors include increased carbon dioxide production because of pain and stress, impairment of ventilation by pain and surgical incision site, and potential for airway obstruction, at both the upper airway and bronchial levels.

Other problems include increases in secretions and added worsening in V/Q distribution because of the tendency to take small breaths. This patient population, perhaps more than any other, is likely to require a period of postoperative ventilation to compensate for their many problems. The decision to continue postoperative ventilation may actually be made preoperatively, if the patient is sufficiently compromised and the procedure judged to be of great magnitude and impact. For example, a patient with a resting P_aCO_2 of 55 who is having emergency surgery for an acute abdomen that turns out to be caused by mesenteric ischemia, almost certainly will require continued ventilation postoperatively. For a larger number of patients, the decision to continue mechanical ventilation is made on the basis of patient observation and the analysis of ABGs in the early postoperative period. After ventilation is discontinued, and again after extubation, the patient must be carefully monitored for signs of hypoxemia or excessive carbon dioxide retention such as agitation, sedation, or hemodynamic abnormalities. In general, these patients deserve a relatively long stay in an area in which they can be closely observed, whether it be in the recovery room, special step-down unit, or even in an ICU.

BIBLIOGRAPHY

Bishop MJ, Cheney FW: Respiratory complications of anesthesia and surgery, *Semin Anesth* 2:91–99, 1983.

Celli BR, Rodriguez KS, Snider GS: A controlled trial of intermittent positive pressure breathing, incentive spirometry, and deep breathing exercises in preventing pulmonary complications after abdominal surgery, *Am Rev Respir Dis* 130:12–15, 1984.

Craig DB: Postoperative recovery of pulmonary function, *Anesth Analg* 60:46–52, 1981.

Gaskell DV, Webber BA: *The Brompton hospital guide to chest physiotherapy*, Oxford, 1973, Blackwell.

Hedley-Whyte J, et al: *Applied physiology of respiratory care*, Boston, 1976, Little, Brown and Co.

Peters RM, Turnier E: Physical therapy—indications for and effects in surgical patients, *Am Rev Respir Dis* 122 (5 Pt2):147–154, 1980.

Pontoppidan H: Mechanical aids to lung expansion in non-intubated surgical patients, *Am Rev Respir Dis* 122 (5 Pt2):109–119, 1980.

Stock MC, et al: Prevention of postoperative pulmonary complications with CPAP, incentive spirometry, and conservative therapy, *Chest* 87:151–157, 1985.

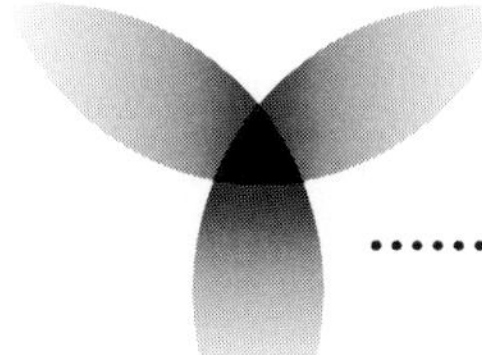

Chapter 14

Anesthesia for the Patient with Neurologic Disease

George S. Leisure, MD, Lawrence Phillips II, MD

Perioperative care of the patient with neurologic disease presents a challenge to the clinician. These illnesses often have associated cardiopulmonary and neuromuscular pathology that is of special concern in the perioperative period. In addition, these patients may be taking medications that have important anesthetic interactions. A thorough understanding of these disorders is essential to avoid postoperative morbidity and ensure an optimal outcome.

• DUCHENNE MUSCULAR DYSTROPHY (DMD)

Duchenne muscular dystrophy is the most common and most severe form of all the muscular dystrophies. It occurs with an incidence of 3/10,000 live births, and is inherited as an X-linked recessive disorder. Although males are primarily affected by this disease, some female carriers may have mild symptoms. The affected patients produce a structural protein, dystrophin, which is found under the sarcolemma of muscle fibers. Plasma creatine kinase (CK) levels are elevated, which possibly reflects an abnormal increase in the permeability of muscle cell membranes. Female carriers may also have elevated plasma CK levels.

The condition is usually clinically suspected around the age of 3 years when the child presents with proximal muscle weakness, pseudohypertrophy of the calf muscles caused by fatty infiltration, and an abnormal waddling gait. Intellectual impairment is common. Muscle biopsy confirms the diagnosis.

The predictable sequelae of this disease includes a relentlessly progressive kyphoscoliosis leading to a severe, restrictive pulmonary disease. The progressive wasting of the respiratory and pharyngeal muscles interferes with effective coughing, leading to frequent episodes of pneumonia. Cardiac muscle degeneration is common, but a congestive cardiomyopathy may occur in only 10% of affected individuals. Papillary muscle dysfunction with mitral regurgitation can be shown in 25% of cases. Death usually occurs by the third decade and is often the result of either myocardial insufficiency or recurrent pulmonary infections and respiratory failure.

Two of the primary perioperative considerations for the patient with DMD include cardiopulmonary dysfunction and an abnormal response to depolarizing muscle relaxants. Dystrophic cardiomyopathy may occur in these patients and is characterized by a loss of myocardium with near-normal performance of the remaining sarcomeres. Histopathologic findings include myofibrillar loss with fibrous replacement. Intraoperative cardiac arrest and death caused by dystrophic cardiomyopathy have been reported. Teenagers with DMD undergoing general anesthesia, especially for spinal fusion, should be evaluated preoperatively for myocardial dysfunction. Clinical evidence of cardiac disease may be difficult to detect in the wheelchair-bound patient. However, Doppler and two-dimensional echocardiography may be helpful in determining the need for a thermodilution-flow-directed pulmonary artery catheter. Myocardial depressants such as halothane and thiopental should be used with caution. In addition, prolonged postoperative ventilatory support may be required in those with advanced stages of the disease, especially in those with vital capacities (VCs) less than 30% of predicted. Diminution of respiratory function in DMD has been related to both thoracic scoliosis and respiratory muscle weakness, with muscle weakness being the major determinant of worsening respiratory function.

The administration of intravenous succinylcholine has led to massive hyperkalemia in patients with DMD, leading to cardiac arrest, rhabdomyolysis, hypermetabolism, and a syndrome similar to malignant hyperthermia. As a result, although succinylcholine has been used safely in some of these patients, it is best avoided in this population. The link between this hyperkalemic response and the syndrome of malignant hyperthermia is suggested in halothane-caffeine contracture testing. However, it remains unknown whether the structural protein abnormalities found in DMD are equivalent to those of malignant hyperthermia.

• AMYOTROPHIC LATERAL SCLEROSIS (ALS)

Jean Martin Charcot is credited with the original description of amyotrophic lateral sclerosis (ALS) around 1872. It is also commonly referred to as Lou Gehrig's disease, so-named after the famous New York Yankees third baseman. It is the most common progressive disease of motor neurons with an annual incidence rate of 0.4 to

1.76 per 100,000 population. Males are affected more frequently than females. Most patients are older than 55 years when symptoms begin. About 10% of cases are familial in an autosomal-dominantly inherited pattern.

The principal pathologic finding is loss of nerve cells in the anterior horns of the spinal cord and motor nuclei of the lower brainstem and cortical motoneurons. These lost cells are then replaced by fibrous astrocytes. The subsequent degeneration of the corticospinal tract is most evident in the lower parts of the spinal cord but can be traced up through the brainstem to the posterior limb of the internal capsule and corona radiata.

The pathogenesis of this disease is unclear. Some postulate a relationship between an attack of paralytic poliomyelitis and the subsequent development of ALS. However, this occurrence is probably a chance event and does not represent the reactivation of the polio virus or any other slow virus. Trauma, disordered immune function, and intoxication with heavy metals such as lead, mercury, and aluminum have all been linked to the development of ALS but the relationship is not understood. Current theories also include the neurotoxic effects of glutamate, an excitatory neurotransmitter. For unclear reasons, an excess of glutamate activity in motor neurons, may literally excite cells to death. Emerging treatments directed toward inhibiting glutamate production, or its effect on cells, have shown some efficacy in slowing the course of the disease; but the overall natural history is of relentless progression to death in 2 to 4 years after diagnosis.

The clinical manifestations of ALS include both upper and lower motor neuron symptoms. The initial signs are often asymmetrical, with the patient complaining of weakness in one extremity. Tasks requiring fine motor control may become difficult. Atrophy of the muscles, as well as fasciculations may be evident. The disease progresses to other extremities, and the triad of atrophic weakness, spasticity, and generalized hyperreflexia in the absence of sensory changes makes the diagnosis. In later stages, the atrophic weakness spreads to the neck, tongue, pharyngeal, and laryngeal muscles and, finally, to muscles in the trunk and lower extremities. As a result of the truncal and pharyngeal muscle weakness, respiratory insufficiency and aspiration are common complications. The heart is unaffected by ALS, but autonomic dysfunction can be present. In approximately one third of patients, the onset of symptoms is in a bulbar distribution. Disease progression and death typically occur more rapidly in such patients.

Perioperative considerations in the patient with ALS involve primarily judicious respiratory care. General anesthetics depress the swallowing reflex in a dose-related manner, which may further predispose these patients to aspiration and airway obstruction, especially if bulbar involvement is profound. Many anesthetics also depress ventilation, which may predispose to alveolar hypoventilation, making weaning and extubation difficult. In one study, 86% of patients with ALS at the time of presentation had evidence of respiratory muscle weakness as shown by pulmonary function studies, although only 19% were symptomatic. There is one case report of a patient with ALS whose initial symptoms were those of obesity-hypoventilation syndrome. If a patient has any respiratory muscle weakness or bulbar dysfunction, endotracheal intubation and mechanical ventilation, even for brief periods, is risky. Once intubated, such patients are difficult or impossible to wean from the ventilator. Because many patients with ALS have prepared advanced directives indicating their wish to not be subjected to long-term mechanical ventilation, they should be fully informed of the risk for its necessity prior to any procedure requiring general anesthesia.

The potential for massive hyperkalemia and cardiac arrest in patients with lower motor-neuron disease receiving succinylcholine is well known. Succinylcholine should, therefore, be avoided. In addition, the patient with ALS may be sensitive to the effects of nondepolarizing muscle relaxants. These agents should be used carefully, titrating to clinical effect with a nerve stimulator.

Epidural anesthesia has been used safely in patients with ALS. The main advantage of a regional technique is that many of the potential hazards of general anesthesia can be avoided. However, if the sensory level rises above T6, ventilatory impairment may occur because of both decreases in expiratory reserve volume and difficulty clearing secretions caused by the absence of an effective cough. Although no data exists to suggest that regional anesthesia causes exacerbations of neurologic disease in patients with ALS, it is prudent to discuss the risks and benefits of regional versus general anesthesia with the patient before proceeding, as well as to document neurologic deficits.

FREIDREICH'S ATAXIA (FA)

In 1861, Freidreich of Heidelberg described a type of familial progressive ataxia that he observed among nearby villagers, and by 1882, this new clinical entity bore his name. Freidreich's ataxia is a familial neuromuscular disorder characterized by degeneration of the posterior columns and the corticospinal and spinocerebellar tracts. The disease exhibits two inheritance patterns. The most common one is autosomal-recessive, with an average age of onset at 11.75 years, and the other dominant, with an average age of onset at 20.4 years. The disease is steadily progressive with a median age at death of 26.5 years for those with the recessive form, and 39.5 years for those with the dominant form.

The initial presentation is ataxia of gait, which usually affects both lower extremities simultaneously. Early symptoms include difficulty with standing steady and running. As is consistent with the pathologic findings in the disease, the ataxia is of mixed sensory and cerebellar type. In many cases, walking is no longer possible within 5 years of the onset of symptoms. The hands become clumsy months or years after the gait disorder. Dysarthria, impaired deglutition, tremor, pes cavus, emotional lability, diabetes mellitus, and kyphoscoliosis are all features of the disease.

Cardiomyopathy is an important aspect of FA. Freidreich recognized an associated heart disease in his original description of the disorder. A form of cardiomyopathy develops in 50% to 90% of patients, and represents the most common cause of death in these patients. In fact, long-term follow-up shows cardiac involvement in 100% of cases. Cardiomyopathy may be the presenting feature of the disease, without ataxia or other neurologic symptoms. The severity of the cardiomyopathy may not correlate with that of the neurologic condition. Cardiac symptoms include palpitations, chest pain, and progressive heart failure.

The most common echocardiographic finding in FA is that of concentric, left ventricular thickening. Thickening was found in 68% of patients in one study. The histologic findings are mainly of diffuse myocardial fibrosis, cellular hypertrophy, and necrosis of cardiac muscle fibers. Patients with FA who have left ventricular hypertrophy (LVH) may exhibit diastolic function abnormalities. Other cardiac defects have also been described in this disease. A small proportion of patients have a hypertrophic obstructive cardiomyopathy with asymmetric septal hypertrophy and LV outflow obstruction. Also rarely reported is a group of patients with a nondilated, globally hypofunctional left ventricle, or so-called "dystrophic" heart. It is interesting to note that a cardiomyopathy seems specifically associated with FA and not with other spinocerebellar-posterior, column-corticospinal, degenerative diseases.

In the perioperative period, attention should be focused primarily on the cardiovascular system. No correlation has been found between the duration or severity of the disease and the degree of LVH. Finley and Campbell suggest performing an echocardiogram as a minimum investigation before general or major regional anesthesia in patients with FA. Furthermore, an electrocardiogram may be important because in a study of fatal cases of FA, atrial dysrhythmias were found in 50% of the patients before death. Furthermore, Alboliras et al. reported that the presence of atrial dysrhythmias in FA is a marker of LV dysfunction and has negative, prognostic implications. The use of invasive monitoring and choice of specific anesthetic techniques must be based on the patient's full cardiac evaluation.

Kyphoscoliosis is present in up to 80% of cases, progressing rapidly once the patient becomes wheelchair-bound. The result is a progressive, restrictive, pulmonary disease pattern with a decrease in vital and total lung capacities. Consequently, respiratory failure in the perioperative period is a hazard. In the advanced form of the disease, when deglutition becomes impaired, aspiration may also become a concern.

Response to muscle relaxants in FA is not fully understood. There are reports describing hypersensitivity to nondepolarizing muscle relaxants, as well as reports describing a normal response to these agents. It is best to administer these agents judiciously while monitoring response with a nerve stimulator. As with any disease that involves denervation, there exists the possibility of massive hyperkalemia after succinylcholine administration.

Finally, diabetes mellitus may occur in up to 18% of patients, with as many as 40% exhibiting abnormal glucose tolerance tests. Both insulin-dependent and noninsulin-dependent types are reported and can be managed in the usual careful manner.

MULTIPLE SCLEROSIS (MS)

Multiple sclerosis is a demyelinating disease of the brain and spinal cord, which remits and recurs over a period of many years. The diagnosis is usually secured by this history of a relapsing and remitting course, as well as evidence on examination of more than one discrete lesion in the central nervous system (CNS). The lesions, or plaques, that characterize this disease affect principally the white matter of the brain and spinal cord and do not extend beyond the root entry zone of the cranial and spinal nerves. The lesions show no special preference for a particular system of fibers but, rather, are randomly spread throughout the brainstem, spinal cord, and cerebellar peduncles. These plaques destroy the myelin but usually leave nerve cells essentially intact.

The etiology of MS is unclear. It may be an autoimmune disease that is initiated by an environmental insult, such as a viral infection. There does exist, however, an epidemiologic association with geographic location. The risk of developing MS rises with increasing latitude in this northern hemisphere. For example, the disease has a prevalence of less than 1 per 100,000 in equatorial areas, 6 to 14 per 100,000 in the southern United States and southern Europe, and 30 to 80 per 100,000 in the northern United States, northern Europe, and Canada. Curiously, a similar pattern has not been found in the southern hemisphere. A familial tendency towards MS is also well established.

The clinical presentation of MS is variable. Some patients exhibit an acute onset and others, a more insidious onset. About two thirds of cases have their onset between the ages of 20 and 40 years. Weakness and/or numbness of one or more extremities are the initial complaints in approximately one-half of patients. Nearly 25% of cases will present with an episode of retrobulbar or optic neuritis, characterized by partial or total loss of vision in one eye. Other presentations and symptoms include transverse myelitis, gait ataxia, brainstem symptoms such as diplopia, vertigo and vomiting, trigeminal neuralgia, and disorders of micturition, as well as impotence. Progression of the disease is variable. Long-term follow-up studies show that 20% to 35% of MS patients have a benign course with minimal disability, 3% to 12% have a malignant course with a rapid and severe disability, and the majority have a course somewhere in between. Relapses have been associated with surgery, anesthesia, fever, emotional or physical trauma, and pregnancy.

Perioperative care of the patient with MS is a challenge. The preoperative neurologic condition of the patient should be documented. Pulmonary function needs to be addressed because kyphoscoliosis may be present, causing restrictive pulmonary disease. Furthermore, acute respiratory failure and respiratory weakness caused by diaphragmatic paralysis have been reported rarely in MS. Lability of the autonomic nervous system has also been reported. Consequently, special attention is required in anesthetic drug selection and during patient movement in order to avoid severe hypotension. In advanced forms of the disease, succinylcholine may need to be avoided because of the possibility of massive hyperkalemia.

There is no evidence that any of the drugs used to induce general anesthesia cause exacerbations of MS. However, a rise in temperature may be associated with a temporary clinical deterioration. The mechanism of this deterioration is uncertain. It has been shown that demyelinated axons are capable of conduction but function optimally at a certain temperature. An increase in temperature may inhibit optimal function. Consequently, it may be advisable to avoid agents with anticholinergic properties such as glycopyrrolate, which may increase the possibility of a temperature rise. Furthermore, antipyretics should be administered when indicated and causes of infection should be treated promptly.

The issue of regional anesthesia remains controversial. Numerous reports exist of exacerbations of MS after spinal anesthesia. The mechanism of this reaction is unclear but may relate to the potential neurotoxic effect of a drug exposed to a spinal cord lacking the protective nerve sheath because of demyelination. It does not appear that diagnostic lumbar puncture induces relapses. Successful lumbar epidural anesthesia has been reported in patients with MS; but, again, there exists the possibility of exacerbation of symptoms. Epidural anesthesia is not contraindicated in those with MS, but a full discussion of risks/benefits should be made with the patient before proceeding. The pregnant patient with MS may be at even higher risk of developing relapse in the puerperium. Labor epidural anesthesia may be approached but only with caution.

PARKINSON'S DISEASE (PD)

This relatively common disease was first described by James Parkinson in 1817 and is also known as paralysis agitans. It is a disease that usually begins between the ages of 40 and 70 years and is uncommon under 30 years of age. It is estimated that 1% of the U.S. population over 50 is affected, males more commonly than females. The pathogenesis of the disease involves a loss of pigmented cells in the substantia nigra and other pigmented nuclei such as the locus ceruleus and dorsal motor nucleus of the vagus. Dopaminergic nerve fibers in the basal ganglia degenerate, leading to a depletion of dopamine in the basal ganglia of the brain. Dopamine acts by inhibiting the rate of firing of neurons that control the extrapyramidal motor system. Consequently, depletion of dopamine leads to decreased inhibition of this system, leading to many of the clinical signs that will be discussed. Although many predisposing factors have been suggested, the etiology of the malady remains obscure.

The clinical picture is characterized by expressionless facies, slowness and poverty of voluntary movement, festinating gait, a resting tremor, stooped posture, soft and monotonous voice, and cog-wheel rigidity. Some of the early symptoms may be difficult to recognize because they may simply be attributed to advancing age. Resting tremor is the most characteristic abnormality in PD and is the presenting symptom in 70% of cases. The tremor, often referred to as a "pill-rolling" tremor, is noted to be prominent in the resting extremity, disappearing briefly with intentional movement. Bradykinesia, or slowness in both the initiation and execution of movement, is a hallmark of the disease. Patients are also noted to have facial immobility characterized by infrequent blinking and little emotional response. As the disease progresses, micrographia develops, the voice becomes progressively less audible, walking is reduced to shuffling, and the patient frequently loses balance. Dementia is commonly associated with PD, occurring in 10% to 20% of advanced cases.

The primary perioperative concerns for these patients involve fully understanding the medications used in PD and the side effects of these agents. Levodopa, an immediate precursor of dopamine, is commonly used in an effort to increase brain concentrations of dopamine. Levodopa is used because dopamine does not cross the blood-brain barrier. The side effects of levodopa may involve the cardiovascular, gastrointestinal, and central nervous systems. Dopamine that results from levodopa administration can augment cardiac rate and contractility, possibly predisposing to cardiac irritability. Consequently, ketamine, halothane, and local anesthetic solutions containing epinephrine should be used with caution. Orthostatic hypotension may also occur in those treated with levodopa for several reasons. First, dopamine inhibits renin release and promotes increases in renal blood flow, glomerular filtration rate, and sodium excretion. Second, dopamine inhibits norepinephrine production in the sympathetic nervous system through a negative-feedback loop. In addition, dopamine replaces norepinephrine at some sites, and because of its weaker pressor action, fails to support the blood pressure adequately. Lastly, patients with PD often have intrinsic autonomic insufficiency. Significant hypotension during anesthesia should be treated with small doses of a direct-acting vasopressor, such as phenylephrine.

Levodopa causes nausea and vomiting, probably through dopaminergic stimulation of the chemoreceptor trigger zone. This is especially prominent when beginning treatment. Consequently, if patients are symptomatic, the usual considerations apply to decreasing the risk of aspiration on induction of general anesthesia. Chronic levodopa treatment can also cause CNS dysfunction, such as dyskinesia. Agitation, confusion, and overt psychosis have been reported in the postoperative period, with an increased incidence in those with PD. It is important to continue treatment with levodopa throughout the perioperative period to avoid skeletal muscle rigidity, including the morning of surgery, because the half-life of levodopa is short. Drugs with dopamine-antagonizing properties, such as phenothiazines and butyrophenones, should be avoided.

Bromocriptine, lisuride, and pergolide are all drugs that may be used in PD. The side-effect profile is similar to levodopa with nausea, vomiting, hallucinations, and hypotension all possible. Amantadine is sometimes used, and side effects are rare. Anticholinergics are also used, and are especially useful for reducing tremor, but less effective for treating bradykinesia and postural instability. The side effects of dry mouth, urinary retention, and confusion can be troublesome. Selegiline, a selective monoamine oxidase (MAO) B inhibitor, has also been used with some success. It does not cause a potentially life-threatening potentiation of catecholamines, as do the nonselective MAO inhibitors.

The choice of muscle relaxants does not seem to be influenced by the presence of PD. However, succinylcholine should be used with caution because one case report of succinylcholine-induced hyperkalemia in a patient with PD exists. Finally, one case report exists of an exacerbation of PD after alfentanil administration. It was suggested that alfentanil may have precipitated this reaction through a dopaminergic-blocking action in the nigrostriatal system.

MYASTHENIA GRAVIS (MG)

Myasthenia gravis is an autoimmune disease resulting from the production of antibodies against the acetylcholine receptors (AChRs) of the motor end-plate. The prevalence of the disease is approximately 1 in every 20,000 adults. It may occur in any age group, but the incidence in those under 10 years of age is low, representing about 10% of all cases. The peak onset for females is between the ages of 20 to 30 years, whereas the peak onset for males is in the sixth to seventh decade.

The trigger for this autoimmune disease is unknown. However, a genetic predisposition exists, as well as an association with other autoimmune disorders such as systemic lupus erythematosus, thyrotoxicosis, polymyositis, and rheumatoid arthritis. The disease is frequently associated with morphologic abnormalities of the thymus gland, such as thymoma and thymic hyperplasia. Hyperplasia occurs more often in younger patients, and thymomas are more common in those over age 30. In fact, 10% of patients with MG have thymomas, especially older males.

Antibodies to the AChR protein are present in the sera of approximately 85% of patients with MG. The majority of these antibodies are of the IgG class and bind to the main immunogenic region of the alpha subunit of the AChR. These antibodies reduce the number of active receptors, either by a functional block of the receptor, by increasing the rate of receptor degradation, or by a complement-mediated lysis of the postsynaptic membrane. The level of circulating receptor antibody does not correlate well with clinical severity of the disease. Furthermore, those patients with MG who fail to show AChR antibodies may possess different antibodies that bind to other, yet to be identified, end-plate determinants.

A clinical hallmark of this disease is that repeated or persistent activity of a skeletal muscle group leads to exhaustion of its contractile power. Rest partially restores the power. The onset of the disease is insidious, and the progression is marked by periods of exacerbations and remissions. The muscles of the eyes, face, jaws, throat, and neck are affected first. The disease then progresses to involve the muscles of the trunk and limbs, proximal muscles being more affected than distal ones. Patients may complain of drooping eyelids and diplopia, as well as altered facial mobility and expression. With bulbar involvement, weakness of pharyngeal and laryngeal muscles results in dysarthria, dysphasia, and difficulty with clearing of secretions. Weakness tends to increase as the day progresses, and temporary increases in weakness have been reported with vaccinations, infections, stress, surgery, menstruation, pregnancy, and extremes of temperature. Smooth and cardiac muscles are not involved. Neonates born to mothers with MG exhibit transient myasthenia in 15% to 20% of cases. This is caused by the passage of AChR antibodies across the placenta and may last for 1 to 3 weeks, sometimes necessitating controlled mechanical ventilation.

Treatment of MG may include immunosuppressants, glucocorticoids, plasmapheresis, thymectomy, and, most commonly, anticholinesterase drugs. These last medications inhibit the breakdown of acetylcholine by tissue cholinesterase, thereby increasing the amount of acetylcholine at the neuromuscular junction. Excessive doses of an anticholinesterase can precipitate a cholinergic crisis, which is marked by increased weakness and excessive muscarinic effects, such as diarrhea, salivation, miosis, and bradycardia.

Perioperative care of the patient with MG begins with adequate preoperative preparation. The severity of myasthenia and involvement of respiratory and bulbar muscles must be assessed. Pulmonary function studies can be done to identify those with poor respiratory reserve and to help predict the need for postoperative respiratory support. If the patient is responding well to the use of pyridostigmine, no further therapy may be needed. However, if the response is poor, preoperative plasmapheresis should be considered. It has been suggested that patients with severe forms of the disease who are treated with prethymectomy plasma exchange required less mechanical ventilation and less time in the intensive care unit, postoperatively.

Patients with MG may need postoperative mechanical ventilation because of respiratory failure. Four risk factors associated with the need for postoperative ventilation have been identified:

1. Duration of MG for longer than 6 years.
2. A history of chronic respiratory disease other than respiratory dysfunction because of MG.
3. A dose of pyridostigmine greater than 750 mg per day.
4. A preoperative vital capacity less than 2.9 l. The location of surgery may be important because only 7.4% of patients undergoing transcervical thymectomy required prolonged postoperative ventilation, whereas 33% to 50% of patients required prolonged postoperative ventilation following transsternal thymectomy. Return of adequate muscle strength and ability to protect the airway must be assured by the usual clinical criteria before extubation.

When possible, the use of regional or local anesthesia is certainly prudent. Theoretically, the use of large doses of ester-type local anesthetics should be avoided in those myasthenic patients on anticholinesterase therapy, because plasma cholinesterase activity is decreased and toxicity may be enhanced. The use of tetracaine for spinal anesthesia may be used because only small doses are needed. There is no evidence that the metabolism of amide-type local anesthetics is altered in MG.

Muscle relaxants must be used carefully in MG. Because of a decreased number of functional ACh receptors in MG, patients exhibit a decreased response to depolarizing agents and a significant sensitivity to nondepolarizing relaxants. This abnormal response is seen in patients who have localized ocular myasthenia and even in those in remission. The ED_{50} and ED_{95} for succinylcholine in patients with MG is 2.0 and 2.6 times normal, respectively; so a large dose may be needed for intubation. However, anticholinesterases used preoperatively can reduce plasma cholinesterase activity, causing a delayed hydrolysis of succinylcholine and potentiation of neuromuscular blockade.

Nondepolarizing drugs must be used with extreme caution in MG. The intermediate-acting drugs atracurium and vecuronium can be used; but, despite their rapid elimination, both of these drugs exhibit prolonged effects in those with MG compared to controlled subjects. Response to muscle relaxants must be carefully titrated to clinical effect with the use of a nerve stimulator. Some clinicians avoid muscle relaxants completely. Certain drugs, especially the aminoglycoside antibiotics, potent, inhaled agents, and magnesium can potentiate the neuromuscular-blocking actions of muscle relaxants and should be used cautiously in those with MG.

The myasthenic syndrome or Lambert-Eaton syndrome must be distinguished from MG. It is a paraneoplastic syndrome often associated with small-cell carcinoma of the lung or other metastatic cancers or autoimmune diseases. It is characterized by proximal muscle weakness, which usually affects the lower extremities. Unlike MG, repeated effort actually improves the muscle weakness, and anticholinesterases are of no benefit. The disorder is thought to result from a prejunctional defect in the release of acetylcholine caused by antibodies directed against voltage-sensitive calcium channels. Patients with this disorder are sensitive to both nondepolarizing and depolarizing agents.

SHY-DRAGER SYNDROME (SDS)

In 1960, Shy and Drager described a group of patients with widespread neurologic disease associated with autonomic failure, causing orthostatic hypotension. The syndrome presents between the fifth and seventh decades of life, is more common in males than females, and does not appear to be inherited. It is a slowly progressive illness that leads to death, often as a result of postsyncopal cerebral ischemia.

The principal pathologic finding is degeneration of the preganglionic lateral horn neurons of the thoracic spinal segments. Later, nerve cells in the vagal nuclei, as well as the nuclei of the tractus solitarius, locus ceruleus, and sacral autonomic nuclei degenerate. The etiology of this disease is unknown.

These pathologic findings correlate well with the clinical findings associated with loss of sympathetic and parasympathetic tone. The triad of postural hypotension, anhidrosis, and impotence, as well as urinary and fecal incontinence, is common to most patients. The severity of the hypotension progresses and is associated with blurry vision, dizziness on standing, and fainting on walking. Not only do patients with SDS exhibit a failure of compensatory vasoconstriction, but they also exhibit a minimal heart-rate response to postural changes. Disordered thermoregulation, unequal pupils, stridor, and difficulty with speaking and swallowing are reported in these patients. Eventually, most of the patients will develop parkinsonian symptoms and dementia.

One of the primary concerns in the perioperative period is the autonomic failure associated with SDS. Preoperative preparation and meticulous intraoperative management are essential in these patients to prevent severe hypotension without causing massive volume overload. Management goals are aimed at decreasing venous pooling, increasing systemic vascular resistance, and increasing plasma volume.

Postural training by sleeping with a 25° head-up tilt and elastic stockings can be used to decrease venous pooling in the lower extremities. The application of 50 mm Hg positive pressure through a G-suit has been used. However, the last method is both uncomfortable and impractical. Preoperative use of sympathomimetic drugs to increase systemic vascular resistance has met with variable success. Amphetamine use may actually exacerbate the symptoms of orthostatic hypotension by causing weight loss with subsequent reduction in plasma volume. MAO inhibitors have been used and produce unpredictable responses. Indirect-acting drugs, such as atropine and ephedrine, will provide little clinical response. Direct-acting drugs, such as phenylephrine, will work. However, these drugs need to be used cautiously because of the possible risk of an exaggerated hypertensive response, reflecting denervation hypersensitivity. Finally, the mineralocorticoid, 9-α-fluorohydrocortisone has been used to help maintain plasma volume through its sodium-retaining properties. During chronic administration, it may actually work by increasing the sensitivity of the resistance vessels to the low concentrations of circulating catecholamines. The possibility of steroid dependence and other side effects must be considered in these patients.

Intraoperative management is primarily concerned with avoidance of severe hypotension. Because of the possibility of abrupt blood pressure changes caused by the absence of intact cardiovascular reflexes, placement of an intraarterial catheter should be considered. A central venous pressure monitor may also aid in volume assessment. Induction agents should be chosen that produce minimal cardiovascular changes. Volatile anesthetic agents can cause exaggerated hypotension because compensatory responses, such as vasoconstriction and tachycardia, may fail because of the absence of carotid sinus activity in these patients. Furthermore, positive-pressure ventilation may depress cardiac output by inhibiting venous return. Maintenance of anesthesia may be complicated by the absence of signs of depth of anesthesia, hyperpyrexia because of poor sweating, and sluggish pupillary reflexes or unequal pupils. The latter finding should be recognized preoperatively to avoid making an erroneous diagnosis of a severe neurologic insult.

Vocal cord paralysis has been reported in SDS. The vocal cord lesion is usually a bilateral abductor paralysis with resultant glottic obstruction and ventilatory failure. This may be the presenting feature in some cases. The obstruction is not always total, and the patient may live uneventfully for some time after the diagnosis. A patient with bilateral abductor vocal cord paralysis may have minimal stridor and normal phonation. Consequently, the diagnosis may not be considered in the preoperative evaluation. It may be prudent to arrange a vocal cord examination on any patient with SDS who presents for anesthesia and surgery.

• STROKE

Strokes are caused by cerebral thrombosis, cerebral embolism, or intracranial hemorrhage. Cerebral thrombosis develops most commonly in those with extensive atherosclerosis. Other causes include profound hypotension, inflammatory diseases of the blood vessels, and hematologic conditions that predispose to poor microvascular blood flow, such as polycythemia and sickle cell anemia. Symptoms depend on the blood vessel affected, and the neurologic dysfunction may progress over minutes to hours. Sequelae can be minor and transient or severe and permanent.

Cerebral embolism is most commonly caused by embolization from the heart, especially in the face of bacterial endocarditis, prosthetic heart valves, and atrial fibrillation. Other sources of embolism include tumor cells, air, and fat. A paradoxical cerebral embolism is one in which an embolus passes from the right atrium into the left atrium through a patent foramen ovale, proceeding, then, directly to the brain. In contrast to cerebral thrombosis, the symptoms of embolism usually have an abrupt onset. The type of neurologic deficits depends on the vessel that becomes occluded.

Intracranial hemorrhage is most commonly caused by rupture of small aneurysms. These aneurysms result from a congenital weakness in the media of the cerebral arteries, predisposing them to rupture. Congenital cerebral aneurysms can be single or multiple. Approximately 50% occur in the middle cerebral artery, and 30% are in the region where the anterior communicating artery joins the anterior cerebral arteries. Intracranial hemorrhage also may occur because of an arteriovenous malformation. Symptoms are related to the site and rapidity of bleeding, as well as the development of increased intracranial pressure.

Perioperative care of a patient who has recently had a stroke involves a thorough medical evaluation. Patients suffering from cerebral embolus or thrombosis may require a cardiac evaluation before surgery because significant cardiac pathology may be present. If a serious neurologic deficit exists with profound motor impairment, succinylcholine should not be used because of the possibility of a massive hyperkalemic response.

In the face of a recent stroke, it may be prudent to delay elective surgery. Cerebral blood flow undergoes changes after a stroke. Loss of carbon dioxide responsiveness and autoregulation is common after the insult. These changes may persist beyond a 2-week period. In addition, blood-brain barrier (BBB) abnormalities, as shown by accumulation of CT contrast agents, are still present 4 weeks after the injury. Histologic resolution of large infarcts may not be complete for several months. Consequently, it may be wise to delay elective surgery for a 6-week period to allow recovery of autoregulation, carbon dioxide responsiveness, and BBB integrity.

BIBLIOGRAPHY

Adams RD, Victor M: *Principles of neurology,* ed 5, New York, 1993, McGraw-Hill.

Aisen M, Arlt G, Foster S: Diaphragmatic paralysis without bulbar or limb paralysis in multiple Sclerosis, *Chest* 97:499–501, 1990.

Alboliras ET, et al.: Spectrum of cardiac involvement in Friedreich's ataxia: clinical, electrocardiographic, and echocardiographic observations, *Am J Cardiol* 58:518–524, 1986.

Baraka A: Anaesthesia and myasthenia gravis, *Can J Anaesth* 39:476–486, 1992.

Bell CF, Kelly JM, Jones RS: Anaesthesia for Friedreich's ataxia. *Anaesthesia* 41:296–301, 1986.

Bevan DR: Shy-Drager syndrome, *Anaesthesia* 34:866–873, 1979.

Birk K, et al: The clinical course of multiple sclerosis during pregnancy and the puerperium, *Arch Neurol* 47:738–742, 1990.

Campbell AM, Finley GA: Anesthesia for a patient with Friedreich's ataxia and cardiomyopathy, *Can J Anaesth* 36:89–93, 1989.

Carre PC, et al: Amyotrophic lateral sclerosis presenting with sleep hypopnea syndrome, *Chest* 93:1309–1311, 1988.

Child JS, et al: Cardiac involvement in Friedreich's ataxia: a clinical study of 75 patients, *J Am Coll Cardiol* 7:1370–1376, 1986.

Cote M, et al: Cardiologic signs and symptoms in Friedreich's ataxia, *Can J Neurol Sci* 3:319–321, 1976.

d'Empaire G, et al: Effect of prethymectomy plasma exchange on postoperative respiratory function in myasthenia gravis, *J Thorac Surg* 89:592–596, 1985.

Drury PME, Weg N: Vocal cord paralysis in the Shy-Drager syndrome, *Anaesthesia* 46:466–468, 1991.

Gravlee GP: Succinylcholine-induced hyperkalemia in a patient with Parkinson's disease, *Anesth Analg* 59:444–446, 1980.

Hewer RL: The heart in Friedreich's ataxia, *Br Heart J* 31:5–14, 1969.
Hutchinson RC, Sugden JC: Anaesthesia for Shy-Drager syndrome, *Anaesthesia* 39:1229–1231, 1984.
Kochi T, Oka T, Mizuguchi T: Epidural anesthesia for patients with amyotrophic lateral sclerosis, *Anesth Analg* 68:410–412, 1989.
Kuwahira I, et al: Acute respiratory failure in multiple sclerosis, *Chest* 97:246–248, 1990.
Leventhal SR, Orkin FK, Hirsh RA: Prediction of the need for postoperative mechanical ventilation in myasthenia gravis, *Anesthesiology* 53:26–30, 1980.
Mets B: Acute dystonia after alfentanil in untreated Parkinson's disease, *Anesth Analg* 72:557–558, 1991.
Morvan D, et al: Cardiomyopathy in Friedreich's ataxia; Doppler-echocardiographic study, *Eur Heart J* 13:1393–1398, 1992.
Rosenbaum KJ, Neigh JL, Strobel GE: Sensitivity to nondepolarizing muscle relaxants in amyotrophic lateral sclerosis, *Anesthesiology* 35:638–641, 1971.
Schapira K: Is lumbar puncture harmful in multiple sclerosis? *J Neurol Neurosurg Psychiatry* 22:238, 1959.
Schiffman PL, Belsh JM: Pulmonary function at diagnosis of amyotrophic lateral sclerosis, *Chest* 103:508–513, 1993.
Shapiro F, et al: Spinal fusion in Duchenne muscular dystrophy: a multidisciplinary approach, *Muscle Nerve* 15:604–614, 1992.
Warren TM, Datta S, Ostheimer GW: Lumbar epidural anesthesia in a patient with multiple sclerosis, *Anesth Analg* 61:1022–1023, 1982.

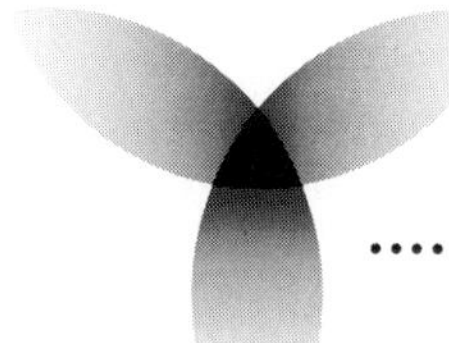

Chapter 15

Management of Acute and Chronic Renal Failure

Donald D. Mathes, MD

PERIOPERATIVE MANAGEMENT OF ACUTE RENAL FAILURE (ARF)

Postoperative acute renal failure (ARF) is the leading cause of acute hospital dialysis. The perioperative physician has a vital role in preventing or decreasing the severity of insult to the kidney during and after surgery. The physician needs to have an understanding of the following in order to prevent ARF in the perioperative period: (1) the predisposing preoperative risk factors for ARF; (2) the physiology of urine production; (3) how to differentiate and manage the causes of ARF; (4) the effects of anesthetic agents and surgery on renal function; and (5) the options available to prevent surgical and anesthetic insults on the kidney.

Risk Factors for Perioperative Renal Failure

Preexisting renal risk factors clearly increase the incidence of perioperative renal failure. Often, the patient may have multiple preexisting renal risk factors, making any further insult in the operating room particularly precarious for the onset of ARF. These risk factors include chronic renal insufficiency, diabetes mellitus, jaundice, poor myocardial function, advanced age, and the recent use of nephrotoxic agents. The patient with chronic renal insufficiency has a decreased ability to compensate and recover from any further renal insult in the operating room.

Patients with diabetes mellitus often have underlying glomerular injury, manifested as glomerular sclerosis and an elevated creatinine. However, diabetic nephropathy during the early stages may be manifested by microalbuminuria alone with otherwise, apparent, normal renal function. In addition, the diabetic with microalbuminuria may not have a urine dipstick positive for protein. Hence, any diabetic should be presumed to have underlying glomerular disease.

Diabetics are often on angiotensin converting enzymes (ACE) inhibitors in order to decrease glomerular perfusion pressure by efferent arteriole vasodilatation and, thus, slow the progression of diabetic nephropathy. Although ACE inhibitors slow the onset of diabetic nephropathy, their use in the perioperative setting can increase the risk of ARF. This risk is because of the efferent arteriole not being able to vasoconstrict to maintain glomerular perfusion pressure during periods of decreased renal perfusion.

Obstructive jaundice patients are at high risk for postoperative ARF. Up to 75% of these patients have been found to have postoperative deterioration of renal function. The etiology of this renal failure is thought to be secondary to increased fibrin deposition in the renal vasculature, caused by increased systemic endotoxin and increased sympathetic activity, causing decreased renal cortical blood flow. Patients with obstructive jaundice are particularly sensitive to decreased renal perfusion and volume depletion. During surgery, they have increased systemic endotoxin release, secondary to a decreased ability of the hepatic reticuloendothelial system to detoxify endotoxin during surgery and anesthesia.

The anesthesiologist should have a low threshold for using invasive monitoring to assess volume status in obstructive jaundice patients. Also, the preoperative use of a 48- to 72-hour course of oral bile salts (sodium deoxycholate) or oral lactulose, lowers the incidence of postoperative renal dysfunction. The mechanism of this renal protection appears to be from decreased systemic absorption of endotoxin in the small intestine during surgery.

The elderly have a linear decrease in renal function by age and, thus, an increased risk of perioperative renal failure. Renal blood flow decreases 1% per year after age 40, with the predominant decrease of blood flow occurring in the renal cortex and resulting in the loss of functioning nephrons in the cortex. Serum creatinine is a less reliable indicator of renal function, given continued loss of muscle mass in the elderly. A better estimate of renal function is the actual glomerular filtration rate (GFR), calculated using the following formula:

$$\text{creatinine clearance} = (140 - \text{age})\ (\text{weight in kg}/72 \times \text{serum creatinine})$$

For women, calculated creatinine clearance should be multiplied by 0.85.

Congestive heart failure (CHF) and poor myocardial function, especially postoperatively, are high-risk factors for the development of ARF from renal insult in surgery. This is especially true in patients after cardiopulmonary bypass (CPB) who have a cardiac index less than 2.5 l/min/m^2 lasting more than 48 hours.

Lastly, the use of nephrotoxic agents, most notably aminoglycosides and radiocontrast material, in the immediate preoperative period increases the vulnerability of the kidney to decreased perfusion during surgery. Often, patients will have several risk factors for perioperative renal failure. Hence, the perioperative physician needs to take an aggressive approach to ensure adequate volume replacement and renal perfusion during the perioperative period in patients with preexisting renal risk factors, including a lower threshold for the placement of invasive monitoring.

The Physiology of Urine Formation

The nephron is the functional unit for urine formation. The nephron is composed of two parts: the glomerulus and tubules. The glomerulus is made of a network of capillaries, which ultrafiltrate approximately 20% of the renal plasma flow into the surrounding Bowman capsule and into the proximal tubule at an average glomerular filtration rate of 125 ml/min in a healthy adult. Renal blood flow (RBF) is delivered to the glomerulus through the afferent arteriole and leaves the glomerulus through the efferent arteriole (Figure 15-1). The glomerular filtration rate is autoregulated by several mechanisms that cause constriction or dilatation of the afferent and efferent arterioles. This allows the glomerulus to maintain a near-constant hydrostatic pressure for ultrafiltration with wide changes in blood pressure and RBF.

The renal tubule is composed of the proximal tubule, the loop of Henle, the distal tubule, and collecting tubule (Figure 15-2). Both the proximal tubule and the loop of Henle have active Na-K-ATPase pumps and, thus, are particularly vulnerable to renal ischemia. The proximal tubule reabsorbs the majority of sodium and other solutes, such as bicarbonate and glucose, by active sodium pumps and cotransport. The proximal tubule can no longer reabsorb all of the ultrafiltrated glucose above a plasma glucose of 180 mg/dl. The glucose will begin to spill into the urine, producing an osmotic diuresis.

The descending loop of Henle is impermeable to sodium and chloride and passively reabsorbs water through a concentration gradient created by the vasa recta and countercurrent exchange. In the thick, ascending loop of Henle active sodium chloride absorption occurs through highly metabolically active pumps. The loop diuretics, such as furosemide, inhibit the Na-K-ATPase pump in the loop of Henle and may have a renal protective effect in times of renal ischemia by decreasing renal tubular workload and oxygen consumption.

In the distal tubule, a simple Na^+Cl^- carrier reabsorbs sodium and chloride. The thiazide diuretics act on the distal tubule by inhibiting the Na^+Cl^- carrier. The distal tubule contains specialized cells involved in tubuloglomerular feedback, called the macula densa. A decrease in the sodium chloride concentration in the distal tubule causes the macula densa to send a signal to dilate the afferent arteriole and increase renin release from the juxtaglomerular cells in the afferent and efferent arterioles. This increased renin release causes the increase in angiotensin II, which in turn,

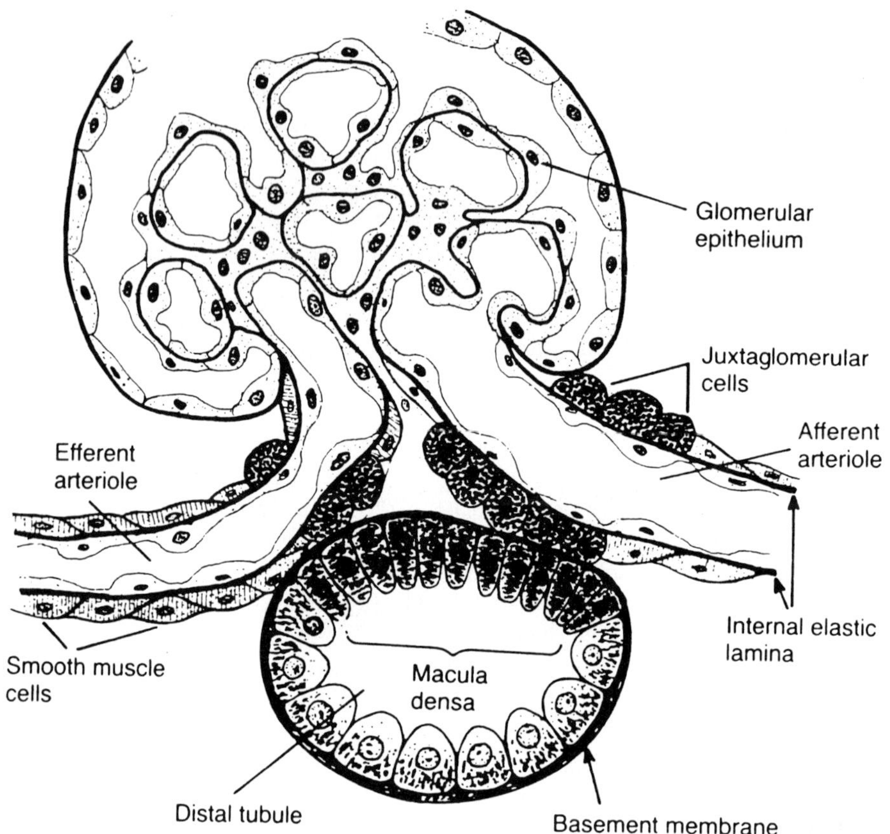

Figure 15-1
The structure of the glomerulus and macula densa. (Used with permission from Guyton AC, Hall JE: *Textbook of medical physiology*, Philadelphia, 1996, WB Saunders.)

causes efferent arteriole constriction. The end result is an increase in glomerular hydrostatic pressure and GFR. Water is impermeable in both the ascending loop of Henle and the first portion of distal tubule; thus, dilute urine is delivered to the collecting tubule.

The collecting tubule is the key portion of the nephron for determination of urine osmolarity. Urine osmolarity can range from 100 mOsm/l to 1200 mOsm/l. Antidiuretic hormone (ADH) is the principal regulator of urine osmolarity. It works directly on the collecting tubule by increasing water permeability. Aldosterone works directly on the Na^+ channels of the collecting tubule to increase sodium reabsorption. Potassium sparing diuretics work in the collecting tubules by either directly inhibit Na^+ channels (amiloride), or by direct competitive inhibition of aldosterone (spironolactone).

Approximately 80% of nephrons are located within the cortex of the kidney with the loop of Henle, reaching the outer medulla only. Greater than 90% of RBF is

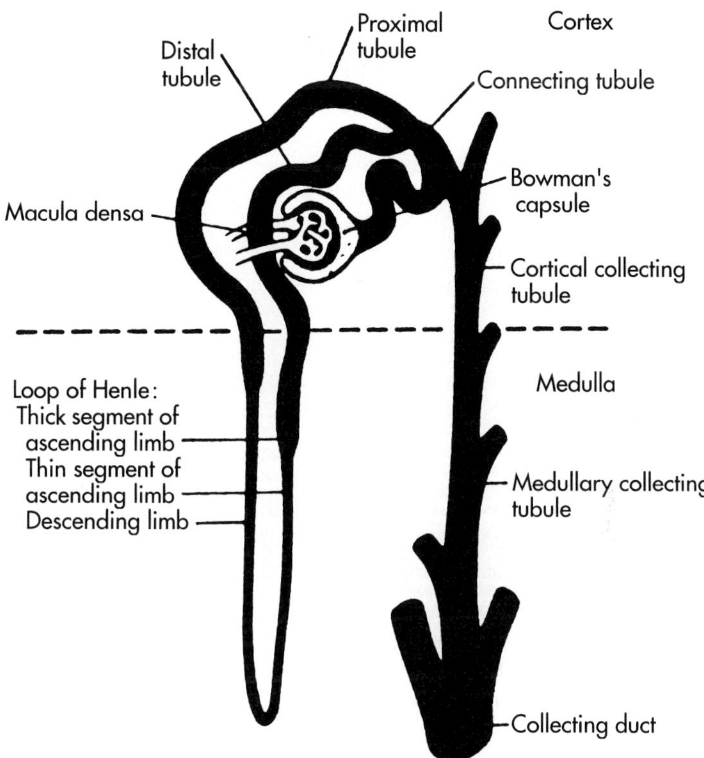

Figure 15-2
Basic tubular segments of the nephron. (Used with permission from Guyton AC, Hall JE: *Textbook of medical physiology,* Philadelphia, 1996, WB Saunders.)

directed to the outer cortex to these nephrons. However, during decreased renal perfusion, blood is shunted from the cortex to the inner medulla, making the cortical nephrons vulnerable to ischemia. Furthermore, after an ischemic insult, blood flow will remain decreased in the outer medullary portion, despite improvement in RBF to the cortex and inner medulla. The remaining nephrons, known as juxtaglomerular nephrons, have long loops of Henle that go deep into the medulla and are more capable of concentrating urine.

The loop of Henle within the medulla is surrounded by a network of capillaries called the vasa recta with a low oxygen tension (8–10 mm Hg). The vasa recta allow countercurrent exchange of water and solutes from the loop of Henle and the maintenance of the concentration gradient. Because of the low oxygen tension in the vasa recta, the loop of Henle is particularly vulnerable to periods of renal ischemia.

Etiology of Acute Renal Failure

By far, the most common cause of perioperative ARF occurs from initial hypoperfusion leading to ischemia of the renal tubules, and if prolonged, development of acute tubular necrosis. However, it is essential for the perioperative physician to examine all potential causes of ARF. Perioperative ARF can be separated into three categories: pre-, post-, and intrinsic renal failure.

PRERENAL FAILURE

Prerenal causes of ARF occur from insufficient renal perfusion. This can be caused by actual hypovolemia or a relative decrease in effective blood volume perfusing the kidney. Hypotension, poor cardiac function, and hepatic failure with ascites can all create a prerenal azotemia, secondary to insufficient blood volume perfusing the kidney. This decrease in RBF causes a whole host of neurohormonal regulators to increase renin-angiotensin, aldosterone, and ADH activity within the kidney; and it thus causes the renal tubules to avidly reabsorb large amounts of sodium and water, leading to urine that is concentrated and low in sodium.

POSTRENAL FAILURE

Postrenal ARF should always be excluded on initial evaluation by placing a Foley catheter and performing renal ultrasound to rule out evidence of urinary tract obstruction. With anuria, the perioperative physician needs to be assured the Foley is patent. The renal ultrasound, besides ruling out upper urinary tract obstruction, is useful to assess the size of the kidney and patency of renal vessels. Small, shrunken kidneys are compatible with long-standing renal disease. Renal ultrasound is especially useful in the elderly in whom serum creatinine may not reflect the extent of renal dysfunction.

INTRINSIC RENAL FAILURE

Damage to the renal tubules causes acute intrinsic renal failure (AIRF), formerly known as acute tubular necrosis (ATN). For purposes of this chapter, AIRF and ATN will be used interchangeably. In the perioperative setting, an ischemic insult to the renal tubules causes most AIRF. This insult develops from an imbalance of oxygen demand and oxygen supply to the metabolically active portions of the renal tubule.

With ischemia and decreased renal perfusion, the renal tubules initially increase solute reabsorption, especially in the medullary thick loop of Henle, through the Na-K-ATPase pump, increasing oxygen demand. This increased oxygen demand occurs at the same time that oxygen delivery to the tubule is decreasing, leaving the renal tubule vulnerable to hypoxic injury, most notably in the outer medullary regions of the kidney. Hypoxic injury to the renal tubule causes swelling of the tubular endothelial cells. Endothelial cell edema causes vascular congestion and a further decrease in perfusion to the already vulnerable hypoxic medullary tubules. After prolonged ischemia, tubular necrosis occurs, causing sloughing of necrotic tubular debris and obstruction of the tubules. Tubular obstruction causes an increase in intratubular pressure, which counteracts the hydrostatic pressure of the glomerules, decreasing GFR and causing oliguria. Furthermore, this increase in intratubular pressure causes increased back-leak of ultrafiltrate and solute across the already damaged tubule endothelial cells, and a further decrease in urine production (Figure 15-3).

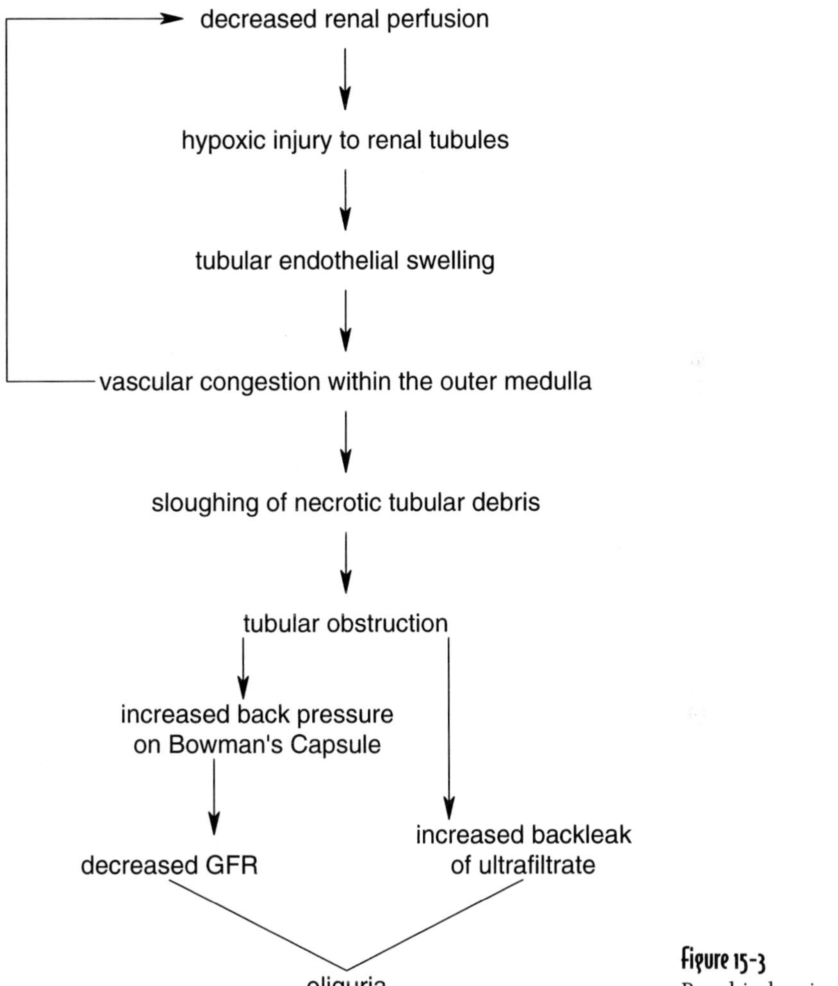

Figure 15-3
Renal ischemia.

Along with the damage to the tubules, decreased renal perfusion stimulates the sympathoadrenal axis. Mild α-adrenergic stimulation causes predominantly efferent arteriole constriction and, thus, helps preserve GFR with a decrease in RBF. However, severe α-adrenergic stimulation predominantly constricts afferent arterioles and decreases GFR. Multiple other intrarenal hormonal changes occur during renal ischemia. These include increases in renin, angiotensin, endothelin, and decreases in endothelial relaxant factor, leading to renal vasoconstriction and decreased perfusion. Also, damage to the proximal tubule and medullary thick loop of Henle with loss of Na-K-ATPase function causes an increase in sodium delivery to the macula densa. This activates the tubuloglomerular feedback causing a further decrease in GFR. This decrease in GFR from tubuloglomerular feedback is hypothesized to be a renal protective mechanism caused by a decrease in solute delivery to the ascending thick loop of Henle, thus, decreasing the oxygen demand on the renal tubule.

Although, in the perioperative setting, an initially prolonged prerenal azotemia most often causes AIRF, other causes must be considered and evaluated from review of the medical history, type of surgery, drugs given in the perioperative period, and examination of the urine (Box 15-1). Often, AIRF may be the result of multiple causes, and occurs from delayed diagnosis and treatment of the initial renal insult in a patient with preexisting renal damage. Therefore, in the perioperative period, it can be difficult to clearly discriminate between the types of ARF.

Diagnosing Etiology of ARF

No single test can be used to clearly distinguish the type of ARF. Instead, the perioperative physician should combine the clinical insults known to have occurred to the kidney with diagnostic testing (Table 15-1). Of the urine laboratory tests, the examination of the urine sediment is useful and should be done in the postoperative setting with ARF. Brown granular casts and cellular debris are compatible with tubular necrosis; whereas, clear urine with only a few granular casts is compatible with prerenal or postrenal azotemia.

In prerenal azotemia, tubular function is intact. The urine will be concentrated with high concentration of nitrogenous waste and low amounts of sodium. In AIRF with tubular damage, the tubule will contain isoosmotic urine with a high amount of sodium. Of the diagnostic tests listed in Table 15-1, the fractional excretion of sodium (FeNa) and renal failure index (RFI) appear to better distinguish prerenal azotemia from acute tubular necrosis of intrinsic renal failure. A FeNa less than 1% is compatible with prerenal azotemia and greater than 2% compatible with ATN. However, several reports have refuted FeNa as potentially misleading during the early periods of ARF. Measurement of urine indices is invalid if a diuretic has recently been given, secondary to an elevation of sodium excretion and a decreased ability to concentrate. Lastly, the measurement of creatinine clearance (CrCl) less than 25 ml/min

Box 15-1 Causes of Perioperative Intrinsic Acute Renal Failure

- Prolonged renal ischemia
- Myoglobinuria
- Hemoglobinuria from transfusion reaction
- Nephrotoxins especially contrast media, aminoglycosides, and nonsteroidals (ketorolac)
- Renal artery thrombosis/embolism
- Renal vein thrombosis
- Interstitial nephritis (most often related to such drugs as penicillin analogues, cephalosporins, and NSAIDs)
- Glomerulonephritis and vasculitis (rare in perioperative setting)

Table 15-1. Urinary Indicies in Acute Renal Failure

	PRERENAL	INTRINSIC
Urine sodium (mEq/l)	<20	>40
Urine osmolality (mOsm/kg)	>500	≤350
Fractional excretion of sodium (FeNa)	<1	>2
Renal failure index (RFI)	<1	>2
Urine sediment	Clear ± few granular casts	Brown granular casts and cellular debris

$$\text{FeNa} = \frac{\text{urine Na / plasma Na}}{\text{urine creatinine / plasma creatinine}} \times 100$$

$$\text{RFI} = \frac{\text{urine Na}}{\text{urine creatinine / plasma creatinine}}$$

in the acute postoperative period, can be used as a predictor of a patient at risk of developing renal failure. However, the measurement of CrCl in the acute postoperative period is limited by requiring a minimum of 2 hours of urine collection and, thus, adds little to rapid assessment and intervention of potential ARF in the perioperative setting.

In the operating room, the anesthesiologist is often limited to what diagnostic tests can be used to assess the etiology of oliguria in a rapid fashion. A spot urine Na and osmolality are rapid diagnostic tests for the anesthesiologist in the operating room if no diuretic has been given. In prerenal azotemia, the tubules avidly reabsorb sodium and water in an attempt to improve renal perfusion. Thus, a urine Na less than 20 mEq/l and urine osmolality greater than 500 mOsm/l is compatible with prerenal azotemia. With surgical stress, ADH levels can increase greatly, thus, causing significant reabsorption of water in the collecting tubules without sodium reabsorption. The anesthesiologist should suspect that excessive ADH is the main cause of oliguria if the urine Na is greater than 40 mEq/l and urine osmolality is greater than 500 mOsm/l. Often, this ADH effect on the collecting tubule can be easily overcome by small amounts of furosemide such as 5 to 10 mg IV. Lastly, in ongoing acute intrinsic renal failure, the tubules lose their ability to reabsorb sodium or concentrate urine because of the loss of the Na-K-ATPase pump. Thus, a urine Na greater than 40 mEq/l and urine osmolality less than or equal to 350 mOsm/l is compatible with AIRF. Brezis et al. noted that during the transition from prerenal azotemia to AIRF, the tubules will first lose the ability to concentrate urine while still reabsorbing sodium. Thus, a low FeNa or low fractional excretion of urine sodium with a low urine osmolality may be a key marker to the early transition from pre-renal ARF to AIRF.

MANAGEMENT OF INTRAOPERATIVE OLIGURIA

The key factor in the prevention and treatment of oliguria in the perioperative setting is the maintenance of the patient in a euvolemic state with stable hemodynamics. The onset of oliguria with urine output less than or equal to 20 ml/hr in an adult may be a serious indication of ongoing tubular damage, which, if prolonged, will lead to ARF and the need for dialysis.

In the initial management of oliguria in the operating room, the anesthesiologist should ensure that the patient has a patent Foley catheter and adequate blood pressure. In high-risk patients, mean arterial pressure (MAP) should not decrease to below 70 to 80 mm Hg. In hemorrhaging patients, RBF was found to decrease 30% when MAP decreased from 80 mm Hg to 62 mm Hg.

The mainstay of treatment of oliguria is aggressive volume loading with isotonic crystalloid, up to the point the anesthesiologist becomes concerned with the patient developing pulmonary edema. Colloid use for oliguria should be avoided because of colloid infusions increasing colloid oncotic pressure. This results in a change in Starling's forces decreasing ultrafiltration. When aggressively volume loading a patient without invasive monitoring, this author places on a low FiO_2 of 25% to 30%, if tolerated, and watches for any decreases in oxygen saturation by pulse oximetry or increases in static airway pressure as early markers of pulmonary edema. Also, if oliguria does not resolve after initial volume challenges, a urine Na and osmolality should be sent to the lab to better differentiate a prerenal state from excessive ADH as the cause of oliguria, as previously discussed. Once the anesthesiologist becomes concerned that the patient may be at risk of developing pulmonary edema, or continues to have unstable hemodynamics, a pulmonary artery catheter should be placed and further volume given as needed, until a pulmonary capillary wedge pressure (PCWP) of 18 mm Hg is reached. If cardiac index is less than 2.5 l/min with adequate PCWP, then inotropes should be administered to increase forward blood flow to the kidneys. The type of inotrope used should depend on whether systemic vascular resistance needs to be increased or decreased (Figure 15-4).

The use of renal-dose dopamine 1 to 3 µg/kg/min with oliguria remains controversial and is discussed later in this chapter. This author would use renal-dose dopamine once adequate volume has been given, secondary to its saluresis effect if low-dose dopamine is not causing any arrhythmias or tachycardia.

RENAL PROTECTIVE AGENTS

Aortic Cross-Clamping

Clearly, one of the highest surgical risks for the development of ARF is the cross-clamping of the aorta, especially above the renal artery. Hence, many studies on perioperative renal protection have been done with aortic cross-clamp procedures. With infrarenal cross-clamping of the aorta, Gamulin et al. found RBF to decrease by 38% and renal vascular resistance to increase by 75%, despite continuous mannitol infusion. These changes persisted for at least 1 hour after cross-clamp was released. Furthermore, the GFR remained diminished for at least the first 4 hours after infrarenal aortic cross-clamp but returned to normal by 24 hours.

With suprarenal aortic cross-clamping, Meyers et al. found postclamp GFR to decrease to 34% of preclamp GFR, compared to 82% for postinfrarenal clamp GFR.

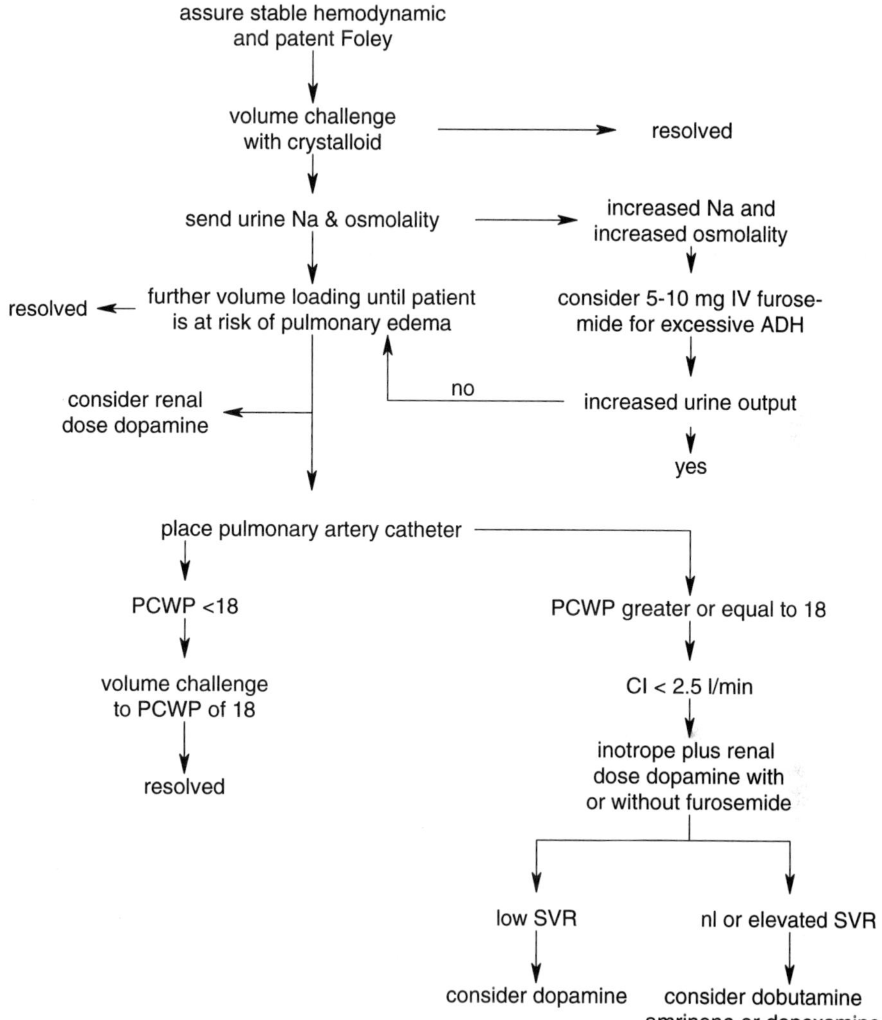

Figure 15-4
Perioperative oliguria.

These changes only slowly improved over the first 4 hours (Figure 15-5). Moreover, the length of suprarenal cross-clamp time directly correlated with the extent and duration of ARF ischemic injury. Those patients with a cross-clamp time of less than 20 minutes had no postoperative drop in GFR. However, those patients with a suprarenal cross-clamp time of more than 50 minutes had the greatest drop in GFR after aortic cross-clamp and had progressive azotemia for 3 to 4 days, with a delayed recovery from the maintenance phase of ARF.

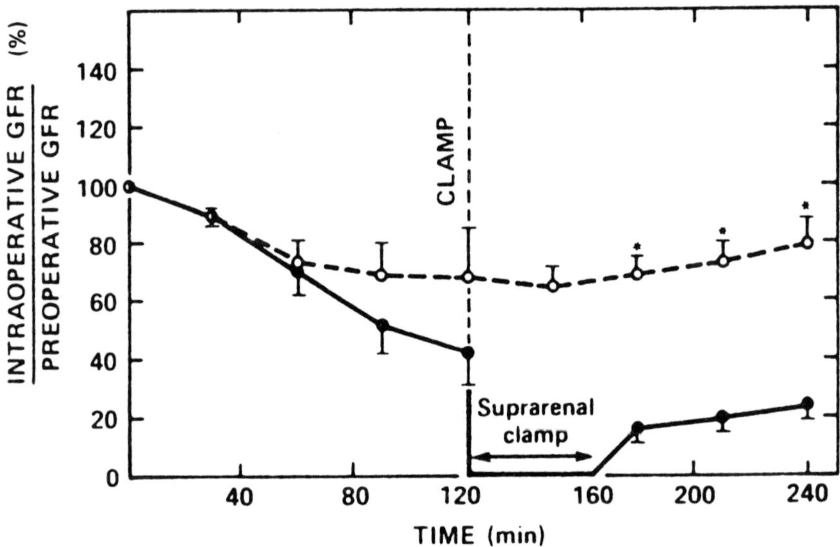

Figure 15-5
Idealized percent GFR vs time curves before and following suprarenal (•) and infrarenal (○) aortic clamping in patients undergoing abdominal aortic surgical repair. *, *P* = <*0.001*. (Used with permission from Meyers BD, et al: Nature of the renal injury following total renal ischemia in man, *J Clin Invest* 73:329–341, 1984.)

Meyers et al. found the decline in GFR after aortic cross-clamping to be far greater than the decrease in RBF. To explain this discrepancy, they found the pressure within Bowman's capsule to be elevated from the back-pressure of proximal tubule obstruction. Hence, this increased back pressure causes a decreased glomerular perfusion pressure and GFR in the postischemic period.

Mechanical

Mechanical means for perioperative renal protection during cross-clamping of the aorta have not been successful. Svensson et al. found no improvement in renal function with cold Ringer's lactate to the kidney during cross-clamp procedures in patients undergoing thoracic or thoracoabdominal aorta repair. Furthermore, renal function actually worsened with distal pump bypass or atrial renal bypass.

Mannitol

Besides assuring adequate extravascular volume and stable hemodynamics, the use of mannitol has been the cornerstone in perioperative renal protection. Despite mannitol's widespread use in vascular surgery, no controlled study has been done in humans showing a decreased incidence of ARF in the perioperative setting. However, mannitol does increase RBF, stimulates intrarenal prostaglandin activity, increases tubular transport, and is a free-radical scavenger associated with reperfusion injury.

In addition, Flores et al. found that mannitol administered to dogs before renal artery occlusion increased GFR and decreased endothelial swelling of the renal tubules. Furthermore, mannitol increases tubular transport, thus preventing increases in tubular back pressure and decreases in GFR.

However, for mannitol to be effective, it should be given before an ischemic insult. Hellberg et al. found mannitol given after renal artery occlusion increased medullary vasocongestion. In contrast, mannitol given before renal artery occlusion decreases postischemic medullary vasocongestion and, therefore, improves oxygen delivery to the ischemic renal tubules. Thus, mannitol helps preserve renal tubule transport and integrity if given before a renal ischemic insult.

Loop Diuretics

Loop diuretics have several potential benefits as renal protective agents. They inhibit the Na-K-ATPase pump in the ascending loop of Henle, and so, decrease oxygen demand during an ischemic insult. They also inhibit tubuloglomerular feedback from the macula densa, possibly preventing afferent arteriole vasoconstriction during renal ischemia. Loop diuretics increase intrarenal prostaglandin activity when given before and during a renal ischemic insult. Lastly, they increase tubular flow and, thus, decrease the back pressure resulting from tubular obstruction.

In control studies, the use of loop diuretics appears to have minimal to no effect in overall outcome in actual, established ARF. In the early stages of AIRF, Levinsky et al. found, upon review of the literature, improved survival in patients in whom urine output increased with furosemide. However, Levinsky commented that a favorable response to furosemide may only have identified a subgroup of patients with less severe tubular damage, and therefore, this subgroup had a better prognosis.

In this author's opinion, loop diuretics as renal protective agents may be beneficial only in the early stages of acute tubular necrosis because of the aforementioned reasons. However, before giving a loop diuretic, one must ensure adequate volume repletion, no longer need further urine indices, and monitor for electrolyte abnormalities if vigorous diuresis occurs.

Dopamine

Low-dose dopamine (1–2 µg/kg/min) has many potentially beneficial effects on renal function. Stimulation of dopamine-1 (D_1) receptors found on the vascular smooth muscle cause vascular smooth muscle relaxation. In addition, dopamine-2 (D_2) receptors are found on the presynaptic terminal of postganglionic sympathetic nerves. Stimulation of these receptors causes decreased norepinephrine release. Dopamine also directly inhibits the Na-K-ATPase pump in the renal tubules and so, inhibits sodium reabsorption. Lastly, dopamine inhibits the tubuloglomerular feedback from the macula densa and, thus, inhibits afferent arteriole vasoconstriction.

Although controversial, it now appears that low-dose dopamine increases RBF more than can be accounted for by increases in cardiac output. Furthermore, low-dose dopamine increases RBF significantly when given with other vasoconstrictors. Schaer et al. found RBF to increase 40% to 50% and lower renal vascular resistance when low-dose dopamine infusion was added to a norepinephrine infusion. This is one subset of patients for whom dopamine likely protects renal function by blunting renal vasoconstriction from systemic vasoconstricting drugs. Lastly, for renal-dose dopamine to be effective, the patient must be euvolemic. Bryan et al. found significant increases in urine output and sodium excretion with 2.5 μg/kg/min of dopamine only in those patients who were euvolemic at the time of infusion. Hypovolemic patients had a minimal response to dopamine.

Hence, it is clear that renal-dose dopamine produces a diuretic and natriuretic effect with adequate hydration. However, it is not clear if renal-dose dopamine has any actual renal protective effect. Several studies have shown little improvement in GFR with dopamine infusion, compared to extracellular volume expansion after aortic cross-clamp, and no change in postoperative renal outcome.

Two studies have shown dopamine to be potentially beneficial if used within the first 24 hours after aortic cross-clamping. Paul et al. found an improved GFR during the immediate period after infrarenal cross-clamp in a subgroup of patients receiving a continuous infusion of mannitol and dopamine that decreased to control levels after discontinuation. Salem et al. found an increased GFR during infrarenal cross-clamp with a dopaminergic infusion. These studies did not show improvement in actual renal outcome. Clearly, if dopamine is going to provide any actual renal protection after aortic cross-clamping, it should be continued for 24 hours postoperatively to offset the normal decrease in RBF during this period. This author would only use renal-dose dopamine in patients with preexisting risk factors for ARF undergoing high-risk surgical procedures and would discontinue dopamine if side effects, such as tachyarrhythmias, present themselves.

Atrial Natriuretic Peptide and Urodilatin

Atrial natriuretic peptide (ANP) is a new, promising renal protective drug currently being studied. It dilates the afferent and constricts the efferent arterioles, causing an increase in the glomerular hydrostatic pressure and an increase in GFR, independent of changes in RBF. When ANP is given either during or after a renal ischemic insult, it has been found to result in better preservation of GFR with less evidence of renal tubule damage.

One serious drawback of ANP is that it also causes hypotension, which limits its usefulness as a renal protective drug. Conger et al. showed improved GFR without hypotension after renal-artery clamping in rats given a combination of ANP and dopamine. Dopamine was titrated to maintain a MAP of 100 to 110 mm Hg. Furthermore, Conger et al. found the combination of ANP and dopamine given 48 hours after a renal ischemic insult and an established ARF, increased the GFR. Most recently, Rahman et al. found improvement in the GFR in established AIRF with ANP alone, without significant accompanying hypotension.

Another promising renal protective drug currently being evaluated is urodilatin. Urodilatin is a peptide isolated from human urine. Urodilatin has a structure and action on the kidney similar to that of ANP but causes less hemodynamic instability. This author anticipates ANP, with or without dopamine, and urodilatin will become viable renal protective drugs for perioperative ARF in the near future.

Vasoactive Renal Protective Drugs

Several vasoactive renal protective drugs are currently being examined in animal and human studies. These drugs include prostaglandin E_1, E_2, and I_2, calcium channel blockers (CCBs), endothelin antagonist, and theophylline. Of the prostaglandins, prostaglandin E_1 may be the most effective. Paller et al., in the rat model, found giving the oral PGE_1 drug misoprostol significantly increased GFR without increasing RBF. Torsello et al. found a significant reduction in postischemic ARF after suprarenal aortic surgery in patients pretreated with PGE_1.

Calcium channel blockers, most notably verapamil and diltiazem, have renal protective effects from renal ischemia. The renal protective effects of CCBs are two-fold. First, CCBs, after renal ischemia, cause afferent preglomerular arterial vasodilatation without efferent arteriole vasodilatation. Thus, CCBs attenuate the preglomerular vasoconstriction seen after ischemia and increase the GFR. Second, they decrease intracellular calcium renal tubule overload from renal ischemia and, thus, preserve renal tubule function and prevent cell death. Several studies have shown improved kidney graft function and a lower incidence of ATN in kidney transplants in which CCBs are flushed into the renal graft and given systematically to the transplant recipient. More clinical studies need to be done before CCBs can be considered absolutely safe and effective. One problem with CCB use during surgery is the potential for cardiac depression and hypotension with anesthesia. Nevertheless, the clinical use of CCBs with renal ischemia is promising.

Endothelin is a potent vasoconstrictor peptide that increases after an ischemic injury to the kidney. Endothelin causes an increase in intracellular calcium and contraction of smooth muscle within the renal arteriole. Hence, endothelin causes a decrease in RBF and GFR. Currently, endothelin antagonists are being developed and studied for use in renal ischemia.

Lastly, theophylline has demonstrated renal protective effects. During renal ischemia, adenosine increases up to six-fold within the kidney. Adenosine constricts the afferent arterioles, which contributes to renal vasoconstriction after renal ischemia. Theophylline antagonizes adenosine and, thus, causes afferent arteriole vasodilatation. Furthermore, theophylline inhibits tubuloglomerular feedback causing afferent arteriole vasodilatation.

In conclusion, the perioperative physician has a direct impact on preventing or decreasing the severity of perioperative ARF. Adequate volume replacement and stable hemodynamics must be maintained during and after a renal ischemic insult. Furthermore, the use of renal protective drugs should strongly be considered. In the near future, the perioperative physician will have many new renal protective drugs for clinical use.

PERIOPERATIVE MANAGEMENT OF CHRONIC RENAL FAILURE

Perioperative morbidity and mortality is higher in patients with end-stage renal disease (ESRD). Besides concerns with the kidney, ESRD patients have multiple end-organ effects from renal failure, which place them at increased perioperative risk.

End Organ Effects of End Stage Renal Disease (ESRD)

NERVOUS SYSTEM

Uremia can lead to sedation, fatigue, and encephalopathy. Furthermore, chronic dialysis can lead to dementia, which is most likely because of aluminum toxicity from chronic dialysis. Also, sedation and confusion are common after dialysis. This is known as dialysis disequilibrium, which is caused by intracellular fluid and electrolyte shifts and can lead to cerebral edema. Hence, ESRD patients can have an increased sensitivity to sedative drugs.

Uremia can also cause both a peripheral and autonomic neuropathy. The peripheral neuropathy can cause severe sensory as well as motor function loss. These neuropathies should clearly be documented before surgery to avoid being confused as a complication of anesthesia. Succinylcholine should be avoided with extensive neuropathy. Patients with autonomic neuropathy may be hemodynamically unstable from an inability to compensate for cardiovascular changes induced with anesthesia.

CARDIAC

End-stage renal disease associated with hyperlipidemia and accelerated atherosclerosis. This, combined with the high incidence of underlying hypertension and diabetes mellitus, places patients with ESRD at higher risk of having ischemic heart disease. The high incidence of hypertension increases the likelihood of left ventricular hypertrophy and left ventricular dysfunction. Uremia can cause both an autonomic neuropathy and pericarditis. These patients have a high incidence of developing CHF, secondary to fluid overload. Furthermore, pulmonary edema can develop despite low-filling pressures, secondary to uremia causing a "leaky pulmonary capillary syndrome."

BLOOD

Normocytic and normochromic anemia and platelet dysfunction are seen in ESRD. Patients with long-standing anemia can often tolerate a hematocrit down to 20% without problems. Hence, many of these patients do not need a blood transfusion preoperatively. Instead, the anesthesiologist needs to ascertain the patient's baseline hemoglobin along with other risk factors, such as coronary artery disease and extent of surgery, before considering transfusion. Today, most ESRD patients have a higher hemoglobin, secondary to recombinant erythropoietin.

Uremic toxins decrease platelet factor III activity and cause abnormal platelet aggregation and adhesiveness. Patients with blood urea nitrogen over 100 mg/dl have a much higher incidence of perioperative bleeding. Preoperative dialysis will improve platelet function if done within a 24-hour period before surgery. If bleeding does occur, desmopressin (DDAVP) 0.4 μg/kg should be given first. Desmopressin increases factor VIII/von Willebrand factor, which improves platelet aggregation. Increasing the hematocrit to 30% will also improve platelet function. At lower hematocrits, platelets will be farther apart from each other and the vessel wall and will not aggregate as easily. Cryoprecipitate with factor VIII/von Willebrand factor will improve platelet function.

ELECTROLYTES

Potassium

Hyperkalemia is the most common complication of ESRD during the perioperative period. Fluid shifts release potassium from damaged cells. Blood products, acidosis, and hypoventilation can all lead to increases in potassium in the anephric patient. Hence, dialysis again should be done within a 24-hour period and potassium checked within a few hours before surgery. Elective surgery should be postponed for a serum potassium above 5.5 mmol/l and 5.0 mmol/l for major surgery. Also the electrocardiogram should confirm before the start of surgery the absence of peaked T waves, and the T waves should be monitored throughout surgery.

Calcium, Phosphorus and Bone

Calcium levels are often low in ESRD as a result of calcium binding to elevated phosphorus levels and decreased absorption of calcium in the gut from lack of 1,25 dihydroxy vitamin D_3. This can cause a significant elevation of PTH from the parathyroid, leading to increased bone reabsorption and renal osteodystrophy. Often ESRD patients will have a parathyroidectomy to prevent the risk of renal osteodystrophy and spontaneous bone fractures. Since elevation of phosphorus is the number one cause of hypocalcemia, the use of phosphate binders, along with dialysis, to keep phosphorus below 5.5 mg/dl is essential.

Acidosis

Chronic metabolic acidosis occurs in ESRD from the inability to excrete inorganic acids. Serum bicarbonate will decrease in an attempt to buffer these acids; monitoring serum bicarbonate can be used as a marker on the need for dialysis. Patients for elective surgery should have a bicarbonate at least 18 mEq/l, because of likely worsening of acidosis during surgery, and postoperatively, from release of hydrogen ions from ischemic cells. Sodium bicarbonate can be given to raise the bicarbonate, but adequate ventilation is needed to compensate for increased carbon dioxide production. Hypoventilation should be avoided.

INFECTION

Infection and sepsis are the leading causes of death in ESRD patients. Leukocyte function is defective with uremia. There is a high incidence of AV graft infections. Thus, strict aseptic technique in the operating room is essential, along with appropriate prophylactic antibiotics. Another concern, especially before erythropoietin, is the high incidence of hepatitis and liver dysfunction resulting from multiple blood products.

Preoperative Concerns of ESRD

1. Besides careful evaluation for other end-organ damage, it is essential that the anesthesiologist review the last dialysis records to determine if the patient is at target weight and whether the patient was hemodynamically stable during dialysis. Hypotension during dialysis is a key marker for the patient being intravascularly volume-depleted. Many nephrologists today

will remove less fluid in the patient going for surgery to help avoid hypotension occurring in the operating room.

2. Review the etiology of renal failure. Causes of renal failure, such as hypertension and diabetes, may place the patient at risk for other organ dysfunction such as ischemic heart disease.
3. Avoid potassium intravenous solutions such as lactated Ringer's solution.
4. Review a recent set of electrolytes, preferably done within a few hours of surgery.
5. Document site and function of any AV fistula, keeping site well-padded and free of any pressure. Avoid any blood draws, intravenous catheters, or blood pressure measurements on any extremity with a functioning AV fistula.

Intraoperative Management of ESRD and Anesthetic Agents

INDUCTION AND NARCOTIC AGENTS

Patients with ESRD have an increased sensitivity to benzodiazepines, barbiturates, and narcotics. The causes of increased sensitivity are multifactorial. Hypoproteinemia causes increased, free drug availability. Uremia and dialysis dementia and disequilibrium cause preexisting central nervous system sedation. Increased sedation can occur from decreased excretion of active renal metabolites. Lastly, metabolic acidosis causes an increase in the unionized fraction of drugs. Thus, drugs such as sodium thiopental have a higher proportion of drug crossing the blood-brain barrier.

Induction drugs such as sodium thiopental and propofol should be reduced because of increased sensitivity and also because of possible underlying intravascular volume depletion, autonomic dysfunction, and left ventricular dysfunction. Morphine and meperidine should not be used for any prolonged period, such as in patient-control analgesia pumps, secondary to the active metabolites morphine glucuronide and normeperidine being excreted by the kidneys.

MUSCLE RELAXANTS

For surgery of short duration, atracurium, cisatracurium, and mivacurium are the ideal muscle relaxants. Atracurium and cisatracurium are eliminated by ester hydrolysis and Hoffman degradation and are unaffected by renal failure. Mivacurium's effect is slightly prolonged because of decreased pseudocholinesterase activity from uremia and dialysis, but the prolongation is not significant, secondary to its short length of activity. Vecuronium is predominately eliminated through bile excretion, but vecuronium's duration will be prolonged, especially with multiple dosing in ESRD. Rocuronium is hepatically eliminated, but the metabolite 17-desacetyl-rocuronium is excreted by the kidney and has one twentieth the neuromuscular-blocking potency of rocuronium. However, with renal failure, rocuronium has, on average, the same duration but more variability in length of neuromuscular blockade, compared to healthy patients. This author has had no problems in using rocuronium in patients with ESRD in cases lasting longer than 45 minutes. Other longer-acting nondepolarizing agents predominantly excreted renally such as pancuronium, D-tubocurare, and metocurine should only be used with utmost vigilance with neuromuscular monitoring. The newer long-acting muscle relaxant pipercuronium and, most notably, doxacurium will also be prolonged with ESRD. Although there continues to be concern about recurization with reversal of muscle relaxants, recurization now appears unlikely because of anticholinesterase action being significantly prolonged in renal failure. Nevertheless, when using long-acting muscle relaxants excreted renally, pyridostigmine may be a prudent choice because of an almost doubled elimination time in anephric patients, compared to edrophonium and neostigmine.

Succinylcholine, a depolarizing agent, can be used safely in ESRD but should be avoided in a patient with elevated potassium over 5.0 mmol/l. Although succinylcholine causes no abnormal potassium increase in ESRD, the normal increased release of potassium of 0.5 mmol/l could be dangerous with preexisting hyperkalemia. The active metabolite succinylmonocholine is excreted renally. Hence, a continuous succinylcholine infusion should be avoided with ESRD.

VOLATILE ANESTHETICS

All the volatile anesthetics, with or without nitrous oxide, will decrease RBF and GFR as a result of myocardial depression and peripheral pooling from vasodilatation. However, these renal effects are normally inconsequential when compared to multiple other effects from the stress of surgery and fluid shifts. Of the volatile anesthetics, enflurane and sevoflurane have the greatest potential for renal toxicity.

Enflurane and sevoflurane are biotransformed by the hepatic cytochrome P450 enzyme system, producing inorganic fluoride. The cytochrome P450 enzyme system can be induced by certain drugs, most notably isoniazid for enflurane and sevoflurane, causing increased fluoride levels. Studies of methoxyflurane found peak fluoride levels above 50 µm inhibited renal tubular ability to concentrate urine. However, it is unclear if 50 µm fluoride levels for sevoflurane or enflurane cause the same nephrotoxicity. Mazze et al. found impaired renal concentrating ability after prolonged enflurane exposure with peak average serum fluoride of only 33 µm. This led Mazze to conclude that the total amount of serum fluoride exposure may be more nephrotoxic than the actual peak fluoride concentrations.

Frink et al. compared the renal concentrating ability of both enflurane and sevoflurane after 9.6 minimal alveolar concentration (MAC) hours. Sevoflurane average peak serum fluoride concentrations were 47 ± 3 µm and 23 ± 1 µm for enflurane. The sevoflurane group was found to have no abnormalities in concentrating ability, whereas two of seven patients given enflurane did, despite lower fluoride levels. Higuchi et al. found impaired concentrating ability in a subgroup of patients with prolonged sevoflurane exposure, with average fluoride levels of 57.5 µm. However, no clinical renal damage was found to have occurred. Thus, it appears that the higher fluoride level is less toxic for sevoflurane than the equivalent or lower fluoride levels seen with enflurane.

Besides the release of fluoride ions, sevoflurane also can cause potential nephrotoxicity through the release of a toxin known as compound A. Compound A is a vinyl ether released from the interaction of sevoflurane with soda lime or baralyme. Significant amounts of compound A can occur with a combination of low-flow anesthesia with baralyme. In rats, exposure to high amounts of compound A caused damage to the renal corticomedullary cells. However, in humans with sevoflurane low-flow anesthesia of more than 10 hours, compound A was found not to cause any changes in renal function. Nevertheless, the FDA currently recommends a minimum of 2 l flow be used with sevoflurane to avoid high levels of compound A. The actual renal toxicity of compound A in humans remains unclear.

The use of sevoflurane and enflurane in patients with preexisting chronic renal insufficiency appears safe if used for moderate duration. However, one has to question why these agents are used in patients with renal insufficiency undergoing prolonged surgery, or in patients undergoing a known, renal ischemic insult such as aortic cross-clamping. Other volatile agents, such as isoflurane, are readily available and cause minimal fluoride levels after prolonged exposure.

In conclusion, the anesthetic management of a patient with ESRD requires an evaluation for other end-organ dysfunction from renal failure, a review of the last dialysis, and a recent electrolyte panel. Furthermore, intravenous anesthetic drugs should be titrated carefully (given the increased sensitivity of ESRD patients to multiple anesthetic drugs), and the type of volatile agent chosen by the length of the case and the potential for elevated fluoride levels.

BIBLIOGRAPHY

Baldwin L, Henderson A, Hickman P: Effect of postoperative low-dose dopamine on renal function after elective major vascular surgery, *Ann Intern Med* 120:744–746, 1994.

Bito H, Ikeda K: Closed-circuit anesthesia with sevoflurane in humans: effects of renal and hepatic function and concentrations of breakdown products with soda lime in the circuit, *Anesthesiology* 80:71–76, 1994.

Bonventre JV: Mechanisms of ischemic acute renal failure. *Kidney Int* 43:1160–1178, 1993.

Brezis M, Rosen SN, Epstein FH: The pathophysiologic implications of medullary hypoxia, *Am J Kidney Dis* 13:253–258, 1989.

Bryan AG, et al: Modification of the diuretic and natriuretic effects of a dopamine infusion by fluid loading in preoperative cardiac surgical patients, *J Cardiothorac Vasc Anesth* 9:158–163, 1995.

Byrick RJ, Rose DK: Pathophysiology and prevention of acute renal failure: the role of the anesthesiologist, *Can J Anaesth* 37:457–467, 1990.

Cahill CJ, Pain JA: Obstructive jaundice renal failure and other endotoxin-related complications, *Surg Annu* 20:17–37, 1988.

Cedidi C, et al: Urodilatin: a new approach for the treatment of therapy-resistant acute renal failure after liver transplantation, *Eur J Clin Invest* 24:632–639, 1994.

Conger JD, Briner VA, Schrier RW: Acute renal failure: pathogenesis, diagnosis, and management. In Lazarus JM, Brenner BM, editors: *Acute renal failure,* ed 3, New York, 1993, Churchill Livingstone.

Conger JD, Falk SA, Hammond WS: Atrial natriuretic peptide and dopamine in established acute renal failure in the rat, *Kidney Int* 40:21–28, 1991.

Conger JD, et al: Atrial natriuretic peptide and dopamine in a rat model of ischemic acute renal failure, *Kidney Int* 35:1126–1132, 1989.

Conzen PF, et al: Renal function and serum fluoride concentrations in patients with stable renal insufficiency after anesthesia with sevoflurane and enflurane, *Anesth Analg* 81:569–575, 1995.

Duke GJ, Bersten AD: Dopamine and renal salvage in the critically ill patient, *Anaesth Intensive Care* 20:277–287, 1992.

Epstein M: Calcium antagonists and the kidney: future therapeutic perspectives, *Am J Kidney Dis* 21:16–25, 1993.

Fischereder M, Trick W, Nath KA: Therapeutic strategies in the prevention of acute renal failure, *Semin Nephrol* 14:41–52, 1994.

Flores J, et al: The role of cell swelling in ischemic renal damage and the protective effect of hypertonic solute, *J Clin Invest* 51:118–126, 1972.

Frink EJ, et al: Renal concentrating function with prolonged sevoflurane or enflurane anesthesia in volunteers, *Anesthesiology* 80:1019–1025, 1994.

Gamulin Z, et al: Effects of infrarenal aortic cross-clamping on renal hemodynamics in humans, *Anesthesiology* 61:394–399, 1984.

Gore DC, Dalton JM, Gehr TWB: Colloid infusions reduce glomerular filtration in resuscitated burn victims, *J Trauma* 40:356–360, 1996.

Guyton AC, Hall JE: Urine formation by the kidneys: glomerular filtration, renal blood flow, and their control. In Guyton AC, Hall JE, editors: *Textbook of medical physiology*, Philadelphia, 1996, WB Saunders.

Hellberg O, et al: Postischemic administration of hyperosmolar mannitol enhances erythrocyte trapping in outer medullary vasculature in the rat kidney, *Renal Physiol Biochem* 13:328–332, 1990.

Higuchi H, et al: Renal function in patients with high serum fluoride concentrations after prolonged sevoflurane anesthesia, *Anesthesiology* 83:449–458, 1995.

Hines R: Dopamine preserves renal function during cardiac surgery, *J Cardiothorac Vasc Anesth* 9:335–336, 1995.

Kellerman PS: Perioperative care of the renal patient, *Arch Intern Med* 154:1674–1688, 1994.

Kentro TB, Lottenberg R, Kitchens CS: Clinical efficacy of desmopressin acetate for hemostatic control in patients with primary platelet disorders undergoing surgery, *Am J Hematol* 24:215–219, 1987.

Lameire N, Verbeke M, Vanholder R: Prevention of clinical acute tubular necrosis with drug therapy, *Nephrol Dial Transplant* 10:1992–2000, 1995.

Lanese DM, et al: Effects of atriopeptin III on isolated rat afferent and efferent arterioles, *Am J Physiol* 261:F1102–1109, 1991.

Lange JW, Aeppli DM, Brown DC: Survival of patients with acute renal failure requiring dialysis after open heart surgery: early prognostic indicators, *Am Heart J* 113:1138–1143, 1987.

Levinsky NG, Bernard DB: Mannitol and loop diuretics in acute renal failure. In Brenner BM, Lazarus JM, editors: *Acute renal failure*, ed 2, New York, 1988, Churchill Livingstone.

Lote CJ, Harper L, Savage CO: Mechanism of acute renal failure, *Br J Anaesth* 77:82–89, 1996.

Luschen TF, Wenzel RR: Endothelin in renal disease: role of endothelin antagonists, *Nephrol Dial Transplant* 10:162–166, 1995.

Mason J, et al: Vascular congestion in ischemic renal failure: the role of cell swelling, *Miner Electrolyte Metab* 15:114–124, 1989.

Mazze RI, Calverly RK, Smith NT: Inorganic fluoride nephrotoxicity: prolonged enflurane and halothane anesthesia in volunteers, *Anesthesiology* 46:265–271, 1977.

Memoli B, et al: Loop diuretics and renal vasodilators in acute renal failure, *Nephrol Dial Transplant* 9:168–171, 1994.

Meyers BD, et al: Nature of the renal injury following total renal ischemia in man, *J Clin Invest* 73:321–341, 1984.

Myers BD, et al: Pathophysiology of hemodynamically mediated acute renal failure in man, *Kidney Int* 18:495–504, 1980.

Moran SM, Myers BD: Pathophysiology of protracted acute renal failure in man, *J Clin Invest* 76:1440–1448, 1985.

Osswald H, Gleiter CH, Muhlbaver B: Therapeutic use of theophylline to antagonize renal effects of adenosine, *Clin Nephrol* 43:533–S37, 1995.

Paul MD, et al: Influence of mannitol and dopamine on renal function during elective infrarenal aortic cross-clamping in man, *Am J Nephrol* 6:427–434, 1986.

Paller MS, Manivel JC: Prostaglandins protect kidneys against ischemic and toxic injury by a cellular effect, *Kidney Int* 42:1345–1354, 1992.

Pass JL, et al: The effect of mannitol and dopamine on the renal response to thoracic aortic cross-clamping, *J Thorac Cardiovasc Surg* 95:608–612, 1988.

Rahman SN, et al: Effects of atrial natriuretic peptide in clinical acute renal failure, *Kidney Int* 45:1731-1738, 1994.

Salem MG, et al: The effect of dopamine on renal function during aortic cross clamping, *Ann R Coll Surg Engl* 70:9–12, 1988.

Schaer GL, Fink MP, Parsillo JE: Norepinepherine alone vs. norepinepherine plus low dose dopamine: enhanced renal blood flow with combination pressor therapy, *Crit Care Med* 13:492–496, 1985.

Shilliday I, Allison ME: Diuretics in acute renal failure, *Ren Fail* 16:3–17, 1994.

Svensson LG, et al: Appraisal of adjuncts to prevent acute renal failure after surgery on the thoracic or thoracoabdominal aorta, *J Vasc Surg* 10:230–239, 1989.

Torsello G, et al: Prevention of acute renal failure in suprarenal aortic surgery. Results of a pilot study, *Zentralbl Chir* 118:390–394, 1993.

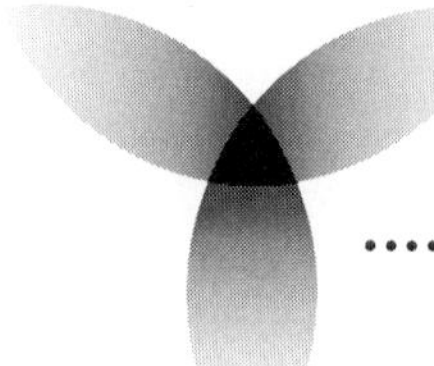

Chapter 16

Management of Common Endocrine Disorders

Donald D. Mathes, MD

DIABETES MELLITUS
- Classification of Diabetes Mellitus
- Metabolism of Diabetes Mellitus
- End-Organ Damage Related to Diabetes Mellitus
- Ketoacidosis and Nonketotic Hyperosmolar Hypoglycemic Coma

PITUITARY DISORDERS
- Hypopituitarism
- Hyperpituitarism
- Prolactinoma
- Diabetes Insipidus
- Syndrome Inappropriate Antidiuretic Hormone

THYROID DISORDERS
- Thyroid Hormone Synthesis and Regulation
- Thyroid Function Tests
- Hyperthyroidism
- Hypothyroidism
- Myxedema Coma

ADRENAL DISORDERS
- Cushing's Syndrome (Excessive Glucocorticoid Activity)
- Primary Hyperaldosteronism (Conn's Syndrome)
- Adrenal Insufficiency (Glucocorticoid Deficiency)
- Stress Steroids
- Acute Adrenal Crisis

PARATHYROID DISORDERS
- Primary Hyperparathyroidism
- Medical Management
- Perioperative Management

BIBLIOGRAPHY

The author acknowledges Mark L. Hartman, MD, from the University of Virginia, Department of Endocrinology, for his valuable assistance on the diabetes mellitus and pituitary subsections.

DIABETES MELLITUS

The perioperative management of the patient with diabetes mellitus can be challenging and unpredictable. Metabolic responses to the stress of surgery can vary greatly, requiring the utmost vigilance of the physician in caring for the diabetic patient during the perioperative period.

Classification of Diabetes Mellitus

Diabetes mellitus is divided into two classes. In type I diabetes mellitus (DM) the pancreatic β cells are unable to secrete insulin because of β-cell destruction, usually occurring from an autoimmune process or viral injury. These patients require insulin injections to prevent the onset of ketoacidosis. Type I DM classically has its onset at a young age. In Type II DM, the insulin production from the pancreas is insufficient to prevent hyperglycemia. This can be caused by decreased production of insulin from the β cells, or more often, insulin resistance associated with obesity. These patients produce enough basal insulin to prevent ketoacidosis but not hyperglycemia. More than 90% of diabetics are type II, and the disease classically occurs in middle age. Often the sulfonylurea agents are used to stimulate β cells of the pancreatic islets to release insulin. These effects can last from 24 to 36 hours, especially with longer-acting agents such as chlorpropamide (Diabinese). Besides the use of sulfonylurea agents, insulin is commonly used in type II DM to counter insulin resistance. Metformin (glucophage) is a biguanide oral hypoglycemic agent recently introduced in the United States for the treatment of type II DM. Metformin is often used in combination with an oral sulfonylurea agent. The mechanism of action of metformin is not completely understood, but it appears to lower insulin resistance by decreasing hepatic glucose production and enhancing insulin-stimulated glucose uptake. Metformin alone does not cause hypoglycemia; but, in combination with exogenous insulin or sulfonylureas, it can increase the risk of hypoglycemia. In patients with cardiac, hepatic and renal insufficiency, there is an increased risk of lactic acidosis with metformin therapy. For this reason it generally should not be used in the perioperative period. In the near future, several diabetic agents with alternative mechanisms of action will be available in the United States. Acarbose (Precose) is an α-glucosidase inhibitor, which lowers glucose by delaying carbohydrate absorption and, hence, decreases postprandial glucose elevation. Troglitazone (Rezulin) is an insulin sensitizing agent, which increases insulin action at the cellular level and inhibits hepatic gluconeogenesis. Again, any of these newer agents should be held during the perioperative period.

The perioperative physician should be aware that patients who have type II DM are a heterogeneous group with various degrees of either insulin resistance or β-cell dysfunction. Over time the type II diabetic can become completely insulin-deficient because of progressive β-cell dysfunction, and so, is prone to ketoacidosis with stressful events. It is often impossible to clinically distinguish this small group of type II diabetics from classic type I patients.

Metabolism of Diabetes Mellitus

Insulin is required for glucose uptake into cells; it also stimulates glycogen formation and suppresses gluconeogenesis and lipolysis. On average, 30 to 40 units of insulin are produced per day in healthy patients. Insulin is metabolized in the liver and kidney. Hence, hepatic or renal dysfunction increases the risk of hypoglycemia from the prolonged action of insulin.

Insulin deficiency leads to a catabolic state. Glucose and potassium uptake by the cells will be limited, leading to hyperglycemia and hyperkalemia if there is coexisting renal dysfunction. Gluconeogenesis will be activated, leading to skeletal muscle protein degradation and worsening hyperglycemia. Lastly, insulin deficiency stimulates lipolysis with free fatty acid formation becoming a primary source of energy. The free fatty acids are oxidized in the liver and ketone bodies, acetoacetic acid, and β-hydroxybutyrate are formed. These ketone bodies can be used for energy but also contribute to metabolic acidosis and electrolyte disorders. Available, routine clinical tests for ketones often only measure acetoacetate. In the presence of vascular collapse, severe hypoxia or alcohol intoxication acetoacetate is reduced to β-hydroxybutyrate and the test for ketones may be negative, masking the presence of true ketoacidosis.

Normally only basal amounts of insulin are needed to prevent lipolysis and ketosis. However, with surgical stress, there is a great increase in secretion of counterregulatory hormones such as catecholamines, cortisol and glucagon. These hormones stimulate hepatic glucose production and lipolysis and, thereby, worsen hyperglycemia, insulin resistance, and ketoacidosis in type I diabetics. In type II diabetics, increased catecholamine release can inhibit insulin secretion by the β cells, and in combination with increased insulin resistance, cause severe hyperglycemia. With the severe stress that often occurs with major surgery, ketoacidosis may occur in type II diabetics. In patients with type I DM, a normal preoperative fasting glucose does not preclude ketoacidosis from developing during surgery or in the postoperative period. Hence, it is essential for the perioperative physician to ensure an adequate basal insulin supply in the fasting type I diabetic patient.

In addition to insulin, a glucose infusion further decreases catabolism. The average fasting patient needs 100 to 125 grams of glucose per day to decrease protein catabolism and ketosis. Giving 5 gm/hr (100 cc/hr of 5% dextrose [D5]) to adults will decrease fat and protein catabolism. Insulin doses should be increased to compensate for a dextrose infusion to avoid an osmotic diuresis from an elevated blood glucose. The combination of insulin and dextrose together will greatly decrease tissue catabolism in the fasting diabetic patient and help preserve metabolic homeostasis.

End-Organ Damage Related to Diabetes Mellitus

The increase in perioperative morbidity and mortality associated with DM is rarely caused by diabetes itself but by end-organ damage from diabetes. Hence, it is essential for the anesthesiologist to have evaluated which end-organ systems have been damaged. Complications of diabetes include cardiovascular disease, peripheral vascular disease, renal insufficiency, stiff joint syndrome, peripheral and autonomic neuropathies, gastroparesis, and decreased granulocyte function (Box 16-1). Basic laboratory examination should include glucose, electrolytes, creatinine, and an electrocardiogram (ECG).

Although the exact etiology of diabetic complications remains unclear, two mechanisms of injury have been supported by substantial experimental evidence. First, in the presence of hyperglycemia, glucose is converted in the polyol pathway to sorbitol by aldose reductase. Increases in cellular sorbitol cause cellular edema and disruption of cellular function. In nervous tissue, demyelination and inhibition of Na-K-ATPase activity occurs from increased intracellular sorbitol and may lead to the development of a neuropathy. Increased intracellular sorbitol levels have been implicated as a potential cause of neuropathy, nephropathy, and aortic disease. Second, hyperglycemia leads to increased nonenzymatic glycosylation of various proteins, including collagen and cholesterol. Abnormal glycosylation of collagen can lead to stiff joints, poor wound healing, and glomerulosclerosis within the kidney. Abnormal glycosylation of low-density lipoprotein (LDL) and high-density lipoprotein (HDL) particles can lead to accelerated atherosclerosis.

NEUROPATHY

Diabetics commonly have somatic and autonomic neuropathies. During preoperative evaluation the anesthesiologist must look for evidence of peripheral neuropathy. Otherwise postoperative neuropathies may be confused as anesthetic related events from positioning or regional anesthesia. Further, 10% to 20% of DM patients have gastroparesis, which can lead to increased risk of aspiration during general anesthesia from delayed gastric emptying.

Diabetic patients with hypertension have a 50% incidence of autonomic neuropathy compared to a 10% incidence in nonhypertensive diabetics. Patients with autonomic neuropathy are at much greater risk for hemodynamic instability (especially after induction), aspiration from gastroparesis, or painless myocardial ischemia and cardiorespiratory arrest. The risk of cardiorespiratory arrest is especially high in the immediate postoperative period.

With autonomic neuropathy, the loss of parasympathetic innervation of the heart is often the earliest manifestation. This results in a resting tachycardia and loss of beat-to-beat heart-rate variability with respiration. The sympathetic nervous system can be affected as well, resulting in an inability to vasoconstrict or increase heart rate to vasodilating effects of anesthetic drugs.

Box 16-1 End-Organ Damage from Diabetes Mellitus

- Cardiovascular
- Renal insufficiency
- Joint-collagen disorders
- Peripheral and autonomic neuropathies
- Decreased granulocyte function
- Microangiopathy causing microvascular and retinal damage

Burgos et al. found a much higher incidence of hypotension and need for vasopressor support after induction in diabetics with autonomic dysfunction, compared to diabetics without autonomic dysfunction. Thus, titrating anesthetic drugs carefully, along with assuring adequate preload before induction is essential for patients with autonomic dysfunction. Furthermore, the anesthesiologist should have a lower threshold for placement of invasive hemodynamic monitoring.

Lastly, there are several case reports of sudden unexplained cardiac and respiratory arrest, especially in the immediate postoperative period in diabetic patients with autonomic neuropathy. Page and Watkins hypothesized that these events were primarily caused by respiratory arrest from an impaired central respiratory center, and from peripheral chemoreceptor dysfunction.

CARDIOVASCULAR

Diabetics have an increased incidence of coronary artery and peripheral vascular disease with an increased risk of myocardial infarction (MI) and stroke. This is caused by accelerated atherosclerosis from abnormal nonenzymatic glycosylation of LDL and HDL. Besides the increased incidence of coronary artery disease, diabetics have a stiffer left ventricle with an elevated left-ventricular diastolic pressure and an increased risk for diastolic dysfunction, compared to age-matched controlled subjects. Furthermore, diabetics have an increased incidence of nondilated cardiomyopathy with systolic and diastolic dysfunction. The etiology of the cardiomyopathy is thought to involve perivascular interstitial fibrosis and increased endothelial thickening of small coronary vessels. The incidence of diabetic cardiomyopathy greatly increases with a combination of diabetes and hypertension.

These cardiac problems, combined with autonomic neuropathy, can lead to significant intraoperative and postoperative hemodynamic instability. In the diabetic patient, the perioperative physician needs to have a lower threshold for performing cardiac-risk stratification tests, such as a dobutamine echocardiography, and using invasive hemodynamic monitoring for major surgery.

NEPHROPATHY

Diabetic nephropathy is the leading cause of end-stage renal disease. Hyperglycemia causes renal hyperperfusion and elevated intraglomerular hypertension. This, along with nonenzymatic glycosylation, leads to increased protein deposition in the mesangium and glomerulosclerosis.

Clinical renal dysfunction from diabetes often does not correlate with actual histologic abnormalities. Diabetic nephropathy may be silent for a long period before one sees an elevation in creatinine. Initially, the diabetic patient may leak small amounts of albumin in the urine, which is not picked up by a routine urine dipstick for protein, but which can be detected by more sensitive methods. The presence of microalbuminuria is highly predictive for the future development of chronic renal insufficiency. Over time, the patient with DM will excrete larger amounts of albumin (macroalbuminuria) with a steady decline in the glomerular filtration rate and elevation of serum creatinine. Hence, the perioperative physician should consider any diabetic patient at increased risk of developing acute renal failure after any renal ischemic event.

STIFF JOINT SYNDROME

Stiff joint syndrome is associated with type I diabetes. Its symptoms are limited joint mobility and tight waxy skin. Initially the syndrome affects the fourth and fifth proximal phalangeal joint and progresses to involve other joints of the finger and hand, the atlantooccipital joint of the neck, and other larger joints. The pathophysiology of the stiff joint syndrome is likely caused by abnormal cross-linking of collagen from nonenzymatic glycosylation. The inability to extend the head because of atlantooccipital immobility can lead to a difficult intubation. Reissell et al. found 31% of type I diabetics to be difficult to intubate. Cervical vertebral mobility often appears normal on physical examination and can mask limited atlantooccipital extension. However, examination of the hands and fingers with the palmar surfaces apposed together, can be used to assess atlantooccipital mobility. This examination of the hands is known as the "prayer sign." The inability of the interphalangeal joints to approximate each other is a useful marker for limited extension of the atlantooccipital joint and should alert the anesthesiologist to the potential of a difficult intubation (Figure 16-1).

INSULIN

In insulin-dependent diabetes, there are several methods for glucose control during the perioperative period. As of yet, no studies have clearly shown that maintaining a glucose level below 200 mg/dl in the perioperative period decreases morbidity or mortality for most surgeries. However, elevated serum glucose concentrations above 250 mg/dl have been implicated as a cause of impaired wound healing, decreased phagocytic activity of granulocytes with increased risk of infections, impaired left-ventricle function upon weaning off bypass, worsened neurologic outcome after a cerebral insult, and increased fetal complications in pregnancy. Hence, this author recommends that serum glucoses be maintained below 200 mg/dl for the following: (1) procedures at risk of cerebral ischemia; (2) open heart surgery; and (3) surgery for infected diabetic wounds or other infection. Normoglycemia should be maintained for procedures involving pregnancy.

Ideally, reasonable glycemic control should be achieved during the 2 to 3 days before surgery. For patients with chronic, poor metabolic control, admission to the hospital for 2 to 3 days to adjust insulin dosage may be necessary. For minor surgery not involving major body cavities, the use of subcutaneous insulin appears adequate. On the morning of surgery, the patient is given one third to two thirds the normal insulin dose subcutaneously, along with 5% dextrose solution at 100 cc/hr/70 kg of body weight. This author gives two thirds the normal insulin dose if fasting glucose is over 250 mg/dl, one half the normal insulin for glucose between 120 to 250 mg/dl, and one third the normal insulin dose for glucose below 120 mg/dl. During surgery, regular insulin intravenous boluses can be given if blood glucoses rise above 200 mg/dl. Patients with low or normal glucose still need small amounts of insulin to offset the increased catabolic effects of the stress of surgery, decreased protein catabolism, and to prevent lipolysis. Without insulin, the type I diabetic is at high risk of developing ketosis with surgery.

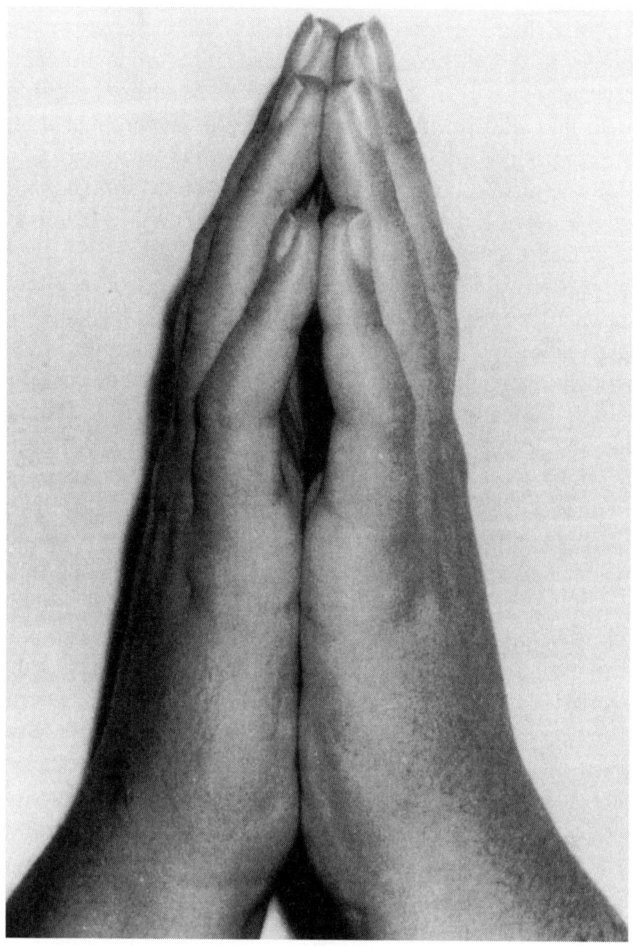

Figure 16-1

The hands of a 31-year-old diabetic woman with a positive prayer sign. Conditions for laryngoscopy were difficult. (Used with permission from Reissel E, et al: Predictability of difficult laryngoscopy in patients with long-term diabetes mellitus, *Anaesthesia* 45:1024–1027, 1990.)

For outpatient surgery, to which the patient is expected to drive in the morning of surgery, the NPH should be reduced by one half the evening before. The morning insulin should be withheld to avoid the risk of hypoglycemia occurring while traveling. The previously described regimen should then begin upon arrival to the hospital. All outpatient diabetics should have surgery done in the early morning to allow better control and less risk of hypoglycemia or ketosis from a prolonged fast.

For major surgery, long-acting insulin injected subcutaneously is likely to be inadequate. The long length of surgery, combined with the stress of major surgery, will likely lead to poorer glucose control and increased metabolic derangement. Classically, the use of regular insulin, glucose, and potassium in the same intravenous infusion has been described for perioperative use. However, this author believes this regimen does not allow rapid adjustment for hypoglycemia or hyperglycemia. Instead, running a separate continuous infusion of regular insulin allows more rapid adjustments. Roizen suggests the insulin infusion rate in units/hr be determined by dividing the blood glucose by 150 or by 100 if the patient is on steroids, is obese, has an ongoing infection, or is already on high amounts of insulin.

The common practice of giving intravenous (IV) boluses of regular insulin alone will provide poorer control for the diabetic. The half-life of IV insulin is 4 to 5 minutes with a biological half-life of 20 minutes. Boluses of regular insulin alone can lead to periods of hypoglycemia, alternating with periods of hyperglycemia, that promotes catabolism with lipolysis and ketogenesis. However, giving small additional IV boluses in combination with a continuous insulin infusion or prior long-acting subcutaneous insulin, can be done safely for rapid control of an elevated glucose, without causing rebound catabolic effects. Nevertheless, the serum glucose should be remeasured 30 minutes after a bolus of insulin.

Lastly, subcutaneous insulin given in the operating room cannot be recommended. The changes in cutaneous blood flow during the operative period will lead to unpredictable insulin absorption. With IV insulin, insulin can be absorbed onto the plastic tubing, leading to unpredictable delivery of insulin. This problem can be rectified easily by flushing the tubing initially with the patient's insulin infusion.

For type II DM patients on oral hypoglycemic agents (OHA), these agents should not be given the night before and the morning of surgery, to avoid hypoglycemia. Patients taking chlorpropamide (Diabinese) are at particularly increased risk of hypoglycemia because of its prolonged hypoglycemic effects (up to 36 hours). This author reduces the chlorpropamide (available as generic now) dosage in half the day before surgery. The more commonly used second-generation sulfonylureas, glipizide and glyburide, have durations of action between 12 to 24 hours. The newest preparation of glipizide, Glucotrol XL, releases glipizide continuously over a 24-hour period. In patients whose serum glucoses are well controlled before surgery, it also is prudent to reduce the dosage of glipizide or glyburide the day before surgery, particularly in elderly patients. Type II DM patients poorly controlled on OHA and undergoing major surgery may benefit from insulin infusion the night before surgery. Metformin (glucophage) also should not be given the morning of surgery because of the increased risk of lactic acidosis from the stress of surgery.

Ketoacidosis and Nonketotic Hyperosmolar Hypoglycemic Coma

The diabetic presenting for emergency surgery in ketoacidosis or hyperosmolar hyperglycemic coma is at much higher risk of perioperative complications. Often the cause for emergency surgery is also the cause of the ketoacidosis or hyperosmolar state. The ability to delay surgery for a short period can significantly improve patient outcome; yet, any further delay in surgery may do more harm to the patient.

The perioperative physician must begin with immediate, aggressive fluid resuscitation with isotonic crystalloid, insulin infusions, and correcting electrolyte abnormalities. Often, the patient will require 5 to 8 liters of crystalloid in the first 12 hours. This author avoids the use of Ringer's lactate in cases of significantly elevated serum glucoses because lactate is converted to glucose by gluconeogenesis. Intravenous insulin bolus of 10 units should be given, along with an insulin infusion calculated by the serum glucose divided by 150 or by 100 if the patient is on steroids, has an ongoing infection, or is already on large amounts of insulin. The insulin infusion can be increased by 50% along with further insulin boluses if the serum glucose does not decline more than 50 mg/dl/hr. Once glucose declines to 250 mg/dl, a dextrose infusion should be started and a reduced insulin infusion continued until ketosis is cleared. The serum glucose should be lowered below approximately 250 mg/dl in the first 24 hours to avoid the rare complication of cerebral edema. For nonketotic hyperosmotic hyperglycemia, the amount of insulin needed to decrease serum glucose is often less, as long as adequate fluid has been given.

Hyperkalemia is often present initially because of leakage of potassium out of the cell from acidosis and lack of insulin. However, total body potassium stores are low caused by intracellular depletion. Hence, potassium should begin to be replaced as soon as the serum potassium is normal and urine output is adequate. Also, serum phosphorus is often low and this can lead to respiratory muscle weakness in the operating room. Both potassium and phosphorus can be replaced together as potassium phosphate. Small amounts of bicarbonate should be given for pH below 7.0 as long as adequate ventilation is assured. Factitious hyponatremia can occur with severe hyperglycemia with the measured sodium decreasing 1.6 mEq/l for every 100 mg/dl increase in glucose. Lastly, all adult patients in ketoacidosis or hyperosmolar states should have a 12-lead ECG performed before surgery. There is a high incidence of silent MIs being the cause of ketoacidosis.

PITUITARY DISORDERS

The pituitary gland is located within the sella turcica underneath the brain. The sella turcica is surrounded laterally and inferiorly by the sphenoid bone and superiorly by a dural sheath called the diaphragm sellae. The hypophyseal stalk connects the hypothalamus to the pituitary gland through the central portion of the diaphragm sellae.

The pituitary gland consists of anterior and posterior lobes. The anterior pituitary gland secretes several hormones that directly stimulate several endocrine glands. These hormones include adrenocorticotropic hormone (ACTH), thyroid stimulating hormone (TSH), follicle stimulating hormone (FSH), luteinizing hormone (LH), growth hormone (GH), and prolactin. The posterior pituitary gland is linked to the hypothalamus through the hypophyseal tract within the pituitary stalk. Vasopressin and oxytocin are synthesized in the hypothalamus and then released through the hypophyseal tract to be stored in the posterior pituitary gland.

Enlargement of the pituitary gland can cause compression of the surrounding structures. The lateral wall of the sella turcica contain the cavernous sinus, internal carotid artery, and cranial nerves III, IV, VI, V_1 and V_2. Therefore, lateral extension of pituitary adenoma can cause ocular motor palsies and facial pain or numbness. The sphenoid sinus is inferior to the sella turcica. Extension of an adenoma inferiorly can lead to erosion of the sphenoid bone and to extension of the adenoma into the sphenoid sinus, which may cause a cerebrospinal fluid (CSF) leak. The optic chiasm is located above the diaphragm sellae, and suprasellar extension of an adenoma can result in visual field deficits, most commonly, a bitemporal hemianopsia. Furthermore, hypopituitarism may develop with suprasellar extension of pituitary adenoma that compresses the pituitary stalk or the hypothalamus or both, which prevents hypothalamic-releasing hormones from reaching the pituitary (Figure 16-2).

Headache is a common symptom of a macroadenoma (adenomas >10 mm in size) and may be caused by stretching of the surrounding dural sheath. For imaging of the pituitary, magnetic resonance imaging (MRI) is superior to other imaging techniques because microadenomas (< 10 mm in size) and the surrounding structures, such as the optic chiasm, may be easily seen.

Hypopituitarism

The most common etiology of hypopituitarism is a pituitary macroadenoma directly compressing the pituitary gland or stalk. Other causes of hypopituitarism include: (1) necrosis from pituitary hemorrhage from either spontaneous direct hemorrhage of an adenoma (pituitary apoplexy) or circulatory collapse after delivery (Sheehan's syndrome), (2) craniopharyngiomas compressing the hypothalamus or pituitary or both, (3) infiltrative and granulomatosis diseases, and (4) surgery or radiation.

The most common presentation of hypopituitarism is impotence and loss of libido in men and secondary amenorrhea in women. Diagnosis can be made from men with low testosterone levels and women with low estrogen levels and inappropriately low or normal FSH and LH levels. A low, free T_4 level with an inappropriately low or normal TSH concentration is diagnostic of secondary hypothyroidism.

The pituitary-adrenal axis can be assessed initially with an 8:00 am cortisol level. Random cortisol levels after 8:00 am are not useful since the normal diurnal rhythm of cortisol results in lower cortisol concentrations later in the day. An 8:00 am plasma cortisol level below 5 µg/dl is diagnostic of adrenal insufficiency; a level above 18 to 20 µg/dl essentially excludes adrenal insufficiency. Intermediate plasma concentration should be followed up with a stimulation test, usually in consultation with an endocrinologist. Three commonly employed tests are: (1) an insulin tolerance test; (2) a corticotropin-releasing hormone (CRH) stimulation test; or (3) a metyrapone test.

The insulin tolerance test is performed by administering 0.15 µ/kg of intravenous regular insulin and measuring plasma cortisol at times of 0, 30, 45, 60, and 90 minutes. If the blood glucose does not decrease to less than 45 mg/dl by 45 minutes, a second dose of insulin (0.3 units/kg) is administered. A peak cortisol concentration above 18 to 20 µg/dl documents a normal pituitary-adrenal axis. This insulin test should not be performed in patients with ischemic heart disease or seizure disorders. The CRH stimulation test will likely replace the insulin tolerance test when CRH becomes approved in the near future; it is better tolerated by patients. The metyrapone test is performed by giving a single 30 mg/kg oral dose of metyrapone at midnight and measuring plasma 11-deoxycortisol and cortisol levels at 8:00 am. Metyrapone prevents the conversion of 11-deoxycortisol to cortisol. With loss of

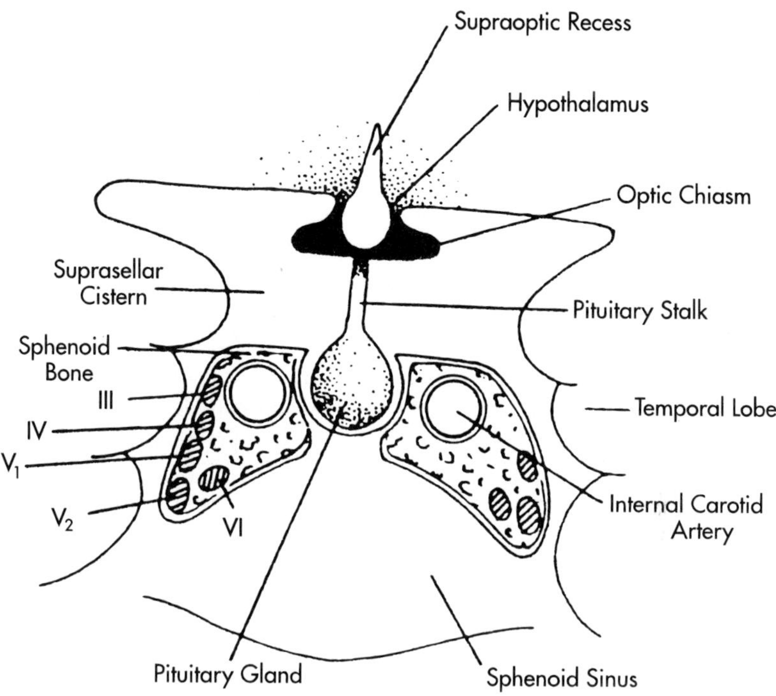

Figure 16-2
Pituitary gland and surrounding structures. (Used with permission from Lechan, RM. Neuroendrocrinology of pituitary hormone regulation, *Endocrinol Metab Clin North Am* 16:475–502, 1987.)

ACTH stimulation, metyrapone will not increase plasma 11-deoxycortisol concentrations. If both 11-deoxycortisol and cortisol levels remain low after metyrapone, this signifies an impaired pituitary-adrenal axis. The metyrapone test can precipitate worsened symptoms of adrenal insufficiency in patients with low ACTH reserve. It should, therefore, be done only in hospitalized patients. The metyrapone test should not be done within 48 hours of a dexamethasone suppression test.

Hyperpituitarism

Hyperpituitarism is caused from either: (1) excessive releasing of GH (acromegaly); (2) excessive ACTH secretion (Cushing's syndrome); or (3) excessive prolactin secretion. Other presentations from excessive secretion of gonadotropins, TSH, or other hypothalamic-releasing hormones are rare.

ACROMEGALY

Acromegaly classically presents with a gradual enlargement of hands, feet, and facial structures from skeletal and soft tissue enlargement. Facial features of acromegaly include frontal bossing, prognathism, and enlargement of nose and tongue. Acromegalic patients will often complain of lethargy, muscle weakness, and paresthesias in the hand from carpal tunnel syndrome. Twenty-five percent of acromegalics will have hypertension, and 15% will have cardiomegaly, most likely from hypertension. Impaired glucose tolerance and DM occur in 30% to 45% and 10% to 20% of acromegalics, respectively. Acromegaly is also associated with a two-fold premature, increased overall mortality rate with excess deaths caused by cardiovascular disease, respiratory disease, and malignancies.

Normally, GH is suppressed after an oral glucose load. Acromegaly is diagnosed by lack of GH suppressibility after an oral-glucose challenge (GH remains >1 ng/ml). Treatment consists of transsphenoidal resection of the adenoma and postoperative radiation therapy if persistent disease is present. Medical therapy, which is often used as an adjunct with surgery or radiation therapy, includes bromocriptine (dopamine agonist) and octreotide (somatostatin analogue), both of which inhibit GH. Of the two agents, octreotide is much more effective and may decrease the size of the adenoma. This is particularly useful for control of GH hypersecretion and symptoms following an incomplete resection. Octreotide and radiation therapy may be used in patients who are not surgical candidates because of other medical illnesses.

PERIOPERATIVE MANAGEMENT

Preoperative evaluation should include an extensive history and physical examination concerning the airway. The new development of snoring, stridor, or sleep apnea should alert the anesthesiologist to significant anatomic alterations in the airway. With acromegaly, extensive encroachment of soft tissue, enlargement of the tongue and epiglottis, involvement of the larynx and subglottic stenosis can occur, making for both a difficult mask ventilation and tracheal intubation. The anesthesiologist should have a low threshold for awake oral intubations for airway securement with a smaller endotracheal tube. Nasal intubation is best avoided because of the increased incidence of nasal turbinate hypertrophy.

An ECG and serum glucose should be obtained preoperatively to look for evidence of left-ventricular hypertrophy and glucose intolerance. If radial arterial line placement is contemplated, adequate ulnar collateral flow must clearly be documented because of a high incidence of inadequate ulnar collateral flow.

CUSHING'S SYNDROME

Cushing's syndrome (hyperadrenocorticism) is caused most commonly by ACTH-secreting pituitary adenomas (70%–75% of cases). Ectopic secretion of ACTH by nonpituitary tumors (usually pulmonary or pancreatic neoplasms) and cortisol-secreting adrenocortical tumors also cause Cushing's syndrome.

The diagnosis of Cushing's syndrome is established by elevated urine-free cortisol in a 24-hour urine collection. If the increase in urine-free cortisol is equivocal, then a low-dose dexamethasone suppression test is performed to confirm the diagnosis. Next plasma ACTH levels are measured in the afternoon. If ACTH levels are undetectable, then an adrenal adenoma or neoplasm is likely and a computed tomography (CT) scan of the adrenal glands is then done. If ACTH levels are normal or elevated, then ACTH-dependent Cushing's is present and a high-dose dexamethasone suppression test is given to distinguish pituitary from ectopic sources (Table 16-1). If

Table 16-1. Test Results in Patients with Cushing's Syndrome of Various Etiologies

ETIOLOGY	LOW-DOSE DEXAMETHASONE	PLASMA ACTH	HIGH-DOSE DEXAMETHASONE
Pituitary	No or partial	Normal or elevated	Suppression
Ectopic ACTH	No suppression	Normal or elevated	No suppression
Adrenal	No suppression	Low	No suppression

(Used with permission from Thorner MO et al: Anterior pituitary. In Wilson JD, Foster DW, editors: *Textbook of endocrinology,* ed 8, Philadelphia, 1992, pp 221–310, WB Saunders.)

the urine-free cortisol is suppressed by over 90%, then a pituitary adenoma is likely. If no suppression occurs, then ectopic ACTH secretion is likely. With intermediate degrees of suppression, inferior petrosal sinus sampling may be necessary to distinguish pituitary from ectopic sources of ACTH secretion. The sensitivity and specificity of this test is enhanced by administration of CRH to enhance the ACTH gradient between the inferior petrosal sinus and peripheral circulation (Figure 16-3).

When a pituitary tumor is suspected, MRI of the pituitary gland should be performed. However, only 50% of pituitary ACTH adenomas will be seen by MRI or CT scan because the majority of these adenomas are very small. Macroadenomas are seen less frequently in Cushing's syndrome.

For Cushing's syndrome caused by a pituitary adenoma, transphenoidal surgical resection is the treatment of choice. Cure rates of 80% for microadenomas can be achieved by experienced surgeons. Radiation therapy has only a 15% to 20% success rate in adults and has the risk of delayed hypopituitarism. For anesthetic management of Cushing's syndrome, see the adrenal subsection.

Prolactinoma

Hyperprolactinemia is the most common anterior pituitary disorder. Prolactin secretion is regulated primarily by inhibition of dopamine secreted by the hypothalamus. Common symptoms of hyperprolactinemia in women include galactorrhea and amenorrhea. However, galactorrhea is not present in all women with elevated prolactin levels because the presence of estradiol is required for lactation. Men typically present with impotence, loss of libido, headache, or visual field abnormalities. Hyperprolactinemia inhibits pulsatile gonadotropin release. This results in hypogonadotrophic hypogonadism. Serum prolactin levels greater than 200 ng/ml are usually the result of a pituitary tumor. Levels between 50 to 200 ng/ml may reflect a large nonsecreting pituitary tumor, which is compressing the pituitary stalk, thus, preventing dopamine from effectively inhibiting prolactin release.

Most prolactinomas can be managed medically with dopamine agonists; bromocriptine and pergolide are the two most commonly used agents in the United States. These agents reduce serum prolactin concentrations and tumor size in the majority of patients. The degree of prolactin suppression varies, but in most series more than 60% of patients achieve normal serum prolactin levels. Some prolactinomas do not respond well to dopamine agonist therapy, probably because of either a decreased number or affinity of dopamine receptors in the tumor. For such patients, surgical

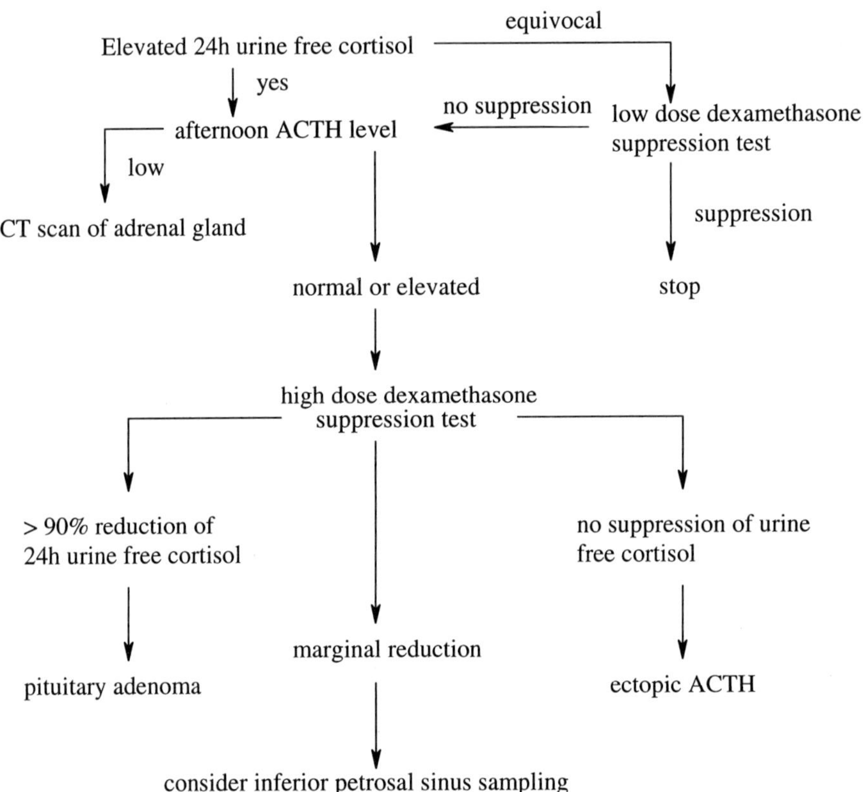

Figure 16-3
Diagnostic flow chart for Cushing's syndrome.

resection is recommended. Transsphenoidal surgery results in normalization of serum prolactin levels in 60% to 80% of microadenomas (<10 mm) but only in 0% to 40% of macroadenomas over 10 mm. In addition, 5-year recurrence rates range from 10% to 50% for microadenomas and are higher for larger tumors. For patients with recurrent disease, either dopamine agonists or radiation therapy or both are used. Although bromocriptine use is not associated with increased risks to a fetus, it is standard practice to discontinue the drug during pregnancy. For this reason, women with macroadenomas may undergo transsphenoidal surgery if tumor reexpansion occurs during pregnancy.

TRANSSPHENOIDAL SURGERY

Any patient scheduled for transsphenoidal resection of a pituitary adenoma should have an assessment of pituitary function done several days before planned surgery.

Neurologic examination should be noted preoperatively, especially cranial nerves II, IV, V, and VI. Magnetic resonance imaging or CT scan should be reviewed for size and any extension of the pituitary tumor. Extension of the tumor near the cavernous sinus greatly increases the risk of significant hemorrhage and air embolism. Routine monitors are usually sufficient; however, an arterial line and precordial doppler may be indicated if there is increased risk of hemorrhage or air embolism caused by the location of the tumor. Stress glucocorticoid coverage should be given upon resection of the adenoma because any manipulation of the pituitary gland may alter normal function for the first few days postoperatively. Thyroid hormone supplementation is not needed in the immediate postoperative period because the half-life of T_4 is approximately 7 days.

In the immediate postoperative period, neurologic examination should be done, particularly examining cranial nerves II, III, IV, V, and VI. Urine output, urine specific gravity, and serum sodium should be followed closely for both diabetes insipidus or syndrome of inappropriate antidiuretic hormone (SIADH). Other less common complications of transsphenoidal surgery include CSF leaks, meningitis, abscess or vascular injury with resultant stroke or hemorrhage, oculomotor palsy, or visual loss.

Diabetes Insipidus

Diabetes insipidus presents with polyuria, elevated plasma osmolality above 295 mosm/kg and low urine osmolality below 200 mosm/kg. Diabetes insipidus left untreated in a patient unable to take fluids by mouth can lead to life-threatening hypernatremia and hypovolemia.

In the perioperative setting, diabetes insipidus is usually caused by diffuse head trauma or surgery near the hypothalamic-pituitary region. Surprisingly, total removal of the posterior pituitary gland usually does not cause permanent diabetes insipidus as long as the hypothalamic-hypophyseal tract remains intact. Transient central diabetes insipidus is not uncommon following transphenoidal surgery. It typically starts abruptly within the first postoperative day and resolves within 2 to 5 days. This is thought to be the result of neuronal shock which is temporary. Permanent diabetes insipidus results only when hypothalamic-hypophyseal injury destroys more than 85% of the neurons in the supraoptic and paraventricular nuclei.

In many cases, transient postoperative diabetes insipidus can be managed with increased IV fluids or oral fluids alone. In more severe cases of central diabetes insipidus, 0.5 to 2.0 µg of DDAVP (1-desamino-8-D arginine vasopressin) can be given intravenously twice a day in the immediate postoperative period, followed by 5 to 10 µg of intranasal DDAVP twice a day. Aqueous vasopressin 5 to 10 units SC or IM every 6 to 8 hours can also be used. An IV aqueous vasopressin drip can be used intraoperatively through an initial IV bolus of 0.1 units, followed by a continuous drip of 0.1 to 0.2 units/hr, as determined by urine output and plasma abnormality and sodium. This author prefers to use DDAVP during the perioperative period because of the potential for significant pressor effects from the use of aqueous vasopressin.

Nephrogenic diabetes insipidus rarely occurs in the perioperative period, but patients may present with long-standing nephrogenic diabetes insipidus from such drugs as lithium. For nephrogenic diabetes insipidus, vasopressin will have no effect because the renal tubules are resistant to ADH. Intraoperatively, the anesthesiologist should have a much lower threshold for central venous pressure monitoring to determine intravascular volume, because urine output will remain elevated. Arterial monitoring also may be helpful for frequent blood withdrawals to closely follow plasma osmolality and sodium.

Syndrome Inappropriate Antidiuretic Hormone

Syndrome inappropriate antidiuretic hormone (SIADH) occurs from multiple etiologies such as paraneoplastic syndromes, brain injury, pulmonary disease, certain drugs, and occasionally after stressful surgery. Classically, SIADH is diagnosed by the combination of hyponatremia, inappropriate elevation of urine osmolality, and sodium with the urine osmolality greater than the plasma osmolality.

The perioperative physician should be cognizant that both hypothyroidism and adrenal insufficiency can mimic SIADH. These endocrine disorders should be excluded by appropriate testing when unexplained hyponatremia occurs. It is especially important to determine the etiology of hyponatremia after transsphenoidal surgery; SIADH often occurs between the sixth to eighth day postoperatively after transsphenoidal surgery. Adrenal insufficiency can also present in this period after initial stress steroids have been discontinued.

Treatment of SIADH consists of fluid restriction of 500 to 1000 cc/day. Any IV fluids should be 0.9% normal saline, avoiding any hypotonic solutions. When the serum sodium is less than 120 mEq/dl in association with neurologic changes, IV hypertonic 3% saline can be given, but at a rate no faster than 6 ml/kg/hr, and should be combined with furosemide to increase free water clearance. Rapid correction of serum sodium (>1–2 mEq/l/h) potentially can cause central pontine myelinolysis. Hypertonic saline should be discontinued when the serum sodium reaches 125 mEq/l, and water restriction alone should be used for further treatment.

THYROID DISORDERS

The thyroid hormones thyroxine (T_4) and triiodothyronine (T_3) are major hormones responsible for initiating cellular activity of multiple organ systems, including cardiovascular, respiratory, and neuromuscular. Furthermore, the thyroid hormones directly affect the cardiac muscle response to sympathetic stimulation at the β and α receptors.

Thyroid Hormone Synthesis and Regulation

The synthesis of thyroid hormone starts with the active transport of iodide from the plasma into the thyroid gland. Iodide is oxidized by a peroxidase reaction to iodine, which binds with tyrosine residues to form monoiodotyrosine (MIT) and diiodotyrosine (DIT). These precursors then undergo oxidation coupling within the thyroglobulin to form T_4 and T_3. The majority of thyroid hormone secreted from the thyroid is T_4, which has lower biologic potency. Eighty percent of the more biologically potent

T_3 is made from the conversion of T_4 to T_3 in the periphery, with the remainder secreted directly from the thyroid.

The thyroid gland is regulated directly by TSH, which is responsible for both stimulating formation and secretion of T_4 and T_3. Secretion of TSH from the pituitary gland is directly influenced by thyrotropin-releasing hormone (TRH), released from the hypothalamus. Thyrotropin-releasing hormone is inhibited by higher amounts of circulating thyroid hormone. Hence, in primary hypothyroidism the TSH level will be elevated because of the lack of negative feedback from low levels of thyroid hormone. An elevated TSH level is the most sensitive marker for hypothyroidism. A new sensitive assay of TSH now allows primary hyperthyroidism to be diagnosed by low levels of TSH.

Thyroid Function Tests

Total serum T_4 level is the most common single diagnostic test. The T_4 level is high in 90% of hyperthyroid patients and low in 85% of hypothyroid patients. Most of the circulating thyroid hormone is bound to thyroid-binding globulin (TBG) with only a small percentage of T_4 and T_3 being free and biologically active. Many conditions that elevate or decrease the level of TBG will elevate or decrease the total T_4 level in euthyroid patients (Table 16-2).

Free T_4 (FT_4) is not affected by changes in the TBG. Most commonly, FT_4 is measured by multiplying total T_4 by the percentage of T_3 resin uptake (T_3RU) to obtain the FT_4 index. T_3 resin uptake is measured by a resin that binds free thyroid hormone. States with an increased number of thyroid-binding globulin sites will have a decrease resin uptake because of decrease availability of free hormone. The T_3RU varies inversely to the number of thyroid-binding sites in the protein and is directly proportional to the amount of free hormone. Hence, states such as pregnancy with elevated TBG and serum T_4 will have a normal FTI but a decreased T_3 resin uptake from decreased availability of T_3 to bind to the resin. Usually, with hyperthyroidism, both total T_4 and T_3RU will be elevated, and with hypothyroidism both will be low. A second method of measuring free T_4 is through an equilibrium dialysis membrane, but this method can be difficult and cumbersome.

Serum T_3 is measured by radioimmunoassay (RIA). Occasionally hyperthyroid patients can have normal T_4 levels but elevated T_3 levels. Serum T_3 levels should be measured when patients suspected of being hyperthyroid are found to have normal FT_4 levels with a suppressed, sensitive TSH assay. Serum T_3 levels are decreased in only 50% of hypothyroid patients. Serum T_3 is also reduced in euthyroid sick syndrome, commonly seen with systemic illness or postoperatively after major surgery. In euthyroid sick syndrome, the conversion of T_4 to T_3 is decreased and the conversion of T_4 to reverse T_3 (RT_3) is increased with normal T_4 and TSH levels. Euthyroid sick syndrome has little clinical significance, but the perioperative physician needs to be aware of it as a cause of decreased total T_3.

Hyperthyroidism

Graves' disease and toxic multinodular goiter are the most common causes of hyperthyroidism. With Graves' disease, most patients present with an enlarged thyroid,

Table 16-2. Levels of Thyroid Binding Globulin

	TBG
Pregnancy	↑
Acute liver disease	↑
Estrogens	↑
Nephrotic syndrome	↓
Chronic liver disease	↓

ophthalmopathy, and dermatopathy. Common manifestations of hyperthyroidism include anxiety, tremor, palpitations, diarrhea, heat tolerance, excessive sweating, and muscle weakness. Cardiovascular symptoms include a hyperdynamic state that can include tachyarrhythmias, atrial fibrillation, and high-output cardiac failure. Ocular signs include exophthalmos in Graves' disease as a result of an infiltrative process of the retrobulbar fat. Skin changes can include pretibial myxedema with raised thickened skin over the tibia and clubbing of fingers.

Toxic multinodular goiter occurs when the thyroid gland becomes autonomous to TSH control. Symptoms of thyrotoxicosis are often less pronounced. In the elderly, apathetic hyperthyroidism may present with arrhythmias, heart failure, weakness, or weight loss.

TREATMENT OF HYPERTHYROIDISM

For elective surgery, such as subtotal thyroidectomy, all hyperthyroid patients should be rendered euthyroid. Standard therapy consists of the antithyroid drugs propylthiouracil at 100 to 200 mg every 6 hours or methimazole. Both these drugs block the oxidation of iodide to iodine, the binding of iodine to tyroxyl residues, and the coupling of iodotyrosyl residues into T_3 and T_4. Furthermore, propylthiouracil will decease the peripheral conversion of T_4 to T_3, hence, it is the most commonly used antithyroid drug. Normally these drugs take 6 to 8 weeks to render a patient euthyroid. Severe reactions of agranulocytosis, skin rashes, and hepatitis occur rarely.

Beta-blockers should be added as needed to blunt sympathetic overactivity with a goal of a heart rate less than 90 beats per minute. Classically, propranolol has been used at doses of 40 to 80 mg every 6 hours. Potassium iodide should be started 7 to 10 days before surgery, especially for subtotal thyroidectomy. Iodide inhibits the release of thyroid hormone and will reduce the vascularity of the thyroid gland for thyroidectomy. Iodide should only be given after antithyroid medication has been given to prevent iodide-stimulating thyroid synthesis by intrathyroidal accumulation of iodine. Two iodide preparations commonly given are Lugol's solution, also known as saturated solution of potassium iodide (SSKI), at 5 drops every 6 hours, and an iodide contrast agent, ipodate, 0.5 to 1.0 gm per day.

ANESTHETIC MANAGEMENT OF HYPERTHYROIDISM

When emergent surgery does not allow for appropriate treatment of hyperthyroidism in advance, then the mainstay of management is to prevent further sympathetic stimulation and to treat the present hyperdynamic state with a β-blocker, such as an esmolol infusion, with a goal of keeping the heart rate below 90 beats per minute. One should avoid all drugs that stimulate sympathetic tone, such as pancuronium or ketamine. Furthermore, an adequate depth of anesthesia should be assured to blunt the surgical stress response and to prevent sympathetic stimulation.

Because of the potential for underlying muscle weakness and increased association with myasthenia gravis, muscle relaxants should be titrated carefully with neuromuscular monitoring. Hypotension should be treated with fluids and direct-acting vasopressors, such as phenylephrine, rather than indirect-acting vasopressors that release catecholamines. Regional anesthesia with adequate volume preload is a good alternative in preventing further sympathetic stimulation. Epinephrine-containing solutions of local anesthetic should be avoided. Lastly, these patients need to be monitored closely in the intraoperative and postoperative period for the development of thyroid storm.

THYROID STORM

Thyroid storm occurs most commonly in the immediate postoperative period. Thyroid storm appears not to be caused by an acute increase of thyroid hormone released from the thyroid gland, but instead, seems to result from an acute increase of free-hormone shifting from being protein-bound. Fever, tachycardia, diaphoresis, and agitation are the key signs and symptoms for the onset of thyroid storm. If not treated, thyroid storm can lead to shock and circulatory collapse (Box 16-2).

The following regimen should be undertaken for treatment of thyroid storm:

1. Propylthiouracil 100 mg by mouth through nasogastric tube every 2 to 6 hours initially.
2. Lugol's solution (potassium iodide), 10 drops initially, then 5 drops every 12 hours. Give first dose at least half an hour after propylthiouracil.
3. Beta blockade with esmolol infusion titrated to heart rate <90 beats per minute.
4. Dexamethasone 2 mg IV every 6 hours to decrease release of thyroid hormone and decrease peripheral conversion of T_4 to T_3.
5. Active cooling.
6. Aggressive volume replacement.

The above regimen will usually stabilize a patient in thyroid storm within a 12- to 24-hour period.

Hypothyroidism

Primary failure of the thyroid gland accounts for over 95% of all causes of hypothyroidism and is marked by an elevation of TSH. Clinical manifestations include

Box 16-2 Signs and Symptoms of Thyroid Storm

- Fever
- Tachycardia
- Diaphoresis
- Agitation
- Shock

lethargy, cold intolerance, dry skin, hair thinning, constipation, and husky voice. Physiologic alterations include depressed myocardial contractility with bradycardia, increased systemic vascular resistance, decreased intravascular volume, decreased baroreceptor reflexes, decreased ventilatory response to hypoxia and hypercarbia, decreased gastric emptying, decreased hepatic drug metabolism, hyponatremia from decreased free water clearance, and hypoglycemia (Box 16-3). Ultimately, periorbital and peripheral edema, tongue enlargement, cardiac dilatation, pleural and pericardial effusion may occur, and lead to myxedema coma with stupor, hypothermia, and cardiovascular instability.

TREATMENT

Initial therapy should begin with 50 µg/day of L-thyroxine (T_4) with a dosage increase to 100 to 150 µg/day over a 2- to 3-month period. In the elderly, and in patients with suspected coronary artery disease, dosage should start at 25 µg/day then slowly increase by 25 µg increments every month. Patients who develop angina with thyroid replacement should not be further treated, but instead, undergo evaluation for coronary revascularization. Becker et al., in a review of the literature, concluded that coronary artery bypass surgery could be safely performed in the hypothyroid patient without preoperative thyroid replacement.

ANESTHETIC MANAGEMENT

Ideally, hypothyroid patients should be made euthyroid before elective surgery. However, several studies found no worse morbidity or mortality in mild or moderate hypothyroid patients undergoing surgery. Weinberg et al. did find an increased incidence of delayed extubation, electrolyte abnormalities, and bleeding, although the differences were not statistically significant nor did the differences affect overall outcome. Clearly, severely hypothyroid patients should be postponed for all elective surgery cases.

Preoperative evaluation of the hypothyroid patient should include a good physical examination for a goiter with a potential for airway obstruction, a lung and cardiac examination for evidence of a pleural and pericardial effusion and cardiomegaly, and examination for delayed return of deep ankle-tendon reflexes, which are likely compatible with at least moderate hypothyroidism. A narrow pulse pressure is compatible with a depressed myocardium and decreased intravascular volume. Laboratory examination should include a hematocrit for anemia and electrolytes, especially looking for hyponatremia and hypoglycemia. An ECG that shows diffuse low voltage should raise the suspicion of a pericardial effusion. With Hashimoto's thyroiditis, other autoimmune disorders, such as adrenal insufficiency and myasthenia gravis, should be considered during preoperative assessment.

In the operating room, the hypothyroid patient may have an exaggerated depressant effect from the anesthetic agents. Hence, reducing the amount of premedication sedatives, induction drugs, narcotics, and volatile agents is recommended, followed by careful titration of drugs as needed to provide adequate anesthesia. Although the anesthesia minimum alveolar concentration (MAC) requirement is not reduced in hypothyroidism, volatile agents can cause significant cardiac depression and vasodilation,

Box 16-3 Physiologic Changes of Hypothyroidism

- Depressed myocardial function
- Bradycardia
- Increased systemic vascular resistance
- Decreased intravascular volume
- Decreased baroreceptor reflexes
- Decreased ventilator response to hypoxia and hypercarbia
- Decreased gastric emptying
- Impaired hepatic drug metabolism
- Decreased free water clearance and hyponatremia
- Hypoglycemia

with a decreased ability to compensate caused by impaired baroreceptor function and decreased intravascular volume. Muscle-relaxant drugs should be titrated with neuromuscular monitoring, keeping in mind the potential for underlying muscle weakness and myasthenia gravis. Active warming should be done to prevent the increased risk of hypothermia. The anesthesiologist should have a lower threshold for invasive monitoring with an arterial line, and cardiac filling pressures for major intraabdominal or vascular surgery. Stress-steroid coverage should be given in the event of prolonged hemodynamic instability for possible adrenal insufficiency.

In the recovery room, delayed awakening and respiratory depression can occur. Besides increased sensitivity to drugs and prolonged hepatic metabolism, other causes such as hypercapnia, hypoxia, hyponatremia, and hypoglycemia should be excluded for delayed awakening and respiratory depression. Lastly, regional anesthesia, which avoids depressant drugs, is an excellent option for the hypothyroid patient. However, adequate volume replacement should be assured before placing central neuroaxis blockade because of a high likelihood of underlying intravascular volume depletion.

Myxedema Coma

For emergency surgery, patients with suspected myxedema coma should be treated before initial thyroid tests have confirmed diagnosis. The use of IV bolus injections of thyroxine (T_4) will rapidly redistribute into storage sites, and, hence, maintain a lower stable plasma level and prevent the risk of excessive cardiovascular stimulation. The disadvantage of IV T_4 is a slow onset time of up to 24 hours and potential for decreased peripheral conversion of T_4 to the more active T_3 because of euthyroid sick syndrome. Using IV T_4 may provide little benefit in the immediate perioperative period. Liothyronine (T_3) has a rapid onset within 2 to 6 hours of being given intravenously but has been known to cause angina and sudden death at dosages of 25 to 50 µg IV because of excessive cardiovascular stimulation.

In the emergency perioperative setting, giving a combination of IV T_3 and T_4 has been recommended. This author advocates giving initially 5 µg of IV T_3 in the elderly or in patients with cardiac risk factors and 10 µg of IV T_3 otherwise, followed by an IV T_4 bolus of 200 to 300 µg. Continuous electrocardiographic monitoring is mandatory because of the potential of tachyarrhythmias and myocardial ischemia. A second small bolus of 5 to 10 µg of IV T_3 can be given at 8 hours and a third after

16 hours if the patient fails to show signs of metabolic improvement and has had no cardiac problems.

This combination of IV T_3 and T_4 allows a rapid onset of thyroid replacement in the perioperative period but lessens the risk of excessive cardiac or metabolic demand. Also, all suspected myxedematous patients should have stress-steroid coverage for the perioperative period until adrenal insufficiency has been excluded. Lastly, a delay in emergency surgery of even a few hours is likely to improve a patient's overall outcome from surgery and anesthesia.

ADRENAL DISORDERS

The adrenal gland is composed of the cortex and medulla. The cortex consists of the (1) zona fasiculata (responsible for glucocorticoid synthesis), (2) zona glomerulosa (responsible for aldosterone synthesis), and (3) zona reticularis (responsible for androgen production). The medulla is responsible for norepinephrine and epinephrine synthesis. Glucocorticoid synthesis is controlled by the hypothalamus-pituitary-adrenal axis. The hypothalamus secretes corticotropic-releasing hormone (CRH) which stimulates the pituitary to secrete ACTH; ACTH then stimulates glucocorticoid secretion in the form of cortisol from the zona fasciculata. Normally, 20 to 30 mg of cortisol is secreted daily in a diurnal pattern. Increases in cortisol cause a negative feedback on CRH and ACTH secretion. Serum cortisol has a half-life of 80 to 110 minutes; yet, by activation of the intracellular receptors, the end-organ effect of cortisol may last for 12 to 24 hours. At doses greater than 30 mg per day, cortisol has increased mineralocorticoid activity with increased salt and water retention. Angiotensin II from the renin-angiotensinogen axis stimulates aldosterone production from the zona glomerulosa.

Cortisol plays a vital role in regulating carbohydrate, protein, and lipid metabolism along with controlling the adrenal medulla and conversion of norepinephrine to epinephrine in the adrenal medulla. Cortisol also acts as a lysosomal membrane stabilizer. At high doses it acts as an antiinflammatory agent by membrane stabilization and inhibition of inflammatory mediators. The mineralocorticoid aldosterone acts on the collecting tubules of the nephron to increase sodium and water absorption and increase elimination of potassium and hydrogen ions.

Cushing's Syndrome (Excessive Glucocorticoid Activity)

Cushing's syndrome is characterized by multiple end-organ effects from excessive glucocorticoid activity. Truncal obesity, muscle weakness, easy bruisability, osteoporosis, hypertension, hypokalemic metabolic alkalosis, hyperglycemia, and hyperpigmented abdominal striae can all occur in Cushing's syndrome. Etiology of Cushing's syndrome occurs from iatrogenic steroid use, excessive activity of the hypothalamic-pituitary axis (most commonly a pituitary adenoma), ectopic-ACTH production from a paraneoplastic syndrome (most commonly bronchogenic, pancreas, kidney and carcinoid tumors), adrenal hyperplasia, or neoplasms. In patients under 40 years of age, a pituitary adenoma is the most common etiology, and in patients over 60 years of age, an adrenal neoplasm or ectopic ACTH is the most common etiology of Cushing's syndrome. In ectopic ACTH, patients can present with an abrupt onset of hypokalemic metabolic alkalosis with few other initial symptoms. For diagnosis of the etiology of Cushing's syndrome, see the Cushing's Syndrome subsection (page 246) and Figure 16-3.

ANESTHETIC MANAGEMENT

The patient with Cushing's syndrome may be scheduled for either a hypophysectomy or adrenalectomy. Adrenal adenomas are treated with adrenalectomy with virtually 100% cure rates. However, cure rates are low with adrenal carcinoma because a complete resection is rarely possible, and metastases are present at the time of diagnosis. Mitotane is used for nonresectable or recurrent disease.

Preoperative assessment should include evaluation for the following: (1) electrolyte disorders, most notably a hypokalemic metabolic alkalosis and hyperglycemia; (2) hypertension; (3) elevated intravascular volume; (4) muscle weakness; and (5) a history of pathologic fractures from osteoporosis. In the operating room, careful positioning is essential because of likely underlying osteoporosis. Muscle relaxants should be titrated carefully because of the potential of underlying muscle weakness. Increased blood loss may occur from tissue friability.

Often, patients with Cushing's syndrome are on such drugs as metyrapone and spironolactone. Patients on steroid inhibitors such as metyrapone or mitotane should be considered adrenally suppressed and receive full stress-steroid coverage perioperatively. For bilateral adrenalectomy or hypophysectomy, full stress-steroid coverage should be implemented upon resection. Patients with bilateral adrenalectomy will also require oral mineralocorticoid supplementation once a low dose of up to 30 to 50 mg/day of hydrocortisone, or the equivalent of prednisone, is used. Giving 0.05 to 0.1 mg/day of fludrocortisone (9-α-fluorocortisone) is considered adequate mineralocorticoid coverage. For unilateral adrenalectomy, stress-steroid coverage should be implemented because of likely continuous suppression of the remaining adrenal gland in the perioperative period.

Primary Hyperaldosteronism (Conn's Syndrome)

One-half to one percent of hypertensive patients without a known etiology have primary hyperaldosteronism. The etiology is most often from a unilateral adrenal adenoma, but bilateral adrenal hyperplasia can also cause hyperaldosteronism. These patients classically have diastolic hypertension, without edema, combined with hypokalemia. The elevated aldosterone levels cause an increase in sodium and water absorption. The combination of low plasma-renin levels combined with failure to suppress elevated aldosterone levels with volume expansion, is diagnostic for primary hyperaldosteronism. Patients with unilateral adenomas can be effectively treated with surgical removal of the adenoma; but patients with bilateral adrenal hyperplasia often do not show improvement in blood pressure with a bilateral adrenalectomy.

ANESTHETIC MANAGEMENT

Preoperatively, these patients often have potassium deficits of 300 to 400 milliequivalents of total body potassium. Severe hypokalemia can cause muscle weakness and tetany, polyuria, and increase ventricular arrhythmias. Correction of hypokalemia should occur over several days, to allow for equilibration of intracellular and extracellular potassium. When severe hypokalemia is diagnosed, hypomagnesemia should be checked and corrected for. Spironolactone is the drug of choice for medical treatment of hyperaldosteronism because spironolactone is a specific aldosterone antagonist. Dosages of 25 to 100 mg every 8 hours should be used; yet, spironolactone may take up to several weeks to correct for the increased intravascular volume and hypokalemia. Intraoperatively, the patients should be managed in the same way as any other hypertensive patient.

Adrenal Insufficiency (Glucocorticoid Deficiency)

The most common cause of primary adrenal failure is autoimmune destruction of the adrenal gland, which is often associated with other autoimmune diseases such as Hashimoto's thyroiditis (Schmidt's syndrome). Other common causes include infection from human immunodeficiency virus (HIV), cytomegalovirus (CMV), tuberculosis, tumor, and hemorrhagic necrosis. In primary adrenal failure, both glucocorticoid and mineralocorticoid production are decreased, and both need to be supplemented. Secondary adrenal failure commonly occurs from withdrawal of glucocorticoid use or failure of the hypothalamic-pituitary axis, such as in panhypopituitary patients. Mineralocorticoid production is normal in these patients because the renin-angiotensin axis is still capable of stimulating aldosterone production.

Classically, these patients present with lethargy, weakness, nausea and vomiting, abdominal pain, hyponatremia, hyperkalemia and hypotension. Patients with primary adrenal insufficiency will have increased pigmentation caused by elevation of ACTH and related peptides from the pituitary gland. The perioperative physician must always consider adrenal insufficiency in any patient presenting for exploratory laparotomy with abdominal pain, nausea, and vomiting. Furthermore, with unexplained shock during the perioperative period, bilateral hemorrhagic necrosis of the adrenal gland should be considered, especially in anticoagulated or septic patients. Hemorrhagic necrosis of the adrenal gland is, often, only diagnosed at autopsy.

Stress Steroids

For primary adrenal failure, no mineralocorticoid supplementation is needed if high doses of hydrocortisone are used. However, the mineralocorticoid fludrocortisone (9-α-fluorocortisone) 0.05 to 0.1 mg should be given for patients on hydrocortisone doses of less than 50 mg/day, or in patients with evidence of salt loss with hyponatremia and hyperkalemia. Other glucocorticoids, such as Decadron, can be given, but the low mineralocorticoid activity of these glucocorticoids should be considered (Table 16-3).

Usually, when stress steroids are given in the perioperative period it is because of prior glucocorticoid use. The patient who has received 2 weeks or more of supraphysiologic glucocorticoids within the past year may be at risk of adrenal suppression. However, many of these patients may have normal adrenal responsiveness to stress. The ACTH-stimulation test is a reliable predictor of an intact hypothalamic-pituitary-adrenal axis and the adrenal cortex ability to increase cortisol production

Table 16-3. Steroid Potency

AGENT (MG)	GLUCOCORTICOID POTENCY	MINERALOCORTICOID POTENCY	DURATION OF ACTION (H)
Hydrocortisone	1	1	8–12
Methylprednisolone	5	0.5	24–36
Prednisone	4	0.8	12–24
Dexamethasone	25	0	72
Fludrocortisone	10	125	20–24

with the stress of surgery. In these cases, cosyntropin (ACTH) 250 µg is given intravenously, and plasma cortisol levels are measured at 30 and 60 minutes after infusion, along with a baseline level. A rise of 7 to 20 µg/dl of cortisol is considered normal. The random measurement of plasma cortisol in general is not diagnostic because of the diurnal pattern, and a normal cortisol level does not assure adequate adrenal reserve to respond to stress. However, under the stress of surgery and the immediate postoperative period, adrenal insufficiency can be excluded with a serum cortisol level above 20 µg/dl. The ACTH-stimulation test is impractical to perform in the immediate preoperative period. Hence, all patients who have been on supraphysiologic glucocorticoids for more than 2 weeks within the prior year should be considered adrenally suppressed during the perioperative period until adrenal response is proven normal.

The adrenal cortex usually excretes between 75 to 150 mg of cortisol in the first 24-hour postoperative period. Maximal adrenal cortex production with maximal ACTH stimulation is now estimated to be 200 mg per day of cortisol. At present, many physicians give 300 mg of hydrocortisone over the first 24-hour intraoperative and postoperative period for stress-steroid coverage and then taper that amount over a 3-day period. A total of 300 mg of hydrocortisone is likely excessive and may cause hyperglycemia and hypertension and inhibit wound healing.

Chernow et al. looked at cortisol response in patients undergoing surgery with no prior glucocorticoid use. Chernow divided the patients into three groups: (1) minor surgery (inguinal hernia repair or laparoscopy), (2) moderate surgery (cholecystectomy, hysterectomy, appendectomy), and (3) severe surgery (major abdominal or vascular). Chernow found negligible cortisol increases with minor surgery but significant increases for 24 hours after moderate or severe surgery; the cortisol levels returned to normal at 5 days. Hence, for minor surgery, only physiologic doses of glucocorticoids are needed for the immediate perioperative period. If the patient already has taken equivalent or higher doses of glucocorticoids the day of surgery, no further glucocorticoid supplementation is needed for minor surgery.

There is little evidence in the literature of actual cardiovascular collapse in the perioperative period from adrenal insufficiency in humans. However, Udelsman et al. studied three groups of previously adrenalectomized primates, placing them on one tenth physiologic, physiologic, and supraphysiologic (10 x physiologic) glucocorticoid dosages, respectively, for 4 days before performing a cholecystectomy, along with a control group. The subphysiologic-dosed primates had a 38% mortality rate and a high incidence of hypotension. However, Udelsman found no difference between physiologic, supraphysiologic, and control groups of primates in hemodynamic monitoring and surgical outcome. Udelsman also found no difference in wound healing or other deleterious effects within the supraphysiologic group. This is in contrast to prior studies on rats which showed delayed wound healing with brief high-dose glucocorticoid administration. Udelsman et al. concluded that there was no clear advantage to giving supraphysiologic glucocorticoids over physiologic replacement.

Symreng et al. in 1981 gave known adrenally suppressed patients undergoing major surgery 25 mg of hydrocortisone IV followed by a continuous 24-hour infusion of 100 mg of hydrocortisone. Symreng then measured subsequent cortisol levels over 24 hours and compared these levels to those in control patients and prior glucocorticoid-treated patients with normal ACTH stimulation tests. The hydrocortisone-replaced patients had higher cortisol levels for the first 4 hours after induction of anesthesia and equivalent, or higher cortisol levels for the remainder of the 24-hour period. Furthermore, the glucocorticoid-treated patients with preserved adrenal function had cortisol levels nearly equal to those in the control group, without any supplementation (Figure 16-4).

In conclusion, a dosage of 200 mg of hydrocortisone should be given in 2 or 3 divided doses over the first 24-hour perioperative period for major surgery. Smaller doses of hydrocortisone, such as recommended by Symreng et al., with a total of 125 mg for the first 24-hour-perioperative period should be more than adequate for such procedures as cholecystectomy or hysterectomy. For minor surgeries, hydrocortisone dosages above 30 to 50 mg during the first 24-hour-period is likely to be excessive, unless the patient is already on higher doses of glucocorticoids.

If supplementing with a lower dose of hydrocortisone, the physician should have a low threshold for giving further hydrocortisone with any evidence of adrenal insufficiency, such as hypotension. The aforementioned stress-steroid regimens should be decreased by 25% per day if no postoperative problems occur. Thus, the perioperative physician must use his or her own judgment in using stress steroids, taking into account the degree of stress of the surgery and the risk that higher doses of corticosteroids will aggravate such conditions as diabetes mellitus, hypertension, or inhibit wound healing.

Acute Adrenal Crisis

In the perioperative period, patients with undiagnosed, but suspected, acute adrenal crisis should receive dexamethasone 4 mg IV plus large amounts of normal saline, followed by an ACTH stimulation test. Dexamethasone does not interfere initially with the testing of the pituitary adrenal axis or the measurement of plasma cortisol levels. Furthermore, the lack of mineralocorticoid activity for dexamethasone is not a problem as long as large amounts of normal saline are given. Once adrenal insufficiency is diagnosed, a maximum of 200 mg/day of hydrocortisone should be given in the immediate postoperative period.

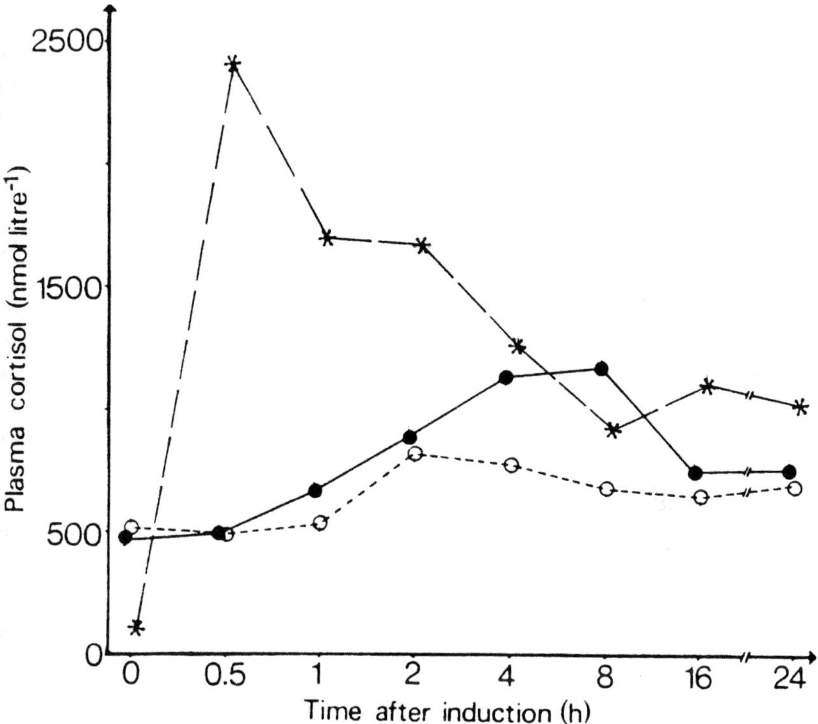

Figure 16-4

Plasma cortisol response to the stress of anaesthesia and surgery. Mean ± SEM. •—•, controls; ∘—∘, patients receiving long-term corticosteroid treatment with normal response to the corticotropin stimulation test (no substitution during surgery); *—*, patients receiving long-term corticosteroids with a subnormal response to the corticotropin test (given low-dose cortisol substitution). (Used with permission from Symreng T, et al: Physiological contisol substitution of long-term steroid-treated patients undergoing major surgery, *Br J Anaesth* 53:949–953, 1981.)

• PARATHYROID DISORDERS

Parathyroid hormone (PTH) interacts directly on bone and kidney and indirectly on the intestine to maintain normal ionized calcium. Low levels of ionized calcium cause an increase in PTH secretion from the parathyroid gland. In bone, PTH acts on the osteoblasts directly, which releases cytokines that activate osteoclasts, thereby releasing calcium from bone. In the kidney, PTH increases renal tubular absorption of calcium. In the intestine, PTH acts indirectly by increasing synthesis of 1,25 $(OH)_2$ D and, hence, calcium absorption in the intestine. Besides calcium, magnesium and phosphorus affect PTH secretion. Chronic hypomagnesemia inhibits release of PTH. Hypophosphatemia increases sensitivity of PTH to bone and increases calcium absorption in the intestine.

Primary Hyperparathyroidism

In primary hyperparathyroidism, there is a loss of normal negative feedback from elevated ionized calcium levels on PTH secretion. The set-point in decreasing PTH production is reset at a higher calcium level before decreasing PTH production. Occasionally, there is complete loss of negative feedback of calcium on the parathyroid gland, leading to acute primary hyperparathyroidism and significant elevations of calcium above 15 mg/dl.

Eighty percent of primary hyperparathyroidism occurs from a single parathyroid adenoma, about 20% from diffuse hyperplasia of the parathyroid gland, and less than 1% from a parathyroid carcinoma. Patients with diffuse parathyroid hyperplasia have a high association with the multiple endocrine neoplasia types I and IIA. Primary hyperparathyroidism is diagnosed by inappropriate elevated levels of PTH with hypercalcemia. Serum calcium can be normal with actual elevated ionized calcium caused by low serum proteins. Serum calcium will decrease 0.8 mg/dl for every 1 g/dl decrease of albumin. Hence, ionized calcium is a more accurate measurement of calcium.

In primary hyperparathyroidism, the main target organs affected are kidney, bone, and muscle. Nephrolithiasis occurs in 20% of patients with primary hyperparathyroidism. Nephrocalcinosis (diffuse renal calcification) with a decrease in creatinine clearance can occur. Also, damage to the collecting tubules from high levels of urinary calcium can lead to an inability to concentrate urine and a clinical picture compatible with nephrogenic diabetes insipidus.

Bone involvement from elevated levels of PTH can lead to subperiosteal bone reabsorption in a process known as osteitis fibrosa cystica. Also, diffuse osteopenia with osteoporosis can occur and lead to pathologic bone fractures. Proximal muscle weakness is commonly seen in primary hyperparathyroidism and is caused by diffuse atrophy of mainly type II muscle fibers. Other clinical manifestations associated with primary hyperparathyroidism are peptic ulcer disease, acute pancreatitis, nausea and vomiting, hypertension, central nervous system (CNS) depression with lethargy, confusion, and psychomotor impairment.

Indications for parathyroidectomy surgery include any symptomatic patient. In asymptomatic patients, serum calcium above 12 mg/dl, significant hypercalciuria, reduced cortical bone density, decreased creatinine clearance without other causes and an age below 50 years are indications for parathyroidectomy. Occasionally, patients can present with acute primary hyperparathyroid crisis with significant elevations in calcium above 15 mg/dl. These patients require immediate surgery and aggressive medical management before surgery. Also, parathyroidectomy can be done for renal osteodystrophy in renal failure. Chronic elevations of phosphorous seen in renal failure can lead to continued hypocalcemia from calcium binding, to elevated phosphate levels. This, along with decreased vitamin D metabolism, can lead to secondary hyperparathyroidism and increased bone reabsorption. Hence, a parathyroidectomy is often done to prevent further renal osteodystrophy.

Medical Management

In the preoperative period, the perioperative physician should make every attempt to decrease serum calcium to below 13 mg/dl. The mainstay of treatment is to restore intravascular volume and increase urinary calcium excretion. Often, these patients are hypovolemic from vomiting and polyuria. Hence, large amounts of normal saline should be given, followed by furosemide once adequate urine output is established. Thiazide diuretics should be avoided secondary to causing increased calcium reabsorption in the distal tubules. Oral phosphates 1 to 2 gms daily can be given to decrease serum calcium. Phosphates inhibit calcium absorption in the gastrointestinal tract, decrease mobilization of calcium from bone, and decrease 1,25 $(OH)_2$ D production. However, in general, phosphates should be given only to patients with serum phosphate levels below 3.0 mg/dl and normal renal function. The product of $Ca^{2+} \times PO_4^{3-}$ of over 40 risks diffuse ectopic calcifications of soft tissues.

Other agents used to treat hypercalcemia are often not effective in primary hyperparathyroidism. The use of glucocorticoids and biphosphonates, such as etidronate and clodrinate, are likely to have minimal effect in primary hyperparathyroidism. New third-generation biphosphonates currently being studied may have short-term effectiveness in lowering serum calcium. Calcitonin, an inhibitor of osteoclastic function, has variable efficacy in treating primary hyperparathyroidism. Nevertheless, because of calcitonin's minimal side effects and rapid onset within 2 to 4 hours, a subcutaneous dose of 4 µg/kg every 12 hours may be beneficial in the preoperative period for serum calcium over 13 mg/dl. Mithramycin (plicamycin) in an IV dose of 25 µg/kg is effective in decreasing serum calcium within 24 to 36 hours by inhibition of osteoclastic bone reabsorption. Mithramycin should be reserved for refractory hypercalcemia because of its renal, bone marrow, and liver toxicity; it should be given under the direction of an endocrinologist or oncologist. Finally, dialysis can be used in life-threatening refractory hypercalcemia.

Perioperative Management

If serum calcium is less than 13 mg/dl and the patient is asymptomatic, the perioperative physician need not delay surgery. Adequate intravascular repletion should be done before the start of surgery. The ECG should be monitored for a shortened PR and QTc interval. The QTc is calculated by dividing the QT interval by the square root of the RR interval. Changes in the QTc interval can be used as a marker for changes in the active ionized calcium levels in the immediate perioperative period. Prolongation of the QTc is a marker of hypocalcemia and indicates the need for postoperative calcium supplementation. In patients with evidence of CNS depression, intravenous anesthetic drugs should be carefully titrated to prevent excessive sedation postoperatively. Muscle relaxants should be titrated with neuromuscular monitoring because of potentially underlying muscle weakness.

In the immediate postoperative period after a parathyroidectomy, compromise of the airway secondary to a hematoma, edema, and recurrent laryngeal injury is of most concern. Severe hypocalcemia usually does not occur within the first 24 hours after a parathyroidectomy. However, in cases of advanced bone disease or in cases of prior residual treatment with such agents as mithramycin, acute hypocalcemia can occur within hours, leading to muscle weakness, tetany, and laryngospasm. Rapid redistribution of calcium and magnesium into bones ("hungry bones") can occur, leading to rapid drops of serum calcium, magnesium, and phosphorus. Hence, starting in the recovery room, serial magnesium, calcium, and phosphate levels should be monitored. Calcium levels generally reach nadir at 3 to 5 days postoperatively. They then slowly normalize as the remaining parathyroid tissue recovers from prolonged suppression, resulting from the overactive parathyroid adenoma and the trauma of surgery. Also, low magnesium levels will lead to continued suppression of PTH production from the remaining parathyroid tissue. Hence, besides calcium replacement, magnesium must also be replaced for hypomagnesemia to establish normal parathyroid homeostasis.

BIBLIOGRAPHY

Alberti KGMM, Thomas DJB: The management of diabetes during surgery, *Br J Anaesth* 51:693–710, 1979.

Becker C: Hypothyroidism and atherosclerotic heart disease: pathogenesis, medical management, and the role of coronary artery bypass surgery, *Endocr Rev* 6:432–440, 1985.

Burgos LG, et al: Increased intraoperative cardiovascular morbidity in diabetics with autonomic neuropathy, *Anesthesiology* 70:591–597, 1989.

Charlson ME, MacKenzie RC, Gold JP: Preoperative autonomic function abnormalities in patients with diabetes mellitus and patients with hypertension, *J Am Coll Surg* 179:1–10, 1994.

Chernow B, et al: Hormonal responses to graded surgical stress, *Arch Intern Med* 147:1273–1278, 1987.

Christiansen CL, et al: Insulin treatment of the insulin-dependent diabetic patient undergoing minor surgery: continuous intravenous infusion compared with subcutaneous administration, *Anaesthesia* 43:533–537, 1988.

Compkin TV: Radial artery cannulation potential hazard in patients with acromegaly, *Anaesthesia* 35:1008–9, 1980.

Drucker DJ, Burrow GN: Cardiovascular surgery in the hypothyroid patient, *Arch Intern Med* 145:1585–1587, 1985.

Ewing DJ, Campbell IW, Clarke BF: Mortality in diabetic autonomic neuropathy, *Lancet* 1:14–16, 1976.

Fein FS, Sonnenblick EH: Diabetic cardiomyopathy, *Prog Cardiovasc Dis* 27:255–270, 1985.

Henriques HF III, Lebovic D: Defining and focusing perioperative steroid supplementation, *Am Surg* 61:809–813, 1995.

Hensel P, Roizen MF: Patients with disorders of parathyroid function, *Anesthesiol Clin N Am* 5:287–297, 1987.

Hirsch IB, et al: Perioperative management of surgical patients with diabetes mellitus, *Anesthesiology* 74:346–359, 1991.

Hogan K, Rusy D, Springman SR: Difficult laryngoscopy and diabetes mellitus, *Anesth Analg* 67:1162–1165, 1988.

Kehlet H: A national approach to dosage and preparation of parenteral glucocorticoid substitution therapy during surgical procedures, *Acta Anaesthesiol Scand* 19:260–264, 1975.

Kehlet H, Binder C: Adrenocortical function and clinical course during and after surgery in unsupplemented glucocorticoid-treated patients, *Br J Anaesth* 45:1043–1048, 1973.

Kehlet H, Binder C: Value of an ACTH test in assessing hypothalamic-pituitary-adrenocortical function in glucocorticoid treated patients, *Br Med J* 2:147–149, 1973.

Knudsen L, Christiansen A, Lorentzen JE: Hypotension during and after operation in glucocorticoid-treated patients, *Br J Anaesth* 53:295–300, 1981.

Ladenson PW, et al: Complications of surgery in hypothyroid patients, *Am J Med* 77:261–266, 1984.

Murkin JM: Anesthesia and hypothyroidism: a review of thyroxine physiology, pharmacology, and anesthetic implications, *Anesth Analg* 61:371–383, 1982.

Page MM, Watkins PJ: Cardiorespiratory arrest and diabetic autonomic neuropathy, *Lancet* 1:14–16, 1978.

Patten BA,et al: The neuromuscular disease of hyperparathyroidism, *Ann Intern Med* 80:182–193, 1974.

Reissell E, et al: Predictability of difficult laryngoscopy in patients with long-term diabetes mellitus, *Anaesthesia* 45:1024–1027, 1990.

Roizen MF: Perioperative management of the diabetic patient. American Society of Anesthesiologists Refresher Course, 412:1–7, 1995.

Salzarulo HH, Taylor LA: Diabetic "stiff joint syndrome" as a cause of difficult endotracheal intubation, *Anesthesiology* 64:366–368, 1985.

Sandberg N: Time relationship between administration of cortisone and wound healing in rats, *Acta Chir Scand* 127:446–455, 1964.

Sane T, et al: Hyponatremia after transsphenoidal surgery for pituitary tumors, *J Clin Endocrinol Metab* 79:1395–1398, 1994.

Silverberg SJ, Fitzpatrick LA, Bilezikian JP: Primary hyperparathyroidism. In Becker KL, editor: *Principles and practice of endocrinology and metabolism*, Philadelphia, 1995, JB Lippincott, pp 512–520.

Silverberg SJ, et al: Nephrolithiasis and bone involvement in primary hyperparathyroidism, *Am J Med* 89:327–334, 1990.

Symreng T, et al: Physiological cortisol substitution of long-term steroid-treated patients undergoing major surgery, *Br J Anaesth* 53:949–953, 1981.

Thomas AN, Pollard BJ: Renal transplantation and diabetic autonomic neuropathy, *Can J Anaesth* 36:590–592, 1989.

Thorner MO, et al: Anterior pituitary. In Wilson JD, Foster DW, editors: *William's textbook of endocrinology*, 8 ed, Philadelphia, 1992, WB Saunders.

Udelsman R, et al: Adaptation during surgical stress: a re-evaluation of the role of glucocorticoids, *J Clin Invest* 77:1377–1381, 1986.

Wartofsky L: Myxedema coma. In Braverman LE, Vtiger RD, editors: *The thyroid. A fundamental and clinical text*, ed 6, Philadelphia, JB Lippincott Co.

Weinberg AD, et al: Outcome of anesthesia and surgery in hypothyroid patients, *Arch Intern Med* 143:893–897, 1983.

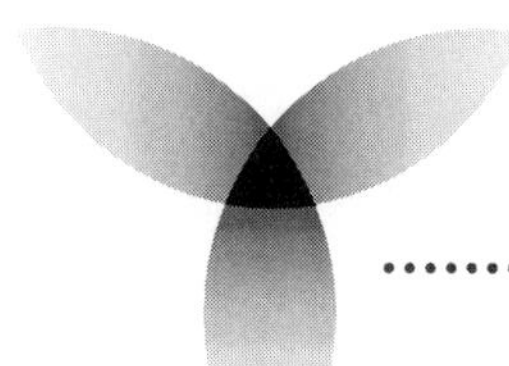

Chapter 17

Uncommon Endocrine Disorders

David L. Bogdonoff, MD, Mary Lee Vance, MD

Two endocrine disorders deserve special mention. Carcinoid syndrome and pheochromocytoma are uncommon conditions that have serious perioperative implications. They require meticulous care before and after surgery, and both are capable of causing an intraoperative catastrophic event. Few practitioners have much experience in managing these conditions. Thus, they will be reviewed separately.

• CARCINOID SYNDROME

Carcinoid syndrome is an uncommon disorder associated with a carcinoid tumor. The syndrome occurs in less than 10% of patients with a carcinoid tumor because these tumors may not be hormonally active enough to cause systemic symptoms. While occasionally resulting from a large solitary tumor, carcinoid syndrome is usually associated with metastatic disease.

Carcinoid tumors originate from primitive stem cells, which differentiate into a variety of neuroendocrine cells throughout the body. Most are derived from enterochromaffin and argentaffin cells within the digestive tract. These neuroendocrine cells are capable of secreting a vast array of peptides and biogenic amines as well as hormones and neurotransmitters. Interestingly, the secretory activity may change over time and metastatic lesions may produce different substances than the parent tumor.

Carcinoid tumors arise from three sites in the body: the foregut, which includes the lungs, the stomach, and first portion of the duodenum; the midgut, from the second half of the duodenum to the right colon; and the hindgut, including the remainder of the colon and rectum. Most tumors are highly differentiated, but, occasionally, they are less well differentiated and can be confused with other carcinomas of the gastrointestinal (GI) tract or with a small cell tumor in the lungs. Various biologic markers aid in identification of these tumors. Nonspecific markers involve heavy metal salt staining, such as silver staining of secretory granules with the argentaffin reaction. Specific markers are available allowing the direct staining of serotonin or other biologic products utilizing radiolabelled or enzyme-linked antibodies in immunocytochemical reactions.

Ninety-five percent of carcinoids arise in the appendix, small bowel, and rectum. Tumors less than 1 cm in diameter rarely metastasize while those larger than 2 cm do so more commonly. Small bowel tumors are more prone to grow larger than 2 cm in size, while appendiceal carcinoids produce obstructive symptoms before they reach that size. Bronchial carcinoids are also likely to become symptomatic and be removed before they reach metastatic-potential size. Hindgut-derived carcinoids are less likely to produce the carcinoid syndrome because these tumors are slow-growing, and metastases are usually necessary for the carcinoid syndrome to be present.

Clinical features of carcinoid syndrome include flushing, sweating, wheezing, diarrhea, and abdominal pain, in addition to blood pressure changes. Patients with carcinoid syndrome may have a myriad of symptoms and often do not manifest the classically described syndrome. It is unclear which substances cause the various symptoms. In addition to serotonin and its precursor 5-HTP, several tachykinins have been implicated. Neuropeptide Y, neurokinin A and substance P are all derived from the common precursor β-preprotachykinin. Other substances such as prostaglandins, dopamine, kallikrein, and histamine have also been suggested as contributory substances.

Flushing is the most common symptom and occurs in over 80% of patients. There are two types of flushing, and they are related to the location of the original carcinoid tumor. Flushing from a foregut tumor is more intense, may last for hours, and is purplish in color. It involves the upper body and acrocyanosis may occur. Flushing may lead to telangectasia and facial skin thickening. Flushing from a midgut tumor, in contrast, is characterized by a light pink or red color, is ephemeral, and does not produce any long-standing skin changes. This flushing involves the face and upper body down to the nipple line and may be provoked by ingestion of alcohol or tyramine-containing foods, or by stress, physical exertion, or an emotional event. It is not unusual for it to occur sporadically without an instigating event.

Abdominal pain and diarrhea occur in approximately 70% of patients. The diarrhea is secretory and does not resolve with fasting. Bronchospasm and dyspnea occur in one third of patients. All other symptoms have an incidence of less than 10%. Myopathy, arthropathy, and pellagra like dermatitis can also be associated with the syndrome. Cardiac involvement historically was also present in one half of patients, although it is probably less common now because diagnosis and intervention occur earlier in the course of disease. Endomyocardial fibrosis of the right side of the heart is classically described with pulmonary stenosis and tricuspid regurgitation occurring together, rather than single valve involvement. Breathlessness and peripheral edema are symptoms of significant cardiac involvement.

Another uncommon and potentially confusing factor is the production of other ectopic hormones. Foregut carcinoids may produce insulin, calcitonin, corticotropin (ACTH), vasopressin, glucagon, secretin, gastrin, growth hormone releasing hormone (GHRH) and other biogenic amines. These multiple hormones contribute to the already confusing situation of the varying clinical presentations.

Foregut carcinoids produce 5-hydroxytryptophan (5-HTP). This is formed in the initial rate-limiting step of serotonin synthesis by a transformation of tryptophan. This is the active product for these foregut carcinoids because they are often deficient in dopa-decarboxylase. Dopa-decarboxylase is present in midgut carcinoids and converts 5-HTP to serotonin (5-HT). Circulating serotonin is converted to 5-hydroxyindoleacetic acid (5-HIAA) by monoamine oxidase (MAO) which is abundant in the kidney. The lack of conversion of 5-HTP in the foregut can lead to a missed diagnosis if the only test performed is the commonly ordered 24-hour-urine screen for 5-HIAA. Thus, measurement of 5-HTP is necessary to exclude a foregut carcinoid.

Screening tests are required if there is a suspicion of disease. Additionally, patients with unexplained, intermittent abdominal pain or irritable bowel may require evaluation because many of these symptoms were present in patients later found to suffer from carcinoid syndrome. Screening involves a search for the aforementioned biochemical products of the carcinoid tumors. A 24-hour-urine measurement of 5-HIAA is the typical screening test. Even so, a number of cases will be missed. Variability is common and, thus, an experienced endocrinologist should be consulted for subtle or unusual cases. Such consultations may involve the use of various provocative tests.

Preoperative Preparation

Most patients with the carcinoid syndrome seen in the perioperative period already carry a biochemical and/or tissue diagnosis of carcinoid and have elements of the various, described clinical syndromes. Surgery remains the best therapeutic option for isolated disease and may be considered for metastatic disease at times. While rarely presenting for a curative resection, it is not uncommon for patients with advanced carcinoid disease to require either a palliative or therapeutic surgical procedure. These patients need to be adequately prepared for surgery.

To some extent, preparation requires an attempt to understand the symptom complex. While some various symptoms are attributed to a predominance of 5-HT in contrast to histamine or the kinins, this determination is likely too simplistic. However, it is important to know if a patient becomes hypertensive or hypotensive when symptomatic. This knowledge may help prepare for identification and treatment of any such perioperative episodes. Known symptomatology is, unfortunately, only partially helpful, because intraoperative events may occur which were not predicted from preoperative observations. For example, only one half of patients suffering intraoperative bronchospasm had any such prior events.

Medical management of carcinoid syndrome involves using antagonist drugs to block the peripheral effects of mediators and, more recently, octreotide or somatostatin to inhibit hormone release. Ketanserin has some effect on the peripheral blockade of serotonin receptors, specifically 5-HT-type 2 receptors. Ketanserin may attenuate some of the systemic effects of the release of a large amount of this hormone. Cyproheptadine has similar blocking effects and may alleviate diarrheal symptoms, along with motility-decreasing drugs like codeine and loperamide. Ondansetron has 5-HT-type 3 receptor-blocking effects and is useful for accompanying symptoms of nausea or vomiting. H1 and H2 blockers can similarly be used to block any potential histamine effects. Steroids have been suggested as adjuncts, although the mechanisms subserving a beneficial effect are speculative. These measures are less than effective because they do nothing to block the instigating mediator release. Recently, the long-acting analog of somatostatin, octreotide, has been shown to be the most effective agent for treatment and for preoperative preparation of the carcinoid syndrome patient.

Somatostatin inhibits the secretion of a number of peptides and is effective in many of these patients. It also antagonizes peripheral effects of the mediators, as well. There is usually a significant diminution in symptomatology with octreotide therapy in patients who respond. Tumor regression and prolongation of life have been reported with octreotide. Various degrees of responsiveness to octreotide is likely related to the number of and type of somatostatin receptors on the tumor. Octreotide is the first-line drug for use in a life-threatening episode of carcinoid crisis and should be kept in the operating room if the patient is suspected of or known to have a carcinoid tumor.

Other nonspecific measures should be taken. They include optimal preoperative hydration and a thorough evaluation of cardiovascular function. Right-sided heart disease must be ruled out and may be done so most easily with noninvasive echocardiography.

Our protocol for preoperative and intraoperative administration of octreotide is shown in Box 17-1. The ideal situation is to operate on a patient who has been treated for several weeks with octreotide and has documented 24-hour urinary 5-HIAA levels in the normal range.

Intraoperative Management

The greatest problem is an intraoperative catastrophe from carcinoid crisis. There are numerous reports of bronchospasm, hypotension, hypertension, and irreversible cardiovascular collapse. These have been associated with the induction of anesthesia but may also be precipitated by preparation of the abdomen or manipulation of the tumor. Recommendations for treatment have been made, although no prospective studies of large numbers of carcinoid-syndrome patients have been performed, and most information is anecdotal or based on small series of patients. It is likely, however, that better drug therapy and patient preparation have actually reduced the mortality and morbidity of these patients in the perioperative period.

Bronchospasm is a potentially troublesome complication. As mentioned, it may be anticipated based on prior patient symptoms. However, just as many events occur in patients without any previous symptoms. Obvious initiators of bronchospasm should be avoided whenever possible; these are predominantly mechanical in the intraoperative period. Propofol is the best induction agent if a patient is at risk for airway reactivity. Avoidance of intubation with the use of face or layrngeal mask

Box 17-1 Preoperative Prophylaxis in Carcinoid Patients

I. Treatment goal is prevention of carcinoid crisis, which may develop on induction or intraoperatively.

II. Ideal situation is extended *preoperative* treatment with octreotide to produce a normal urinary 5-HIAA level.

III. Recommended dose schedule:
   a. 250 μg subcutaneously q8h for 2 to 3 days
   b. 250 μg subcutaneously within 1 to 2 hours preop
   c. 500 μg in OR for IV bolus use, (5000 μg multidose vial in OR for repeated doses as needed)

ventilation is possible for minor procedures. This is impractical for intraabdominal surgery. Careful endotracheal tube placement will avoid unnecessary stimulation of the dense bed of mechanoreceptors near the carinal bifurcation. Anesthetic and analgesic drugs with a propensity to release histamine (morphine, curare, atracurium) are easily avoided, although there is no certainty these drugs are problematic.

Treatment of bronchospasm with the use of adrenergic drugs is controversial. Intravenous use should be avoided because these drugs have been implicated in the release of additional mediator substances. Perhaps inhaled β2 agonists would be less likely to release the substances, but there is no evidence to support or refute this notion. Steroids may be effective but require time to be effective. They are best used prophylactically when there is suspicion of carcinoid. Inhaled anesthetic agents are effective because of their smooth-muscle relaxant effects. Anticholinergic drugs, such as atropine or glycopyrrolate, should also be given prophylactically in case of any contributory muscarinic cholinergic effects.

Hypotension is another potential grave intraoperative event. Hypovolemia, secondary to secretory diarrhea or other causes of dehydration, is easily treated with adequate hydration preoperatively. Invasive monitors should help in this diagnosis. Regardless of the cause, adequate volume repletion is essential in patient management. As with bronchospasm, the use of adrenergic agonists is contraindicated because of their propensity to lead to additional mediator release. A decrease in the level of any inhalational anesthetic may be helpful.

Hypertension is another potential intraoperative problem. It may be associated with bronchospasm and is likely related to serotonin release. Vasodilating drugs can be used without concern for aggravation of mediator release and nitroglycerin or nitroprusside are good choices. Ketanserin has been reported as useful.

Postoperative Care

Continued vigilance for symptoms of carcinoid crisis is necessary, particularly if successful surgical excision or debulking was not accomplished. At times, devascularization of hepatic metastases is a useful therapeutic modality and may be attempted intraoperatively. Necrosis of previously functioning carcinoid tissue is associated with a large release of mediator hormones and should be anticipated. Octreotide therapy should be continued until after complete recovery from surgery if a complete resection is achievable. After discontinuation, a 24-hour urine measurement of 5-HIAA (or 5-HT as indicated) should be performed to confirm complete removal of the tumor. Other patients must have octreotide continued because it is the only drug shown to increase longevity in patients with metastatic disease.

PHEOCHROMOCYTOMA

Pheochromocytoma is another uncommon disorder, which requires meticulous peri- and intraoperative attention to detail. It is a tumor that produces, stores, and releases catecholamines. If correctly diagnosed it is potentially curable; if left untreated, it can cause significant morbidity and mortality.

Pheochromocytomas are derived from chromaffin cells of neural crest origin. Ninety percent of these tumors develop in the adrenal glands. However, there are extra-adrenal locations of these chromaffin cells. Hence, tumors can also be found in the periaortic organ of Zuckerkandl, sympathetic ganglia, carotid body, and aortic chemoreceptors. Extraadrenal tumors occur more commonly in patients with familial disease, particularly associated with von Hippel–Lindau disease. While other names may be used for these extraadrenal tumors (e.g., paraganglionoma, glomus jugulare tumor), they must be treated like pheochromocytomas if they are hormonally active.

Pheochromocytomas are usually encapsulated solitary tumors. Ninety percent are benign, 90% are sporadic in contrast to familial, and 90% are in the adrenal gland. There is a slight predilection for solitary tumors to occur on the right side of the body. One half of familial tumors tend to be bilateral and/or extra-adrenal. Familial pheochromocytoma occurs in patients with multiple endocrine neoplasia (MEN II) and von Hippel–Lindau disease.

Pathologically, these tumors show the chromaffin reaction caused by the oxidation of epinephrine and norepinephrine by chromate staining, hence the derivation of the name. A variety of biochemical markers can be identified in pheochromocytomas, but there is a reduced likelihood of expression in malignant tumors. This means that there is still no effective test for determining which tumors are malignant, short of obvious evidence of clinical spread. A radionuclide scan using metaiodobenzyl guanidine (MIBG) is approximately 94% accurate in identifying a catecholamine-producing tumor and is useful in identifying metastatic disease.

Most of the signs and symptoms of pheochromocytoma are related to the activity of the released catecholamines. Occasionally, poorly differentiated and nonfunctional tumors will arise from the adrenal medulla and be classified as pheochromocytomas, pathologically and histologically. These tumors present as any other neoplastic disease (adrenal mass) and, if truly inactive, will require no special perioperative endocrinologic and pharmacologic attention. Proper care of the pheochromocytoma patient requires a thorough understanding of the sympathoadrenal system and catecholamine metabolism.

The sympathoadrenal system is part of the sympathetic nervous system that is responsible for the "fight or flight" responses of the body. Neural signals from multiple areas of the brain travel to synapses on cell bodies in the intermediolateral-cell columns of the spinal cord. Preganglionic axons leave the spinal cord and synapse in the sympathetic chain ganglia located in prevertebral and periaortic regions. From these ganglia, postganglionic fibers travel to effector organs. Preganglionic synaptic transmission is mediated by acetylcholine while postganglionic effector nerves utilize norepinephrine as their neurotransmitter. Some of the preganglionic axons terminate and innvervate the adrenal medulla where chromaffin cells function as the equivalent of the postganglionic fibers. These effector cells use epinephrine to achieve their systemic effects.

Catecholamines are synthesized from tyrosine only in neural tissues. Tyrosine is obtained from dietary intake or from the conversion of phenylalanine in the liver. Tyrosine hydroxylase synthesizes the conversion of tyrosine to dopa (dihydroxyphenylalanine), which is the rate-limiting step in synthesis. Dopa is decarboxylated to dopamine, which is then taken up into chromaffin granules. Within the granule, dopamine is converted into norepinephrine by β-hydroxylation. In most neural tissue, norepinephrine remains within the granule until the time of its release. In the adrenal medulla, however, norepinephrine returns to the cytosol and is converted to epinephrine by the action of phenylalanine-methyl transferase (PNMT). Epinephrine is then stored in granules for later release. Phenylalanine-methyl transferase is a nonspecific enzyme and is induced by high levels of glucocorticoids. The adrenal medulla is uniquely bathed by high levels of glucocorticoids by the surrounding adrenal cortex. Hence, this forms the basis for the adrenal medulla as the predominant source of epinephrine in the body. While norepinephrine is released from nerve endings and produces local effects, epinephrine is released into the circulation and acts systemically.

The predominant mechanism for termination of catecholamine effects is the reuptake of the catechol molecules into the presynaptic nerve terminals. Reuptake is followed by reincorporation into a vesicle or by oxidation by MAO and conversion to dihydroxyphenylglycol (DHPG). Catechols escaping from the synapse or those released into the circulation are catabolized by catechol-O-methyl transferase (COMT). Norepinephrine is converted to normetanephrine and epinephrine is transformed into metanephrine. Further action by MAO produces vanillylmandelic acid (VMA) and methoxyhydroxyphenylglycol (MHPG). The metanephrines and VMA are used, along with the catechols themselves, for diagnostic measurements as discussed further on.

Catecholamines exert their effects through stimulation of adrenergic receptors. An extensive discussion of these receptors is beyond the scope of this chapter. However, adrenergic receptors are subdivided into α1, α2, β1, and β2 categories. Knowledge of the actions of these receptors, as well as their agonists and blockers, is required for the practitioner caring for these patients in the perioperative setting.

The α1-adrenergic receptors are postsynaptic and located on effector tissues, such as vascular smooth muscle, where they mediate vasoconstriction. They also mediate pupillary dilation, intestinal relaxation, and uterine contraction. Phenylephrine is the classical α1 agonist, and prazosin, a specific receptor blocker. Activation of this receptor leads to increases in cytosolic calcium concentrations mediated by phosphoinositols.

The α2 receptors also cause vasoconstriction through their postsynaptic effects. Complicating the picture, however, is the fact that α2 receptors are mostly found in presynaptic locations in the central nervous system where they actually function to decrease the output of the sympathetic nervous system. Therefore, classical α2 agonists like clonidine, methyldopa, and guanethidine actually reduce blood pressure through their central effects.

β1-adrenergic receptors have diverse effects depending on the target tissue. In the heart they exert positive inotropic and chronotropic effects. They cause lipolysis in adipose tissue and renin release by the kidney. Dobutamine is the classical β1 agonist, while atenolol and metoprolol are specific antagonists. All β adrenergic effects are mediated by an activation of adenyl cyclase and an increase in cyclic AMP.

β2-adrenergic receptors also have diverse functions. They cause bronchodilation in the lungs and vasodilation in skeletal and intestinal smooth muscle. They also cause glycogenolysis in the liver. β2 agonists include metaproterenol, albuterol, terbutaline, and isoetharine. Epinephrine is more stimulatory of the β2 receptor than is norepinephrine. β2 receptors are blocked by propranolol, nadolol, and timolol, though all of these are nonspecific in their blockade and affect β1 receptors as well.

Patients with pheochromocytoma have varied clinical presentations. These tumors are responsible for hypertension in only 0.1% of all patients with hypertension. Pheochromocytoma may be totally asymptomatic or may cause a hypertensive crisis, myocardial infarction, stroke, or death. The latter symptoms are characteristic of a tumor which produces a predominance of norepinephrine. Intermittent or sustained hypertension is found in most pheochromocytoma patients, with an equal likelihood of each. Classically, paroxysms of hypertension are characterized by sudden onset of headache, sweating, palpitations, skin pallor, feelings of impending doom, nausea with or without vomiting, and abdominal and/or chest pain. The combination of headache, sweating, and palpitations occurring with hypertension is highly suggestive for pheochromocytoma and requires evaluation. Furthermore, a tumor that produces predominantly epinephrine does not cause hypertension. Rather, epinephrine-producing tumors cause hypotension and the patient may present with near syncope or orthostatic symptoms.

Postural hypotension is frequently found but may be asymptomatic. It is more common with epinephrine-secreting tumors. Some patients are volume-depleted with a decrease in circulating blood volume. Hyperglycemia is not unusual and glucose can be elevated during a hypertensive crisis; it results from both excess glucose production and inhibition of insulin release by catecholamines. Constipation caused by an inhibition of intestinal activity is also observed. Congestive heart failure, because of downregulation of adrenoreceptors and cardiomyopathy, is a rare but dangerous presenting symptom.

Diagnosis for pheochromocytoma can be problematic and requires a high index of suspicion. There is a long list of alternatives to consider for patients with any of the signs and symptoms. Clearly, the occurrence of other components of a multiple endocrine neoplasia syndrome or a family member with a pheochromocytoma suggests this diagnosis. The following features have been suggested as findings which must lead to a search for pheochromocytoma:

1. Triad of headaches, sweating, and tachycardia.
2. Family history of pheochromocytoma.
3. Accompanying features of multiple endocrine neoplasia type II (medullary carcinoma of the thyroid, hyperparathyroidism, and pheochromocytoma).
4. An incidentally discovered adrenal mass.
5. Hypertension with slightly elevated catecholamine levels.
6. Hypertension poorly responsive to treatment.
7. A history of severe hypertension, tachycardia and/or arrhythmia in response to anesthesia, surgery, or medications known to precipitate pheochromocytoma symptomatology (i.e., sympathomimetic drugs).

Diagnostic evaluation is straightforward if the appropriate studies are obtained. The first test is a 24-hour urine measurement of norepinephrine, epinephrine, metanephrines, and VMA, collected preferably when the patient is hypertensive. Interfering medications must be discontinued before the urine collection. Some patients have only a mild elevation in one or more of the urine tests. Measurement of only one hormone or metabolite (e.g., VMA) is ill-advised. Some tumors have a relatively poor degredative mechanism. Thus, the VMA or metanephrines and normetanephrines may be normal in the setting of significantly elevated catecholamine levels (norepinephrine, epinephrine). Conversely, some tumors are extremely efficient in degrading catecholamines—the norepinephrine and epinephrine levels will be normal with high VMA, metanephrine, and normetanephrine levels. Plasma assays for catecholamines and, possibly, metanephrines are also useful but can be erroneous unless the sample is collected properly. The collection is done through an indwelling venous cannula that has been in place for 30 minutes, with the patient at rest. Additionally, serum measurements are only able to assess physiologic events from a particular moment in time. Timed urine samples, on the other hand, are able to assess the effects of numerous events integrated over several hours.

Suppression tests may be invoked. Clonidine is the most commonly used agent. Plasma catechol levels before and 3 hours after a dose are compared. While patients with essential hypertension have a drop in plasma norepinephrine and epinephrine levels, those with pheochromocytoma will have unchanged or increased levels. Provocative tests have also been used but have become less common because of the danger of precipitating a hypertensive crisis.

Following the biochemical diagnosis of pheochromocytoma, efforts must be made to localize the tumor to enable subsequent definitive surgical treatment. The magnetic resonance imaging (MRI) scan may reveal the characteristic high signal ("light bulb") on T2-weighted images. The MIBG scan is a nuclear procedure which localizes a pheochromocytoma in approximately 94% of patients. A positive scan depends on the ability of the tumor to take up the radiolabeled catechol-like molecule.

Unfortunately the diagnosis of pheochromocytoma is still often missed. Older autopsy studies suggest that the majority of pheochromocytomas are found after death and that this is even more likely in elderly patients. While psychological stress is an unlikely precipitating event, physical stress, trauma, or any other stressor leading to a sympathetic nervous system response are common instigating factors.

Hence, the induction of anesthesia, palpation of the abdomen, or a surgical incision is likely to bring about a hypertensive reaction. Undiagnosed patients are the ones who are likely to die in the operating room. Pheochromocytomas are much less dangerous when one is aware of their existence. In fact, large surgical series of such cases have been recently reported with rare or no mortality. It is imperative that every patient who has an adrenal mass be evaluated for a pheochromocytoma before surgery is performed.

Preoperative Preparation

The mainstay of preparation for surgery is pharmacologic therapy with α- and sometimes β-blockers, and/or metyrosine to block catecholamine synthesis. Other drugs, and even protocols without the use of drugs, have been proposed. Most importantly, if surgery is elective, no patient should undergo an operation until he or she is prepared adequately; the surgical schedule is not inviolate. The management of the patient with pheochromocytoma is best handled by an approach coordinating the efforts of various involved services. Symptom reduction and correction of underlying abnormalities may be achieved but demand meticulous patient monitoring during the preoperative preparatory phase. Unfortunately, there are no controlled studies of preoperative and intraoperative management, making conclusions difficult.

The greatest experience and probably the most conservative approach is with the preoperative use of α-blocking drug, most commonly phenoxybenzamine. Mortality has definitely decreased since the introduction of these drugs, leading some to attribute the improved clinical outcomes purely to adequate preoperative pharmacologic preparation. Whether this is true, or simply the result of parallel improvements in physiologic monitoring and intraoperative anesthetic care, is unclear.

Phenoxybenzamine is a long-acting, nonspecific α-blocking drug. The beginning dose is to 20 mg orally, usually twice a day. It is gradually increased as tolerated and as guided by diminution of symptoms and decrease in blood pressure. Indicators of effectiveness include the elimination of sweating and headache symptoms, and the reduction of blood pressure, preferably to normal. Complaints of nasal stuffiness are not uncommon. Orthostatic hypotension of a moderate degree is to be expected and tolerated. Development of tachycardia is an indication to add a β-blocker. Additionally, one may see a drop in fasting blood sugar from the blockade of the inhibitory effects of catecholamines on insulin secretion. The final dose of medication(s) is titrated to the blood pressure (supine and standing) and heart rate. A β-blocker is *never* started before adequate α-blockade is established if the tumor produces norepinephrine predominantly (the most common situation). Treatment with a β-blocker before α-blockade often precipitates a hypertensive crisis. The only exception to this is the patient with the rare pure epinephrine-producing tumor; in this situation, the treatment of choice is a β-blocker and metyrosine (to block catechol synthesis).

The duration of α-blockade has also been the subject of debate. Some authors have suggested a minimum of 10 to 14 days, while others have suggested longer preoperative treatment. While there have been suggestions of eliminating α-blockade because of an apparent lack of effect on mortality, others have shown additional beneficial effects. Higher than usual doses of phenoxybenzamine resulted in fewer hemodynamic side effects in a recent small controlled study. An increase in intraoperative tissue oxygen delivery was shown when phenoxybenzamine was given and served a protective role against the adverse effects of intraoperative catechol excesses.

Prazosin is a selective α-1-blocking drug which has also been used for preoperative preparation. Its advantages over phenoxybenzamine are theoretical because of selective α-1-blockade, and probably depend on the experience of the clinician following the patient. Initial severe postural hypotension is not uncommon and the initial dose should be low (e.g., 0.5–1 mg) and administered at bedtime. The final dose ranges from 2 to 5 mg, 2 or 3 times daily. Other comparable selective α-1 blockers are now available and include doxazosin and terazosin.

Beta blockade should *only* be instituted *after* α-blockade is established. Tachydysrhythmias or symptomatic tachycardia are the only indications for these drugs and, in fact, most patients may be prepared for surgery without a β-blocker. Beta blockers will inhibit β-2-mediated vasodilation from epinephrine, leading to even more intense vasoconstriction from unopposed α-stimulation. Reports of heart failure and hypertensive crisis caused by unopposed α-adrenergic stimulation, have followed the institution of β-blockade without prior α-blockade.

Perhaps the most elegant method of preoperative preparation involves the use of metyrosine along with α-blockade. This drug blocks the enzyme tyrosine hydroxylase, which is the rate-limiting step in catechol synthesis. Metyrosine lowers catechol levels in the pheochromocytoma itself, in other sympathetic nerve terminals, and, thus, in the urine. Sympathetic neurons may also have higher than normal levels in the untreated state from an increased reuptake of catechols, secondary to the excesses in circulating levels. The initial dosage is 250 mg 2 or 3 times a day. Dosages are increased by 250 to 500 mg every few days, as indicated by urinary catecholamine and VMA levels. The maximum dose is 1.5 to 4 grams per day. Treatment success is apparent by a reduction in circulating catechol levels and decreased urinary excretion of catecholamines and metabolites. Central nervous system actions of the drug result in a diminution of brain catechols with resultant sedation, depression, and nightmares that limit further dose increases. Prolonged use of metyrosine may deplete the myocardium of needed catecholamines and cause heart failure from drug-induced cardiomyopathy. Thus, once adequate lowering of urinary catecholamines and metabolites is accomplished, surgery should be performed without delay.

Preoperative evaluation must include an assessment of cardiovascular function to rule out catecholamine-induced cardiomyopathy. It is diagnosed by history and physical examination, ECG, and echocardiography. Cardiac function and ECG changes may improve over time with α-blockade or some other form of afterload reduction. It is likely that when cardiomyopathy is present, a longer duration of preoperative pharmacologic preparation may prove to be useful.

While classical treatment and most texts insist upon preoperative α-blockade with or without metyrosine and β-blockers, a fairly large collection of cases from one center suggests that this may not be necessary. Of 60 patients undergoing 63 operations, 26 did not receive preoperative α-blockade. Only one death was reported in the series and did not result from a hypertensive crisis; progression of intracranial mass lesions was responsible. This study suggests that knowledge of the existence of pheochromocytoma, combined with expectant pharmacologic therapy and modern invasive and noninvasive intraoperative monitoring, may preclude more meticulous pharmacologic preparations. The conservative approach is still likely to involve both excellent pre- and intraoperative management as the best therapeutic option.

Drug therapy continues up to the time of surgery. Because of their relatively long half-lives, phenoxybenzamine and metyrosine are given at midnight or early on the day of surgery in reduced doses. Heavy premedication with benzodiazepines and narcotics is an essential part of the immediate preoperative preparation en route to the operating room.

Intraoperative Management

Invasive monitoring intraoperatively is a necessity and begins with an arterial line placed in a quiet operating room before induction but after heavy sedation. Central venous cannulation permits access for hemodynamic monitoring of volume status and for the timely administration of vasoactive drugs. It is usually placed following the anesthetic induction. Pulmonary artery catheterization may be chosen, especially if there is any concern about compromised cardiac or pulmonary function.

No large trials of anesthetic administration have been undertaken and use of virtually all possible drugs and techniques have been reported. It is important to minimize patient anxiety and other stresses of the anesthetic induction because hypertensive responses are common, despite the lack of direct tumor manipulation at these times. Induction is usually done with thiopental. Intubation generally follows a documented deepening of anesthesia, accomplished with intravenous narcotics and inhalational agents delivered with gentle mask ventilation. A neuromuscular blocker devoid of hemodynamic effects (rocuronium, vecuronium or, *cis*-atracurium) is a logical choice. Once blood pressure is stable, intubation is accomplished. It is this author's experience that anesthetic induction is usually uneventful in the prepared patient when one takes these simple, gentle steps.

All adrenergic nerve endings have increased catechol levels. Therefore, exaggerated responses may occur as a result of any intervention. This fact has led some to suggest supplemental epidural anesthesia in order to block the sympathetic nervous system. While admirable in its concept, this technique causes venodilation and may complicate unnecessarily volume management. Furthermore, the major challenge which occurs intraoperatively results from the inevitable manipulation of the tumor, and this is not affected by peridural sympathetic blockade.

Tenfold or more increases in circulating catecholamine levels have been measured during surgical manipulation of a pheochromocytoma. Such elevated levels cause significant blood pressure lability and require a means for rapid blood pressure control. Systolic blood pressure should not be allowed to exceed 200 mm Hg. The most commonly used agent to control hypertension is nitroprusside. It is very familiar to anesthesiologists and useful because of its rapidity of action and short half-life. Phentolamine, a short-acting α-blocker, is also useful, particularly when high doses of nitroprusside are required. Inhalational anesthetic agents are also effective for their vasodilatory effects. Usually, a combination of these drugs is used.

Care must be taken not to overshoot and cause dangerous hypotension. Tachycardia and ventricular ectopy are easily treated with esmolol, a rapidly acting β-blocker with a half-life of only 9 minutes. Propranolol or metoprolol can be used if large doses of esmolol are required, but their long half-lives make them less versatile.

It is important to stop or decrease the infusion of vasoactive drugs in anticipation of ligation of the last adrenal veins. Following tumor removal, drastic decreases in serum catecholamines occur and the patient is prone to hypotension and hypovolemia, secondary to vasodilation of both the venous and arterial circulations. Large amounts of isotonic fluid administration (up to 1 or 2 liters) usually suffices and should be administered before tumor removal, especially if large doses of vasodilating drugs have been required intraoperatively. Decreasing the level of inhalational anesthetic at this point is helpful. Occasionally, direct-acting vasopressors are required. It may be difficult to estimate the appropriate dosage of vasopressor because responses vary widely. Patients who have not been treated aggressively preoperatively will likely have some degree of downregulation of adrenergic receptors and may have a subnormal response to adrenergic drugs. Variability in the persistent levels of the long-lasting α-blocker phenoxybenzamine (half-life approximately 12 hours) also complicates the dosing of a vasopressor drug.

Other drugs that have been reported to be helpful in the perioperative period include calcium channel blockers and magnesium. Calcium is necessary for the release of catechols from normal sympathetic axons, and blockade of its channels may decrease catechol release. Additionally, these drugs have antihypertensive actions. Magnesium has some smooth-muscle vasodilatory effects and is particularly helpful in the face of dysrhythmias caused by catecholamine excesses.

Postoperative Care

Hypotension in the postoperative period is not uncommon and may be the result of persistent α-blockade. It is best treated with aggressive volume resuscitation. Hypotension usually resolves within the first 24 hours. Persistent hypertension is also possible and has a few causes which must be considered. Residual pheochromocytoma is a potential cause if high pressure persists for several days. Continued high catecholamine levels are not unusual in the early postoperative period and represent the output from normal sympathetic nervous tissue. These normal sympathetic neurons are overly supplied with catecholamines from their accumulation by reuptake from the circulation during the preoperative period of excessive catecholamine production by the tumor. Any biochemical assessments for residual pheochromocytoma should not be done for 5 to 7 days after surgery, to avoid being misled by this phenomenon. Adequate pain control must be provided. Volume overload, in an attempt to avoid hypotension, may lead to hypertension. This must be considered as well.

Occasionally, one is presented with a patient who has had a failed resection attempt because of difficulty localizing the tumor, anatomic constraints, or, perhaps, because of unresectable metastatic disease. This type of patient will require continuation of antihypertensive therapy. A search for additional disease will need to be undertaken eventually in those patients cases for whom an additional resectional attempt is deemed appropriate.

Surgical resection of a pheochromocytoma is usually curative. This is best achieved by meticulous pre- and intraoperative medical management to avoid complications and the risk of mortality.

BIBLIOGRAPHY

Boutros AR, et al: Perioperative management of 63 patients with pheochromocytoma, *Cleve Clin J Med* 57:613–617, 1990.

DeGroot LJ, et al, eds: *Endocrinology,* ed 3, Philadelphia, 1995, WB Saunders.

Manger WM, Gifford RW Jr, eds: *Clinical and experimental pheochromocytoma,* ed 2, Cambridge, MA, 1996, Blackwell Science.

Mulvihill SJ: Perioperative use of octreotide in gastrointestinal surgery, *Digestion* 54 (suppl 1):33–37, 1993.

Newell KA, et al: Plasma catecholamine changes during excision of pheochromocytoma, *Surgery* 104:1064–1073, 1988.

Perry RR, et al: Surgical management of pheochromocytoma with the use of metyrosine, *Ann Surg* 212:621–628, 1990.

Veall GR, et al: Review of the anaesthetic management of 21 patients undergoing laparotomy for carcinoid syndrome, *Br J Anaesth* 72:335–341, 1994.

Warner RR, et al: Octreotide treatment of carcinoid hypertensive crisis, *Mt Sinai J Med* 61:349–355, 1994.

Williams RH, Wilson JD, Foster DW, eds: *Williams' textbook of endocrinology,* ed 8, Philadelphia, 1992, WB Saunders.

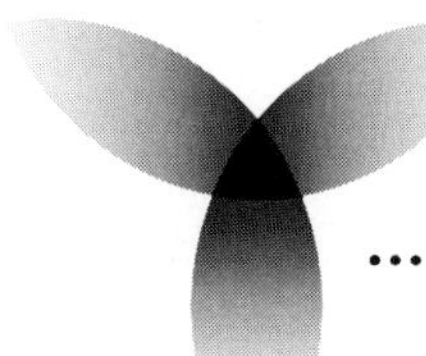

Chapter 18

Perioperative Management of Hematologic and Platelet Disorders

Donald D. Mathes, MD, Daniel J. Kennedy, MD

The perioperative management of hematologic and platelet disorders requires a multidisciplinary effort between hematology, anesthesiology, and surgery to prevent complications. The perioperative period increases the risk of complications because of both the stress of surgery and direct insult to hematologic homeostasis from surgical trauma and bleeding. This chapter will focus on the perioperative management of common hematologic and platelet disorders or rarer disorders that pose particular risk of complications during the perioperative period.

• HEMATOLOGIC DISORDERS

Sickle Cell Disease

Sickle cell disease is inherited in a codominant pattern of hemoglobin S (Hgb S) with either hemoglobin A, S, C, β-thalassemia, or other rarer hemoglobin abnormalities.

Homozygous SS (sickle cell anemia), Hgb SC, or Hgb SB (sickle-thalassemia) is classically grouped as sickle cell disease; Hgb AS is classified as sickle cell trait. In the United States, 1 in 625 African-Americans has Hgb SS and 1 in 833 has Hgb SC.

PATHOPHYSIOLOGY

Hemoglobin S occurs because of an abnormal substitution of valine for glutamic acid in the sixth amino acid position of the β-globulin chain. This substitution causes an intramolecular rearrangement in which deoxygenated hemoglobin increases weak intermolecular forces, triggering polymerization and sickling of red blood cells. Hemoglobin S begins to sickle at oxygen saturation levels of 85% and sickling is usually complete by 40% oxygen saturation. Sickle-cell-trait (Hgb AS) patients do not begin to sickle until a PaO_2 of 25 to 30 mm Hg; hence, sickle-cell-trait patients remain asymptomatic except under extremely hypoxic conditions. Hemoglobin F inhibits deoxyhemoglobin S polymerization. Patients with higher amounts of hemoglobin F, such as infants or people of Middle Eastern or Indian descent, often have minimal sequelae because of the protective effects of hemoglobin F preventing polymerization.

In the case of sickle cell disease, there are numerous other factors besides oxygen saturation levels, which increase the risk of erythrocytes sickling. These factors include the following: acidosis, hypothermia, hypovolemia, increased blood viscosity, venous stasis, the concentration of hemoglobin S, and the concentration of hemoglobin within the erythrocyte. The mean corpuscular hemoglobin concentration (MCHC) is the hemoglobin concentration within the red blood cell. An elevated MCHC makes the red blood cells rigid and more prone to stasis and sickling in the microcirculation. Conditions that cause red blood cell dehydration, such as the hyperosmolar portion of the renal medulla, cause an increase in the MCHC and a decrease in red blood cell deformability.

The oxygen dissociation curve is shifted to the right in sickle cell disease because of an increase in 2,3-DPG. Although this right shift improves oxygen unloading to the tissues, it also causes lower oxygen saturation for a given PaO_2 further increasing the amount of deoxygenated hemoglobin. Acidosis can cause a further shift to the right on the dissociation curve, hence exacerbating the amount of deoxyhemoglobin with decreases in PaO_2. Hypothermia, although causing a left shift on the oxygen dissociation curve, will cause increased sickling in the microcirculation from stasis, because of increased blood viscosity and peripheral vasoconstriction. Stasis in the microcirculation prolongs the time hemoglobin remains deoxygenated and, hence, increases the risk of hemoglobin S polymerization.

Homozygotes (Hgb SS) have a chronic hemolytic anemia caused by the distorted red blood cells being eliminated in the reticuloendothelial system. This chronic hemolysis can lead to chronic elevation of bilirubin with jaundice and cholelithiasis, and end-organ damage from iron deposition. The average hemoglobin is 6 to 9 gm/dl with an average red blood cell lifespan of 10 to 12 days.

The hemoglobin-SC or S-thalassemia patient has many of the same pathophysiologic and clinical manifestations of SS disease, but the condition is usually less severe and better tolerated. Hemoglobin SA (sickle-cell-trait) patients are usually asymptomatic, with minimal or no end-organ damage.

Clinical Manifestations

Nearly every organ system is affected from vasoocclusion in sickle cell disease. Preoperatively, the perioperative physician must evaluate for end-organ damage and determine if the sickle-cell patient is stable at the time of surgery. Patients with any recent, ongoing acute vasoocclusive problems are likely to have significantly more postoperative problems (see preoperative subsection).

Musculoskeletal

Acute vasoocclusive crises cause both muscle and bone pain. Bone pain occurs from infarction of the bone marrow. Radiographs of the skull and spine reveal enlarged bone-marrow spaces, cortical thinning, and increased trabecular markings.

Neurologic

Multiple neurologic sequelae can occur from sickle cell disease, including cerebral thrombosis, hemorrhage, seizures, transient ischemic attacks, and spinal cord infarctions. Cerebral thromboses occur most commonly in children, while cerebral hemorrhage occurs most commonly in adults. Any patient with a recent history of a cerebrovascular accident (CVA) should have aggressive, partial-exchange transfusions to keep the Hgb S to less than 30% because of the high risk of a recurrent CVA without exchange transfusion. This is especially important in the perioperative period, in which further stresses will increase the risk of an acute vasoocclusive neurologic event.

Pulmonary

Acute chest syndrome usually presents with cough, dyspnea, and chest pain along with the less common symptoms of fever, tachypnea, chest radiograph infiltrates, and leukocytosis. The etiology of acute chest syndrome is usually vasoocclusion, infection, or both. Acute chest syndrome is a common serious postoperative complication because of the high incidence of hypoxia causing systemic vasoocclusion. Chronically, an increased ventilation-perfusion mismatch occurs from recurrent pulmonary vascular vasoocclusion, leading to an increased incidence of hypoxia, pulmonary hypertension, and eventually, cor pulmonale.

Cardiac

In sickle cell disease, chronically elevated cardiac outputs occur because of chronic anemia. Approximately 50% of adults with sickle cell disease will have left ventricular hypertrophy, and 15% to 20% will have right ventricular hypertrophy. Although the cardiac output is elevated, adults have decreased cardiac reserve and are at risk for congestive heart failure from excessive transfusion and fluid administration. Furthermore, underlying cardiac structural damage occurs from excess iron deposition from repeat transfusions and chronic hemolysis. Lastly, cor pulmonale can occur from long-standing pulmonary hypertension and hypoxia.

Liver and Biliary

Cholelithiasis is a common complication of sickle cell disease because of the formation of biliary gallstones from increased bilirubin production from chronic hemolysis.

Often, laparoscopic cholecystectomy is done to prevent confusion of acute cholecystitis from other causes of abdominal pain. Hepatic complications include viral hepatitis from blood transfusion, cirrhosis from iron deposition, hepatic infarcts, and hepatic sequestration causing sudden liver enlargement and a sudden decrease in hemoglobin.

SPLEEN

The spleen becomes nonfunctional in early childhood because of autoinfarction from vasoocclusion. Hence, the patient with sickle cell disease has a higher incidence of infections from encapsulated organisms, such as *Streptococcus pneumoniae, Haemophilus influenzae,* and *Salmonella*. The perioperative physician should make sure the sickle cell patient has had both pneumococcal and *H. influenzae* vaccines and continue any prophylactic penicillin, or similar antibiotics, in the perioperative period.

RENAL

The kidney is particularly vulnerable to vasoocclusive damage because of the medullary portions of the vasa recta, being both hypoxic to PO_2 to 10 mm Hg and hyperosmotic to 1200 mOsm/L. This often leads to hematuria, papillary necrosis, and an inability to concentrate urine (isothenuria). Isothenuria can lead to rapid volume depletion with inadequate hydration such as a prolonged preoperative fast from fluid. The glomerular filtration rate decreases steadily with age from glomerulosclerosis and glomerular dropout. By age 40, approximately 20% of homozygotes will have significant renal insufficiency.

BLOOD

Chronic anemia results from both extravascular and intravascular hemolysis of deformed red blood cells. This chronic hemolysis is partially compensated for by an increased erythropoieses with elevated reticulocytosis. Chronic folic-acid supplementation is essential to assure an adequate erythropoiesis.

Hemolytic crisis is often seen with a vasoocclusive crisis, secondary to the increased destruction of irreversible sickled cells. This can lead to further decreases in the hemoglobin because of inadequate compensation of erythropoieses. Aplastic crisis of the bone marrow can cause a precipitous decline in hemoglobin, platelets, and white blood cells. Aplastic crisis should be suspected with a decreasing blood count with an inappropriate low reticulocyte count. In children, acute sequestration of blood can occur in the liver or spleen and cause a large decrease in the hemoglobin and intravascular volume depletion.

PREOPERATIVE MANAGEMENT

Any patient with sickle cell disease undergoing elective surgery should be seen by an anesthesiologist, surgeon, and hematologist several weeks before surgery. This will allow the perioperative team of physicians to determine if the patient is medically stable and if a preoperative blood transfusion is needed. Any patient with a recent or ongoing vasoocclusive crisis should likely be postponed for any elective surgery, given the greater likelihood of increased postoperative complications from the stress of surgery.

Preoperative assessment should include evaluation of end-organ damage from sickle cell disease. A complete blood count should be obtained to assure an adequate hemoglobin. Any unexpected low hemoglobin (<7 gm/dl) should have further evaluation, including a reticulocyte count to assure adequate erythropoietic activity. Folic-acid administration up to 5 mg per day should be continued in the preoperative period. Other screening tests should include serum glutamic oxaloacetic transaminase (SGOT), bilirubin, and creatinine as baseline for any moderate or major surgery, as well as an electrocardiogram (ECG) in older patients looking for evidence of left or right ventricular hypertrophy. Evidence of hypertrophy on ECG is a likely marker of decreased cardiac reserve and should alert the anesthesiologist to have a lower threshold for placing invasive monitors for major surgery.

The decision to give a preoperative blood transfusion should be a multispecialty decision between the hematologist, anesthesiologist, and surgeon. In 1995 Vichinsky et al. found aggressive partial exchange transfusion to offer no further benefit over simple transfusions to a hemoglobin of 10 g/dl for most surgeries. Koshy et al. found little to no association between Hgb A levels and complication rates. Koshy et al. also found a significant higher complication rate in adults compared to children. Although it is difficult to infer any definite overall conclusions from Koshy's study, sickle-cell patients with a hemoglobin below 10 g/dl had fewer overall complications with a simple transfusion to a hemoglobin of 10 to 11 g/dl. However, patients with Hgb SS with a baseline hemoglobin of 10 to 11 g/dl who did not receive a perioperative transfusion, did as well as patients with a preoperative transfusion to a hemoglobin of 10 to 11 g/dl.

Unfortunately, no good, randomized control study has been done looking at overall perioperative outcome in sickle-cell patients receiving or not receiving a perioperative transfusion. Several older studies have shown minimal complication rates for stable sickle-cell patients not receiving perioperative transfusion. Griffin and Buchanan found minimal perioperative complications for children with sickle cell disease receiving no perioperative transfusion, except for a subgroup of patients undergoing laparotomy, thoracotomy, and tonsillectomy. Although no definite conclusions can be drawn at this time on the need for perioperative transfusion, this author has the following recommendations:

1. Children younger than age 14 with sickle cell disease have a lower perioperative complication rate. Perioperative transfusions are normally not needed for most minor surgeries. However, a preoperative transfusion should be given for severe anemia, thoracotomy, laparotomy, tonsillectomy and adenoidectomy, or for any other major stressful surgery.
2. Adults with sickle cell disease have a higher perioperative complication rate and likely will benefit from simple transfusion preoperatively to a hemoglobin of 10 g/dl for most surgeries. Simple transfusions to a hemoglobin greater than 11 g/dl are likely harmful because of increased blood viscosity. If preexisting hemoglobin is 10 g/dl or higher in sickle cell disease, then transfusion is not needed. However, patients with a Hgb SC are still likely to benefit with preoperative transfusion to a hemoglobin of 12 g/dl.

3. The percentage of Hgb S is not a factor in perioperative outcome for most surgeries. Hence, simple transfusions should be done over partial exchange transfusions because there is less risk of alloimmunizations, transfusion reactions and blood infection transmission.
4. Any preoperative transfusion should be given ideally 2 to 3 weeks in advance of surgery to decrease erythropoiesis and, hence, further decrease Hgb S caused by the short life of Hgb S erythrocytes.
5. Minor surgeries, such as myringotomy or other surgeries not requiring general anesthesia, or central neuraxis blockade, do not normally need preoperative transfusions.
6. The decision to transfuse a patient preoperatively should be a multidisciplinary team decision between the hematologist and the perioperative physician. The potential benefits of a transfusion should be considered against the risks of alloimmunization, transfusion reactions, and viral hepatitis, as well as other blood-related infections.

INTRAOPERATIVE MANAGEMENT

Before the start of any anesthetic, the patient should be euvolemic. Patients arriving the same day of surgery should have clear liquids up to 3 hours before surgery to minimize fasting-fluid deficits. Furthermore, any fluid deficits should be rapidly corrected before the start of anesthesia. Preoperative sedation should be limited to avoid respiratory depression and the risk of hypoxia.

The goals of anesthesia are to avoid hypoxia, hypotension, hypovolemia, venous stasis, and either hypothermia or hyperthermia. The method of achieving these goals under general anesthesia or regional anesthesia is not as important as maintaining homeostasis throughout the perioperative period. Although regional anesthesia may appear to be the better choice, by creating a sympathectomy and increased blood flow, it can cause a compensatory vasoconstriction in nonblocked areas and increase the risk of microcirculatory stasis in the nonblocked areas.

Intraoperative blood loss should be replaced without allowing the patient to have significant drops in hemoglobin. Transfusions should not be above 11 gm/dl to prevent increased viscosity of blood. High amounts of FiO_2 for general anesthesia, or supplemental oxygen for regional anesthesia, is prudent to avoid any occurrence of hypoxia. Careful positioning of the patient should be done to minimize any pooling and stasis of blood in any one region of the body.

No particular drugs, such as prophylactic bicarbonate infusions or dextran infusions, have been found to be beneficial in the perioperative period. However, bicarbonate along with adequate ventilation should be used to correct for metabolic acidosis. Theoretically, slight hyponatremia may be beneficial by decreasing the concentration of hemoglobin within the red blood cell and MCHC. Hence, this author prefers to use lactated ringers if there is no lactic acidosis over normal saline because of the lower sodium content of lactated ringers. Lastly, mannitol or hypertonic saline should be used with great caution in the sickle-cell-disease patient because increased serum osmolality may cause red blood cell dehydration.

POSTOPERATIVE MANAGEMENT

Postoperative management goals are the same as those for intraoperative management. These goals include continuous liberal intravenous hydration, supplemental oxygen, normothermia, and good pain control for the first 24 to 48 hours. Furthermore, patients should be monitored closely for any vasoocclusive crisis. Acute chest syndrome is one of the most common vasoocclusive complications, and can lead to hypoxia and systemic vasoocclusive crisis. Treatment of any vasoocclusive postoperative complications should involve consultation with a hematologist. The hematologist can determine the need for any further simple or partial-exchange transfusions to prevent further vasoocclusion.

Maintaining adequate oxygenation is essential and can be difficult, especially in abdominal or thoracic cases in which atelectasis, splinting, and a decrease in the functional-reserve capacity cause increased ventilation-perfusion mismatch. Such measures as sitting up, early mobilization, incentive spirometry, and good pain control with epidural analgesia can lessen the severity of the ventilation-perfusion mismatch. The use of continuous-pulse oximetry or spot-pulse oximetry can help anticipate and prevent hypoxia after the patient is discharged from the recovery room.

Thalassemia

Thalassemia includes a broad spectrum of inherited hemoglobinopathies caused by abnormal α- and β-chain synthesis. The presentation can vary from causing in utero death to being asymptomatic. Classically, diagnosis should be suspected when microcytosis is found on a complete blood count with a mean corpuscular volume (MCV) of less than 75 fl with a nearly normal red cell count of greater than 5 million cells/μl.

BETA-THALASSEMIAS

The β-thalassemias occur generally in people of Middle Eastern, Mediterranean, and African heritage. Beta-globin-chain synthesis is determined by two genes, each located on chromosome 6. Defects in one or both of these genes cause decreased β-chain production. This decrease leads to different degrees of an imbalance of excessive α-chain to β-chains. Free-α chains are unstable and are readily destroyed, causing accelerated hematopoiesis and chronic hemolysis.

Beta-thalassemia major (Cooley's anemia) is one of the most serious thalassemias. These patients are transfusion-dependent with ineffective erythropoiesis, despite significant hyperplastic bone marrow. Most of the erythroblasts are destroyed within the bone marrow because of free α-globin accumulation and aggregation. The few erythrocytes released into the blood are readily destroyed in the reticuloendothelial system within the spleen and liver. Significant expansion of the bone marrow can occur in the vertebral bodies and thorax, causing spinal-cord compression; Expansion in the upper facies causes frontal bossing and maxillary bone hypertrophy, creating a chipmunk facies appearance (Figure 18-1). The combination of hemolysis and chronic transfusions causes hemosiderosis to occur in the heart, liver, and pancreas leading to a cardiomyopathy, arrhythmias, cirrhosis, and diabetes mellitus. Iron chelation therapy now has allowed improved survival into adulthood. Splenectomy is

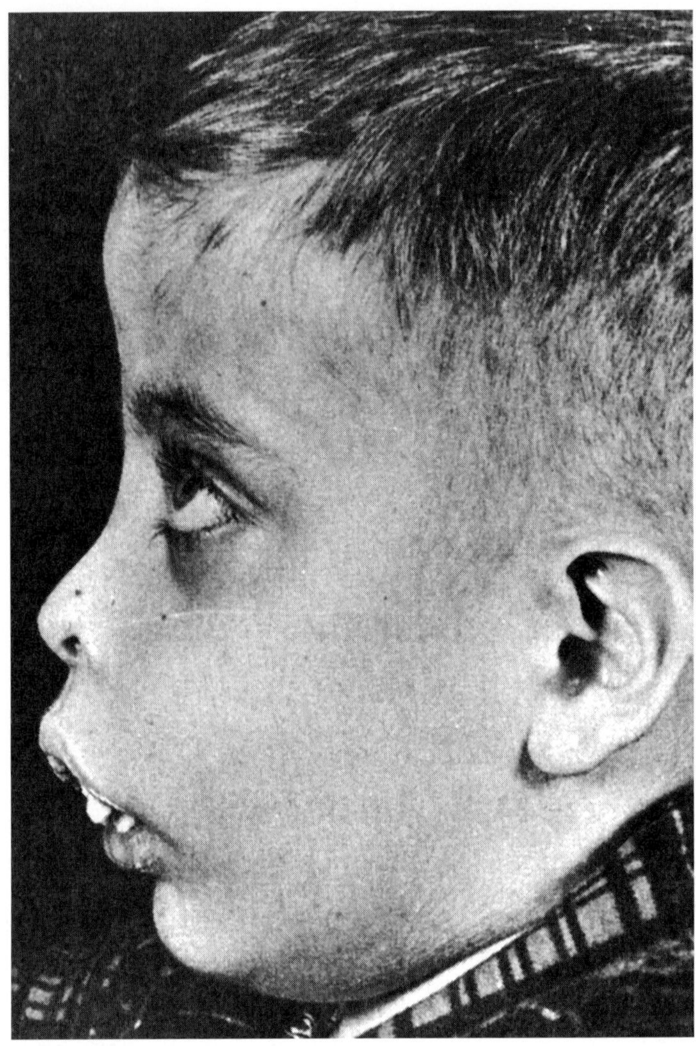

Figure 18-1
Facial morphologic changes as a result of β-Thalassemia major. (Used with permission from Jurkewicz et al: *Ann N Y Acad Sci* 165:437–42, 1969)

rarely performed because of persistent pancytopenia. Bone-marrow transplantation is now being done with good success.

Thalassemia intermedia is caused by various defects of β-chain synthesis; however, the coupling of β and α chains is improved in these patients, allowing more effective erythropoiesis and significantly fewer symptoms. Under stressful conditions, such as major surgery or infections, erythropoiesis can become ineffective rendering the patients transfusion-dependent. These patients still may have problems with iron overload because of chronic hemolysis and increased gastrointestinal iron absorption. Moderate degrees of splenomegaly are common and a splenectomy may be needed with serious anemia to decrease hemolysis and prevent the thalassemia-intermedia patient from being transfusion-dependent.

Beta-thalassemia-minor (trait) patients are usually asymptomatic with minimal end-organ damage. Typically, these patients have a mild anemia with a low MCV on a complete blood cell count (CBC) but a normal number of red blood cells.

ALPHA THALASSEMIA

Alpha thalassemias occur primarily in people of Asian or African heritage. Alpha-chain synthesis is dependent upon four genes, with two genes located on each chromosome 16. The type of α-thalassemia depends on the number of abnormal genes. Alpha thalassemia minor is caused by two dysfunctional genes. Alpha thalassemia minor normally presents with mild microcytic anemia with splenomegaly and elevated erythropoiesis. Alpha thalassemia major occurs from a defect in three of the four genes. This causes a significant imbalance of free β chains which can lead to production of β-chain tetramers known as Hgb H. Hemoglobin H is unstable and is readily hemolyzed. Although α-major-thalassemia patients are anemic, they do not normally require transfusions except under stressful conditions. Dysfunction of all four α-chain genes is incompatible with life (hydrops fetalis), and these individuals die in utero because of the formation of a tetramer of γ-chains called Hgb Bart, which is incapable of unloading oxygen to the tissues in utero.

ANESTHETIC MANAGEMENT

The β- and α-thalassemia-minor patients should be managed perioperatively as any other patient with mild anemia. Patients with β- or α-thalassemia major or β-thalassemia intermedia should likely have preoperative transfusions to increase hemoglobin levels to at least 10 g/dl for any moderate or major surgery. Although α-thalassemia-major or β-thalassemia-intermedia patients are not transfusion-dependent under normal conditions, the stress of major or moderate surgery may increase hemolysis without adequate compensatory erythropoiesis. Preoperatively, the physician should be aware of the high incidence of hemochromatosis. The perioperative physician should examine the patient for any evidence of a cardiomyopathy, arrhythmias, cirrhosis, and diabetes mellitus caused by hemochromatosis.

With β-thalassemia major, the hypertrophy of the cranial facial bones can lead to a difficult mask fit and intubation because of enlargement of the maxillary structures (see Figure 18-1). Intraoperatively, the anesthesiologist should have a lower threshold for placing invasive monitors for major surgery because of decreased cardiac reserve and increased likelihood of cardiac structural damage from iron deposition. Blood transfusions should be given for any significant blood loss for thalassemia major or intermedia patients, because these patients have little ability to compensate for blood loss with increased erythropoiesis.

Postoperatively, hemoglobin levels should be followed closely because of the risk for inadequate erythropoiesis and increased hemolysis. Decreases in hemoglobin below baseline should be replaced with blood transfusions.

Glucose-6-Phosphate Dehydrogenase Deficiency (G-6PD)

The G-6PD gene is located on the X chromosome; hence, G-6PD deficiency is sex-linked and predominantly affects males and the rare homozygote female. The deficiency is the most common of the red blood cell enzyme disorders affecting approximately 10% of African-American males.

Normally, red blood cells are able to protect against oxidative stresses by increasing reduced glutathione by the hexose-monophosphate shunt. Reduced glutathione prevents the sulfhydryl group on hemoglobin from oxidizing and causing precipitation of hemoglobin within the red blood cell. In G-6PD deficiency, the red blood cell is not able to regenerate reduced glutathione with oxidative stresses and hemoglobin precipitates, causing primarily extravascular hemolysis within the reticuloendothelial system. Younger red blood cells are more resistant to oxidative stresses in G-6PD deficiency; hence, hemolysis usually occurs first in the older red blood cells. The G-6PD A-variant is found in the majority of African-American males and is less severe than many other variants. In these patients, hemolysis is usually limited to periods following an oxidative stress, such as drug exposure or infection, with hemoglobin levels stabilizing within 1 week.

Intraoperatively, most anesthetic drugs are safe and no special intraoperative management needs to be done besides avoiding drugs known to cause an oxidative stress (Table 18-1). Many drugs in the past were associated with hemolysis with G-6PD deficiency. Most of these drugs were proven to be safe with further investigation. The initial reports of drug-induced hemolysis were actually caused by an infection for which the drug was used for treatment. The most notable of these drugs, aspirin and acetaminophen, are now considered safe in moderate doses for most variants of G-6PD deficiency (Table 18-2). Postoperatively, G-6PD deficiency should be strongly considered in any unexplained drops in hemoglobin and elevations in indirect bilirubin.

Pyruvate Kinase Deficiency

Pyruvate kinase deficiency is the second most common red blood cell enzymopathy next to G-6PD deficiency. Pyruvate kinase deficiency results in a decreased ATP production and increased concentration of 2,3-DPG, causing a right shift of the oxyhemoglobin dissociation curve. Chronic hemolysis occurs because of decreased ATP and Na-K-ATPase pump activity, causing dehydrated cells. The incidence of splenomegaly, bone-marrow hyperplasia and, indirect hyperbilirubinemia occurs in direct proportion to the severity of hemolysis. Stresses such as surgery or infection can cause an aplastic crisis and dramatic reduction in blood counts. Perioperatively, these patients' blood counts should be followed closely by monitoring for aplastic crisis. Splenectomy often significantly increases hemoglobin and reticulocytes and can eliminate the need for transfusions.

Hereditary Spherocytosis

Hereditary spherocytosis is an autosomal-dominant inherited disease with a prevalence of 1:4500. The red-blood-cell cytoskeleton is deficient in spectrin which causes the red blood cells to become spheroidal and rigid. The spherocytes cannot deform

Table 18-1. Common Drugs that Can Induce Hemolytic Anemia in Persons with G-6PD Deficiency

Acetanilid	Niridazole
Doxorubicin	Nitrofurantoin
Furazolidone	Phenazopyridine
Methylene blue	Primaquine
Nalidixic acid	Sulfamethoxazole

(Used with permission from Beutler E: *N Engl J Med* 324:169, 1991.)

readily in the spleen and become damaged and hemolyzed within the spleen. The spherocytes have an increased osmotic fragility and hemolyze more readily in a hypotonic environment.

Splenomegaly, indirect hyperbilirubinemia, anemia, and cholelithiasis are common clinical manifestations. Hemolysis is normally compensated for by increased erythrocytosis. However, under stressful conditions such as infection or surgery, increased hemolysis can occur, complicated by bone-marrow hypoplasia and aplastic crisis, requiring blood transfusions. Splenectomy normally eradicates hemolysis, but should be reserved for children over 3 years of age to lessen the risk of severe infections. Any patient scheduled for splenectomy should have had a full set of vaccinations against encapsulated organisms, most notably *Streptococcus pneumoniae* and *Haemophilus influenzae*. Postoperatively, patients who have not had a splenectomy should be monitored closely for aplastic crisis.

Paroxysmal Nocturnal Hemoglobinuria (PNH)

Paroxysmal nocturnal hemoglobinuria is a disease affecting all the hematologic lines within the bone marrow. Cell membranes have an increased sensitivity to complement fixation. This increased sensitivity to complement can lead to intravascular hemolysis, leukopenia, and intravascular thrombosis from complement-activating platelets. Classic symptoms include nocturnal hemoglobinuria, jaundice, malaise, fever, and infection. Intravascular thrombosis can present as abdominal and back pain from hepatic, portal, or mesenteric vein thrombosis. Deficient granulocytes can predispose these patients to infection, in which the infection can further activate complement and cause hemolysis.

Perioperative management poses a significant challenge because the stress of surgery has a higher proclivity to activate complement, thus, predisposing these patients to intravascular hemolysis and thrombosis. Upon consultation with a hematologist, these patients will likely benefit from preoperative blood transfusions of washed or frozen-thawed deglycerolized cells. Preoperative blood transfusions provide perioperative protection by decreasing bone-marrow production of abnormal erythrocytes and by diluting the number of abnormal erythrocytes. Washed or deglycerolized cells should be used to limit transfusion of any complement factors.

Intraoperatively, providing stress-free anesthesia to avoid activating complement should be the goal of the anesthesiologist. Appropriate broad spectrum prophylactic antibiotics and strict aseptic measures should be implemented intraoperatively,

Table 18-2. Common Drugs that Can Safely be Given in Therapeutic Doses to Most Variants of G-6PD Deficiency

Acetaminophen	Probenecid
Ascorbic acid	Procainamide
Aspirin	Pyrimethamine
Chloramphenicol	Quinidine
Chloroquine	Quinine
Colchicine	Streptomycin
Diphenhydramine	Sulfamethoxypyridazine
Isoniazid	Sulfisoxazole
Menadione sodium bisulfite	Trimethoprim
Phenacetin	Tripelennamine
Phenylbutazone	Vitamin K
Phenytoin	

(Used with permission from Beutler E: *N Engl J Med* 324:169, 1991.)

because of the increased risk of infection. Bladder catheterization is advisable for any significant surgery to monitor for evidence of intravascular hemolysis from hemoglobinuria. If hemoglobinuria occurs, then corticosteroids, such as 1 mg/kg of methylprednisolone, should be given to decrease complement activity and hemolysis. Furthermore, aggressive hydration and mannitol should be given to increase urine output to prevent renal tubular damage.

Aggressive measures should be implemented to avoid thrombosis intraoperatively and postoperatively. Such measures as the use of low-molecular-weight dextran, adequate hydration, and avoidance of venous stasis is beneficial intraoperatively. Postoperatively, early mobilization along with use of heparin or coumadin should be used, if not contraindicated. If anticoagulation drugs are not used, then a postoperative epidural for thoracic, abdominal, and lower-extremity surgery is a valuable adjunct to decrease the postoperative stress response, complement activation, and, thus, the risk of thrombosis. Complement activation normally peaks at the fourth postoperative day; hence, epidural use for anticoagulation measures should likely be continued at least 4 to 5 days postoperatively.

Immune Hemolytic Anemia

Immune hemolytic anemia occurs when antibodies IgG, IgM, or complement bind to the red blood cells, leading to extravascular or intravascular hemolysis. The etiology of an immune hemolytic anemia can be idiopathic but is usually associated with the following: (1) disease processes such as chronic lymphocytic leukemia, systemic lupus erythematosus (SLE), or lymphoma; (2) drug exposure; or (3) sensitization of erythrocytes from a transfusion or pregnancy.

Classically, IgG antibodies coat the erythrocytes in which splenic macrophages attach to the IgG and damage the erythrocyte membrane. The damaged erythrocyte is then trapped and destroyed in the reticuloendothelial system of the spleen. Intravascular hemolysis can occur when IgG antibodies activate the complement system, which can directly lyse the red cell membrane, causing release of free hemoglobin.

Specific drugs can cause an immune hemolytic anemia through different mechanisms. First, drugs such as α-methyldopa or procainamide can produce direct antibodies against red blood cells. Approximately 10% to 20% of patients on α-methyldopa will have a positive direct antiglobulin (Coombs) test, in which the results will remain positive for up to 1 year after discontinuing α-methyldopa. Most patients with a positive direct Coombs will not actually undergo hemolysis because of a low level of IgG coating the red blood cells. Secondly, large amounts of a penicillin or cephalosporin antibiotic can bind to the red blood cells, forming a hapten complex. This hapten complex can induce the formation of antibodies against the hapten complex and red blood cell and cause extravascular hemolysis. Thirdly, quinidine-type drugs can form a complex with a protein in the plasma, in which antibodies are produced that bind to red blood cells. This phenomenon is often referred to as the "innocent bystander effect." Other drugs implemented in the innocent bystander effect include the sulfonamides and aminosalicylic acid.

Drug-induced hemolysis normally can be managed conservatively with supportive care and by discontinuing the offending drug. Idiopathic autoimmune hemolytic anemia or hemolysis from a disease process should be managed initially with corticosteroids, such as prednisone 1 mg/kg. Prednisone decreases the amount of antibody coating of red blood cells and decreases macrophage phagocytic activity. Alternative immunosuppressives, such as cyclophosphamide or azathioprine, can be used with good success.

Splenectomy is indicated for the following: (1) failure to respond to corticosteroids or other immunosuppressives; (2) significant side effects of corticosteroids or immunosuppressives; or (3) continued need to use large doses of prednisone more than 10 to 20 mg/day. Splenectomy removes much of the reticuloendothelial system, decreasing phagocytosing macrophages, and decreasing antibody production from B cells.

Perioperatively, anticipated blood products should be ordered well in advance of surgery because of anticipated difficulty with crossmatching from antibodies. Immunosuppressants should be continued perioperatively and, perhaps, increased under the direction of a hematologist, to decrease the risk of further hemolysis from the stress of surgery. Any patient scheduled for splenectomy should have appropriate vaccinations against encapsulated organisms. Patients receiving blood transfusions should be monitored carefully for a transfusion reaction, given the increased risk of alloimmunization (see subsection on transfusion reactions).

Cold Agglutinin Disease

Cold agglutinin disease is a disease process in which autoantibodies bind to erythrocytes at cold temperatures, and reversibly unbind from erythrocytes at warm temperatures. Classic presentation is a mild, stable, chronic hemolytic anemia with acrocyanosis of the nose, ear lobes, fingers, and feet upon exposure to cold. The majority of cold agglutinin disease is caused by a B-cell lymphoma or chronic lymphocytic leukemia, producing a monoclonal band of IgM antibodies. These IgM antibodies form cold agglutinins with erythrocytes upon exposure to cold and activate the classic complement pathway. Self-limited cold agglutinin disease is associated with certain infectious diseases, such as *Mycoplasma pneumoniae* and infectious mononucleosis.

High doses of immunosuppressants and splenectomy are not usually an effective treatment for IgM cold agglutinins. Occasionally, high-dose corticosteroids are effective for IgM cold agglutinins. Splenectomy is not effective because the liver is the dominant site of hemolysis with cold agglutinins. Plasma exchange and plasmapheresis may be effective with acute severe hemolysis.

Intraoperatively, normothermia should be strictly maintained. Extremities should be prevented from cooling with such measures as warming blankets. All blood transfusions and fluids should be given through warmers heated at 37°C. Cardiopulmonary bypass poses a special challenge for patients with cold agglutinins. Various anesthetic management plans have been described in the literature. Park and Weiss described the following regimen:

1. Determine the thermal reactivity of the cold antibody, at which either hemagglutination or complement activation occurs.
2. Perform plasmapheresis the day before surgery, decreasing antibody titer 8- to 10-fold.
3. Intraoperatively, warm all fluids and blood products to 37°C. Maintain systemic temperature above critical temperatures of the cold antibody during bypass.
4. Use warm crystalloid or blood potassium cardioplegia.
5. Postoperatively, continue to warm all fluids and blood products and maintain normothermia. Patient should be monitored for evidence of ongoing hemolysis.
6. Consider using only washed donor cells for blood transfusions to limit complement transfusion. Unwashed donor cells lack the complement inhibitor C_3d and could potentiate complement activation and hemolysis by the cold antibodies.

Transfusion Reactions

HEMOLYTIC TRANSFUSION REACTION

Hemolytic transfusion reactions are caused by intravascular and extravascular hemolysis, and may be acute or delayed in onset. Most acute, life-threatening reactions occur from ABO incompatible blood being given, such as type B–positive blood to an O-positive patient. When ABO incompatible blood is given, the patient has significant antibodies that bind to donor red blood cells and activate the complement cascade. Fixation of C_5b-9 complement to the red blood cell membrane causes cell-membrane lysis and intravascular hemolysis. Furthermore, the complement cascade releases C_3a and C_5a that cause hypotension, bronchospasm, and pulmonary dysfunction with increased ventilation-perfusion mismatch.

Acute intravascular hemolysis will present with both hemoglobinemia and hemoglobinuria, with pink- to red-tinged plasma and urine. The free hemoglobin stroma causes renal vasoconstriction, leading to renal ischemia. This insult, combined with the toxicity of free hemoglobin on the renal tubules, can lead to acute tubular necrosis. One third to one half of patients with major intravascular hemolysis will develop disseminated intravascular coagulation (DIC).

Awake patients classically complain of a feeling of impending doom with shortness of breath, chest pain, hypotension, bronchospasm, nausea, and low-back pain. Many of these symptoms are caused by activation of the complement cascade and release of cytokines. Under general anesthesia, an acute hemolytic transfusion reaction may initially present as a change in urine color or diffuse, unexplained surgical bleeding.

Initial management of a suspected acute transfusion reaction should begin with stopping the blood transfusion, followed by aggressive hydration with isotonic crystalloid and possible inotropic support to assure adequate renal perfusion. Patients not intubated should be followed closely for evidence of stridor, laryngeal edema, or pulmonary edema. Patients should be intubated early for any suspected airway difficulty. Any untransfused blood should be sent directly to the blood bank with paperwork rechecked, along with blood and urine samples, for a transfusion workup. Tests should include a direct antiglobulin test (direct Coombs), urine and plasma hemoglobin, and repeat cross-matching tests with the transfused blood.

Once a transfusion reaction is confirmed then the prothrombin time (PT), partial thromboplastin time (PTT), fibrinogen, and platelet count are followed for potential DIC. The creatinine and blood urea nitrogen (BUN) should be followed daily and a urine output of 100 cc/hr maintained by continued intravenous fluids and possible mannitol or furosemide. If the initial workup does not reveal evidence of hemolysis, but the patient has continued hemodynamic instability, then other possibilities, such as sepsis from contaminated blood or an allergic reaction, should be considered.

Patients with a confirmed hemolytic reaction should be monitored closely for 24 hours with repeat coagulation, hemoglobin, and creatinine laboratory tests. If the patient remains hemodynamically stable with good urine output for 24 hours without worsening laboratory abnormalities, then the patient will likely have no further sequelae from the initial transfusion reaction.

EXTRAVASCULAR HEMOLYTIC TRANSFUSION REACTION

Extravascular hemolytic transfusion reactions occur when the complement cascade is not activated. Hence, the red blood cell membrane remains intact, but coated with antibodies or C_3b. These antibodies or C_3b-coated red blood cells are then destroyed by the reticuloendothelial system within the spleen and liver. Extravascular hemolysis is usually caused by antibodies from the Rh, Kell, Duffy, or Kidd systems.

These patients usually remain hemodynamically stable without hemoglobinemia, hemoglobinuria, or other outward sequelae. The diagnosis is made by a positive, direct antiglobulin test from the donor red blood cells being coated with the patient's antibody, and an elevation of indirect bilirubin and lactate dehydrogenase (LDH). Usually, no intervention is needed. The patient should have no further hemolysis after a few days because the donor red blood cells are destroyed.

DELAY TRANSFUSION REACTION

Both intravascular and extravascular hemolytic transfusion reactions can be delayed up to 4 to 14 days after a transfusion. This occurs because, initially, the levels of antibody titer that exist are low and then gradually increase with exposure to donor blood. Patients typically have minimal sequelae, except for an inappropriate drop in hemoglobin, elevation of indirect bilirubin and LDH, and possible malaise and low-grade fever. The donor blood is hemolyzed slowly and gradually removed. Diagnosis is made by a new, positive-direct antiglobulin test.

Febrile Nonhemolytic Transfusion Reaction

A febrile nonhemolytic transfusion reaction (FNHTR) occurs from agglutinating antibodies in patients' plasma reacting against antigens located on donor platelets and leukocytes. Classically, FNHTRs present with a temperature elevation of more than 1°C and shaking chills during or immediately after a transfusion. The fever and shaking chills are caused by release of cytokines such as interleukin, and tumor-necrosis factor from antibody platelet or leukocyte interaction.

Initial management includes ruling out a hemolytic reaction by stopping the transfusion, rechecking paperwork and cross-match, and checking a new direct antiglobulin test. A negative-direct antiglobulin test confirms the likely diagnosis of FNHTR. However, sepsis from bacterial contaminated blood should be considered and blood cultures should be obtained from the transfused blood and patient if a patient appears clinically septic.

Patients with a history of one febrile reaction have a 1:8 chance of future febrile reactions with a blood transfusion. These patients likely benefit from prophylactic treatment with acetaminophen and 100 mg of intravenous hydrocortisone before a transfusion. Patients with a history of recurrent febrile reactions should get leukocyte-poor blood, either from washed or frozen deglycerolized red blood cells. The leukocytes need to be removed at the time of donation to prevent cytokine release in stored blood. Hence, leukocyte filters at the time of transfusion will likely not prevent a febrile reaction.

Allergic Transfusion Reaction

Allergic reactions from transfusion of blood products result from infusion of plasma proteins. Patients' antibodies are directed against the donor-plasma proteins. Most allergic reactions consist, initially, of pruritus and a rash or hives. Less often, severe urticaria, hemodynamic instability, bronchospasm, and anaphylaxis can occur. The most severe anaphylaxis can occur in patients who are IgA-deficient.

One in 650 patients is IgA-deficient and may have anti-IgA antibodies. The IgA present in the donor plasma reacts with anti-IgA antibodies, causing an anaphylactoid reaction. Reactions are preventable by using washed or frozen deglycerolized red blood cells. Plasma-protein components such as fresh frozen plasma, albumin, or platelets should only come from IgA-deficient patients.

Treatment for patients who develop mild allergic symptoms of pruritus and hives consists of stopping the transfusion and giving 25 to 50 mg of diphenhydramine. The patient should then be monitored for any worsening allergic manifestations. The blood transfusion may be restarted only if the patient's allergic symptoms are resolving. Patients who have had repeated allergic reactions or a severe allergic reaction should receive washed red blood cells. Leukocyte filters will not prevent plasma proteins from being transferred and, hence, will not prevent an allergic reaction.

• PLATELET DISORDERS

The platelet disorders of most concern to the perioperative physician consist of either platelet dysfunction or low platelet number (thrombocytopenia). Platelet counts as low as 50,000/mm^3 may cause no increased surgical bleeding if platelet function is normal; but normal platelet counts with dysfunctional platelets can cause significant surgical bleeding. Therefore, the perioperative physician must have an understanding of the actual platelet disorder and treatment options to prevent excessive surgical bleeding.

Thrombocytopenia

The normal platelet count is between 150,000 to 450,000/mm^3. A platelet count below 150,000/mm^3 is defined as thrombocytopenia. Spontaneous hemorrhage from thrombocytopenia usually does not occur until the platelet count is below 20,000/mm^3. For surgical hemostasis, platelet counts between 50,000/mm^3 and 100,000/mm^3 are usually adequate if platelet function is normal. No single platelet number can serve as the sole basis for transfusing platelets perioperatively. Instead, the decision to transfuse platelets perioperatively depends on the individual case and the risk of significant surgical bleeding or serious consequence from surgical bleeding or poor surgical hemostasis. In patients with borderline platelet counts, the bleeding time may be useful, preoperatively, in deciding whether to transfuse platelets or perform regional anesthesia. The bleeding time has a low, positive-predictive value in asymptomatic patients without suspected platelet abnormalities. However, the bleeding time is of value with a good sensitivity and predictive value for suspected platelet abnormalities.

Thrombocytopenia is caused by sequestration of platelets, decreased platelet production, or accelerated platelet destruction (Figure 18-2). This subsection will not discuss all the possible causes of thrombocytopenia, but instead focus on the common causes of thrombocytopenia and different perioperative management issues of these causes.

PLATELET SEQUESTRATION

One third of the platelets are normally sequestered in the spleen. With splenomegaly, up to 90% of platelets are sequestered in the spleen, causing thrombocytopenia. Diseases such as liver cirrhosis with portal hypertension or tumor infiltration of the spleen, can cause significant platelet sequestration from splenomegaly. Perioperative management is usually conservative unless significant thrombocytopenia less than 50,000/mm^3 exists. Splenectomy is effective for disorders such as Gaucher disease or chronic hemolytic disorders but relatively contraindicated for most leukemias or in portal hypertension. Although the platelet count may be decreased, platelet function usually remains intact from splenic sequestration unless there is bone-marrow involvement from a hematologic or malignancy disorder.

PLATELET PRODUCTION DEFECT

A bone-marrow biopsy revealing decreased megakaryocytes is compatible with a platelet production defect. Typically this is associated with leukemia, other hematologic

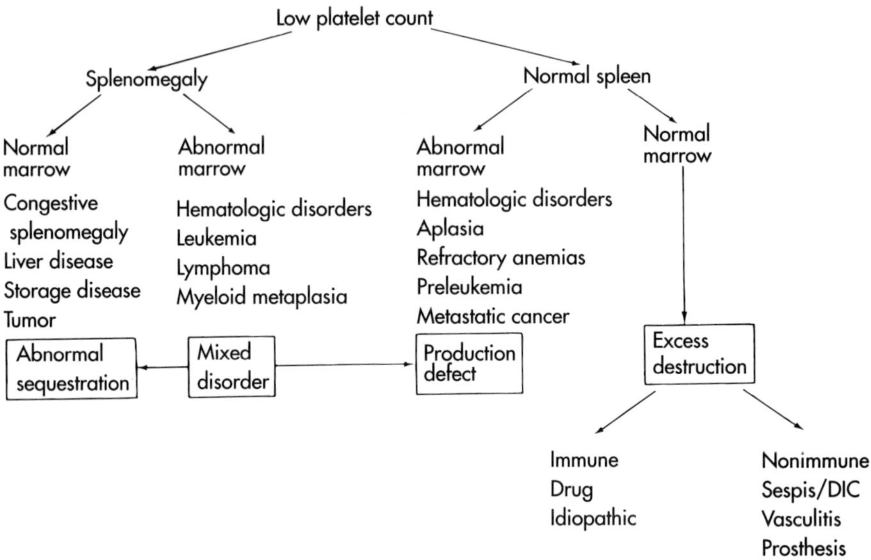

Figure 18-2
A schematic approach to the clinical evaluation of patients with thrombocytopenia. (Used with permission from Handin RI. In Beck W, editors: *Hematology,* ed 4, Cambridge, MA, 1985, MIT Press, p. 442.)

disorders, metastatic cancer, or myelosuppressive chemotherapy agents. Also, certain drugs, most notably the thiazide diuretics, ethanol, gold, and sulfa drugs can selectively inhibit platelet production alone. Treatment consists of treating the underlying hematologic disorder or malignancy, or discontinuing the suspected drug.

ACCELERATED PLATELET DESTRUCTION

Accelerated platelet destruction is caused by nonimmune or immune causes. The nonimmune causes include DIC, vasculitis, and cardiac prosthetic valves. The immune causes are related to platelet antibodies from drugs, infections, prior transfusions of platelets, or from autoantibodies related to SLE, idiopathic thrombocytopenia purpura (ITP), or Evans' syndrome (ITP and hemolytic anemia). The immune-thrombocytopenic patient will usually have a normal spleen, and normal bone marrow with increased megakaryocyte production. The normal platelet lifespan of 7 to 10 days may be reduced to less than 1 hour in immune thrombocytopenia.

Drug-Induced Immune Thrombocytopenia

Many drugs may cause severe thrombocytopenia and mimic ITP. Drug-induced thrombocytopenia is usually caused by the drug or its metabolite binding to the platelet forming an antigen, to which platelet antibodies then bind. This trimolecular complex is then destroyed in the reticuloendothelial system. Most noted drugs

Table 18-3. Common Drugs Causing Immune Thrombocytopenia

Heparin	Penicillins
Thiazide diuretics	Cephalosporins
Aspirin	Sulfa antibiotics
NSAIDs	Quinidine
Phenytoin	Quinine
Carbamazepine	Gold
Valproic acid	Cimetidine

causing platelet antibodies include heparin, thiazide diuretics, aspirin, phenytoin, carbamazepine, penicillin, cephalosporin and sulfa antibiotics, quinidine and quinine (Table 18-3).

Treatment consists of discontinuing any suspected drug. Platelet counts usually begin to increase in a few days, but thrombocytopenia may persist several weeks because of prolonged tissue storage of such drugs as phenytoin. Platelet transfusion should be reserved for life-threatening bleeding or emergency surgery because of the short half-life of transfused platelets from platelet antibodies. High-dose intravenous γ-globulin at a dose of 0.4 to 1.0 g/kg given before a platelet transfusion can prolong platelet survival. The γ-globulin inhibits the reticuloendothelial phagocytic activity.

Heparin-Induced Thrombocytopenia

In the first few days of heparin exposure, most patients will have a mild decrease in platelets. This phenomenon is likely caused by the platelet proaggregatory effect of heparin itself, and is not related to heparin antibodies. Heparin-induced thrombocytopenia (HIT) typically occurs after 5 days of heparin treatment and occurs in 2% to 5% of patients. The thrombocytopenia caused by the heparin is not usually of any risk to the patient. However, thrombotic events are often associated with the thrombocytopenia. These thrombotic events include deep venous thrombosis, pulmonary embolism, cerebral thrombosis, myocardial infarction, and thrombotic ischemic injury to the extremities.

The etiology of HIT and thrombosis is caused by platelet-activating antibodies binding to complexes of heparin and platelet factor 4, a heparin-binding protein found on platelets. This immune complex activates platelets to aggregate, decreasing the platelet count. Furthermore, the vascular endothelium contains a heparin-like substance that, upon exposure to heparin and platelet-activating antibodies, leads to immune complexes binding to the vascular endothelial wall. These immune complexes combine with platelet activation and aggregation and can lead to life-threatening thrombosis.

Optimal management of HIT, perioperatively, remains unclear and should be done with consultation of a hematologist. Treatment options for a patient with a history of HIT and undergoing vascular or cardiac surgery, include the use of iloprost (a prostacyclin analogue), Orgaran (a low-molecular-weight heparinoid), ancrod (a defibrinogenating agent), and low-molecular-weight fractionated heparin. Iloprost (a stable prostacyclin analogue) prevents heparin-induced platelet aggregation. In HIT patients, iloprost infusions of 10 to 48 ng/kg/min started after the induction of anesthesia, allowed full-dose porcine heparin to be used for extracorporeal circulation, and heparin to be reversed with protamine without platelet aggregation. The disadvantage of iloprost infusions is systemic vasodilatation, requiring phenylephrine infusions to prevent hypotension.

Orgaran is a low-molecular-weight heparinoid with a 10% cross-reactivity with heparin-induced antibodies. Before Orgaran is used as an alternative to heparin for HIT, Orgaran should be laboratory tested for cross-reactivity of heparin antibodies. Measurement of adequate anticoagulation can only be done through Orgaran (antiXa) plasma levels; not standard coagulation parameters which are not reliable. For extracorporeal circulation, bolus dosages of 5000 U before bypass has prevented thromboembolic events with plasma levels between 1.0 to 1.5 U/ml.

The manufacturer of Orgaran also has recommended priming the heart-lung machine with 7500 U of Organon; but the priming increases the risk of postoperative bleeding. Orgaran has antiXa activity and can only be partially antagonized by protamine or fresh-frozen plasma; no specific antidote is currently available. For vascular surgery or postoperative anticoagulation, drug levels (antiXa levels) of 0.4 to 0.8 U/ml provides adequate anticoagulation. This can be accomplished by a bolus injection of 400 U/hr x 2 to 4 hr followed by 300 U/hr x 2 to 4 hrs, then a maintenance infusion of 150 to 200 U/hr.

Ancrod, derived from the Malayan pit viper, is a defibrinogenating agent with no cross-reactivity with heparin. Ancrod is usually given by a continuous, intravenous infusion to maintain fibrinogen concentrations of 0.2 to 0.7 g/l during extracorporeal circulation. The activated clotting time (ACT) is not a reliable measurement of anticoagulation. Instead, fibrinogen concentrations should be measured directly. For anticoagulation postoperatively, ancrod should start at 1 to 2 U/kg given over 6 hours intravenously. Then, additional doses of 1 to 2 U/kg should be given subcutaneously or intravenously once a day to achieve a fibrinogen level of 0.5 to 1.0 g/l. Ancrod-induced hypofibrinogenemia can be reversed by infusion of fibrinogen from cryoprecipitate.

Low-molecular-weight heparin (enoxaparin) can potentially be used instead of heparin, but enoxaparin can cause thrombocytopenia in patients with a history of HIT. Slocum et al. found 34% of patients with HIT had positive platelet aggregation upon exposure to low-molecular-weight heparin. However, Slocum et al. also concluded that low-molecular-weight heparin could be used safely in HIT patients who had negative-platelet aggregometry tests with exposure to low-molecular-weight heparin. Enoxaparin is a viable option for anticoagulation in HIT patients only after appropriate negative-platelet aggregometry testing.

Idiopathic Thrombocytopenia Purpura (ITP)

Idiopathic thrombocytopenia purpura (ITP) is classically defined as thrombocytopenia without any other etiologies and a normal bone marrow and spleen. In children, the onset of thrombocytopenia is abrupt and severe and often preceded by a viral exanthem or upper respiratory illness. Ninety percent of children will fully recover by 4 months. In adults, ITP presents with a less acute onset. The disease course is chronic with a low, spontaneous remission rate. The thrombocytopenia is caused by platelet destruction from autoantibodies against platelet-membrane glycoproteins.

Management of ITP

Platelet counts above 30,000/mm^3 are usually adequate to prevent spontaneous bleeding; patients are often observed without treatment. For most surgeries, platelet counts above 50,000/mm^3 are safe. Although thrombocytopenia exists, platelet function is normal. For surgery with risk for significant bleeding, the adequacy of the existing platelet count can be investigated with a bleeding time.

Treatment options include prednisone, IV immunoglobulin, azathioprine, cyclophosphamide, and splenectomy. First-line therapy consists of prednisone 1 mg/kg for 2 to 3 weeks, in which two-thirds of patients will have a significant increase in platelet count. However, the majority of patients will relapse when the prednisone is tapered. Intravenous immunoglobulin used intermittently can quickly increase platelet count within a few days. Cyclophosphamide and azathioprine are used for chronic management to avoid long-term corticosteroid toxicity.

Splenectomy resolves ITP in two thirds of patients. Splenectomy is preserved in adults with an acute, severe onset unresponsive to prednisone, or patients requiring chronic prednisone dosages of 10 mg or more for several months. Platelet counts begin to rise within a few days of a splenectomy. As mentioned previously, all patients undergoing a splenectomy should have at least *S. pneumoniae* and possibly *H. influenzae B* vaccine 2 weeks or more before surgery.

Platelet transfusions should be avoided before a splenectomy or other surgeries. Any platelets transfused will have a life span potentially of less than 1 hour. Instead, significant thrombocytopenia should be treated with larger dosages of prednisone (1 mg/kg), starting at least 1 week before surgery or IV immunoglobulin 1 g/kg for 2 days given 3 days before surgery.

Splenectomies have been done with platelet counts as low as 10,000/mm^3. Platelets should be available in the operating room, but only given for significant bleeding. If a platelet transfusion must be given, then IV immunoglobulin at 1 g/kg should be given before platelet administration, and, for a splenectomy, platelet transfusions should be given after the splenic pedicle is clamped.

Platelet Dysfunction

Platelet dysfunction is characterized by a normal platelet count but inadequate primary hemostasis because of a defect in the platelet itself or a defect in a coagulation component interacting with platelets. These disorders include Von Willebrand's disease, Bernard-Soulier, Glanzmann's thrombasthenia, platelet granular disorders, and drug-acquired platelet dysfunction.

VON WILLEBRAND'S DISEASE (VWD)

Von Willebrand's disease (VWD) is the most common inherited bleeding disorder, with an estimated prevalence of 1 in 1000 individuals. Von Willebrand's disease is inherited in an autosomal-dominant pattern with a penetrance of 60% to 90%, but, occasionally, it may have an autosomal-recessive pattern or be acquired. Classically, VWD presents with bleeding from mucocutaneous sites and, only rarely, with hemarthrosis, as seen in hemophiliacs. The disease is caused by a deficiency or abnormal structure of Von Willebrand's factor (VWf). Von Willebrand's factor causes platelet adhesion to the vascular submatrix, under high-shear stress conditions, by binding platelet-membrane receptors to the vascular endothelium. Most of VWf is synthesized by the vascular endothelium and lesser amounts by megakaryocytes. It is composed of a heterogeneous mixture of large, medium and small multimers. The high-molecular-weight (large) multimers of VWf are the key components for platelet aggregation and primary hemostasis. In the plasma, VWf acts as a carrier for factor VIII and forms a noncovalent complex with factor VIII, which allows factor VIII activation by thrombin.

The diagnosis of VWD is made by a combination of a prolonged bleeding time, reduced VWf concentration (VWf:Ag), reduced factor-VIII activity, and reduced ristocetin cofactor-activity. Reduction in factor-VIII activity is not universal in all forms of VWD. Factor VIII activity may be normal or only moderately reduced in milder forms of VWD. Hence, the activated PTT may be normal in VWD, and is not a good screening test for VWD. Ristocetin is an antibiotic that induces platelet agglutination in the presence of normal amounts of VWf in the plasma. The ristocetin cofactor test (VWfR:Co) is a quantitative assay, using formalin-fixed normal platelets which agglutinate in the presence of various concentrations of VWf. The assay is a measure of both function and amount of VWf and usually is directly proportional to VWf levels (VWf:Ag) in the majority of VWD patients. The ristocetin cofactor assay is done in a shorter time than directly measuring VWf levels (VWf:Ag), and, therefore, the VWfR:Co assay is most often used to determine efficacy of various treatments.

VWD may be subdivided into three types. Types I and III are quantitative disorders with reduction of plasma VWf, but usually no abnormalities in structure or function of VWf. Type II is a qualitative disorder of VWf with structural or functional abnormalities.

Type I

Type I VWD is the most common type of VWD with a 60% to 70% incidence. Clinical symptoms are variable but often mild. Laboratory tests reveal concurrent reduction of VWf concentration, ristocetin-cofactor activity, and factor VIII levels. Structure and function of VWf is normal with a full range of multimers. The quantitative concentration of VWf is directly measured by VWf:Ag levels measured by various immunoassays; VWf:Ag levels of 15 to 35 U/dl are considered mild. Levels below 5 U/dl are severe, and often associated with a significant bleeding diathesis.

Type II

Type II VWD is caused by a qualitative disorder with either structural and functional abnormalities of VWf. Type IIA is the second most common variant. It is caused by a deficiency of higher-molecular-weight (HMW) multimers, leading to an abnormal VWf function. Platelet agglutination and aggregation is diminished and laboratory studies reveal a greater reduction in VWfR:Co activity, compared to VWf:Ag. The VWf levels may be normal.

Type IIB is the third most common variant. These patients have loss of only the HMW multimers derived from endothelium. However, platelet-derived VWf multimers are normal. This discrepancy between VWf structures from the endothelium and platelets, can lead to spontaneous binding of VWf to platelets and increase platelet aggregation. This increased platelet aggregation can lead to increased clearance of platelets and HMW multimers from the plasma and thrombocytopenia. Laboratory tests reveal mild reduction of VWf:Ag, loss of HMW multimers on electrophoresis, and a relatively greater ristocetin-cofactor activity, compared to VWf:Ag, because of increased platelet aggregation.

Type III

Type III VWD is rare. Yet, it is the most serious type of VWD, with an estimated occurrence of 1 in 1,000,000. Patients have no detectable levels of VWf:Ag or VWfR:Co, and have low-factor-VIII levels less than 5 U/dl. Because of the need for frequent transfusions with plasma fractions, these patients often have antibodies that make perioperative management difficult.

Treatment Goals and Options

Goals of preoperative treatment for VWD in the case of major surgery, is to correct the VWf levels to 80 to 100 U/dl (normal = 100 U/dl) immediately before surgery, and then keep VWf levels above 40 U/dl for the initial 3 days postoperatively. The factor VIII levels should be kept at 50 U/dl (50% activity) during the perioperative period. For minor or moderate surgery with lower risk of bleeding, maintaining VWf levels, as measured by VWfR:Co, above 50 U/dl is sufficient. Bleeding times can be used as a measure of adequate therapy and usually normalize when VWf exceeds 50 U/dl. A VWfR:Co at 50 U/dl will often only partially correct the bleeding time, but is usually adequate for surgical hemostasis for low-bleeding risk surgery. Normalization of the bleeding time correlates with VWfR:Co greater than 50 U/dl and adequacy of treatment for high-risk surgery.

For plasma-derived products, there is approximately 1 unit of VWf per unit of factor VIII. Both VWf and factor VIII have a half-life of 12 hours and the dosing is similar to treatment for hemophilia A. A dose of 40 U/kg will increase VWf levels to 80 to 100 U/dl if no antibodies exist. Cryoprecipitate is the traditional therapy for exogenous von Willebrand factor. Typical dosing of cryoprecipitate is 1 U/10 kg every 12 to 24 hours and continuous transfusions for 2 to 3 days. The disadvantage of cryoprecipitate is the risk of viral transmission.

Factor-VIII concentrate is heat or solvent/detergent-treated to reduce infection risk and is used for treatment of VWD with variable success. The main problem with most factor-VIII concentrates is diminished VWf amounts or dysfunctional VWf with decrease HMW multimers or both. Factor VIII made from monoclonal antibodies or recombinant factor VIII contains only small amounts of VWf. However, Humate-P, an intermediate purity concentration, is used effectively because of increased VWf with HMW multimers. Humate-P should only be used with the realization that not all patients get a predictable correction of a bleeding time. This variability is caused by HMW multimers being partially damaged in the purification process.

1-Desamino-8-D-arginine vasopressin (DDAVP) is an analogue of the antidiuretic hormone (vasopressin) with a reduced vasopressor response. Also known as desmopressin, DDAVP causes a 2- to 6-fold increase in factor VIII and VWf from release of stored factors in the vascular endothelium. Most of the released VWf consists of HMW multimers, which are particularly effective in promoting platelet adhesion to the vascular endothelium. Tachyphylaxis to DDAVP can occur with more than two doses within a 24-hour period because of depletion of stored factors. If a patient undergoes repeat dosing of DDAVP every 12 to 24 hours for more than a single day, then a postinfusion VWfR:Co should be monitored for evidence of tachyphylaxis. Responsiveness to DDAVP will return after a treatment-free interval. Preoperatively, a VWfR:Co assay should be checked after a DDAVP dosing, if one has not been checked previously, to document an adequate response.

The usual dosage of DDAVP is 0.3 μg/kg given intravenously over 20 to 30 minutes. Dosages above 0.3 μg/kg will not further increase release of VWf. Peak response is within 30 to 60 minutes and half-life of the release of VWf is 12 hours. Side effects of DDAVP include vasodilatation, hypotension, and facial flushing which are reduced with slow administration. Hyponatremia is usually only a risk with repeat dosing.

PERIOPERATIVE MANAGEMENT OF VON WILLEBRAND'S DISEASE TYPES

Type I

Type I VWD is a deficiency in the amount, but not function, of VWf. Hence, DDAVP is the mainstay of treatment in the immediate perioperative period. Most patients with Type I VWD will have an adequate response from DDAVP. A small subset of patients, especially with low baseline levels of VWf (i.e., <15 U/dl) or diminished levels of platelet-associated VWf, may have an inadequate response to DDAVP. Therefore, documentation of adequate response to DDAVP should be done 1 hour after infusion. VWf levels of 40 to 50 U/dl after DDAVP is considered an adequate response. For low-bleeding-risk surgery, DDAVP alone is often adequate treatment given every 12 hours for 48 hours. However, cryoprecipitate or Humate-P should be available because of the risk of tachyphylaxis to DDAVP.

For high-bleeding-risk surgery, 30 to 40 U/kg of plasma concentrate should be given to increase VWf levels to 80 to 100 U/dl during surgery, then 15 to 20 U/kg every 12 hours to keep VWf above 50 U/dl for 3 days postoperatively. This can be followed by once a day DDAVP-dosing for postoperative days 4 to 7. Any repeat dosing of DDAVP should have serum sodium checked daily for hyponatremia (Table 18-4).

Type IIA

Type IIA VWD is marked by a discordantly greater decrease in VWf:Co compared to VWf levels. This signifies dysfunctional VWf caused by absent high- and intermediate-molecular-weight multimers. Desmopressin is often inadequate because the released VWf is lacking the HMW multimers. It should only be given with prior documentation of adequate VWfR:Co activity above 50 U/dl.

The majority of patients will require cryoprecipitate or Humate-P. For minor surgery, 15 to 20 U/kg is adequate for one or two dosings, with repeat dosing given as needed for bleeding. For major surgery with risk of significant bleeding, initial

Table 18-4. Treatment of VWD

TYPE	TYPE OF HEMORRHAGE	THERAPY	DOSE AND DURATION
I Moderate/severe	Minor	DDAVP	0.3 μg/kg* daily for 1–2 doses 15–20 μ/kg
	Major/surgical		30–40 U/kg bolus then 15–20 U/kg every 12 hr to maintain VWf activity >50 U/dL for 3 days, then DDAVP once daily for 3–7 days in patients who respond to DDVAP.[†] For patients who do not respond, continue Humate P, 15–25 U/kg for 3–7 days.
I Mild	Minor	DDAVP	0.3 μg/kg* daily for 1–2 doses
	Major/surgical	DDAVP	0.3 μg/kg every 12 hr for 2–3 days in patients who achieve VWf activity >100 U/dL after DDAVP, then 0.3 μg/kg once daily for 3–5 days. 20–30 U/kg every 12 hr to maintain VWf activity >50 U/dL for 3 days, then DDAVP once daily for 3–5 days in patients who respond to DDAVP
IIA	Minor	DDAVP	15–20 U/kg; 0.3 μg/kg* daily for 1–2 doses
	Major/surgical		30–40 U/kg bolus, then 15–25 U/kg every 12 hrs to maintain VWf activity >50 U/dL for 3 days, then 15–25 U/kg every day for 3–5 days
IIB	Minor		15–20 U/kg
	Major/surgical		30–40 U/kg, bolus then 15–25 U/kg every 12 hrs to maintain VWf activity 50 U/dL for 3 days, then 15–25 U/kg every day for 3–5 days
III	Minor		10–20 U/kg
	Major/surgical		30–50 U/kg bolus, then 15–25 U/kg every 12 hr to maintain VWf/FVIII >50 U/dL for 3 days, then 15–25 U/kg every day for 3–5 days

* The use of DDAVP in this circumstance is dependent on knowing that the patient previously had a good response to DDAVP. For minor and moderate bleeding, a VWf level of 40–50 U/dL or normalization of the bleeding time 1 hr after infusion usually represents an adequate response.

[†] Patients receiving repetitive doses of DDAVP should be monitored for hyponatremia and for the development of tachyphylaxis with serial measurements of VWf activity.

(Adapted with permission from Montgomery RR, Coller BS. In *Hemostasis and Thrombosis Basic Principles and Clinical Practice*, ed 3, Colman RW, et al, eds: Philadelphia, 1994, JB Lippincott Co.)

dosing of 30 to 40 U/kg should be given. This is followed by 15 to 25 U/kg every 12 hours for 3 days to maintain VWfR:Co activity greater than 50 U/dL; then a dosage of 15 to 25 U/kg per day should be given for postoperative days 4 to 7 (see Table 18-4).

Type IIB

Type-IIB patients are missing only the highest molecular-weight multimer from endothelium-derived VWf. This dysfunctional VWf causes increased platelet aggregation and so, will have a discordantly greater increase VWfR:Co activity, compared to VWf levels.

Desmopressin is relatively contraindicated because the increased release of abnormal endothelium VWf leads to further increases in platelet aggregation, and further exacerbation of thrombocytopenia. For minor surgery, plasma concentrate of 15 to 20 U/kg should be given for 1 or 2 doses. For major high-risk-bleeding surgery, an initial dosage of 30 to 40 U/kg should be given, followed by 15 to 25 U/kg every 12 hours for 3 days maintaining VWf levels above 50 U/dl, then 15 to 25 U/kg for postoperative days 4 to 7. The VWfR:Co assay, which is normally done after infusions, is likely not an accurate marker of actual VWf level because of the VWfR:Co being disproportionately higher than the VWf level (see Table 18-4).

Type III

Type III-VWD patients have almost absent extracellular VWf and intracellular endothelium and platelet stores of VWf. Hence, DDAVP will not raise VWf levels. For minor surgery, 15 to 20 U/kg of plasma concentrate should be given for 1 or 2 doses. For major surgery, 40 U/kg should be bolused, followed by 15 to 25 U/kg every 12 hours to maintain VWfR:Co activity above 50 U/dl for 3 days. Then 15 to 25 U/kg per day should be given for postoperative days 4 to 7. Patients with Type-III disease are likely to have received multiple, prior plasma-concentrate infusions. They are at increased risk for having antiVWf antibodies which complicate therapy. Therefore, appropriate responsiveness to plasma concentrate should be documented before surgery. Platelet transfusions can be used with good success in patients with VWf antibodies. The platelet transfusion provides an additional source of VWf not affected by alloantibodies (see Table 18-4).

Platelet Hereditary Abnormalities

Many rare platelet hereditary abnormalities exist that increase the risk of significant perioperative bleeding. In contrast to VWD, these platelet abnormalities usually can only be treated by transfusion of platelets because the primary defect is the platelet itself and not a certain component interacting with platelets.

Bernard-Soulier disease is an autosomal-recessive disorder manifesting with a prolonged bleeding time, giant platelets, and thrombocytopenia. Bernard-Soulier platelets are deficient in the glycoprotein GPIb-IX, the binding site of VWf. Therefore, platelet adhesion to the subendothelial matrix under high-shear conditions is decreased. This abnormality perioperatively can only be corrected with a platelet transfusion of normal platelets.

Glanzmann's thrombasthenia is an autosomal-recessive disorder manifested by a prolonged bleeding time but with normal platelet morphology and count. Platelet dysfunction is caused by absent platelet aggregation with collagen. Perioperatively, patients should receive an infusion of HLA-matched platelets before surgery. HLA-matched platelets should be used for all platelet defect disorders to limit platelet alloimmunization for future platelet transfusions.

PLATELET GRANULE DISORDERS

Gray platelet and dense-granule-deficiency syndromes result in deficiencies in certain key granular components on platelets responsible for platelet adhesion and aggregation. This subgroup of platelet disorders is unique because DDAVP at 0.3 µg/kg in one or two doses likely can be used alone for surgeries with low risk of bleeding. An appropriate correction of the bleeding time should be documented before surgery, because not all patients with platelet granular disorders respond to DDAVP. Instead, they may require platelet transfusions.

DRUG-ACQUIRED PLATELET DYSFUNCTION

Aspirin, nonsteroidal antiinflammatory drugs (NSAIDs), ticlopidine, β-lactam antibiotics, and plasma expanders can all cause platelet dysfunction. Aspirin causes irreversible inhibition of platelet cyclooxygenase, leading to a deficiency in thromboxane A_2, the final product of the platelet arachidonic metabolism. Thromboxane A_2 activates platelet membrane receptors and increases aggregation by promoting platelet granular secretion. Hence, platelets exposed to aspirin have impaired aggregation, increasing the risk of surgical bleeding.

Perioperatively, aspirin should be discontinued for at least 5 days before surgery. This period of 5 days without aspirin exposure is sufficient to allow one half the platelets to be replaced with normal platelets, given the normal platelet lifespan of 10 days. Patients with normal platelet function and count should have adequate surgical hemostasis after 5 days from last aspirin exposure.

Most patients with recent aspirin exposure do not have significantly increased blood loss from most surgeries, unless there is an additional insult to platelet dysfunction, such as cardiopulmonary bypass or heparinization. Patients with significant surgical bleeding from suspected aspirin-induced platelet dysfunction should initially be treated with DDAVP. Platelet transfusions are effective but should only be used as a last course of treatment for excessive bleeding.

Ticlopidine causes a dose-dependent inhibition of platelet aggregation by inhibiting adenosine diphosphate–induced, platelet-fibrinogen binding. Ticlopidine causes irreversible platelet dysfunction. The terminal elimination half-life of ticlopidine is 4 to 5 days with chronic use. Because of ticlopidine's long elimination half-life and causing irreversible platelet dysfunction, ticlopidine should be discontinued 10 to 14 days prior to surgery. For emergency surgery, 20 mg of intravenous methylprednisolone will normalize a prolong bleeding time from ticlopidine within hours. Methylprednisolone administration is a viable treatment to limit potential excessive bleeding from ticlopidine exposure during the perioperative period.

Other NSAIDs cause temporary cyclooxygenase inhibition only as long as the NSAID is present in the circulation. Platelet dysfunction usually only lasts for 4 to 8 hours after the NSAID is stopped. For elective surgery, an NSAID should be stopped the evening before surgery.

Plasma Expanders

The dextrans are branched polysaccharides of glucose. Dextran 70 or dextran 40 (low-molecular-weight dextran) is used in the perioperative period. Besides both dextrans being plasma expanders, the dextrans also affect platelet function. Dextran infusions impair platelet aggregation and reduce VWf concentration. Dextran infusions are particularly useful for perioperative deep venous thrombosis prevention because of altering platelet function without an increased risk of bleeding.

Hydroxyethyl starch (hetastarch) is a plasma expander used perioperatively for rapid volume expansion. Hydroxyethyl starch does decrease factor VIII, fibrinogen, Von Willebrand's factor and platelet aggregation. The significance of these changes in the case of perioperative bleeding remains unclear due to multiple conflicting studies. The literature does show an increased tendency for a prolongation of the bleeding time, PT, and PTT when large amounts of hydroxyethyl starch are given in the presence of another hemostatic defect, such as a dilutional coagulopathy, caused by a massive transfusion. However, Warren and Durieux upon review of the literature noted an idiosyncratic response to hydroxyethyl starch. They found that small amounts of hydroxyethyl starch may cause a coagulopathy, yet in other patients large amounts of hydroxyethyl starch caused no coagulopathy. They concluded that it is difficult to recommend a maximum safe dose of hydroxyethyl starch and that hydroxyethyl starch should not be used in a patient with a known coagulopathy.

BIBLIOGRAPHY

Aster RH: Heparin-induced thrombocytopenia and thrombosis, *N Engl J Med* 332:1374–1376, 1995.

Berchtold P, McMillan R: Therapy of chronic idiopathic thrombocytopenic purpura in adults, *Blood* 74:2309–2317, 1989.

Beutler E: Glucose-6-phosphate dehydrogenase deficiency, *N Engl J Med* 324:169–174, 1991.

Cole CW, et al: Ancrod versus heparin for anticoagulation during vascular surgical procedures, *J Vasc Surg* 17:288–293, 1993.

Desager JP: Clinical pharmacokinetics of ticlopidine, *Clin Pharmacokin* 26:347–355, 1994.

Embury SH: Sickle cell disease. In Hoffman R, et al, editors: *Hematology: basic principles and practice*, ed 2, New York, 1995, Churchill Livingstone. 648.

Fox MA, Abbott TR: Hypothermic cardiopulmonary bypass in a patient with sickle-cell trait, *Anaesthesia* 39:1121–1123, 1984.

George JN, el-Harke MA, Raskob GE: Chronic idiopathic thrombocytopenia purpura, *N Engl J Med* 331:1207–1211, 1994.

George JN, Shattil SJ: Acquired disorders of platelet function. In Hoffman R, et al, editors: *Hematology: basic principles and practice*, ed 2, New York, 1995, Churchill-Livingstone.

Griffin TC, Buchanan GR: Elective surgery in children with sickle cell disease without preoperative blood transfusion, *J Pediatr Surg* 28:681–685, 1993.

Kappa JR, et al: Intraoperative management of patients with heparin-induced thrombocytopenia, *Ann Thorac Surg* 49:714–723, 1990.

Koshy M, et al: Surgery and anesthesia in sickle cell disease, *Blood* 86:3676–3684, 1995.

Logan LJ: Treatment of von Willebrand's disease, *Hematol Oncol Clin North Am* 6:1079–1094, 1992.

Montgomery RR, Coller BS: Von Willebrand disease. In Colman RW, et al, editors: *Hemostasis and thrombosis: basic principles and clinical practice,* Philadelphia, 1994, JB Lippincott Co.

Ogin GA: Cholecystectomy in a patient with paroxysmal nocturnal hemoglobinuria: anesthetic implications and management in the perioperative period, *Anesthesiology* 72:761–764, 1990.

Paglia DE: Enzymopathies. In Hoffman R, et al, editors: *Hematology: basic principles and practice*, ed 2, New York, 1995, Churchill-Livingstone.

Park JV, Weiss CI: Cardiopulmonary bypass and myocardial protection: management problems in cardiac surgical patients with cold autoimmune disease, *Anesth Analg* 67:75–78, 1988.

Reithmuller R, Grundy EM, Radley-Smith R: Open heart surgery in a patient with homozygous sickle cell disease, *Anaesthesia* 37:324–327, 1982.

Schrier SL: *Anemia: hemolysis, scientific american medicine.* In Rubenstein E, Federman DD. 5:IV, New York, 1995, Scientific American Incorporated.

Schwartz E, Benz EJ Jr, Forget BG: Thalassemia syndromes. In Hoffman R, Benz EJ Jr, Shattil SJ, et al, editors: *Hematology: basic principles and practice*, ed 2, New York, 1995, Churchill Livingstone.

Schwartz RS, Silberstein LE, Berkman EM: Autoimmune hemolytic anemias. In Hoffman R, et al, editors: *Hematology: basic principles and practice*, New York, 1995, Churchill-Livingstone.

Slocum MM, et al: Use of enoxaparin in patients with heparin-induced thrombocytopenia syndrome, *J Vasc Surg* 23:839–843, 1996.

Snyder EL: Transfusion reactions. In Hoffman R, et al, editors: *Hematology: basic principles and practice*, ed. New York, 1995, Churchill-Livingstone.

Sokol RJ, et al: Patients with red cell autoantibodies: selection of blood for transfusion, *Clin Lab Haematol* 10:257–264, 1988.

Sokol RJ, Booker DJ, Stamps R: The pathology of autoimmune haemolytic anaemia, *J Clin Pathol* 45:1047–1052, 1992.

Spiekermann BF, et al: Normal activated clotting time despite adequate anticoagulation with ancrod in a patient with heparin-associated thrombocytopenia and thrombosis undergoing cardiopulmonary bypass, *Anesthesiology* 80:686–688, 1994.

Vichinsky EP, et al: A comparison of conservative and aggressive transfusion regimens in the perioperative management of sickle cell disease, *N Engl J Med* 333:206–213, 1995.

Warkentin TE, et al: Heparin-induced thrombocytopenia in patients treated with low-molecular-weight heparin or unfractionated heparin, *N Engl J Med* 332:1330–1335, 1995.

Warkentin TE, Trimble MS, Kelton JG: Thrombocytopenia due to platelet destruction and hypersplenism. In Hoffman R, et al, editors: *Hematology: basic principles and practice*, ed 2, New York, 1995, Churchill-Livingstone.

Warren BB, Durieux ME: Hydroxyethyl starch: Safe or not? *Anesth Analg* 84:206–212, 1997.

Wilhelm MJ, et al: Cardiopulmonary bypass in patients with heparin-induced thrombocytopenia using Org 10172, *Ann Thorac Surg* 61:920–924, 1996.

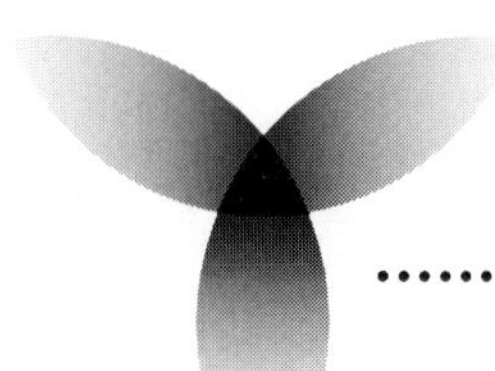

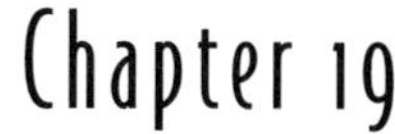

Perioperative Management of the Oncology Patient

Donald D. Mathes, MD

Perioperative management of the oncology patient can be challenging for the physician. Multiple problems, resulting directly from cancer or treatment of cancer, increase the potential for morbidity in the perioperative period. The perioperative physician

Parts of this chapter were adapted from Mathes DD, Bogdonoff DL: Preoperative evaluation of the cancer patient. In Lefor AT, editor: Surgical problems affecting the patient with cancer: Interdisciplinary Management, Philadelphia, 1996, Lippincott-Raven Press, pp. 273–304.

needs to have an understanding of what potential problems are associated with the oncology patient to anticipate and decrease the incidence of perioperative complications. This chapter will focus on the management of potential perioperative problems, resulting from cancer itself, and the treatment of cancer.

HEAD AND NECK CANCER

Perioperative management of patients with head and neck cancer can be particularly challenging because of the ever-present potential for severely distorted airway anatomy. In addition, these patients often have other pathologic sequelae from associated long-standing alcohol and tobacco abuse.

Of utmost concern to the anesthesiologist is airway management in patients undergoing head- and neck-tumor resection. Obviously, large tumors encroaching near the larynx usually require an awake fiberoptic intubation or awake tracheostomy before induction of general anesthesia. However, patients with apparently normal airway anatomy on examination still may be difficult to intubate. Distortion of airway anatomy from a tumor can occur insidiously in an asymptomatic patient and not be recognized until after induction of general anesthesia and direct laryngoscopy. Review of the neck computed tomography (CT) scans and good communication with a surgeon, who has previously visualized the airway by indirect laryngoscopy or fiberoptic visualization, is helpful in determining the safest mode of securing the airway.

Besides tumor invasion of the airway, prior radiation therapy to the head and neck can lead to further distortion of airway anatomy. Edema and swelling of airway tissue can occur acutely after radiation treatment but normally resolves shortly after radiation therapy. Fibrosis of the soft tissue of the airway and neck can also occur from prior radiation therapy. This fibrosis can cause loss of mobility and displacement of airway tissue, leading to a difficult or impossible intubation. Examination of the external neck anatomy, including the mobility of the mental to hyoid soft tissue, often will allow the perioperative physician to be forewarned of a difficult airway from radiation therapy.

Hence, the anesthesiologist should approach airway securement in a patient with head and neck cancer with utmost caution. The anesthesiologist should have a low threshold for proceeding with an awake intubation or tracheostomy before the induction of anesthesia.

Postoperatively, the perioperative physician can have further difficulty maintaining the airway because of edema of the larynx and other structures. The trauma of surgery on the airway and adjacent structures can lead to severe edema. Often, dosages of 0.5 mg/kg of dexamethasone are given to limit the extent of airway edema. In addition, prior radiation therapy can obliterate the lymphatic and venous channels within the airway and further worsen airway edema, postoperatively. The prudent perioperative physician will often allow the patient to remain intubated and sitting up during the initial postoperative period, as well as document an adequate cuff leak before extubation.

• MEDIASTINAL MASSES

Anatomy of the Mediastinum

The mediastinum is composed of anterior, middle, and posterior compartments (Figure 19-1). The anterior compartment is the space in front of and superior to the heart shadow, and contains the thymus gland, any substernal extension of the thyroid gland, the aortic arch, and innominate vein and lymphatic tissues. The middle compartment contains the pericardium, heart, tracheobronchial tree, and lymphatic tissue. The posterior compartment is defined as the area from the posterior vertebral body to an imaginary line just anterior to the vertebral bodies. The posterior compartment contains the esophagus, descending aorta, and paravertebral lymph nodes.

Preoperative Evaluation

Perioperative management of a patient with an anterior or middle mediastinal mass is associated with significant risk of serious intraoperative and postoperative complications. These masses can encroach and obstruct the tracheobronchial tree, pulmonary artery, superior vena cava, and heart. Large posterior mediastinal masses still need to be managed cautiously intraoperatively because of the potential encroachment into the middle mediastinal space. In adults, the majority of anterior and middle mediastinal masses are metastatic-bronchogenic carcinomas or lymphomas; but teratomas, enlarged retrosternal thyroids, thymomas, bronchogenic cysts, or pericardial cysts are among a list of many possible sources (Box 19-1).

Definitive treatment is dependent upon tissue diagnosis of the mass. A specimen of the mass should be obtained before treatment to make an accurate pathologic diagnosis and determine the type of treatment plan. Before considering a biopsy of a mediastinal mass, other noninvasive locations, such as axillary or supraclavicular lymph nodes, need to be excluded as possible biopsy sites.

A thorough preoperative evaluation is essential for seeking evidence of compression of any vital structures within the mediastinum. Patients with anterior or middle mediastinal masses may be at high risk for complete airway obstruction or cardiopulmonary arrest upon induction of general anesthesia. Under general anesthesia, extrinsic tracheobronchial compression, distal to the tip of the endotracheal tube, can lead to the inability to ventilate. Furthermore, compression of the pulmonary artery and heart from the mediastinal mass can lead to cardiopulmonary arrest under general anesthesia.

A history of postural dyspnea in any position, stridor, or wheezing should warn the physician of potential airway obstruction. In addition, postural cyanosis or syncope are compatible with pulmonary artery or cardiac compression. Upper extremity and facial swelling with jugular venous distention strongly suggest superior-vena-cava syndrome. General anesthesia should be avoided, if at all possible, if there are any positive findings on history and physical examination of possible mediastinal compression of vital structures.

In the asymptomatic patient, a CT scan of the chest, inspiratory and expiratory flow volume loops, and possible echocardiography should be performed on patients

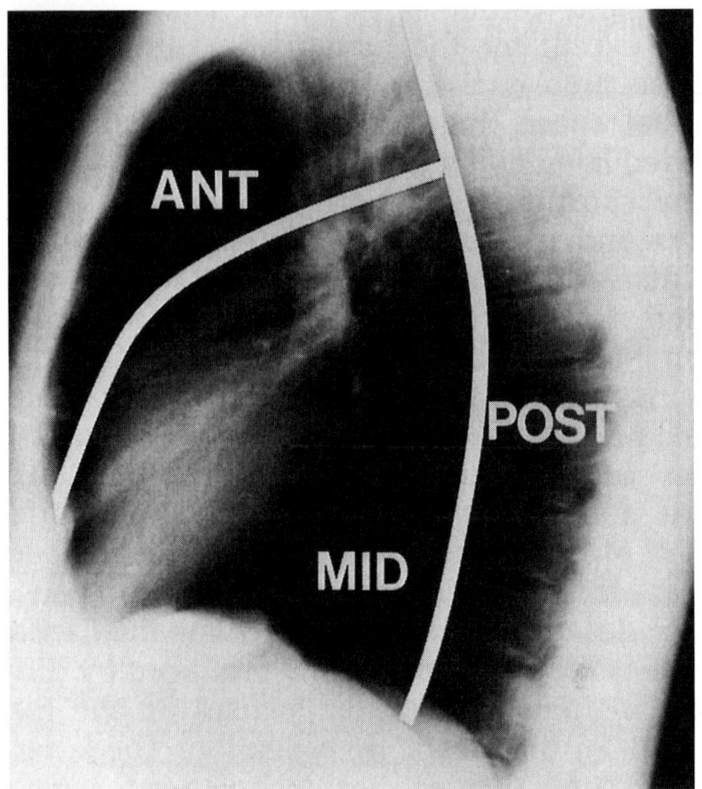

Figure 19-1
The mediastinum is divided into anterior (*ANT*), middle (*MID*), and posterior (*POST*) compartments as seen on a lateral chest radiograph. (Used with permission from Pierson DJ: Disorders of the mediastinum. In Murray JF, Nadel JA, editors: *Textbook of respiratory medicine*, Philadelphia, 1988, WB Saunders, p. 1782.)

with any large anterior or middle mediastinal mass, to rule out occult tracheobronchial, pulmonary artery, or cardiac compression. The CT scan of the mediastinum should be reviewed closely for tracheobronchial compression or encroachment of the pulmonary artery (Figure 19-2). In the pediatric population, Azizkhan et al. found over 30% extrinsic compression of the trachea on CT scan to be an accurate predictor of severe airway problems under general anesthesia.

Expiratory and inspiratory flow-volume loops are considered the most sensitive test for diagnosing occult airway compression. This test should be done in both supine and upright positions. Most often with intrathoracic airway impingement, a prolonged expiratory plateau is found with the patient in the supine position, which improves in the upright position (Figure 19-3). A large reduction of maximal expi-

Box 19-1 Mediastinal Masses

ANTERIOR	MIDDLE	POSTERIOR
Metastatic cancer	Metastatic cancer	Neurogenic tumor
Lymphoma	Lymphoma	Lymphoma
Retrosternal thyroid	Bronchogenic cyst	Aortic aneurysm
Thymoma	Pericardial cyst	Diaphragmatic hernia
Teratoma	Teratoma	
Cystic hygroma	Aortic aneurysm	
Aortic aneurysm		
Diaphragmatic hernia		

ratory flow should alert the perioperative physician to possible tracheomalacia and potential further difficulty of tracheal collapse upon extubation.

Echocardiography should be performed in both the supine and upright position if a CT scan reveals the mediastinal mass to be near any cardiac structure or pulmonary vessels, or if a patient has positive findings on history and physical examination. Echocardiography can be used to identify decreased cardiac filling and function from encroachment of the pericardium, heart, or pulmonary vessel by a mediastinal mass.

Intraoperative Management

If there are any positive findings on the noninvasive tests or on history and physical examination, then a biopsy should be done under local anesthesia. If local anesthesia cannot be performed, then the patient should begin treatment in an attempt to decrease the compression caused by the mediastinal mass. Radiation to the thorax can be used sparingly to leave a small window of unradiated tumor mass for biopsy. Also, pathologic diagnosis often can be made if obtained within a few days after beginning steroid or chemotherapy treatment. Again, before undergoing general anesthesia, the aforementioned noninvasive tests should be performed (Figure 19-4).

If general anesthesia is indicated, despite continued positive symptoms or findings after treatment of the mediastinal mass, then the following should be implemented: (1) an awake fiberoptic intubation; (2) continuous spontaneous ventilation throughout the general anesthetic; (3) rigid bronchoscope immediately available for placement to stent open a collapsed airway; (4) the ability to quickly change the patient to a lateral, prone, or sitting position if airway obstruction or cardiovascular collapse does occur; and (5) femoral-to-femoral cardiopulmonary bypass on immediate standby in the operating room, with the femoral area prepped and the pump primed in the event of cardiopulmonary collapse.

With general anesthesia, airway caliber is reduced because of the loss of the normal tethering effect on the airway and decreased tension of inspiratory smooth muscle. Also, under general anesthesia, there is loss of physiologic positive end-expiratory pressure (PEEP), and cephalad movement of the diaphragm. All these physiologic

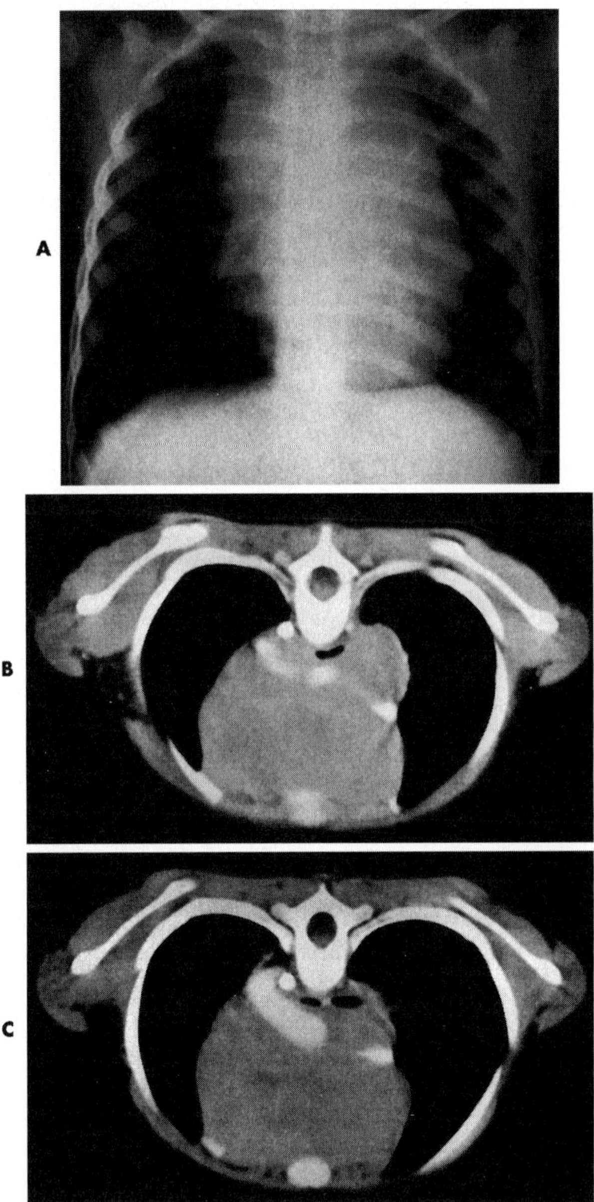

Figure 19-2

A. Chest radiograph showing widening of the mediastinum. B.CT scan of chest at the third thoracic vertebra level showing tracheal compression by the anterior mediastinal mass. C. CT scan of chest at fifth thoracic vertebra level showing bronchial compression. (Used with permission from Akhtar TM, Ridley S, Best CJ: Unusual presentation of acute upper airway obstruction caused by an anterior mediastinal mass, *Br J Anaesth* 67:632, 1991.)

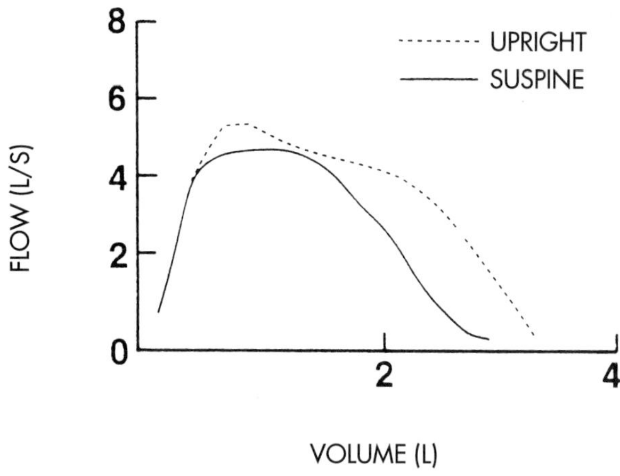

Figure 19-3
Flow-volume loop before radiation therapy in upright and supine positions with significant reduction in vital capacity and expiratory flow rates. The expiratory flow rate plateau is indicative of intrathoracic airway obstruction. (Used with permission from Neuman GG, et al: The anesthetic management of the patient with an anterior mediastinal mass, *Anesthesiology* 60:144, 1984.)

changes under general anesthesia can cause complete airway collapse from extrinsic compression. Furthermore, positive-pressure ventilation and muscle relaxation will cause loss of the negative, transpleural pressure gradient that normally helps keep the airway open. Hence, under general anesthesia, both positive-pressure ventilation and muscle relaxants should be avoided. If awake fiberoptic intubation is not feasible (i.e., in the pediatric population) induction of anesthesia should be with spontaneous mask ventilation.

With awake fiberoptic intubation, examination of the entire trachea and major bronchi should be performed, looking for evidence of extrinsic compression. If extrinsic compression is seen in the trachea, then a single-lumen-armored endotracheal-tube tip should be placed beyond the compression site above the carina. If significant compression occurs at or just above the carina or mainstem bronchi, then elective endobronchial intubation should be performed in the unaffected bronchi before induction of anesthesia through a single- or double-lumen endotracheal tube.

Positioning can greatly exacerbate mediastinal mass compression of vital structures. Supine positioning causes a decrease in thoracic-cavity size and increases mediastinal mass compression from gravity. Placing the patient in the lateral decubitus position for a thoracotomy, with the affected side up, can cause cardiopulmonary collapse because of gravity of the compressing mass. Therefore, the anesthesiologist must be prepared to change position quickly to a prone, lateral position with the mediastinal mass side down or a semi-sitting position. Induction of anesthesia should be performed in a semi-sitting position.

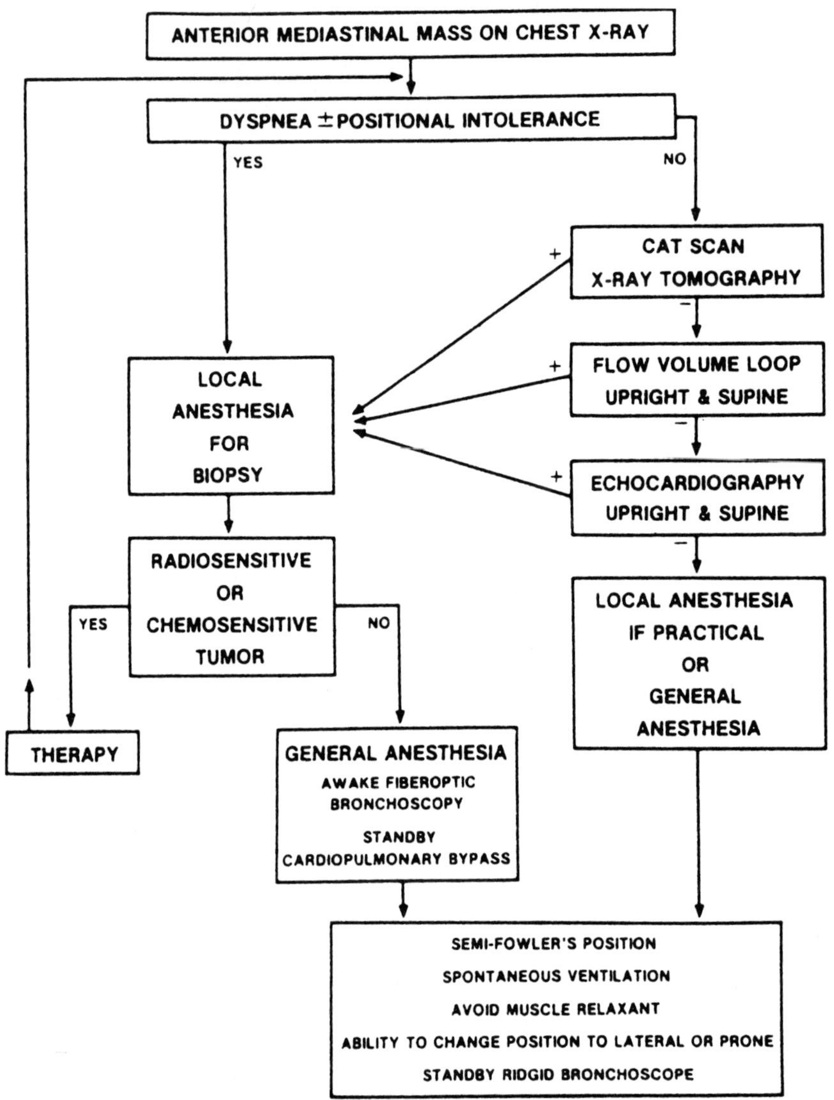

Figure 19-4
Algorithm for the preoperative evaluation of the patient with an anterior mediastinal mass, +, positive findings; –, negative workup. (Used with permission from Neuman GG, et al: The anesthetic management of the patient with an anterior mediastinal mass, *Anesthesiology* 60:144, 1984.)

Postoperative Management

Emergence from general anesthesia and the immediate postoperative period is a high-risk time for complete airway collapse. Coughing and bucking while intubated can lead to airway collapse caused by a rise in intrathoracic pressure. Tracheomalacia can cause dynamic airway collapse after extubation. After biopsy, manipulation or resection of a mediastinal mass, swelling, and hemorrhage can occur, causing further airway compression. Hence, extubation should be approached with utmost caution.

Before extubating, reexamination of the trachea and major bronchi should be done with the patient spontaneously ventilating. Evidence of significant extrinsic-airway compression, prior evidence of significant compression above the end of the endotracheal tube, or any difficulties with airway collapse intraoperatively, should be an indication for the patient to remain intubated until initial therapy can decrease the mediastinal-mass size. Extubation in the operating room can be performed with a deep extubation or, as this author prefers, with an intravenous lidocaine bolus of 1.0 to 1.5 mg/kg, followed by a lidocaine infusion of 3 to 5 mg/min in an adult, during the initial postoperative period to prevent coughing and dynamic-airway collapse upon extubating.

SUPERIOR VENA CAVA SYNDROME (SVCS)

Obstruction of the superior vena cava most often occurs from lung cancer. Preoperative evaluation should be the same as for mediastinal masses. SVCS can cause severe airway edema, distortion of airway anatomy, and vocal-cord paralysis. The anesthesiologist should have a low threshold for performing an awake intubation with any suspected airway abnormality. An arterial catheter should be placed in patients undergoing general anesthesia. All intravenous access should be in the lower extremity, and any central line should be placed from the femoral vein.

Any patient undergoing surgery on or near the affected structures is at high risk for significant bleeding from elevated venous pressures. Extubation should be performed cautiously because of the risk of significant airway edema and laryngospasm. The perioperative physician will, wisely, often leave the patient intubated until such treatment as radiation therapy or chemotherapy can decrease facial and airway edema.

HEMATOLOGIC ABNORMALITIES

The oncology patient can have multiple hematologic abnormalities ranging from anemia and thrombocytopenia to polycythemia vera, thrombocytosis, and hypercoagulable states. Anemia and thrombocytopenia are often caused by bone-marrow suppression from chemotherapy, radiation therapy, or direct infiltration of the tumor into the bone marrow. Often, these patients are already transfusion-dependent with little to no ability to increase bone-marrow production with further blood loss. For those patients, the perioperative physician should have a lower threshold for transfusing blood products during the perioperative period.

Blood Transfusions

Blood transfusions may increase cancer recurrence rates. Schriemer et al. in a review of the literature, found several studies showing a higher recurrence rate of colon, rectal, breast, cervical carcinomas, and soft-tissue sarcomas with perioperative blood transfusions in surgically treated oncology patients. The risk of recurrence appears to increase significantly in surgical patients who have received whole blood, or more than 3 units of homologous-packed red blood cells. The etiology of this higher recurrence rate appears to be from an unknown mediator in the plasma of transfused blood causing immunosuppression, especially the decrease of natural-killer cell activity. If blood is needed in the surgical oncology patient, it should be limited to packed red blood cells to reduce the amount of plasma transfused to the patient.

The use of prior-donated autologous blood is an effective method to limit the amount of homologous blood transfusions. There is no evidence that receiving autologous blood in the perioperative period increases the recurrence rate of cancer. However, for autologous blood to be effective, the patient needs to have normal bone-marrow function.

The use of cell-saver blood intraoperatively in the oncology patient remains controversial. Several studies have found no higher recurrence rate of malignancy in cell-saver blood used in urologic-cancer resections. Karczewski et al. found that filtration of cell-saver blood from leiomyosarcoma resection and radial cystectomy, filtered 94% of cancer cells from the blood. Of the remaining cancer cells in the cell-saver blood, none of these cancer cells was viable. Salsbury, in reviewing the literature, found circulating cancer cells in blood had minimal or no prognostic significance.

The risk of the hematogenous spread of cancer cells from cell-saver blood is likely less than the hematogenous spread from tumor resection itself. No definite recommendations can be made on the use of cell-saver blood from tumor resection at this time. The perioperative physician must weigh the known risk of immunosuppression and increased recurrence rate with large amounts of homologous blood versus the unclear risk of giving cell-saver blood.

Polycythemia Vera

Polycythemia vera is associated with certain malignancies: most notably, renal, adrenal, ovarian, uterine, and hepatic cancers. These tumors can secrete excessive erythropoietin. Hemoglobins should be reduced to below 15 g/dl to decrease risk of perioperative complications from both bleeding and thrombosis. It is important for perioperative physician to assure adequate intravascular repletion before surgery to decrease blood viscosity. Furthermore, during surgery, hypotension and venous stasis should be avoided. Postoperatively, aggressive measures to prevent deep-venous thrombosis should begin immediately in the recovery room.

Thrombocytosis

Thrombocytosis with platelet counts greater than 1,000,000/mm^3 may be caused by a reactive thrombocytosis associated with a solid malignancy, or an essential thrombocytosis associated with myeloproliferative disorders. When thrombocytosis is associated with either a solid tumor or a myeloproliferative disorder, the platelet count should be lowered below 1,000,000/mm^3 by either chemotherapy or platelet pheresis. In a patient with a malignancy, platelet counts above 1,000,000/mm^3 during the perioperative period are associated with both increased bleeding and thrombosis. Again, in the postoperative period, these patients should be treated with aggressive deep-venous thrombosis prevention.

COAGULATION ABNORMALITIES

Multiple coagulation abnormalities are associated with malignancy which can worsen during the perioperative period. Trousseu, in 1865, reported a strong association between thrombosis and malignancy. Increases in fibrinogen, fibrinogen turnover, and factors V, VIII, IX, and XI have been reported with malignancy. The oncology patient is at particular risk for deep-venous thrombosis postoperatively, which may occur from decreased antithrombin-III levels, along with preexisting elevation of several coagulation factors. Again, aggressive measures should be implemented in both the operating room and immediate postoperative period to prevent venous thrombosis.

Subclinical disseminated intravascular coagulopathy (DIC) is often found with malignancies. Clinically significant DIC is associated with mucin-secreting adenocarcinomas, especially of the prostate, pancreas, and stomach. During the perioperative period, surgical manipulation of these adenocarcinomas can release tissue thromboplastin, causing significant DIC. This is most notable after a prostatectomy for prostate cancer.

Acute promyelocytic leukemia often is associated with DIC, most notably after chemotherapy induction, from release of tissue thromboplastin. If clinical bleeding is not seen during DIC, low-dose heparin at approximately 7.5 U/kg/hr, along with replacement of coagulation factors and fibrinogen, may be used to control DIC.

Except for thrombocytopenia, hypocoagulable states are not usually seen in the oncology patient. An elevation in the prothrombin time (PT) or partial thromboplastin time (PTT) can be caused from among the following multiple etiologies: (1) a consumptive coagulopathy (DIC); (2) direct liver damage from the malignancy or chemotherapy; and (3) malabsorption or poor nutritional intake, leading to a vitamin K deficiency. Furthermore, certain malignancies such as multiple myeloma can produce paraproteins that surround coagulation factors, preventing normal function. Lastly, a lupus anticoagulant factor can be associated with malignancy. This factor causes a prolonged PT but paradoxically is associated more often with thrombosis.

MANAGEMENT OF THE BONE-MARROW-TRANSPLANT PATIENT

The perioperative care of a patient who is undergoing or has received a bone-marrow transplant, can be complicated by multiple problems. These include immunodeficiency, bone-marrow suppression, graft versus host disease, interstitial pneumonitis, and direct complications from high-dose chemotherapy and total-body irradiation.

Direct Toxicity of High-Dose Chemotherapy and Total-Body Irradiation

Much higher dosages of chemotherapy drugs and total-body irradiation are used as pretransplant treatment, compared to normal drug therapy. This results in severe pancytopenia, lasting approximately 3 weeks. After 3 weeks, the transplanted bone-marrow cells begin to restore bone-marrow function. Direct toxicity to other organs results in conditions including potentially fatal hepatic venoocclusive disease, severe cardiac toxicity from high-dose cyclophosphamide, and interstitial pneumonitis from high-dose *N,N*-bis(2-chloroethyl)-N-nitrosourea (BCNU) and other chemotherapy drugs (see subsection on chemotherapy toxicities). In addition, hypothyroidism caused by total-body irradiation occurs in almost 50% of patients within 6 to 24 months of bone-marrow transplant.

Immunodeficiency

Allogeneic bone-marrow-transplant patients continue to have abnormal B- and T-cell function for up to 1 year posttransplant. Furthermore, with chronic graft versus host disease (GVHD), T-cell function will continue to remain abnormal. Hence, these patients have a high incidence of opportunistic infections, especially during the first year after transplant. Interstitial pneumonitis is a common complication within the first year with cytomegalovirus (CMV) being the etiology in the majority of patients. Therefore, the perioperative physician must use sterile technique in all procedures, including delivery of drugs. Furthermore, the physician must be aware of the potential of concurrent, ongoing infection during the perioperative period.

Graft Vs Host Disease

Graft versus host disease occurs when the cells from the donor bone marrow react against the recipient tissue. Acute GVHD typically occurs within the first 100 days after a bone-marrow transplant and is often fatal. The skin, liver, and gastrointestinal (GI) tract are the predominant organs affected. Skin involvement ranges from a macular papular rash to diffuse erythroderma with desquamation. Nausea, vomiting, diarrhea, and abdominal pain are common GI symptoms. Liver involvement can range from mild elevation of transaminases to fulminant liver failure. A combination of cyclosporine, methotrexate, and corticosteroids are often used prophylactically in allogeneic transplants for the first 6 months to prevent acute GVHD.

Chronic GVHD occurs in approximately 25% of transplant patients who survive beyond 6 months. Generally, chronic GVHD presents similarly to other autoimmune diseases such as systemic lupus erythematosus with initial skin involvement, and can intensify to involve eyes, mouth, esophagus, large and small intestine, lungs, and liver. Furthermore, chronic GVHD patients remain immunocompromised with deficient T-cell function and have a higher incidence of severe infections. Treatment usually consists of a combination of azathioprine and corticosteroids. The perioperative physician must be aware of preexisting end-organ damage from GVHD during the perioperative period.

Blood Products in the Bone-Marrow-Transplant Patient

Seronegative-cytomegalovirus (CMV) patients should only receive CMV-seronegative-blood products. Infections with CMV can be prevented in CMV-seronegative patients by transfusion of CMV-free blood products. Many institutions have a paucity of CMV-negative blood and are now giving CMV-positive blood with leukocyte filter to CMV-negative patients. With a leukocyte filter, the risk of CMV transmission appears to be minimal.

All bone-marrow transplant or severe, immunocompromised patients should receive irradiated blood and platelets only. Irradiation prevents lymphocyte transmission and, thus, prevents the risk of GVHD activation from the transfusion of lymphocytes.

A potential, significant risk of giving irradiated blood is hyperkalemia from damage to the red blood cells from irradiation. Potassium levels have been found to be 2 to 3 times higher in blood that has been irradiated with 2000 to 3000 rads and stored for 5 days. The perioperative physician should strive to give freshly irradiated blood and be aware of an increased risk of significant hyperkalemia after transfusion, especially for irradiated blood stored for several days.

PARANEOPLASTIC SYNDROMES

Paraneoplastic syndromes include a wide spectrum of problems which may have important implications in the perioperative care of the oncology patient. These paraneoplastic syndromes can include fever, weight loss, and cachexia. They may also include connective tissue disorders such as polymyositis, dermatomyositis and scleroderma, and multiple neurologic and endocrine disorders. The perioperative physician should have a keen awareness of a paraneoplastic syndrome being the possible cause of all abnormalities found on history, physical, and laboratory examination. Neurologic and endocrine paraneoplastic syndromes are of the most concern to the perioperative physician, intraoperatively and postoperatively.

Neurologic

Oncology patients may have neurologic abnormalities to the central or peripheral nervous system, not related to metastatic lesions. These include muscle weakness from Eaton-Lambert syndrome, peripheral neuropathies, radiculopathies, as well as brain stem, cerebellar, and cerebral degeneration.

Eaton-Lambert syndrome presents in much the same way as myasthenia gravis, with muscle weakness. However, with Eaton-Lambert, extremity and pelvic muscle weakness may be the initial presentation instead of ocular-bulbar weakness. Also, muscle strength may improve with repetitive motion. Eaton-Lambert syndrome most often is associated with small-cell (oat-cell) bronchogenic carcinoma, but multiple other types of malignancy are associated with Eaton-Lambert syndrome.

The anesthesiologist should examine the oncology patient for any evidence of the multiple neurologic problems associated with malignancies. Any positive finding, such as a neuropathy, should have a thorough evaluation for possible metastatic spread to either the central or peripheral nervous system before surgery. In addition, patients with suspected Eaton-Lambert syndrome should not receive muscle relaxants or receive careful titration of short-acting muscle relaxants to a neuromuscular monitor because of the potential for underlying, prolonged muscle weakness.

Endocrine

Multiple endocrine disorders can arise from potential, abnormal hormonal productions, resulting from tumors. A screening electrolyte panel, along with history and physical examination, should be done preoperatively, to screen for associated endocrine disorders. The most common paraneoplastic endocrinopathies include excessive ACTH, ADH, and calcium-mobilizing substances. Other less common paraneoplastic endocrinopathies include hypoglycemia, hyperthyroidism, excessive renin, and erythropoietin production.

Ectopic corticotropin (ACTH) production is most commonly associated with oat-cell (small-cell) carcinoma of the lung. Thymic tumors, pancreatic carcinoma (usually, islet-cell), and bronchial adenoma (carcinoid), also have been associated with ectopic ACTH. Ectopic-ACTH syndrome does not normally present as typical Cushing's syndrome. Instead, patients with ectopic ACTH present with weight loss, muscle weakness, hyperpigmentation from excessive ACTH and melanotropic substances, and hypokalemic-metabolic alkalosis (see Chapter 16 on how to diagnose ectopic ACTH). Treatment consists of steroid inhibitors, usually a combination of metyrapone (11-β-hydroxylase enzyme inhibitor) and aminoglutethimide (which blocks the conversion of cholesterol to pregnenolone). Patients on steroid inhibitors should receive stress-steroid coverage during the perioperative period.

The syndrome of inappropriate secretion of antidiuretic hormone (SIADH) is known to be associated with oat-cell (small-cell) carcinoma, large-cell carcinoma, and adenocarcinoma of the lung. The syndrome of inappropriate secretion of antidiuretic hormone SIADH has been found in approximately 7% of patients with oat-cell carcinoma of the lung. It also has been associated with duodenal and pancreatic carcinoma (see Chapter 16 on how to diagnose SIADH). Any oncology patient found to have hyponatremia preoperatively should be suspected of having SIADH. Perioperative management includes fluid restriction and fluid replacements with 0.9 normal saline in the operating room.

Hypercalcemia, secondary to malignancy, can occur from several etiologies. Metastatic invasion of the bone, ectopic PTH-like substance, production of other calcium-mobilizing substances such as osteoclast-activating factor, and prostaglandins can all cause hypercalcemia. Treatment, as discussed in the chapter on common endocrine disorders, consists of hydration and loop diuretics. For severe hypercalcemia, mithramycin combined with phosphates are most effective. Osteolytic lesions causing hypercalcemia often are improved by local radiation therapy.

Besides islet-cell carcinoma, fasting hypoglycemia is associated with several other tumors. These tumors include the following: (1) large mesenchymal tumors such as rhabdomyosarcomas, neurofibromas and mesotheliomas; (2) hepatocellular carcinomas; (3) adrenal cortical carcinomas; (4) pancreatic nonislet cell; and (5) other GI tumors. The etiology of fasting hypoglycemia from these noninsulin-producing tumors remains unclear. Possible causes of hypoglycemia include production of an insulinlike substance and insulin receptors by the tumor, and increased glucose consumption by the tumor. Those patients with tumors associated with hypoglycemia should have dextrose-maintenance fluid, along with glucometer checks during the perioperative fasting period.

Hyperthyroidism is associated with patients with trophoblastic tumors such as choriocarcinoma and hydatiform mole. These tumors appear to secrete a trophoblastic thyroid-stimulator hormone, which increases thyroid-hormone secretion and suppresses pituitary thyroid stimulating hormone (TSH). Preoperatively, these patients need to have thyroid-function tests done if there is any evidence on history and physical examination of possible hyperthyroidism.

Excessive renin production is associated with tumors of the kidney, particularly of the juxtaglomerular apparatus, along with several other tumors: most notably Wilms' tumor and hepatocellular carcinoma. These patients may present with severe hypertension, and hyperaldosteronism with hypokalemia. Angiotensin-converting-enzyme inhibitors and aldosterone antagonists may blunt the effects of excessive renin and should be continued during the perioperative period.

CHEMOTHERAPY INTERACTIONS WITH ANESTHESIA

Most oncology patients who have undergone chemotherapy have received multiple cytotoxic agents. These patients are subject to multiple end-organ sites of damage. The preoperative evaluation should always begin with a complete history and physical examination, determining the cytotoxic agents the patient has received, the total amount of certain key cytotoxic agents (such as adriamycin, daunorubicin, and bleomycin), and the last cycle of any chemotherapy agent. Laboratory testing should be based on the known toxic effects of the chemotherapy. Bone-marrow suppression, cardiac, pulmonary, and hepatic damage, coagulation dysfunction, renal and electrolyte abnormalities, and neurologic dysfunction can all occur from chemotherapy. The majority of chemotherapeutic agents cause bone-marrow suppression, with the nadir of blood counts usually occurring within 7 to 14 days, and starting to return to normal within 21 to 28 days. Other problems from chemotherapy include multiple GI disturbances, causing the patient to be hypovolemic and in poor nutritional status during the perioperative period, as well as tumor lysis syndrome from tumor destruction from chemotherapy.

Chemotherapy Agents

ANTIBIOTICS

Antibiotic chemotherapy drugs include the anthracyclines (adriamycin, daunorubicin, and mitoxantrone), bleomycin, mitomycin C, actinomycin D, and mithramycin. The antibiotic chemotherapy drugs are often of most concern to the perioperative physician, because of the known cardiac and pulmonary toxicities (Table 19-1).

ANTHRACYCLINES

The anthracyclines, especially adriamycin (doxorubicin) and daunorubicin (daunomycin) are well-known cardiac toxic agents. The most sensitive test for identifying underlying cardiac damage is a right-sided endomyocardial biopsy. These biopsies show myocyte necrosis with mitochondria and nuclear degeneration. These changes,

Table 19-1. Toxicity of Chemotherapy Agents

CHEMOTHERAPY AGENT	MAJOR TOXICITY
Antibiotics	
Actinomycin D	Myelosuppression
Adriamycin	Cardiomyopathy; myelosuppression
Bleomycin	Pulmonary fibrosis
Daunorubicin	Cardiomyopathy; myelosuppression
Mithramycin	Myelosuppression; hepatic dysfunction; hemorrhagic diathesis
Mitoxantrone	Myelosuppression; cardiomyopathy
Alkylating Agents	
Busulfan	Pulmonary fibrosis; myelosuppression
Chlorambucil	Myelosuppression
Cyclophosphamide	Myelosuppression; hemorrhagic cystitis; SIADH; pseudocholinesterase inhibition
Dacarbazine (DTIC)	Refractory nausea, vomiting; flulike illness
Ifosfamide	Myelosuppression; hemorrhagic cystitis
Mechlorethamine (nitrogen mustard)	Myelosuppression
Melphalan	Myelosuppression
Nitrosoureas	
Carmustine (BCNU)	Myelosuppression; pulmonary fibrosis; renal toxicity
Lomustine (CCNU)	Myelosuppression
Semustine (methyl-CCNU)	Myelosuppression; renal toxicity
Streptozocin	Myelosuppression; hepatotoxicity; renal tubular damage; hyperglycemia
Antimetabolites	
Cytosine arabinoside (ARA-C)	Myelosuppression; elevated liver enzymes
5-Fluorouracil (5-FU)	Myelosuppression; stomatitis; angina; cerebellar dysfunction
6-Mercaptopurine	Myelosuppression; cholestatic jaundice
Methotrexate	Myelosuppression; hepatic and renal tubular damage; interstitial pneumonitis
Thioguanine	Myelosuppression
Mitotic Inhibitors	
Vinblastine	Myelosuppression
Vincristine	Neurotoxicity; SIADH
VP-16 (etoposide)	Myelosuppression
Miscellaneous Agents	
Cis-platinum	Myelosuppression; renal tubular damage; hypomagnesemia; neuropathies
Procarbazine	CNS depression or excitability; neuropathies; weak monoamine oxidase inhibitor
L-Asparaginase	Liver and pancreatic abnormalities; coagulopathy; hyperglycemia; CNS depression

seen on endomyocardial biopsy, are identifiable much earlier than any changes on echocardiography or radionuclide ventriculography.

Adriamycin and daunorubicin have two different cardiotoxic effects. Acutely, these drugs can cause electrocardiographic changes, whereas, chronically, these drugs cause a cumulative dose-dependent cardiomyopathy. Common electrocardiographic changes include nonspecific ST-T wave changes, sinus tachycardia, premature atrial and ventricular contractions, and low voltage of the QRS complex. Only a decreased voltage of the QRS complex of at least 30% is significant as a possible harbinger for the development of a cardiomyopathy.

The anthracycline-induced cardiomyopathy is dose-dependent. A total dosage of at least 550 mg/m^2 for adriamycin and a total dosage over 600 mg/m^2 for daunorubicin increase the risk of developing a cardiomyopathy (Figures 19-5 and 19-6). The development of a cardiomyopathy can be delayed several months or years after the last dose of an anthracycline; usually, the cardiomyopathy is not reversible.

Mitoxantrone is a newer anthracycline developed in hopes of decreasing cardiotoxicity. Mitoxantrone has been used primarily to treat acute leukemias in the pediatric population. Patients treated with mitoxantrone are still at risk for a dose-dependent cardiomyopathy. Mather et al. reported a 15% incidence of cardiomyopathy with total dosages of 120 mg/m^2 versus 6% at 60 mg/m^2 of mitoxantrone.

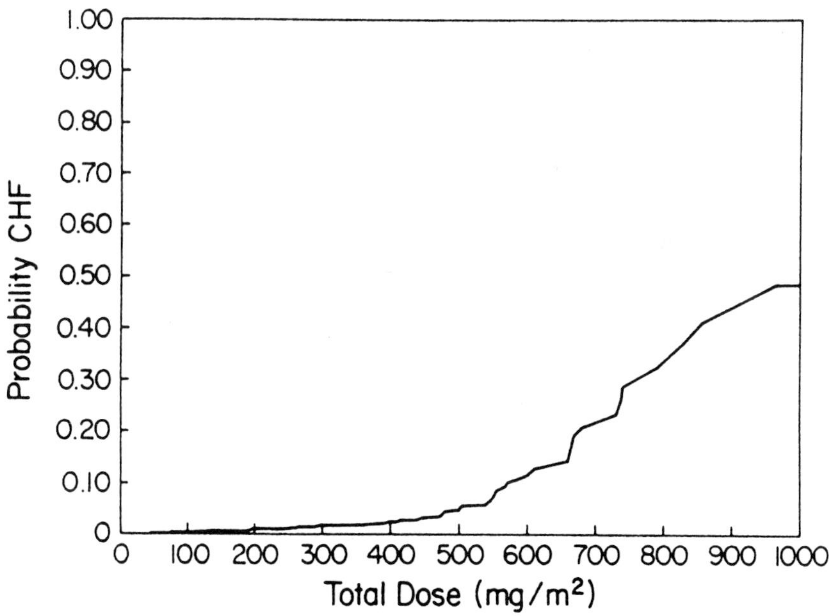

Figure 19-5

Probability of developing adriamycin-induced congestive heart failure (CHF) versus total cumulative dose of adriamycin. (Used with permission from Von Hoff DD, Layard MW, Basa P, et al.: Risk factors for doxorubicin-induced congestive heart failure, *Ann Intern Med* 91:710, 1979.)

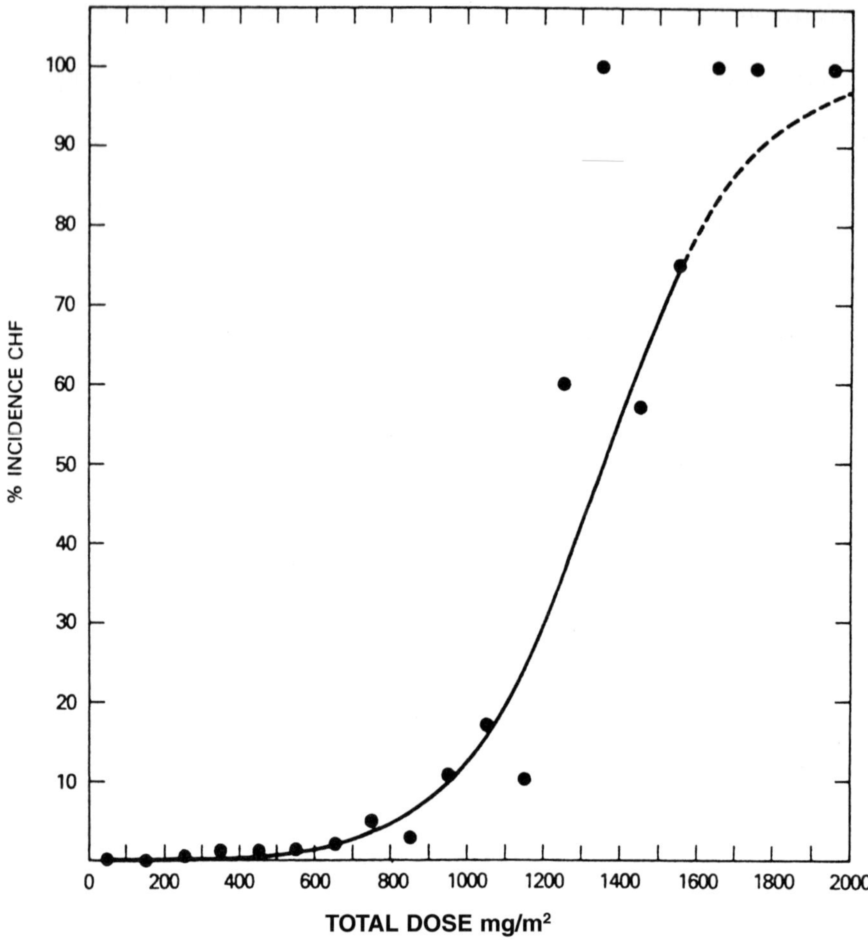

Figure 19-6
The percent incidence of congestive heart failure (CHF) vs total dose of daunorubicin. (Used with permission from Von Hoff DD, et al: Daunomycin-induced cardiotoxicity in children and adults: a review of 110 cases, *Am J Med* 62:200, 1977.)

There are other risk factors increasing the incidence of anthracycline-induced cardiomyopathy at lower total dosages of anthracyclines (Box 19-2). For adriamycin, prior or concurrent radiation therapy to the mediastinum, preexisting heart disease, concurrent use of cyclophosphamide or mitomycin, and elderly and pediatric age are known additional risk factors for cardiomyopathy. Prior or concurrent radiation therapy is a particular high-risk factor for a cardiomyopathy, even at much lower doses of adriamycin. For daunorubicin, only total dosage and elderly or pediatric age have been shown as risk factors for cardiomyopathy. Other risk factors for daunorubicin have not been verified. For mitoxantrone, radiation therapy and prior

Box 19-2 Risk Factors for Anthracycline-Induced Cardiomyopathy

ADRIAMYCIN	DAUNORUBICIN	MITOXANTRONE
1. Total dose ≥ 550 mg/m^2 2. Radiation therapy to mediastinum 3. Preexisting heart disease 4. Concurrent use of cyclophosphamide or mitomycin C 5. Age ≥ 70 or ≤ 4	1. Total dose ≥ 600 mg/m^2 2. Age ≥ 65 and ≤ 15	1. Total dose ≥ 100mg/m^2 2. Radiation therapy to mediastinum 3. Prior use of adriamycin

use of adriamycin are risk factors. Initially, mitoxantrone often was given after adriamycin use, in hopes of decreasing the total adriamycin dosage and risk of cardiomyopathy, without decreasing efficacy of treatment. However, the cardiac-toxic effects of adriamycin and mitoxantrone were found to be additive, and most oncologists no longer combine both adriamycin and mitoxantrone.

Multiple cardiac-protective agents currently are being investigated to decrease anthracycline toxicity. Most of these agents work by preventing the anthracycline–iron complex within the myocardium, thereby, decreasing cardiac toxicity. The United States Food and Drug Administration (FDA) recently approved dexrazoxane (Zinecard) to be used with adriamycin for metastatic breast cancer. Adriamycin cardiac toxicity appears to be much lower with dexrazoxane. However, the side effects of dexrazoxane are increased myelotoxicity when combined with other chemotherapy agents. One study found a statistically significant lower responsiveness for metastatic breast cancer with dexrazoxane use, compared to placebo.

ANTHRACYCLINES AND PERIOPERATIVE MANAGEMENT

The preoperative evaluation of a patient with a previous history of anthracycline use requires evaluation of several aspects to determine if further preoperative risk stratification needs to be done before surgery. Besides obtaining the total dosage of agent and looking for the other risk factors described previously, the physician must obtain a good history and physical examination, looking for evidence of an underlying cardiomyopathy. Signs or symptoms such as an unexplained resting tachycardia, decreased exercise tolerance, or upper-abdominal fullness should raise suspicions of underlying cardiac damage.

Whether every patient with a history of anthracycline exposure should have further evaluation of ventricular function before surgery, often is not an issue, since many oncologists will have already obtained echocardiography or radionuclide ventriculography (also known as multiple-gated acquisition [MUGA]) in patients with higher cumulative-anthracycline dosages. However, the perioperative physician must remain cognizant that a normal echocardiography or MUGA scan does not mean the patient will have normal ventricular function during the perioperative period. The appearance of a cardiomyopathy can be delayed several months after a dosage of an anthracycline. Furthermore, a large percentage of patients with a normal resting echocardiography or MUGA scan still will have underlying heart damage, as seen on endomyocardial biopsy, and an abnormal exercise echocardiography or MUGA scan (Figure 19-7).

Burrows et al. examined the question of whether preoperative echocardiography is needed for anthracycline-treated patients with no prior assessment of ventricular function. Burrows et al. retrospectively studied 111 anesthetics in patients who had received adriamycin. All of these patients had echocardiography done preoperatively. Eighteen patients were found to have a cardiomyopathy. In 7 of 111 anesthetics, the patients had intraoperative hypotension, in which three of these patients had a positive history of congestive heart failure (CHF). The remaining four patients who had intraoperative hypotension had normal echocardiography. No patient with an abnormal echocardiography, but no evidence of CHF on history and physical examination, had any complications. Burrows concluded that preoperative echocardiography is only needed in those patients with a clinical history of CHF or physical examination compatible with CHF.

In asymptomatic anthracycline-treated patients, preoperative ventricular assessment is usually not warranted for minimal or moderate surgery. However, in those asymptomatic patients who have received larger doses of anthracyclines, or have other risk factors for cardiac toxicity, such as radiation therapy, and are undergoing major surgery with large fluid shifts, assessment of preoperative ventricular function is warranted. This is particularly true if the results of echocardiography or MUGA scan will determine the extent of invasive monitors placed or change the anesthetic management. Lastly, exercise echocardiography or exercise-MUGA scan may be the best predictor of ventricular function under the stress of surgery, and provide better information to the anesthesiologist for intraoperative management.

Bleomycin

Bleomycin is an antitumor antibiotic often used in the treatment of testicular and squamous-cell cancers and lymphomas. Bleomycin has minimal myelotoxicity and, thus, is an excellent adjuvant to other combinations of chemotherapy agents, limited by bone-marrow toxicity.

Bleomycin partially intercalates with DNA within the cell and is dependent upon iron and oxygen to become activated. Upon exposure to oxygen, the ferrous state of bleomycin is oxidized to an activated, ferric-bleomycin state in which oxygen is reduced to free-oxygen radicals. This combination of activated-ferric bleomycin and the release of oxygen-free radicals in close proximity to the already partially intercalated bleomycin and DNA complex, causes DNA cleavage and subsequent cell damage.

Bleomycin is inactivated by the enzyme-bleomycin hydrolase, which prevents the oxidation of the bleomycin-iron complex. Bleomycin hydrolase is found in low concentrations within the alveolar cells of the lung and in high concentrations in the bone marrow. The low concentration of bleomycin hydrolase and the increased oxygen exposure within the lung, combine to make the lung the principle organ damaged by bleomycin.

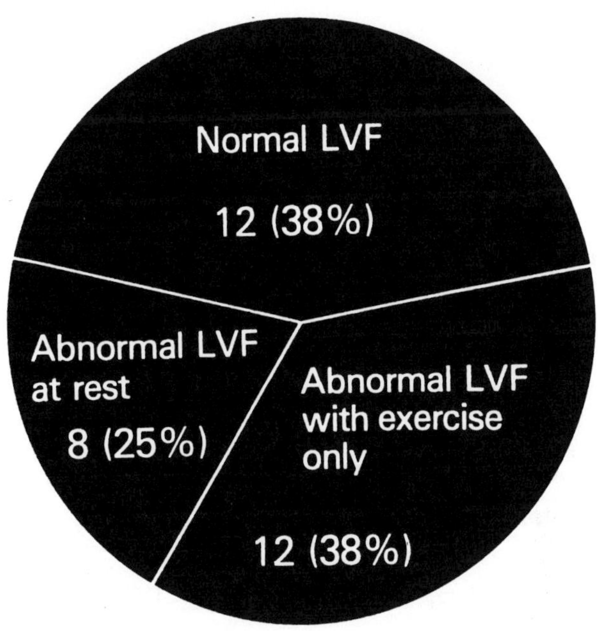

Figure 19-7
Distribution of rest and exercise left ventricular function (LVF) abnormalities in 32 patients after adriamycin. (Used with permission from Gottdiener JS, et al: Exercise increases detection of LVF abnormalities, *Ann Intern Med* 94:433, 1981.)

Lung damage from bleomycin results in pulmonary fibrosis. Bleomycin-induced pulmonary fibrosis has been reported in 3% to 11% of patients. Pulmonary fibrosis can develop insidiously and continue to occur several months after the last dose of bleomycin. Clinical symptoms and signs of pulmonary fibrosis, such as dyspnea, nonproductive cough, fever, and bibasilar crackles, often precede radiographic changes. A decrease in the single-breath carbon monoxide diffusion capacity (DLCO) is considered the earliest and most sensitive marker of pulmonary damage. Later changes seen on pulmonary function tests (PFTs) include an increase in the alveolar-arterial oxygen gradient and restrictive findings on spirometry. The DLCO usually is followed serially by the oncologist using bleomycin. Thus, the DLCO is a valuable marker for the perioperative physician in identifying underlying lung damage.

Several factors increase the risk of bleomycin-pulmonary toxicity. Total cumulative dosages of at least 450 mg (units) in adults, greatly increase the incidence of pulmonary toxicity (Figure 19-8). Prior or concurrent radiation therapy to the chest enhances the pulmonary toxicity of bleomycin, with a reported incidence of 35% to 55%. Other risk factors include the following: (1) renal dysfunction with a creatinine clearance less than 35 ml/min, decreasing bleomycin elimination; (2) concomitant chemotherapy with cyclophosphamide; (3) the elderly over 70 years of age; (4) possible hyperoxia exposure greater than or equal to an FiO_2 of 30%.

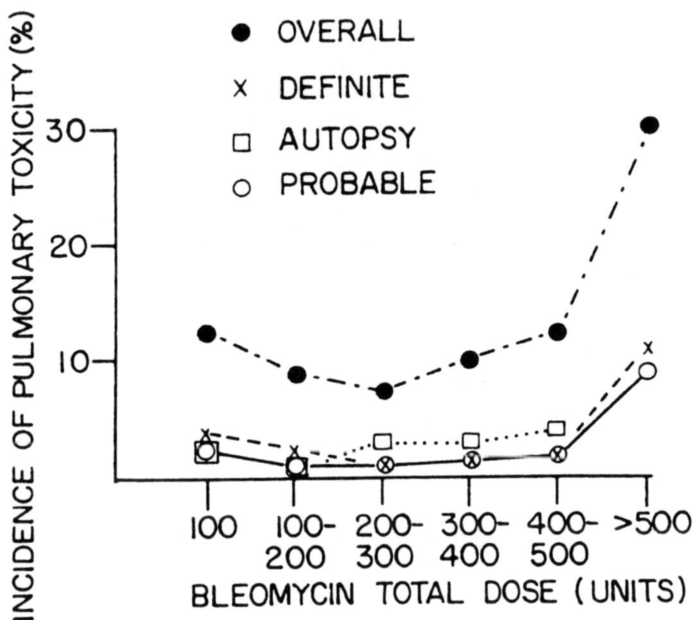

Figure 19-8
The incidence of pulmonary toxicity and total cumulative bleomycin dose. (Used with permission from Ginsberg SJ, Comis RL: *Semin Oncol* 9:35, 1982.)

Hyperoxia Exposure and Bleomycin

Is hyperoxia exposure with an FiO_2 greater than 30% in a patient previously treated with bleomycin safe? This question remains controversial because of many conflicting case reports and studies. Several studies have reported the development of adult respiratory distress syndrome (ARDS) and pulmonary fibrosis, related to exposure to FiO_2 concentrations greater than 30%, intraoperatively and postoperatively, in patients treated with prior bleomycin. Initial studies by Goldiner et al. also concluded that administration of excessive crystalloid contributed to ARDS, but other studies only identified hyperoxia exposure as a risk factor for ARDS in bleomycin-treated patients. However, later retrospective studies reported no respiratory problems in previously treated bleomycin patients exposed to several hours of an FiO_2 over 30%.

Mathes, after extensive review of the animal and human studies and case reports, identified two significant risks in bleomycin-treated patients developing ARDS with hyperoxia exposure perioperatively. These risk factors are the following: (1) preexisting pulmonary injury from bleomycin, especially a decrease in the diffusion capacity of carbon monoxide; and (2) prior exposure to bleomycin within a 1- to 2-month period. The bleomycin patients, described to have hyperoxia-pulmonary damage in the literature, were found to have one or both of these risk factors. Other risk factors for bleomycin-pulmonary damage, such as a high-total dosage of bleomycin over 450 mg or renal insufficiency, were not found in themselves to be risk factors for hyperoxia-pulmonary damage, except for increasing the risk of having underlying preexisting pulmonary damage (Box 19-3).

The perioperative physician should make every attempt to keep FiO_2 exposure below 30% in bleomycin-treated patients found to have risk factors for hyperoxia-pulmonary damage. Such measures as the use of PEEP intraoperatively and CPAP postoperatively can limit FiO_2 exposure. In surgeries where high amounts of FiO_2 are likely needed (i.e., one lung ventilation), continuous, mixed-venous monitoring may be useful to limit the amount of oxygen exposure. Although no controlled studies have been done, a few authors have recommended giving prophylactic high-dose steroids before surgery in bleomycin-treated patients likely to be exposed to higher amounts of FiO_2 during surgery. Several case reports have documented improvement with high-dose corticosteroids when ARDS occurred postoperatively from bleomycin-hyperoxia exposure, but again, no controlled studies have been done.

MITOMYCIN C

Mitomycin C is commonly used in lung, breast, and GI cancers. It is now being used as the primary agent for intraperitoneal hyperthermic perfusion chemotherapy in the operating room. Besides myelosuppression, pulmonary fibrosis is another common, serious toxic effect of mitomycin. Risk factors for the development of pulmonary fibrosis appear to be related to prior or concurrent radiation therapy to the lungs. Concurrent use of other chemotherapy drugs, such as 5-fluorouracil (5-FU). FiO_2 exposure over 30%, has been speculated but not definitively proved to increase the risk of pulmonary fibrosis occurring from mitomycin C. Several authors have recommended minimizing oxygen exposure to less than 30%, unless higher concentrations are needed to provide adequate oxygenation. Surprisingly, the total dosage of mitomycin C appears not to be a risk factor for pulmonary toxicity.

ACTINOMYCIN D (DACTINOMYCIN)

Actinomycin D (dactinomycin) is an antitumor antibiotic used primarily in pediatric solid tumors, such as Wilms' tumor, and in various sarcomas. Primary toxicity is myelosuppression, with nadir occurring 1 to 2 weeks after treatment. Cardiac and pulmonary toxicity is minimal, except for a rare incidence of pericarditis.

MITHRAMYCIN

Mithramycin is used today, primarily for severe refractory hypercalcemia. Mithramycin toxic effects can have a major impact on the perioperative care of a patient. Besides causing myelosuppression with thrombocytopenia and platelet dysfunction, mithramycin can cause hepatic dysfunction and severe hemorrhagic diathesis. Hence,

Box 19-3 Risk Factors for Bleomycin Hyperoxia Pulmonary Damage

1. Preexisting pulmonary injury from bleomycin.
2. Prior exposure to bleomycin within a 1- to 2-month period.

a complete blood count, liver enzyme, and coagulation screenings should be performed preoperatively.

Alkylating Agents

The alkylating agents are among the most commonly used chemotherapy agents. Cyclophosphamide (Cytoxan), ifosfamide, mechlorethamine (nitrogen mustard), melphalan, busulfan, chlorambucil, and dacarbazine (DTIC) are common alkylating agents in use today. All these agents cause myelosuppression and varying degrees of GI disturbances, most notably nausea and vomiting.

These agents are often used to treat lymphomas and other hematologic malignancies. Tumor-lysis syndrome can occur when alkylating agents are used on rapidly growing lymphomas, such as Burkitt's or large-cell lymphoma. The result is a release of multiple breakdown products causing hyperkalemia, hyperphosphatemia, hypocalcemia, and uric acid nephropathy. It is essential that these patients be kept on allopurinol, along with aggressive hydration and mannitol, furosemide, and sodium bicarbonate during the perioperative period to prevent uric-acid nephropathy.

CYCLOPHOSPHAMIDE AND IFOSFAMIDE

Cyclophosphamide has many adverse effects that have direct bearing on perioperative management. Acrolein and other breakdown products of cyclophosphamide can cause severe hemorrhagic cystitis, requiring surgical intervention. It is important during cyclophosphamide use to maintain a high-urine output with good hydration. However, cyclophosphamide exerts an ADH-like effect on the kidney, in which aggressive hydration to prevent hemorrhagic cystitis can cause severe hyponatremia and seizures. Cyclophosphamide also inhibits pseudocholinesterase activity and can prolong the effects of succinylcholine and mivacurium in the operating room.

Cyclophosphamide rarely causes an interstitial pneumonitis when given concurrently with bleomycin and carmustine (BCNU). Cyclophosphamide, when given in high doses, such as 200 mg/m^2 for bone-marrow transplantation, can cause fulminate acute heart failure and hepatic venoocclusive disease.

Ifosfamide is an isomer of cyclophosphamide used in the treatment of testicular cancers, sarcomas, and hematologic malignancies. Besides myelosuppression, the side effects of ifosfamide include hemorrhagic cystitis, renal tubular damage, and neurotoxicity. Mesna (2-mercaptoethane sulfonate) is usually administered with ifosfamide and high-dose cyclophosphamide. Mesna prevents the metabolites of ifosfamide and cyclophosphamide from harming the bladder.

BUSULFAN, CHLORAMBUCIL, AND MELPHALAN

Busulfan, chlorambucil, and melphalan are used most often to treat the hematologic malignancies. All three agents cause myelosuppression and interstitial pneumonitis. Of the three, busulfan is the most likely to result in pulmonary toxicity. Busulfan-pulmonary toxicity is enhanced with prior or future radiation therapy to the chest. Total dosages of busulfan do not appear associated with pulmonary toxicity, but there are no reported cases below total dosages of 500 mg. Melphalan and chlorambucil only rarely are reported to cause pulmonary toxicity.

DACARBAZINE

Dacarbazine is used as a primary agent in the treatment of malignant melanoma, and in combination therapy for sarcomas and Hodgkin's disease. The toxicity of dacarbazine is refractory nausea and vomiting. Other problems include bone-marrow suppression, mild liver-enzyme abnormalities, and a flu-like illness.

Nitrosoureas

BCNU, CCNU, METHYL-CCNU, AND STREPTOZOCIN

Nitrosurea agents include carmustine (BCNU), lomustine (CCNU), semustine (methyl-CCNU), and streptozocin. BCNU, CCNU, and methyl-CCNU all cause myelosuppression, in which the nadir for myelosuppression can be delayed 4 to 6 weeks. BCNU in high doses causes a significant incidence of interstitial pneumonitis. The following factors are associated with BCNU-pulmonary toxicity: (1) cumulative doses greater than 1000 mg/m^2 and an approximate 50% pulmonary-toxicity occurrence at cumulative doses of 1500 mg/m^2; (2) tobacco use; (3) radiation therapy; and (4) concurrent cyclophosphamide use.

Streptozocin is most often used in the treatment of pancreatic islet-cell carcinoma and malignant carcinoid. Streptozocin can cause hypoglycemia after infusion, but chronically; streptozocin can cause hyperglycemia because of the toxicity to the β-islet cells of the pancreas. Other toxic effects include myelosuppression, transient hepatotoxicity, and renal-tubular damage with proteinuria.

Antimetabolites

The common antimetabolites in use today include methotrexate, 5-fluorouracil (5-FU), cytosine arabinoside (ARA-6), 6-mercaptopurine, thioguanine, and hydroxyurea. These agents are commonly used in GI and lung malignancies as well as various leukemias. Major toxicities of the antimetabolites are myelosuppression and GI disturbances, often leading to stomatitis, diarrhea, nausea, and vomiting.

METHOTREXATE

Methotrexate inhibits the enzyme dihydrofolate reductase, which causes the conversion of dihydrofolate to tetrahydrofolate and, hence, inhibits nucleic-acid production. The toxic bone-marrow effects can quickly be reversed with leucovorin (folinic acid). Intrathecal methotrexate can lead to severe meningeal irritation for up to 72 hours after injection. Chronically, intrathecal or intravenous methotrexate can cause an encephalopathy, especially when combined with cranial irradiation. High-dose methotrexate, combined with low urine output, can lead to crystallization of methotrexate within the renal tubule and thus, acute renal failure. A hypersensitivity interstitial pneumonitis, responsive to corticosteroids, can develop from methotrexate. Acutely, methotrexate often causes a transient rise in liver enzyme tests which normally return to normal 1 to 2 weeks after the last exposure. Chronic methotrexate exposure, such as used in the treatment of rheumatoid arthritis, can lead to hepatic cirrhosis with periportal fibrosis. Hence, preoperatively, patients treated with methotrexate should have a creatinine and liver-function test as well as careful evaluation for possible interstitial pneumonitis. In the operating room, nitrous oxide should not be used for any extended period in those patients with recent exposure to large dosages of methotrexate. Nitrous oxide inhibits the enzyme, methionine synthetase, involved in thymidine synthesis from B_{12}. Nitrous oxide could potentiate methotrexate toxicity.

6-MERCAPTOPURINE AND CYTOSINE ARABINOSIDE (ARA-C)

Besides myelosuppression, both 6-mercaptopurine and cytosine arabinoside (ARA-C) can be hepatotoxic. 6-mercaptopurine can cause cholestatic jaundice, which is normally reversible. Cytosine arabinoside causes an elevation of liver enzymes in 25% of patients, and rarely, hepatic venoocclusive disease in high doses used for bone-marrow transplantation.

5-FLUOROURACIL

5 Fluorouracil is used predominantly in the treatment of GI adenocarcinomas, and in combination with cis-platinum for head and neck cancers. Toxicity of 5-FU is primarily myelosuppression and mucositis, in which severe stomatitis can occur. Angina after infusion of 5-FU is reported to occur between 1% to 4% and can lead to myocardial infarction. The etiology of the angina appears to be from 5-FU, causing coronary vasospasm. High doses of 5-FU can cause acute cerebellar dysfunction with ataxia and slurred speech, which usually resolves with discontinuing 5-FU.

Mitotic Inhibitors

VINCRISTINE, VINBLASTINE, AND VP-16

Vincristine, vinblastine, and VP-16 (etoposide) are mitotic inhibitors commonly used in the treatment of testicular cancers, lymphomas, and oat-cell lung cancer. Vinblastine and VP-16 dose-limiting toxicity is myelosuppression. Vinblastine can cause mild neurotoxicity with paresthesias.

Vincristine is used with multiple combinations of chemotherapy regimens because vincristine causes minimal myelosuppression. Vincristine's major toxicity is neurologic. Vincristine can cause severe sensory and motor neuropathies with muscle weakness, loss of deep tendon reflexes, abdominal pain, ileus, and constipation. Few authors have advised against the use of succinylcholine in patients with vincristine-induced neuropathies. Vincristine also can potentiate the release of antidiuretic hormone, leading to the development of hyponatremia. Hence, the perioperative physician should preoperatively check a serum sodium and document any neuropathies in a patient with recent vincristine exposure.

MISCELLANEOUS AGENTS

Cis-Platinum

Cis-platinum is a heavy metal compound often used in the treatment of testicular, ovarian, bladder, and head and neck cancer. Dose-limiting toxicity is secondary to nephrotoxicity and myelosuppression. Cis-platinum can cause a decrease in renal-blood flow and glomerular filtration, and cause renal-tubular necrosis. The extent of renal damage can be decreased greatly with continuous diuresis with normal saline hydration, mannitol, and furosemide. Severe, prolonged magnesium wasting in the urine from renal-tubular damage can occur from cis-platinum, leading to chronic hypomagnesemia. Hypomagnesemia can lead to hypokalemia. Thus, in patients receiving *cis*-platinum, it is essential that magnesium, potassium, and creatinine be checked preoperatively. *Cis*-platinum also can cause neurotoxicity, with ototoxicity and peripheral neuropathies being the most common neurologic side effects.

Procarbazine

Procarbazine is used to treat lymphomas, brain tumors, melanomas, and oat-cell carcinoma. Myelosuppression is the dose-limiting toxicity. Commonly, central nervous system depression occurs with lethargy and drowsiness, which can be greatly potentiated with sedative drugs such as phenothiazine or barbiturates. Thus, procarbazine-treated patients may have delayed arousal after general anesthesia. The use of such drugs as propofol, instead of sodium thiopental for induction of general anesthesia and limiting other sedative drugs, may be helpful in minimizing postoperative sedation. Other less common neurologic toxicities include a 10% to 20% incidence of reversible peripheral neuropathies, muscle myalgias, and, rarely, CNS excitability and convulsion.

Procarbazine is a weak monamine oxidase inhibitor. Monamine oxidase inhibition from procarbazine is reversible, with peak inhibition lasting 3 days after dosing. Thus, the perioperative physician must use caution in using indirect sympathomimetic drugs, such as ephedrine, within 3 to 5 days of procarbazine being given. This is because of the potential for an exaggerated hypertensive response.

L-Asparaginase

L-Asparaginase is used commonly in acute lymphocytic leukemia. With drug administration, hypersensitivity reaction can occur, ranging from urticaria to anaphylaxis. L-Asparaginase commonly causes drowsiness and confusion after administration, and, rarely, can cause a severe stupor or coma to occur. These central nervous system symptoms are usually reversible within days of discontinuing L-asparaginase. L-Asparaginase inhibits protein synthesis in the liver and pancreas. This can lead to elevated liver enzymes, coagulopathy with either bleeding or thrombosis caused by an imbalance of various coagulation factors, and hyperglycemia from decreased insulin production. Acute pancreatitis occurs in 1% to 2% of patients treated with L-asparaginase. Thus, patients on preoperative assessment should be evaluated for hyperglycemia, liver-function abnormalities, elevated amylase, and coagulopathies.

SUMMARY

Perioperative care of the oncology patient requires integration by the physician of the multiple complex problems and treatment, each oncology patient may have in the preoperative period. An understanding of the end-organ damage from malignancy and its treatment, combined with knowledge of how anesthesia and surgery interact with the affected end organs, is vital to providing safe perioperative care.

Indeed, the care of the oncology patient in the perioperative period exemplifies the specialty of perioperative medicine, combining the skills and knowledge of anesthesiologists, internists, oncologists, and surgeons.

BIBLIOGRAPHY

Azizkhan RG, et al: Life-threatening airway obstruction as a complication to the management of mediastinal masses in children, *J Pediatr Surg* 20:816–822, 1985.

Burrows FA, Hickey PR, Colan S: Perioperative complications in patients with anthracycline chemotherapeutic agents, *Can J Anaesth* 32:149–157, 1985.

Cundy J: The perioperative management of patients with polycythemia. *Ann R Coll Surg Engl* 62:470, 1980.

Goldiner PL, et al: Factors influencing postoperative morbidity and mortality in patients treated with bleomycin, *Br Med J* 1:1664–1667, 1978.

Gottdiener JS, et al: Doxorubicin cardiotoxicity: assessment of late left ventricular dysfunction by radionuclide cineangiography, *Ann Intern Med* 94:430–435, 1981.

Karczewski DM, Lema MJ, Glaves-Rapp D: The efficacy of using an autotransfusion system for removal of tumor cells from blood harvested during cancer surgery, *Anesthesiology* 71:A87, 1989.

Kempin S, Gould-Rossbach P, Howland WS: Disorders of hemostasis in the critically ill cancer patient. In Howland WS, Carlon GC, editors: *Critical care of the cancer patient*, Chicago, 1985, Year Book Medical Publishers.

Klimberg I, et al: Intraoperative auto-transfusion in urologic oncology, *Arch Surg* 121:1326–1329, 1986.

Mather FJ, et al: Cardiotoxicity in patients treated with mitoxantrone: Southwest oncology group phase II studies, *Canc Treat Rep* 71:609–613, 1987.

Mathes DD: Bleomycin and hyperoxia exposure in the operating room, *Anesth Analg* 81:624–629, 1995.

Mathes DD, Bogdonoff DL: Preoperative evaluation of the cancer patient. In Lefor AT, editor: *Surgical problems affecting the patient with cancer: interdisciplinary management*, Philadelphia, 1996, Lippincott-Raven Publishers.

Neuman GG, et al: The anesthetic management of the patient with an anterior mediastinal mass, *Anesthesiology* 60:144–147, 1984.

Rinder CS: Cancer therapy and its anesthetic implications. In Barash PG, Cullen BF, Stoelting RK, editors: *Clinical anesthesia*, ed 2. Philadelphia, 1992, JB Lippincott Company.

Salsburg AJ: The significance of the circulating cancer cell, *Cancer Treat Rev* 2:55–72, 1975.

Schriemer PA, Longnecker DE, Mintz PD: The possible immunosuppressive effects of perioperative blood transfusion in cancer patients, *Anesthesiology* 68:422–428, 1988.

Sherwood LM: Paraneoplastic endocrine disorders (ectopic hormone syndromes). In Degroot LJ, et al, editors: *Endocrinology*, ed 3, Philadelphia, 1995, WB Saunders Company.

Von Hoff DD, et al: Risk factors for doxorubicin-induced congestive heart failure, *Ann Intern Med* 91:710–717, 1979.

Von Hoff DD, Rozencweig M, Layard M: Daunomycin-induced cardiotoxicity in children and adults. A review of 110 cases. *Am J Med* 62:200–208, 1977.

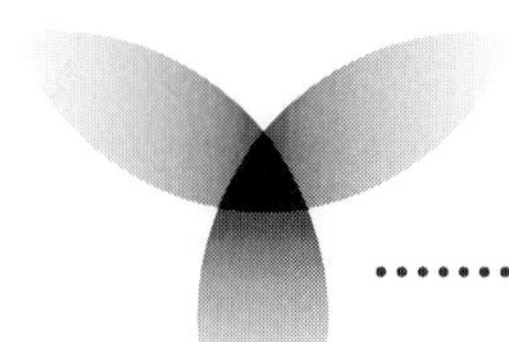

Chapter 20

Coagulation Disorders

Daniel J. Kennedy, MD

The perioperative management of patients with coagulation disorders requires an appreciation of the normal mechanisms of hemostasis, the pathophysiology of the particular disorder, and a knowledge of the treatment options, including the risk-to-benefit ratio of each particular therapeutic intervention. A comprehensive understanding of this complex and ever-expanding field of medicine is beyond the scope of most nonhematologists, and, thus, close communication and consultation with a hematologist is recommended when caring for patients with a known or suspected coagulopathy. This chapter covers the pathophysiology and perioperative management of the most common inherited and acquired disorders of hemostasis.

CONGENITAL DISORDERS OF COAGULATION

Factor VIII Deficiency (Hemophilia A)

Factor VIII deficiency (hemophilia A, classic hemophilia) is one of the most common disorders of coagulation. It is inherited as an X-linked recessive trait, with males affected almost exclusively. Approximately one third of factor VIII deficiency cases have no family history and are the result of spontaneous mutations in the gene coding for factor VIII production. The incidence of affected males is estimated at approximately 1 in 5000 to 1 in 10,000 live births. The underlying pathology involves production of either inadequate amounts of factor VIII (antihemophilia factor [AHF]) or production of an abnormal variant with inadequate hemostatic function. The majority of patients with hemophilia A have inadequate production of the normal functioning factor VIII protein, while approximately 10% to 15% of patients have the qualitative defect. Clinically, the two forms are indistinguishable.

Factor VIII is required as a cofactor, along with factor V, to accelerate the rate of activation of factor X by activated factor IX. Factor VIII circulates in the plasma in a noncovalently bonded complex with von Willebrand factor (vWF), which protects factor VIII from proteolytic degradation and enhances delivery of factor VIII to sites of endothelial damage or clot formation. Factor VIII is also known as factor VIII:c to differentiate the clotting factor from vWF, which is sometimes called factor VIII:vWF. The absence of vWF, or presence of an abnormal vWF, as seen with von Willebrand's Disease, will impair the ability of factor VIII to participate in normal hemostasis. (See von Willebrand's Disease, Chapter 18.)

Factor-VIII activity in the plasma is expressed as units (U), with one U representing the amount of factor VIII activity present in one milliliter of normal plasma. Factor-VIII activity may also be expressed as a percentage of normal factor VIII activity. Factor-VIII levels of greater than 30% of normal (activity >0.3 U/ml) are usually asymptomatic, and are not associated with clinical bleeding or laboratory abnormalities. When the plasma factor VIII activity falls below 20% to 25% of normal, the activated partial thromboplastin time (aPTT) is prolonged, with a normal prothrombin time (PT) and thrombin time (TT). Specific assays for factor-VIII activity are readily available and should be utilized to quantify the degree of factor-VIII activity deficiency.

The severity of bleeding and hemorrhagic complications correlates well with the degree of factor-VIII activity. Patients with factor-VIII levels greater than 5% to 7% of normal are considered to have *mild* disease. These patients generally have few spontaneous bleeding episodes, but may bleed excessively following surgery or trauma. Patients with factor-VIII activity levels of 2% to 5% of normal have *moderate* disease, and occasionally, suffer spontaneous hemorrhage, as well as excessive postoperative bleeding. Patients in whom factor-VIII activity is less than 2% of normal (>0.02 U/ml factor-VIII activity) are considered to have *severe* factor-VIII deficiency. These patients suffer frequent, spontaneous, and often repeated bleeding episodes, especially hemarthroses, subcutaneous and intramuscular hematomas, epistaxis, mucosal and gastrointestinal (GI) bleeding, as well as life-threatening intracranial hemorrhages. Hemophilia (both hemophilia A and B) should be suspected when a patient relates a history of excessive bleeding after minor trauma or surgery such as dental extractions, when there is a family history of excessive bleeding in any male family member, or when laboratory values demonstrate a prolonged aPTT in the presence of a normal PT, TT, platelet count, and bleeding time. The diagnosis should be confirmed by measuring factor-VIII and factor-IX activity in the plasma.

PERIOPERATIVE MANAGEMENT OF PATIENTS WITH FACTOR-VIII DEFICIENCY

For patients with known factor-VIII deficiency, preoperative consultation with the patient's hematologist is recommended. Effective communication between the hematologist, anesthesiologist, and surgeon is essential for optimal patient preparation and timing of surgery, and to assure adequate postoperative care. A factor-VIII activity assay should be performed preoperatively, as well as an assay for the presence of an inhibitor to factor VIII. Approximately 5% to 10% of patients treated with factor-VIII replacement will develop antibodies to factor VIII, making administration of additional factor-VIII concentrates of little value. Perioperative management of patients with factor VIII-inhibitor is problematic and may require use of porcine-derived factor-VIII concentrates, "activated" factor-IX concentrates, antifibrinolytic agents, intravenous immunoglobulins, corticosteroid administration, plasmapheresis with exchange transfusion or other novel approaches, and should be undertaken under the close supervision of a hematologist.

The cornerstone of perioperative management of patients with factor-VIII deficiency is the determination and correction of factor-VIII activity. For minor bleeding such as epistaxis, subcutaneous bleeding, or minor trauma, factor-VIII levels of 15% to 25% are usually sufficient to control bleeding. For more severe bleeding, such as GI bleeding, hematuria, deep soft-tissue hematoma formation, or for minor trauma, factor-VIII levels of 25% to 50% are required to prevent excessive bleeding. Factor-VIII activity between 50% to 75% may be required to control life-threatening bleeding, such as bleeding associated with major trauma, massive soft-tissue hematoma formation, or overwhelming GI or urologic bleeding. Factor-VIII levels of between 25% to 50% are probably adequate to prevent excessive postoperative bleeding associated with minor surgery, but for major surgical procedures, especially those involving the central nervous system, factor-VIII activity should be increased to 75% to 100% of normal.

Various formulas have been proposed to calculate the amount of factor VIII required for replacement, but the factor-VIII activity should always be measured after administration of factor VIII to document adequacy of replacement before surgery. One unit of factor-VIII activity represents the amount of factor-VIII activity present in one milliliter of normal plasma. Plasma volume averages approximately 50 milliliters per kilogram of body weight. Therefore, infusion of one unit per kilogram body weight will raise the factor-VIII activity by approximately 2% or 0.02 U/ml. For an 80-kilogram patient, the amount of factor VIII required to increase the plasma factor-VIII activity by 50% would be 2000 units (80 kg x 50 ml/kg plasma volume = 4000 ml plasma; 4000 ml plasma x 50% increase in activity = 2000 units factor VIII required.) The biologic half-life of factor VIII in the plasma is approximately 8 to 12 hours, requiring administration of factor-VIII replacement 2 to 3 times daily, or by continuous infusion. Factor-VIII activity should be assayed approximately 15 minutes following administration of factor-VIII replacement to document adequacy of the amount of factor VIII infused, and 8 to 12 hours later to help determine the factor-VIII dosage and interval required for ongoing replacement. Duration of replacement therapy depends on the severity of the factor-VIII deficiency and the magnitude of the surgery or trauma. Factor-VIII replacement may be required for several weeks following surgery.

Until recently, fresh frozen plasma (FFP) and cryoprecipitate were used for factor-VIII replacement therapy. Fresh frozen plasma contains one unit factor-VIII activity per milliliter, while cryoprecipitate contains 80 to 120 units of factor VIII activity per 10- to 15-milliliter bag, as well as 200 to 300 mg of fibrinogen, and smaller amounts of vWF and factor XIII. Therefore, usefulness of FFP in factor-VIII replacement therapy is limited by the volume required (for example, to affect a 50% increase in factor-VIII activity in an 80-kilogram patient would require 2000 milliliters of FFP infusion). Factor-VIII concentrates, harvested from pooled plasma obtained from hundreds to thousands of donors, contain up to 200 units per milliliter, but may carry a higher risk of viral-disease transmission than single donor cryoprecipitate. However, with improved donor screening, and protein purification and sterilization methods, the risk of viral transmission is now negligible. Recombinant technology has now been utilized to produce factor-VIII concentrates which should carry no risk of disease transmission. Four such products are now available for clinical use (Table 20-1).

Some patients with mild factor-VIII deficiency may increase circulating factor-VIII concentrations in response to desmopressin (1-desamino-8-D-arginine vasopressin [DDAVP]) administration, although the response can be variable. Desmopressin increases release of vWF from endothelial storage sites, resulting in an increase in factor-VIII carrying capacity, and, hence, increased factor-VIII activity in the plasma. Patients who show a response may increase factor-VIII activity 2 to 5 times baseline levels within 30 to 60 minutes in response to 0.3 μ/kg of DDAVP infused intravenously. Desmopressin may be administered once or twice daily, but tachyphylaxis develops after 2 to 3 days. Most patients with moderate or severe factor-VIII deficiency, however, show little response to DDAVP administration.

Hemophiliacs undergoing dental extraction, intraoral surgery, or oral trauma often have a particular problem with bleeding because saliva has a high concentration of plasminogen activators, resulting in rapid clot degradation. Hemorrhage following dental extractions is reduced or prevented by administration of antifibrinolytic agents such as epsilon aminocaproic acid (Amicar) or tranexamic acid (Cyklokapron), in addition to factor-VIII activity correction. The current recommendations for severe hemophiliacs undergoing dental procedures is to administer 25 mg/kg of tranexamic acid intravenously with factor VIII (or factor IX for patients with hemophilia B) before surgery. Postoperatively, 25 mg/kg of tranexamic acid is given orally 3 to 4 times a day for 7 to 10 days. Epsilon aminocaproic acid may also be used in a similar fashion. In addition, some authors also advocate packing of epsilon aminocaproic acid-soaked sponges into tooth sockets following dental extractions. Aminocaproic acid and tranexamic acid are almost totally renally excreted, and oral dosages should be reduced to 2 to 3 times a day in patients with renal insufficiency. Thrombotic complications have been reported in patients treated with aminocaproic acid or tranexamic acid for upper urinary tract bleeding. These agents should be avoided or used cautiously in patients with hematuria if an upper urinary tract source is suspected.

Many patients with factor-VIII deficiency are infected with viral hepatitis and the human immunodeficiency virus (HIV) as a result of factor-VIII-replacement therapy, especially those who received cryoprecipitate and pooled factor-VIII concentrates between 1979 and 1984. The prevalence of HIV infection in patients with factor-VIII deficiency is estimated to be 33% to 90%, and more than 3000 patients have

Table 20-1. Factor VIII Concentrates

NAME	MANUFACTURER	SOURCE
Alphanate	Alpha	Human Plasma
Humate-P	Armour	Human Plasma
HemoFil M	Baxter	Human Plasma
Koāte-HP	Bayer	Human Plasma
Monoclate-P	Armour	Human Plasma
HYATE:C	Speywood	Porcine Plasma
Bioclate	Armour	Recombinant (Chinese hamster ovary cell line)
Helixate	Armour	Recombinant (baby hamster kidney cells)
KOGENATE	Bayer	Recombinant (baby hamster kidney cells)
Recombinate	Baxter	Recombinant (Chinese hamster ovary cell line)

developed acquired immunodeficiency syndrome (AIDS). With mandatory screening of donors for hepatitis B, hepatitis C, syphilis, human T-cell leukemia/lymphoma virus I and II (HTLV-I, HTLV-II), HIV-1 and HIV-2, the risk of transmission of these infectious agents is greatly reduced, although a small risk likely remains. Improvements in sterilization, protein purification, and virus-inactivation methods have also added to the safety of human-derived factor-VIII concentrates.

Intraoperatively, patients with factor-VIII deficiency may have positioning difficulties related to recurrent hemarthroses and subsequent arthritis with limitation of joint mobility, neurovascular compromise from bleeding into closed spaces, and the potential for airway compromise from airway trauma, central-venous access attempts, and so on.

Factor IX Deficiency (Hemophilia B)

Factor-IX deficiency (hemophilia B, Christmas disease) is an X-linked recessive bleeding disorder, clinically similar to factor-VIII deficiency (hemophilia A). The incidence is approximately 1:30,000 live male births. Factor IX (dependent upon vitamin K for posttranslational completion of synthesis through carboxylation of the γ-carbon in key glutamic acid residues), plays a pivotal role in the intrinsic clotting pathway. Once activated by activated factor XI, factor IX activates factor X in the presence of factor VIII, calcium and platelet phospholipid. Activated factor X is responsible for the conversion of prothrombin to thrombin, which ultimately converts fibrinogen into fibrin. Factor IX can also be activated by activated tissue factor (factor VIIa) and, thus, factor IX represents one of the common links between the intrinsic and extrinsic pathways. A quantitative deficiency in factor IX production accounts for 60% to 80% of cases, while 20% to 40% of patients produce a factor-IX protein with abnormal hemostatic function. The clinical bleeding seen with this disorder is usually indistinguishable from that seen with factor-VIII deficiency, and patients with factor-IX deficiency also have a prolongation of the aPTT with a normal PT, TT, and template bleeding time. Definitive diagnosis is made by assaying factor-IX activity in the plasma.

Mild hemophilia B (factor-IX levels of 6% to 30% of normal) is associated with a slight increase in the risk of postoperative bleeding, but spontaneous hemorrhage is rare. Moderate disease (factor-IX activity 1% to 5% of normal) is associated with increased postoperative bleeding and occasional spontaneous bleeding episodes, while patients with severe disease (factor IX activity < 1% of normal) are subject to frequent, recurrent, and occasionally life-threatening hemorrhagic episodes. As with Hemophilia A, bleeding seen with factor-IX deficiency is primarily intraarticular, intramuscular, and soft-tissue bleeding. Life-threatening intracranial, GI, and retroperitoneal bleeding can also be seen.

Factor-IX activity of 20% to 30% of normal is usually sufficient to control minor bleeding, such as superficial subcutaneous, muscular, or soft tissue bleeding, or uncomplicated hemarthroses. For moderate injuries, more extensive hemorrhaging, dental extractions, or hematuria, factor-IX activity of 25% to 50% of normal may be required to control bleeding. Major bleeding associated with trauma, bleeding into the pharynx, upper airway, retroperitoneum, central nervous system, or bleeding associated with surgical procedures may require 50% to 100% of normal factor IX activity to assure adequate hemostasis. The duration of treatment is a matter of judgment, based on the severity of the injury or magnitude of surgery, as well as the underlying level of factor-IX deficiency. Several days to weeks of replacement therapy may be required, and it is probably better to err on the side of treating too long, rather than too short. Consultation with a hematologist may be helpful in determining the duration of replacement therapy required.

Administration of one unit of factor IX per kilogram of body weight will increase the factor-IX activity in the plasma by approximately 1%. To raise the factor-IX activity level by 50% requires the infusion of 50 Units per kilogram, approximately 3500 Units in a 70-kilogram patient. The half-life of factor IX is roughly 18 to 30 hours, so subsequent doses of one-half the original dose should be given every 12 to 24 hours, as determined by factor-IX-activity assays. Fresh frozen plasma has one Unit factor IX activity per milliliter, requiring an excessive volume administration to achieve adequate factor-IX replacement. Currently, several factor-IX concentrates are available, all of which are derived from pooled human plasma (Table 20-2). The older products, known as prothrombin complex concentrates (PCCs) also contain variable amounts of the other vitamin-K-dependent factors, such as factors II, VII, X, protein C, and protein S. Newer, more highly purified factor-IX concentrates are also available, and contain negligible amounts of other clotting factors. The older PCCs have been associated with thrombotic and embolic complications including DIC, perhaps caused by impurities or contamination by activated clotting factors. These complications have not been seen with the use of the highly purified factor-IX concentrates. Recombinant factor IX is being developed, but is not yet commercially available for clinical use.

Activated prothrombin complex concentrates (APCCs) are indicated for use in patients in whom antibodies to factor IX have developed. These APCCs contain

Table 20-2. Characteristics of Commercially Available Factor IX Products

	UNITS/100 UNITS OF FACTOR IX			
PRODUCT (MANUFACTURER)	II	VII	IX	X
Prothrombin Complex Concentrates				
Bebulin VH (Immuno)	120	13	100	139
Proplex T (Baxter-Hyland)	50	400	100	50
Profilnine HT (Alpha)	148	11	100	64
Konyne 80 (Cutter)*	100	20	100	140
Highly Purified Factor IX Concentrates				
AlphaNine (Alpha)†	<5	<5	100	<20
Mononine (Rorer)	0	0	100	0
Activated Prothrombin Complex Concentrates				
Autoplex T (Baxter-Hyland)	Variable amounts of factors II, VII, IX, and X activated factors VIIa, IXa, and Xa			
FEIBA (Immuno)				

(Used with permission from Roberts HR, Eberst ME: *Hematol Oncol Clin North Am* 7(6):1269-1280, 1993.)

* Estimated based on original data from Konine.

† AlphaNine SD is available and is derived from plasma that is "solvent-detergent" treated to inactivate certain viruses.

variable amounts of the vitamin-K-dependent factors in both the precursor and activated forms, thus, bypassing the need for functional factor IX in the plasma. Intravenous gamma globulins, corticosteroids, plasmapheresis, immunosuppression with cyclophosphamide, and immunoadsorption of the inhibitor antibody have all been utilized in patients with factor-IX inhibitors, but are best undertaken under the guidance of a hematologist. Antifibrinolytic agents, such as epsilon aminocaproic acid or tranexamic acid, are useful adjuvant agents for patients undergoing dental extractions (see factor-VIII deficiency). Like hemophilia A, many patients with factor IX deficiency have contracted viral hepatitis, HIV, and AIDS as a result of factor-IX-replacement therapy using human-derived factor IX concentrates. As discussed in the previous section, improvements in virus inactivation, sterilization, and protein purification have all but eliminated this risk.

Antithrombin III Deficiency

Antithrombin III (ATIII) is the primary inhibitor in plasma of thrombin (factor IIa), as well as factors IXa, Xa, and XIa. Antithrombin III binds in a 1:1 complex with these factors in a reaction which proceeds slowly. However, when ATIII binds first to a specific pentasaccharide sequence on certain glycoproteins such as heparin, a conformational change occurs which serves to accelerate the binding of ATIII to thrombin by 10,000-fold. Endothelial cells express heparinlike glycoproteins on their surface membranes, contributing to the antithrombogenic properties of the vascular endothelium. Antithrombin III deficiency is inherited as an autosomal-dominant trait with a prevalence in the general population of 1:250 to 500.

Two major types of ATIII deficiency have been identified. Type I ATIII deficiency is the result of reduced synthesis of biologically normal ATIII molecules, whereas type II is characterized by production of an abnormally functioning ATIII protein. Both types of ATIII deficiency are associated with an increased risk of thromboembolic complications, especially when ATIII levels are below 40% to 50% of normal. The normal level of ATIII in plasma is approximately 120 to 250 µg/ml. Deep venous thromboses are seen in up to 55% to 60% of patients with ATIII deficiency. Recurrent pulmonary emboli may lead to impaired pulmonary-gas exchange and pulmonary hypertension. An acquired form of ATIII deficiency has been reported to occur in association with acute venous thrombosis, liver disease, disseminated intravascular coagulation (DIC), and with the use of oral contraceptives.

Chronic anticoagulation with coumarin to prevent further venous thrombosis, and replacement therapy with ATIII concentrates are the cornerstones of therapy for patients with ATIII deficiency. Patients should have the coumarin discontinued for 4 to 7 days before surgery, and should have coagulation studies performed immediately preoperatively. Patients with recent thromboembolic episodes, for whom complete withdrawal of anticoagulant therapy would not be advisable, should be anticoagulated with heparin in the preoperative and postoperative periods. Heparin has limited efficacy as an anticoagulant in the absence of adequate, functioning ATIII. Thus, unusually high doses of heparin, or supplementation with ATIII concentrates may also be required. Administration of ATIII concentrate also corrects the original underlying pathology. Infusion of one unit of ATIII per kilogram of body weight should increase the ATIII activity in the plasma by 1.5%. The biologic half-life of ATIII in the plasma is approximately 48 hours, so subsequent doses of 50% to 60% of the original dose should be given at 24- to 48-hour intervals. Plasma levels should be monitored to assure that the ATIII activity remains 80% to 100% of normal throughout the perioperative period. However, clinical evidence that increasing and maintaining normal ATIII levels results in improved outcome or decreased perioperative morbidity is lacking.

Protein C and Protein S Deficiency

Protein C is a serine protease enzyme, dependent upon Vitamin K for posttranslational completion of synthesis. Protein C is manufactured in the liver, and circulates in a precursor or inactive form. It is activated by thrombomodulin, a protein residing on the endothelial cell surface, with thrombin acting as a cofactor. Activated protein C, along with another vitamin-K dependent cofactor called protein S, inactivates factors Va and VIIIa, and activates tissue plasminogen activator (tPA). Normal plasma also contains an enzyme which inhibits protein-C activity, known as protein C Inhibitor. Patients with either a diminished Protein C production (type I or classic protein C deficiency), or production of an abnormal Protein C (type II Protein-C deficiency), are at significant risk of thrombosis.

Congenital protein C and protein S deficiencies are autosomal-dominant traits, and patients with the homozygous disease usually present in infancy with recurrent thrombotic episodes. Patients who are heterozygous for the abnormality may or may not suffer spontaneous thrombosis but are probably at an increased risk of thrombotic complications related to surgery, trauma, and immobility in the postoperative period. An acquired deficiency of protein C or protein S may be seen with pregnancy, liver disease, malabsorption, vitamin-K deficiency, severe infection, septic shock, DIC, or the respiratory distress syndrome.

Chronic anticoagulation with heparin or coumarin decreases the risk of recurrent thromboembolic complications in patients with protein-C or S deficiency. Administration of the deficient proteins, in the form of fresh frozen plasma, has been advocated by some authors, especially when coumarin or heparin therapy is contraindicated. Protein-C concentrate is only available as an investigational drug, but experience with this form of therapy is limited. The half-life of protein C in the plasma is approximately 6 to 12 hours, requiring frequent redosing, or continuous infusion. Protein-S concentrate is not yet available for clinical use. Anticoagulation with coumarin should be discontinued several days before anticipated surgery, and consideration given to anticoagulation with heparin, allowing more rapid reversal of anticoagulation at the time of surgery. Care should be taken to minimize potential thrombogenic factors, such as dehydration, arterial or venous compression, or stasis resulting from patient positioning. Anticoagulation should be reinstituted as soon as possible after surgery to prevent deep venous-thrombosis formation. As proteins C and S are vitamin K-dependent factors, initiating therapy with coumarin alone carries the potential for inducing a transient hypercoagulable state by suppressing protein C and S production before suppression of the other vitamin K–dependent factors. Therefore, the reinstitution of coumarin should be undertaken with the patient fully heparinized.

• ACQUIRED DISORDERS OF COAGULATION

Vitamin K Deficiency

Vitamin K plays an important role in the synthesis of several clotting factors and cofactors. Vitamin K serves as a cofactor for the hepatic microsomal enzyme system responsible for posttranslational modification of several glutamic acid residues on factors II, VII, IX, X, protein C and protein S. A carboxyl group is inserted into the γ-carbon. This site is where calcium binds to the factor, allowing attachment to platelet membrane phospholipid. In the absence of this carboxylation, the vitamin K–dependent factors cannot localize to areas of active clot formation.

Vitamin K is furnished by dietary intake of leafy green vegetables, and by synthesis of intestinal bacterial flora. Vitamin K is lipid soluble and absorbed primarily in the small intestine. Poor dietary intake, malabsorption, and decreased intestinal production, all lead to a deficiency state. Antibiotic administration, especially when prolonged or with nonabsorbable agents such as neomycin, can impair the synthetic capability of the intestinal flora. Vitamin K absorption can be impaired by intestinal disease or as a result of surgical resection, biliary obstruction, or cholestyramine therapy. Warfarin derivatives inhibit the hepatic enzymes vitamin K_1 reductase and vitamin K_1 epoxide reductase, effectively inhibiting production of the biologically active form of vitamin K, and leading to decreased production of all the vitamin K–dependent factors and cofactors.

The PT is the most sensitive test for the presence of vitamin K–deficiency states, reflecting the short half-life and rapid turnover of factor VII in plasma. In more severe deficiency states, the aPTT will also become prolonged because of decreased activity of factors II, IX, and X, while the TT and fibrinogen levels remain normal. In the absence of significant liver parenchymal dysfunction, administration of exogenous vitamin K should quickly correct the deficiency.

Phytadione, the natural fat-soluble vitamin K_1 is the preferred form of vitamin-K replacement, with administration by subcutaneous, intramuscular, or intravenous routes being more reliable than oral administration. Intramuscular injections may be associated with significant hematoma formation when clotting factors are deficient, and, thus, should be avoided, if possible. Intravenous administration of phytadione may be associated with anaphylactic reactions, which may be lessened if the drug is administered slowly and in a dilute solution. Oral-phytadione administration will correct vitamin K deficiency states, except when malabsorption limits uptake of fat-soluble vitamins, in which case the water-soluble form, vitamin K_3 (menadione), may be used. In the absence of liver parenchymal disease, a single dose of phytadione should result in shortening or correction of the PT within 6 to 12 hours, but the aPTT may not fully correct for 1 or 2 days. If more rapid correction is required, such as for emergent procedures, administration of 2 to 3 units of fresh frozen plasma, or infusion of prothrombin-complex concentrates should be used until the parenteral vitamin K is effective. Frequent PT determinations should be performed to gauge the efficacy of vitamin K replacement, and help determine the timing of elective surgical procedures.

Correction of the PT and aPTT merely requires clotting-factor levels of greater than roughly 25% to 30% of normal. Therefore, correction of the PT and aPTT does not imply normal levels of vitamin K-dependent clotting factors, and the patient may still be at risk for excessive bleeding following surgery. Vitamin K replacement should be continued for several days to provide adequate vitamin K required for production of those factors with a slower rate of synthesis, such as factors II and X. If large quantities of vitamin K antagonists such as coumarin have been ingested, large doses of phytadione (up to 50 mg per day) may be required for 7 to 10 days. A careful search for the cause of the underlying vitamin-K deficiency should always be undertaken, once the clinical situation is stabilized.

Liver Disease

All of the factors and cofactors involved in the coagulation and fibrinolytic cascades are synthesized in the liver, with the exception of von Willebrand factor (vWF), which is manufactured and stored in vascular endothelial cells. Progressive hepatic disease results in decreased synthetic function, and a complex, multifactor deficiency state ensues. In addition, decreased hepatic clearance of activated clotting factors and plasminogen activator adds to the coagulopathy seen with advanced liver disease. Decreased synthesis of prekallikrein impairs the initial contact activation phase of coagulation. Thrombocytopenia may ensue from splenic sequestration and decreased platelet survival time. Decreased synthesis of α_2-antiplasmin encourages fibrinolysis. Decreased production of antithrombin III can induce abnormal coagulation, leading to DIC. In the absence of overt DIC, fibrinogen levels in the plasma are not usually decreased; however, an abnormal variant of fibrinogen is often produced. Factor VIII levels, as well as vWF levels, are often normal or elevated in patients with liver disease, suggesting that factor may be an acute-phase reactant in liver disease. As many as 85% of patients with liver disease have one or more coagulation defect, and 10% to 20% have clinically apparent coagulopathies with bleeding. The majority of bleeding episodes in patients with liver disease, however, are from anatomic sites, such as esophageal varices, peptic ulcers, or trauma.

The PT is usually the first laboratory test to become abnormal in patients with liver disease, caused by the short half-life of factor VII and decreased production of factor V. As the liver disease progresses, abnormalities in the aPTT, TT, platelet count, and occasionally, the template bleeding time, ensue. Fibrinolysis and DIC will be reflected by a decrease in plasma fibrinogen and an increase in fibrin and fibrinogen split products, such as D-dimers and fibrinopeptides A and B.

Patients with moderate liver dysfunction may respond to parental vitamin-K administration, but therapy may be discontinued after three daily doses in patients showing no improvement in PT values. Fresh frozen plasma provides clotting factors as well as the normal inhibitors of coagulation and fibrinolysis, but many patients with severe liver disease are unable to tolerate the large volume required to correct the factor deficiencies. Plasma infusions, in combination with plasmapheresis, have been used with some success in patients with severe liver disease and clinically significant bleeding. Prothrombin concentrates and activated prothrombin-complex concentrates should be avoided in patients with severe liver disease. These products do not contain all of the deficient factors, may contain variable amounts of activated factors, and have been associated with thrombotic complications and initiation of DIC.

Uremia

Renal insufficiency is associated with a multifactorial coagulopathy, which contributes greatly to the morbidity and, perhaps the mortality of, patients with uremic renal failure. The primary hemostatic disturbance is a qualitative platelet defect. Defective platelet factor-3 generation and impaired platelet aggregation are reflected in a prolongation of the template bleeding time, and an increased risk of mucosal bleeding. The defect in aggregation is at least partially reversible with dialysis, suggesting one or more dialyzable metabolites is responsible for the qualitative defect; however, the exact substance or substances have not yet been definitively identified. Prostacyclin production may be increased, or its degradation impaired, in patients with uremic renal failure, further impairing the ability of platelets to adhere to damaged endothelium. Severe anemia also impairs normal platelet function. As the hematocrit progressively falls, there is a decrease in the rheologic forces displacing the platelets toward the periphery of the vascular lumen, resulting in less frequent platelet-endothelial interaction.

Perioperative management of uremic patients is aimed at improving platelet function. Hemodialysis shortly before and immediately after any proposed surgical procedure will lessen the uremic-induced decrease in platelet aggregation. Desmopressin administration increases the plasma concentration of large vWF multimers, and shortens or normalizes the abnormal bleeding time. Desmopressin 0.3 μ/kg body weight infused shortly before commencement of any surgical procedure, shortens bleeding time for at least 4 to 6 hours, and has been shown to decrease perioperative blood loss in uremic patients. Intranasal DDAVP at a dose of 3 μ/kg appears to be effective, although the peak effect is slightly delayed. Peak response occurs in 30 to 60 minutes when DDAVP is given intravenously, whereas the peak effect is approximately 90 minutes with the intranasal form. An intranasal preparation containing 100 μ/ml is available. The decrease in perioperative bleeding seen in uremic patients treated with DDAVP seems to be independent of complete normalization of the bleeding time. Repeat doses should be given after 8 to 12 hours as needed, but subsequent vWF increases will be less than the original increase, because of depletion of vascular endothelial vWF stores. Cryoprecipitate has been used to correct the bleeding tendency in uremic platelets, by supplying vWF and factor VIII. However, the risk of transmission of infectious diseases has made this form of therapy less attractive. Uremic renal failure is also associated with an increased risk of thrombotic complications. Increased levels of some clotting factors, such as factors V, VIII, and fibrinogen, coupled with decreased plasma levels of antithrombin III and proteins C and S, render the uremic patient susceptible to thrombosis. Infusion of cryoprecipitate may further increase this thrombotic tendency.

Disseminated Intravascular Coagulation (DIC)

Disseminated intravascular coagulation (DIC) is a pathologic process which is associated with many systemic illnesses, complicating management, and contributing greatly to the morbidity and mortality of many critically ill patients. The pathophysiology of DIC is complex, with involvement of the clotting, inhibitory, and fibrinolytic pathways. Patients may exhibit hemorrhage, thrombosis or frequently, simultaneous bleeding and thromboembolic complications. Disseminated intravascular coagulation is usually initiated by exposure of blood to a procoagulant substance, such as tissue thromboplastin, snake venom, bacterial endotoxin, or subendothelial structures as a result of endothelial injury (Table 20-3). Tumor necrosis factor (TNF) or other cytokines may play a role in amplification of clot initiation. Intravascular coagulation leads to small-vessel occlusion and end-organ dysfunction. Myocardial and cerebral infarction, mesenteric ischemia, and renal dysfunction are all common sequelae of this small-vessel obstruction.

Conversion of prothrombin to thrombin is normally limited to areas of damaged endothelium, with resultant platelet-plug formation and platelet-associated coagulation-factor binding. In DIC, however, thrombin generation in the intravascular lumen occurs in the liquid, free-flowing plasma component. Activation of either the intrinsic or extrinsic pathway, ultimately leads to thrombin activation through activated factor Xa. Thrombin catalyzes the cleavage of fibrinopeptides A and B from fibrinogen, generating soluble fibrin monomers. Polymerization and cross-linking of these soluble fibrin monomers leads to fibrin-rich thrombus formation in small blood vessels. Thrombin also activates platelets, and activates factors V, VII, VIII, and XI, which may further propagate the generation of thrombin through the intrinsic pathway.

Table 20-3. Disease Entities Associated with Disseminated Intravascular Coagulation

Exposure to Procoagulant Material
Amnionic fluid embolism
Retained fetal material
Placental abruption
Eclampsia
Snake venom
Fat embolism
Ascitic fluid absorption
Head injury (brain thromboplastin)
Malignancies (promyelocytic leukemia, etc.)
Endotoxemia
Vascular Endothelial Injury
Infectious disease
Rocky Mountain Spotted Fever
Bacterial sepsis (meningococcus, etc.)
Fungal sepsis
Viral illness (herpes, CMV, hepatitis, etc.)
Vasculitis
Heat stroke
Rhabdomyolysis
Malignant hyperthermia
Toxin ingestion

The fibrinolytic system is also activated by tPA, factor XII, and other factors involved in the contact activation phase such as prekallikrein and high-molecular-weight kininogen (HMWK). Plasmin is not usually present in its active form in plasma, but circulates as the precursor plasminogen. Conversion of plasminogen to plasmin occurs in the plasma and on the surface of the small vessel thrombi, as a result of increased amounts of circulating activated clotting factors and plasminogen activators. Activated plasmin is capable of enzymatically degrading fibrinogen, fibrin, as well as factors V and VIII. Fibrin and fibrinogen-degradation products exert negative feedback on many of the clotting factors, and also have direct inhibitory effects on platelets. Thrombin also activates protein C, leading to increased destruction of factors V and VIII. Increased levels of circulating thrombin rapidly saturate the available antithrombin-III pool, and other factors are consumed by unchecked coagulation and fibrinolysis. Platelets are incorporated into the fibrin-rich thrombi to such a degree that thrombocytopenia is almost always present in severe cases of DIC. Hemolysis and red-cell fragmentation (schistocytes) are common as a result of erythrocyte damage on intravascular fibrin strands and plugs.

Laboratory abnormalities associated with DIC include prolongation of the PT, aPTT, and template bleeding time, decreased fibrinogen levels, elevated fibrin and fibrinogen-degradation products, decreased ATIII levels, and thrombocytopenia. Hemolysis may be seen on a peripheral blood smear. Assays of specific factor activity usually reveal significant decreases in factors V and VIII, and variable decreases in other factors.

Treatment of patients with DIC involves a careful search for the underlying pathologic process with the primary focus of therapy aimed at removing the inciting agent. Support may be required for the patient's cardiopulmonary, hemodynamic, and coagulation systems. Significant bleeding should be treated with red cell administration, and consideration of platelet and fresh-frozen plasma infusions. Cryoprecipitate may be required if plasma-fibrinogen levels are low. Low-dose heparin, at a rate of 500 units per hour, is usually sufficient to interrupt the ongoing consumptive coagulation, and should be considered if there are no major contraindications such as central nervous system trauma or heparin-induced thrombocytopenia.

Many patients will exhibit a shortening of the aPTT and PT, and an increase in fibrinogen and platelet count following institution of heparin therapy. Antithrombin-III depletion can be corrected with the use of antithrombin-III concentrates, and has been shown in several studies to be of value in decreasing thrombotic complications. Activated prothrombin complex concentrates should be avoided because they can potentiate the ongoing coagulation. Likewise, antifibrinolytic agents such as epsilon aminocaproic acid or tranexamic acid, should be used with caution in patients with known or suspected DIC. Inhibition of fibrinolysis leads to progressive small-vessel occlusion with an increase in end-organ damage. Life-threatening and fatal thromboses have been reported with their use. If the decision has been made to use an antifibrinolytic agent, it is imperative that the patient be anticoagulated with heparin before initiating the antifibrinolytic agent.

Fibrinolysis

Primary fibrinolysis is an uncommon clinical entity, most frequently associated with the use of thrombolytic therapy such as tPA or streptokinase. Patients who have recently received a thrombolytic agent and require surgical intervention, such as a patient treated with tPA for an acute myocardial infarction who now requires emergent coronary bypass, are at an increased risk of perioperative hemorrhage. Antifibrinolytic agents, such as epsilon aminocaproic acid, tranexamic acid, or aprotinin have been used in this clinical situation, and have limited excessive perioperative blood loss.

Secondary fibrinolysis may be seen with a number of clinical conditions, including promyelocytic leukemia, aortic aneurysms, and neoplastic disease, especially metastatic carcinoma of the prostate, and pancreatic carcinoma. Inherited or acquired deficiencies of α_2-antiplasmin allow uncontrolled fibrinolysis by plasmin to occur. A deficiency of plasminogen activator inhibitor (PAI-1) has been described, allowing excessive tPA activity and fibrinolysis to occur.

Fibrinolysis is diagnosed by confirming decreased fibrinogen levels with significantly elevated D-dimers (reflecting breakdown of cross-linked fibrin). It is important to differentiate primary fibrinolysis from fibrinolysis secondary to intravascular clotting, a distinction which is difficult to make at times. Factors supporting fibrinolysis, secondary to intravascular clotting, include depletion of clotting factors, especially antithrombin III, thrombocytopenia, and increased levels of fibrinopeptides A and B, reflecting increased fibrinogen degradation, and increased circulating thrombin-antithrombin (TAT) complexes. The finding of elevated D-dimers without increased levels of fibrinogen-degradation products, fibrinopeptides A and B, and a normal platelet count, support the diagnosis of primary fibrinolysis.

Once DIC has been eliminated as a cause of fibrinolysis, infusion of an antifibrinolytic agent in the perioperative period, with close monitoring of the patient's fibrinogen, D-dimers, and platelet count should be performed. Epsilon aminocaproic acid (Amicar) is the most common antifibrinolytic agent used for primary fibrinolysis. Epsilon aminocaproic acid is a competitive inhibitor of plasminogen activation and plasmin activity, and hence, decreases the breakdown of fibrinogen and fibrin. Typical Epsilon aminocaproic acid dosages in adults without renal failure include a slow, intravenous loading dose of 100 to 150 mg/kg (approximately 5–10 grams), followed by an infusion of 10 to 15 mg/kg/hr (about 1 gram per hour). Tranexamic acid (Cyklokapron), like Epsilon aminocaproic acid, is also a lysine analog which acts as a competitive inhibitor of plasminogen activation and plasmin activity. It is approximately 10 times more potent than Epsilon aminocaproic acid. Oral therapy consists of 10 mg/kg of body weight 3 to 4 times a day, with dosage reduced to once or twice daily for patients with renal failure. When the possibility exists that fibrinolysis is secondary to either disseminated intravascular coagulation or a more localized intravascular coagulation, consultation with a hematologist is recommended before antifibrinolytic administration, because severe, life-threatening and, frequently, fatal systemic thrombosis may occur.

BIBLIOGRAPHY

Aledort L: Inhibitors in hemophilia patients: current status and management, *Am J Hematol* 47: 208–217, 1994.

Bennett B, Ogston D: Fibrinolytic bleeding syndromes. In Ratnoff OD, Forbes CD, editors: *Disorders of hemostasis*, ed 3, Philadelphia, 1996, WB Saunders.

Bick RL: Disseminated intravascular coagulation: objective criteria for clinical and laboratory diagnosis and assessment of therapeutic response, *Clin Appl Thrombosis/Hemostasis* 1:3–23, 1995.

Esmon CT: The roles of protein C and thrombomodulin in the regulation of blood coagulation, *J Biol Chem* 264:4743–4746, 1989.

Evatt BL: AIDS and hemophilia—current issues, *Thromb Haemost* 74:36–39, 1995.

Forbes CD: Clinical aspects of the genetic disorders of coagulation. In Ratnoff OD, Forbes CD, editors: *Disorders of hemostasis*, ed 3, Philadelphia, 1996, WB Saunders.

Fourrier F, et al: Double-blind placebo-controlled trial of antithrombin III concentrates in septic shock with disseminated intravascular coagulation, *Chest* 104:882–888, 1993.

Furie B, Limentani SA, Rosenfield CG: A practical guide to the evaluation and treatment of hemophilia, *Blood* 84:3–9, 1995.

George JN: Disorders of hemostasis or thrombosis. In Stein JH, editor: *Internal medicine*, Boston, 1983, Little, Brown, pp 1528–1536.

Gill JC: Therapy of Factor VIII deficiency, *Semin Thromb Hemost* 19:1–12, 1993.

Gralnick HR: Acquired disorders of blood coagulation. In Kelley WN, editor: *Textbook of internal medicine*, Philadelphia, 1989, JB Lippincott, pp 1397–1400.

Hathaway WE: Clinical aspects of antithrombin III deficiency, *Semin Hematol* 28:19–23, 1991.

Hedner U, Glazer S: Management of hemophilia patients with inhibitors, *Hematol Oncol Clin North Am* 6:1035–1046, 1992.

Hoyer LW: Hemophilia A, *N Engl J Med* 330:38–47, 1994.

Katz JO, Terezhalmy GT: Dental management of the patient with hemophilia, *Oral Surg Oral Med Oral Pathol* 66:139–144, 1988.
Lechner K, Kyrle PA: Antithrombin III concentrates—are they clinically useful? *Thromb Haemost* 73:340–8, 1995.
Levi M, et al: Pathogenesis of disseminated intravascular coagulation in sepsis, *JAMA* 270:975–979, 1993.
Lusher JM: Thrombogenicity associated with Factor IX complex concentrates, *Semin Hematol* 28(3 Suppl 6):3–5, July 1991.
Mannucci PM, Gringeri A, Cattaneo M: Use of recombinant Factor VIII in the management of hemophilia, *Curr Stud Hematol Blood Transfus* 58:46–51, 1991.
Marlar RA, Mastovich S: Hereditary protein C deficiency: a review of the genetics, clinical presentation, diagnosis and treatment, *Blood Coagul Fibrinolysis* 1:319–330, 1990.
McIntyre AJ: Blood transfusion and haemostatic management in the perioperative period, *Can J Anesth* 39(5Pt2):R101–114, 1992.
Menache D: Antithrombin III concentrates, *Hematol Oncol Clin North Am* 6:1115–1120, 1992.
Menache D: Replacement therapy in patients with hereditary antithrombin III deficiency, *Semin Hematol* 28:31–38, 1991.
Mudad R, Kane WH: DDAVP in acquired Hemophilia A: case report and review of the literature, *Am J Hematol* 43:295–299, 1993.
Ratnoff OD: Disseminated intravascular coagulation. In Ratnoff OD, Forbes CD, editors: *Disorders of hemostasis*, ed 3, Philadelphia, 1996, WB Saunders.
Ratnoff OD: Hemostatic defects in liver and biliary tract disease and disorders of vitamin K metabolism. In Ratnoff OD, Forbes CD, editors: *Disorders of hemostasis,* ed 3, Philadelphia, 1996, WB Saunders, pp 422–442.
Rick ME, Gralnick HR: Inherited disorders of blood coagulation. In Kelley WN, editor: *Textbook of internal medicine*, Philadelphia, 1989, JB Lippincott, pp 1391–1396.
Roberts HR, Eberst ME: Current management of Hemophilia B, *Hematol Oncol Clin North Am* 7:1269–1280, 1993.
Schuster HP: AT III in septicemia with DIC, *Intensive Care Med* 19(suppl 1):S16–18, 1993.
Sloand EM, Pitt E, Klein HG: Safety of the blood supply, *JAMA* 274:1368–1373, 1995.
Spero JA: Complications of the treatment of hemostatic disorders. In Ratnoff OD, Forbes CD, editors: *Disorders of hemostasis*, ed 3, Philadelphia, 1996, WB Saunders, pp 510–535.
Thompson AR: Faxtor IX concentrates for clinical use, *Semin Thromb Hemost* 19:25–36, 1993.
Verstraete M: Clinical application of inhibitors of fibrinolysis, *Drugs* 29:236–261, 1985.
Zimmerman TS, Plow EF: Disorders of coagulation. In Stein JH, editor: *Internal medicine*. Boston, 1983, Little, Brown, pp 1607–1617.

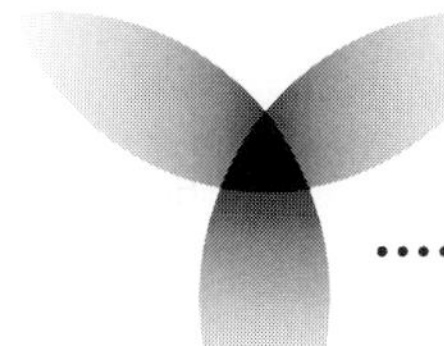

Chapter 21

Liver Disease in the Surgical Patient

Stephen H. Caldwell, MD, Carolyn Driscoll, RN, MSN

Over the past 10 to 15 years, much has changed in the field of hepatology and the approach to surgical patients with liver diseases. There are a number of newly recognized liver disorders and our understanding of previously recognized types of liver disease has changed. In addition, with improvements in minimally invasive surgery and anesthesia, more intervention is often considered in patients who previously may not have been considered candidates for aggressive therapy. We will briefly review some of the fundamental aspects of liver disease and address several specific topics relevant to surgical intervention in these patients.

MECHANISMS OF LIVER DISEASE

The overt clinical expression of liver disease represents potential dysfunction at several different levels. The major underlying mechanism is usually one of three problems: dysfunction of the individual hepatocytes, architectural destruction of the hepatic vasculature resulting in portal hypertension, or an inadequate number of hepatocytes (Figure 21-1). While there is much overlap between these three, there are diseases in which one or another of these plays a more or less dominant role.

For instance, drug toxicity as in acetaminophen or FIAU (a nucleoside analogue that can cause a fatal hepatitis), involves primarily liver-cell dysfunction. Liver failure in this setting may involve the development of portal hypertension, but is more related to impairment at the cellular level. In contrast, many of the hepatocytes in cirrhosis often function normally on an individual basis (the "intact hepatocyte theory"), but scar formation and nodular regeneration cause destruction of the overall liver architecture, so that the normal pathway through which blood percolates through the liver is destroyed and portal hypertension ensues with all its attendant problems. Even if the inciting mechanism, which leads to cirrhosis can be controlled, there may be such a compromise of blood flow that atrophy (often an asymmetrical process of focal and diffuse atrophy) develops. This leads to the third major mechanism of liver disease, that is, loss of liver mass. The shrinking liver of cirrhosis is well-known, especially in clinically advanced stages.

PORTAL HYPERTENSION AND ITS SEQUELAE

Portal hypertension (Box 21-1) is defined as an elevation of the portal vein pressure greater than 10 mm Hg, or an elevation of the gradient from portal vein to vena cava of greater than 5 mm Hg. Portal hypertension can develop as a result of pressure elevation in the hepatic vein (posthepatic portal hypertension as in right-heart failure or Budd-Chiari syndrome), various diseases within the liver at the presinusoidal, postsinusoidal, or sinusoidal levels, and from obstruction of the portal vein itself (prehepatic portal hypertension). Cirrhosis, one of the most common causes of portal hypertension, causes elevation of the portal vein pressure, primarily through distortion of the microvasculature within the lobules of the liver. Mechanically, the development of portal hypertension causes the opening of a collateral system of veins, which connect the portal system to central venous system. The loss of portal blood flow eventually results in hepatic atrophy.

The most clinically apparent complications of liver disease often stem from portal hypertension. These include the development of the "hyperdynamic state" of cirrhosis, wherein there is significant systemic vasodilation, a lowering of peripheral

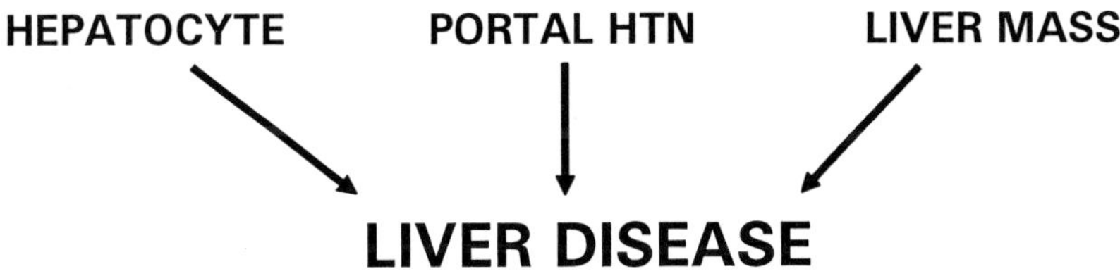

Figure 21-1
The mechanisms of liver disease. Although these often overlap, it is conceptually useful to think of these three underlying problems: (1) dysfunction of the hepatocyte as seen in some forms of drug-induced liver disease and Reye's syndrome, (2) portal hypertension caused by loss of the normal hepatic vascular architecture, and (3) loss of liver mass caused by atrophy itself often because of loss of portal blood inflow, which is rich in trophic factors.

vascular resistance, and increase in cardiac output. The exact mechanism involved is uncertain, but likely involves activation of nitric oxide through gut-derived mediators that are inadequately cleared because of the opening of the collateral pathways and ensuing portosystemic shunts. Significant vasodilation of the pulmonary vasculature, with loss of vascular tone, is seen in approximately 5% of cirrhotic patients who develop the hepatopulmonary syndrome.

Portosystemic encephalopathy, likely mediated in large part by ammonia, also results from portosystemic shunting. The shunt pathways often involve thin-walled veins in the intestinal tract, especially around the stomach and distal esophagus leading to varices in many cirrhotic patients. Ascites forms from excess hepatic lymph which weeps off the surface of the liver when compensatory pathways (primarily, thoracic duct-lymph flow) are overwhelmed. The accumulation of this fluid is usually not clinically apparent until the lymphatics of the peritoneal cavity, which serve to resorb the fluid, are overwhelmed, as well. Thus, there are a number of factors set in motion by portal hypertension, which result, eventually, in clinically apparent disease.

• CIRRHOSIS: MANY CAUSES

Although the term *cirrhosis* often conjures up the image of an alcoholic with the "arachnoid" body habitus, we are all aware that there are numerous and sometimes coexisting causes of this common disorder. The outward appearance of such patients ranges from fully ambulatory and productive individuals to those who are completely incapacitated and at death's door. The subtlety with which cirrhosis can develop and exist is sometimes not appreciated by those less familiar with the field. Following is a brief review of some of the currently recognized causes of chronic liver disease (Figure 21-2).

Box 21-1 Portal Pressures

- Low-resistance venous system
- Perfusion: 1.5 liters per minute
  - 70% portal
  - Driving pressure = 5 mm Hg
- Portal hypertension*
  - Portal vein >10 mm Hg
  - Gradient >5 mm Hg
  - 1 mm Hg = 1.36 cm H_2O
- Hemodynamic derangement
  - Encephalopathy (portosystemic)
  - Intestinal varices
  - Ascites
  - Metabolic abnormalities

* Portal Hypertension. Unlike most other inflowing blood systems, the liver is perfused largely by the relatively low-pressure portal venous system. It is most remarkable because of the size of the organ, the volume of blood which percolates through it, and the low driving pressures in the portal vein. Thus, the normal system is analogous to a river delta that spreads out and then recollects before pouring into the vena cava.

Alcohol-Related

The term *alcohol-related liver disease* avoids the stigma associated with *alcoholic liver disease* and, perhaps, increases awareness of the spectrum of alcohol-induced liver injury and the variable susceptibility among alcohol users—both "social" users and abusers. This variable susceptibility is most striking when comparing threshold exposure between males and females. Daily consumption of 20 to 40 g ethanol in women can lead to significant injury while the range is higher, 60 to 80 g per day, in men. In terms of common measures, it is helpful to remember that 12 oz beer, 4 oz wine, and 1 oz of liquor contain approximately 13 g of ethanol. It is debated whether lower daily exposures over a long period of time (i.e., over decades) are as injurious as higher daily dosages over a shorter period of time. The commonly accepted range to place a male at risk is usually said to be 60 to 80 g/day for approximately 10 years. More recent data has suggested much lower threshold ranges, expressed in weekly dosages; approximately 70 g/week for females and 140 g/week for males. This translates into risk amounts over many years of 10 g/day for females and 20 g/day for males.

In addition to the variable susceptibility between males and females, there is individual variation, some of which may be inherited. Different isoforms of alcohol-metabolizing enzymes, such as alcohol dehydrogenase and the p450 enzymes, may explain some of this variation. Coexisting liver diseases such as hepatitis C, hemochromatosis (possibly heterozygosity, as well as homozygosity), and α-1-antitrypsin deficiency, may also influence the course of alcohol-related liver disease.

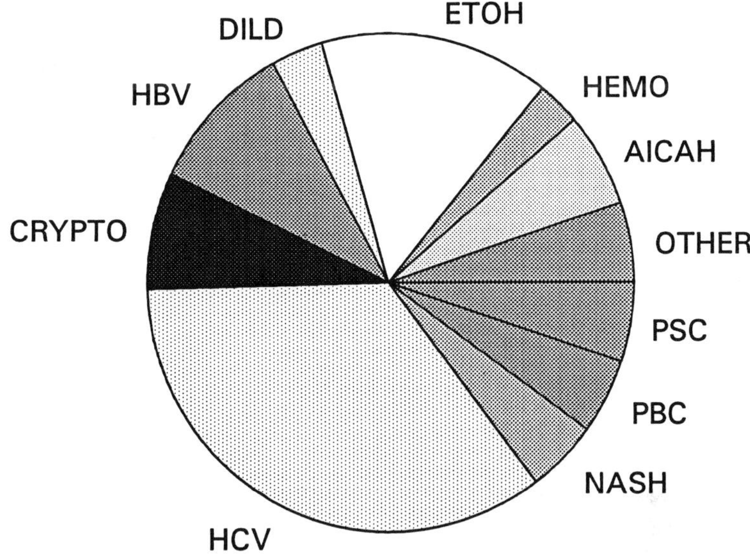

Figure 21-2
The spectrum of liver diseases seen in the University of Virginia Liver Clinics. Data from the UVa Liver Registry. Relative proportions are shown. Abbreviations as follows: DILD, drug-induced liver disease; ETOH, alcohol-related liver disease; HEMO, hemochromatosis; AICAH, autoimmune chronic active hepatitis; PSC, primary sclerosing cholangitis; PBC, primary biliary cirrhosis; NASH, nonalcoholic steatohepatitis; HCV, hepatitis C; Crypto, cryptogenic cirrhosis; HBV, hepatitis B.

Alcohol-related liver disease can be broadly divided into acute and chronic forms (Figure 21-3). Chronic injury is more subtle and usually involves steatosis and fibrosis in the peri-central vein areas and sinusoids. These can lead, eventually, to cirrhosis and atrophy. Acute alcohol-related hepatitis is usually seen in heavy abusers, and is associated with a high mortality. The diagnosis is often made clinically, but biopsy is necessary to conclusively prove the diagnosis. Aside from general supportive measures, corticosteroids have been proven to reduce mortality in patients with high-risk indices—the "discriminant score"—based on bilirubin, prothrombin time, and degree of encephalopathy. Almost all patients with acute alcohol-related hepatitis develop this disorder in the setting of underlying chronic injury, usually cirrhosis. The degree of cirrhosis and, especially, the degree of associated atrophy, likely plays a role in determining survival beyond the acute phase.

Chronic alcohol-related liver disease usually develops without an acute phase. These patients are generally not jaundiced when they come to medical attention. However, ascites and malnutrition are almost always present. Most of these patients present with either ascites or variceal bleeding or both. Jaundice and refractory encephalopathy are usually late findings. Many of these patients will have had long

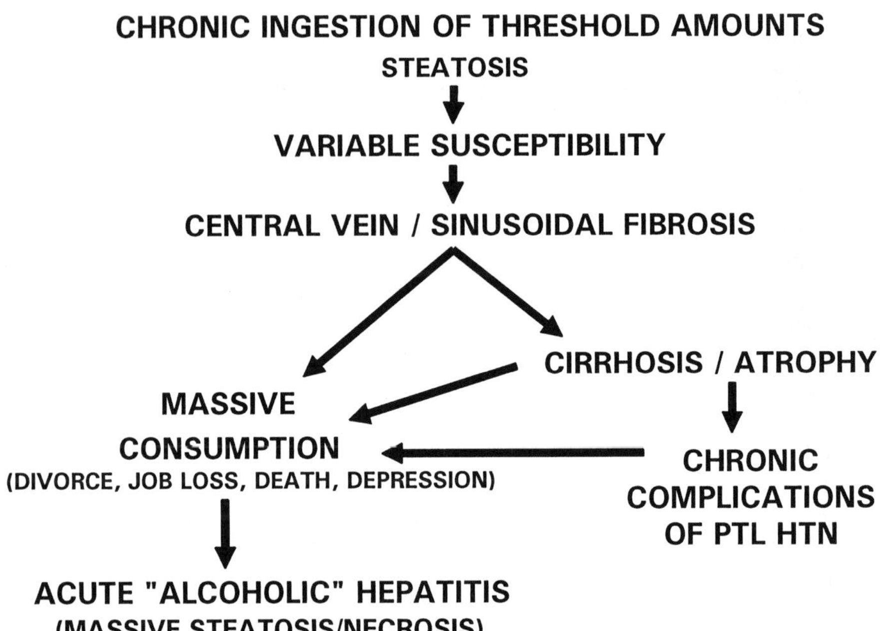

Figure 21-3
Hypothetical relationship between chronic and acute alcohol-related liver disease. The chronic forms afflicts approximately 20% of drinkers consuming threshold amounts (see text). The threshold amount can vary significantly and, for some individuals, falls within what may be accepted as "social" drinking. Chronic disease is characterized by steatosis, mild necroinflammatory changes, and, eventually, heavy fibrosis. The acute form usually follows heavy consumption, often precipitated by major life-occurrences such as death, loss of job, or major depression. It can occur at any point along the path to chronic disease; hence, the degree of background cirrhosis and atrophy can vary widely.

periods of abstinence preceding their deterioration. This presumably represents progressive atrophy of the liver set in motion by the prior development of cirrhosis.

Nonalcoholic Steatohepatitis (NASH)

This is a very common, and as yet, incompletely understood form of liver disease. It is notable for its often silent existence. Although it is associated with both obesity and diabetes, it can exist in the absence of these disorders. Progression to cirrhosis is thought to occur in roughly 10% of patients over approximately 10 years. Natural history studies that have included serial biopsies over years have shown that, once cirrhosis develops, biopsy may fail to show substantial fat accumulation which characterizes early NASH. This is perhaps caused by changes in regional blood flow (portosystemic shunting) and changes in lipoprotein metabolism. Thus, patients who present with cirrhosis may fall into the category of cryptogenic cirrhosis (see following section). As a result, advanced NASH may be underdiagnosed.

Unfortunately, with early NASH there is no entirely satisfactory treatment except dietary weight loss, which is often not successful. Weight loss of even a modest amount, is often associated with normalization of the liver enzymes. Whether this alters histologic disease remains unproven, but is suspected. Jejunoileal bypass, seldom performed now, is associated with severe progression of the disease. Other forms of surgical bypass procedures for weight loss, such as gastric bypass, are probably less injurious, but there is little written experience. Ursodeoxycholic acid (a tertiary-bile acid) has been reported to improve liver enzymes in one small study. This remains under investigation. Antioxidant medications, such as vitamin E, may also play a role, but these too remain unproved.

Cryptogenic Cirrhosis

Cryptogenic cirrhosis is a term that is often used to describe patients with cirrhosis of uncertain cause. It is best applied only after an extensive workup, usually including liver biopsy. These patients are characteristically female and usually older than age 50 (Figure 21-4). While no clear diagnosis can be made regarding etiology, many of these patients have risks for either viral hepatitis (usually from a prior blood transfusion), NASH (history of obesity or diabetes), and/or autoimmune hepatitis markers (such as ANA) in the absence of other defining features. Some, no doubt, have occult-alcohol exposure. Conceptually, one may view this disease as an endpoint of this spectrum (Figure 21-5). With further definition of various forms of liver disease, this diagnosis will continue to shrink as the ability to better define various, underlying diseases grows.

"Autoimmune" Liver Diseases

This broad group includes autoimmune hepatitis (AIH), primary biliary cirrhosis (PBC), and primary sclerosing cholangitis (PSC). There are now several forms of AIH characterized by various autoantibody profiles (antinuclear antibody, anti-smooth muscle antibody, antiliver-kidney microsomal antibody, and antisoluble liver antigen). Although there is overlap with chronic viral hepatitis (especially hepatitis C), this disease can usually be defined serologically and histologically. It is remarkable for frequent, severe presentation and striking response to coriticosteroids. Young females are most frequently afflicted.

Primary biliary cirrhosis is a disease largely of young to middle-aged females. It is associated with cholestatic hepatitis (relatively higher elevation of alkaline phosphatase), antimitochondrial antibody, pruritus, and slow progression to cirrhosis. Antimitochondrial antibody is now known to be directed at epitopes of the pyruvate dehydrogenase enzyme complex located in the mitochondria. The role of this antigen, possibly through mistaken insertion into the plasma membrane rather than the mitochondrial membrane, continues to be debated. Primary sclerosing cholangitis is a disease usually of young to middle-aged males. It is characterized by obliterative sclerosis of the biliary tree and is often (but not invariably) associated with inflammatory bowel disease. It is also a cholestatic illness characterized by recurrent

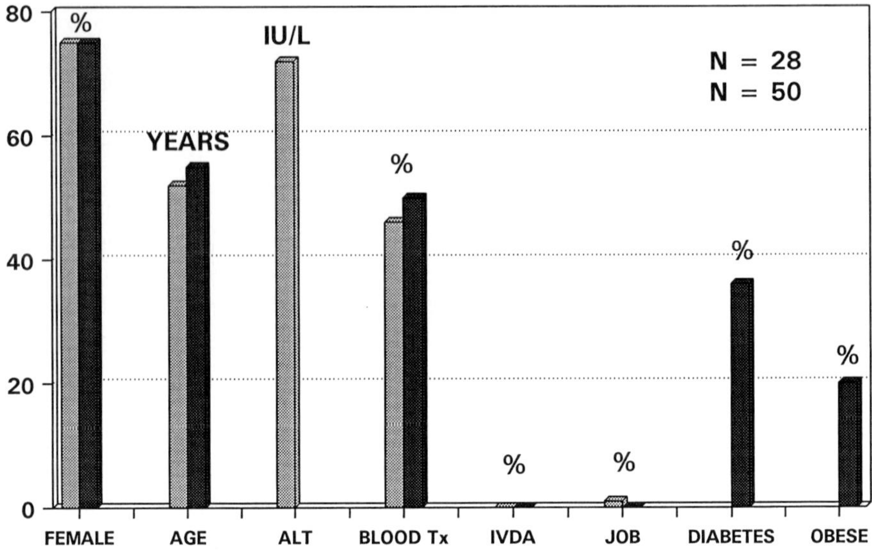

Figure 21-4
The characteristics of cryptogenic cirrhosis. The patients are often female, over the age of 50, have characteristically low (near-normal) liver enzymes, and a mixed picture of autoimmune markers such as ANA, history of risk factors for viral hepatitis (blood transfusion), and often, a history of obesity and diabetes. Risk factors for viral hepatitis are indicated as Blood Tx (for blood transfusion), IVDA (for intravenous drug use), and JOB (for work-related accidental needle exposure). (Data from the University of Virginia Liver Registry N = 50 and Kodali et al: *Am J Gastroenterol* 89:1836-1839, 1994, N = 28).

bouts of cholangitis and slow progression to cirrhosis. Secondary forms of sclerosing cholangitis, such as those associated with hepatic artery occlusion and acquired immunodeficiency syndrome (AIDS) cholangiopathies, are increasingly recognized. They are indistinguishable from the *primary* form by cholangiography.

Viral and Other Forms of Chronic Liver Disease

Viral hepatitis is discussed further on. In general, it is worth noting that hepatitis A and E are both acute, enteric forms of hepatitis, and neither is associated with chronic liver disease, although hepatitis A exposure has been proposed as a trigger for later AIH. Chronic disease and progression to cirrhosis is seen with hepatitis C, B, and D. The recently described hepatitis G does not appear to cause significant liver injury, even among chronic carriers. Metabolic-liver diseases include inherited diseases such as α-1-antitrypsin deficiency, Wilson's disease, and the more common hemochromatosis. Although the gene for primary hemochromatosis (autosomal-recessive) is one of the most common abnormal genes, abnormal iron studies in a patient with liver disease is more often secondary to either hepatitis C or alcohol exposure. However, biopsy is often necessary to exclude hemochromatosis.

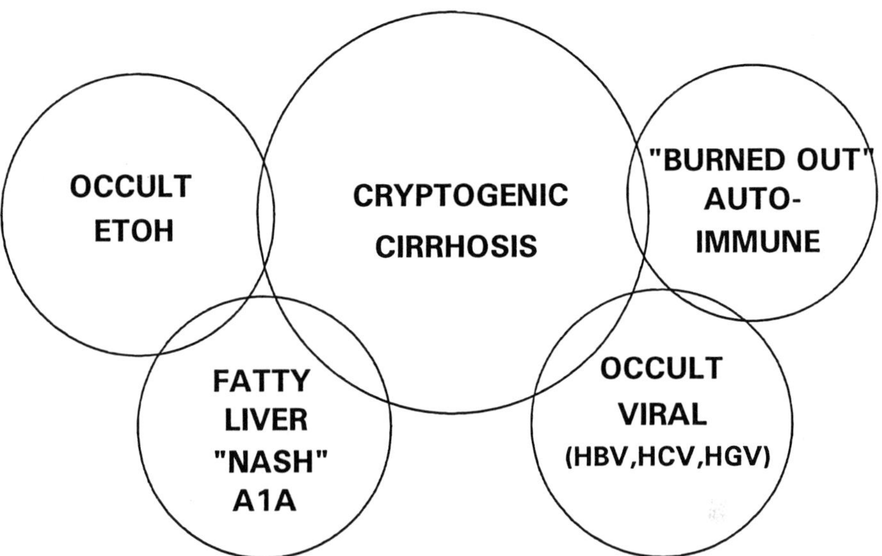

Figure 21-5
Concept of cryptogenic cirrhosis. There are likely many ways to arrive at the endpoint of cryptogenic cirrhosis. Based on the common clinical features of these patients, the dominant groups appear to be advanced steatohepatitis or "NASH" (which loses the histologic hallmarks with cirrhosis), autoimmune hepatitis which has never had an overt flare of active hepatitis, occult, as yet unidentified hepatotropic viruses and, no doubt, occult-heavy alcohol consumption; although this is far less frequent than may be commonly perceived.

ESTIMATING SEVERITY OF CIRRHOSIS AND LIVER DISEASE: PROGNOSIS

Various interventions, including surgical procedures, in chronic liver disease are, in part, based on the expected natural history of the disease and expected outcome of the procedure. The easiest prognostic system for cirrhosis is that originally derived for predicting survival in portocaval shunt surgery—the Child-Pugh-Turcotte class (with Pugh modification) (Table 21-1). This simple scheme has proved to be a durable means of developing prognosis in patients with established cirrhosis. It is nondisease-specific in that it can be used in most forms of cirrhosis, and has been shown to predict long-term survival outside of those patients undergoing shunt surgery. The three classes, A, B, and C, are based on numerical scores from assessing or measuring encephalopathy, amount of ascites, coagulopathy, albumin level, and bilirubin level (score 1 to 3 for each for a total score of 5 to 15). Although often used because of its simplicity, the score lacks linearity over the score range, and does not take into account features of the underlying liver disease such as hepatitis C, alcohol-related causes or PBC. Thus, a number of disease-specific prognostic scores have been developed.

Table 21-1. Child-Turcotte Class Pugh Modification

	CLASS		
	A	B	C
Ascites	Absent	Moderate	Tense
Encephalopathy	None	Grade 1–2	Grade 3–4
Albumin	>3.5	3–3.5	<3.0
Bilirubin	<2.0	2–3	>3
PT (sec)	<4	4–6	>6
Score:* 5–6 = A, 7–9 = B, 10–15 = C			

* The Child-Turcotte score as modified by Pugh. In clinical practice, the formal score is often omitted and patients are broadly classified into classes. This is generally satisfactory for day-to-day practice. Investigative studies generally require more formal scoring. In addition to the broadly applied Child-Pugh Class, disease-specific prognostic scores are often used (see text).

The prognosis of alcohol-related liver disease can be broadly related to the presence or absence of major complications of portal hypertension, such as ascites or variceal bleeding and abstinence. Several more detailed scoring systems have also been utilized, including the Combined Clinical and Laboratory Index (CCLI), which provide a score that has a linear relation to long-term prognosis. Disease-specific scores have also been developed for PBC and PSC which are helpful in estimating the need and timing for liver transplantation in those conditions. Unfortunately, no such prognostic score exists for autoimmune hepatitis. The natural history of chronic viral hepatitis has been studied extensively, and the course and estimated rate of progression can be predicted from these studies. With hepatitis C, it has become evident that 30% to 50% of untreated patients will progress to *histologic* cirrhosis over a period of 5 to 10 years. However, the rate of progression to complicated cirrhosis is much lower, and often difficult to predict. None of these prognostic assessments take into account the risk of cancer; hepatoma in all forms of cirrhosis (especially hepatitis C), and cholangiocarcinoma in PSC.

True tests of liver function have been developed to further complement the existing prognostic systems. These are usually tests of hepatic metabolism, including lidocaine metabolism (MEGX test), indocyanin green clearance, galactose elimination, caffeine metabolism, and aminopyrine breath tests. These tests vary, depending on the hepatic extraction of the test material, and in some cases, the state of the cytochrome p450 system. For instance, the MEGX test, because it is blood-flow-dependent, represents an indirect measure of the degree of portosystemic shunting and is also influenced by inducers of p450. Nonetheless, a number of articles have shown the utility of these tests as complements to the more common clinical scores. The MEGX test has been used to help predict the development of complications (and, hence, the need for early transplantation) in otherwise stable hepatitis C.

• COMMON MEDICATIONS IN PATIENTS WITH CIRRHOSIS

Several medications commonly used in cirrhotic patients are well established and generally known to most practitioners. These include diuretics, especially spironolactone which increases urinary sodium and lowers portal pressure, lactulose which promotes ammonia excretion, and neomycin, which suppresses ammonia formation. In addition, there are now many newer treatment strategies commonly used in these patients.

For instance, β-blockers and nitrates, either alone or in combination, reduce portal pressure, and are often used to prevent initial variceal bleeding in patients with high-risk endoscopic scores of esophageal varices (primary prophylaxis). They are also used to prevent rebleeding in patients who have previously bled from varices (secondary prophylaxis). These medications may further be combined with endoscopic therapy, as with band ligation, to treat varices. Likewise, octreotide has emerged as the major medicinal agent for treating acute variceal hemorrhage. It is thought to act by lowering portal pressure through an inhibitory effect on vasoactive-gut peptides.

Newer antiviral agents, in addition to interferon, include interferon-ribavirin combinations for hepatitis C and interferon-lamivudine therapy for hepatitis B. Other drugs and combinations for chronic viral hepatitis are under study to further improve efficacy and reduce side effects. Cholestatic liver diseases, such as PSC and PBC, are now often treated with a form of bile salt called ursodeoxycholic acid. This medication may also be useful in other settings such as cholestatic hepatitis in the patient with postoperative cholestasis and jaundice. Corticosteroids are now known to be useful in some (but not all) patients with acute, alcohol-related hepatitis. Especially when combined with azathioprine, these medications are extraordinarily effective in autoimmune hepatitis.

• UNEXPECTED CIRRHOSIS IN SURGERY

Unexpected cirrhosis holds many pitfalls for the surgical patient. Although figures are not available to estimate the frequency of this occurrence, it is fairly common in clinical practice. This is usually because of the sometimes subtle nature of cirrhosis and portal hypertension. Typical examples include gallbladder surgery in patients with occult cirrhosis from hepatitis C, in whom the common occurrence of right-upper-quadrant pain leads to confusion. In the era of laparoscopic cholecystectomy, this has been a relatively common occurrence in my practice. Another example is seen in patients undergoing weight-loss surgery (gastric bypass or stapling), in whom there has been the development of cirrhosis usually caused by NASH. Finally, the development of ascites in a female without a history of known liver disease, often prompts a search for ovarian malignancy and measurement of tumor markers such as Ca 125. Ca 125 is elevated in some ovarian cancers, but is also elevated in cirrhosis. Exploratory surgery or resective procedures in the pelvis, in patients with unrecognized cirrhosis and spurious elevation of Ca 125, can lead to severe complications, decompensated cirrhosis with ascites, and poor wound healing.

Unrecognized cirrhosis can have many repercussions, both during the surgery itself (from unexpected collateral blood vessels) and in the postoperative period (see following). This is especially true of abdominal surgery. However, other surgery undertaken in this setting can also tip these patients into a decompensated state. To prevent this situation, the preoperative evaluation should always take into account the possibility of occult liver disease. The general examination can provide simple and useful information, such as the detection of spider angiomas, palmar erythema, or a firm liver border. Mild elevation of the liver enzymes should be investigated further with viral profiles, and, at least, consideration of more extensive evaluations. This especially applies to patients with known risk factors for liver disease such as obesity, diabetes, risks for viral hepatitis, or a family or personal history of autoimmune diseases. We have often noted low preoperative platelets to be a useful marker for occult-portal hypertension and hypersplenism.

• VIRAL HEPATITIS

Disease Activity and Flares

In general, the commonly measured liver enzymes are a good (although imperfect) indicator of the presence of inflammation in chronic viral hepatitis. In hepatitis C, minimal enzyme elevations may, however, be associated with significant underlying disease such as cirrhosis. In both hepatitis B and C, patients may sometimes have cirrhosis with completely normal ALT (alanine aminotransferase) and AST (aspartate aminotransferase). Nonetheless, ALT and AST provide useful markers for these illnesses. Hepatitis C is usually characterized by mild-to-moderate elevations in the 70 to 120 U/l range for ALT and levels often fluctuate 10 to 20 U/l when serially measured over time. Hepatitis C seldom resolves without therapy, although it is unusual to have severe flares of this disease. The effect of short courses of corticosteroids such as those that may be given to treat other intercurrent disorders, is variable. Sometimes, there may be significant improvement in the enzyme levels. However, exacerbation, especially with steroid withdrawal, may also be seen.

In contrast, chronic hepatitis B is associated with wide swings in disease activity. Corticosteroids and other immunosuppressors significantly exacerbate this tendency, especially when these medications are withdrawn; at that time the patient can experience a severe flare of hepatitis. However, flares of chronic hepatitis B can also be seen "spontaneously" presumably caused by mutations of the virus. Seroconversion from an active carrier to a so-called "healthy carrier" (i.e., one with minimal or no viral replication and no inflammation) is also associated with a transient flare of hepatitis, which can be severe.

Spectrum of Associated Diseases with Hepatitis C

Since its identification in 1989, hepatitis C has emerged as one of the most common causes of liver disease. It has become increasingly apparent that this virus causes much more injury than simply chronic hepatitis. However, before discussing these disorders, some nuances of chronic hepatitis C bear mention. Pain is seen in roughly

60% of these patients, commonly in the right-upper quadrant. Most often, the pain is described as a "catching" sharp pain especially with movement. It is often reproducible on physical examination when the edge of the liver is palpated (pseudo-Murphy's sign). If gallstones are present, there is often confusion as to the exact source of the pain, although the pain associated with chronic hepatitis is usually not meal-related. Because the liver-enzyme abnormalities associated with hepatitis C may be mild, this clinical picture often results in cholecystectomy, at which time, the liver is noted to be abnormal, often cirrhotic. In general, the pain does not resolve after cholecystectomy.

"Extrahepatic" manifestations of hepatitis C have been increasingly recognized over the past few years. The most severe of these include mixed essential cryoglobulinemia, which causes a vasculitis characterized by rash and glomerulonephritis. The mechanism is uncertain but appears to directly relate to hepatitis C. Perhaps, this is as a result of hypersensitivity to viral antigens. The spectrum of this disorder is wide and ranges from asymptomatic cryoglobulinemia, to renal failure, to frank and, sometimes fatal, systemic vasculitis. The response to interferon is variable. In addition to cryoglobulinemia, hepatitis C is now closely associated with porphyria cutanea tarda, characterized by skin blisters and other changes on the dorsum of the hand, (the common triad is hepatitis C, variable iron overload, and regular use of alcohol), lichen planus, and a rare form of corneal ulceration. For unknown reasons, abnormalities of iron indices such as ferritin, serum iron, and iron-binding capacity are common in hepatitis C, and sometimes lead to confusion with hemochromatosis. Occasionally, hepatitis C and genetic hemochromatosis coexist.

Recommendations for Surgeons Regarding Viral Hepatitis

The growing recognition of various forms of blood-borne viral hepatitis has increased awareness of the potential for transmission, both from patients to surgeons and vice versa. The latter should remind us of the need for hepatitis B vaccination of all health-care providers, especially those with high risks for blood exposure and the need for practicing universal precautions for hepatitis C prevention. Although uncommon, both hepatitis C and B have been reported to be transmitted from surgeons to patients. Indeed, the presence of past major surgical procedures (apart from blood transfusion) has been observed in epidemiologic studies to be a risk factor for hepatitis C (albeit, far less a risk than blood transfusion or intravenous-drug use). The exact vector often cannot be determined but is thought to involve injury to the surgeon's fingertips during the operation. Sweat has been inadequately studied as a potential vector.

Formal recommendations from the Center for Disease Control (CDC) and Prevention exist for surgeons discovered to have chronic viral hepatitis. These recommendations are now undergoing additional study, in light of more recent transmission reports. Currently, for physicians with chronic hepatitis C, the risk for transmission is thought to be relatively low. Universal precautions for all blood-borne pathogens are all that are recommended, without restrictions on specific activities. With hepatitis B, the recommendations vary depending on the proliferative activity of the virus. Universal precautions without specific restrictions are recommended if hepatitis B E antigen is absent (i.e., the virus is in a low-proliferative state). If the E antigen is present, the risks are higher because of increased levels of viremia. In this situation, the local institution has the responsibility to review the individual case and consider restrictions for high-risk procedures such as cardiothoracic surgery. (More information regarding these matters can be obtained from the Center for Disease Control and Prevention at 404-332-4555.)

Exposure to hepatitis B or C should be handled according to the policy at the local institution. In general, hepatitis B infection is preventable and the algorithm for addressing this problem is fairly well established. For hepatitis C, because dependable, preventive measures are lacking, the course is not as clear. In general, the healthcare provider should be tested for hepatitis C by the standard antibody tests. Unfortunately, these tests will not detect early viremia. We usually recommend early hepatitis C RNA testing if there was a definite exposure to positive blood. Early detection allows closer monitoring and possible institution of antiviral medications such as interferon.

Treatment within the first few months following exposure is thought to be relatively more effective than delayed treatment. However, it is not known just how early this should be instituted, nor whether or not especially early intervention, within weeks or days, is helpful or potentially harmful (possibly by selecting for resistant strains during the time of early, rapid-viral replication, or by hampering natural immunity which is seen in approximately 20% of patients). These recommendations will undoubtedly change as we learn more about this virus.

HEPATOPULMONARY SYNDROME

The hepatopulmonary syndrome (HPS) is a recently described entity, characterized by pulmonary vasodilation and loss of vascular tone in the pulmonary bed in the portal hypertension setting. As such, patients with HPS develop hypoxia and relative pulmonary *hypotension*. Clinical features include finger clubbing, prominent spider angiomata, dyspnea, platypnea, and orthodeoxia (lower-blood oxygen in the upright position). The last findings are caused by the loss of vascular tone so that when the patient is upright, there is pooling of blood in the lower-lung fields. The mechanism of hepatopulmonary syndrome involves nitric oxide, perhaps triggered by gut peptides which increase along with portosystemic shunting.

The syndrome appears to fall within the spectrum of the portal hypertensive-hyperdynamic state (the marked peripheral vasodilation of cirrhosis). Portal hypertension is essential but not sufficient to produce the disorder. The full-blown form is seen in approximately 5% of cirrhotic patients, while 15% of cirrhotic patients can be shown to have subclinical HPS. Why only a fraction of patients develop the syndrome is unknown. It can be postulated that these patients lack some pulmonary-compensatory mechanism. Lung-function tests show normal volumes and mechanics, but the diffusion capacity is characteristically low ("perfusion diffusion defect"). Severely afflicted patients are cyanotic. Not infrequently, these patients have been misdiagnosed as having various forms of intrinsic lung disease, such as COPD or interstitial disease, in spite of the paucity of findings to support the diagnosis.

Hepatopulmonary syndrome has several significant clinical ramifications for the surgeon and anesthesiologist, aside from the obvious hypoxia and incapacitation in severely afflicted patients. Cirrhosis (or other causes of portal hypertension) in these patients may be subtle. Thus, the correct diagnosis may not be evident in postoperative patients experiencing difficulty with oxygenation. In addition, if not recognized, patients may be felt to not be candidates for various treatments, based on the presence of advanced lung disease. However, HPS is reversible in many cases with liver transplantation. More recently transvenous intrahepatic portosystemic shunts (TIPS) have been shown to have a surprisingly beneficial palliative effect in many patients. Perhaps the most relevant point for anesthesiologists and surgeons is to consider and recognize the disorder to best direct further management of these patients.

PORTAL HYPERTENSION: THE ROLE OF PREOPERATIVE DECOMPRESSION

With the emergence of TIPS as a relatively mild but highly effective intervention in chronic portal hypertension, its role in various clinical situations has become a frequent topic of discussion. The most obvious situation is that of hernia repair in the setting of cirrhosis with ascites (Figure 21-6). Abdominal-wall hernias are common in patients with ascites because of the pressure of the ascitic fluid. These hernias can be inguinal, umbilical, or ventral. Repair is usually considered if these are symptomatic or large and at risk for incarceration. If ascites cannot be controlled with diet and diuretic use, the recurrence rate after repair is high. In addition, depending on the type of repair undertaken, there is a risk of collateral-vessel injury (portal hypertension) and postoperative wound-ascites leak.

Large-volume paracentesis may allow transient control of ascites to permit a safer procedure, but reaccumulation of the ascites can be rapid and reduce the success of the repair (incarceration after large-volume paracentesis has also been noted). Such patients may be considered for TIPS to decompress the portal vein and control the ascites. In selected patients, the TIPS can produce remarkable control of ascites and allow elective surgical repair. Patients must have adequate cardiac and renal function and have sufficient liver reserve to tolerate safe placement of the shunt. When the liver is small, the risk of TIPS placement (because of hemoperitoneum) becomes prohibitive in many patients. In addition, TIPS occlusion remains a problem and is usually associated with recurrence of the ascites and, possibly, recurrence of the hernia.

The utility of TIPS as a preoperative measure in other situations has been little explored. The risks of the procedure are substantial, but in selected patients (as noted previously) the results can be remarkable. As a prelude to liver transplantation, TIPS has been variably received by transplant surgeons. While decompression of the portal collateral system may be desirable, there may be technical difficulties with the metal mesh extending into the portal vein, especially if the shunt extends too far into the portal vein. We have had one case of fingertip injury from the exposed end of the metal TIPS mesh in a hepatitis C-positive-transplant recipient, who had previously undergone TIPS placement.

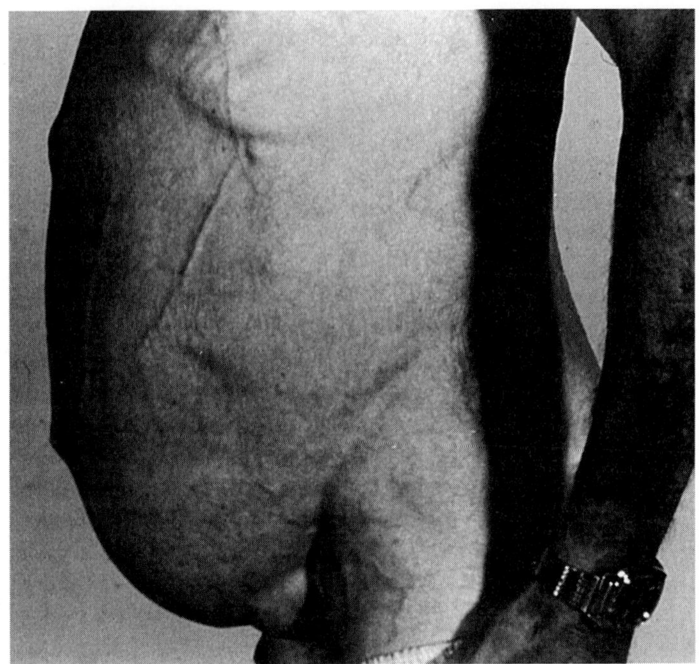

Figure 21-6
An inguinal hernia in a patient with cirrhosis and recurrent ascites.

• PERITONEOVENOUS SHUNTS: A HEPATOLOGIST'S PERSPECTIVE

The popularity of peritoneovenous shunts (PV), either Denver or LeVeen, for refractory ascites has waxed and waned over the years. These devices serve to route ascites fluid from the peritoneal cavity to the central venous system through plastic tubes tunneled under the skin from the right- or left-upper abdomen to the right- or left-jugular vein. Patients must have relatively low central-venous pressures (we usually assess cardiopulmonary function by echocardiography), and minimal or no prior abdominal surgery to ensure free flow of ascites fluid within the peritoneal cavity. Potential complications include pulmonary congestion, infection (we usually recommend postoperative prophylactic antibiotics), disseminated intravascular coagulation, and shunt failure. Any of these may be severe and require removal of the device.

Although less popular now than in the past, we occasionally find a role for PV shunts in patients who have failed diuretic therapy, require frequent large-volume paracenteses (usually greater than one per month), and who are not candidates for either orthotopic liver transplantation (OLT) or TIPS. Thus, the patients are usually older and have more advanced liver disease. Although a number of relatively positive reports are in the literature, we have observed limited success in about one third, worsening of their condition in about one third, and little change in their overall condition in the remaining patients. Nonetheless, there are patients in whom these devices provide one of the few available alternatives to help palliate their condition.

POSTOPERATIVE CARE IN CIRRHOTIC PATIENTS: PITFALLS

Patients with underlying liver disease are at increased risk for complications when undergoing just about any type of surgical procedure. Elective procedures may allow at least some degree of preventive intervention, such as preoperative correction of coagulopathy, consideration of bleeding risks, and close postoperative monitoring of electrolytes. They also allow fluid balance, early resumption of diuretics such as spironolactone, and avoidance of certain medications which can potentiate complications. Unexpected cirrhosis or urgent surgery in a cirrhotic patient often hampers care and further increases the risk of complications.

Ascites

The presence of ascites following abdominal procedures offers obvious potential problems in postoperative care. These include poor wound healing, ascites leakage, and wound infection. For these reasons, abdominal surgery is often avoided in patients with known advanced liver disease. The problem, however, is more likely to be evident in patients without known antecedent cirrhosis, and in those requiring urgent abdominal surgery. Exacerbation of ascites may also be seen following non-abdominal surgery such as hip repair (often in older females with cryptogenic cirrhosis), or intracranial procedures following subdural hematomas in cirrhotic patients with coagulopathy.

In general, ascites in this setting results from salt loading of the cirrhotic patient, usually through intravenous fluids. Hypoalbuminemia from cirrhosis and malnutrition may also contribute to the ascites, as well as generalized edema. Although hemodynamic monitoring may occasionally be useful, particularly if the ascites is complicated by renal insufficiency, it is seldom needed and, indeed, may be difficult to interpret because of the hemodynamic derangements that accompany cirrhosis. The treatment involves judicious use of saline solutions, avoidance of nonsteroidal anti-inflammatory analgesics (NSAIDs), which cause significant sodium retention in these patients, large-volume paracentesis with subsequent colloid (albumin) if the ascites is tense, and gentle diuretic use. We usually recommend beginning therapy with spironolactone as soon as the patient is taking oral medicines. In refractory cases, TIPS may serve to decompress the portal vein and reduce ascites sufficiently to allow complete wound healing.

Bleeding

The presence of portal hypertension is always associated with the formation of a rich collateral-vascular bed within the peritoneal cavity. The exact pattern varies from individual to individual. It may involve primarily upper-portosystemic connections (around the stomach, esophagus, gall bladder, spleen, and umbilical vein), lower portosystemic connections around the rectum and lower-abdominal wall, or both of these systems. Collaterals may also extend into the chest. Thus, the risk of injuring an unexpected and often large vein is substantial. Coagulopathy and thrombocytopenia may also be present. The coagulopathy of cirrhosis may involve simply inadequate production of clotting factors, or there may be greater complexity in the form of dysfibrinogenemia or hyperfibrinolysis. These clotting disorders are often difficult to correct, even with generous infusions of plasma or concentrated factors. Recently, recombinant factor VII (activated) has been shown to be a potentially powerful tool in this situation, although it currently remains under investigation in the United States.

Jaundice

Although jaundice may develop for many reasons following surgery, many of the potential scenarios are beyond the scope of this chapter. However, jaundice in the patient with underlying liver disease deserved a few relevant comments. The development of postoperative jaundice in previously well-compensated patients with liver disease could be caused by resorption of hematoma, blood transfusion, progressive liver dysfunction, renal failure, or hemolysis. As an initial step in the evaluation, liver enzymes and fractionation of bilirubin should be undertaken. A high unconjugated fraction suggests that hemolysis (usually of transfused blood) or resorption of hematoma is the underlying problem. Near-normal liver enzymes in the setting of postoperative jaundice is often seen with the cholestasis of parenteral nutrition and sepsis. Disproportionate elevation of alkaline phosphatase suggests either biliary tract disease, or drug-induced cholestasis. Significant elevation of liver enzymes suggests an acute superimposed hepatitis, often ischemic, in the postoperative setting. This is especially so in trauma cases, for patients who may have experienced significant hypotension. Any of these conditions, in the patients with underlying chronic liver disease, may herald the onset of severe, and often fatal, liver and multiorgan failure (the commonly observed "downward spiral" of the liver patient).

Encephalopathy

Encephalopathy may be multifactorial in these patients. If present, a recheck of the liver enzymes to make certain that there is not an unexpected exacerbation of the underlying liver disease (for example from drug-induced hepatitis) is warranted early during the evaluation. Withdrawal syndromes may play a role in some patients, especially alcoholics. More often, the problem is caused or exacerbated by constipation, which results in severe hyperammonemia. Constipation may result from immobilization, narcotic use, or abdominal surgery. Narcotic use is a particularly difficult problem. Lactulose is a synthetic disaccharide that serves to increase bowel movements and acidify the stool slightly, which favors ammonia excretion (caused by formation of ammonium ion). Although it is quite effective, too much use can cause excessive free-water loss and potentially fatal hypernatremia or trigger renal failure which quickly progresses to hepatorenal syndrome. In addition, the use of lactulose especially with poor gut motility can lead to excessive gas formation and secondary abdominal distention; in this setting, it may be easily mistaken for ascites. Alternatives to lactulose include neomycin and sometimes oral metronidazole. Both of these medications also lower ammonia. Sodium benzoate is rarely used to promote excretion of ammonia in the urine.

Bone Disease

Bone disease, especially osteoporosis in chronic cholestatic liver diseases like PBC or steroid-treated autoimmune hepatitis, is common. These patients are not only at high risk for fractures leading to the need for various forms of surgery, but also for progressive bone dissolution in the postoperative period for any type of surgery that leads to a period of immobilization. Early mobilization is obviously helpful. All patients should resume calcium supplements as soon as possible. Consideration should be given to other forms of treatment aimed at osteoporosis such as vitamin D supplementation and bisphosphonates (such as etidronate).

PAIN MEDICATIONS IN CIRRHOSIS

Pain medication can become a difficult issue in patients with underlying liver disease. The use of sedating medications may hide or imitate worsening encephalopathy. In addition, narcotics have the double strike of decreasing gut motility, which exacerbates hyperammonemia and encephalopathy. Acetaminophen is often avoided because of concerns for potential hepatotoxicity. This may often represent overconcern, however. Acetaminophen metabolism *is* induced in regular consumers of alcohol (also with phenobarbital use). This can lead to high levels of the toxic metabolite and acute hepatitis, at even low doses of the medication. In other patients, this is less of a concern. Acetaminophen may actually be the lesser of potential "evils" when compared to narcotics, which can imitate worsening encephalopathy or cause constipation and actually induce hepatic encephalopathy or NSAIDs. The NSAIDs (any class) can induce severe fluid retention and ascites in cirrhotic patients because of inhibition of renal-prostaglandin formation. In addition, if portal gastropathy is present, there may be an increased risk of bleeding.

SUMMARY

The need for surgical intervention in a patient with underlying liver disease or the discovery of unexpected cirrhosis in a patient undergoing elective surgery, can present the surgeon and anesthesiologist with many difficult problems. We have touched on some of these issues and attempted to briefly review some newer aspects of hepatology. The ability to bring these patients through difficult procedures has improved over the past several decades. That is because some of the early literature dealt, to a large extent, with either shunt or gallbladder surgery in these patients. Increased awareness of the subtlety with which cirrhosis can exist and influence the postoperative course, will further improve the care of these often difficult patients.

BIBLIOGRAPHY

Angelico M, et al: Isosorbide-5-mononitrate versus propranolol in the prevention of first bleeding in cirrhosis, *Gastroenterology* 104:1460–1465, 1993.

Ferenci P, Herneth A, Steindl P: Newer approaches to therapy of hepatic encephalopathy, *Semin Liver Dis* 16:329–338, 1996.

Fernandez-Rodriguez C, et al: Arteriovenous shunting, hemodynamic changes, and renal sodium retention in liver cirrhosis, *Gastroenterology* 104:1139–1145, 1993.

Kaplan MM: Primary biliary cirrhosis, *New Engl J Med* 335:1570–1580, 1996.

Kodali VP, et al: Cryptogenic liver disease in the United States: further evidence for non-A, non-B, non-C hepatitis, *Am J Gastroenterol* 89:1836–1839, 1994.

Krawitt EL: Autoimmune hepatitis, *New Engl J Med* 334(14):897–903, 1996.

Krowka M, Cortese D: Hepatopulmonary syndrome: An evolving perspective in the era of liver transplantation, *Hepatology* 11:138–142, 1990.

Lee Y-M, Kaplan MM: Primary sclerosing cholangitis, *N Engl J Med* 332:924–932, 1995.

Lieber CS: Medical disorders of alcoholism, *N Engl J Med* 333(16):1058–1065, 1995.

Matsumoto A, et al: Increased nitric oxide in the exhaled air of patients with decompensated liver cirrhosis, *Ann Intern Med* 123:110–113, 1995.

Meyer B, et al: Quantitation of intrinsic drug-metabolizing capacity in human liver biopsy specimens: support for the intact-hepatocyte theory, *Hepatology* 13:475–481, 1991.

MMWR. Recommendations for preventing transmission of human immunodeficiency virus and hepatitis B virus to patients during exposure-prone invasive procedures, *MMWR* 40:1–9, 1991.

Ochs A, et al: The transjugular intrahepatic portosystemic stent-shunt procedure for refractory ascites, *N Engl J Med* 332:1192–1197, 1995.

Sharara Al, Hunt CM, Hamilton JD: Hepatitis C, *Ann Intern Med* 125(8):658–668, 1996.

Sheth SG, Gordon FD, Chopra S: Nonalcoholic steatohepatitis, *Ann Intern Med* 127:137–145, 1997.

Vallance P, Moncada S: Hyperdynamic oxide? *Lancet* 337:776–778, 1991.

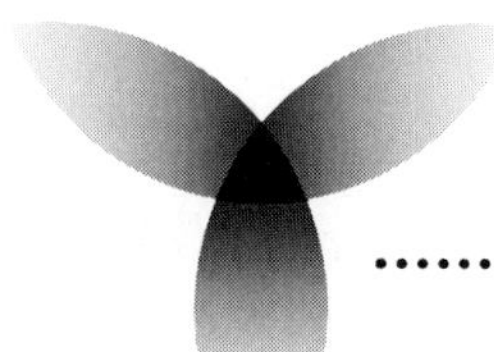

Chapter 22

Rheumatologic, Infectious, and Immunologic Diseases

George S. Leisure, MD, Brian Wispelway, MD

• RHEUMATOLOGIC DISEASES

Systemic Lupus Erythematosus (SLE)

Systemic lupus erythematosus is a multisystem disease that can produce variable manifestations including rashes, alopecia, fever, arthritis, leukopenia, thrombocytopenia, pleuritis, pericarditis, anemia, nephritis, and central nervous system (CNS) effects. The disease can occur at any age, but its onset is primarily between the ages of 16 and 55 years, occuring more frequently in women. The etiology of SLE remains unknown. However, a role for immune, environmental, hormonal, and genetic influences have all been suggested. These patients develop antibodies to a number of nuclear and other cellular antigens. As a result, antibodies can be directed at red blood cells, white blood cells, platelets, endothelial cells, and neuronal cells, leading to many of the clinical manifestations of the illness. The disease may also be induced by drugs such as isoniazid, D-penicillamine, hydralazine, procainamide, and α-methyldopa. The clinical manifestations of the drug-induced form of SLE are similar to those of the spontaneous form of the illness, but the symptoms are more mild and progression of the disease is slower.

The clinical course is characterized by periods of remissions, alternating with acute or chronic relapses. The disease may be exacerbated by stresses such as infection, surgery, or pregnancy. The initial symptoms may be nonspecific and include fatigue, fever, myalgias, depression, arthralgias, nausea and vomiting, headaches, and easy bruising. Photosensitivity is common in these patients after exposure to ultraviolet B light, occurring in over 50% of patients. Many other cutaneous manifestations are common, and Raynaud's phenomenon occurs in 17% to 30% of patients.

Pulmonary manifestations are common in SLE, manifesting as cough, dyspnea, pleuritis, and pleural effusions. Interstitial infiltrates can form and fibrosis may develop, leading to pulmonary hypertension, hypoxemia, and a restrictive lung disease.

Cardiovascular manifestations include pericardial effusions, which can be seen echocardiographically in many of these patients, and pericarditis. However, tamponade and restrictive pericarditis are rare. Myocarditis and unexplained cardiomyopathy with congestive heart failure have been reported. Myocarditis may cause cardiac conduction abnormalities. Premature atherosclerosis causing coronary artery disease is also increasingly recognized. This phenomenon may be the result of a combination of factors including steroid-induced lipid abnormalities, immune-complex deposition along blood vessels, and hypertension caused by lupus nephritis. Mitral valve prolapse is common, and Libman-Sachs verrucous endocarditis can also occur, affecting the mitral and aortic valves.

Hematologic manifestations include abnormalities of all the formed elements of blood, as well as abnormalities of the clotting and fibrinolytic systems. Lupus nephritis can lead to hypertension and renal failure. In addition, proteinuria and hypoalbuminemia may be seen. Cranial or peripheral neuropathies, seizures, and psychoses are all possible neurologic sequelae of this disease. Strokes also occur and are usually related to vascular thrombosis. Abnormal liver-function tests are common, and severe lupoid hepatitis can occur.

PERIOPERATIVE CONCERNS

As a result of the multisystem nature of SLE, many of the complications may require surgical intervention. Prolonged steroid use can lead to avascular necrosis of the femoral head, requiring joint reconstruction. Many of the disease manifestations such as peritonitis, mesenteric ischemia, and renal-vein thrombosis can either mimic or represent true surgical emergencies. Patients with acute relapses of the disease should probably not undergo elective surgery.

An elevation of the partial thromboplastin time (PTT) should prompt a search for a coagulation factor deficiency. However, this may be caused by the presence of a lupus anticoagulant, an antibody that reacts with the prothrombin activator complex, leading to a prolongation of the PTT. The presence of a lupus anticoagulant has been associated with thrombocytopenia, frequent miscarriages, pulmonary artery hypertension, and thrombotic stroke. It is rarely associated with bleeding unless profound thrombocytopenia is present. The presence of a lupus anticoagulant should not interfere with surgery.

Rashes and vasculitic lesions are common, and only local care is required to avoid breakdown and secondary infection. Nasal ulcers can occur and should be documented before nasal intubation. A cold operating room and the stress of surgery can precipitate Raynaud's phenomenon. Care should be taken to keep the extremities warm. In addition, these patients may be receiving postganglionic α-blockers or calcium channel blockers to ameliorate the symptoms of Raynaud's phenomenon. Laryngeal involvement including recurrent laryngeal nerve palsy, cricoarytenoid arthritis, and mucosal ulceration may also be present.

The spectrum of renal involvement in SLE ranges from asymptomatic to hypertension from nephritis or edema from nephrosis, or depressed glomerular filtration. Nephrotoxic drugs should be used with extreme caution because a normal serum creatinine may not represent a completely normal glomerular filtration rate.

Cardiopulmonary involvement must be looked for in the perioperative period. Patients with a long history of SLE may have restrictive pulmonary hypertension, or diaphragmatic dysfunction. Cardiac involvement is common but usually not of great clinical significance. Libman-Sachs valvular disease may predispose to bacterial endocarditis, so the use of prophylactic antibiotics should be considered.

Patients may also require stress dosages of steroids in the perioperative period to avoid the effects of decreased adrenal reserve, especially if they have been on steroids chronically. In addition, it has been postulated that the stress of surgery may precipitate an exacerbation of SLE. Consequently, some clinicians advocate increasing the baseline dosage of corticosteroids for a few weeks postoperatively.

Scleroderma

Scleroderma, or progressive systemic sclerosis, is a rare disease characterized by fibrosis of skin and several visceral organs including the gastointestinal (GI) tract, lungs, heart, and kidneys. Scleroderma is an autoimmune disorder. Endothelial cell injury causes vascular destruction and leakage of serum proteins into the interstitium, resulting in tissue edema, lymphatic obstruction, and fibrosis. The disease varies significantly in its extent and severity. Some patients develop the CREST syndrome (calcinosis, Raynaud's phenomenon, esophageal hypomotility, sclerodactyly, and telangiectasias). The etiology of scleroderma is unknown, and there is no cure for the disease, although penicillamine is often used for skin involvement.

The distinction between limited cutaneous scleroderma and diffuse cutaneous scleroderma is important. If the disease is limited to the hands, fingers, and face, limited cutaneous scleroderma is present and visceral involvement is unlikely. If truncal skin changes are present, then diffuse cutaneous scleroderma is present and surveillance of visceral function is indicated. Prognosis is related to the extent of visceral involvement, rather than to cutaneous involvement. The skin is described as "hidebound," and skin tautness can limit movement of the wrists, elbows, shoulders, mouth, and thorax. Severe Raynaud's phenomenon may be present. In about one half of patients, pregnancy leads to an exacerbation of the disease.

Pulmonary involvement is the major threat to life in scleroderma. Pleural effusions, pulmonary hypertension, interstitial lung disease with fibrosis and obstructive pulmonary disease may all play a role in the pulmonary insult in scleroderma. Dyspnea may be a late complaint in the patient who is sedentary because of skin and joint restrictions. Pleural effusions may need to be drained to improve ventilation.

Renal involvement in scleroderma can lead to accelerated hypertension and oliguria, previously accounting for the majority of deaths in scleroderma. Fewer patients now develop renal failure because of improved agents used to control the hypertension, especially angiotensin converting enzyme inhibitors.

Cardiac manifestations include pericardial effusions, congestive heart failure, and conduction system disorders leading to cardiac dysrhythmias. Cor pulmonale may result from pulmonary hypertension. Gastrointestinal manifestations include esophageal hypomotility and small intestinal hypomotility. Lower esophageal sphincter tone is decreased resulting in gastric reflux. Abdominal pains that mimic mechanical obstruction can lead to laparotomy.

PERIOPERATIVE CONSIDERATIONS

As a result of the many organ systems that are potentially involved in this disease, a thorough, perioperative medical evaluation is essential. Venous access may be difficult in the patient with scleroderma because of fibrosis. Chest wall involvement may result in restrictive pulmonary function. In the presence of severe pulmonary disease, postoperative ventilatory support may be needed. Factors known to increase pulmonary vascular resistance such as respiratory acidosis and hypoxemia should be avoided. Oral endotracheal intubation may be difficult because of a restricted mouth opening, necessitating fiberoptic intubation. Oral or nasal telangiectasias can be traumatized during intubation, causing profuse bleeding.

Chronic hypertension and vasomotor instability may make hypotension more likely on induction of anesthesia. In addition, the decrease in lower esophageal sphincter tone may make regurgitation of gastric contents and subsequent pulmonary aspiration more likely in these patients. Nephrotoxic drugs must be used with caution. The eyes should be well-protected during surgery because of the possibility of coexisting keratoconjunctivitis. These patients should also be kept warm to minimize peripheral vasoconstriction by maintaining a warm operating room environment and administering warm intravenous fluids. The extremities must be well padded during surgery to avoid damage to peripheral nerves.

Rheumatoid Arthritis

Rheumatoid arthritis (RA) is a chronic systemic inflammatory disease characterized by symmetric polyarthropathy and extensive systemic involvement. The peak incidence of onset is between the ages of 40 and 60 years, but it can occur from childhood to later life. Females are 2 to 3 times more likely to be affected by this disease than males. The etiology of this disease is unknown. Genetic susceptibility has been clearly demonstrated. Rheumatoid arthritis also appears to be an "autoimmune" disease. The rheumatoid factor, an autoantibody to the Fc portion of immunoglobulin G molecules, is present in 80% to 90% of patients with RA. However, it does not cause the disease because it is present in other disorders such as SLE, pulmonary fibrosis, and viral hepatitis. An infectious cause has also been postulated. It may be that all of these factors play a role, so that an infectious agent activates the cellular immune response in a genetically susceptible patient.

The clinical presentation of RA is highly variable, and its course is marked by exacerbations and remissions. In the majority of cases, joint stiffness and/or pain develops insidiously over weeks to months. However, the onset can be abrupt, sometimes coinciding with a stressful event. Rheumatoid nodules may be present at pressure points, particularly below the elbow. The disease can be distinguished from osteoarthritis because in RA, the terminal interphalangeal joints are spared. The joints of the hands, elbows, knees, and wrists all may be involved, with morning stiffness being a hallmark of the illness. Mandibular motion may be limited by involvement of the temporomandibular joint. The cervical spine may be involved in RA, whereas the thoracic, lumbar, and sacral spines are spared. Atlantoaxial subluxation, with separation of the atantoodontoid articulation can be seen radiographically in 30% of cases. When this separation is profound, the odontoid process can protrude into the foramen magnum. This may result in compression of the spinal cord. Vertebral arteries can also be compressed, leading to vertebrobasilar insufficiency with vertigo or syncope, especially with downward gaze. The odontoid process may itself be eroded, which will pose less of a threat to the spinal cord. The cricoarytenoid joints may also be involved, resulting in dysphagia, anterior neck pain, hoarseness, stridor, and dyspnea.

The systemic manifestations of RA are caused by a diffuse vasculitis. Pleural effusions are a common pulmonary manifestation, and rheumatoid nodules can occur in the lungs. These nodules are usually asymptomatic, but they can become infected and cavitate, or rupture into the pleural space causing a pneumothorax. Diffuse, interstitial fibrosis can also result.

Pericardial disease is the most common cardiac manifestation of RA. However, clinically relevant pericarditis and large pericardial effusions with tamponade are rare in RA. Constrictive pericarditis is more common, and it presents as right-sided heart failure, peripheral edema, and dyspnea. Rarely, rheumatoid nodules can occur on heart valves or in the myocardium, and vasculitis can involve the coronary arteries.

Peripheral neuropathies are produced by proliferating synovium, causing nerve compression. Carpal tunnel syndrome caused by a median neuropathy and tarsal tunnel syndrome caused by tibial neuropathy are common. Sjögren's syndrome can lead to corneal damage because of dryness of the eyes. Mild anemia and mild liver-function abnormalities are common in RA.

PERIOPERATIVE CONSIDERATIONS

As with many other rheumatologic diseases, the multiorgan involvement of RA must be understood to ensure the safety of the patient in the perioperative period. A thorough cardiopulmonary evaluation is essential to uncover any involvement of these systems with RA. The medications to treat this disease must also be appreciated. Aspirin is often used to provide analgesia, and its use is limited by unwanted effects such as GI bleeding and interference with platelet function. Other nonsteroidal antiinflammatory medications are commonly used. Corticosteroids are also frequently used. Large doses may be associated with poor wound healing, adrenal supression, myopathy, and GI bleeding. Stress dosages of corticosteroids may be required in the perioperative period. Gold salts are used, and the side effects of their parenteral use includes leukopenia, thrombocytopenia, eosinophilia, and proteinuria. The oral gold preparation, auranofin, may have fewer adverse effects. Cyclophosphamide, azathioprine, and methotrexate may be used. All three may be limited by hematologic toxicity.

The airway is a major consideration for those patients with RA needing surgery. The restricted motion of the temporomandibular joint may limit mouth opening, making oral-endotracheal intubation difficult. Atlantoaxial subluxation may be present, predisposing the patient to compression of the spinal cord or vertebral arteries. The preoperative physical examination should evaluate the patient for the presence of symptoms related to flexion, extension, or rotation of the head. If intubation is necessary, direct laryngoscopy should be performed in a manner to avoid extreme movements of the neck. If the cricoarytenoid joints are involved, the glottic opening may be narrowed. If necessary, fiberoptic intubation should be performed.

• IMMUNOLOGIC DISEASES

Allergic Reactions

Allergic reactions imply an immunologically mediated response and must not be confused with direct drug toxicity or overdosage. These reactions can be classified as either anaphylactic or anaphylactoid. The distinction between these two reactions is based on the mechanism of the response, but the clinical presentations may be similar.

Anaphylaxis is a life-threatening manifestation of an antibody-antigen interaction. It is a type 1, or immediate hypersensitivity, reaction which is produced by immunoglobulin E–mediated (IgE) release of chemical mediators. This reaction may occur whenever prior exposure to an antigen has elicited the production of antigen-specific IgE antibodies. Subsequent exposure of the patient to this antigen results in an antibody-antigen complex that causes degranulation of mast cells and basophils. The effects these mediators have on the end organs produce the clinical syndrome of anaphylaxia.

Urticaria can be seen in the skin, bronchospasm and upper-airway edema in the respiratory system, vasodilation and cardiac depression caused by leukotrienes, and increased capillary permeability in the cardiovascular system. Indeed, capillary permeability can be so profound that massive fluid resuscitation is required. The onset of symptoms is usually immediate, but can be delayed up to 15 minutes. The reaction has been reported to occur as late as 2.5 hours after the parenteral administration of the antigen. Manifestations occur at more unpredictable times after oral administration. In a patient under general anesthesia, hypotension may be the only clinical manifestation of anaphylaxis. Bronchospasm and urticaria may not be present.

In contrast, anaphylactoid reactions are not mediated by IgE or an antigen-antibody complex. This reaction occurs as a result of administration of certain drugs that cause the release of histamine from basophils and mast cells. Since this reaction does not depend on an antigen-antibody interaction, it can occur in a patient exposed to a drug for the first time.

Although it is not usually possible to predict which patient will have an allergic reaction to a drug, certain patient characteristics may make such a reaction more likely. Patients with a history of atopy or allergic rhinitis may be at increased risk for having an allergic reaction in the perioperative period. In addition, patients allergic to penicillin have a 3- to 4-fold increased risk of experiencing an allergic reaction to any medication. Allergic reactions have been reported with almost all injectable drugs used during the administration of anesthesia. Muscle relaxants, however, are most commonly associated with drug-induced allergic reactions in this period. Allergic reactions can also occur to blood and plasma-volume expanders, vascular-graft material, intravascular-contrast material, and latex-containing medical devices.

Treatment of anaphylaxis includes ensuring adequacy of arterial oxygenation, inhibition of further mediator release, and aggressive fluid resuscitation. Above all, the condition must be recognized and treated promptly. Early intervention with epinephrine is essential. Epinephrine increases intracellular concentrations of cyclic adenosine monophosphate (cAMP) which serves to restore membrane permeability, and its β-agonist effects serve to relax bronchial smooth muscle. An antihistamine such as diphenhydramine can be administered, but once mediators have been released, it may be of limited value. In addition, it will not reverse the bronchospasm or negative inotropic effects produced by leukotrienes. Corticosteroids should be administered as they may enhance the β-effects of other medications, and inhibit the release of arachidonic acid. Beta-2 agonists should be administered by inhalation to treat bronchospasm.

Cryoglobulinemia

Cryoglobulinemia is a disease characterized by abnormal circulating proteins that precipitate when cooled and dissolve when heated. These proteins can be cryoglobulins or cold agglutinins, and they usually do not precipitate unless blood temperatures decrease below 33°C. Precipitation of these proteins leads to platelet aggregation, plasma hyperviscocity, clotting-factor consumption, and activation of the complement pathway. Microvascular thrombosis may lead to renal impairment, which is a frequent occurence in these patients.

PERIOPERATIVE CONSIDERATIONS

Body temperature of those with cryoglobulinemia must be maintained above the thermal reactivity of the cryoglobulin throughout the perioperative period. Patients requiring cardiopulmonary bypass, in which the technique of deliberate hypothermia is commonly used, present a unique perioperative challenge. Cold cardioplegia can result in intracoronary precipitation, resulting in obstruction with resultant ischemia, infarction, or poor myocardial preservation. Preoperative plasmapharesis should be considered which can significantly decrease the level of circulating cryoglobulins.

Hypothermia in the operating room environment can be avoided by increasing the ambient temperature in the room, humidifying and warming the inspired gases, warming the intravenous fluids, and using a warming blanket.

Hereditary Angioedema

Hereditary angioedema (HAE) is a relatively rare autosomal-dominant disorder, affecting 50% of the offspring of a patient and occuring with equal frequency in males and females. The disorder is caused by either low levels or a decreased functional activity of the plasma-protein C1-esterase inhibitor. This protein controls activation of the complement pathway. As a result of the absence of this inhibitor, when the complement pathway is activated, it is not adequately regulated, leading to the release of vasoactive mediators. Hereditary angioedema is characterized by episodic, painless attacks of nonpitting edema involving the skin of the extremities and face, as well as mucosal membranes. The GI tract may be involved, causing severe abdominal pain. Rarely, the attack can cause laryngeal edema, producing respiratory obstruction and asphyxiation. Attacks are often sporadic, but approximately 50% of patients note an increase in attack frequency with emotional stress. Local trauma may also precipitate an attack. Attacks last approximately 48 to 72 hours. The disorder is usually mild in childhood, becoming more severe with the onset of puberty.

Attacks of HAE often respond poorly to epinephrine, glucocorticoids, and antihistamines. However, these medications are still used. Patients undergoing surgery should receive 2 units of fresh frozen plasma (FFP) preoperatively to prevent attacks. Fresh frozen plasma may help by supplying missing inhibitor proteins. There are some reports of FFP helping to terminate an attack. However, reports also exist of FFP exacerbating edema. Consequently, FFP is not recommended to treat life-threatening laryngeal edema. In the perioperative period, overzealous suctioning of the airway should be avoided. Regional anesthesia appears safe, and the choice of medications to produce regional or general anesthesia should not be affected by the presence of HAE. For long-term prophylaxis, many of these patients will be taking acetylated, artificial androgens which increase the levels of C1 inhibitor.

• INFECTIOUS DISEASES

Hepatitis A

Hepatitis A is referred to as infectious or short-incubation hepatitis. It is caused by a 27-nm diameter RNA virus that is transmitted almost exclusively by the fecal–oral route. It may be transmitted by handling food, in drinking water, and by fomites. Parenteral transmission is rare but has been documented. There is no evidence that a chronic form or a carrier state of hepatitis A exists. Clinically inapparent acute cases seem to serve as the "reservoir" for the virus.

The infection has an incubation period of 2 to 6 weeks. Serum antibody is initially predominantly of the IgM class, but an IgG antibody soon appears and persists for many years. The presence of the IgM antibody almost always indicates infection within the past few months. The presence of the IgG antibody indicates prior exposure and immunity.

The acute illness is often clinically inapparent, presenting with flu-like symptoms. Jaundice is mild if present at all. Liver-function test abnormalities return to normal and symptoms abate usually within a 3- to 4-month period. Systemic immune reactions such as vasculitis, purpura, nephritis, and cryoglobulinemia have been reported. The syndrome of cholestatic hepatitis occurs occasionally and may last for several months. These patients have cholestatic features such as dark urine, light stools, pruritus, direct-acting hyperbilirubinemia, and elevated alkaline phosphatase. The prognosis for this is almost always favorable. Rarely, massive hepatic necrosis and fulminant hepatic failure have been reported.

Prevention of this illness is primarily through strict attention to hygiene, by both caregivers and patients alike. Careful handwashing is important and the wearing of gloves by caregivers is appropriate. The virus is inactivated by boiling and exposure to formalin, chlorine, or ultraviolet irradiation. For cooperative and informed patients in the hospital setting, strict isolation is not usually required. Close contacts of patients with hepatitis A should receive immunization with immune-serum globulin, preferably within the first few days of exposure. A formalin-inactivated vaccine may soon be available.

Hepatitis B

Hepatitis B virus (HBV) differs significantly from the hepatitis A virus. The complete infective virion, or Dane particle, is a DNA virus which consists of antigenically distinct surface and core components. The inner, protein core, hepatitis B core antigen (HBcAg), contains a circular, partially double-stranded DNA molecule, and the outer core consists of hepatitis B surface antigen (HBsAg). Unlike hepatitis A viral infection, hepatitis B can have a myriad of acute or chronic hepatic and extrahepatic manifestations, as well as a chronic-carrier state. The hepatocellular injury and necrosis that result from HBV infection is thought to be caused by a host-immune reaction against hepatocytes that express HBV antigens, especially HBcAg, in conjunction with class I HLA determinants on their surface.

Hepatitis B virus is present in virtually all secretions and body fluids. Transmission is primarily by the parenteral route, such as through transfusion of infected blood, sharing of infected needles, through intimate sexual contact, or at birth. Blood is the most effective vehicle for HBV infection because the concentration of viral particles in blood is significantly greater than in other body fluids, such as semen or saliva. Unlike hepatitis A, transmission of HBV by the fecal-oral route is relatively unimportant. Infection may result after oral ingestion, but a large inoculation is required.

The diagnosis of HBV infection can be made by examination of the serologic markers for this infection. Hepatitis B surface antigen may be detected in the serum as soon as 2 weeks, especially after a large parenteral exposure. The presence of this antigen in the blood indicates infectivity. It can be measured in the serum before the onset of symptoms or the increase in alanine aminotransferase (ALT) levels, which may take between 4 weeks and 6 months to occur. Hepatitis B surface antigen usually becomes undetectable in the serum before antibody to HBsAg appears. At about the time of clinical onset and the rise in ALT level antibody to HBcAg becomes detectable. The presence of HBcAg indicates a high risk of HBV infectivity. Initially, an IgM antibody to the HBcAg is found in acute HBV infection and it can persist for several months to 1 year. Thereafter, IgG antibody to the HBcAg predominates, persisting for up to several years after acute hepatitis and being present indefinitely in all chronic carriers. Immunity to HBV infection is usually confirmed by the presence of antibody to the HBsAg. Unfortunately, several HBV mutants have been identified, and infection has occurred despite active immunization.

Hepatitis B virus infection resolves in 95% of healthy adults. Fewer than 1% develop massive hepatic necrosis. However, some patients will become chronic carriers as indicated by the presence of HBsAg in the serum for greater than 6 months without antibody formation. These patients are chronic carriers who can possibly infect others. About 25% of chronic carriers develop chronic active hepatitis, which can progress to cirrhosis. In addition, primary hepatocellular carcinoma is more likely to develop in chronic carriers of HBV infection. In addition, HBV infection is associated with extrahepatic manifestations such as urticaria, arthritis, and, less commonly, glomerulonephritis and vasculitis.

An effective and safe vaccine exists for the prevention of HBV infection, consisting either of a highly purified and triple-inactivated HBsAg obtained from the serum of chronic carriers, or a recombinant preparation using HBsAg synthesized in microorganisms. The vaccine is administered in three doses, initially, at 1 month, and at 6 months. The vaccine elicits antibody to the HBsAg in over 90% of healthy recipients. Unfortunately, immunosuppressed individuals exhibit a poor antibody response to immunization. The duration of protection varies, but by 5 years, 20% to 30% of people who were successfully immunized lack protective levels. Official recommendations concerning booster doses have not been made. The vaccine should be administered intramuscularly, and is more likely to be effective in the deltoid than the gluteal muscles. Pregnant women can safely receive the recombinant vaccine.

If an individual has been exposed to HBV and has completed hepatitis vaccination, additional immunization is not waranted if the titer of antiHBs is protective; that is, 10 mIU/ml. If the titer is too low, passive immunization with hepatitis B immune globulin (HBIG) should be instituted as soon as possible and a booster dose of vaccine given. If the individual has not been immunized, HBIG should be administered, combined with simultaneous initiation of active immunization with the HBV vaccination. Ideally, the rational approach to postexposure prophylaxis depends on documenting the serologic status of both the "donor" and "recipient" so that the appropriate decision to administer HBIG and/or vaccine can be made.

Hepatitis C

Hepatitis C virus (HCV) accounts for most of the cases of hepatitis previously referred to as non-A, non-B hepatitis. It is an RNA virus related to the virus family which includes flaviviruses and pestiviruses. There appears to be a large degree of variability in the HCV genome, and these genotypic variations can be generated rapidly during the course of acute and chronic infection. This is important because the primers and probes used in the laboratory to identify HCV may fail to recognize the nucleotide sequences of the particular isolate, leading to false-negative testing for either host antibody to HCV or for viral RNA by means of polymerase chain reaction (PCR) assays. In addition, multiple infections with different HCV strains can occur. These characteristics of HCV infection may influence the efficacy of treatment for chronic HCV infection, and make vaccine development difficult.

Hepatitis C virus can be detected in the serum of infected patients, but the viral concentrations are usually lower than those found in HBV infection. In addition, HCV concentrations are even lower or undetectable in other body fluids such as stool, semen, vaginal secretions, urine, and saliva. Consequently, the infection can be transmitted by means of a large volume innoculation such as a transfusion, but it is much less likely than HBV to be spread among family members or by perinatal or sexual contacts.

Hepatitis C virus has been the major cause of posttransfusion hepatitis. The incidence of this complication has declined over the past two decades because of screening for antibodies to HCV, HBsAg, and other surrogate markers of non-A, non-B hepatitis, and as a result of eliminating paid donors. Hepatitis C virus infection is also seen in renal dialysis patients, in recipients of untreated commercial preparations of clotting-factor concentrates, intravenous drug abusers who share needles, and recipients of organ transplants from HCV-positive donors.

After exposure, the incubation period is 5 to 7 weeks. The acute illness cannot be distinguished on clinical or general laboratory examination from other causes of acute hepatitis. Hepatitis C virus infection is rarely associated with massive hepatic necrosis and fulminant hepatic failure. However, HCV has a higher propensity than HBV to cause a chronic infection, occurring in 50% of patients with HCV infection. There is, at present, no vaccine against HCV, and the value of pooled gamma globulin in prophylaxis against hepatitis C is not documented.

Tuberculosis

Approximately 1.7 billion people, one-third of the world's population, are infected with *Mycobacterium tuberculosis (M. tb)*. From this pool, an estimated 8 million new cases of tuberculosis (TB) develop each year, resulting in 3 million deaths. In the United States, there are an estimated 10 to 15 million people with latent TB infection.

Tuberculosis was a leading cause of death in the United States at the turn of the century. The incidence of TB began to decline in 1944, largely because of improvements in sanitation and housing, and later, because of the introduction of specific antituberculous medications. The decrease continued until 1984, when a dramatic reversal in this trend occurred. From 1984 to 1992, the number of TB cases in the United States increased by 20% to over 26,000/year. While this increase was primarily caused by the rise of HIV infection, additional factors that contributed included increased immigration from countries with a high incidence of TB, transmission among persons residing in congregate settings (prisons, shelters, nursing homes), and a decline in resources for TB-control programs. The increased incidence of TB in the mid-80s was disturbingly associated with an increase in the percentage of isolates found to be resistant to either isoniazid (INH) alone or to the multiple standard agents. The term *multidrug-resistant TB* (MDR-TB), by definition, implies resistance to at least INH and rifampin. In 1995, a total of 37 states reported drug susceptibility results and 7.6% of isolates were found to be resistant to at least INH, and 1.4% were resistant to at least INH and rifampin. The rates clearly vary be region with rates of MDR-TB approaching 20% of cases in New York in the early 90s.

M. tuberculosis is spread by airborne droplet nuclei. Particles which are 1 to 10 microns in size are able to reach the terminal bronchioles and produce infection. Larger particles are trapped in the upper airway and eliminated from the body. Initially, *M. tb* multiplies without resistance, but within 2 to 6 weeks, an intact cell-mediated immunity limits further multiplication in approximately 95% of persons. At this point, the person is usually asymptomatic and may remain so for life. Most persons will have a positive ppd at this point and may have a healed, calcified lesion on chest radiograph. Between 5% to 15% of HIV-negative persons develop active TB with most of this risk confined to the first 3 years after infection. Isoniazid prophylaxis can significantly decrease this risk. HIV-infected persons are at increased risk of developing active TB. This risk may be as high as 50% in the first year following infection, with risk roughly correlating with declining CD4 counts.

Tubercle bacilli can subsequently spread from the primary complex though the blood stream to multiple sites. If a large number of organisms are involved, miliary disease may develop. Small numbers may result in scattered foci that may remain inactive for life, or reactivate and produce clinical disease. The tubercle bacilli multiply at sites where oxygen tension is the greatest including apices of the lungs, the kidneys, and growing ends of long bones. In the normal host, the immunologic response to infection with *M. tb* provides protection against subsequent exposure to organisms and, therefore, reinfection is rare.

The current recommendations for empiric antituberculous therapy reflect the previously described trends. A four-drug regimen including INH, rifampin, pyrazinamide, and either ethambutol or streptomycin is suggested as initial therapy for patients in areas of INH resistance of at least 4%. Considering the current prevalence and characteristics of drug resistance, at least 95% of patients will receive adequate initial therapy, which can subsequently be modified pending the outcome of susceptibility testing.

PERIOPERATIVE CONCERNS

One out of every eight hospitals responding to a survey by the Centers for Disease Control (CDC) in 1992 reported that at least one employee had developed active TB as the result of a nosocomial exposure. Additionally, a survey of 359 U.S. hospitals found an average TB-skin-test conversion rate among health care workers of 0.65% in 1992. Those individuals at highest risk for infection include nurses, pathologists, laboratory workers, and pulmonologists. Effective hospital control programs are essential to prevent nosocomial transmission and require mechanisms for early identification of infected patients and staff, rapid and effective isolation procedures, and aggressive treatment of documented cases. The degree of infectiousness of a given case is determined by the anatomic site of infection, the presence of a cough, positive sputum smears for *M. tb*, the ability of the patient to cover the mouth while coughing, the presence of a cavity on chest radiograph, timing of therapy, and the use of cough-inducing procedures. A person with documented TB who has been on adequate therapy for at least 2 to 3 weeks and has had definite clinical and bacteriologic (three consecutive, negative, sputum smears) is probably no longer infectious.

TB should at least be considered a possibility in patients with respiratory symptoms and the appropriate risks previously discussed. Documented or high-likelihood cases should be isolated in a private room with appropriate ventilation. The best systems result in a negative-pressure ventilation and yield greater than six air exchanges per hour. While the newer, personally fit HEPA-filtration masks may yield the best personal respiratory protection, the increased filtering capacity may not be worth the increased cost. Proper isolation, ventilation, and appropriate antibiotic therapy have proved to be the most important components of any control program. Class "C" masks, which provide a greater than 95% filtering capacity offer significant, personal respiratory protection.

In summary, tuberculosis remains a significant medical problem in the United States and significant risk to health care workers. We must again think about TB as the first step in controlling it.

Acquired Immunodeficiency Syndrome (AIDS)

HUMAN IMMUNODEFICIENCY VIRUS (HIV) EPIDEMIOLOGY

As of July 1996, the World Health Organization estimated that approximately 28 million people, 25.5 million adults and 2.4 million children, had been infected with human immunodeficiency virus (HIV) since the start of the global epidemic. An estimated 7.7 million people have either progressed to full-blown acquired immunodeficiency syndrome (AIDS) or died of AIDS-related illnesses. Heterosexual transmission now accounts for an estimated 70% of all HIV infection worldwide. Those currently at greatest risk of infection are poor and socially deprived, and young people between the ages of 15 and 24, especially women. More than 90% of all infections in infants and children are caused by vertical transmission (transmission from mother either *in utero* or by perinatal transmission).

Data from North America and Western Europe show that the United States has, by far, the highest reported number of AIDS cases in the industrialized world. More than 1.2 million adults in North America and Western Europe are living with HIV/AIDS (6% of the global total). Adult-HIV prevalence ranges from 2 per 1000 in Western Europe and 5 per 1000 in North America.

In the early 1980s, HIV infection principally affected homosexual and bisexual men, and intravenous drug users. Over time, additional groups emerged, including transfusion patients, hemophiliacs, and other individuals receiving infected blood or blood products. In recent years, the incidence of HIV infection among heterosexuals has grown, particularly in urban areas with high rates of intravenous drug use and sexually transmitted diseases. The increase in HIV incidence among women of childbearing age means that newborns are also at increased risk of acquiring HIV infection.

The high incidence of HIV infection in these various groups reflects the major routes of transmission of the virus: sexual intercourse, contact with contaminated blood and other body substances, and vertical transmission from mother to child. Transmission from patient to health care worker has been well documented, as well.

HIV TESTING

The type of test routinely used for diagnosis of HIV infection is an HIV-antibody test, which reveals infection only after seroconversion, when antibodies become detectable. Seropositivity can be detected usually between 6 to 12 weeks after infection. Before seroconversion, infected individuals who do not yet have detectable antibodies can, nevertheless, transmit HIV to others. Tests are available to detect the virus, the viral genome, or viral particles in blood before the appearance of antibodies, but are currently too expensive and labor-intensive for routine diagnostic use.

THE COURSE OF HIV INFECTION

The clinical course of HIV infection reflects a continuous battle between the virus and the immune system. Human immunodeficiency virus replicates predominantly in the cells and tissues of the immune system, especially in CD4+ cells. It attaches to CD4 molecules on T cells, as well as to a recently identified group of coreceptors, both of which have implications for the natural history and transmissibility of the disease. These coreceptors for HIV, termed "CXCR4" and "CCR5" are, like CD4, linked to the immune system. They serve as receptors for chemokines, a large family of polypeptide chemoattractants with roles in the inflammatory process. Interestingly, the absence of expression of CCR5 by a cell is associated with reduced sensitivity to HIV infection. A genetic variant causing a deletion of CCR5 has been linked to resistance to HIV infection in some people at high risk who are exposed to the virus, and possibly linked also with a delay in the progression of the disease.

The primary phase of HIV infection involves rapid, viral replication of high "viral load," or concentration of virus in the blood. In roughly one half of infected individuals, this phase is accompanied by an acute clinical syndrome, which starts between 2 to 6 weeks after infection, and lasts approximately 2 weeks. Symptoms include fever and lymphadenopathy, skin rash, GI and neurologic symptoms, and general malaise. This initial phase, when viral load is high but antibodies are not yet detectable, is called the "window period." The body then begins to mount an immune response, during which HIV antibodies appear and the concentration of whole virus in the blood is dramatically reduced. A clinically asymptomatic phase follows, which may last for several years.

Current detection techniques show that infectious HIV is nearly always present in blood of infected individuals, whether or not they show any symptoms. The viral load is greatest during the first few weeks after infection, and, again, months to years later after the onset of AIDS. The large quantities of infectious virus present in the early phase of infection is highly significant in terms of transmission risk, since the individual may not yet be aware that he or she is infected.

PROGNOSIS

The course of HIV infection can vary considerably among individuals, with a mean interval from infection to the development of AIDS of 10 to 11 years. There are many variables that can affect the rate of progression from HIV infection to AIDS in HIV-infected individuals, including the strain of HIV, host-immune factors, and environmental factors; it is, therefore, difficult to make an accurate prognosis. A decrease in CD4+-cell count has proved to be a good predictor of AIDS onset, but has the disadvantage of only being measurable relatively late in infection. There is mounting evidence that the viral load in blood shortly after seroconversion is highly predictive of progression to AIDS. Individuals with acute retroviral illness and higher viral loads following seroconversion have a greater risk of rapid progression, while those with low-viral loads have a better chance of long-term survival.

Since the availability of zidovudine (ZDV), there has been optimism, but little evidence, that specific antiretroviral therapy could significantly alter an HIV-infected person's prognosis. While ZDV was found to prolong life in a person who had already progressed to AIDS, there is no evidence that it could prolong life in individuals with lesser degrees of immunosuppression. This appeared to be caused by ZDV's minimal and transient effect on viral load, as a result of rapid emergence of ZDV-resistant HIV variants. Recent studies of combined drug therapies have caused renewed optimism, however. For example, the combination of ZDV and didanosine (ddI) is more effective than ZDV alone in slowing clinical progression and reducing mortality when given to asymptomatic patients. The combination of ZDV and 3TC (lamivudine) has resulted in suppression of viral load for periods greater than 1 year. This has recently been shown to correlate with improved outcome. Finally, combinations to two nucleosides, such as ZDV and 3TC, with recently approved protease inhibitors (ritonavir, indinavir), are capable of suppressing viral loads to undetectable levels for prolonged periods. These results have already been shown to prolong life in patients with advanced AIDS. The apparent capacity of these protease inhibitor-based regimens to totally suppress viral replication (at least in the bloodstream), has led some investigators to raise the possibility of a "suppressive" cure. This hypothesis is now being tested in persons newly infected with HIV.

PERIOPERATIVE CONCERNS

Health care workers are continually at risk of acquiring bloodborne infections, particularly HBV, HCV, and HIV, all of which are associated with high morbidity or mortality. During the AIDS epidemic, concern has also grown over the increased risk to health care workers of acquiring respiratory diseases, mainly tuberculosis. The risk of occupational infection by bloodborne pathogens is related to the prevalence of infection in the patient population, and the frequency and type of exposure events.

The prevalence of HIV in the patient population is one determinant of occupational risk of HIV infection. In one U.S. study, the CDC evaluated the risk of HIV infection in emergency department workers, comparing suburban hospitals with inner-city hospitals where AIDS incidence is high. From January to September 1989, seroprevalence ranged from 4.1 to 8.9 per 100 patient visits in 3 inner-city hospitals, and from 0.2 to 6.1 per 100 patient visits in 3 suburban hospitals. Seroprevalence rates were greatest in the 15- to 44-year-old age group, in males, in blacks and Hispanics, and in patients with pneumonia.

The Sentinel Hospital Surveillance System, established by the CDC, provides information on HIV seroprevalence among patients in U.S. hospitals. Seroprevalence data collected between January 1988 and October 1991 show a wide variation in the rate of HIV-1 infection. The high seroprevalence rates reported at some sentinel hospitals suggest a need for routine voluntary counseling and testing of patients. It is estimated that a national program offering voluntary counseling and testing to people between the ages of 15 and 54 in the U.S. hospitals with AIDS diagnosis rates of 1.0 or more per 1,000 discharges, could potentially identify as many as 110,000 patients with unsuspected HIV infections per year.

An anonymous seroprevalence survey of HIV infection in British Columbia, Canada, which involved the testing of laboratory specimens, found an HIV seroprevalence of 0.88% among men and 0.07% among women from a total of 66,658 outpatients aged 15 to 55.

The following body fluids, tissues, and substances are potential sources of HIV exposure and should be taken into consideration in the postexposure risk assessment:

1. Blood or bloody body fluids, tissues, or substances.
2. Cerebrospinal, amniotic, peritoneal, pleural, synovial, and pericardial fluids.
3. Inflammatory exudates.
4. Semen or vaginal secretions.
5. Human milk.
6. Viral cultures, regardless of the age of the specimens.

The principal routes of exposure to substances that carry a potential risk of HIV transmission are:

1. Percutaneous injuries, i.e., skin puncture from contaminated needles or lacerations from sharp objects.
2. Exposure of mucous membranes.
3. Exposure of nonintact skin.

In addition to these principal routes of transmission, there are reports of cases in which HIV appears to have been transmitted by prolonged contact with contaminated blood over large areas of intact skin by bites, and by blood contact during bloody fights. When health care workers are exposed to HIV by these rare routes of transmission, a case-by-case assessment should be carried out.

The major determinant of HIV transmission from occupational exposures appears to be the size of the viral inoculum. This is a function of the concentration of virus in the source patient's blood or other body substances, and the volume of the inoculum introduced into the health care worker. A higher viral load in patients is observed in the early phase of HIV infection and in terminal illness. Quantification of HIV-RNA, when feasible, is useful in better defining transmission risk. Although definitive data are not available, patients with more than 30,000 HIV-RNA copies/ml can be considered highly infective even when they are asymptomatic. Therefore, the risk of transmission from an occupational exposure is directly related to the type of exposure and the clinical stage of the source patient's HIV infection.

U.S. Public Health Service recommendations for HIV postexposure chemoprophylaxis are also based on a hierarchy of risk, taking into consideration both the exposure severity and the concentration of virus in the source material.

As described earlier, HIV is present and continuously replicating at all stages of infection, with the amount of HIV in blood and other body fluids highest during the primary acute infection and later, when the symptoms of AIDS are present. Most documented cases of occupational HIV transmission involve source patients with AIDS, but there are also a few cases involving asymptomatic source patients, even source patients in the window period of infection.

HIV TRANSMISSION RATES

Approximately two thirds of reported worldwide cases of occupational HIV infection are in the United States. Despite an active surveillance program, case identification is known to be incomplete. As of June 1996, the CDC reported 51 documented and 108 possible causes of occupational HIV transmission. The rate of HIV transmission following occupational exposure has been the subject of several studies. The estimated average is a 0.3% transmission rate per exposure. However, individual exposures are rarely "average." For instance, the probability of transmission following a needle stick from a blood-drawing needle and involving a source patient with high HIV titers, would greatly exceed the average 0.3%.

The average risk of transmission after mucous membrane or skin contact with HIV-infected blood has been estimated at 0.1% or less. Again, the risk depends on the size of the viral inoculum, with a higher risk when blood contains high HIV titers, where there is prolonged skin contact, when a large surface areas is affected, or when visible skin lesions are present on the health care worker. In addition, there is accumulating evidence indicating that blood exposure of conjunctivae is an efficient route of transmission of HIV and other bloodborne pathogens.

According to a CDC surveillance study, in which HIV-exposed health care workers were followed, the average risk of acquiring HIV infection following percutaneous injury was 0.36%. In a case-controlled study also conducted by the CDC, it was shown that the risk of HIV seroconversion was higher for exposures involving:

1. Deep injuries.
2. Visible blood on the device causing injury.
3. A hollow-bore needle that had been in the source patient's vein or artery.
4. A source patient who died of AIDS within 60 days of the occupational exposure.

The CDC has used mathematical modeling to estimate transmission risks in the presence or absence of specific risk factors. Preliminary calculations suggest that the risk from percutaneous exposures to HIV can range from 0.05%, if none of the above four risk factors are present to more than 5% if three or four are present.

POSTEXPOSURE PROPHYLAXIS—AN URGENT DECISION

The decision of the exposed health care workers to accept or decline postexposure–HIV prophylaxis is an urgent one, since it is recommended that prophylaxis starts within 1 hour of exposure. The current CDC recommendations for postexposure–HIV chemoprophylaxis should be observed and explained to the health care worker. In particular, the health care worker should be:

1. Provided with a risk assessment and counseled on the transmission risk associated with the specific exposure.
2. Informed of current data regarding the efficacy and toxicity of post-exposure prophylaxis, and also of the limited nature of these data.

3. Informed that he or she has the option to decline consent for post-exposure prophylaxis.

The CDC now recommends lamivudine in combination with ZDV for postexposure prophylaxis because such a combination:

1. Provides greater antiviral activity than ZDV alone.
2. Is active against ZDV-resistant strains of HIV.
3. Results in no significant increases in toxicity compared with ZDV alone.

The protease inhibitor indinavir is also a recommended component of postexposure prophylaxis in cases of high-risk exposure. Other drugs licensed for the treatment of HIV infection, such as didanosine, zalcitabine and some protease inhibitors, are not as suitable for use in combination with ZDV in postexposure prophylaxis, because of their unacceptable levels of toxicity. The stavudine-ZDV combination has been shown to be antagonistic when its activity against ZDV-resistant HIV was assessed in cell culture.

The implementation of new post-exposure protocols incorporating chemoprophylactic regimens has necessarily led to an increase in the cost of, and effort required for, a comprehensive post-exposure follow-up program. The potential effectiveness of new prophylaxis drug regimens in preventing the transmission of HIV makes the effort and the cost worthwhile, and is an important step forward in reducing the risk of occupational HIV transmission. Unfortunately, there is still no intervention proven to completely eliminate the risk of HIV transmission after an exposure, and the continuing spread of HIV in the general population means that HIV prevalence in patient populations is not likely to decline in the foreseeable future. As a result of these factors, and because of the continued risk of exposure to other bloodborne pathogens, exposure prevention remains a top priority. The added expense of the new chemoprophylaxis regimens also means that prevention has become more cost-effective than ever, in relation to the high cost of follow-up.

BIBLIOGRAPHY

Frank MM, Gelfand JA, Atkinson JP: Hereditary angioedema: the clinical syndrome and its management, *Ann Intern Med* 84:580,1976.

Harris ED Jr: Rheumatoid arthritis: pathophysiology and implications for therapy, *N Engl J Med* 322:1277, 1990.

LeRoy EC: A brief overview of the pathogenesis of scleroderma, *Ann Rheum Dis* 51:286, 1992.

McGowan JE Jr: Nosocomial tuberculosis: new progress in control and prevention, *Clin Infect Dis* 21:489, 1995.

Sharara AL, Hunt CM, Hamilton JD: Hepatitis C, *Ann Intern Med* 125:658, 1996.

Wainright RE, et al: Duration of immunogenicity and efficacy of hepatitis B vaccine in a Yupik Eskimo population, *JAMA* 261:2362–2368, 1989.

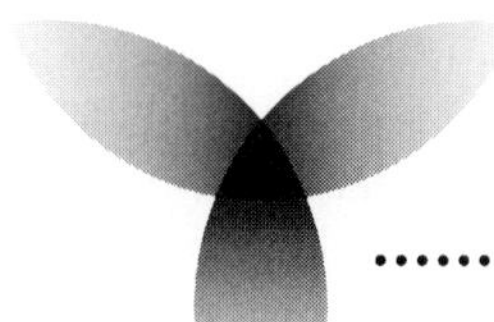

Chapter 23

Pregnancy

Burkhard F. Spiekermann, MD, Cosmo DiFazio, MD, PhD

In the United Kingdom, before 1957, pregnancy accounted for 4% of women's deaths between the ages of 15 and 44. Between 1957 and 1987 this number decreased to 0.7%. Undoubtedly, improved peripartum care and an understanding of the physiologic alterations associated with pregnancy, played a major role in the reduction of mortality associated with pregnancy. In reality, the physician caring for a pregnant patient automatically assumes responsibility for at least two patients, namely, the mother and the unborn fetus. Interventions performed for the benefit of the mother should not harm the fetus and vice versa. As a general rule, the statement holds that "whatever harms the mother will also harm the child."

Pregnant patients may require surgical interventions related to their pregnancies, such as cesarean sections (C-sections) or cervical cerclage, but each year between 0.75% to 2% of pregnant patients will undergo a surgical procedure that is not directly pregnancy-related, for example, trauma, cholecystectomy, and appendectomy. To make rational decisions regarding the pregnant patient's perioperative care, an understanding of the altered physiology and the potential complications associated with the pregnant state is necessary. This chapter reviews the physiologic alterations of pregnancy and their implications. In addition, it discusses uteroplacental circulation, the effects of anesthesia on labor and delivery, the special concerns for the patient with preeclampsia-eclampsia, the patient with massive bleeding, and the patient with fetal distress. Concerns regarding the pregnant patient with cardiac and pulmonary disease, and/or diabetes mellitus are also addressed. At the end of the chapter, we will outline the perioperative issues in the pregnant patient undergoing nonobstetric surgery. Excellent textbooks on the anesthetic management of obstetric patients are available. Thus, we will not specifically discuss intraoperative management.

• PHYSIOLOGIC CHANGES DURING PREGNANCY AND EVALUATION OF THE PREGNANT PATIENT

In a sense, pregnancy is a multiorgan process. The early physiologic alterations seen in the pregnant patient are largely caused by hormonal influences. Later in pregnancy, the growing uterus has mechanical implications, affecting primarily the cardiovascular and respiratory system. These alterations need to be appreciated because they will influence the response to any planned surgical and anesthetic intervention.

Cardiovascular Changes and Perioperative Implications

In the term parturient, cardiac output (CO) is increased by 40% primarily because of an increase in stroke volume (30%), and to a smaller degree, because of an increase in heart rate (15%). Most of the increase in CO is delivered to the placenta. During labor, CO may increase another 45% above prelabor values. The greatest increase in CO occurs immediately after delivery, where it can exceed prelabor values by 80%. This is secondary to autotransfusion from the uterine vasculature, with an associated increase in preload.

Approximately 10% to 15% of term patients may develop the so-called "supine hypotension syndrome," characterized by severe hypotension with and without changes in mental status, diaphoresis, nausea, and vomiting, when the patient assumes the supine position. This is most likely caused by an obstruction of the vena cava by the gravid uterus, when lying supine, that precipitates a severe decrease in preload and CO.

Intravascular volume in term pregnancy is increased by 1000 to 1500 ml. Plasma volume increases by approximately 40%, while red blood cell volume increases by only 20%. This explains the decrease in the hemoglobin concentration to approximately 11 g/dl (physiologic anemia of pregnancy). In contrast, a hemoglobin level over 14 g/dl is abnormal and should be seen as a sign of hemoconcentration and hypovolemia, as for example, seen in the preeclamptic patient. The increase in intravascular volume compensates for the average blood loss of 500 ml and 1200 ml, during vaginal and cesarean-section delivery, respectively. A dilutional effect from the increase in plasma volume is also responsible for a reduction in the total plasma-protein concentration.

Mean arterial blood pressure is decreased by 15 mm Hg in the parturient, and hypertension in the previously normotensive patient should always be considered abnormal. Since CO is increased in the face of a decreased blood pressure, systemic vascular resistance has to be lower. In fact, total peripheral resistance is decreased by roughly 15%. Central venous pressure is not changed in the healthy parturient. However, if femoral venous pressures (and uterine venous pressures) are measured, an increase of 15 mm Hg is noted. This is a result of flow resistance through the vena cava. Table 23-1 summarizes the changes in the cardiovascular parameters seen during pregnancy.

When evaluating the pregnant patient, a systolic murmur is commonly heard on auscultation that is caused by an increase in blood flow, secondary to the increase in CO per unit time and the decrease in vascular resistance. Diaphragmatic shifts will displace the heart leftward, which moves the point of maximum impulse to the left and may enlarge the cardiac silhouette on chest radiograph. The electrocardiogram shows a left-axis deviation for the same reason. Fatigue, dyspnea, and pedal edema are common complaints in the parturient; these do not necessarily reflect cardiac compromise. Generalized edema, a high hematocrit, a diastolic murmur, high blood pressure, and pronounced cardiorespiratory symptoms, however, warrant further investigations.

The supine position should be avoided in the term parturient. Even if there is no history of supine hypotension syndrome, caval compression will occur to a certain degree in this position and will cause an increase in uterine-venous pressure and a decrease in uterine-perfusion pressure. The latter is the difference between uterine-artery and uterine-vein pressure. If patients need to be positioned supine, a soft wedge should be placed under the right lateral thoracolumbar area that will shift the uterus off the vena cava.

Patients without cardiac disease usually have no significant problems handling the stress imposed on the cardiovascular system during the peripartum period. Conversely, the large increases in intravascular volume and CO, especially immediately postpartum, may present a significant insult to the patient with preexisting cardiovascular disease, as discussed in the following.

Respiratory Changes and Perioperative Implications

Minute ventilation is increased by 50% in term pregnancy as a result of a 40% increase in tidal volume and a 15% increase in respiratory rate. The increase in tidal volume is at the expense of a 15% to 20% decrease in the functional residual capacity (FRC). Total lung volume remains the same or is slightly decreased. In up to one third of the pregnant patients closing capacity will actually exceed FRC in the supine position, thus, predisposing pregnant women to airway closure and hypoxemia. Figure 23-1 illustrates the changes in lung volumes in the pregnant state.

Table 23-1. Cardiovascular Changes Associated with Pregnancy

VARIABLE	AVERAGE CHANGE
Blood volume	35% increase
Plasma volume	45% increase
Red blood cell volume	20% increase
Cardiac output	40% increase
Stroke volume	30% increase
Heart rate	15% increase
Femoral venous pressure	15 mm Hg increase
Total peripheral resistance	15% decrease
Mean arterial pressure	15 mm Hg decrease
Systolic blood pressure	0–15 mm Hg decrease
Diastolic blood pressure	10–20 mm Hg decrease
Central venous pressure	No change

With the increase in minute ventilation, a compensated respiratory alkalosis (pCO_2 30 mm Hg and serum bicarbonate 20 mEq/l) is present in the parturient. During contractions minute ventilation can increase by an additional 300%. The developing hypocarbia and alkalosis may result in compensatory hypoventilation after a contraction, possibly causing hypoxemia.

Oxygen consumption is increased by 20%, secondary to an increase in maternal metabolism. During labor the oxygen consumption may increase another 60% above prelabor values. The high oxygen demand, in combination with the low FRC, is another reason why pregnancy predisposes the parturient to hypoxemia. A summary of the respiratory changes seen in pregnancy is shown in Table 23-2.

Of interest to the anesthesiologist is that the high progesterone levels of pregnancy also induce dilatation of capillary beds, including the nasopharyngeal mucosa. Thus, swelling of airway structures may make laryngoscopy and intubation more difficult and mucosal bleeding with airway instrumentation more common.

The patient should be examined for any signs of respiratory compromise. Wheezing is not a normal finding in pregnancy. Recent upper-respiratory-tract infections may worsen edema of upper airway structures. Severe edema of the oropharynx, with or without pulmonary edema, may be present in the preeclamptic or eclamptic patient. Beta agonists used as tocolytics to abort preterm labor may precipitate cardiac failure and pulmonary edema. Because pulmonary reserve is decreased considerably with pregnancy, every effort should be made to treat additional reversible causes of airway compromise. Supplemental oxygen should be administered with any sign of distress, and to avoid airway closure, patients should not be positioned supine. If intubation and mechanical ventilation is necessary, difficulty in airway management should be anticipated. As discussed, pregnancy increases minute ventilation and causes the normal pCO_2 with pregnancy to be approximately 30 to 32. Maintaining normocarbia (pCO_2 of 40 mm Hg) with mechanical ventilation would, in effect, create a respiratory acidosis in the pregnant patient. However, excessive hyperventilation ($pCO_2 < 30$ mm Hg) should be avoided. That is because, in addition

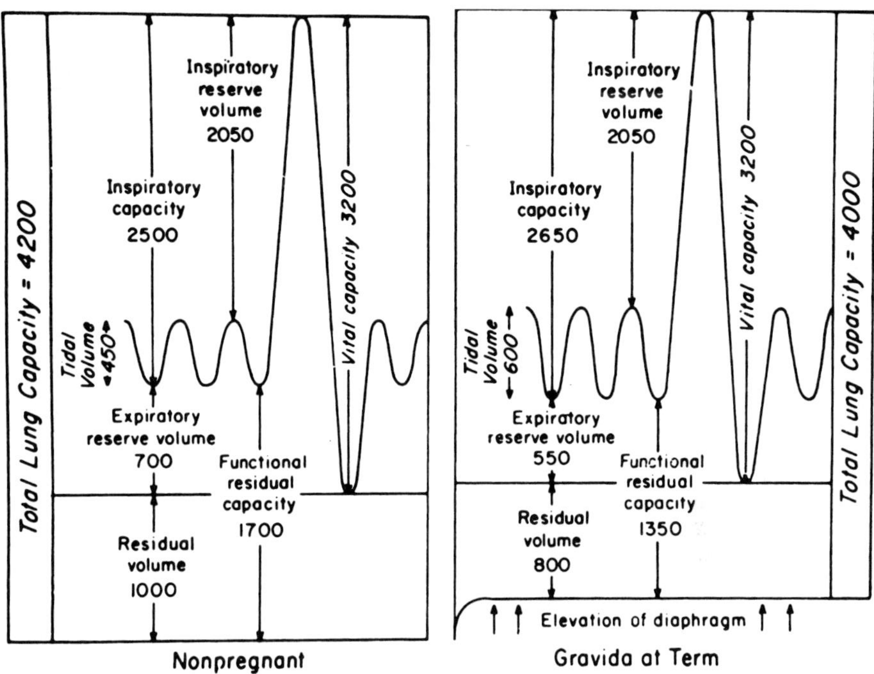

Figure 23-1
Changes in lung volumes associated with pregnancy. See text for details (Reprinted with Permission from Bonica, JS, McDonald, JS: *Principles and practice of obstetric analgesia,* Baltimore, 1995, Williams & Wilkins.)

to the mechanical effects of positive pressure ventilation, uterine vascular constriction secondary to alkalosis, in combination with a left shift of the hemoglobin–oxygen dissociation curve, all lead to a decreased placental-oxygen exchange.

Gastrointestinal Changes and Perioperative Implications

More than 50% of pregnant women develop heartburn and symptoms of gastroesophageal reflux during their pregnancy. Mechanical and hormonal alterations are responsible for esophageal-sphincter incompetency, delayed gastric emptying, and increased gastric acid production. Positional shifts of the stomach caused by the gravid uterus also decrease esophageal sphincter competency and delays passage of gastric contents past the pylorus. Progesterone decreases esophageal-sphincter tone. Placenta-produced gastrin decreases gastric motility and increases gastric acid production. Additionally, gastric emptying may be further delayed by the administration of narcotic analgesics used during labor.

A pregnant patient is at higher risk for acid aspiration of gastric contents (the so-called "Mendelson's syndrome") and extra precautions should be taken to avoid pulmonary aspiration when the patient's protective airway reflexes are disrupted with heavy sedation and the induction of general anesthesia. The usual precautionary

Table 23-2. Respiratory Changes Associated With Pregnancy

VARIABLE	AVERAGE CHANGE
Minute ventilation	50% increase
Alveolar ventilation	70% increase
Tidal volume	40% increase
Total lung capacity	0–5% decrease
Vital capacity	No change
Functional residual capacity	20% decrease
Expiratory reserve volume	20% decrease
Residual volume	20% decrease
Respiratory rate	15% increase
Arterial PO_2	10 mm Hg increase
Arterial PCO_2	10 mm Hg decrease
Serum bicarbonate	4 mEq decrease
Arterial pH	No change
Oxygen consumption	20% increase

measures taken include no oral food intake after the onset of labor, the administration of a nonparticulate antacid (sodium citrate) before a general anesthetic, and extra precautions, such as the Sellick maneuver during airway management and intubation. A rapid-sequence induction is indicated, as described in the chapter on airway management. Administration of H_2 blockers and metoclopramide have also been recommended to decrease gastric acid production and to improve gastric emptying. However, because of time constraints required to produce the desired effects, many clinicians, including physicians at this institution, do not routinely use these drugs. The mortality of a significant pulmonary aspiration is high and prevention remains the best therapy.

Renal Changes and Perioperative Implications

During the first trimester glomerular filtration rate (GFR) and renal blood flow increase by 50% to 60%, and lead to an increase in creatinine clearance and a decrease in serum creatinine values. A normal serum-creatinine concentration is generally less than 0.5 mg/dl in the pregnant patient. Higher values should be considered abnormal and may be suggestive of dehydration or intrinsic renal dysfunction. Over the last trimester, GFR gradually decreases to prepregnancy values. Progesterone induces dilatation and atony of the renal collecting system, which, in turn, can cause urinary stasis and an increased frequency of urinary tract infections.

Hepatic Changes and Perioperative Implications

Total hepatic blood flow and overall hepatic function are not significantly changed during pregnancy. However, the values for serum transaminases, lactate dehydrogenase, and alkaline phosphatase are commonly increased. One should remember that an increase of these enzymes does not necessarily indicate hepatic disease. However, a rapid rise may be a marker of disease in patients with preeclampsia-eclampsia or in patients with "HELLP syndrome." (HELLP is an acronym for **h**emolysis, **e**levated **l**iver enzymes, and **l**ow **p**latelet count.) Total serum-protein concentration is decreased during pregnancy, which may cause an increase in the free-drug concentrations of highly protein bound drugs and require a decrease in the drug-dosage requirements.

Neurologic Changes and Perioperative Implications

The minimum alveolar concentration (MAC) for inhalational anesthetic agents is decreased by approximately 30% in the pregnant patient. The increase in central nervous system (CNS) sensitivity to anesthetics is thought to be mediated by hormonal (progesterone) changes and by an increase in the concentration of endogenous opioids. An increased sensitivity of the axonal membrane to local anesthetics is also present. Therefore, an epidural block will require only two thirds of the usual amount of local anesthetic to achieve the same degree of neural blockade as in a nonpregnant woman. Increased spread of epidurally placed local anesthetics also occurs, and is caused by engorgement of the epidural veins during pregnancy which decreases the volume within the epidural space into which the local anesthetic is injected. Thus, smaller doses of local anesthetic volume is required to block as many nerve root segments as in the nonpregnant woman.

The anesthetic concentrations of inhalational anesthetics required to produce surgical anesthesia are decreased 15% to 25% during pregnancy. The concentration that may only produce mild sedation in the nonpregnant patient may actually produce unconsciousness and loss of protective airway reflexes in the pregnant patient. Likewise, cardiovascular instability may result from high thoracic blocks when the dosage of lumbar-epidural local anesthetic is not reduced from that used in the nonpregnant patient. Continuous monitoring and careful titration of anesthetic agents are essential.

• UTEROPLACENTAL CIRCULATION AND THE EFFECTS OF ANESTHETIC AGENTS

Blood is carried from the mother to the placenta through the uterine arteries and returns to the maternal venous circulation through the uterine veins. Uterine-blood flow (UBF) in the term parturient is approximately 700 ml/min. Unlike blood flow to the kidney or the brain, UBF is not autoregulated. This implies that UBF is directly proportional to the mean perfusion pressure (uterine artery minus uterine vein pressure) and inversely proportional to uterine vascular resistance:

$$\text{UBF} = \frac{\text{uterine artery pressure} - \text{uterine vein pressure}}{\text{uterine vascular resistance}}$$

Anything affecting one or more of the three variables in this equation directly impacts on UBF and, subsequently, can affect fetal oxygenation. Box 23-1 summarizes the most common endogenous and exogenous etiologies causing decreased UBF. By far, the most important variable that controls UBF is maternal mean systemic arterial pressure. Prolonged periods of hypotension (less than a systolic pressure of 100 mm Hg for more than 10 minutes) are associated with fetal acidosis.

Box 23-1 Causes for Decreased Uterine Blood Flow

Decreased uterine perfusion pressure
- Hypotension
  - Hypovolemia
  - Sympathetic blockade
  - Supine hypotensive syndrome
- Increased uterine vein pressure
  - Vena cava compression from the gravid uterus in the supine position

Increased uterine vascular resistance
- Uterine contractions
  - Abruptio placentae
  - Oxytocin
- Sympathomimetics
  - Endogenous sympathetic discharge from pain
  - Exogenous vasoconstrictors with predominantly α-adrenergic effects

Before the administration of any medication, a knowledge of its effect on UBF is essential. This is especially true in patients in whom uteroplacental exchange is already compromised from other causes (e.g., preeclampsia) and the functional reserve is minimal.

Intravenous Anesthetic Agents

As long as systemic arterial pressure is maintained, barbiturates, narcotics, propofol, and benzodiazepines do not adversely affect UBF. Ketamine at doses of less than 1 mg/kg does not decrease UBF. However, at higher doses uterine vascular resistance increases and UBF may decrease.

Inhalational Anesthetic Agents

All commonly used inhalational anesthetics have a dose-dependent effect on UBF. At lower doses (up to 1 MAC) they produce no adverse effects on UBF. While they decrease mean arterial pressure, a concomitant decrease in uterine vascular resistance maintains UBF at normal levels. High concentrations of inhalational anesthetics, however, will decrease UBF, primarily because of excessive reductions in maternal blood pressure and CO. For this reason, high concentrations of inhalational anesthetics should be avoided.

Local Anesthetics

Except for cocaine, which is a potent uterine-vasculature vasoconstrictor, the effect of local anesthetic agents on UBF is primarily indirect through their effect on maternal blood pressure during epidural or spinal blockade. If regional anesthesia precipitates hypotension, UBF will be compromised. For this reason, many clinicians advocate a fluid bolus of 500 to 1000 ml of crystalloid before instituting regional anesthesia in the parturient. However, if hemodynamics are unaltered, regional anesthesia may increase UBF. While pain of labor decreases UBF, attenuation of labor-pain induced maternal-catecholamine-release with epidural analgesia, improves intervillous blood flow through the placenta.

Vasopressors

High doses of vasoactive agents with predominantly α-adrenergic effects (phenylephrine, methoxamine) decrease UBF by increasing uterine-vasculature resistance. Low doses of an α-agonist will minimally affect UBF. Mixed and indirect-acting agents like ephedrine and metaraminol increase systemic blood pressure without negatively affecting UBF. If vasopressors are required to restore maternal blood pressure, ephedrine is the agent of choice in the healthy parturient.

EFFECTS OF ANESTHETICS ON LABOR AND DELIVERY

The progress of labor and delivery is inherently very variable. In addition to its intrinsic variability, its time course depends primarily on the patient's parity, her pelvic anatomy, and obstetric management practice. The anesthetic management during labor may also influence its progress, but probably to a lesser degree than previously suggested.

At present, the main controversy focuses on the effects of regional (epidural) analgesia on labor and the rate of C-sections performed. Recent prospective studies do not support the previously held belief that epidural analgesia increases the length of the first stage of labor, the incidence of fetal malpresentation, instrumental, or cesarean delivery. However, the second stage of labor (the "expulsive phase" after full-cervical dilatation) may be prolonged, especially if epidural blockade is dense and affects motor function of the abdominal and perineal muscles. If patients choose epidural analgesia for labor, it should be pointed out that a prolongation of the second stage is possible. Adverse effects secondary to epidural analgesia have never been documented and most women with uncomplicated epidural analgesia would prefer the possibility of a somewhat prolonged but "comfortable" labor, over a shorter, painful labor. It is important that the obstetric team is aware of and allows an increase in the duration of the second stage of labor. The decision as to the appropriate analgesic should be discussed with all parties involved.

COMPLICATIONS ASSOCIATED WITH EPIDURAL ANALGESIA

At the University of Virginia, more than 50% of laboring women request epidural analgesia for pain relief. Continuous epidural analgesia is, by far, the most effective way to control labor pain. However, it is not without potential hazards and complications as described in Chapter 40, Regional Anesthesia. The most important factor in preventing adverse complications associated with continuous epidural analgesia, is providing a "continuous anesthesia service" along with the procedure. The safe conduct of continuous epidural analgesia is not possible without a dedicated team of trained personnel available at all times. The long-term administration of epidural drugs is clearly different from an epidural or spinal administered by the obstetrician at the time of delivery.

During labor, hypotension secondary to sympathetic blockade caused by an epidural should be treated even more aggressively than in the nonparturient to prevent prolonged decreases of UBF. To decrease the severity of hypotension, intravenous infusions should be started and the patient should receive 500 ml to 1000 ml of a balanced salt solution before institution of the block. Ephedrine (5–10 mg IV) should be administered when systolic blood pressure falls below 90.

A postdural puncture headache (PDPH) from an accidental dural puncture with an epidural needle is much more common (up to 85%) in the pregnant patient, as compared to the nonpregnant woman in the same age group. Diagnosis and treatment of PDPH is described in Chapter 40. It should always be suspected in women developing a postpartum headache who received epidural (or spinal) analgesia. However, a postpartum headache is common and may have many other etiologies. For example, over 14% of postpartum women who never received an epidural will complain of a headache. If a postural component is not present with the headache (see Chapter 40), dural puncture and PDPH is an unlikely cause.

Backache is another common postpartum complaint. More than 25% of women, regardless of whether epidural analgesia is administered or not, will have back complaints. In the majority of cases, this is related to positioning during delivery, as well as preexisting back problems that can be amplified by straining with expulsive efforts during delivery. If epidural analgesia was administered, a careful examination of the epidural site and a quick neurologic examination will rule out serious complications secondary to the epidural: for example, epidural hematoma, or an epidural infection or nerve injury.

• COMPLICATIONS ASSOCIATED WITH GENERAL ANESTHESIA FOR CESAREAN SECTION

General anesthesia (GA) in the pregnant patient carries a higher risk than in any other healthy patient group. This is one reason why there has been a dramatic shift in the last decade from GA to regional anesthesia as the anesthetic technique of choice for C-section delivery. Most anesthetic practices in this country reserve GA for so-called "crash C-sections"; those that are emergent sections because of imminent maternal or fetal compromise.

Inability to intubate the trachea in a patient who has a much higher likelihood of gastric aspiration during general anesthesia, is the area of greatest concern. Delayed or difficult intubation is more frequent in the parturient because of airway edema, as discussed previously in this chapter. Additional airway management equipment should be available in the operating room, including different laryngoscopy blades, a laryngeal mask airway (LMA), and a setup for transtracheal jet ventilation (see Chapter 37, Airway Management and the Induction of Anesthesia.) If intubation of the anesthetized patient is impossible, but mask ventilation is possible, letting the patient emerge and then proceeding with an awake intubation technique may be the safest route to follow. If ventilation is not possible, an LMA may provide a manageable airway. However, it does not protect the airway from aspiration. Only under dire emergencies should a patient undergo a C-section under general anesthesia without a cuffed endotracheal tube in place. Aspiration pneumonitis carries a high morbidity, especially when caused by acidic particulate matter. As mentioned, the administration of a nonparticulate antacid is commonly used and a classic rapid-sequence induction is always performed in the parturient who requires a GA. If aspiration does occur, supportive management is the goal. The oropharynx should be immediately suctioned vigorously and the patient should be ventilated with 100% oxygen. Unless large particles obstruct major airways, bronchoscopy is unnecessary and the prophylactic administration of steroids and antibiotics appears to be of no benefit.

Awareness under GA is rare. However, the patient group that has the highest incidence of recall includes women undergoing a cesarean section with low anesthetic concentrations. A fear of compromising the fetus or causing excessive uterine vasodilation prevents some practitioners from using potent inhalational agents as part of their anesthetic. Many studies have shown that adding 0.5% halothane or 0.6% isoflurane to 50% nitrous oxide will effectively abolish recall under GA, without any harm to the mother or the fetus.

THE HIGH-RISK OBSTETRIC PATIENT

High-risk obstetric patients can be classified into two categories: the patient with pregnancy-related complications, and the patient with preexisting underlying medical conditions that may be exacerbated by the pregnant state. Common pregnancy-related complications include preeclampsia-eclampsia, placenta previa, abruptio placenta, and fetal distress requiring emergent delivery. Underlying medical problems that require careful assessment include cardiovascular disease, diabetes, and asthma. The specific considerations regarding perioperative care of these patients will be highlighted. The reader is referred to the bibliography references at the end of this chapter for more in-depth discussion of the specific disease states.

Obstetric Complications

PREECLAMPSIA-ECLAMPSIA

Preeclampsia-eclampsia occurs with the highest frequency in young primigravid women and does not usually manifest itself before 20 weeks of gestation. Preeclampsia is defined by the triad of hypertension (systolic blood pressure >140 mm Hg or diastolic blood pressure >90 mm Hg), proteinuria (>500 mg day^{-1}), and generalized edema. When a seizure occurs, preeclampsia becomes eclampsia by definition. The etiology of preeclampsia-eclampsia remains unclear but it is thought to be related to placental ischemia that may cause, or be the result of, increased thromboxane and decreased prostacyclin production. It is accompanied by uterine and generalized vasoconstriction, endothelial-cell damage, activation of procoagulant factors with platelet aggregation, and, ultimately, injury to the kidney, hearts, brain, liver, and other vascular organs. Plasma volume in the preeclamptic is often reduced, secondary to a state of generalized vasoconstriction. Cardiovascular compromise, in association with pulmonary endothelial damage and decreased colloid-oncotic pressure, may lead to pulmonary edema. Oliguria or anuria may be present from low blood volume or renal causes. A low platelet count may lead to bleeding tendencies. If the liver is also involved, or if preeclampsia-eclampsia is complicated by the HELLP syndrome, progressive fulminant-liver failure and disseminated intravascular coagulation may develop. Approximately 90% of patients with HELLP develop epigastric pain, secondary to liver engorgement and liver capsule distention; hepatic rupture becomes a major concern.

Untreated, maternal and fetal mortality is high in the rapidly progressing preeclamptic. Preeclampsia and eclampsia are thought to contribute to or cause 20% to 40% of the maternal deaths and 20% of the perinatal fetal deaths. Medical therapy for hypertension and seizure prevention includes the administration of IV magnesium sulfate and antihypertensive therapy with hydralazine, methyldopa, β-adrenergic blockers, and/or calcium-channel blockers, but the only definite therapy is delivery of the infant.

The physician taking care of the preeclamptic patient should have a clear picture of the urgency and rate of progression of the clinical situation. Communication between the anesthesiologist and the obstetric team is essential. Often, serial laboratory tests (platelet count, liver-function studies, serum creatinine) are indicators for progression of the disease and may help in deciding whether delivery of the fetus is urgent or can be delayed. A low or rapidly falling platelet count may also indicate that epidural analgesia/anesthesia for labor or C-section is not indicated.

Patient preparation before either lumbar-epidural anesthesia or GA for labor or for cesarean section includes blood pressure control to attain a diastolic blood pressure of less than 110 mm Hg. The presence of a coagulopathy should be ruled out if an epidural block is planned. This is most easily accomplished by taking the patient's history (for example, determining if easy bleeding occurs when brushing teeth). The documentation of a recent acceptable platelet count is also useful. The bleeding time has not been shown to be of practical diagnostic value, however.

Severe preeclampsia (blood pressure >160/110 mm Hg), proteinuria in excess of 5 g/day, and oliguria (<500 ml/day) all greatly increase both maternal and fetal morbidity and mortality. Invasive cardiovascular monitoring is indicated in these patients, including an arterial catheter, a central venous pressure monitor and, if there is evidence of myocardial dysfunction, a pulmonary artery catheter. With the large amount of fluid shifts after delivery, invasive monitoring may be even more important for postpartum management.

If time permits and there is no contraindication from a coagulation standpoint, we prefer to institute epidural analgesia early in the course of labor for two main reasons: (1) adequate analgesia during labor decreases circulating catecholamine levels in the preeclamptic, thereby facilitating blood pressure control and improving uterine blood flow; and (2) if a cesarean delivery is required, the epidural catheter that is in place can be used to institute surgical levels of anesthesia. Epidural anesthesia in the preeclamptic is associated with better hemodynamic control than with general anesthesia, and avoids the manipulation of a potentially very edematous airway that may present a challenge on intubation.

If epidural anesthesia is contraindicated or general anesthesia is required because of the urgency of the situation, a thorough airway examination is mandatory, and expert help in managing the airway should be available. One should be prepared to treat severe hyper- and hypotension, especially on induction to minimize maternal and fetal morbidity. Clinically, the use of magnesium sulfate produces and potentiates the action of neuromuscular blockers and dosage adjustment, and careful monitoring of neuromuscular blockade is necessary. As already mentioned, the preeclamptics' cardiovascular status frequently worsens within the first 24 to 48 hours postpartum. Therefore, monitoring in a critical-care environment with appropriately trained nurses is a must.

MASSIVE HEMORRHAGE

There are many etiologies responsible for peripartum hemorrhage, some as benign as cervicitis, some as potentially fatal as uterine rupture. In general, peripartum bleeding is much more dangerous for the fetus than for the mother. Placenta previa and placental abruption, two of the more common reasons for massive hemorrhage in the obstetric patient, have perinatal mortality rates up to 22% and 37%. Early diagnosis and proper management is critical.

Placenta Previa

Placenta previa is present when the placenta lies close to (marginal placenta previa), partially covers the cervical os (incomplete placenta previa) or completely (complete placenta previa) covers the cervical os. The incidence of placenta previa is approximately 1 in 200 pregnancies. These patients classically present with painless bleeding in the second or third trimester. The diagnosis is confirmed by ultrasound.

Patients with placenta previa should be admitted and urgently evaluated by the obstetrician and the anesthesiologist. With this diagnosis, the incidence of an emergent cesarean section is high. Although initial episodes of bleeding rarely cause severe hypotension and shock, priorities in the perioperative care include an assessment of the patient's volume status, including a recent hematocrit value. Adequate volume access (2 large-bore IVs) should be established and a blood sample for a type and crossmatch should be sent to the blood bank. A vaginal examination should only be performed in the operating room, with all arrangements made for an emergent C-section under general anesthesia (the so-called "double setup.") Two units of packed red blood cells and a blood warmer should also be available because the onset of bleeding can be sudden and dramatic. If the placenta does not separate easily from the myometrium (placenta accreta), blood loss may be massive and a dilutional thrombocytopenia may result which may require platelet transfusion. Unlike with placental abruption, disseminated intravascular coagulation (DIC) is rare.

Abruptio Placentae

Placental separation from the decidua basalis may cause concealed or frank vaginal bleeding and is usually associated with pain and fetal distress. The incidence is approximately 1% and the diagnosis is made clinically and confirmed by ultrasound. The incidence is higher in diabetic patients, patients with preeclampsia, and smokers. Unlike placenta previa, blood loss may be concealed and a large retroplacental hematoma (up to 2500 ml) may be present without any overt evidence of bleeding. Intravascular volume may be severely decreased and preparation and precautions, as outlined in the section on placenta previa, are required.

In addition to hemorrhagic shock, other complications seen in patients with abruptio placenta include acute renal failure and DIC. Expedient delivery is the cure. Uterine atony is common after delivery and when coupled with a coagulopathy may be the cause for persistent postpartum bleeding. Admission to an intensive care unit (ICU) is mandatory for patients who require large amounts of blood products and/or who have a persistent coagulopathy and are hemodynamic unstable.

FETAL DISTRESS

Fetal distress is sometimes a loosely used term describing any signs of compromised utero placental circulation. Fetal monitoring throughout labor is helpful in identifying which babies are at risk and in need of immediate delivery. It is not uncommon that parturients who are incompletely prepared and evaluated are rushed to the operating room for an emergency C-section for one or two episodes of fetal heart rate decelerations. In some of these cases, a hurried general anesthetic is administered, intubation is unsuccessful, the patient aspirates, and hypoxia results in morbidity to both the mother and the newborn. In 1992, the American College of Obstetricians and Gynecologists (ACOG) recommended "the development of strategies to minimize the need for emergency induction of general anesthesia in women for whom this would be especially hazardous." If fetal monitoring shows concerning patterns, early involvement of the anesthesiologist will prevent hurried, and potentially lethal, decisions. Many times an epidural catheter for analgesia can be placed early during labor, when fetal parameters become worrisome, but not critical. If rapid delivery through a C-section becomes necessary, the epidural analgesia can be converted to epidural anesthesia, and general anesthesia can frequently be avoided. If a general anesthetic is necessary, adequate help and assistance is needed to prevent and overcome airway difficulties. The mother's life should never be at risk to deliver a distressed fetus.

Nonobstetric Complications

THE PARTURIENT WITH CARDIAC DISEASE

With improved medical and surgical care, many women with cardiovascular disease will carry out a pregnancy. Today, up to 3% of all pregnancies are complicated by the presence of maternal heart disease. This includes patients with surgically repaired complex, congenital cardiac lesions, ischemic heart disease, valvular disorders, and patients with heart transplants. We will not discuss the specific implications regarding the many different lesions, because these are discussed in excellent detail in major textbooks on obstetric anesthesia. What characterizes all of these diseases is that physiologic, cardiovascular changes associated with pregnancy may stress the delicate, compensated state to the point of rapid deterioration in the peripartum period. The goal is anticipation of these superimposed stresses and adequate medical intervention. The obstetrician, the anesthesiologist, and the cardiologist need to develop a plan that allows safe delivery of the infant. At no other time is early cooperation among the members of the health-care team more important than it is in this patient population.

Ideally, patients with cardiovascular disease are followed by a cardiologist before conception. If this is not the case, it is the obstetrician's duty to refer the patient to a consultant as quickly as possible. It is unwise to manage patients with significant cardiac disease without the input of a cardiologist. Hopefully, the anesthesiologist will never be in the situation where he/she has to be involved in the obstetric care of a parturient who has been inadequately diagnosed and treated for cardiovascular disease.

While cardiac lesions are a concern, not many cardiac lesions present an absolute contraindication to epidural analgesia/anesthesia for labor and delivery. Patients with aortic stenosis (AS), asymmetric septal hypertrophy (ASH) and patients with Eisenmenger physiology will not tolerate any acute changes in afterload from a sympathectomy secondary to neuroaxial blockade. However, regional analgesia anesthesia has been used successfully in such patients. Adequate prehydration and a slow incremental onset of the epidural block will prevent precipitous decreases in systemic vascular resistance (SVR). Administration of neuraxial opioids for analgesia can be an excellent choice for labor analgesia because epidurally or spinally administered narcotics will produce analgesia for a vaginal delivery without changing SVR.

Patients with an expected, complicated vaginal delivery or those requiring C-sections who have cardiac lesions that place them at risk for infective endocarditis, should receive prophylactic antibiotics as recommended by the American Heart Association (Table 23-3).

Hemodynamic changes and cardiovascular stress may be at their peak immediately after delivery because of autotransfusion of blood from the placenta; hence, it is prudent to monitor such patients postpartum in an ICU.

THE DIABETIC PATIENT

Diabetes mellitus is one of the most common medical problems associated with pregnancy. Glucose intolerance may be induced by pregnancy in the previously nondiabetic person (gestational diabetes), or pregnancy may further complicate glucose homeostasis in the known diabetic patient. Pregnancy induces β-cell hyperplasia in the pancreas and a state of increased insulin secretion. However, the antiinsulin effect from increased concentrations of human placental lactogen, cortisol, and progesterone may produce hyperglycemia in spite of increased insulin levels. Adequate glucose control is desired during pregnancy because glucose readily crosses the placenta through facilitated diffusion and may cause fetal hyperglycemia, which in turn, will cause fetal hyperinsulinemia. Severe hypoglycemia may then develop in the newborn, when glucose supply through the placenta stops but high-insulin levels are still present. In addition, poor glucose control is associated with more complications during pregnancy for both the mother and the fetus.

Table 23-3. Antibiotic Prophylaxis for Subacute Bacterial Endocarditis in the Susceptible Patient Undergoing Genitourinary Procedures

PATIENT CATEGORY	ANTIBIOTIC REGIMEN
High-risk patient	Ampicillin 2 g IV or IM 30 min before procedure Gentamicin 1.5 mg/kg IV or IM 30 min before procedure repeat 8 hrs after procedure, or give amoxicillin, 1.5 g PO 6 hours after procedure
High-risk penicillin allergic	Vancomycin, 1 g IV 1 hour before patient procedure Gentamicin 1.5 mg/kg IV or IM 1 hour before procedure; may repeat once, 8 hours later
Low-risk patient	Amoxicillin, 3 g PO 1 hour before procedure Amoxicillin, 1.5 g PO 6 hours later

The peripartum care of the diabetic patient includes a careful assessment for any signs of end-organ disease, secondary to long-standing diabetes, especially in the heart and kidneys (as discussed in Chapter 16, Common Endocrine Diseases). An endocrinology consult may help with insulin management, but as a general rule one third to one half the usual dose of regular insulin should be administered on the day of the expected delivery. Long-acting preparations should be avoided, because insulin sensitivity increases dramatically after delivery, and insulin shock may be precipitated with the use of long-acting agents. Serum glucose levels should be monitored regularly (at least every 4 hours) and small doses of intravenous, regular insulin can be administered if serum glucose levels are undesirably high. The newborn infant should also be monitored closely for hypoglycemia.

Earlier observations suggested that spinal anesthesia for C-section in the diabetic patient may cause an increased incidence of fetal acidosis, when compared to general anesthesia. It was suggested that spinal anesthesia be avoided in the diabetic parturient. These findings have not been substantiated and regional anesthesia is not contraindicated in the woman with diabetes mellitus.

THE ASTHMATIC PATIENT

Asthma is a common and seemingly increasing condition in otherwise healthy young women. The incidence of asthma during pregnancy is estimated to be 1% to 7%, with the highest prevalence in the 15- to 17-year-old age group. Pregnancy has variable effects on the course of asthma, with some women improving, some getting worse, and some remaining the same with regard to their subjective feelings of airway obstruction. The unpredictability is probably caused by opposing hormonal effects secondary to the pregnancy, with increased progesterone and prostaglandins having a bronchodilator effect, other prostaglandins and a reduced sensitivity to circulating cortisols having a bronchoconstrictor effect.

Severe asthma, causing prolonged or repeated episodes of hypoxia, may have an obvious negative effect on the fetus. It is the general opinion that medical therapy, with the possible exception of methylxanthines and high-dose intravenous steroids, should be maintained during pregnancy. Inhaled β-adrenergic agonists, the mainstay of chronic asthma therapy, do not produce a tocolytic effect and are not teratogenic. If theophylline preparations are required for adequate medical therapy, serum concentrations should be carefully monitored. Theophylline clearance is decreased during the third trimester and alterations in protein binding may also influence theophylline pharmacokinetics. The administration of systemic steroids is associated with hyperglycemia, and hyperglycemia has been associated with increased perinatal morbidity. However, if the severity of the asthma dictates the use of steroids they should not be withheld. In this case, serum glucose levels should be monitored.

A history and physical examination will give the physician all necessary information in the stable asthmatic patient. A chest radiograph and an arterial blood-gas sample will rarely provide additional clues, unless an acute exacerbation or an additional problem, like a pneumonia, is suspected. One must also consider the effects of a chest radiograph on the fetus, especially in the first trimester. If an induction of labor is planned in a patient with asthma, prostaglandins should be used with caution, if at all. Severe bronchoconstriction can be caused by such agents. Beta blockers for the treatment of hypertension should also be used carefully, as should the use of ergot alkaloids for the treatment of postpartum hemorrhage. Again, bronchospasm may occur with the use of such drugs.

One of the most potent stimuli for bronchoconstriction is airway manipulation during laryngoscopy. In general, in patients with severe reactive-airway disease endotracheal intubation should be avoided, if possible. If general anesthesia is the only option, laryngoscopy and intubation should be performed as quickly and as smoothly as possible in a well-anesthetized patient following tracheal topicalization with a local anesthetic. All the potent inhalational agents are excellent bronchodilators and severe bronchospasm may be "broken" with depending levels of inhalational anesthetics. If bronchospasm persists, despite maximal medical therapy, the patient may need to remain intubated and mechanically ventilated in the ICU.

THE PREGNANT PATIENT UNDERGOING NONOBSTETRIC SURGERY

Besides maternal safety, fetal safety with regards to teratogenicity of drugs administered and the possibility of inducing preterm labor with surgery are the two most concerning issues that need to be addressed in the pregnant patient who presents to the operating room. In general, only *emergent* or *urgent* operations should be performed during pregnancy. It is astounding that every so often, pregnant women are scheduled for purely elective surgical cases without having been told by anyone that surgical procedures and anesthesia carry risks for fetal development and fetal wastage. In our opinion, elective surgery should be postponed until after delivery. If pregnant patients do require operative interventions, a consultation by the obstetric team is mandatory.

Teratogenicity of Anesthetics

Virtually every drug has been shown to produce teratogenic effects if given in doses high enough in animal models. The period of highest vulnerability to the teratogenic effects of drugs is the period of organogenesis, which is the first 13 weeks of intrauterine development. Nitrous oxide and benzodiazepines have been associated with neural tube defects, and the latter have also been thought to cause cleft-palate anomalies in animals. However, no human study ever produced convincing data that anesthetic agents (except cocaine), when given in clinically relevant doses, produce teratogenic effects in humans. This should be reassuring to the patients who need surgery during pregnancy, as well as to the anesthesiologist administering the anesthetic. As a general rule, only agents with a long "track record" should be used. Fetal heart-rate monitoring during the operation should be considered to recognize and potentially treat signs of fetal distress. If the surgical procedure lends itself to an epidural, subarachnoid block, or a peripheral nerve block, this may be preferred over general anesthesia: Drug exposure to the fetus is minimal, especially if a subarachnoid block is used. However, it is much more important also to avoid hypoxia, hypercarbia, and hypotension than any specific anesthetic agent. The former can all impact directly on fetal oxygenation and are known to cause fetal malformation and even fetal death.

Preterm Labor

Preterm labor is more common after intraabdominal procedures. There does not seem to be an association with the anesthetic technique used, but there is a direct correlation between preterm labor and the proximity of the operative site to the gravid uterus and the amount of intraoperative uterine manipulation. Statistically, the risk of a first trimester miscarriage increases from 5% without surgery to 8% with surgery. The risk of preterm labor increases from 5% to 7.5% with surgery. The need for prophylactic tocolytic therapy and the need for intra- and postoperative monitoring should be discussed with the obstetric consultant. The pediatric service should also be advised, especially if the patient's pregnancy is less than 32-weeks' gestation. This avoids unnecessary confusion and stress if preterm labor ensues in the recovery room and delivery is expected. If the fetal lung is immature and the likelihood of preterm labor high, preoperative administration of steroids to the mother should be considered.

SUMMARY

The physiologic alterations associated with pregnancy and the needs of the fetus will influence every planned medical and surgical intervention. Perioperative care of the pregnant patient requires close communication and cooperation between members of the different health-care teams. We hope this chapter highlights some of the concerns and will facilitate such cooperation, so that optimal outcome for both the mother and the unborn child is assured.

BIBLIOGRAPHY

Bonica JJ, McDonald JS: *Principles and practice of obstetric analgesia and anesthesia*, Baltimore, 1995, Williams & Wilkins.

Chestnut DH: *Obstetric anesthesia: principles and practice*, St. Louis, 1994, Mosby-Year Book.
Shnider SM, Levinson G: *Anesthesia for obstetrics*, ed 3, Baltimore, 1993, Williams & Wilkins.
Stoelting RK, Dierdorf SF: Physiologic changes and diseases unique to the parturient. In Stoelting RK, Dierdorf SF, editors: *Anesthesia and coexisting disease*, ed 3 New York, 1993, Churchill Livingstone.

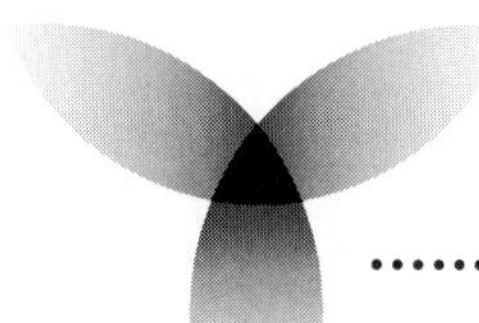

Chapter 24

Perioperative Care of Genetic Disease

Guy Weinberg, MD

PERIOPERATIVE CONSIDERATIONS IN GENETIC DISEASE

The importance of studying genetics may not be immediately apparent to the anesthesiologist, surgeon, or other physician involved in the operative care of patients. Conditions like malignant hyperthermia, or pseudocholinesterase deficiency that confer sensitivity to specific pharmacologic agents might first come to mind, but aside from these unusual diseases, genetics doesn't seem, to many physicians, to have a role in the operating room. However, genetic diseases, though individually rare, are collectively quite common. Genetic disease is also far more common among the population of operative patients than one might initially expect. This derives from the fact that people with inherited disease are more likely to need surgery than the population at large. Furthermore, genetic disease puts these patients at greater operative risk than a healthy population. Patients with sickle cell disease or trisomy 21, for instance, are commonly seen in the operating suite and their disease puts them at much greater risk for perioperative morbidity than healthy peers. These and other genetic diseases require special consideration in the perioperative period to offset this increased risk.

There are literally thousands of single gene disorders, making it virtually impossible for even the most experienced clinical geneticist to have a comprehensive familiarity with even a sizable fraction of them. This makes the task of preparing an anesthetic plan for such patients all the more daunting to the perioperative physician. However, there are guidelines that are generally applicable to assessing these patients and common principles that can guide their care. The main goal of this chapter is to review those principles and the necessary resources that will aid the physician in the preoperative evaluation and perioperative management of any patient with an inherited illness. Finally, examples of several important genetic diseases are provided to illustrate these general principles and their specific application to the perioperative care of these diseases.

Structure of the Genetic Substrate

Understanding the mechanisms of genetic disease requires a basic appreciation of the normal structure and flow of genetic information. The two most important biologic discoveries of this century were the determination by Avery, McLeod, and McCarty that DNA is the primary molecular agent of inheritance and the publication by Watson and Crick of the structure of DNA. These findings together provide the basis of the fundamental paradigm of molecular biology, which states that genetic information is encoded in the nucleotide sequence of DNA and that the flow of genetic information is from DNA to RNA through transcription, and then by translation to the synthesis of a protein molecule to whose amino-acid sequence is directed unambiguously, according to the original DNA nucleotide code. An important principle that springs from the double helical structure of the DNA molecule is complementarity: the fact that the nucleotide sequence of one strand of the DNA molecule demands a specific, complementary sequence in the sister strand. Complementarity is the basis of the ability of DNA to replicate itself faithfully and is the necessary underpinning of virtually every aspect of recombinant technology.

The human genome comprises 22 pairs of autosomal chromosomes and 2 sex chromosomes. Each chromosome contains a single, tightly coiled DNA molecule and together, these 46 chromosomes contain roughly 3 billion base pairs, and 50 thousand to 100 thousand genes encoded in their sequences. Each gene contains a coding sequence that defines, in turn, the amino-acid sequence of the corresponding protein. However, the coding sequences, or exons, of almost all eukaryotic genes are interrupted by several noncoding regions of DNA called introns. Synthesis of RNA from the DNA template requires binding of the transcription machinery to promoters, regions of DNA upstream (in the 5′ direction), to the gene whose normal function is necessary for expression of the gene product. The initial RNA transcript contains the noncoding intron nucleotide sequences, as well as sequences downstream from the gene's coding regions. Normal function of the transcript requires processing, which involves removing the intron sequences by splicing and further modifying both the 5′ and 3′ regions of the transcript (capping and adding a poly A tail, respectively) to increase stability and allow transport of the mature messenger RNA.

The best definition of a gene is that it includes the sum of all sequences upstream, downstream, and including the coding sequence proper, that are necessary for normal expression of the protein product. Mutation or alteration of any of these sequence elements can prevent production of the corresponding protein.

In addition to the noncolinear relation of nucleotide sequence to protein sequence required by the presence of introns, modern recombinant technology has discovered another unanticipated, nonintuitive aspect of genomic structure: junk DNA. The actual coding sequences of DNA responsible for directing the synthesis of a protein comprise only approximately 1% of the genome. The remaining 99%, including both intragenic introns and noncoding extragenic regions, has no known function, as yet. Roughly 25% of this junk DNA occurs as repetitive sequences, seen as either tandem repeats or repeats that are widely dispersed throughout the genome. Some of these repeats are known to be mobile genetic elements, transposons. The remaining junk DNA occurs as single, nonrepetitive sequences.

• TYPES OF GENETIC DISEASE: MODES OF INHERITANCE

Genetic diseases are classically divided into three broad categories: mendelian, or single gene diseases; chromosomal abnormalities; and polygenic, or multifactorial disease. This classification is useful in counseling families with inherited disease about recurrence risk and, to some extent, the natural history of a disease. Logically, however, the best information regarding outcome, progression, and the possibilities for treating an ailment, genetic or otherwise, derive from accurate diagnosis and knowledge of the best reference sources.

Mendelian Disease

The single-gene disease derives from mutation at a single genetic locus. The autosomal genes of diploid organisms like humans occur in two copies, or alleles. Those on the X chromosome without a sister allele on the Y chromosome are effectively haploid, occuring in one copy only. Thus, single-gene diseases are divided into recessive or dominant and autosomal versus sex-linked. Gregor Mendel coined the terms *recessive* and *dominant* in the 19th century to describe and predict the outcomes of crossings of various traits among common garden peas. We now understand that recessive disorders occur when both alleles of a given gene are altered, while dominant traits require a mutation at only one allele to cause disease. A good example of an autosomal-recessive disease that impacts anesthetic care is given by mutation at the gene coding for pseudocholinesterase. A person who harbors mutation in one of their two pseudocholinesterase genes is considered heterozygous for the mutation, and this defect may be detectable by an abnormal dibucaine number. However, in most heterozgotes, the remaining normal gene provides enough functional gene product, in this case pseudocholinesterase, that they are not affected to a clinically significant degree. Conversely, someone with the same mutation in both pseudocholinesterase genes is homozygous for the mutation and, depending on the type of mutation, may not generate sufficient pseudocholinesterase activity to hydrolyze a typical dose of succinylcholine. This person will have prolonged paralysis after treatment with succinlycholine.

A special case occurs when both alleles of a gene are mutant but are affected by different mutations. This patient is considered a compound, or double, heterozygote, and the clinical severity of the resulting disease is usually in-between those of the corresponding homozygotes. Thus, hemoglobin SC (HbSC) disease results from double heterozygosity at the β-globin locus and clinical severity is roughly between that of sickle cell anemia (HbSS), and hemoglobin C disease (HbCC), a mild hemoglobinopathy caused by a different mutation at the same site as the sickle-cell-anemia mutation: replacement of the sixth amino acid in the β-globin chain.

Expressivity is the geneticist's term for the clinical severity of a disease. The expressivity of any genetic disease is the distillation of the interaction of genetic as well as nongenetic factors. Genetic factors involved in the process of determining expressivity include the primary mutation, as well as other aspects of the patient's genetic makeup, that affect the internal milieu in which the disease develops. Nongenetic factors include environmental and nutritional contributions to this same milieu. These factors account for variability of clinical severity among different patients with the same disease. Generally, autosomal-recessive diseases show only minimal variation in expressivity from one individual and one family to another. Nevertheless, even a disease like sickle cell anemia occurs within a spectrum, as there are examples of mildly affected patients with sickle cell disease and others who die at an early age from infarction of a vital organ. Expressivity, to some extent, is subject to modification by the application and availability of medical treatment.

Pedigrees of families with an autosomal-recessive disease typically show multiple affected members in one sibship but no vertical transmission. That is, though both parents of affected children are usually heterozygous, or carriers, for the mutation, the disease does not typically occur in both parents and children. Given carrier status of both parents, the recurrence risk for each offspring is 25%. There is also a higher than expected incidence of consanguinity among parents of patients affected by an autosomal-recessive disease.

Dominant diseases occur in persons heterozygous for mutation at a given locus. The resulting clinical phenotype is the result of a balance between the abnormal and normal genes' expression, as well as the same genetic and nongenetic factors that influence the expressivity of all genetic disease. Dominant disorders, in contrast to the relative uniformity of recessive disease, typically have greatly variable expressivity among affected individuals. A good example is given by neurofibromatosis 1, a dominant disease caused by mutation in the gene coding for neurofibromin, a tumor suppressor. Classical neurofibromatosis patients have cutaneous lumps and bumps as well as hyperpigmented regions of skin, called café au lait spots. In some cases, these may be the only signs of disease and might minimally or negligibly alter the patient's life and longevity. However, other patient's with neurofibromatosis have severe disease with large disfiguring neurofibromas, or neurofibromas that disable by compressing structures in the central nervous system, or a shortened life span caused by malignant transformation of a neurofibroma.

Penetrance is the term geneticists use to describe the probability that, with a given mutation, clinically detectable disease will occur. Penetrance is typically reserved for describing dominant disease, and in a mildly affected patient, is often a function of how hard the clinician is willing to look for some sign of disease. Penetrance can be age-dependent, as in Huntington's disease in which patients are usually asymptomatic until middle age. Penetrance can also be conditional, as in both malignant hyperthermia and pseudocholinesterase, in which patients are typically asymptomatic until exposed to a trigger or succinlycholine. Penetrance can also be idiosyncratic, since not every exposure to a classical trigger results in a hyperthermic crisis among susceptible individuals. Obviously, the concepts of conditional and idiosyncratic penetrance are relevant to perioperative care.

Pedigrees of dominant diseases typically show vertical transmission; that is, affected members appear in sequential generations of a family. The recurrence risk for each offspring of an affected individual is 50%. Obviously, assessing risk among offspring of a questionably affected individual in a family with an autosomal-dominant disease having extremely variable expressivity requires careful examination to exclude the possibility of mild expression. The difference in recurrence risk for each offspring of a person who is not a carrier vs those of a mildly affected heterozygote is 0% vs 50%!

X-Linked Disease

Classical X-linked recessive diseases exhibit significant differential expressivity between female and males carriers of an X chromosome containing a disease-causing mutation. The bulk of genetic material on the X chromosome has no counterpart in the Y chromosome. Thus, males are functionally hemizygous for most X-chromosome genes, and mutation in these genes leaves no normally functioning allele to produce gene product. Females have two X chromosomes in each somatic cell; however, random inactivation of one X chromosome in each cell during early development leaves the individual having a genetic mutation on an X chromosome functionally mosaic for that mutation. Males harboring mutation in their dystrophin gene, have muscular dystrophy with a severity that depends on the specific type of mutation, and the resulting amount and functional characteristics of the mutant protein produced. Females having an X chromosome with the same mutation are likely to be asymptomatic, or mildly symptomatic, depending on the physical distribution of cells whose normal X chromosome is inactivated.

The typical pedigree in a family with an X-linked disease shows the so-called "knight's move" in which affected males appear in alternate generations, and carrier females appear in the intervening generations. Male-to-male transmission generally excludes X-linked inheritance. Roughly one third of cases of any lethal X-linked disease are sporadic, occurring by spontaneous mutation. Some X-linked diseases are dominant in that female carriers are predictably affected, regardless of their pattern of X inactivation.

Chromosomal Disease

Another class of genetic diseases results from derangement, by deletion or duplication, of chromosomal material. As a group, chromosomal diseases typically have extremely diverse, multisystem effects. This phenomenon, called pleiotropy, is described in the section dealing with principles of genetic disease. It seems logical that any abnormality in chromosome number or content is likely to cause significant dysfunction of genetic material, that will, in turn, severely alter organ function as well as development. Generally, it is thought that the loss or gain of chromosomal material causes disease by a relatively simple, gene-dose effect. Either excessive or inadequate production of the genes included in the affected region can cause disease.

Chromosomal disease includes a spectrum from an abnormal number of chromosomes, or aneuploidy, at one end, to barely detectable, small deletions or duplications of genetic material, called aneusomy, at the other. DiGeorge's syndrome, for example, is caused by a microdeletion at 22q11 (geimsa band 11 on the long arm of chromosome 22), which leaves affected persons functionally hemizygous for this locus, called the DiGeorge critical region (see CATCH-22 following). "Critical region" refers to a specific karyotypic locus responsible for a given phenotype. Down's syndrome for instance is caused by trisomy 21, but the entire phenotype is mapped to a small Down's critical region on chromosome 21.

Traditionally, aneuploidies and aneusomies are detected by various techniques of chromosome preparation, staining, and light microscopy, collectively referred to as karyotyping. Recombinant technology can be applied to complement classical karyotyping techniques. Molecular probes are now available for many chromosome regions, so that fluorescent *in situ* hybridization (FISH) can detect with high degrees of specificity and sensitivity small derangements of particular chromosome regions. Revisiting DiGeorge's syndrome as an example, this diagnosis can be established by using a FISH probe to detect deletion of the DiGeorge critical region.

Genetic disease can also result from rearrangement of chromosomes when the breakpoints of such rearrangements disrupt normal gene structure or expression. However, some chromosome rearrangements retain the normal complement and function of genetic material and are referred to as "balanced." Balanced translocations, for instance, of one part or all of one chromosome to another, can leave a person entirely asymptomatic. Such individuals, however, are at risk for passing on an unbalanced, symptomatic, or possibly lethal, chromosome complement to offspring. Though most chromosome abnormalities result from nondisjunction of chromosome material during meiosis, and are, therefore, sporadic, such unbalanced translocations can be inherited in a fashion similar to single-gene traits from an unaffected or mildly affected, carrier parent.

Polygenic Disease

One reason to study the various modes of inheritance and mechanisms of genetic disease is to achieve a better understanding of the spectrum of ways and means by which the genetic substrate affects our clinical status. On one end of the spectrum lie the chromosome abnormality and single-gene trait: a specific defect underlying the disease, oftentimes, a direct connection either proved or inferred between genotype and phenotype and a predictable and, in many instances high, probability of recurrence among relatives of affected individuals. At the other end of the spectrum of genetic disease are those ailments with a genetic component that is statistically apparent, but lack both a specific defect and a precise mechanism to describe how the disease occurs. The statistical evidence for a genetic basis of these diseases is provided by a higher incidence of these diseases among the first-degree relatives of affected individuals than the population at large and a higher rate of concordance among monozygotic twins than fraternal twins. These diseases each occur within a spectrum of severity and include many common malformations such as cleft lip and pyloric stenosis, as well as other common ailments like schizophrenia and adult-onset diabetes.

Such diseases are also referred to as multifactorial or "complex" traits, to reflect the popular view that they occur as the result of an interaction between diverse genetic and environmental factors. A person's genetic makeup may predispose him or her to one of these diseases, but current belief holds that the ailment becomes manifest only if a certain threshold is exceeded by the additive affects of these many genetic and nongenetic factors. Currently, considerable scientific effort is being applied to elucidate the specific genetic factors involved in these complex traits.

Other Modes

Two additional modes of inheriting genetic disease deserve note. First is the inheritance of mutation in the mitochondrial genome. Since mitochondria are present in ova but not sperm, any mutation in the circular mitochondrial chromosome results in a purely maternal pattern of inheritance: affected mother to son and daughter, affected father to neither. Leiber's hereditary optic neuropathy is a classical example of mitochondrial inheritance. Second, is somatic mutation. That is, mutation occurring after fertilization, often in advanced age, that may result in disease. The best examples of this pattern are provided by inherited and noninherited forms of cancer. In inherited forms, such as inherited retinoblastoma, the patient inherits a mutation in a tumor suppressor gene that in itself is harmless, because the product of the normal allele is able to suppress malignant transformation. However, when a somatic mutation occurs in the normal allele of a given cell, the so-called "second hit," the cell is not prone to malignant transformation. Children with this form of retinoblastoma are prone to develop the cancer early and in both eyes. Retinoblastoma that is not inherited occurs when somatic mutation affects both alleles in a given cell. This is a rare event, and these children do not usually develop cancer in both eyes.

• TYPES OF GENETIC DISEASE: MECHANISMS OF MUTATION

The revolution in recombinant technology has allowed a clearer grasp of the correlation of genotype to phenotype. This, in turn, provides the basis for a better understanding of what and how mutations result in clinically apparent disease. Finally, elucidating the mechanisms of genetic disease offers a means for understanding the molecular basis of normal biologic and physiologic function of the entire organism. The classical types of mutation describe alterations in gene structure and in humans; the hemoglobinopathies as a group provided the fertile pathologic soil on which much of this research grew.

A transition mutation is the single nucleotide substitution of a purine for another purine or pyrimidine for another pyrimidine; a transversion occurs when a purine is switched for a pyrimidine or vice versa. A missense mutation occurs when an alteration in a gene's coding sequence causes a codon to code for a different amino acid. Nonsense mutation occurs when this alteration causes the new codon to become a stop codon, thereby resulting in a truncated protein. Deletions and insertions in a coding region can be in-frame if they don't alter the reading frame, or cause a frame shift if they do. Generally, frameshift mutations result in grossly abnormal or nonfunctional gene product. Mutations in virtually any component of a gene have been described, and each can cause dysfunction of the corresponding protein. Null mutations completely prevent synthesis of the gene product. Mutations can occur in coding regions as described earlier, but mutations outside the reading frame can also alter gene expression. They can affect upstream promotor regions necessary for transcription of normal message, resulting in reduced transcription rates; or alter intro-exon consensus sequences necessary for normal message processing; or affect regions within or downstream from the coding sequences, necessary for normal protein processing and cell extrusion. Any of these mutations, within or outside the coding regions, can alter function or synthesis of the protein product, causing disease.

Unstable triplet repeats are an important, recently described mutational mechanism responsible for a variety of neuronal degenerative diseases. The "repeats" refer to a tandem repeating sequence of three nucleotides that occurs in noncoding regions of the normal gene, and is expanded to a much larger number of repeats in the mutant gene. Examples of diseases caused by this mutational mechanism include myotonic dystrophy and Huntington's disease. The number of such repeats is often directly proportional to the clinical severity of the disease. These repeats are considered unstable because DNA replicative machinery is prone to slip while copying these segments and the number of repeats can then vary significantly between generations in a given family. This apparently accounts for the peculiar phenomenon of "anticipation" in certain dominant diseases, where successive generations of a pedigree can appear to be more severely affected than members of preceding generations.

Another important mechanism in dominant diseases is the "dominant-negative" mutation. This refers to the phenomenon whereby a heterozygote for a mutation that produces an abnormal gene product is more severely affected than the heterozygote for a null mutation. This occurs when the protein in question is normally part of a multimer whose function is altered by presence of an abnormal subunit. In this case, the smaller quantity of protein synthesized by the null heterozygote is less detrimental than the abnormal, presumably nonfunctional protein synthesized by incorporating the mutant, "poison" protein into the multimer.

FOUR TRADITIONAL PRINCIPLES OF GENETIC DISEASE

The value in finding universal features of genetic disease comes in the clinically useful inferences they allow in assessing such disease. Already addressed in the section on autosomal disease, both variable expressivity and penetrance can apply to all forms of inherited disease. Simply stated, these principles imply that all genetic diseases occur within a spectrum of clinical severity, and that at the mild end of that spectrum, the mutation underlying some genetic diseases may not always result in clinically detectable disease. The value of these principles to the evaluation of the operative patient is to recognize that all patients with a given disease are not equally affected and that one's ability to safely extrapolate from literature reports or previous experience, is limited in genetic disease.

Heterogeneity refers to the fact that apparently similar genetic diseases can have very different underlying genetic causes and, therefore, different outcomes and clinical concerns. This is an important principle to the geneticist when predicting a disease's recurrence risks or natural history for a patient. There are two basic types of heterogeneity. Allelic heterogeneity describes the different forms a disease can take, depending on which particular mutation or mutations of a given gene are at work. The previous examples of the different diseases corresponding to the presence of HbSS versus HbSC versus HbCC provide equally good examples of alleleic heterogeneity since all these mutations affect the same gene but cause disease with widely differing outcomes. Locus heterogeneity refers to the phenomenon in which diseases that appear similar are caused by mutation in entirely different genes. For instance, Marfan disease and homocystinuria both produce a long, slim body habitus and patients with both diseases are susceptible to dislocation of the ocular lens. However, these diseases result from mutation in entirely different genes and have very different natural histories and treatments. Skeletal dysplasias are another good example of genetic heterogeneity. There are literally hundreds of different causes of disproportionate short stature. Many appear similar to one another, though their underlying mutations differ and result in very different patterns of inheritance and clinical outcomes. The relevance of heterogeneity to the preoperative evaluation of the patient with genetic disease comes in retaining a healthy doubt when assessing a patient's diagnosis because understanding the relevant patient-care issues depends on having an accurate diagnosis.

Pleiotropy is the principle that most genetic diseases have multiple clinical effects. This is by far the most important of the traditional, clinical genetic principles to the care and evaluation of the operative patient. Just as pathology in virtually any organ system can impact the operative course, virtually every genetic disease can affect multiple organ systems. Pleiotropy also occurs in degrees, varying from one disease to another. Plasma cholinesterase deficiency, for instance, is not highly pleiotropic since the only clinically significant effect is prolonged paralysis after receiving a dose of succinylcholine. Sickle cell anemia, on the other hand, is a highly pleiotropic disease that can affect virtually any vital organ. In this instance, the pleiotropic effects of the disease are nearly all secondary to a single process: hemoglobin gel formation, leading to red cell deformation and sludging that ultimately causes organ infarction.

In the same way that safe driving requires constantly scanning the road to get the big picture, pleiotropy demands the anesthesiologist consider the broadest possible scope of clinical pathology in assessing the patient with a genetic disease. Finally, note that heterogeneity and pleiotropy are nearly the inverse of one another; heterogeneity results from many different genotypes mapping into a single phenotype, while pleiotropy refers to one genotype having many phenotypic effects.

• PERIOPERATIVE ASSESSMENT OF GENETIC DISEASE

Major advances in molecular biology and recombinant technology have yielded astounding new insights in the pathogenesis of an ever-increasing number of genetic diseases and other complex traits lacking a simple genetic origin. This progress has led to innovation in the treatment of a wide variety of ailments, and a significant, parallel impact of genetics in all of the many corresponding medical specialties. Genetic disease can imperil the operative patient in a variety of ways. The patient's well-being, and the anesthesiologists' tranquility, depend on knowing how to anticipate, prevent and, when necessary, treat perioperative complications among these patients.

Pleiotropism dictates that virtually any organ system can be affected by genetic disease. Organ systems and effects particularly relevant to the perioperative specialist that genetic diseases can alter, by either malformation or metabolic aberration, include: pharmacodynamic responses to anesthetic agents, airway maintenance, cardiopulmonary function, oxygen transport, blood coagulation, skin fragility, skeletal muscle strength and response to pharmacologic agents, joint laxity, and range of motion. In each case, it is important to be aware that there are a variety of ways a genetic disease can affect an organ or system. I refer to this as pathogenic heterogeneity. Genetic disease can affect the heart, for instance, in many forms: structural malformation, congestive, restrictive, obstructive or ischemic cardiomyopathies, valvular disease, arrhythmias, or aortic root dissection. Similarly, airway management can be complicated by tumor (neurofibromatosis), torsion of the larynx (hemifacial microsomia), mandibular hypoplasia (Treacher Collins syndrome), large tongue (Trisomy 21 or Hurler's syndrome), cervical spine instability (Trisomy 21 or Morquio's syndrome), reduced range of cervical motion (Klippel-Feil syndrome), and so on. Thus, it is useful to know what organ systems are affected by a given disease but also important to know how the pathologies are manifest.

Preoperative evaluation of a patient with a genetic disease must, like any patient, require careful history, physical examination, and assessment of laboratory data. In addition, a family history is helpful if there is a previous history of a family member with an anesthetic complicated by a prolonged intubation or intensive care admission; a muscle biopsy; early deaths in the family; or, any trait or medical problem common to several family members. Note that a negative family history does not rule out any genetic disease. Finally, it is useful to become familiar with available clinical genetic references, including on-line resources (see following), to quickly scan for the most clinically relevant features likely to be seen in a particular disease.

SEVEN ILLUSTRATIVE GENETIC DISEASES

The following are brief clinical summaries of several genetic diseases. These conditions are chosen to emphasize and illustrate clinical principles important to the perioperative specialist. The examples include one aneuploidy and one aneusomy, both remarkably pleiotropic. There are also two classical pharmacogenetic diseases, one dominant, one recessive. One lethal X-linked disease with substantial perioperative implications is presented. Two hematologic diseases commonly seen in the operating suite are also described: one a recessive disease that alters oxygen delivery, and the other, a heterogeneous, dominant coagulopathy.

Next to each single-gene condition is its McKusick number. This number corresponds to the relevant genetic locus (autosomal-dominant conditions begin with "1," autosomal-recessive with "2," and X-linked start with "3") and is a key to finding the disease in the comprehensive catalogue of single-gene traits: Mendelian Inheritance in Man. It is important to note that the MIM is now maintained by the National Center for Biotechnology Information and is continuously updated online. One can now search the entire national gene data bank for information about any genetic disease. A particularly easy and useful way to do this is by the on-line MIM, available at: *http://www3.ncbi.nlm.nih.gov/Omim/*

At the appropriate point on this screen just type in the disease you would like to have information about, and click the search button to receive comprehensive clinical descriptions with extensive scientific background.

Trisomy 21

Trisomy 21 is the most common genetic malformation syndrome. The familiar phenotype of Down's syndrome is thought to result from triplication of a critical region of chromosome 21; the subsequent gene-dose effect causes a 50% overproduction of genes in this region. Trisomy 21, like all autosomal aneuploidies, is highly pleiotropic, affecting nearly every organ system. The clinical features of trisomy 21 most relevant to their perioperative care are cardiac defects present in roughly 40%, and cervical instability seen in 20% of cases. Conotruncal abnormalities and ventricular septal defects are the most common congenital heart defects in trisomy 21. Though a large tongue might make the airway of trisomy 21 patients appear difficult to intubate, visualization is rarely a problem. However, ligamentous laxity and muscular hypotonia increase the risk of mask ventilation and instrumenting the airway in those patients with cervical spine instability. Tracheal hypoplasia is not uncommon in trisomy 21, so it is important to select the correct tube size and carefully evaluate for the degree of leak after intubation with an uncuffed tube.

CATCH-22

CATCH-22 refers to a group of closely related dysmorphic syndromes that have in common a microdeletion at chromosome 22q11. CATCH is an acronym for cardiac defect, abnormal face, thymic aplasia, cleft palate, and hypocalcemia, and includes the classical DiGeorge's syndrome. The deletion is usually sporadic but can be inherited resulting in pedigrees with multiple affected individuals.

Strictly speaking, CATCH-22 is considered a sequence by clinical geneticists, rather than a syndrome, because all the resulting features can be traced to developmental defects in a single anatomic region: pharyngeal pouches III and IV and the intervening branchial arch IV. The parathyroids and thymus arise from these pharyngeal pouches, while the left branchial arch IV contributes to the aortic arch and the right to the right subclavian artery. The classic DiGeorge sequence includes neonatal hypocalcemia caused by parathyroid hypoplasia, and immunodeficiency caused by T-cell deficiency. A variety of cardiac defects are possible, aortic arch abnormalities are most common. The facial abnormalities include hypertelorism, short upper lip, downslanting eyes, and ear anomalies. Short stature and mild mental retardation can also occur, as well as a series of other midline defects including choanal or esophageal atresia, and diaphragmatic hernia.

However, before the DiGeorge sequence was correlated with a microdeletion, two related syndromes were described with features that overlapped with DiGeorge. These include the velocardiofacial syndrome of Shprintzen in which cleft palate, ventricular septal defect, short stature, mild retardation and abnormal facies predominate, and Takao syndrome in which cardiac defects, particularly conotruncal abnormalities, are most common. These three syndromes are now recognized as variable expressions of microdeletion in the same chromosome region. Clinical variation between and among the different syndromes may result from differences in the actual deletion and other nongenetic factors.

These patients are likely to come to the operating room for correction of either a congenital heart defect or cleft patate. Their extreme pleiotropy and clinical variability make their operative care challenging. The submucous cleft often occurs with glossoptosis and associated Robin sequence. Thus, airway obstruction during mask ventilation and difficult visualization during laryngoscopy are possible. Induction and control of the airway is even more challenging when such patients are developmentally delayed and uncooperative. Patients should be evaluated for hypocalcemia, particularly when there is a history of neonatal tetany. Evaluating the patient's cardiac status is obviously essential; this includes assessing exertional tolerance, a history of previous surgery, and determining the precise of nature of any defect.

The CATCH-22 syndromes are both clinically and scientifically fascinating. To the clinical geneticist, they are an elegant illustration of the principles of heterogeneity, variable expressivity, and pleiotropy. They are challenging to the anesthesiologist because metabolic derangements accompany an array of structural alterations. Scientifically, there is much to be learned from the CATCH-22 group in correlating gene expression of a specific critical chromosome region, to development of a particular set of rostral midline structures.

Malignant Hyperthermia

Malignant hyperthermia (MH) is the quintessential anesthetic-genetic disease: a potentially fatal inherited sensitivity to certain, commonly used anesthetic agents, collectively referred to as "triggers." The incontrovertible MH triggers among commonly used agents are succinylcholine and all the potent inhalational agents. Malignant hyperthermia usually has an autosomal-dominant pattern of inheritance and sporadic occurrences are common. It is a highly heterogeneous disease, with variable expressivity and penetrance that is both conditional and idiosyncratic.

The classic MH response to a triggering agent is sustained skeletal muscle contracture, resulting in an extreme, hypermetabolic state, rhabdomyolysis, hyperkalemia, increased oxygen consumption and carbon dioxide production, metabolic acidosis, hyperthermia, arrhythmias, pulmonary edema, renal failure, disseminated intravascular coagulation and, if untreated, death. The most sensitive indicator of an MH reaction is an abnormally elevated arterial carbon dioxide tension (end-tidal tension greater than 55 mm Hg or arterial tension greater than 60 mm Hg). This may conceivably be masked by progressively increasing the patient's minute ventilation, but a supervising physician should consider this diagnosis when ventilator settings seem significantly beyond those expected for a given patient. The most specific indicator for an MH reaction is generalized muscle rigidity. The classic response to a trigger most frequently occurs within minutes of the exposure, but delay of as much as 11 hours is reported. In all cases, the most important factor in reducing morbidity and mortality is to consider the diagnosis.

The typical MH response results from exaggerated, unregulated, and sustained release of calcium ions from the skeletal muscle sarcoplasmic reticulum into the cytoplasm. This release is through the calcium-dependent calcium release channel (CRC), also called the ryanodine receptor. Once released, calcium triggers the normal ratcheting of the actin-myosin complex, thus, generating the muscular contractile force which represents the last step in excitation-contraction coupling. Relaxation then requires the active pumping of calcium ions into the sarcoplasmic reticulum, reducing the free-cytoplasmic calcium ion concentration. A single mutation in the gene coding for the CRC protein is found in all pigs with the porcine version of MH. The same mutant nucleotide substitution is rare in human MH; however, linked mutations, possibly in the same gene, are present in approximately 30% of human MH pedigrees. An equal percentage of families with MH have mutations that map to the adult muscle sodium channel alpha subunit. A variety of other mutations, mostly involving ion channels or other modes of signal transduction, are proposed to account for the remaining families with MH.

Once suspect, the diagnosis of MH susceptibility is best made by the caffeine-halothane contracture test. This involves incubating fresh specimens of skeletal muscle, attached to a strain guage, in baths containing standardized concentrations of either halothane or caffeine. An abnormal degree or duration of contracture during this exposure is taken as a positive test, indicating susceptibility. This test is highly specific and nearly 100% sensitive, as cases of false-negatives are reportable.

Treatment of MH is based on a combination of intravenous dantrolene and supportive care. It is important for the perioperative physician to have a well worked-out plan of attack before such an occurrence, since there is little time available to consider and weigh various options at that moment. First, begin hyperventilating the patient with 100% oxygen, and inform the surgeon that the operation must end immediately. Next, call for assistance, and when help arrives, give each person one of the following specific tasks: get the MH cart and begin diluting dantrolene; start an arterial cannula and send an arterial specimen for blood gas determination; draw venous blood for electrolyte, creatinine, creatine phosphokinase, myoglobin, and clotting tests; place an nasogastric tube and do cold saline gavage; put ice in plastic bags to pack the patient in an effort to lower body temperature; acquire a cooling blanket and cold intravenous solution; possibly, place a central venous line. As soon as the drug is available, begin infusion of dantrolene, 2.5 mg/kg initially, then 2.0 mg/kg every few minutes until the symptoms of MH resolve. In addition to intravenous dantrolene and cooling measures, supportive care includes bicarbonate therapy to treat the metabolic acidosis and alkalinize the urine which improves solubility of myoglobin, and treatment of hyperkalemia with either insulin-glucose or ionized calcium, as dictated by the electrocardiogram (ECG). Once recovered, patients must be monitored in an intensive care setting for at least 24 hours and receive additional doses of dantrolene, intravenously every 6 hours for 24 hours and orally for another day.

Two controversies deserve discussion. First is the question of how to prepare the possibly or definitely susceptible patient for a general anesthetic. Many years ago, such patients were given preoperative dantrolene orally for days. Now, no preoperative dantrolene is recommended. Similarly, in the past, if a clean machine wasn't available, it was recommended to run high-flow oxygen through the anesthesia machine for 24 hours before surgery. Now it is recommended to flush the machine and ventilator with 100% oxygen at 10 liters per minute for 10 minutes, and replace the common gas outlet, reservoir bag, circuit, and absorbent. This individual should receive an anesthetic with no trigger agents. Thiopental and propofol are good agents for induction of anesthesia and general anesthesia is safely maintained in the MH-susceptible patient with nitrous oxide/oxygen, narcotics, and propofol or nondepolarizing muscle relaxants, as needed.

The other controversy arises in evaluating cases of masseter spasm in otherwise healthy children following a dose of succinylcholine. The problem is determining, acutely, whether masseter spasm in such cases represents a prodrome to MH, a crisis in which the operation must be cancelled and preparations made for intensive intervention, or merely a nonlifethreatening, variant pharmacodynamic response. Given that as many as one half the patients with a history of masseter spasm have positive halothane-caffeine contracture tests, the first course seems more prudent. However, the fact that as many as 1% of pediatric patients experience this response indicates most aren't prodromes to MH because the overall incidence of MH reactions is on the order of 1 per 10,000 anesthetics, not 1 in 200. The current belief is that masseter spasm occurs in a spectrum and that mild or moderated examples, where the jaw is opened with difficulty, are not suggestive of MH, but cases where the jaw is locked and cannot be opened may represent an MH prodrome. It is prudent to continue cases in the first set with nontrigger agents, maintaining vigilance for signs of MH; those with severe masseter spasm are cases that should probably be cancelled and dantrolene given if further monitoring reveals any signs of MH. Patients in this group should be monitored overnight in any case, and have determinations of their serum creatine phosphokinase. Muscle biopsy at a later date for halothane-caffeine contracture test is also a consideration for the severe case of masseter spasm.

Plasma Cholinesterase Deficiency

Plasma cholinesterase is an enzyme without a known naturally occurring substrate. Homozygosity for a mutation that eliminates the enzyme's hydrolytic activity is entirely asymptomatic, until the patient receives a dose of succinylcholine. The resulting prolonged paralysis was first described by Kalow in 1957 and the field of pharmacogenetics was born with this report. Since then, the gene for plasma cholinesterase has been mapped and sequenced and a wide variety of mutants with varying degrees of clinical significance are well-characterized. However, it is useful to know that of all the many known mutations in this gene, the classic atypical variant is, by far, the most common of those that can result in significantly prolonged paralysis after succinylcholine treatment. This gene produces normal quantities of an enzyme with no hydrolytic activity. Heterozygote frequency among caucasians for this gene is roughly 1 in 25 and homozygotes occur at 1 in 2500. Homozygosity for the often-discussed fluoride variant, by comparison, occurs in roughly 1 in 200,000 among the same population.

Kalow also determined an early method for detecting this defect by showing that the atypical variant, while possessing no hydrolytic activity for succinylcholine, was more susceptible to inhibition by the local anesthetic dibucaine, than was the normal gene product. The percent of inhibition of the enzyme's activity by dibucaine gives the dibucaine number: roughly 80 for normal homozygotes, 20 for atypical homozygotes (those with sensitivity to succinylcholine), and approximately 50 for heterozygotes.

Without a previous history of prolonged paralysis or intubation after an anesthetic, it is impossible to anticipate this type of sensitivity to succinylcholine. A negative family history provides no assurance because this is an autosomal-recessive disease and unaffected first-degree relatives are expected. The best advice is to delay the use of nondepolarizing muscle relaxants following a dose of succinylcholine, until evidence of twitch recovery. Plasma cholinesterase deficiency usually presents as prolonged postoperative weakness that is unresponsive to standard reversal agents. It is a diagnosis of exclusion, however, and it is important to consider this condition in your differential diagnosis of failure to reverse paralysis or failure to tolerate extubation. Notably, mivicurium is normally metabolized by plasma cholinesterase and homozygotes for the atypical variants also show prolonged paralysis after treatment with this drug.

Treatment of paralysis following a dose of succinylcholine or mivacurium is supportive, comprising mechanical ventilation until strength returns. Liver transplantation repairs the defect in these patients. It is also worth noting that sufficient succinylcholine passes the placental barrier and that an affected infant could develop prolonged weakness if the mother was given a dose before delivery.

Duchenne Muscular Dystrophy

Duchenne muscular dystrophy is the most common X-linked lethal disease. It is a progressive disease of skeletal and cardiac muscle, usually first presenting as weakness and gait disturbance in the toddler years, leading to the wheelchair by adolescence and death in the second or third decade, typically from respiratory or cardiac failure. The disease results from mutation in the gene coding for dystrophin. Allelic heterogeneity accounts for milder forms, such as Becker's dystrophy, as well as a version that affects the heart predominantly, X-linked dilated cardiomyopathy.

Dystrophin is the actin-binding protein that connects the contractile apparatus to the muscle cell membrane, the sarcolemma. Actually, this connection extends to the extracellular matrix through large glycoprotein molecules that transit the sarcolemma. This dystrophin-glycoprotein complex anchors the contractile apparatus, providing a structural base against which the actin-myosin fibers can efficiently and effectively exert force without damaging the cell membrane. Fluorescent antibody staining of dystrophin shows no illumination of muscle biopsy from those with Duchenne muscular dystrophy and patchy staining in muscle from those affected by the much milder Becker dystrophy.

Perioperative care requires accurate evaluation of the patient's cardiac function and pulmonary reserve. Chest radiographs, echocardiography, and room-air arterial-blood gas determinations are helpful in this regard. In addition to skeletal muscle weakness, severe scoliosis is common and can impair spontaneous and controlled ventilation.

There is a risk of hyperkalemic response to succinylcholine in patients with muscular dystrophy, and this agent is certainly contraindicated in the Duchenne and Becker types. Nondepolarizing muscle relaxants will have prolonged effects in Duchenne muscular dystrophy and should only be used when absolutely required, and then, only in small doses, carefully titrated to an endpoint from which reversal of blockade is expected to be rapid and complete. Nondepolarizing muscle relaxants, though not strictly contraindicated, are rarely needed during surgery for these patients, given their underlying weakness and the mild, muscle-relaxant effects of most inhalational agents. Regional anesthesia is a good alternative in peripheral and limb procedures in these patients. However, when the degree of sedation and height of a conduction blockade impair the patients' oxygenation, it is obviously preferable to induce general anesthesia to control or assist ventilation and use a more reliably enriched oxygen supply.

Sickle Cell Anemia

Sickle cell is the most common structural hemoglobin mutation and nearly 10% of African-Americans are heterozygotes. This autosomal-recessive disease results from a transversion mutation causing a substitution of valine for glutamic acid in the sixth position of in the β-globin molecule. The predominant hemoglobin of homozygotes comprises two α and two sickle β molecules: HbSS. Reduced forms of this hemoglobin tend to polymerize, creating a gel which deforms red cells into the characteristic sickle shape. These cells are much less deformable than normal red cells and are prone to sludging in the capillary bed. Propagation of this process results in the vasoocclusion and organ infarction that underly both acute and chronic manifestations of the disease.

Acute disease in sickle cell anemia can take the form of pain crisis, priapism, chest crisis, sequestration of blood cellular elements in spleen and liver, bone marrow aplasia, or infarction of a vital organ. Crises are precipitated and worsened by hypothermia, hypoxia, acidosis, stress, and infection. Treatment consists of reversing these reversible factors, oxygen therapy and, when necessary, transfusion or exchange transfusion to reduce the fraction of sicklable hemoglobin.

Chronic disease takes the form of impairment of those organs subject to recurrent bouts of vasoocclusion: lung, kidney, spleen, central nervous system, skeletal system, joints, and skin. Long-term therapy now includes oral hydroxyurea, a mild marrow toxin that promotes synthesis of fetal hemoglobin. This interferes with HbSS polymerization by dilution of HbSS and by formation of hybrids like HbBF. Another important advance in therapy for sickle cell disease is bone marrow transplantation which holds potential for offering a cure from symptomatic vascular occlusion.

Preoperative evaluation requires assessing the natural history of the patient's disease. Is the patient taking hydroxyurea? What are the frequency and severity of symptoms, and what is the date of last transfusion or hospitalization for crisis? Laboratory evidence of end-organ damage, will also help ascertain where a patient is on the clinical spectrum.

Recent studies suggest that transfusion to a preoperative hemoglobin of 10g/dl is equally as effective at preventing perioperative morbidity for most operations, as is the more traditional, aggressive regimen of exchange transfusion to a HbAA of greater than 50%. The latter also has an increased risk of excessive alloimmunization. The most important factors in intraoperative care of the HbSS patient are keeping the patient, the room, and the intravenous fluids warmed. Generous hydration is also beneficial. The selection of general versus regional or local anesthesia should be based on which method will sustain the best arterial oxygen saturation. Thus, when monitored care will require sedation that puts the patient at risk for hypoventilation, low saturation, and respiratory acidosis, it is better to opt for general anesthesia in which minute ventilation and inspired oxygen concentration are easily controlled.

Finally, none of the commonly available autologous transfusion options is appropriate for the HbSS patient, because the methodologies of cell salvage and presurgical donation result in significant gel formation and loss of functional red cells.

von Willebrand Disease

Von Willebrand disease is a common heterogeneous group of coagulopathies presenting with recurrent mucocutaneous hemorrhage. All have deficient function of von Willebrand factor and the clinical effects of such deficiency are predictable from the normal function of this protein. Von Willebrand factor plays two important roles in coagulation. It is a very large multimer, comprising more than 20 von-Willebrand-factor monomers per molecule, and possessing binding sites for both collagen and platelets. These let it form a bridge, linking platelets with the subendothelial connective tissue exposed in an injured blood vessel. Von Willebrand factor is also the serum carrier protein for factor VIII, which is highly unstable in blood in its unbound form. Thus, defects in von-Willebrand-factor function result in abnormalities of both platelet aggregation and fibrin-clot formation.

Type I von Willebrand disease accounts for roughly 75% of cases. It is autosomal-dominant and results in reduced production of qualitatively normal von Willebrand factor. Type III is also a quantitative defect. It is recessive and results in virtually absent von Willebrand factor synthesis, producing a coagulopathic phenotype much more severe than type I and similar to hemophilia. Type II comprises the qualitative von-Willebrand-factor defects and has several subtypes.

Von-Willebrand-factor activity in Type I von Willebrand disease increases dramatically in response to deamino-8-D-arginine vasopressin (DDAVP). Thus, preoperative treatment with intravenous DDAVP (0.3 micrograms per kilogram) is appropriate for patients with type I disease undergoing a procedure where blood loss is likely. DDAVP is ineffective in all type-II subtypes and in type-III disease. These patients are best treated with cryoprecipitate or factor-VIII concentrate which both contain large multimer von Willebrand factor. Notably, DDAVP is specifically contraindicated in type IIB von Willebrand disease. Their von Willebrand factor possesses abnormally high affinity for platelet surface receptors and they can suffer severe, acute thrombocytopenia following DDAVP treatment.

BIBLIOGRAPHY

Abboud MR, et al: Neurologic complications following bone marrow transplantation for sickle cell disease, *Bone Marrow Transplant* 17:405–407, 1996.

Adu-Gyamfi Y, Sankarankutty M, Marwa S: Use of a tourniquet in patients with sickle-cell disease, *Can J Anaesth* 40:24–27, 1993.

Alusi GH, et al: Bleeding after tonsillectomy in severe von Willebrand's disease, *J Laryngol Otol* 109:437–439, 1995.

Bhattacharyya N, et al: Perioperative management for cholecystectomy in sickle cell disease, *J Pediatr Surg* 28:72–75, 1993.

Borowski A, et al: Down syndrome as a factor influencing hemodynamic response to pulmonary artery banding, *Pediatr Cardiol* 17:375–381, 1996.

Budarf M, et al: Cloning a balanced translocation associated with DiGeorge syndrome and identification of a disrupted candidate gene, *Natue Genet* 10:269–278, 1995.

Byrick RJ, Rose DK, Ranganathan N: Management of a malignant hyperthermia patient during cardiopulmonary bypass, *Can Anaesth Soc J* 29:50–54, 1982.

Carr AS, et al: Incidence of malignant hyperthermia reactions in 2,214 patients undergoing muscle biopsy, *Can J Anaesth* 42:281–286, 1995.

Charache S: Experimental therapy of sickle cell disease. Use of hydroxyurea, *Am J Pediatr Hematol Oncol* 16:62–6, 1994.

Christiaens F, et al: Malignant hyperthermia suggestive hypermetabolic syndrome at emergence from anesthesia [see comments], *Acta Anaesthesiol Belg* 46:93–97, 1995.

Christian AS, Ellis FR, Halsall PJ: Is there a relationship between masseteric muscle spasm and malignant hyperpyrexia? *Br J Anaesth* 62:540–544, 1989.

Denborough MA, Lovell RRH: Anaesthetic deaths in a family, *Lancet* 2:45, 1960.

Embury SH: New treatments of sickle cell disease, *West J Med* 164:444, 1996.

Favaloro EJ, Facey D, Grispo L: Laboratory assessment of von Willebrand factor. Use of different assays can influence the diagnosis of von Willebrand's disease, dependent on differing sensitivity to sample preparation and differential recognition of high molecular weight VWF forms, *Am J Clin Pathol* 104:264–271, 1995.

Ferster A, et al: Transplanted sickle-cell disease patients with autologous bone marrow recovery after graft failure develop increased levels of fetal haemoglobin which corrects disease severity, *Br J Haematol* 90:804–808, 1995.

Franke U, et al: Interstitial deletion of 22q11 in DiGeorge syndrome detected by high resolution and molecular analysis, *Clin Genet* 46:187–192, 1994.

Goertzen M, Baltzer A, Voit T: Clinical results of early orthopaedic management in Duchenne muscular dystrophy, *Neuropediatrics* 26:257–259, 1995.

Jacobs IN, Gray RF, Todd NW: Upper airway obstruction in children with Down syndrome, *Arch Otolaryngol Head Neck Surg* 122:945–950, 1996.

Jones K: *Recognizable patterns of human malformation*, ed 4 Philadelphia, 1988, WB Saunders.

Kalow W, Genest K: A method for the detection of atypical forms of human serum cholinesterase. Determination of dibucaine numbers, *Can J Biochem Physiol* 35:339–346, 1957.

Karpati G, Acsadi G: The principles of gene therapy in DuChenne muscular dystrophy, *Clin Invest Med* 17:499–509, 1994.

Katsanis N, Fisher EM: The gene encoding the p60 subunit of chromatin assembly factor I (CAF1P60) maps to human chromosome 21q22.2, a region associated with some of the major features of Down syndrome, *Hum Genet* 98:497–499, 1996.

Koshy M, et al: Surgery and anesthesia in sickle cell disease. Cooperative Study of Sickle Cell Diseases, *Blood* 86:3676–3684, 1995.

Lane PA: Sickle cell disease, *Pediatr Clin North Am* 43:639–664, 1996.

Larach MG, et al: A clinical grading scale to predict malignant hyperthermia susceptibility, *Anesthesiology* 80:771–779, 1994.

Larsen UT, et al: Complications during anaesthesia in patients with Duchenne's muscular dystrophy (a retrospective study) [see comments], *Can J Anaesth* 36:418–422, 1989.

Law PK, et al: Feasibility, safety, and efficacy of myoblast transfer therapy on Duchenne muscular dystrophy boys, *Cell Transplant* 1:235–244, 1992.

Levitt RC, et al: Evidence for genetic heterogeneity in malignant hyperthermia susceptibility, *Genomics* 11:543–547, 1991.

Litman RS, Zerngast BA, Perkins FM: Preoperative evaluation of the cervical spine in children with trisomy-21: results of a questionnaire study, *Paediatr Anaesth* 5:355–361, 1995.

Littleford JA, et al: Masseter muscle spasm in children: implications of continuing the triggering anesthetic [see comments], *Anesth Analg* 72:151–160, 1991.

MacLennan DH, Phillips MS: Malignant hyperthermia, *Science* 256:789–794, 1992.

Milaskiewicz RM, Holdcroft A, Letsky E: Epidural anaesthesia and von Willebrand's disease, *Anaesthesia* 45:462–464, 1990.

Mitchell V, Howard R, Facer E: Down's syndrome and anaesthesia, *Paediatr Anaesth* 5:379–384, 1995.

Morgan PG, Sedensky MM: A review of molecular genetics for the anaesthetist, *Eur J Anaesthesiol* 12:221–247, 1995.

Motegi Y, et al: Malignant hyperthermia during epidural anesthesia, *J Clin Anesth* 8:157–60, 1996.

Ohkoshi N, et al: Malignant hyperthermia in a patient with Becker muscular dystrophy: dystrophin analysis and caffeine contracture study, *Neuromuscul Disord* 5:53–8, 1995.

Ording H, Hedengran AM, Skovgaard LT: Evaluation of 119 anaesthetics received after investigation for susceptibility to malignant hyperthermia, *Acta Anaesthesiol Scand* 35:711–716, 1991.

Pantuck E: Plasma cholinesterase: gene and variations, *Anesth Analg* 77:380–386, 1993.

Petersen R, et al: Prolonged neuromuscular block after mivicurium, *Anesth Analg* 76:194–196, 1993.

Platt OS, Guinan EC: Bone marrow transplantation in sickle cell anemia—the dilemma of choice [editorial; comment], *N Engl J Med* 335:426–428, 1996.

Rittoo DB, Morris P: Tracheal occlusion in the prone position in an intubated patient with Duchenne muscular dystrophy, *Anaesthesia* 50:719–721, 1995.

Rizzolo S, Lemos MJ, Mason DE: Posterior spinal arthrodesis for atlantoaxial instability in Down syndrome, *J Pediatr Orthop* 15:543–548, 1995.

Rosenberg H, Gronert G: Intractable cardiac arrest in children given succinylcholine, *Anesthesiology* 77:1054, 1992.

Scriver CR, editors: *The metabolic basis of inherited disease*, ed 7, New York, 1995, McGraw-Hill.

Serfas KD, et al: Comparison of the segregation of the RYR1 C1840T mutation with segregation of the caffeine/halothane contracture test results for malignant hyperthermia susceptibility in a large Manitoba Mennonite family [see comments], *Anesthesiology* 84:322–329, 1996.

Sloand EM, et al: 1-Deamino-8-D-arginine vasopressin (DDAVP) increases platelet membrane expression of glycoprotein Ib in patients with disorders of platelet function and after cardiopulmonary bypass, *Am J Hematol* 46:199–207, 1994.

Svensson EC, Tripathy SK, Leiden JM: Muscle-based gene therapy: realistic possibilities for the future, *Mol Med Today* 2:166–172, 1996.

Turpin IM, Manino J: Malignant hyperthermia in an office surgery suite: a case report, *Aesthetic Plast Surg* 13:121–123, 1989.

Tinsley JM, et al: Amelioration of the dystrophic phenotype of mdx mice using a truncated utrophin transgene, *Nature* 384:349–352, 1996.

Weinberg G: *Genetics in anesthesiology: Syndromes and science,* Boston, 1996, Butterworth-Heinemann.

Ware RE, et al: A human chimera for von Willebrand disease following bone marrow transplantation, *Am J Pediatr Hematol Oncol* 15:338–342, 1993.

Wilson D, et al: DiGeorge syndrome: part of CATCH-22, *J Med Genet* 30:852–856, 1993.

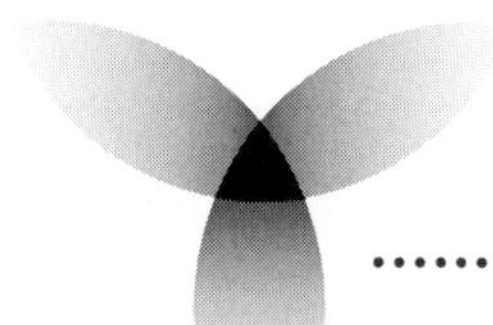

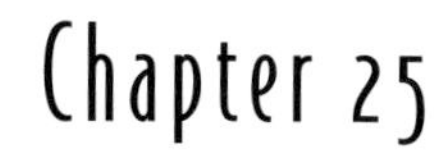

Chapter 25

Geriatrics

Tim Harwood, MD

Perioperative care for the elderly has changed greatly since Albert John Ochsner declared that no elective inguinal herniorraphy should be considered in patients older than 50 years. In the United States, 33.2 million people were 65 years of age or older in 1994. This represents 12.7% of the U.S. population. Since 1990, the number of older Americans has increased by 7%, compared to an increase of 4% for the under-65 population. The older population itself is getting older. In 1994, the 65 to 74 age group (18.7 million) was 8 times larger than in 1900, but the 75 to 84 group (10.9 million) was 14 times larger and the 85+ group (3.5 million) was 28 times larger. By 2030, there will be approximately 70 million persons age 65 or older, more than twice their number in 1990. By the year 2000, people older than 65 are projected to represent 14% to 15% of the population, and by the year 2030 they will constitute 20% of the total population.

Given the estimate that over one half of Americans older than 65 will undergo a surgical procedure before death, one may predict that 15 million elderly patients living today will have surgery before dying. Assuming a perioperative mortality rate of roughly 6% for the group as a whole, an improvement of 50% in that mortality figure would postpone the deaths of almost 500,000 of those individuals. This area certainly has to be one of the greatest challenges ahead for the perioperative physician in the next century.

The perioperative physician must understand the multiple complex interactions of the changes involved with aging in the perioperative care setting. Care of the geriatric patient is not the same as that for a younger adult in the perioperative period. This chapter will focus on the biologic and pharmacologic changes associated with aging, and the preoperative, intraoperative, and postoperative management of these patients.

• CHANGES OF AGING

Central Nervous System

ANATOMIC, PHYSIOLOGIC, AND CHEMICAL CHANGES

Although significant variation exists within our population, it is generally thought that the central nervous system in humans steadily deteriorates after the age of 50 years. A variety of changes occur with aging (Box 25-1).

Beginning at 40 years of age, brain mass gradually decreases, with an ultimate loss of approximately 7% to 8% of its initial adult mass in the aged. Consequently, widening of the sulci and decreased width of gyri with an increase in ventricular size occur. Brain degeneration takes place primarily in the temporal and frontal lobes, where emotional, affective, and memory domains primarily reside. Cerebral blood flow and oxygenation decrease by 25% to 30% by the age of 80. Although these decreases generally match one another, the normal increase in regional cerebral blood flow that occurs with cerebral neuronal activity is blunted. This is thought to be primarily caused by the high prevalence of atherosclerotic disease that occurs in the elderly.

NEUROLOGIC DISEASES

Neurologic diseases account for approximately one-half of elderly disabilities. The most prevalent among these are dementia, Alzheimer's disease, and Parkinson's disease. Dementia is probably the most serious pathologic process and appears to be a strong predictor of perioperative mortality. The early stages of dementia can be difficult to diagnose. The majority of patients with dementia show no personality changes. In approximately one half of patients with dementia, atherosclerosis of the cerebral vasculature is the primary cause of dementia. Other causes of dementia include hypothyroidism, anemia, renal failure, and drug effects.

Alzheimer's disease is differentiated from typical dementia by specific pathologic changes. These changes include frontotemporal atrophy with plaques and neurofibrillary tangles. Cholinergic activity decreases significantly within the central nervous system (CNS) eventually leading to poorer cognitive abilities. This decrease in cognitive ability is exacerbated by a loss of glutamate receptors and a decrease in the dopamine neurotransmitter system.

Calcium activity within the neuron diminishes with age. This leads to alterations in sodium and potassium, and a decrease in neurotransmitter release. This decreased

Box 25-1 CNS Changes in Biochemistry and Physiology

Decreased brain mass
Decreased cerebral oxygen consumption
Decreased cerebral blood flow
Decreased vascular autoregulation
Changes in Na, K, Ca homeostasis
Reduced neurotransmitter release

release of neurotransmitter is exacerbated by a reduced production of neurotransmitters with aging. Changes in calcium activity, sodium and potassium transport, and neurotransmitter release and production result in decreased cognitive abilities, memory, cardiovascular reflexes, and endocrine responses. Furthermore, both the motor changes of parkinsonism (tremor, senile gait, etc.) and depression occur in the elderly from decreased neurotransmitter release.

COGNITIVE CHANGES ASSOCIATED WITH AGING

Research on the human brain has documented dramatic decreases in brain size and efficiency throughout our lives, beginning virtually from the time of birth. Yet, in spite of these anatomic and physiologic declines, studies have found evidence of only limited decrements in actual intellectual functioning associated with the aging process. This section examines the changes of aging in two fundamental domains of cognitive functioning: intelligence and learning and memory. The fact that most older persons experience little functional impairment, despite their cognitive limitations, is a testimony to the redundancy built into the human brain, as well as the ability of humans to find ways to compensate for potential cognitive limitations. It also reflects the fact that intellectual ability is only one of many factors affecting functioning in later life. Ultimately, intellect may be considerably less important than self-care ability and social competence in determining an older person's ability to function independently.

Intelligence

Intelligence includes a range of abilities that allow us to make sense of our experiences: the ability to learn new information, think abstractly, to make rational decisions, spatial ability, numerical ability, verbal fluency, and so forth. Some abilities (e.g., the ability to think abstractly) are genetically determined and are relatively independent of particular applications, reflecting what has been called "fluid intelligence." Other intellectual abilities (e.g., verbal fluency) tend to reflect the knowledge and skills a person has gained throughout life (crystallized intelligence). Intelligence tests have demonstrated a pattern of age-related changes in intellectual functioning beginning after the age of 60. Typical testing of the aged demonstrates slightly poorer performance on tests of fluid intelligence, but minimal difference on tests of crystallized intelligence. The fact that older persons appear to perform more poorly on tests of fluid intelligence is partially caused by reduced efficiency of nerve transmission in the brain, resulting in slower information processing, and greater loss of information during transmission. However, performance decrements may also be caused by a variety of noncognitive factors, including impairments in motor ability and sensation. When making decisions, older persons sacrifice speed for accuracy, rejecting quick and simplistic solutions to problems, and preferring to work slowly and methodically. In general, older adults can perform about as well as younger persons on tasks which provide sufficient opportunity to compensate for slower physical and cognitive functioning. Finally, many of the health problems which are more common in later life (e.g., cardiovascular problems) can significantly affect cognitive functioning as well as test-taking ability.

Learning and Memory

A modest increase in memory problems occur in the elderly, particularly in regard to recent memory. Decrements are found both in the ability to accumulate new information and in the ability to retrieve existing information from memory storage. Because of the reduced efficiency of neural transmission and because of sensory deficits that limit the ability to quickly and accurately perceive information to be learned, the process of learning new information and storing it, requires more time as individuals get older. In the rapidly changing and unknown territory of the hospital, this may prevent elderly patients from giving the attention needed for complete encoding into secondary memory. The elderly also have difficulty identifying the correct information from the large store of information they have gathered over a lifetime of experiences. This can be particularly difficult when the new information resembles previously learned information (e.g., when one is trying to recall instructions given in the office from those given in the hospital).

Older persons have better memory for certain events that occurred in the distant past than for recent experiences. To a large extent, this is because the distant events that are remembered have special personal significance (e.g., a spousal relationship), or are so unique that they are not affected by later experiences (e.g., special childhood occurrences). These experiences have been recalled mentally numerous times throughout life, increasing their familiarity and making them easier to recall than routine details of day-to-day life. Finally, it is important to note that cognitive processes such as learning, memory, and intellectual functioning are extremely responsive to a person's physical and psychologic state. Physical illnesses and medications can affect neuronal function and also reduce the energy available for cognitive processes.

SENSORY CHANGES WITH AGING

Senses play a central role in our ability to gather information and to interact with others. Along with a variety of physiological changes which accompany the aging process, changes in the sensorium also occur. The effects of the sensory changes on the individual's perceptions and social interaction depend upon many factors, such as the specific sense affected, the nature of the change, and the extent to which reversal of the changes can be accomplished.

Beginning in the fourth decade, the pupil begins to decrease in size and in response time to light. Because of these changes, it is estimated that older adults require 3 times the amount of illumination to see as a younger person. Also, focusing takes longer with an increase in presbyopia, making small print harder to read. Another normal change is thickening and yellowing of the lens of the eye. This results in light diffraction, increased sensitivity to glare, decreased depth perception, and more difficulty distinguishing pastel colors, especially blues and greens. Pathologic changes of the eye include cataracts or significant opacification of the lens, glaucoma, and various retinal disorders such as macular degeneration and diabetic retinopathy.

Hearing changes associated with aging include a decrease in sensitivity to high frequency tones and decreased discrimination of similar pitches. These changes are usually the result of normal changes to the bones and cochlear hair cells of the inner ear. Significant hearing loss, while relatively common in the elderly population, is not a normal part of the aging process. Approximately 30% of all elderly persons have some hearing impairment. Such loss is usually the result of damage to the ear, the peripheral nervous system, the CNS, or a combination of the three. This may result in poor communicative abilities between these individuals and health care personnel, leading to withdrawal of the patient and ignoring of the patient on the part of health care providers.

Taste and smell are interrelated and important for eating. Older adults experience some decline in the ability to taste resulting from a reduction in the total number of taste buds, especially after age 80. This decline in taste may impact upon the elderly not attaining adequate nutritional status, particularly when multiple medications may alter taste postoperatively.

With advanced age, the skin becomes somewhat less sensitive to all modalities of sensation. This may influence the ability of the elderly patient to recognize pressured areas on dependent portions of their bodies and encourage the formation of pressure sores. With regard to pain, it appears that nociperception may decrease somewhat with advancing age. Although it has been well-documented that elderly surgical patients require a lower total dose of analgesics for incisional pain, it remains unclear whether this is caused by pharmacokinetic or pharmacodynamic changes, or from decreased efferent pain input to the CNS.

In elderly patients with intact cognition and psychomotor abilities, visual analogue pain scores appear to correlate well with those of younger adults for similar surgical procedures. The well-recognized clinical observation that older patients "need" less analgesia is probably because of the following factors: (1) the elderly clear analgesics more slowly, (2) the elderly, particularly those with mental status changes, tend to be less verbal in their response to pain, and (3) the elderly may feel they are a "brother" to health care personnel in requesting analgesia.

Cardiovascular System

ANATOMIC

The heart undergoes ventricular enlargement, primarily because of myocardial cell hypertrophy, and build up of collagen, fibrous tissue, and lipid substance. The cellular hypertrophy is caused by the normal increase in systemic vascular resistance that occurs with aging. Conversely, end-diastolic and end-systolic ventricular volumes change little with aging. Because of the high pressures the aortic outflow area is subjected to, calcification and fibrosis commonly occur in the aortic valve. Aortic sclerosis occurs in approximately 20% of those over the age of 65.

Starting within the aorta, elastic fibers in the arterial system begin to decrease in number by age 30, and be replaced by calcium deposits. As the aortic becomes less compliant, systemic blood pressure increases. Further distally in the arterial tree, hyaline degeneration occurs within the media layer of arterioles, increasing vascular resistance.

PHYSIOLOGIC

Cardiac output drops with aging at a rate of roughly 1%/year past the age of 30. This occurs as a result of decreased stroke volume, increased afterload, lower sympathetic nervous system activity, and decreased total body oxygen consumption. Reduced diastolic compliance can result in delayed diastolic filling and diastolic dysfunction. These factors, in turn, lower stroke volume. The altered diastolic filling makes the atrial systolic contribution to ventricular filling a greater percentage (40% vs 20%) of end-diastolic ventricular volume. This creates a greater need for proper atrial-ventricular systolic timing in the aged patient.

PATHOLOGIC

Coronary Artery Disease

The majority of American men over the age of 60 have at least one coronary artery significantly blocked (>75%). Although the onset of coronary artery disease is slowed in women, by the age of 70, the incidence of significant disease approaches that of men. Coronary artery disease (CAD) remains the major cause of death in persons over the age of 65. In elderly patients undergoing surgery, CAD accounts for one third to one half of all perioperative deaths.

Valvular Disease

Calcification of the heart valves can lead to valvular sclerosis. Valvular sclerosis, in some cases, leads to stenosis or insufficiency. This most commonly occurs in the aortic valve, which can result in aortic stenosis or insufficiency or both. Identifying this process is vital because significant aortic stenosis leads to higher morbidity and mortality in the perioperative period.

Calcification of the mitral annulus also occurs with aging, observed in almost one-half of patients over the age of 90. This may lead to the occurrence of mitral regurgitation or stenosis with subsequent atrial fibrillation. Because of the importance of atrial contraction to ventricular filling in the elderly, processes involving the mitral valve and the presence of atrial fibrillation can have a great impact on cardiac output.

Pulmonary System

VOLUMES AND CAPACITIES

With aging, pulmonary changes are characterized by deterioration of gas exchange and changes in breathing mechanics. P_aO_2 decreases approximately 0.5 mm Hg/yr after age 20, and the alveolar-arterial oxygen gradient increases. This decrease in

P_aO_2 is caused by V/Q mismatching that results from decreased cardiac output and degenerative changes (loss of alveolar septae) in the lungs. Aging alone does not alter P_aCO_2, although the alveolar-arterial carbon dioxide gradient may increase because of increased physiologic dead space. Mechanical ventilatory function is impaired because of decreased elasticity of the lungs and increased stiffness of the thorax. Vital capacity and the forced expired volume (FEV_1) decrease (roughly 1%/yr) with aging, while residual volume (RV) and functional residual capacity (FRC) increase. Maximum breathing capacity is substantially reduced. Pneumonia occurs with increased frequency. In the elderly, there is an increased incidence of aspiration of secretions, probably because of decreased airway protective reflexes.

As with tissues in other parts of the body, lung tissue tends to lose elasticity with age. This results in collapse of small airways with greater air trapping, resulting in the increase in both RV and FRC. Although total lung capacity remains somewhat stationary, this results in a higher RV/TLC ratio. As a result, vital capacity is impinged upon, falling from a median value of 1.7 to 1.2 liters per m^2 of body surface area. The FEV_1 follows the decrease in vital capacity, allowing a constant FEV_1/FVC ratio.

Respiratory muscle function also decreases with age, lessening the ability of the elderly to inspire and expire forcibly. Moreover, the diaphragm tends to flatten, inhibiting its function to contract and expand the thoracic volume as fully. These factors contribute to a fall in ventilatory reserve. By the age of 70, the ventilatory drive in response to hypoxemia or hypercarbia is reduced by almost one half. This decrease in ventilatory drive, in combination with pharmacologic inhibition of ventilation (from residual volatile anesthetic and opiates) and decreased respiratory muscle function, can lead to profound decreases in P_aO_2. This may, as a consequence, put the elderly patient at risk for cerebral hypoxia, potentially leading to myocardial ischemia or mental status changes.

Genitourinary System

As with other vital organ systems, age also takes it toll on the kidney. Glomerular filtration rate reduces linearly with age (from 80 ml/min/m^2 at age 30 to 58 at age 80) in subjects considered in normal health. Glomerular filtration rate can be estimated from the following equation:

$$\text{Creatinine clearance (ml/min)} = \frac{140 - \text{age } \varepsilon \text{ yrs)} \times \text{lean body mass } \varepsilon \text{ kg}}{72 \times \text{serum creatinine } \varepsilon \text{ men}}$$

For women, multiply this formula by 0.85.

Renal blood flow also diminishes progressively with age to approximately 50% of normal by age 65. This loss occurs primarily in the cortex, causing a paradoxic increase in juxtamedullary flow. This decrease in renal blood flow, coupled with a decrease in length, number, and thickness of renal tubules, results in an impaired concentrating ability and electrolyte regulation. With this diminution of renal function, the elderly patient is more susceptible to intravascular fluid overload, dehydration, and electrolyte imbalance. Maximal acid excretion and base reabsorption also are reduced, leading to the potential for altered plasma acid-base balance when presented with an increased acid load from increased metabolic acids or reduced ventilation.

In addition to changes in the renal aspect of the genitourinary system, the prostate also changes greatly with age. By the age of 65, the majority of men have some prostatic hypertrophy. Underlying bladder outlet obstruction is exacerbated by the effects of anesthetics, analgesics, and the anticholinergic effects of medications, and can lead to postoperative urinary retention. If the need for bladder catheterization arises, ambulation may be impaired, and the incidence of urinary tract infection rises significantly.

Gastrointestinal/Metabolic System

As we age, we experience a reduction in the production of hydrochloric acid, digestive enzymes, and saliva. These changes can result in gastrointestinal (GI) distress, impaired swallowing, and delayed emptying of the stomach. Perhaps more importantly, the breakdown and absorption of foods may also be impaired, potentially resulting in vitamin deficiencies of B, C, and K vitamins, and malnutrition in severe cases. If left untreated, these deficiencies may result in capillary weakening, easy bruising, muscle cramping, reduced appetite, weakness, mental confusion, and illness.

Overall metabolic activity also decreases with aging. Because of lower levels of sympathetic activity, metabolic hormones, and decreased muscle mass, the basal metabolic rate decreases by approximately 1% per year after age 30. This decreased metabolic demand should be considered when administering perioperative supplemental nutrition. Conversely, adequate protein intake to prevent a negative nitrogen balance and enough carbohydrate to supply metabolic energy needs should be calculated and provided.

Diabetes is the most common endocrine abnormality in the elderly. This is generally caused by inadequate insulin release or receptor activity. Because of the stress response in the perioperative period, blood glucose levels usually rise, even without the provision of enteral or parenteral dextrose. Because of the altered levels of consciousness observed immediately in the postoperative period, mental status may not be a good guide to hypoglycemia or extreme hyperglycemia. Blood glucose levels should be closely monitored in these patients.

Hepatic System

Total liver blood flow falls to roughly two thirds of its normal flow with aging, primarily in the portal system. This will influence the effect of orally administered drugs more than intravenous medications. Conventional liver function tests show no change with aging, although serum albumin levels may drop slightly. More importantly, the "quality" of the albumin, as judged by its binding ability, appears to be altered, leading to higher unbound levels of protein-bound drugs. Although it seems that microsomal hydroxylation and oxidation are not impaired with aging, demethylation decreases. This may explain the prolonged effect of drugs, such as diazepam, in the elderly.

• PHARMACOLOGIC CHANGES IN THE ELDERLY

Pharmacologic changes in the elderly are caused by changes in both pharmacokinetics and pharmacodynamics. The metabolism and distribution of many drugs change with aging. Likewise, the cellular response to drugs commonly used in the perioperative period that affect the CNS (benzodiazepines, anesthetics, metoclopramide, narcotics) and the cardiovascular system (β-blockers, calcium channel blockers, diuretics), are frequently altered in older adults.

No generalizations concerning potential age-related alterations in pharmacodynamics, however, can be made since the elderly patient's pharmacologic response is increased for certain drugs, reduced for others, and unchanged for still others. Both the physiologic changes of aging, as well as altered homeostatic mechanisms in the elderly, may cause an increased sensitivity to drug response. The effect of pharmacodynamic alterations may range from therapeutic failure to major drug toxicity. Age-related alterations in metabolism of drugs are a complicated interaction of aging, genetics, disease, and environment. Common age-related pathophysiologic changes and the medications that may exacerbate them are listed in Table 25-1.

Pharmacodynamic Changes

ABSORPTION

Absorption of drugs into the systemic circulation from the GI route is accompanied by greater variability in an elderly patient as compared to intravenous administration. This is caused by age-related changes in absorption including increased gastric pH and decreased GI motility and absorptive surface. These changes may increase or decrease absorption of various drugs, depending upon the drug's pharmacokinetic properties.

DISTRIBUTION

Drug distribution is affected by several age-related changes: (1) decreased cardiac output (as in congestive heart failure [CHF]), (2) total body water, (3) change in serum proteins, (4) alterations in lean mass/fat ratio, and (5) increased body fat. For example, phenytoin, an anticonvulsant, is highly bound to albumin. The age-related decrease in albumin results in less albumin available to which phenytoin may bind. As a result, "free" (unbound) phenytoin increases, which leads to increased phenytoin effect and toxicity.

METABOLISM

Metabolism is the process of chemical alteration of a drug by the body. Metabolism usually takes place in the liver where the chemical structures of drug molecules are altered so that they no longer have any pharmacologic activity. It is frequently necessary for a drug to be metabolized before it can be eliminated from the body by way of the liver or kidney, or other means. Changes in drug metabolism can result from decreased liver blood flow, severe liver disease, disease states common in the elderly (thyroid disease, CHF, cancer), smoking, and drug interactions. Drug-related metabolic changes are especially significant in the elderly because of the increased amount of drug therapy used in this age group, which, thereby, increases the chance of an interaction of various drugs and drug metabolites.

First-phase hepatic enzymatic transformation of drug (oxidation, reduction, and hydrolysis) changes more with aging than second-phase reactions (conjugation and

Table 25-1. Changes in Autonomic Function

PATHOPHYSIOLOGIC EVENT	DRUG
Orthostatic hypotension	Phenothiazines, tricyclic antidepressants, centrally acting antihypertensives
Bladder and bowel dysfunction	Anticholinergics
Thermoregulation impairment	Phenothiazines, alcohol, aspirin
Cognitive function reduction	Psychoactive agents
Glucose intolerance	Glucocorticoids, insulin
Immune-response reduction	Hepatitis B vaccine

synthesis) do. Most evidence indicates that there is an age-related decline in the clearance of drugs that are metabolized by first-phase reactions. This places more importance on the renal system for cessation of pharmacologic activity by eliminating drugs.

EXCRETION

Excretion is the removal of intact drug or drug metabolites from the body by the kidneys, or in some instances, the liver. In most older adults, renal and hepatobiliary function decreases with aging. This can result in the accumulation of drugs or their active metabolites.

Renal function, however, is the primary determinant of drug elimination. Most renal excretion involves the free portion of the drug, with a balance of glomerular filtration and tubular secretion/reabsorption. The extent to which aging affects renal excretion depends upon the fraction of drug mass that is eliminated by the kidney. For example, aminoglycosides are virtually entirely eliminated by the kidney while many β-adrenergic blockers are primarily removed from the circulation by the hepatobiliary system.

The effect of age-related changes on pharmacokinetics is illustrated by the action of benzodiazepines in the elderly. Their elimination half-life is longest in the newborn and in older adults. In these populations, the half-life of diazepam is 3 to 4 times longer than in young adults. Moreover, diazepam can be metabolized to nordazepam and oxazepam. Nordazepam has a half-life of up to 100 hours. Thus, the reduction in renal and hepatic excretion of both unmetabolized and metabolized drug will drastically prolong the clinical effect.

A 20% to 30% reduction in blood volume occurs by age 75. Therefore, injection of anesthetic drugs will initially be dispersed in a contracted blood volume in the elderly, producing a higher than expected initial plasma-drug concentration. Furthermore, because binding to serum protein is reduced for some agents in the elderly, an exaggerated clinical effect may be expected. The brain concentration of the drug more closely approaches the plasma concentration if a lesser degree of plasma-protein binding exists.

Age-related changes in body composition are a loss of skeletal muscle and an increase in percentage of body fat. The latter results in a greater availability of lipid storage sites and a larger reservoir for deposition of lipid-soluble anesthetics. The greater sequestration of anesthetics in the lipid storage sites of the elderly results in a more gradual and protracted release of anesthetics from these areas. This increases elimination time and results in greater residual plasma concentrations, which contribute further to prolonged anesthetic effects.

A pharmacodynamic-related characteristic of advancing age is a continual loss of CNS neurons, accompanied by a parallel reduction in cerebral blood flow and cerebral oxygen consumption. This may be one reason why, as people age, anesthetic requirements generally decrease. In general, pharmacodynamic alterations in drug action in various elderly patients reflect greater sensitivity to drug effect. This is particularly true with medications affecting the CNS. At given free-drug levels in plasma, the sedative effect of benzodiazepines tends to affect psychomotor test results more in aged subjects. This phenomenon holds true for other anesthetic-related drugs, such as inhaled anesthetics and opioids. The converse is the case for sympathetic nervous system agonists. A decrease in both β- and α-2 receptor activity occurs with advancing age. This phenomenon results in: (1) a decreased dose-response to intravenous β-adrenergic agonists such as isoproterenol, and (2) a reduction in the efficacy of β-adrenergic blockers such as propranolol. The latter result is complicated by diminished autonomic reflexes in the elderly. A summary of drugs that have their pharmacodynamic activity altered by aging are listed in Box 25-2.

• PERIOPERATIVE PRINCIPLES OF CARE OF THE ELDERLY PATIENT

Clinicians generally acknowledge that an elderly patient is at higher risk for developing postoperative complications than one who is younger. Most older persons have at least one chronic condition and many have multiple conditions. The most frequently occurring conditions are arthritis (49%), hypertension (35%), heart disease and hearing impairments (31%), orthopedic impairments (18%), cataracts and sinusitis (15%), and diabetes, tinnitus, and visual impairments (10%).

Studies have implicated age as a contributing factor to postoperative morbidity and mortality, although the association of age with more severe diseases complicates determining the cause for this increase in perioperative risk. Careful elicitation of the patient's history and a detailed examination will put the practitioner on alert for the higher-risk patient. In addition, knowledge of the specific needs of the debilitated

Box 25-2 Drugs that Have Their Pharmacodynamic Activity Altered by Aging

MORE PHARMACODYNAMIC ACTIVITY	LESS PHARMACODYNAMIC ACTIVITY
Benzodiazepines	β-adrenergic agonists
Opioids	α-2 adrenergic agonists
Inhaled anesthetics	
Coumadin	

elderly patient will add to the effectiveness of care for this group. Because of the improved education of clinicians concerning care of the elderly, perioperative complications have fallen to the point that in patients over the age of 90, elective surgical mortality is approximately 2%.

Preoperative Assessment and Management

Preparation for a surgical procedure should begin at the time that the procedure is first planned. Preoperative teaching of patients and their support figures helps reduce anxiety, stress, and incorrect expectations. The patient and family members should recognize that functional impairment may be possible and that perioperative complications will be anticipated and dealt with if they occur.

CONSENT FOR PROCEDURES

Historically, full legal consent to undergo a surgical or anesthetic procedure depended only on the patient agreeing that the surgeon or anesthesia provider could perform the recommended procedure. Since the 1960s, however, courts began to require physicians to not only specify the procedure but also to explain the reasons for the procedure, the consequences of performing it, and the alternatives to it. In most elderly patients, this is not a particular problem. For the older patient who may have subtle, or even overt cognitive dysfunction, however, obtaining legal informed consent for undergoing procedures may be intricately difficult. For the patient undergoing a life-threatening procedure, mental status is moot. Those patients may be treated without consent, if in the usual judgment of the medical community, delay of the procedure would put their lives at risk.

Also, the presence of advanced directives or legally binding documents specifying measures of medical care should be sought. These documents can either be living wills or provisions for power of attorney. Living will leave instructions for caregivers concerning what treatment measures patients do, or do not, wish to have performed on them if they do not have the ability to provide consent for a procedure. The power of attorney is a document that enables a third party, such as a spouse, to take legal actions on behalf of the person executing the document (testator) if that person has become incapable of making decisions. The decision to provide consent for the patient then rests with the individual who has been granted power of attorney. This is called durable power of attorney. With ordinary power of attorney, decision-making ability does not transfer to the third party if the testator becomes incapacitated.

Without advanced directive or the consent of the person with power of attorney, nonemergent treatment should not be started until after advice from the institution's risk management or general counsel is obtained. Practically, of course, procedures are frequently performed on patients considered to be incompetent to make decisions. This usually depends upon the consent of the closest available relative. Legally, however, obtaining consent of the closest available relative who does not have power of attorney, may open the physician to liability for failure to obtain legal informed consent if harm comes to the patient as a result of the procedures provided.

The elderly patient may have a greater fear of death or significant organ damage either from the surgical procedure or the anesthetic. These fears should be solicited in a tactful manner and addressed as appropriate for the individual case. A frequent mistake is to casually respond to these fears with "you have nothing to worry about." These patients know that their age group is more ill and more prone to complications. An assurance that their surgical conditions and vital signs will be continually monitored and that you are aware of specialized issues in geriatric care will do a great deal to allay their fears.

MEDICAL ASSESSMENT AND PREOPERATIVE READINESS

The decision whether to operate for a specific condition rests upon two considerations. The first is the likelihood that the patient will live long enough, based on preexisting diseases, to obtain meaningful benefit if the operation is successful. The second is the probability that the patient will survive the operation without significantly disabling sequelae. Most of the information needed to predict this perioperative risk can be gleaned from a good history and physical.

Associated diseases are the most significant predictor of postoperative morbidity and mortality. In patients over the age of 70, cardiovascular, pulmonary, and renal diseases are the most commonly occurring comorbid processes. The qualitative assessment of pulmonary (accessory muscle use, breath sounds, degree of dyspnea, and cough), cardiac (orthopnea, chest pain, dyspnea on exertion, jugular venous distention, and abnormal heart sounds), and neurologic (mental status, neurologic deficits) signs and symptoms can lead the clinician to an adequate classification of risk. Farrow et al. found 16% of the deaths in the elderly occurring postoperatively, were in patients with preexisting CHF and 11% of deaths in those with preoperative renal impairment.

Some advocate technologic measurements to more quantitatively assess degree of disability. Although many studies have indicated good correlation of the results of these tests (pulmonary function testing, cardiac stress testing, echocardiography, and so forth) with morbidity in the postoperative period, it is unclear whether the information obtained from these tests actually alters anesthetic and postoperative management. One could argue that the quantitative severity of the results can put the busy clinician on alert for problems and influence the use of more intensive therapeutics perioperatively. Whether this phenomenon occurs and influences outcome must be judged by the particular clinicians involved for specific cases.

For example, administering intensive pulmonary care to all patients undergoing colectomy would not be cost-effective in significantly reducing morbidity in groups taken as a whole, considering that the overall pulmonary complication rate is less than 3%. But treating the identified high-risk pulmonary patient with intensive preoperative smoking-cessation, postoperative pulmonary preparation with deep-breathing incentive spirometry and bronchodilators, and postoperative epidural analgesia will probably reduce morbidity within that specific group.

Knowledge of the specific sites where morbidity and mortality occur helps the busy clinician focus where it is most important. Cardiovascular complications amount to one half of the total, while pulmonary complications contribute approximately 20% of perioperative mortality. Attention to these two organ systems will, thus, help diminish complications in over two thirds of affected patients.

PSYCHIATRIC EVALUATION

Studies examining the incidence of mental impairment in the elderly varies greatly, probably because of differences in methodology and definition of the dependent variable. The range indicates mental impairment at 1% or less in those aged 65 to 70 but occurring in up to 40% in those over the age of 90 years. The presence of subtle cognitive changes is probably higher, although less well-studied. Several studies have shown that preexisting cognitive impairment in the elderly is a risk factor for postoperative decline in mental status testing and an increased incidence of delirium. Depression has been determined to be the most important psychologic symptom contributing to poor memory and learning scores postoperatively.

In a large prospective cohort study of 1341 patients, examiners found an incidence of postoperative delirium of 9%. Independent correlates included the following: (1) age over 70 years, (2) alcohol abuse, (3) poor preoperative cognitive status, (4) poor functional status, (5) significantly abnormal preoperative serum sodium, potassium, or glucose levels, (6) noncardiac thoracic surgery, and (7) aortic aneurysm surgery. Using a point-scale system as shown in Table 25-2, a risk stratification predictor was developed. Also, the authors discovered that patients who developed postoperative delirium also had higher rates of major complications, longer lengths of stay, and higher rates of discharge to long-term care or rehabilitative facilities.

Preoperative Drugs

Medications are often implicated in the causation of mental confusion in the elderly. The elderly, who are starting with reduced cholinergic activity, may be particularly sensitive to medication with anticholinergic activity that penetrates the CNS. Several antidepressant and antipsychotic drugs have significant anticholinergic side effects. Box 25-3 lists several of the most commonly used drugs with anticholinergic activity.

NUTRITIONAL STATUS

The nutritional status of the aged frequently shows some degree of malnourishment. Reasons include: (1) an altered taste sensation leading to decreased appetite for many foods, (2) the higher prevalence of depression, (3) less income for buying food, (4) lesser ability to absorb nutrients through the GI tract, and (5) frequent institutionalization and dependence on institutional food. Malnourishment will impair recovery from surgical procedures through: (1) inadequate protein stores or intake to prevent muscle wasting, (2) altered electrolytes leading to muscle weakness and altered wound healing, (3) inhibited osteoblastic activity, and (4) decreased metabolic activity.

ANESTHETIC PREOPERATIVE ASSESSMENT

After specific medical and surgical conditions are assessed, evaluation of the elderly patient then is guided toward specific anesthetic-related conditions. The airway in the elderly patient is frequently different because of lack of dentition and gum resorption, leading to poor mask-fitting and the potential for difficult mask ventilation. In

Table 25-2. Point Scale System for Postoperative Dementia Risk Factors

RISK FACTOR	POINTS
Age >70 yr	1
Alcohol abuse	1
TICS score <30*	1
SAS class IV†	1
Na <130 or >150 mEq/L	
K <3.0 or >6.0 mEq/L	
Glucose <60 or >300 mg/dl	1
Aortic aneurysm surgery	2
Noncardiac thoracic surgery	1

TOTAL POINTS	RISK OF DELIRIUM, %
0	2
1–2	11
>2	50

* TICS indicates Telephone Interview for Cognitive Status (scores <30 suggest cognitive impairment).
† SAS indicates Specific Activity Scale (class IV indicates severe physical impairment).

addition, osteoarthritic changes in the cervical spine may lead to inability to adequately extend the head and expose the larynx during laryngoscopy. Arthritic changes may also lead to greater inflexibility in the spine and extremities, leading to a higher number of body areas requiring padding during the surgical procedure.

Osteoarthritic changes in the spine can cause more difficulty in placement of spinal or epidural needles used in regional anesthesia or analgesia. Positioning should be optimized to facilitate placement of these needles. Generally, with adequate skill, placement of these blocks should be successful in the majority of elderly patients.

In patients with vascular disease, atherosclerosis may be widespread. Auscultation for bruits in the carotid arteries should be performed. If present, the clinician should definitely determine if there is a history of any occurrence of cerebral ischemic events. If present, further angiographic or flow studies should be obtained. If not, determining if head and neck positioning elicits ischemic or preischemic events is important. Because of the possibility of stenosis in arterial flow to the arms, brachial artery blood pressure should be compared in both upper extremities.

As mentioned earlier, testing for pulmonary and cardiac dysfunction must be made in the context of whether it will alter anesthetic management. One of the most commonly discussed and studied areas is preoperative cardiac assessment. Many studies indicate that preoperative myocardial ischemia is a predictor of postoperative ischemia and, therefore, a predictor of postoperative myocardial infarction. It remains unclear, however, whether screening patients for preoperative ischemia with technologic means and then subjecting some of them to cardiac catheterization, some of whom will go on to coronary-artery revascularization, improves overall group outcome. For the symptomatic individual (unstable angina, ischemia with

Box 25-3 Drugs Commonly Used in the Perioperative Period That Have Anticholinergic Activity

Amitriptyline
Imipramine
Nortriptyline
Chlorpromazine
Prochlorpromazine
Meperidine
Morphine
Diphenhydramine

failure) for whom the planned surgical procedure is elective, coronary assessment and therapy has certainly been proven to be advantageous in terms of outcome. For the majority of individuals who are asymptomatic, however, there are no proven scientific grounds for recommending testing for CAD.

Intraoperative Care

ANESTHETIC MANAGEMENT

After preoperative risk factors have been delineated and reduced to a minimum, the anesthetic plan is then considered. In most cases, the anesthesiologist involved with the intraoperative care of the patient (or the preoperative evaluation clinic, in the case of outpatients) should be consulted at least the day before surgery, and anesthetic options discussed. If the physical and mental status of the patient is relatively normal, however, the patient may be brought in the day of surgery and assessed at that point.

The types of anesthetic options include either general, regional, or a local anesthetic with or without the provision of sedation. For most elderly patients, the determination of what type of anesthetic is given is affected by patient, anesthesiologist, and surgeon preference for the type of procedure that is taking place. For the majority of patients, however, it appears that the primary determinant of morbidity and mortality depends on the skill and attentiveness of the care providers, not on the mode of anesthetic.

A database large enough to examine differences in outcome in a general, elderly surgical population has not yet been developed. Aging and disease produce a less homogeneous population because the rate of damage to various organ systems varies greatly from patient to patient. A minority of high-risk patients, however, will be optimally cared for by either one technique or another. For example, the replacement of a cataract with an artificial lens in an 80-year-old patient with mild memory deficits, would certainly benefit from the use of a peribulbar block, accompanied with minimal short-acting sedation. This technique would result in the least perturbation of the patient's mental and physical status, and should lead to a short stay within the surgical center. Conversely, the moderately demented patient with severely compromised left ventricular function undergoing upper-abdominal surgery would likely be best served by general anesthesia with a short-acting anesthetic, pulmonary artery catheterization, and an epidural analgesic postoperatively, to provide an optimal level of analgesia, postoperative cardiopulmonary function, and minimal CNS alterations.

GENERAL ANESTHESIA

Induction

The typical induction agent used for most general anesthetics is sodium thiopental. With increasing age, sodium-thiopental serum levels are higher for a given dose than in younger patients because of a decreased volume of distribution and a diminished rapid-clearance rate. When dosing thiopental, the physician should expect a slower induction time, because the elderly patient may have decreased cardiac output, leading to a prolonged arm-to-brain circulation time.

For the patient with compromised cardiovascular function, other induction agents that are useful include etomidate and ketamine. Both drugs depress cardiac contractility and arterial tone to a minimal extent. The disadvantages of etomidate include a higher incidence of postoperative nausea and vomiting and vein irritation upon injection. Ketamine has the more potentially severe disadvantages of causing tachycardia, hypertension, increased cerebral blood flow, and postoperative hallucinations. Ketamine, classified as a neuroleptic drug, may also create limbic-cortical disassociation, leading to postoperative mental status changes (confusion, disorientation, altered speech/motor ability).

The benzodiazepines, primarily midazolam, lorazepam, and diazepam, are occasionally used for induction in long cases in which the patient remains on ventilatory support in the postoperative period (such as heart surgery). The benzodiazepines, particularly longer-acting lorazepam and diazepam, cause prolonged sedation and amnesia, thus, leading to unwanted effects in the patient who is expected to recover to baseline mental status during the immediate postoperative day, up to the second or third day. The use of benzodiazepines has also been implicated in an increased rate of falls in the elderly. Midazolam, however, can be used in small doses to provide conscious-to-deep sedation in the awake patient. Because the effect of benzodiazepines varies significantly from patient to patient, the range of dosages can vary a great deal. Since midazolam has a fairly rapid onset, however, starting sedation with 0.5 to 1.0 mg and then adding additional 0.5 to 2.0 mg doses, as needed, can produce titrated, yet rapid, results. If midazolam is used as a primary general anesthetic agent, it has been shown that its reversal by an antagonist may improve postoperative mental status. Flumazenil reverses sedation and is associated with improved alertness and better comprehension, cooperation, and recall during transport and during the first 15 minutes in the recovery room.

Propofol is another induction agent that has gained popularity since its appearance on the market in 1989. The major advantage of propofol is its rapid onset, short-acting nature coupled with a much lower incidence of nausea and vomiting. Its titratability lends itself to usefulness in the elderly patient, in whom a rapid return to preoperative mental status is desired. As with the other induction agents, propofol has a lower volume of distribution and a lower clearance rate in the elderly patient. This leads to a diminished dose requirement (1.5–1.75 mg/kg vs

2.25–2.5 mg/kg) in the patient over 65 years of age. The primary disadvantage of propofol is its significant depression of the cardiovascular system. Although propofol normally decreases mean arterial blood pressure by about 20%, in the patient with compromised ventricular function, sympathetic nervous system function, or hypovolemia, the blood pressure may drop up to 50% or 60%, particularly if propofol is given in conjunction with opioids or benzodiazepines. Therefore, the use of propofol in the unhealthy elderly patient should be used only as a lower-dose adjunct to other anesthetic agents, or as a low-dose (5–30 mcg/kg/min) infusion agent for conscious sedation.

Maintenance

For the majority of cases, maintenance of anesthesia is provided by a varied combination of an inhaled volatile anesthetic, intravenous opioids, and a neuromuscular blocking drug. The proportion of the three changes depend on the patient, the duration of the anesthetic, and the surgical procedure being performed. Five inhaled volatile anesthetics exist on the American market today: halothane, enflurane, isoflurane, sevoflurane, and desflurane. They are listed in decreasing rank of blood solubility. The rapidity of uptake and elimination is inversely proportional to the solubility of anesthetics in blood. Therefore, the less soluble an inhaled anesthetic is, the greater the titratability and more rapid the onset and elimination are. This factor gives potential advantages to sevoflurane and desflurane, which also happen to be the newest agents on the market. As of yet, however, in studies of small groups of subjects, the difference in psychometric testing between groups exposed to the older and the newer anesthetics is small in the early postoperative period, and is insignificant after a few hours. If overall outcome of mental status is unchanged, there remains the potential advantage of earlier return of baseline mental status, particularly in the elderly patient. For the patient in whom early analysis of mental status is needed (postcraniotomy, patients with cognitive dysfunction, outpatients), desflurane and sevoflurane may be useful agents.

NEUROMUSCULAR BLOCKING AGENTS

Succinylcholine

As with other rapidly acting intravenous drugs, succinylcholine may have a prolonged onset in patients with slow circulation times. Although plasma cholinesterase levels are somewhat lower in the elderly, the duration of action is relatively unchanged.

Nondepolarizing Muscle Relaxants

Generally, the initial dose required for endotracheal intubation does not change with aging, although the time to peak effect may be slightly prolonged because of decreases in cardiac output. Because most of these drugs are primarily metabolized by the liver and their slightly active metabolites are excreted by the kidney, their duration of action tends to be prolonged in the aged patient. A few studies have determined that recovery from pancuronium, a longer-acting agent, can be prolonged as much as 80%. Even the intermediate-acting agents, such as vecuronium, have significantly reduced clearance rates (less than one half the rate in younger adults).

The benzylisoquinoline muscle relaxants (atracurium, *cis*-atracurium, and mivacurium) are primarily metabolized by spontaneous degradation (Hofmann elimination) and by plasma cholinesterase. These drugs, therefore, do not have the prolonged clinical activity in elderly patients who have either hepatic or renal dysfunction, as seen with the other nondepolarizing muscle relaxants. For the elderly patient with compromised liver or kidney function, these drugs have a more predictable duration of action. In the clinical situation, these drugs may be the drugs of choice for procedures lasting less than 1 hour.

In terms of pharmacodynamics, the activity of all neuromuscular relaxants remains relatively unchanged in the healthy elderly patient. As with all patients with electrolyte disorders or preexisting neuromuscular disease, however, the effect of a given plasma level of drug may be exacerbated and result in residual neuromuscular blockade during the early postoperative period. Patients with extremes of electrolyte imbalance, particularly calcium, phosphate, and magnesium, are particularly prone to muscle weakness. Alcoholism, chronically poor nutrition, and renal disease all contribute to these abnormalities.

Reversal of neuromuscular blockade is usually accomplished with neostigmine. The activity, onset, and duration of neostigmine appears to be unchanged in the elderly patient. The peripheral cholinergic activity of neostigmine is balanced with the use of glycopyrrolate. Because both neostigmine and glycopyrrolate cross the blood-brain barrier to a negligible extent, mental status should not be greatly affected by these drugs. Neostigmine should be used as in any other patient under similar clinical circumstances. Its use, however, may increase the incidence of postoperative nausea and vomiting. In the elderly, the use of atropine to balance the cholinergic effects of neostigmine or edrophonium may increase the risk of postoperative delirium.

Opiates

Elderly patients are more sensitive to the effects of narcotics. At specific plasma levels, all opiates have increased effects on perceived analgesia, respiratory depression, and sedation. In terms of pharmacokinetics, morphine has prolonged activity in some older patients, probably because of altered hepatic blood flow and metabolism of the drug. Studies of the synthetic opioids such as fentanyl, sufentanil, and alfentanil have demonstrated variable pharmacokinetics. A few studies have showed that the clearance of fentanyl and alfentanil is prolonged with aging. One group demonstrated an unchanged clearance and elimination of sufentanil. Because the elderly patient is at higher risk of hepatic dysfunction, it is prudent to titrate all opiates to the desired effect in this patient population. A specific dose cannot be recommended for an entire group. The clinician must take into consideration the pathologic processes ongoing in the patient, hepatic function, and the duration and type of surgical procedure.

REGIONAL ANESTHESIA

A common question faced by anesthesiologists is whether a general or regional anesthetic technique is most appropriate for a specific patient. Although a few studies indicate minor differences in the incidence of postoperative confusion, most studies have revealed no overall difference in outcome in terms of neurologic, cardiac, or pulmonary morbidity or mortality. The analysis of these studies reveal several problems. First is the lack of power inherent in studies performed in single institutions. To determine whether small differences exist between groups, it can take hundreds, or sometimes thousands of subjects to discover these differences. This lack of power is also caused by, in part, the inherent uncontrolled nature of clinical studies.

Only a few contraindications to regional anesthesia exist. Absolute contraindications include coagulopathy, informed patient refusal, infection in the area of the block, and increased intracranial pressure. Relative contraindications include sepsis (particularly if untreated), severe cardiovascular compromise (in the case of moderate-to-high-level spinal or epidural blockade), or an uncooperative patient who cannot be sedated using pharmacologic means. Preexisting neurologic disease is considered by some to be a contraindication, but must be assessed for the potential risk of exacerbation of symptoms on an individual basis. Again, individual details of each patient will dictate the best choice of anesthetic. The stable 80-year-old patient with chronic obstructive lung disease undergoing a total hip replacement would be served well with either a spinal or epidural anesthetic. The delirious 65-year-old patient with bacteremia from a septic gangrenous leg and a blood pressure of 90/50 undergoing above-knee amputation would not be a good candidate for a spinal anesthetic.

Although not scientifically proven to change outcome, some potentially advantageous qualities from regional anesthesia exist. One is the ability to maintain consciousness in the patient, thereby allowing mental status to be a monitor of cerebral function, and attenuating the usual postoperative decrement in cortical function. Another proven benefit is the inhibition of the perioperative hypercoagulable state. With regional anesthesia, a decrease in deep venous thrombosis is observed in patients given regional anesthesia for joint replacements, compared to those who receive general anesthesia for the same procedures. Another observation noted in some studies of vascular surgery patients is a decrease in graft thrombosis occurring in the postoperative period. Other studies have not corroborated this action of regional anesthetics. It is unknown whether other pharmacologic forms of anticoagulation would provide the same benefit observed with regional anesthesia in preventing thrombosis.

FLUID THERAPY

Although fluid requirements in the elderly are the same as those in younger patients, the accompanying changes in cardiovascular, nervous system, pulmonary, and renal function in older patients have a great impact on perioperative fluid therapy. Because of poorer cardiovascular reflexes in the older patient, the hypotensive effect of anesthetic agents is enhanced. A common response from the anesthetist intraoperatively, and the surgeon postoperatively, is to administer additional fluid therapy for suspected hypovolemia. Instead, residual vasodilation, myocardial compromise, or lack of chronotropic response is the actual cause of hypotension. With aging, decrements in the autonomic nervous system decrease the ability to adjust for changes in volume status, perioperatively. In addition, medications can exacerbate the diminution of autonomic responsiveness in the elderly.

Because of decreased sympathetic responsiveness to vasodilation or hypovolemia, many elderly patients rely on intrinsic myocardial changes in contractility (Frank-Starling mechanism) to maintain or increase their cardiac output. Because of decreased ventricular compliance (higher incidence of cardiomyopathies, fibrotic changes, and hypertrophy), however, aged patients may exhibit steeper pressure-volume curves. This leads to a smaller zone of optimal contractility in response to preload, increasing the risk of left ventricular overload if too much fluid is administered. Therefore, in elderly patients in whom ventricular function is compromised and significant fluid shifts (blood loss, third-space losses) are expected, central-venous or pulmonary-artery monitoring is helpful.

Normally, because of the catabolic state encountered in the postoperative period, the osmotic load to the kidney is increased. Because of decreased renal tubular function in the elderly, this increase in osmotic load is not handled as easily as in the younger patient. Renal blood flow also decreases as the stress response to surgery increases norepinephrine levels. Either of these circumstances may lead to fluid overload and resulting CHF and pulmonary edema. The increased antidiuretic hormone (ADH) response to stress in the elderly also predisposes them to fluid overload in the postoperative period. Conversely, sodium deprivation is also not handled as well because of the poor responsiveness of the aldosterone response in the aged.

Fluid requirements intraoperatively are generally estimated from several sources. First, preoperative fluid status is estimated. This is a combination of the disease process (poor oral intake, blood loss leading to anemia, low-serum protein levels, and so on), bowel preparation (cathartics), and NPO duration. In addition, maintenance requirements, replacement for blood loss, losses from visceral evaporation or tissue disruption, and sequestration of electrolytes and water (third-space) need to be considered. Estimates for surgical losses of fluid and third-spacing vary from none to 15 or 20 ml/kg/hr in major abdominal or thoracic cases. Because these are only estimates, in the severely compromised geriatric patient, intraoperative guidance of fluid administration (urine output, central-pressure monitoring, cardiac-output measurements) may be warranted.

States of hyponatremia and free-water excess are more common in the elderly. This may, in part, be caused by relatively excessive ADH release and an attenuated release of aldosterone in this age group. In particular, elderly patients taking diuretic therapy or on sodium-restricted diets frequently will demonstrate the phenomenon of hyponatremia caused by the relative excess of water to sodium. Although mild hyponatremia appears to have no significant adverse effects, serum-sodium levels below 125 mEq/l lead to a higher incidence of altered cerebral function and dysrhythmias.

ANEMIA AND BLOOD REPLACEMENT

Although healthy elderly patients may tolerate hematocrits in the mid-20% range, (particularly if chronic in nature) estimates of optimal red cell mass depends on the individual's ability to increase oxygen delivery in other ways (increased cardiac output) and the oxygen demand of that individual. Both of these factors are difficult to accurately estimate in the compromised or seriously ill patient. Although it has been estimated that optimal oxygen delivery occurs at a hematrocrit of approximately 30% because of rheologic and cardiovascular workload factors, this may not be an optimal figure in every patient. For example, in the patient with significantly compromised left ventricular function, a hematrocrit closer to 35% to 40% may be needed to provide adequate oxygen delivery. Likewise, the 70-year-old individual with an increased oxygen demand (>5 cc/kg/min) because of trauma or sepsis, may require a higher hematocrit to avoid anaerobic conditions and lactic acidosis. Because of the limitations to a cardiovascular response, whether caused by normal aging or an imposed pathologic process, aging is a factor that hinders the compensation for anemia.

Specific illnesses associated with aging put the elderly patient at risk for detrimental effects from anemia (Box 25-4).

Atherosclerotic disease in vessels leading to organs with critical oxygen demand (heart, brain) puts those organs at risk for ischemia and infarction. A hematocrit less than 28% leads to an increase in myocardial ischemia in patients at such risk perioperatively. It is not clear whether a hematocrit below a specific level increases the risk of cerebrovascular compromise. In addition, to lower oxygen delivery to the myocardium, lower hematocrits may also exacerbate myocardial ischemia through compensatory mechanisms needed to increase cardiac output. The compensatory increase in heart rate and stroke volume may increase myocardial oxygen consumption enough to outstrip regional coronary oxygen delivery, thus, creating zones of ischemia.

THERMAL REGULATION

Elderly surgical patients become hypothermic more easily intraoperatively, than younger patients. Because of a lower metabolic rate, poorer sympathetic tone (resulting in less peripheral vasoconstriction), and in some cases, less subcutaneous fat, thermal homeostasis is generally more compromised in the older patient. The secondary effects of hypothermia include increased myocardial ischemia, diminished postoperative cognitive function, dysfunction of coagulation, postoperative shivering with increased oxygen consumption, and an increased stress response.

When providing a combined regional and general technique, patients become more hypothermic than with either technique alone. In the recent past, intraoperative core temperatures of 34°C were a common occurrence, particularly in the elderly patient with multitrauma or undergoing an intrathoracic or abdominal procedure. With the increased usage of actively warmed intravenous fluids and the advent of active warming blankets, hypothermia below 35°C is preventable. Studies now indicating an improved perioperative morbidity and mortality rate may be reflecting the much lower incidence of hypothermia, now occurring in the elderly surgical population.

Box 25-4 Conditions That Increase Risk from Anemia

Coronary artery disease
Congestive heart failure (or any cardiac output-limiting process)
Hypoxemia
Cerebrovascular disease

Postoperative Assessment and Management

POSTOPERATIVE COMPLICATIONS IN THE ELDERLY PATIENT

Postoperative Cardiovascular Complications

Most elderly patients who die perioperatively do so after the second postoperative day. Myocardial ischemia, one of the major causes of morbidity and mortality, occurs much more frequently postoperatively than either preoperatively or intraoperatively. Moreover, myocardial ischemia peaks on the third to fifth postoperative day. Another likely cause of increased postoperative morbidity and mortality is the relocation of extravascular fluid to the intravascular space, beginning during the second postoperative day. This phenomenon may lead to CHF, pulmonary edema, and hypoxemia.

Measures to prevent myocardial ischemia perioperatively include avoidance of tachycardia, hypotension, hypertension, and anemia. While β-adrenergic blockade therapy has not been proven to prevent ischemia, patients on β-adrenergic blockers preoperatively should have this therapy resumed as soon as possible postoperatively. Blood pressure should optimally be maintained within 20% of the patient's normal preoperative blood pressure values. Also, hematrocrits less than 28% should be avoided in those with risk factors for coronary artery disease because even moderate anemia may increase the likelihood of myocardial ischemia.

Postoperative Delirium

Mental status changes in the immediate postoperative period are a concern of many clinicians and are the subject of increasing study. In nondemented older adults, a decline in cognitive function 3 days after elective surgery predicts a decline of cognitive function 10 months later, as measured by the Mini-Mental Status Exam (MMSE). The incidence of postoperative delirium varies from 2% to roughly 50%, depending on the sample population, diagnostic criteria, and case-discovery methods. Delirium, as diagnosed by DSM-III-R criteria or isolated postoperative mental status changes (such as inability to sustain attention), continue to be underdetected and inadequately documented.

Previous reports on acute delirium in geriatric patients have found that patients experiencing delirium have an increased risk of other serious complications, including progression to severe permanent cognitive dysfunction and death. Keating et al. studied long-term nursing home residents and the resultant in-hospital morbidity and mortality. Deterioration in mental function occurred in 28% of subjects at the time of discharge from the hospital. Major complications associated with deterioration of mental function included a high rate of psychiatric decompensation (e.g., profound depression). Neuropsychiatric complications occurred in 25%, acute delirium in 9%, and profound involutional melancholia in 13%.

A 1990 meta-analysis of 18 studies of perioperative mental status changes in the elderly discovered 4 items: (1) surgery has a significantly decompensating impact on the mental status of the elderly, although the average effect is slight, (2) for cognition, delirium, and affect, age appears to be a significant influence, (3) women tend to experience delirium while men develop cognitive decompensation, and (4) most research in this area is purely descriptive or anecdotal.

Many clinicians believe that delirium resolves within a few weeks if no complications occur postoperatively. There is no research, however, that verifies this clinical observation. In fact, one study indicates that the implementation of an intensive perioperative care policy for elderly patients with hip fractures can significantly reduce the incidence of postoperative acute confusional states. Postoperative delirium results in increased morbidity, delayed functional recovery, and prolonged hospital stay.

The features of postoperative delirium include its transient nature, an altered sleep pattern, impaired cognition, altered psychomotor activity, and fluctuating levels of consciousness. It is usually observed within the first 2 postoperative days and tends to worsen nocturnally. Historically, studies indicate that physicians or nurses detect only about one-half the cases of delirium diagnosed by testing. Testing for cognitive changes postoperatively basically hinges on brief examinations. A rapidly administered test that can be used for gross screening is the Short Portable Mental Status Questionnaire (SPMSQ) (Box 25-5).

One of the most popular and well-studied tests is the MMSE. This examination has been widely used and has shown to have good reliability (Table 25-3). Orientation, registration, attention, concentration, language memory, and graphomotor skills are assessed. The primary drawback is its lack of sensitivity to mild cognitive changes. To assess for mild changes, other extensive testing should be used, such as the Halstead-Reitan, Luria-Nebraska, and Michigan Neuropsychological Test Battery.

Various studies have separately implicated age, gender, pharmacologic agents, alcohol abuse, preoperative cognitive dysfunction, hypoxemia, type of surgical procedure, sepsis, and hypotension as contributors to postoperative delirium. In a sample of 234 medical and surgical inpatients, Schor et al. found an inhospital prevalence of delirium (tested for by the Delirium Symptom Interview) of 38%. Independent risk factors included prior cognitive impairment, age over 80 years, fracture on admission,

Box 25-5 The Short Portable Mental Status Questionnaire

QUESTIONS
What is the date, month, year?
What is the day of the week?
What is the name of this place?
What is your phone number (or address)?
How old are you?
When were you born?
Who is the current President of the United States?
Who is the past President of the United States?
What was your mother's maiden name?
Can you count backward from 20 by 3s?

SCORING
0–2 errors: normal
3–4 errors: mild impairment
5–7 errors: moderate impairment
≥8 errors: severe impairment

Table 25-3. The Mini-Mental State Examination

COGNITIVE FUNCTION	QUESTIONS OR TASKS	SCORE
Orientation	What is the year? Season? Date? Day? Month?	_____ of 5
Orientation	Where are we? State? County? Town? Hospital? Floor?	_____ of 5
Registration	Name three objects. Have patient repeat them afterwards.	_____ of 3 (# of trials needed to learn all three names)
Attention and Calculation	Begin with 100 and subtract backward by 7 (stop after five answers).	_____ of 5
Recall	Repeat the three objects named earlier.	_____ of 3 names
Language	Show patient a pencil and a watch. Ask him to name them.	_____ of 2
Language	Repeat the following: "no ifs, ands, or buts."	_____ of 1
Language	Ask the patient to do this three-stage command; take this piece of paper in your right hand, fold it in half, and put it on the floor.	_____ of 3
Language	Read this and do what it says, "Close your eyes."	_____ of 1
Language	Write a sentence.	_____ of 1
Language	Copy this design:	_____ of 1

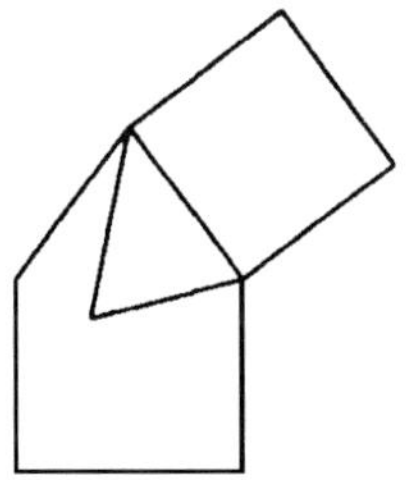

Threshold score for assessing cognitive impairment:

YEARS OF EDUCATION	SCORE
0–4	<20
5–8	<24
9–12	<28
>12	<30

symptomatic infection, male gender, and neuroleptic or narcotic use. In a 1989 study done at the Brigham & Women's Hospital (Boston, MA), investigators examined elderly orthopedic patients to determine the incidence of natural history and risk factors associated with postoperative delirium. Preoperatively, subjects were given multiple neuropsychiatric tests and a health assessment questionnaire. Findings show that 26% of the subjects were possibly or definitely delirious following surgery. Treatment with propanolol, scopolamine, or flurazepam conferred a relative risk of almost 12 times greater than those not receiving these drugs. Also, delirium was associated with increased postoperative complications, poorer postoperative mood, and an increase of approximately 1 and one-half days in length of stay. In another study of patients undergoing coronary artery bypass surgery, those with a higher level of depression preoperatively had a significantly higher risk of postoperative cognitive dysfunction, as tested for by the MMSE. The presence of preoperative cognitive dysfunction reduces the amount of postoperative decrement needed to reach the clinically obvious threshold of delirium. Preoperative dysfunction also reduces the personal psychologic resources available to combat delirium.

Drugs in the benzodiazepine class and those with anticholinergic activity appear to be specific offenders in regard to postoperative cognitive dysfunction and delirium. The pharmacologic basis for the association with anticholinergic drugs is that older patients have reduced CNS concentrations of cholinergic fibers. Because a loss of memory coincides with a decrease of cholinergic synaptic activity, the elderly may be particularly sensitive to these medications. Other drugs associated with this condition include CNS depressants, H_2-antagonists, digitalis, phenytoin, lidocaine, and aminophylline.

Alcohol abuse can lead to delirium through either acute intoxication, withdrawal, or chronic anatomic and neurochemical changes resulting in Korsakoff's psychosis or Wernicke's encephalopathy. Hypoxemia is potentially a problem through its reduction in cerebral oxygenation. Hypoxemia is more common in the elderly because of their decrement in pulmonary and cardiac function, and the decreased responsiveness of their CNS ventilatory control to hypoxemia. Studies indicate that postoperative hypoxemia has no independent effect on the incidence of delirium. This may have to do with the threshold for defining hypoxemia and the time of measurement of arterial oxygen tension.

The surgical procedure itself, whether it is valvular surgery leading to emboli to the CNS, or a hip replacement leading to fatty pulmonary emboli, may play a role in the incidence of delirium. Hypotension, again through reduction in cerebral oxygenation and glucose delivery, can theoretically affect the establishment of postoperative delirium, but studies of mean arterial pressure (MAP) in which patients' MAP was brought down to 50 mm Hg (in the absence of profound hypocarbia) show no decrement in postoperative psychomotor testing.

POSTOPERATIVE ANALGESIA

Analgesia is one of the most important interventional areas during the postoperative period. The authors of a study in 1992 compared the effects of using either epidural or intravenous infusions for postoperative analgesia on the incidence of delirium after bilateral knee replacement surgery in elderly patients. No patient had dementia preoperatively. The overall incidence of acute delirium was 41%, with no difference between types of postoperative analgesia. Predictors of delirium were age, gender, and preoperative alcohol use. All cases of delirium resolved within 1 week.

NUTRITION

Almost one half of elderly patients undergoing GI resection have at least a 10% weight loss preoperatively with an associated functional impairment. Perioperative nutritional replenishment in these patients contributes toward lower postoperative morbidity and shorter hospitalization time. Up to one half of patients hospitalized for greater than 2 weeks, experience protein malnutrition. Hence, in the elderly, aggressive nutritional replenishment is essential during the preoperative and postoperative period.

PRESSURE SORES

Over 1.5 million persons over the age of 70 are affected by pressure sores, with the majority of these occurring in the hospital. Overall national expenditures for pressure ulcers exceeds 5 billion dollars annually. The average inhospital prevalence is estimated to be approximately 10%. With the development of pressure sores, inhospital mortality quadruples and hospitalization time can more than double.

Surgical procedures lasting longer than 5 hours, particularly when coupled with hypotension, may predispose to areas of pressure ischemia. Postoperatively, patient motion is important in preventing the establishment of pressure ulcers. Patient movement can be a problem because of pain and limited nursing care. Results of one study indicate that those who can move more than 20 times per night have a negligible incidence of developing sores. The following lists some of the risk factors for the development of pressure sores (Box 25-6).

Ambulatory Surgery

A remarkable trend during the past 15 years has been the rapid growth in the number of patients undergoing surgical procedures on an outpatient basis. The elderly have not been left out of this trend. In 1995, more than 5 million patients over the age of 65 underwent a surgical procedure on an outpatient basis. The establishment of lower-cost overnight stay in-hospital units has helped give surgeons the ability to

Box 25-6 Risk Factors for Pressure Sores

Age
Dehydration
Depressed consciousness
Dementia
Extremely high or low body weight
Fracture
Incontinence
Major surgery
Vascular disease

admit their patients the morning of surgery, place them in a low-severity inhospital unit, and discharge them the next day.

A major advantage to placing elderly patients in the outpatient setting is that they lose autonomy to a lesser extent and for a shorter period of time. Returning older patients to familiar surroundings as soon as possible helps reduce the incidence of postoperative confusional and anxiety states. Although this method of care tends to place more care responsibilities on family (or other support group) members, the advantage to the patient obviously outweighs the increased duties of the family.

Elderly surgical outpatients have a higher incidence 2 to 3 times those of younger patients) of unplanned admissions to the hospital. This probably occurs because of the concurrent diseases frequently encountered in the aged patient. Because of this phenomenon, the patient and family should be aware of the possibility of hospital admission should perioperative complications occur.

CONCLUSION

Perioperative care of the elderly has improved a great deal over the past 50 years. Because of the increasing number of elderly in our country, this improvement is crucial to the overall safety of providing surgical and anesthetic care to hospitalized patients. Particularly at this time, and into the next century, the perioperative physician must understand the structural and physiologic changes in the aging patient to provide optimal care. Many changes occur as the body ages, with significant potential ramifications for perioperative morbidity and mortality. The importance of understanding the peculiarities of perioperative medical care for the elderly continues to grow.

BIBLIOGRAPHY

Farrow SC, et al: Epidemiology in anaesthesia II: factors affecting mortality in hospital, *Br J Anaesth* 54:811–817, 1982.

Felts JA, guest editor: *Anesthesia and the geriatric patient*, Philadelphia, 1986, WB Saunders.

Johnson JC: Surgical assessment in the elderly, *Geriatrics* 43(suppl):83–90, 1988.

Katlic MR, editor: *Geriatric surgery: comprehensive care of the elderly patient*, Baltimore, 1990, Urban & Schwarzenberg.

Hall MRP, MacLennan WJ, Lye MDW, editors: *Medical care of the elderly*, ed 3, New York, 1993, Wiley.

Marcantonio ER, et al: A clinical prediction rule for delirium after elective noncardiac surgery, *JAMA* 271:134–139, 1994.

Reichel W, editor: *Care of the elderly—clinical aspects of aging*, ed 4, Baltimore, 1995, Williams & Wilkins.

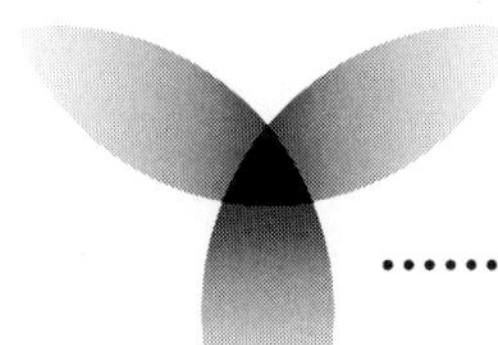

Chapter 26

Perioperative Pharmacology

Nicholas C. Gagliano, MD, George S. Leisure, MD

Many health care providers are responsible for the perioperative care of patients. The perioperative period is complicated by the variety of medications a patient receives while in the operating suite. A thorough understanding of the pharmacology of anesthetic agents and medications used during this time period is essential to provide responsible care.

In this chapter, we will discuss many medications that are specific to the practice of anesthesiology. These drugs include anesthetic induction agents (intravenous, intramuscular, and inhalational), narcotics, and muscle relaxants. The use of these medications allows a smooth transition from the conscious to anesthetized state.

Specifically, general anesthesia should provide lack of awareness, amnesia, analgesia, and various degrees of muscle relaxation.

We will also discuss many other medications that are often used in the perioperative period. Prophylactic antibiotics for surgery and subacute bacterial endocarditis will be reviewed. Local anesthetics will be discussed in detail in Chapter 40.

BASIC PHARMACOLOGIC TERMS

In order to discuss pharmacology, knowledge and understanding of basic pharmacologic principles is essential. Pharmacokinetics refers to the absorption, distribution, metabolism, and elimination of a drug, whether inhaled, ingested, or injected. Volume of distribution is an approximation of the presence of a drug relative to its movement in tissues (mathematically represented as total amount of drug divided by drug concentration). Bioavailability refers to the amount of drug available to exert its end-organ effects. Redistribution denotes the rapid transport of drugs from highly perfused or vessel-rich organs (brain, heart, lungs, liver) to less active tissue sites (fat, muscle, bone). Clearance (l/min) refers to the removal of a drug from the blood usually in a given time period. Elimination half-time is the time necessary to decrease the plasma drug concentration by 50%. Redistribution to inactive tissue sites is responsible for the initial plasma drug-concentration decrease (α-elimination half-life) after parenteral administration. Repeat boluses or continuous infusions depend on drug metabolism and clearance (β-elimination half-life).

Pharmacodynamics refers to the physiologic or receptor-mediated effect of an inhaled, ingested, or injected drug. Agonists are drugs that bind to and activate a particular receptor; whereas antagonists are drugs that bind to a receptor and prevent agonist-binding.

INDUCTION AGENTS

Induction agents refer to those drugs that provide a relatively fast, safe, and effective transition from the awake state to unconsciousness. These drugs can be inhalational, intravenous, or intramuscular. The relative potency of inhalational agents is defined by the minimum alveolar concentration (MAC), the alveolar concentration at 1 atmosphere, necessary to prevent movement to a noxious stimulus (surgical incision in humans) in 50% of subjects at a steady-state level; the MAC for surgical anesthesia is 25% to 30% higher. The MAC for laryngoscopy is approximately 1.5 MAC for surgical incision.

Many of these drugs are also useful and effective for the maintenance of general anesthesia, either alone or in combination with other agents.

Inhalational Agents

Inhalational anesthetic agents enter the body through the lungs during spontaneous or controlled ventilation. Inhalation induction of anesthesia is achieved, in a pharmacodynamic sense, when an adequate partial pressure of anesthetic has been achieved in the brain. Anesthetic gas uptake and equilibrium is determined by: delivered concentration > alveolar > tissue. Box 26-1 shows various physiologic and pharmacologic factors that can influence the MAC of any given agent.

NITROUS OXIDE

Nitrous oxide is a simple, relatively inexpensive and easy inhalational agent to deliver to the awake or unconscious patient. This gas does not cause airway irritation and is a pleasant way to begin an awake inhalation induction, especially in pediatric patients.

Nitrous oxide, however, cannot provide complete anesthesia when used alone (MAC is 104%). It is commonly used as an adjunct to a potent inhalation agent (in oxygen) for anesthesia, or as a nitrous oxide–oxygen combination for sedation/monitored anesthesia care. At concentrations greater than 50%, nitrous oxide should provide sedation and loss of awareness. It has a low blood and tissue solubility. This low solubility is partially responsible for the fast onset of and recovery from the anesthetic state (within minutes upon discontinuation).

Nitrous oxide has a blood:gas partition coefficient that is 34 times that of nitrogen. As a result, nitrous oxide can diffuse from blood into a closed air space 34 times faster than nitrogen can leave the space to enter blood. Because of this differential solubility, nitrous oxide should be used with caution in surgical cases involving potential or actual closed air spaces (middle ear cavity, pneumothorax, intestinal obstruction, pulmonary blebs). For example, commonly used concentrations of nitrous oxide (70%) can rapidly expand the volume of a pneumothorax and lead to hemodynamic compromise. Animal models have shown that high-inspired nitrous oxide concentrations (75%) can double the size of the pneumothorax in 10 minutes. In comparison, the rate of rise in bowel-gas volume from nitrous-oxide administration is slow. The doubling time in this situation may take hours and is usually not a significant factor. However, the minimal to moderate amount of bowel-gas-volume increase may complicate surgical exposure or abdominal closure, and nitrous oxide's use may need to be limited or avoided. For middle ear surgery, nitrous oxide should be avoided or discontinued at least 15 minutes before middle-ear-cavity closure (e.g., tympanoplasty graft placement) to prevent negative-pressure effects (serious otitis, graft displacement) in the middle ear as nitrous oxide is rapidly absorbed when its use is discontinued.

Similar to all inhaled anesthetics, nitrous oxide increases the frequency and decreases the tidal volume of breathing as anesthetic concentrations increase. This gas does not have a consistent effect on the cardiovascular system or pulmonary vasculature. Inhaled nitrous oxide tends to be a direct myocardial depressant, but it also activates the sympathetic nervous system, leading to variable increases in systemic vascular resistance. In general, it also tends to increase pulmonary vascular resistance.

The central-nervous-system (CNS) effects of nitrous oxide include cerebral vasodilation and a minimal increase in cerebral blood flow and cerebral metabolic rate of oxygen consumption ($CMRO_2$). During operations at high risk for venous air embolism

Box 26-1 Physiologic and Pharmacologic Factors That Affect Minimum Alveolar Concentration (MAC)

INCREASED MAC REQUIREMENTS
- Infants
- Chronic ethanol use
- Chronic stimulant drug use
- Monoamine oxidase inhibitors, tricyclic antidepressants
- Hyperthermia (>42°C), hypernatremia

DECREASED MAC REQUIREMENTS
- Newborns/premature infants
- Elderly
- Pregnancy
- Acute ethanol/depressant drug use
- Concomitant use of central nervous system depressants (barbiturates, benzodiazepines, opioids)
- Concomitant use of intravenous anesthetic agents (e.g., propofol, etomidate, ketamine, neuroleptics)
- Lithium carbonate
- Hypothermia, severe hypoxia, hyponatremia
- Mean arterial pressure <40 mm Hg
- Clonidine

(e.g., sitting craniotomies) nitrous oxide should be used with caution. If an air embolism is suspected, nitrous oxide use should be discontinued immediately.

The most common side effect of nitrous oxide administration is postoperative nausea and vomiting. The mechanism of this effect is not fully understood. It has been shown that prolonged exposure to nitrous oxide is teratogenic in laboratory animals.

HALOTHANE

Halothane is a volatile, liquid anesthetic that was developed during the 1950s. Its nonflammability is a feature that was welcome during the era of ether as the primary maintenance anesthetic and necessary in the electrically sophisticated operating suites of today.

Halothane is a relatively pleasant, nonirritating, and highly soluble anesthetic gas. It is a potent anesthetic agent with a MAC of 0.75%. When used for inhalation induction of anesthesia, it allows a rather fast and smooth transition to unconsciousness. This characteristic is desirable and advantageous in the pediatric or anxious patient without intravenous access.

Halothane produces bronchodilation, probably because of a decrease in vagal tone. Because of its bronchodilating effects, it is the inhalation anesthetic of choice for patients with reactive airway disease at values less than 1 MAC. Like all anesthetic agents, halothane is a potent respiratory depressant that results in increased end-tital carbon-dioxide concentration in the spontaneously breathing patient. This agent tends to cause shallow and frequent breaths from a presumed central effect on the respiratory centers.

Halothane is a myocardial depressant with dose-dependent reductions in cardiac output. Heart rate and contractility are both affected, presumably because of a direct effect on nodal tissues and an indirect effect on calcium availability to the sarcoplasmic reticulum of cardiac muscle, respectively. It is common to see sinus arrhythmias (sinus bradycardia, junctional rhythms) during halothane anesthesia. Halothane may also cause an increase in the arrhythmogenicity of cardiac muscle cells, especially in the presence of endogenous or exogenously administered epinephrine. Epinephrine in local anesthetic solutions should be limited to 1:100,000 or less when used for hemostatic purposes in the presence of halothane.

Halothane is a cerebral vasodilator and results in a significant increase in cerebral blood flow while interfering with cerebral autoregulation. However, it does reduce the cerebral metabolic rate of oxygen consumption ($CMRO_2$). As the anesthetic state is deepened with halothane, the electroencephalogram (EEG) shows a progression from fast, low-amplitude voltages to slow, greater amplitude waves. As a result of its effects on the cerebral vasculature, halothane is not the inhalational agent of choice for the patient with increased intracranial pressure.

Halothane, like the other inhalational anesthetics, potentiates the effects of nondepolarizing muscle relaxants. Halothane causes a dose-related decrease in renal blood flow, glomerular filtration rate, and urine production.

The hepatotoxic effects of halothane should be understood. Halothane causes a decrease in hepatic blood flow that is probably related to its overall decrease in systemic blood pressure. It causes a reversible decrease in hepatocellular function. These factors do not cause postoperative problems in the majority of patients. However, halothane has been linked to postoperative hepatitis and fulminant hepatic necrosis in 1 in 20,000 to 35,000 administrations. The mild form of hepatitis is usually self-limited with transient increases in liver enzymes. The more severe form of halothane hepatitis or hepatotoxicity appears to be an immune-mediated reaction. Autoantibodies attack the liver and can result in fulminant hepatic failure. This reaction tends to occur on reexposure to halothane. Risk factors for this reaction include female sex, obesity, and age greater than 40 years. Halothane should be avoided in any patient with unexplained hepatic dysfunction after halothane anesthesia.

ISOFLURANE

Isoflurane is an inhalation anesthetic gas that has been used extensively since its introduction to clinical practice in 1981. However, it is generally not used as an induction agent because of its pungent odor and the significant amount of upper airway irritation. Isoflurane undergoes little biotransformation and, therefore, generates small quantities of inorganic fluoride.

Isoflurane causes a dose-dependent decrease in arterial blood pressure caused by a decrease in systemic vascular resistance with preservation of myocardial blood flow. Cardiac output is maintained at 1 to 1.5 MAC levels. Isoflurane causes an increase in heart rate, especially in younger patients, which is usually seen at higher concentrations and with prolonged exposure. It does not appear to alter myocardial conduction or increase arrhythmogenicity.

Isoflurane is a respiratory depressant whose effects lead to rapid, shallow breathing and an altered response to hypercarbia or hypoxia. Similar to halothane, isoflurane causes bronchodilation. Its effects on pulmonary vascular resistance tend to be small in the normal state. However, isoflurane does interfere with hypoxic pulmonary vasoconstriction.

Isoflurane causes a slight increase in cerebral blood flow and a decrease in $CMRO_2$ (as great as 50%). This increase in cerebral blood flow can be prevented by hyperventilation. Slow-wave EEG activity prevails at 1 MAC with burst suppression and isoelectricity at 1.5 and 2.0 MAC, respectively. This agent does not cause an increase in epileptogenic foci (e.g., a decrease in the seizure threshold). These favorable characteristics make isoflurane an ideal choice for neuroanesthesia.

Kidney blood flow is decreased. The low concentration of fluoride ion produced does not appear to cause permanent renal damage or limit its usefulness in renal insufficiency. Isoflurane produces a degree of muscle relaxation similar to halothane.

Overall, hepatic blood flow is reduced with increasing concentrations of isoflurane, but hepatic arterial flow is preserved. Because of its relative sparing of hepatic arterial flow and low risk of hepatic toxicity, isoflurane is useful for patients with hepatic dysfunction.

SEVOFLURANE

Sevoflurane is a newly developed inhalation anesthetic that began widespread clinical use in 1995. This agent offers a rapid onset of and emergence from general anesthesia because of its relatively low-blood solubility. Sevoflurane is a nonpungent, pleasant smelling gas that is easily used for inhalation induction, especially in the pediatric population. Airway irritation is minimal. These characteristics support its extensive use in the ambulatory surgical setting.

The pharmacodynamic impact of sevoflurane on all major organ systems is similar to isoflurane. However, because of the small number of patients with renal insufficiency studied, caution should be exercised with the use of sevoflurane in the presence of renal insufficiency.

Sevoflurane is a chemically stable liquid anesthetic. Its low-blood solubility and rapid pulmonary excretion significantly limit the amount of agent available for hepatic metabolism. Biodegradation of sevoflurane through direct contact with carbon dioxide absorbers (soda lime and Baralyme) produces a potentially toxic metabolite known as pentafluoroisopropenyl fluoromethyl ether, or Compound A. Compound A is produced in higher quantities with closed-circuit anesthesia systems (circle systems), elevated temperatures in the absorbent, and when Baralyme is used instead of soda lime. Fresh gas flows of greater than 2 l/min decrease the production and rebreathing of this metabolite. Compound A has been shown to be nephrotoxic in laboratory rats. The low concentrations present during clinical use in humans have not been linked to renal failure or death. Continued clinical investigations into the effects of Compound A are needed to support its safety in clinical use.

DESFLURANE

Desflurane is also a relatively new inhalation anesthetic that differs from isoflurane by the substitution of fluorine for the chlorine atom found at carbon number 1. This halogen substitution causes a decrease in potency, an increase in vapor pressure, and increased molecular stability. Desflurane's increased vapor pressure requires a heated and pressurized vaporizer for gas delivery. The increased stability results in little metabolism of the gas (<0.02%) and, potentially, less hepatic or renal toxicity.

Desflurane, like isoflurane, is a pungent gas that causes significant airway irritation to the awake patient and limits its usefulness for inhalation induction. However, its low-blood solubility makes it an ideal agent for maintenance of anesthesia with the ability to change anesthetic levels rapidly with low gas flows. This characteristic allows fast induction of and emergence from anesthesia.

The hemodynamic effects of desflurane are similar to isoflurane. In contrast, desflurane produces a dose-dependent increase in heart rate, usually seen with sudden increases in the delivered concentration.

Desflurane depresses the EEG in a dose-dependent manner and does not promote seizures. Its effects on cerebral blood flow and intracranial pressure are comparable to isoflurane. Its hepatic and renal effect are similar to isoflurane. The extremely minimal metabolism of desflurane decreases the likelihood of organ toxicity.

These characteristics make desflurane a good choice for anesthetic use in the outpatient setting.

Malignant Hyperthermia

In susceptible individuals, malignant hyperthermia (MH) is a rare condition triggered by all inhalational anesthetics, and the neuromuscular blocker succinylcholine. It is an inherited disorder characterized by a hypermetabolic state that includes muscle rigidity, hypercarbia, hyperthermia, hyperkalemia, tachycardia, and metabolic and respiratory acidosis. The proposed mechanism is a defect in the calcium-release channel of striated muscle sarcoplasmic reticulum. Susceptible patients should be identified by preoperative screening; a family history of adverse reactions to anesthetic agents should be sought. A negative family history, however, does not preclude sensitivity to MH.

Prevention of this condition in susceptible patients is the goal. Regional anesthesia (if possible), or general anesthesia with agents that do not trigger MH, is prudent. Agents that have not been linked to malignant hyperthermia include barbiturates, opioids, propofol, etomidate, nondepolarizing muscle relaxants, benzodiazepines, nitrous oxide, and local anesthetics.

Treatment of MH includes immediate cessation of all inhalational anesthetics, hyperventilation with 100% oxygen, active cooling of all accessible body cavities, and surface cooling. The drug of choice for treatment of MH is dantrolene (2–3 mg/kg IV every 5 minutes, up to a maximum dose of 10 mg/kg). Intravenous sodium bicarbonate may correct the metabolic acidosis. Kidney function may be preserved by forced diuresis with furosemide or mannitol. Dialysis may be required for correction of metabolic derangements or preservation of function.

Other Agents

Intravenous medications are most commonly used for the induction of general anesthesia. They are easy to administer, have a quick onset, and have relatively few untolerable side effects.

BARBITURATES

The most commonly used barbiturate for induction of general anesthesia is thiopental. It is prepared as a 2.5% alkaline solution (pH 10.5) of the water-soluble sodium salt. Methohexital (2.5% solution) and thiamylal (1% solution) are other commonly used barbiturates. Methohexital can be administered rectally in the child without intravenous access and provide profound sedation in 5 to 10 minutes.

Barbiturates depress the reticular activating system. This response is based on their effect on the gamma-aminobutyric acid (GABA) receptor, an inhibitory receptor located in the CNS that increases chloride-ion conductance with consequent cellular hyperpolarization. Barbiturates decrease the rate at which GABA (an inhibitory neurotransmitter) dissociates from its receptor, thereby, potentiating its inhibitory effects.

When given as a single intravenous-induction dose, barbiturates cause unconsciousness within 20 to 30 seconds. This rapid induction of anesthesia is related to the rapid brain uptake of these highly lipid-soluble drugs. These agents undergo rapid redistribution from the brain to muscle and fat which is responsible for the rapid recovery (3–5 minutes) to the awake state after barbiturate induction. Prolonged awakening from barbiturates will occur after the administration of large doses (1–2 g total) because saturation of inactive tissue sites, such as muscle and fat, allow the storage and subsequent rerelease of these agents into the blood. Barbiturates undergo hepatic metabolism, and less than 1% is excreted in the urine as the parent compound.

Barbiturates cause a transient decrease in blood pressure because of vasodilation of capacitance vessels. This decrease in preload translates to a decrease in cardiac output that is partially corrected by the baroreceptor-mediated increase in heart rate. Although these effects are minimal in euvolemic patients, they can be pronounced in hypovolemic patients or those with advanced cardiovascular disease.

Respiratory depression is caused by barbiturate action on the medullary respiratory center. Cough and laryngospasm may still occur, necessitating the need for muscle relaxation to facilitate tracheal intubation. The respiratory depressant effects of barbiturates are enhanced by concomitant use of opioids or other sedatives. Barbiturates are not analgesic and may even be hyperalgesic in moderate doses. Barbiturates provide little muscle relaxation.

Barbiturates cause profound cerebral vasoconstriction which decreases cerebral blood flow (CBF), cerebral blood volume (CBV), and intracranial pressure (ICP). This cerebral vasoconstriction occurs in normal areas of brain with intact blood-brain barriers (but little or no effect in ischemic areas that are maximally vasodilated in response to injury). These agents significantly decrease $CMRO_2$. In large doses, barbiturates are capable of EEG burst-suppression to the point of isoelectricity. In clinical neuroanesthesia practice, thiopental is the most commonly used barbiturate and is often used for cerebral protection during episodes of regional cerebral ischemia.

Methohexital can enhance epileptogenic foci in patients with epilepsy. Because of its enhancement of epileptiform activity, methohexital is an ideal intravenous sedative/anesthetic for electroconvulsive shock therapy.

Side effects associated with barbiturates include headache, nausea, vomiting, and the prolonged sedative effects that may persist in the early postoperative period. Barbiturates can cause venous thrombophlebitis if used in concentrations greater than 2.5% for thiopental and thiamylal, or 1% for methohexital. Inadvertent arterial injection of barbiturates is extremely toxic to vascular endothelium, causing intense vasoconstriction and, possibly, thrombosis as well as resultant tissue ischemia or gangrene. Acute intermittent porphyria and porphyria variegata are absolute contraindications to the use of barbiturates because barbiturates enhance porphyrin synthesis and may trigger a porphyrin crisis.

OTHER INDUCTION AGENTS

Etomidate

Etomidate is an imidazole derivative that causes unconsciousness within 30 to 45 seconds after an intravenous-induction dose. Unconsciousness is followed by rapid recovery within 5 to 10 minutes. It is commonly used for induction of general anesthesia in critically ill patients. It acts at the neurosteroid site of the GABA receptor, potentiating its inhibitory effects. Hepatic metabolism occurs with renal excretion of the inactive metabolites. Like barbiturates, etomidate has no analgesic potency. A dose of 0.2 to 0.4 mg/kg is used for intravenous induction.

Etomidate maintains cardiovascular stability. Preload, cardiac output, and heart rate show little change with a minimal decrease in afterload. It is, therefore, an ideal induction agent for patients with significant cardiovascular disease.

Etomidate decreases $CMRO_2$, CBF, and ICP secondary to cerebral vasoconstriction. An EEG pattern of delta waves followed by burst-suppression is characteristic after an induction dose of etomidate. Like methohexital, etomidate activates epileptogenic foci.

Side effects of etomidate include pain on injection. Etomidate also increases the incidence of postoperative nausea and vomiting. Myoclonus following intravenous injection is common. Etomidate suppresses 11β-hydroxylase, an enzyme necessary for adrenal steroidogenesis. This effect may compromise adrenal reserve for several hours following an induction dose, and prevent compensatory adrenal hormone production in the postoperative period. Etomidate should be used cautiously, if at all, for prolonged periods.

Propofol

Propofol is 2,6-diisopropylphenol. It is lipid-soluble and prepared in soybean oil, glycerol, and purified egg lecithin as the commonly recognized white-colored solution. Propofol should not be administered to patients with egg yolk (lecithin) allergies.

Propofol is used for intravenous induction (1.5–2.5 mg/kg) and maintenance (100 to 200 μg/kg/min) of general anesthesia, and for sedation (25–50 μg/kg/min) during monitored anesthesia care or regional anesthesia procedures. Unconsciousness occurs within 30 seconds of an administered induction dose with rapid recovery to the awake state in 4 to 8 minutes. This recovery is more complete than that following barbiturate or etomidate use. Efficient metabolism by conjugation within the liver, and rapid plasma clearance of inactive metabolites by the kidney, allow rapid and complete awakening. Delayed awakening may occur with large intermittent doses or prolonged continuous intravenous use because of propofol accumulation in inactive tissue sites.

Propofol causes myocardial and respiratory depression. Blood pressure and cardiac output/index are decreased in a dose-dependent fashion, with little changes in heart rate. These changes are caused by vasodilation and a direct myocardial-depressant effect.

The respiratory depressant effects of propofol are similar to those of barbiturates, with a decreased responsiveness to hypoxia and hypercarbia. A short period of apnea tends to occur in response to a single intravenous induction dose, and may persist for minutes.

Propofol use is associated with an extremely low incidence of postoperative nausea and vomiting. Pain on injection can be minimized by the prior or concomitant administration of lidocaine. Strict aseptic technique must be exercised when propofol is administered because its preservative-free preparation permits rapid bacterial growth. Opened vials of propofol should be used within 4 to 6 hours.

Ketamine

Ketamine, a phencyclidine (PCP) derivative, is the only intravenous (IV) anesthetic induction agent with profound analgesic properties. It is called a dissociative anesthetic because of its ability to interfere with sensory input and processing between the thalamus and the limbic system. Voluntary movements or myoclonus may occur. Patients appear to be awake, with their eyes usually open, but they do not respond normally to sensory input.

Induction of anesthesia usually occurs within 45 to 60 seconds from intravenous administration (1–2 mg/kg) or 2 to 4 minutes from intramuscular (IM) injection (2–4 mg/kg). These rapid induction times are related to ketamine's high lipid-solubility, relatively low protein-binding, and increases in CBF that allow rapid brain uptake. Extensive hepatic metabolism and redistribution to peripheral sites is responsible for its short duration of action. Because of its similarity to PCP, patients often experience psychomimetic side effects (disturbing visual and auditory illusions, bizarre dreams, emergence delirium). These unpleasant effects can be decreased by the preinduction or intraoperative use of benzodiazepines.

Ketamine is a centrally acting, sympathetic-nervous-system stimulant. It causes an increase in heart rate, blood pressure, and cardiac output. These changes are associated with an increase in pulmonary vascular pressures and increased myocardial-oxygen demand. These characteristics are useful for patients in hypovolemic shock, but may be harmful to the patient with ischemic heart disease, cerebral or peripheral arterial aneurysms, or uncontrolled hypertension. Furthermore, ketamine is a direct myocardial depressant in large doses. This effect can be disastrous in the patient with depleted catecholamine stores or sympathetic blockade (prolonged congestive heart failure, long-standing β-blockade, severe or prolonged shock).

Ketamine causes minimal respiratory depression. Ketamine decreases airway resistance and may be indicated in the asthmatic patient. Respiratory secretions are increased but can be minimized by premedication with an anticholinergic agent (atropine or glycopyrrolate).

Ketamine is a potent cerebral vasodilator that increases CBF, intracranial blood volume, and ICP. As a result, its usefulness in patients with space-occupying intracranial lesions, or increased ICP for any reason, is limited. $CMRO_2$ is not reliably changed.

This agent can be useful for short, painful procedures. The ability to induce anesthesia with IM administration is particularly helpful in the uncooperative patient. Prolonged use of ketamine for repetitive procedures can result in tolerance.

Benzodiazepines

Benzodiazepines are highly lipid-soluble drugs that exert their effect at the GABA receptor complex, primarily in the cerebral cortex. They preferentially bind to the α subunits on the receptor and promote chloride conductance and cellular hyperpolarization similar to barbiturates. The three commonly used benzodiazepines are lorazepam, diazepam, and midazolam. Benzodiazepines are excellent sedative-hypnotics and are used for induction of general anesthesia, perioperative sedation or premedication, or treatment of seizures. This class of drugs can be administered intravenously, intramuscularly, orally, or rectally.

Their high lipid solubility results in a rapid brain uptake and onset of effect. They undergo extensive hepatic metabolism with renal elimination of metabolites. Diazepam, lorazepam, and midazolam are highly protein-bound.

Benzodiazepines exert their effects primarily in the CNS and display few peripheral effects. They exhibit cardiovascular stability with minimal decreases in systemic vascular resistance, blood pressure, and cardiac output. Heart rate may increase slightly. As a result, these drugs are useful for induction of general anesthesia in patients with extensive cardiac disease.

Hypercarbic responses are decreased and apnea can result from the administration of benzodiazepines. Careful observation of the patient's respiratory status is important, especially during IV sedation for diagnostic procedures or monitored anesthesia care. The respiratory depression can be magnified by the administration of opioids.

Benzodiazepines decrease CBF, ICP, and $CMRO_2$. They are also excellent anticonvulsants.

Midazolam is the most commonly used benzodiazepine for premedication or the induction of general anesthesia. Midazolam is water-soluble at low pH, but its imidazole ring closes at physiologic pH and increases its lipid solubility. Midazolam's volume of distribution is similar to diazepam; however, its high-hepatic extraction results in a significantly shorter elimination half-life. The hepatic metabolites of midazolam are biologically inactive.

Intravenous midazolam results in a peak effect within minutes. Intramuscular injection results in peak plasma drug levels in 30 to 90 minutes. Oral administration (0.5–0.75 mg/kg) is helpful for premedication of the pediatric patient before general anesthesia or diagnostic procedures. Midazolam is an excellent choice when a rapid onset and relatively short duration of action are required. Furthermore, this drug provides significant anterograde amnesia.

Diazepam is less potent than midazolam. It is lipid-soluble and prepared in propylene glycol for parenteral administration. Although useful as an IV premedication (5–10 mg IV), IM injection is painful and absorption is unpredictable. It produces a lesser degree of amnesia and longer onset to general anesthesia than midazolam. Diazepam is hepatically metabolized to active metabolites with a slow hepatic clearance and an elimination half-time of approximately 24 to 36 hours. As a result, use of this drug is limited when rapid and complete awakening without neurologic depression is required or desired at the end of surgery. Diazepam is a useful anticonvulsant (IV or pr) for the treatment and control of grand mal seizures.

Lorazepam exhibits a significantly slower onset and prolonged duration of action because of its decreased lipid solubility and low hepatic extraction ratio. Lorazepam is useful in the prophylaxis and treatment of delirium tremens related to alcohol withdrawal.

Erythromycin prolongs the action of benzodiazepines by interfering with their metabolism. Heparin can displace diazepam from plasma proteins and increase the amount of free drug available. Concomitant administration of opioids can potentiate the respiratory depressant effects of benzodiazepines. Benzodiazepine effects can be reversed with the benzodiazepine-receptor antagonist, flumazenil (0.5 mg increments, repeated every 5 minutes to a maximum dose of 2.0 mg). This agent effectively reverses the majority of CNS side effects caused by benzodiazepines.

Neuroleptics

Neuroleptic agents are dopamine-receptor antagonists that also possess α-adrenergic blocking, antihistaminic, and anticholinergic properties. The two classes of neuroleptic drugs are the phenothiazines and butyrophenones. As anesthetic adjuvants, neuroleptics are able to produce variable degrees of analgesia, amnesia, and unconsciousness when combined with narcotics or nitrous oxide.

Another potentially dangerous side effect of neuroleptic agents is hematopoeitic stem-cell suppression manifested as anemia, leukopenia, or thrombocytopenia. This reaction usually occurs within weeks of initiation of chronic treatment with neuroleptics and resolves upon discontinuation of therapy.

DROPERIDOL

Droperidol is a butyrophenone that is structurally similar to haloperidol. It is a dopamine-receptor antagonist. Neurosynaptic transmission is affected by droperidol, with resultant CNS-sedative effects. Dopamine-receptor blockade at the chemoreceptor trigger zone is the mechanism of its antiemetic effect.

Patients who receive droperidol appear relaxed but are often frightened and express a fear of death. Droperidol as a sole agent does not produce analgesia, amnesia, or unconsciousness. In fact, many patients experience dysphoria and agitation. These CNS side effects can be minimized by the concomitant administration of opioids.

It is usually given intramuscularly as a premedicant (0.04–0.07 mg/kg), and intravenously as a sedative (0.02–0.07 mg/kg) or antiemetic (0.05 mg/kg or

0.625–1.25 mg). Rapid redistribution after administration results in a short plasma half-life, but, its sedative effects can be prolonged because of its large size, high degree of protein binding, and high receptor affinity. Rapid clearance and metabolism by hepatic enzymes yields inactive metabolites that are renally excreted.

Few cardiovascular or respiratory side effects are evident. A moderate decrease in arterial blood pressure may occur, especially in hypovolemic patients, because of droperidol's peripheral α-adrenergic blockade. Cerebral vasoconstriction results in a decrease in CBF and ICP with little or no effect on $CMRO_2$.

Because of its antidopaminergic property, droperidol may cause extrapyramidal reactions, especially in patients with Parkinson's disease and should not be used in these patients. These CNS effects on dopamine receptors can be antagonized by the parenteral administration of diphenhydramine.

NEUROLEPTIC MALIGNANT SYNDROME

Neuroleptic malignant syndrome is a rare disorder characterized by a hypermetabolic state that can occur hours or weeks after a patient receives antipsychotic (neuroleptic) medications. Dopamine-receptor blockade at various CNS sites is the reported mechanism. Hyperthermia, rhabdomyolysis, muscle rigidity, altered mental status, and hemodynamic instability are often seen, and can mimic malignant hyperthermia. The mortality rate can approach 30% to 40%. Treatment with dantrolene (a direct muscle relaxant) or bromocriptine (a dopamine agonist) can be effective and life-saving.

Other commonly used neuroleptics include the phenothiazines: chlorpromazine (Thorazine), thioridazine (Mellaril), perphenazine (Trilafon), and trifluoperazine (Stelazine).

OPIOIDS

Opioids are drugs that bind to specific receptors located primarily in the CNS. Opioid receptors are classified as μ (subtypes μ-1 and μ-2), κ, δ, σ, and ε.

The clinical effects of specific opioid-receptor activation are shown in Table 26-1. Opioid-receptor binding and activation by agonists prevents the presynaptic release of, and postsynaptic response to, neurotransmitters (norepinephrine, substance P, acetylcholine) from nociceptive neurons. Agonist binding and receptor activation also cause an inhibition of adenyl-cyclase activity, which results in cellular hyperpolarization. Hyperpolarization prevents the neuron from generating an action potential and the resultant transmission of information (for example, a painful sensation). The administration of opioids before a painful stimulus may decrease the subsequent amount of opioid necessary for analgesia in the postprocedure period. This concept is known as preemptive analgesia. Repeated use of opioids can lead to tolerance or physical and psychological dependence.

Morphine Sulfate

Morphine is a hydrophilic drug with a low-lipid solubility. The low-lipid solubility of morphine slows its movement across the blood-brain barrier and its resultant

Table 26-1. Opioid Receptor Location and Specific Receptor-Mediated Effects

OPIOID RECEPTOR	LOCATION	RECEPTOR-MEDIATED EFFECTS
Mu-1	Cerebral cortex	Analgesia (supraspinal)
Mu-2	Brainstem and spinal cord	Analgesia (spinal) Sympathetic suppression Muscle rigidity
Delta	Brainstem, cortex, and spinal cord	Analgesia (mostly spinal) Respiratory depression
Kappa	Cortex and spinal cord	Sedative Analgesia (mild to moderate) with limited respiratory depression
Sigma	Cortex, limbic system	Dysphoria Hallucinations Tachycardia, hypertension

effects on the CNS. Approximately one third of the plasma concentration of morphine is protein-bound. The plasma half-life of morphine is 2.5 to 3 hours, but the redistribution half-life is significantly shorter (10–15 minutes). Peak analgesic effects occur 20 to 60 minutes after parenteral administration. Parenteral administration results in higher plasma concentrations than the oral route because of first-pass metabolism by the liver (parenteral:oral potency ratio of 3:1). Morphine undergoes rapid hepatic extraction and metabolism to active forms. Renal excretion is responsible for approximately 90% of the elimination of morphine and its metabolites. As a result, patients with renal insufficiency may exhibit prolonged effects for several hours to days after analgesic doses of morphine.

Morphine is available in parenteral and oral preparations. As an instant-release oral preparation, morphine has an analgesic onset time of 45 minutes and a peak effect within 60 to 90 minutes. Sustained-release morphine preparations (dosed every 8–12 hours) exert their analgesic effects within 2 to 4 hours and peak in 6 to 8 hours.

Meperidine

Meperidine is a synthetic opioid that was originally studied for its atropine-like effects. At physiologic pH, meperidine has a low-ionized fraction, moderate lipid solubility and high degree of protein binding. The analgesic effects of meperidine occur 10 or 20 minutes after parenteral or oral administration, respectively. Meperidine undergoes rapid redistribution (within minutes) and has a plasma half-life of 3 to 4 hours. After parenteral administration, peak analgesia occurs within 60 minutes, compared to 2 hours after oral administration.

Meperidine has a high hepatic-extraction ratio. Hepatic metabolism by N-demethylation yields the metabolite, normeperidine. Normeperidine causes excitatory effects on the CNS and has a plasma half-life of 15 to 20 hours. Seizures can occur with the accumulation of normeperidine. Patients with renal insufficiency are particularly susceptible to normeperidine's excitatory CNS effects because renal excretion is responsible for normeperidine's elimination. Meperidine should be used cautiously in patients requiring prolonged administration of opioids for chronic pain syndromes.

For parenteral administration, approximately 100 mg of meperidine is equivalent to 10 mg of morphine. The parenteral:oral potency ratio of meperidine is approximately 2:1. In other words, oral administration requires a doubling of the planned parenteral dose for equipotent analgesia.

Fentanyl, Sufentanil, Alfentanil

Fentanyl, sufentanil, and alfentanil are synthetic opioids. Fentanyl is approximately 100 times more potent than morphine, whereas alfentanil and sufentanil are 10 and 1000 times more potent than morphine, respectively.

Synthetic opioids differ with respect to lipid solubility, protein binding, nonionized fraction, and volume of distribution at physiologic pH. Knowledge of these characteristics is important to understand the different pharmacologic effects of these opioids.

The high-lipid solubility of fentanyl and sufentanil results in a rapid onset and short duration of action. The high hepatic-extraction ratio and metabolism of fentanyl and sufentanil yield inactive metabolites.

Alfentanil's high-nonionized fraction and small volume of distribution translates into a more rapid onset and shorter duration of action, despite its lower-lipid solubility with respect to fentanyl or sufentanil. High hepatic extraction and metabolism of alfentanil result in short plasma half-life and yield inactive metabolites.

Fentanyl is useful for intraoperative and postoperative analgesia, as well as for anesthetic induction, or to blunt the hemodynamic responses to intubation. Fentanyl may be delivered by a transdermal patch for patients with chronic pain syndromes. Sufentanil can be used for induction and maintenance of anesthesia. Alfentanil is useful for brief procedures because of its potent analgesic effects and short duration of action.

As a class, opioids minimally affect cardiovascular function when given to normovolemic patients. Meperidine may cause tachycardia because of its structural similarity to atropine. Morphine and meperidine are associated with dose-related histamine release. Histamine release caused by morphine and meperidine administration can lead to significant decreases in systemic vascular resistance, but may be minimized by slow intravenous administration. Fentanyl, sufentanil, and alfentanil can cause significant bradycardia. Myocardial contractility is classically preserved with opioid administration (except with meperidine). As a result, these agents are useful for anesthetic induction in patients with impaired myocardial function.

Opioids are respiratory depressants. Administration of opioids produces a decrease in respiratory rate with elevation of $PaCO_2$. The respiratory drive in response to hypoxia or hypercarbia is blunted by direct effects on brainstem respiratory centers. Chest wall stiffness with decreased compliance is often seen with rapid administration of fentanyl, sufentanil, or alfentanil. This rigidity may interfere with adequate mask ventilation during anesthetic induction but can be prevented by the use of neuromuscular blockers. Opioids can blunt the hemodynamic and bronchial responses to intubation. Finally, histamine release associated with meperidine and morphine use can cause bronchoconstriction.

Opioid administration can reduce CBF, ICP, and $CMRO_2$. However, hypercapnia from respiratory depression may result in ICP increases, which can be avoided by prior hyperventilation. Opioids cause sedation but do not reliably produce amnesia. Opioids cause a dose-dependent slowing of the EEG but not burst-suppression or EEG silence. These CNS-protective effects are variable and significantly less than the protective effects of barbiturates or benzodiazepines.

Opioid stimulation of the chemoreceptor trigger zone causes nausea and vomiting. Opioid-induced decreases in gastric motility may predispose a patient to aspiration because of delayed gastric emptying and sedation with decreased protective airway reflexes. Sphincter of Oddi spasm is possible with opioid administration and may mimic biliary colic.

Opioid usage is also associated with pruritus that can be annoying to the patient. This side effect is most commonly seen with intrathecal or epidural opioid use.

Opioid-receptor effects can be reversed by the pure opioid antagonist, naloxone. Naloxone should be titrated in small doses (40 μg increments) to decrease the possibility of hypertension, severe pain, and pulmonary edema that can accompany narcotic reversal. Because of its short duration of action (30–45 minutes), naloxone may require redosing for continued reversal of opioid-induced respiratory or CNS depression.

NEUROMUSCULAR BLOCKERS

These quaternary ammonium compounds are capable of interfering with normal nerve impulse transmission across the synaptic cleft at the neuromuscular junction. Normally, acetylcholine (ACh) is released by the presynaptic nerve terminal in response to depolarization. The ACh molecules diffuse across the synaptic cleft and bind to nicotinic cholinergic receptors on the motor end-plate of the muscle fiber. If sufficient receptor-binding occurs, the summation of miniature end-plate potentials will cause action potential generation (opening of voltage-dependent sodium channels) of the muscle fiber, and resultant muscle contraction (by intracellular calcium release and actin/myosin contractile protein interaction). After depolarization, ACh is rapidly hydrolyzed to acetate and choline by acetylcholinesterase (AChE) present in the synaptic cleft.

There are two distinct classes of neuromuscular blocking agents, known as depolarizing and nondepolarizing muscle relaxants. Depolarizing agents bind to the ACh receptor and lead to action potential generation (depolarization of the muscle fiber) by mimicking the effects of ACh. Nondepolarizing agents bind to ACh receptors, but do not cause depolarization of the muscle fiber; these agents are competitive antagonists of ACh.

Reversal of muscle relaxation depends on the class of agent used and degree of neuromuscular blockade. Depolarizing muscle relaxants cause prolonged depolarization (minutes) and do not allow repolarization of the muscle fiber until they diffuse away from the ACh receptor. Pseudocholinesterase present in plasma and the liver is the enzyme responsible for the breakdown of depolarizing agents. This enzyme differs from acetylcholinesterase (true cholinesterase) described earlier. Nondepolarizing muscle relaxants are not metabolized by acetylcholinesterase or pseudocholinesterase; the exception to this rule is mivacurium, a nondepolarizing agent hydrolyzed by pseudocholinesterase. Reversal of nondepolarizing blockade depends upon metabolism and excretion of the drug. Acetylcholinesterase inhibitors are used to speed the reversal of nondepolarizing blockade by decreasing the hydrolysis of ACh. The increased concentrations of ACh can then compete with nondepolarizing agents for binding to the ACh receptor. Acetylcholinesterase inhibitors do not reverse but prolong a depolarizing block, since they also decrease metabolism of succinylcholine.

Depolarizing Muscle Relaxants

SUCCINYLCHOLINE

Succinylcholine is the only clinically useful depolarizing neuromuscular blocker. Structurally, succinylcholine is composed of two, joined acetylcholine molecules. Succinylcholine provides muscle relaxation for tracheal intubation in 30 to 60 seconds, and its duration of action is approximately 5 to 10 minutes. This depolarizing agent is highly water-soluble. As a result, dosages required for pediatric patients are usually higher because of the relatively larger, extracellular water compartment in neonates/children. Succinylcholine undergoes rapid metabolism by pseudocholinesterase. Pseudocholinesterase function from two normal genes results in rapid hydrolysis of succinylcholine. Individuals who inherit one normal and one abnormal gene (heterozygous atypical, 2% of the population) exhibit a prolonged duration of action for succinylcholine (usually 15–30 minutes). Rarely, individuals inherit two abnormal genes (homozygous atypical, <0.04% of the population) for pseudocholinesterase, with succinylcholine blockade that lasts hours and requires prolonged postoperative ventilation. Nondepolarizing muscle relaxants should not be given until return of neuromuscular function from succinylcholine blockade is observed. Succinylcholine should be avoided in individuals who have a history (or family history) of prolonged paralysis following succinylcholine use.

Succinylcholine is commonly used for rapid sequence anesthetic inductions to facilitate tracheal intubation. The rapid onset of muscle paralysis is a unique characteristics of succinylcholine that allows fast and reliable intubating conditions in those requiring rapid tracheal intubation for airway control. Although succinylcholine's action at nicotinic receptors is responsible for its mechanism of neuromuscular blockade, side effects are often related to muscarinic cholinergic-receptor activation.

Cardiovascular effects of succinylcholine are related to its effects on parasympathetic and sympathetic ganglia that innervate the heart. Increases or decreases in heart rate and blood pressure can be observed. Furthermore, succinylmonocholine is a succinylcholine metabolite, capable of causing significant bradycardia, secondary to mimicking ACh's effect at the sinoatrial node.

Neuromuscular blockade from succinylcholine is characterized by fasciculations. This effect is believed to be the cause of postoperative myalgias, sometimes related to succinylcholine use. Pretreatment with a small dose of a nondepolarizing muscle relaxant (10% of an intubating dose) before succinylcholine use, may decrease the incidence of fasciculations and postoperative myalgias.

Normal depolarizing blockade by succinylcholine causes a small, transient rise in serum potassium (0.5–1.0 mEq/L). Problems with hyperkalemia may arise in individuals with renal insufficiency or those with extrajunctional nicotinic receptors on muscle fibers. Extrajunctional receptors develop in individuals with neurologic conditions (Guillain-Barré syndrome, stroke, spinal cord injury, prolonged immobilization, major burns, prolonged sepsis, closed head injuries, and myopathies or muscular dystrophies) that lead to denervation of large segments of the peripheral nervous system. Succinylcholine-induced potassium release in these individuals can be significant, and may cause life-threatening, cardiac arrythmias that are often refractory to conventional treatments. Treatment aimed at rapid lowering of the serum potassium level (calcium, epinephrine, glucose, insulin, and sodium bicarbonate) is essential. In severe cases, dialysis may be required to acutely lower the serum potassium. Routine succinylcholine use should be avoided in the pediatric population because of the risk of life-threatening hyperkalemia and cardiac arrest in children with undiagnosed muscular dystrophies.

Since succinylcholine can trigger MH in susceptible individuals, succinylcholine should be avoided in patients with a family history of MH.

Nondepolarizing Muscle Relaxants

Nondepolarizing muscle relaxants are usually categorized by their duration of action and unique characteristics. These agents interfere with the ability of ACh to bind to postjunctional receptors. Muscle paralysis develops without fasciculations. Nondepolarizing agents are highly ionized at physiologic pH and relatively water-soluble. Their volume of distribution is small and confined to the extracellular space. Metabolism and clearance from the plasma depend upon the agent used, and affect duration of action. Many nondepolarizers rely on renal excretion for a large portion of their elimination.

Various physiologic variables affect the duration of action of nondepolarizing agents. Hypothermia and acidosis potentiate most nondepolarizers, probably by decreasing metabolism and excretion. Hypocalcemia, hypokalemia, and hypermagnesemia (often seen in preeclamptic patients on magnesium sulfate [$MgSO_4$]) may prolong nondepolarizing blockade. Renal or hepatic insufficiency can decrease the metabolism and excretion of nondepolarizers and augment nondepolarizing blockade. Patients with neuromuscular diseases (Guillain-Barré, amyotrophic lateral sclerosis, myasthenia gravis or myasthenic syndrome, cerebral palsy, cerebrovascular accidents) demonstrate variable responses to nondepolarizing muscle relaxants. Concomitant medical therapy may prolong the duration of action of nondepolarizers (calcium channel blockers, local anesthetics, cardiac antidysrhythmics, aminoglycoside antibiotics, and volatile anesthetics).

LONG-ACTING AGENTS

Tubocurarine

Tubocurarine (curare) is a nondepolarizing relaxant that undergoes minimal metabolism. An intubating dose of 0.5 to 0.6 mg/kg, administered over 1 to 2 minutes, produces conditions for intubation within 3 to 5 minutes and lasts for 40 to 70 minutes. Maintenance of neuromuscular blockade is guided by a peripheral nerve stimulator. Tubocurarine produces autonomic ganglia blockade and histamine release that may manifest as hypotension. Slow administration or antihistamines may decrease the degree of histamine release and resultant hypotension. Caution must be exercised when administering this agent to patients with asthma because of the potential for histamine-induced bronchospasm.

Primary excretion is renal (approximately 50%), with variable degrees of biliary excretion (10%–40%). As a result, curare's duration of action may be prolonged in patients with renal insufficiency.

Curare is useful for neuromuscular blockade in long surgical procedures because of its relatively low cost, long duration of action, and infrequent redosing schedule.

Pancuronium

Pancuronium has a steroid nucleus with two modified ACh molecules attached, which are responsible for its binding to the nicotinic ACh receptor. Limited deacetylation by the liver is responsible for metabolites excreted primarily by the kidneys (40%) and minimally by biliary excretion (10%). Renal insufficiency may prolong pancuronium's duration of action.

An intubating dose of 0.08 to 0.10 mg/kg produces neuromuscular blockade for intubation in 3 to 4 minutes and lasts for 50 to 80 minutes. Additional doses are given to maintain intraoperative relaxation.

Pancuronium causes vagal blockade and stimulates the sympathetic nervous system, which can result in hypertension and tachycardia. It is a useful agent for neuromuscular blockade in trauma or hypotensive patients. However, this sympathetic stimulation may be dangerous in patients with cardiovascular compromise. Furthermore, ventricular irritability may be caused by the heightened adrenergic state, especially in the presence of agents known to enhance arrhythmogenicity.

INTERMEDIATE-ACTING AGENTS

Vecuronium

Vecuronium is an analog of pancuronium, which lacks vagolytic properties and does not depend on renal function for its clearance from plasma. Rapid clearance and elimination are responsible for its shorter half-life. Metabolites from deacetylation in the liver primarily undergo biliary excretion (40%–60%), with a limited amount of renal excretion (10%–25%). However, dosage adjustment may be necessary in renal insufficiency. Accumulation of vecuronium's metabolites can result in prolonged neuromuscular blockade which should be monitored during prolonged use. An intubating dose of 0.08 to 0.12 mg/kg produces muscle relaxation within 2 to 4 minutes that lasts 30 to 45 minutes.

Vecuronium causes minimal or no significant hemodynamic changes, unlike other nondepolarizing muscle relaxants. Dosages should be decreased, or vecuronium should be avoided, in patients with hepatic insufficiency.

Rocuronium

Rocuronium is a new, nondepolarizing muscle relaxant that is an analog of vecuronium. Unlike vecuronium, rocuronium can produce muscle relaxation 60 to 90 seconds following an intubating dose of 0.9 mg/kg (normal intubating doses are 0.5–0.6 mg/kg). This rapid onset of action makes rocuronium the nondepolarizer of choice for rapid sequence induction in patients who should not receive succinylcholine. Rocuronium's duration of action is similar to vecuronium.

In normal dosages, rocuronium causes tachycardia by vagal blockade. Blood pressure is usually not affected. Rocuronium is not metabolized, and excretion is primarily hepatic (50%–70%). Dosages should be decreased in patients with hepatic insufficiency. Renal excretion is minimal.

Rocuronium can precipitate in the intravenous line if it is given simultaneously with thiopental. This effect can be avoided by flushing the intravenous line after barbiturate administration.

Atracurium/*cis*-Atracurium

Atracurium has a benzyl isoquinolone structure that is responsible for many of its pharmacologic effects. Near-complete hydrolysis by nonspecific esterases and Hoffman elimination are responsible for its degradation in plasma. Pseudocholinesterase and acetylcholinesterase do not affect atracurium's metabolism. The nonenzymatic Hoffman elimination process is a chemical reaction that is pH- and temperature-dependent; acidosis or hypothermia can prolong this elimination process. Minimal amounts of atracurium are excreted unchanged in urine or bile. An intubating dose of 0.4 to 0.5 mg/kg produces relaxation in 3 to 4 minutes, and lasts 20 to 30 minutes.

Atracurium may cause histamine release. Slow administration of the drug can minimize this effect. Hypotension caused by vasodilation can be significant. Severe bronchospasm may also be precipitated in asthmatics and necessitate the use of another nondepolarizer.

A potential problem with prolonged atracurium use is the accumulation of its toxic metabolite, laudanosine. Laudanosine is a CNS stimulant that may cause seizures at high plasma concentrations. Hepatic metabolism of laudanosine avoids this accumulation in normal patients, but atracurium use should be carefully monitored in patients with hepatic insufficiency. No dosage adjustment is required for renal insufficiency. In fact, atracurium is often used for muscle relaxation in patients with renal failure.

Cis-atracurium, like atracurium, undergoes Hoffman elimination with the production of laudanosine but does not undergo ester hydrolysis to any measurable degree. Intubating doses of 0.1 to 0.15 mg/kg produce muscle relaxation within 3 minutes and are associated with minimal histamine release.

SHORT-ACTING AGENTS

Mivacurium

Mivacurium is a benzyl isoquinolone derivative, similar to atracurium and *cis*-atracurium. Metabolism of mivacurium by pseudocholinesterase is similar to succinylcholine. Individuals with abnormal pseudocholinesterase function may experience prolonged neuromuscular blockade following normal doses of mivacurium. Decreased plasma cholinesterase levels can result from renal and hepatic insufficiency and may alter mivacurium's duration of blockade.

An intubating dose of 0.15 to 0.20 mg/kg produces conditions for intubation within 2 to 4 minutes and usually lasts 12 to 20 minutes. Because of its short duration of action, mivacurium is especially useful for brief surgical procedures.

Histamine release from mivacurium administration is similar to that seen with atracurium use. As expected, this effect can be minimized by slow intravenous administration and is usually not problematic.

Cholinesterase Inhibitors

Cholinesterase inhibitors (AChE inhibitors) are used to reverse nondepolarizing muscle blockade. These inhibitors reversibly bind to acetylcholinesterase and inhibit ACh metabolism in the synaptic cleft. As a result, more ACh is available for binding to the motor end-plate receptor to restore normal neuromuscular transmission. Reversal should not be attempted unless peripheral nerve monitoring shows some return of neuromuscular function (usually twitch responses to train-of-four stimulation). Otherwise, inadequate reversal of neuromuscular blockade may occur.

The duration of action of various cholinesterase inhibitors depends on their binding characteristics to acetylcholinesterase, and their metabolism and clearance from the plasma. Neostigmine and edrophonium are commonly used for reversal of nondepolarizing blockade. Physostigmine is the only cholinesterase inhibitor that is a tertiary amine. This structure allows lipid-solubility and movement across the blood-brain barrier, which makes physostigmine useful to treat the central cholinergic effects of atropine or scopolamine overdose.

The increase in available ACh caused by acetylcholinesterase inhibitors can have profound effects on both nicotinic and muscarinic ACh receptors. Cardiac muscarinic effects may cause profound bradycardia. Bronchospasm from bronchial smooth muscle contraction, as well as increased respiratory tract secretions, may adversely affect pulmonary function. Gastrointestinal effects include increased gastric and intestinal motility with increased luminal secretions. These gastrointestinal changes may cause cramping, nausea and vomiting, or compromise of intestinal anastomoses. Increased bladder tone may also occur and cause problems in the postanesthesia care unit. Coadministration of an anticholinergic agent (atropine or glycopyrrolate) may lessen the undesirable muscarinic side effects of cholinesterase inhibitors.

NEOSTIGMINE

Neostigmine is a cholinesterase inhibitor that covalently binds to AChE. A quaternary ammonium group renders neostigmine extremely lipid-insoluble and unable to cross the blood-brain barrier.

Clinical effects of neostigmine occur within 5 to 10 minutes and can last longer than 60 minutes. Coadministration of an anticholinergic, usually glycopyrrolate, can lessen muscarinic side effects. Glycopyrrolate is useful because it has a similar rate of onset as neostigmine. Neostigmine is useful for reversal of intense neuromuscular blockade, because its strong covalent bonding to AChE and relatively long duration of action decrease the probability of reblockade by long-acting muscle relaxants.

EDROPHONIUM

Edrophonium noncovalently binds to AChE and is, therefore, much less potent than neostigmine. Like neostigmine, edrophonium is lipid-insoluble and cannot cross the blood-brain barrier.

The onset of action of edrophonium is within 2 minutes. Edrophonium is useful for rapid reversal of nondepolarizing blockade when return of neuromuscular function is advanced (four twitches on train-of-four peripheral nerve stimulation). Since edrophonium's cholinesterase inhibition usually lasts less than 45 minutes, this agent is not ideal for reversal of intense neuromuscular blockade by long-acting nondepolarizers. Edrophonium is coadministered with atropine because the onset of atropine's anticholinergic effects parallels the onset of edrophonium's muscarinic effects.

ANTICOAGULATION

The perioperative physician must understand the pharmacology of anticoagulants and the management of patients receiving short- and long-term anticoagulant therapy. For medical anticoagulant therapy, the most common medications are warfarin (coumadin) and heparin. However, many patients also receive aspirin, dipyridamole, and the nonsteroidal antiinflammatory drugs, which can significantly interfere with coagulation. Long-term antithrombotic therapy is usually recommended for patients with atrial fibrillation, prior or recurrent thromboemboli, coronary artery disease, cardiomyopathy, valvular heart disease, left-atrial dilation or thrombus, and prosthetic heart valves.

Warfarin

Warfarin is a vitamin-K antagonist that interferes with the γ-glutamate carboxylations of coagulation factors II, VII, IX, X, and proteins C and S. These factors, synthesized in the liver, are biologically inactive unless certain glutamic acid residues are carboxylated. Therapeutic doses of warfarin can decrease synthesis of these coagulation factors by 30% to 50%. The half-life of these factors varies from approximately 6 hours for factor VII to 50 hours for factor II and predicts the time required for return of normal coagulation after discontinuation of coumadin. Warfarin is 99% bound to plasma proteins and freely crosses the placenta.

A decreased effect of warfarin may be seen in patients with low-protein states (nephrotic syndrome, cirrhosis), high dietary vitamin-K intake, increased metabolism by hepatic enzyme induction (secondary to barbiturates, phenytoin, rifampin, chronic alcohol use), or concomitant cholesterol-binding resin therapy. An increased effect may be seen with decreased metabolic clearance or protein binding of warfarin (coadministration of cimetidine, metronidazole, allopurinol, or amiodarone), acute ethanol use, or decreased dietary vitamin-K intake.

A patient's prothrombin time (PT) is used to monitor coumadin therapy. Recently, an International Normalized Ratio (INR) has been adopted in the United States to standardize anticoagulant therapy with warfarin. The INR target range is guided by the specific medical condition and its risk of thromboembolism.

Heparin

Heparin is a naturally occurring human glycoprotein synthesized in the liver. Heparin increases the activity of antithrombin III 1000-fold. Antithrombin III is a circulating anticoagulant which inhibits activated coagulation factors IXa, Xa, XIa, XIIa, thrombin, and kallikrein. Heparin has an immediate onset and a half-life that is dependent upon the dosage administered. The anticogulant effect of heparin usually disappears within hours, but can be rapidly reversed with protamine. Full anticoagulation with heparin requires continuous, intravenous infusions aimed at prolonging the activated partial thromboplastin time (aPTT) to 1.5 to 2.0 times (50–70 seconds) the normal mean aPTT. Subcutaneous heparin, (5000 units) every 12 hours, should not significantly affect the aPTT. Heparin does not cross the placenta.

Heparin-associated thrombotic thrombocytopenia (HATT) is a condition that may occur within 7 to 14 days of the onset of heparin anticoagulant therapy. Thrombotic complications from arterial thrombosis, such as stroke or myocardial infarction, can occur.

Recently, low-molecular-weight heparin (LMWH) preparations have been developed. These fragments of (unfractionated) heparin have a higher bioavailability (100%), longer half-life (4–8 hours), and minimal effect on platelets when compared to unfractionated heparin. Presently, more information is needed regarding the anticoagulant effects of LMWH and its perioperative management.

Perioperative Management of Anticoagulation

Perioperative management of the anticoagulated patient requires knowledge of the underlying medical condition, its risk of thromboembolism, and the surgical procedure planned. Interruption of anticoagulant therapy is often necessary for noncardiac surgery. Historically, discontinuation of warfarin therapy 3 to 5 days before major elective surgery, with immediate reinstitution of coumadin therapy as soon as feasible in the postoperative period, was recommended. This practice increases the risk of thromboembolism for anticoagulated patients in the immediate, perioperative period. A safe, but impractical, alternative for all anticoagulated patients, is to stop oral anticoagulant therapy 3 to 5 days before surgery and begin continuous intravenous anticoagulation with heparin to an aPTT level that corresponds to a blood heparin level of 0.2 to 0.4 U/ml (Fourth American College of Chest Physicians [ACCP] Consensus Conference on Antithrombotic Therapy, 1992). Heparin can then be discontinued 2 to 4 hours before noncardiac surgery to allow normalization of coagulation. Perioperative heparin therapy requires hospitalization (unless the patient is already hospitalized) with a significant increase in hospital costs. So, who should discontinue warfarin 3 to 5 days before surgery with no further treatment, and who should be switched to heparin anticoagulation (3 days preoperatively) until immediately before surgery? Also, can anticoagulation be maintained for patients who require minor surgical procedures?

Clearly, patients at high risk for thromboembolism upon discontinuation of anticoagulant therapy should remain anticoagulated until immediately before surgery. According to the ACCP, higher-risk patients include those with atrial fibrillation and associated medical problems (known coronary artery disease, diabetes mellitus, age >65), prior thromboembolism, significant coronary artery disease, left-atrial thrombus or dilation, caged-ball valves, more than one prosthetic heart valve, and patients with a mechanical prosthetic valve in the mitral position. For patients who require minimally invasive procedures (dental extractions, superficial biopsies and procedures), the ACCP recommends briefly reducing the INR to the low or subtherapeutic range, with immediate resumption of the normal, oral anticoagulant dose immediately following the procedure. In patients with a high risk of operative bleeding (major surgery) and a high risk of thromboembolism without anticoagulant therapy, the ACCP recommends perioperative heparin therapy. Patients between these extremes require a risk/benefit assessment of decreased oral anticoagulant therapy versus perioperative heparin therapy. These decisions require the collaborative input of the patient's anesthesiologist, surgeon, primary care physician, and cardiologist.

Once decided, reversal of oral anticoagulant therapy with small parenteral doses of vitamin K (0.5–1.0 mg IV), with normal liver function, should reduce the INR to near normal levels in 12 to 24 hours. Heparin anticoagulation can be started and continued until 2 to 4 hours preoperatively, and reinstituted postoperatively when considered safe. Warfarin therapy can be reinstituted with return of oral intake. If reversal of oral anticoagulation is required for emergent surgery, fresh frozen plasma can be administered parenterally.

Finally, what risk does the anticoagulated patient present to the regional anesthetist? Epidural or subarachnoid hematoma following neuraxial blockade can have catastrophic consequences. Most experts agree that central neuraxial blockade (spinal or epidural) should be avoided in patients with significantly elevated prothrombin or partial thromboplastin times. A thorough history, with attention to abnormal bleeding and preoperative laboratory evaluation of the patient's PT and aPTT, is essential for the anesthesiologist. A preoperative risk/benefit assessment of general versus regional anesthesia should be individualized to the patient, planned surgery, hemostatic defect, and concomitant medical problems. When possible, heparin or warfarin anticoagulation should be discontinued or reversed to allow normalization of coagulation parameters. Similarly, indwelling epidural catheters should be removed before the reinstitution of anticoagulation, or before the patient's PT or aPTT are significantly elevated.

No definitive clinical studies have evaluated the safety of central neuraxial blockade in the setting of hemostatic platelet defects or thrombocytopenia.

Recently, numerous studies have addressed the risk of spinal/epidural hematoma in patients receiving LMWH and central neuraxial blockade. Bergquist reviewed over 9000 patients who received LMWH and central neuraxial blockade, and reported no hematomas. However, case reports of spinal/epidural hematoma in patients receiving LMWH and central neuraxial blockade continue to appear. At present, recommendations for patients receiving LMWH preparations and spinal/epidural anesthesia include: delaying spinal or epidural anesthesia until 10 to 12 hours after the last dose of enoxaparin (LMWH preparation); delaying the first postoperative enoxaparin dose until 10 to 12 hours after surgery; and delaying indwelling epidural catheter removal until 10 to 12 hours after the last enoxaparin dose, with subsequent enoxaparin redosing 2 hours after catheter removal.

PROPHYLACTIC ANTIBIOTICS

The beneficial use of prophylactic antibiotics has been well established. Since the 1950s, numerous studies have evaluated the use of antibiotics for prophylaxis of wound infections, as well as for bacterial endocarditis. These studies have included prospective, randomized, double-blinded, and placebo-controlled designs.

Antibiotics for Prophylaxis of Wound Infections

ANTIBIOTIC SELECTION AND ADMINISTRATION

In choosing a prophylactic antibiotic, one must understand the planned procedure, incidence of postprocedural infection, pathogens most often encountered, and the patient's risk factors for infection. Since the majority of wound infections are caused by bacteria, an ideal prophylactic antibiotic would be bacteriocidal, or at least bacteriostatic, against the pathogens most likely encountered. Table 26-2 shows the pathogens commonly encountered for specific surgical sites.

A prophylactic antibiotic should also be nontoxic, easy to administer (oral or parenteral), with high-resultant tissue concentrations, and useful for repetitive procedures. It should require no specialized monitoring, have few side effects or contraindications, and be relatively inexpensive. Realistically, no single antibiotic can be useful for infection prophylaxis in all procedures, nor do all procedures warrant the use of prophylactic antibiotics.

Prophylactic antibiotics should be given at least 20 minutes before, and preferably, within 2 hours of, surgical incision to provide adequate plasma and tissue antibiotic levels. Depending on the pharmacokinetics of the chosen antibiotic, redosing should be considered during lengthy procedures or after two half-lives of the specific antibiotic. One may also consider redosing the antibiotic if significant blood loss occurs, which results in lower plasma antibiotic levels. Prophylactic antibiotics should be continued only for a short time period, usually for 24 hours or less. Prolonged or inappropriate administration of broad-spectrum antibiotics may lead to selection of resistant organisms. When considering the use of prophylactic antibiotics, the clinician should weigh the risks of treatment vs nontreatment. Finally, prophylactic antibiotic therapy must be distinguished from therapeutic or empiric antibiotic therapy, aimed at a known or suspected infectious source, respectively.

Table 26-2. Pathogens Commonly Encountered for Specific Surgical Sites

SURGICAL SITE	PATHOGENS COMMONLY ENCOUNTERED
Skin, superficial	*Staphylococcus aureus/epidermidis, Propionobacterium acnes*
Nose, mouth, pharynx, upper airway	Streptococci (esp. *Pneumococcus*), *S. aureus/epidermidis,* meningococci, *Hemophilus influenzae,* diptheroids, peptostreptococci, *Bacteroides melaninogenicus*
Biliary tract	*Escherichia coli, Proteus* sp., *Klebsiella pneumoniae, Clostridia* sp.
Lower gastrointestinal tract and colon	*E. coli, Bacteroides* sp. (esp. *B. fragilis*), *Clostridia, Klebsiella, Enterobacter, Proteus,* peptostreptococci
Genitourinary tract	*E. coli, Enterobacter, Proteus, Klebsiella,* peptostreptococci, staphylococci and streptococci, gonococcus

The cephalosporins are ideal choices for prophylaxis of wound infection. These antibiotics are bactericidal, offer a broad spectrum of activity against gram-positive (streptococci, *S. aureus*) and gram-negative (*Escherichia coli, Klebsiella pneumoniae, Proteus mirabilis*) bacteria, and result in high-tissue concentrations. Cephalosporins are easy to administer, have a high therapeutic to toxicity ratio, and a low incidence of allergic reactions. The most widely used first-generation cephalosporin for prophylaxis is cefazolin. This antibiotic provides excellent tissue levels when given 20 to 60 minutes before surgical incision. If prophylaxis against anaerobic bacteria (especially *Bacteroides fragilis*) is planned, a second-generation cephalosporin (e.g., cefoxitin) should be chosen or clindamycin should be added. If a patient is allergic to cephalosporins, vancomycin is an effective, though costly, substitute. Vancomycin is especially effective against methicillin-resistant staphylococci or enterococci.

In addition to prophylactic antibiotics, mechanical cleansing of the surgical area (iodinated preparation solutions, 70% alcohol, or chlorhexidine gluconate), strict adherence to sterile technique, and minimizing tissue trauma and operative time, collectively decrease the rate of wound infection.

Although prophylactic antibiotics are generally safe, complications include allergic reactions, selection of resistant organisms, pseudomembranous colitis, and drug interactions; toxic reactions (nephrotoxicity or ototoxicity) may also occur.

In the following sections, we will review the appropriate use of antibiotics for prophylaxis of wound infections and subacute bacterial endocarditis.

CLASSIFICATION OF OPERATIVE WOUNDS

In 1964, the U.S. National Research Council of Medical Sciences detailed a surgical case classification system that continues to guide our choices for antibiotic prophylaxis today. This case classification system categorizes all operative wounds as clean, clean-contaminated, contaminated, or dirty.

Clean wounds usually include elective cases that are closed primarily and not drained; there is no tissue trauma or active inflammatory process; the respiratory, gastrointestinal, or genitourinary tracts are not entered; and there is no break in sterile technique. The wound-infection rate is approximately 2% to 5%. Clean-contaminated cases are nontraumatic cases in which the respiratory, gastrointestinal, or genitourinary tract are entered under controlled circumstances, without gross spillage of their contents (appendectomy, vaginal examination, biliary or bladder procedures without infected bile or urine); minor breaks in sterile technique may occur. The risk of wound infection is less than 10%. Contaminated cases have major breaks in sterile technique; traumatic, fresh injuries or gross spillage from the gastrointestinal tract occurs; and the biliary or genitourinary tract are entered, in the presence of infected bile or urine. The infection rate for contaminated cases is approximately 20%. Dirty or infected cases include traumatic wounds with retained devitalized tissue or foreign bodies, fecal contamination, delayed treatment or trauma from a dirty source; acute bacterial inflammation or a perforated viscus is encountered; and clean tissue may be opened for drainage of an abscess. The wound-infection rate for dirty procedures exceeds 30%.

Clean Procedures

Clean procedures do not generally require antibiotic prophylaxis. However, if the result of postoperative infection would be disastrous, prophylaxis should be instituted.

Cardiothoracic and Vascular Surgery. Many vascular and cardiac procedures involve the insertion of prosthetic or graft material in clean cases. Since the effect of postoperative infection would be catastrophic, antibiotic prophylaxis is recommended. The most common pathogen encountered is *S. aureus*. Intravenous cefazolin is the prophylactic antibiotic often recommended. Alternatively, some institutions successfully use second-generation cephalosporins for antimicrobial prophylaxis in these patients. In patients with cephalosporin allergies, or in hospitals with a high incidence of methicillin-resistant staphylococcal infections, vancomycin (1 g, IV) should be used. The length of prophylactic therapy is controversial. Many surgeons prefer to continue antibiotic prophylaxis until thoracostomy tubes or mediastinal drains are removed. However, the efficacy of therapy beyond 48 hours has not been proved.

Prophylactic antibiotics are not routinely indicated for pacemaker or chest tube insertion.

Orthopedic Surgery. The majority of orthopedic procedures can be classified as clean cases, and the routine use of prophylactic antibiotics is not indicated. However, procedures which require insertion of prostheses are clean cases in which postoperative infection would be catastrophic. Antimicrobial prophylaxis is justified for orthopedic prosthetic material insertion, as in cardiothoracic/vascular procedures.

The most common pathogen in postoperative orthopedic infections is *S. aureus*. Staphylococci, *S. epidermidis*, and gram-negative rods are less frequently encountered. A first-generation cephalosporin, specifically cefazolin, is the preferred prophylactic agent. Cefazolin has a longer half-life and higher peak level in bone and serum than other first-generation cephalosporins. Furthermore, cefazolin has been shown to concentrate in postoperative hematomas. Vancomycin should be used in hospitals with a high incidence of methicillin-resistant staphylococci, or in patients with cephalosporin allergies.

Open fractures are generally considered clean-contaminated or contaminated cases in which antibiotic use is empiric or therapeutic.

Neurologic Surgery. Neurosurgical cases are classified as clean cases, and the effect of postoperative infection can be severe (meningitis, encephalitis, abscess formation). The benefit of prophylactic antibiotic use has been controversial. However, most neurosurgeons elect to use antimicrobial prophylaxis for craniotomies. Gram-positive organisms are responsible for the majority of postoperative infections, but gram-negative organisms may be encountered in ventriculo-peritoneal shunt procedures. The chosen prophylactic antibiotic (usually cefazolin or vancomycin) should be active against gram-positive cocci, and achieve high cerebrospinal fluid levels after IV administration.

Superficial and Other Surgery. Breast procedures, hernia repairs, and superficial lesion excisions have shown a greatly reduced incidence of wound infection after a single dose (or 24-hour course) of a first-generation cephalosporin. Clean, uncontaminated neck dissections demonstrate a reduced incidence of wound infection after a short course of antibiotic prophylaxis (aimed predominantly at gram-positive organisms).

Clean-Contaminated Procedures

Gastroduodenal and Biliary Tract Surgery. In normal individuals, the gastroduodenal and biliary tracts are sterile environments. However, many individuals who undergo gastroduodenal- or biliary-tract surgery have risk factors that increase the probability of colonization or infection of these areas, and the subsequent rate of postoperative infection. Patients who are treated with H_2 antagonists, antacids, or antimotility agents have a higher incidence of bacterial colonization of the upper gastrointestinal tract. Patients with obstructive jaundice, cholelithiasis, or cholecystitis/cholangitis have a high incidence of infected bile, and are at risk for postoperative infection. Infectious complications are usually caused by gram-negative rods and anaerobic bacteria.

Prophylactic antibiotics usually include cefazolin, or a second-generation cephalosporin (cefoxitin). Intraoperative Gram stain and cultures can be used to guide the use of therapeutic antibiotics.

Colorectal Surgery. Colorectal surgery involves operative areas with a high bacterial content at high risk for postoperative infection. Preoperative mechanical cleansing of the bowel with osmotic agents and poorly-absorbed oral antibiotics (erythromycin and neomycin) is essential to reduce the risk of infection.

Pathogens encountered include gram-negative rods and anaerobic bacteria (especially *B. fragilis*). Prophylaxis with a second-generation cephalosporin (with or without metronidazole) is effective.

Gynecologic Surgery. The use of prophylactic antibiotics for abdominal hysterectomy has not been consistently proven to reduce the incidence of postoperative infection. Although the infection rate for abdominal hysterctomy remains low, most gynecologists elect to use preoperative antibiotic prophylaxis. Vaginal hysterectomy has a significantly higher infection rate and warrants the use of prophylactic antibiotics. A single preoperative dose of a first- or second-generation cephalosporin is the antimicrobial of choice. Elective abortion procedures should receive a similar regimen.

Since the 1970s, many studies have addressed the use prophylactic antibiotics for Cesarean section. At present, true prophylaxis does not occur in Cesarean sections because the antibiotics are usually given after surgical incision, specifically after umbilical-cord clamping to reduce the exposure of the newborn to antibiotics. Yet, the risk of postoperative infection in Cesarean section is relatively high because of the incidence of premature rupture of amniotic membranes, and the emergency nature of many cases. Prophylaxis for emergent cases should include a broad-spectrum cephalosporin because of the potential for anaerobic infection; whereas prophylaxis for elective procedures is generally not indicated.

Genitourinary Surgery. Antibiotic prophylaxis in cases with sterile urine is probably not indicated. Prophylaxis for prostate resection, or when an indwelling Foley catheter is present without bacturia, remains unclear. Patients with an indwelling catheter and significant bacturia should receive prophylaxis against infection caused primarily by aerobic gram-negative bacteria (see Table 26-2). Single-dose prophylaxis with a third-generation cephalosporin is often sufficient.

Head and Neck Surgery. Prophylaxis for extensive head and neck procedures is prudent to decrease the risk of wound infection and skin flap failure. Infection is usually caused by gram-positive cocci and upper airway anaerobes. Cefazolin, with or without anaerobic coverage, or a third-generation cephalosporin is effective.

Contaminated or Dirty Procedures

Contaminated or dirty procedures require antibiotics for empiric or therapeutic uses. These cases include open, traumatic orthopedic injuries, and blunt or penetrating abdominal trauma with gastrointestinal injury or disruption, in addition to those scenarios discussed earlier. Antibiotics should be tailored against the pathogens most often encountered.

Prophylaxis of Subacute Bacterial Endocarditis

Endocarditis is a serious illness which is uniformally fatal if untreated, and can result in significant morbidity and mortality, even if successfully treated.

The yearly incidence of endocarditis in the United States is 4000 to 8000 cases, the majority of which occur in patients with preexisting cardiac abnormalities. Bacterial endocarditis follows bacteremia. Bacterial attachment to damaged or congenitally abnormal heart valves, or on endothelium near congenital cardiac shunts, may result in endocarditis. Many diagnostic and therapeutic procedures result in transient bacteremias with organisms that are responsible for the development of endocarditis in susceptible individuals. The incidence of bacteremia is highest for oral and dental procedures, intermediate for genitourinary procedures, and lowest for diagnostic gastrointestinal procedures.

Only a small percentage of cases of bacterial endocarditis can be attributed to dental, diagnostic, or surgical procedures. Knowledge of the specific procedure and its risk for bacterial endocarditis is essential to endocarditis prophylaxis. Because of the catastrophic nature of endocarditis, antibiotic prophylaxis seems prudent for intermediate and high-risk lesions or procedures. Intermediate-risk lesions include congenital heart disease, rheumatic valvular disease, mitral valve prolapse with regurgitation, acquired valvular disease, hypertrophic cardiomyopathy, hemodialysis shunts, and indwelling, transvalvular central venous catheters. High-risk lesions include prosthetic heart valves, previous history of endocarditis, or surgically created systemic-pulmonary shunts (Box 26-2). Low-risk lesions are categorized in Box 26-2 as cardiac conditions for which endocarditis prophylaxis is not recommended. Box 26-3 lists procedures for which prophylaxis is recommended (intermediate and high-risk) and not recommended (low-risk).

It is important to remember that no prospective, randomized, or placebo-controlled study has been performed to evaluate the effectiveness of endocarditis prophylaxis.

Box 26-2 Cardiac Conditions*

ENDOCARDITIS PROPHYLAXIS RECOMMENDED
- Prosthetic cardiac valves, including bioprosthetic and homograft valves
- Previous bacterial endocarditis, even in the absence of heart disease
- Most congenital cardiac malformations
- Rheumatic and other acquired valvular dysfunction, even after valvular surgery
- Hypertrophic cardiomyopathy
- Mitral valve prolapse with valvular regurgitation

ENDOCARDITIS PROPHYLAXIS NOT RECOMMENDED
- Isolated secundum atrial septal defect
- Surgical repair without residua beyond 6 months of secundum atrial septal defect, ventricular septal defect, or patent ductus arteriosus
- Previous coronary artery bypass graft surgery
- Mitral valve prolapse without valvular regurgitation†
- Physiologic, functional, or innocent heart murmurs
- Previous Kawasaki disease without valvular dysfunction
- Previous rheumatic fever without valvular dysfunction
- Cardiac pacemakers and implanted defibrillators

* This table lists selected conditions but is not meant to be all-inclusive.

† Individuals who have a mitral valve prolapse associated with thickening and/or redundancy of the valve leaflets may be at increased risk for bacterial endocarditis, particularly men who are 45 years of age or older.

Box 26-3 Dental or Surgical Procedures*

ENDOCARDITIS PROPHYLAXIS RECOMMENDED

- Dental procedures known to induce gingival or mucosal bleeding, including professional cleaning
- Tonsillectomy and/or adenoidectomy
- Surgical operations that involve intestinal or respiratory mucosa
- Bronchoscopy with a rigid bronchoscope
- Sclerotherapy for esophageal varices
- Esophageal dilatation
- Gallbladder surgery
- Cystoscopy
- Urethral dilatation
- Urethral catheterization if urinary tract infection is present†
- Urinary tract surgery if urinary tract infection is present†
- Prostatic surgery
- Incision and drainage of infected tissue†
- Vaginal hysterectomy
- Vaginal delivery in the presence of infection†

ENDOCARDITIS PROPHYLAXIS NOT RECOMMENDED‡

- Dental procedures not likely to induce gingival bleeding, such as simple adjustment of orthodontic appliances or fillings above the gum line
- Injection of local intraoral anesthetic (except intraligamentary injections)
- Shedding of primary teeth
- Tympanostomy tube insertion
- Endotracheal intubation
- Bronchoscopy with a flexible bronchoscope, with or without biopsy
- Cardiac catheterization
- Endoscopy with or without gastrointestinal biopsy
- Cesarean section
- In the absence of infection for urethral catheterization, dilatation and curettage, uncomplicated vaginal delivery, therapeutic abortion, sterilization procedures, or insertion or removal of intrauterine devices

---

* This box lists selected procedures but is not meant to be all-inclusive.

† In addition to prophylactic regimen for genitourinary procedures, antibiotic therapy should be directed against the most likely bacterial pathogen.

‡ In patients who have prosthetic heart valves, a previous history of endocarditis, or surgically constructed systemic-pulmonary shunts or conduits, physicians may choose to administer prophylactic antibiotics even for low-risk procedures that involve the lower respiratory, genitourinary, or gastrointestinal tracts.

PROPHYLAXIS FOR DENTAL, ORAL, AND UPPER AIRWAY PROCEDURES

Dental, oral, and upper-airway procedures are commonly associated with endocarditis. Any dental procedure that causes gingival or mucosal bleeding, including teeth cleanings, should receive antibiotic prophylaxis. Prophylaxis is not recommended for spontaneous shedding of primary teeth or simple orthodontic manipulations.

Upper-airway procedures including tonsillectomy and adenoidectomy, rigid bronchoscopy, and manipulation of respiratory mucosa require endocarditis prophylaxis. *Streptococcus viridans* is the most common cause of endocarditis following these procedures. Amoxicillin is the recommended standard prophylactic regimen; erythromycin or clindamycin can be used for penicillin-allergic patients (Table 26-3).

Table 26-4 shows an alternative prophylactic regimen for patients who are unable to take oral medications, or who are considered high risk and not candidates for standard therapy.

PROPHYLAXIS FOR GASTROINTESTINAL AND GENITOURINARY PROCEDURES

Diagnostic and surgical procedures involving the gastrointestinal and genitourinary tracts are responsible for a high incidence of transient bacteremia, especially when infection is present. Table 26-5 lists gastrointestinal and genitourinary procedures for which endocarditis prophylaxis is essential. *Enterococcus faecalis* is the most common cause of endocarditis following these procedures.

The standard prophylactic regimen uses ampicillin and gentamicin before the procedure, followed by amoxicillin after the procedure. The standard regimen and

Table 26-3. Recommended Standard Prophylactic Regimen for Dental, Oral, or Upper Respiratory Tract Procedures in Patients Who Are at Risk

DRUG	DOSAGE REGIMEN*
Standard Regimen	
Ampicillin, gentamicin, and amoxicillin	Intravenous or intramuscular administration of ampicillin, 2.0 g, plus gentamicin, 1.5 mg/kg (not to exceed 80 mg), 30 min before procedure; followed by amoxicillin, 1.5 g, orally 6 h after initial dose; alternatively, the parenteral regimen may be repeated once 8 h after initial dose
Ampicillin/Amoxicillin/Penicillin-Allergic Patient Regimen	
Vancomycin and gentamicin	Intravenous administration of vancomycin, 1.0 g, over 1 h plus intravenous or intramuscular administration of gentamicin, 1.5 mg/kg (not to exceed 80 mg), 1 h before procedure; may be repeated once 8 h after initial dose
Alternative Low-Risk Patient Regimen	
Amoxicillin	3.0 g orally 1 h before procedure; then 1.5 g 6 h after initial dose

* Initial pediatric doses are as follows: ampicillin, 50 mg/kg; amoxicillin, 50 mg/kg; gentamicin, 2.0 mg/kg; and vancomycin, 20 mg/kg. Follow-up doses should be one half the initial dose. **Total pediatric dose should not exceed total adult dose.**

Table 26-4. Alternative Prophylactic Regimen for Dental, Oral, or Upper Respiratory Tract Procedures in Patients Who Are at Risk

DRUG	DOSING REGIMEN*
Patients Unable to Take Oral Medications	
Ampicillin	Intravenous or intramuscular administration of ampicillin, 2.0 g, 30 min before procedure; then intravenous or intramuscular administration of ampicillin, 1.0 g, or oral administration of amoxicillin, 1.5 g, 6 h after initial dose
Ampicillin/Amoxicillin/Penicillin-Allergic Patients Unable to Take Oral Medications	
Clindamycin	Intravenous administration of 300 mg 30 min before procedure and an intravenous or oral administration of 150 mg 6 h after initial dose
Patients Considered High Risk and Not Candidates for Standard Regimen	
Ampicillin, gentamicin, and amoxicillin	Intravenous or intramuscular administration of ampicillin, 2.0 g, plus gentamicin, 1.5 mg/kg (not to exceed 80 mg), 30 min before procedure; followed by amoxicillin, 1.5 g, orally 6 h after initial dose; alternatively, the parenteral regimen may be repeated 8 h after initial dose
Ampicillin/Amoxicillin/Penicillin-Allergic Patients Considered High Risk	
Vancomycin	Intravenous administration of 1.0 g over 1 h, starting 1 h before procedure; no repeated dose necessary

* Initial pediatric doses are as follows: ampicillin, 50 mg/kg; clindamycin, 10 mg/kg; gentamicin, 2.0 mg/kg; and vancomycin, 20 mg/kg. Follow-up doses should be one half the initial dose. **Total pediatric dose should not exceed total adult dose.** No initial dose is recommended in this table for amoxicillin (25 mg/kg is the follow-up dose).

alternative regimens for penicillin-allergic and low-risk patients are shown in Table 26-5. Gentamicin dosages may need to be adjusted in patients with renal insufficiency.

SUMMARY

Patients receive a variety of medications in the perioperative period. Knowledge of the pharmacology of anesthetic-induction agents, opioids, neuromuscular blockers, and their reversal agents will help the health care professional with perioperative patient care. This knowledge will smooth the patient's transition from the nursing unit to the operating room and the patient's return after postanesthesia recovery.

Table 26-5. Regimens for Genitourinary/Gastrointestinal Procedures*

DRUG	DOSING REGIMEN[†]
	Standard Regimen
Amoxicillin	3.0 g orally 1 h before procedure; then 1.5 g 6 h after initial dose
	Amoxicillin/Penicillin-Allergic Patients
Erythromycin	Erythromycin ethylsuccinate, 800 mg, or erythromycin stearate, 1.0 g, orally 2 h before procedure; then one-half the dose 6 h after initial dose
or	
Clindamycin	300 mg orally 1 h before procedure and 150 mg 6 h after initial dose

* Includes those with prosthetic heart valves and other high-risk patients.
† Initial pediatric doses are as follows: amoxicillin, 50 mg/kg; erythromycin ethylsuccinate or erythromycin stearate, 20 mg/kg; and clindamycin, 10 mg/kg. Follow-up doses should be one half the initial dose. **Total pediatric dose should not exceed total adult dose.** The following weight ranges may also be used for the initial pediatric dose of amoxicillin: <15 kg, 750 mg; 15 to 30 kg, 1500 mg; and >30 kg, 3000 mg (full adult dose).

Prophylactic antibiotics decrease the incidence of postoperative wound infection for many clean and clean-contaminated diagnostic and surgical procedures. Cefazolin is usually the antibiotic of choice in patients without a cephalosporin allergy. Empiric or therapeutic antibiotics are often used to treat suspected or confirmed infection in contaminated or dirty procedures. Endocarditis prophylaxis is recommended for patients with intermediate or high-risk cardiac lesions who undergo intermediate or high-risk diagnostic or surgical procedures. Antibiotic prophylaxis of endocarditis will hopefully reduce the postprocedural incidence of bacterial endocarditis.

BIBLIOGRAPHY

Bergquist D: Review of clinical trials of low molecular weight heparins, *Eur J Surg* 158:67–78, 1992.

Bergquist D, Lindblad B, Matzsch T: Low molecular weight heparin for thromboprophylaxis and epidural/spinal anesthesia: is there a risk? *Acta Anesthesiol Scand* 36:605–606, 1992.

Classen DC, et al: The timing of prophylactic administration of antibiotics and the risk of surgical-wound infection, *N Engl J Med* 326(5):281–285, 1992.

Dajani AS, et al: Prevention of bacterial endocarditis, *JAMA* 264(22):2919–2922, 1990.

Durack DT: Prevention of infective endocarditis, *N Engl J Med* 332(1)38–43, 1995.

Gilman AG, et al: *Goodman and Gilman's The pharmacological basis of therapeutics*, ed 8, New York, 1990, McGraw Hill.

Paradisi F, Corti G: Which prophylactic regimen for which surgical procedure? *Am J Surg* 164(suppl 45):2s–5s, 1992.

Rauck, Richard L: The anticoagulated patient, *Reg Anesth* 21(6S):51–56, 1996.

Sheridan RL, Tompkins RG, Burke JF: Prophylactic antibiotics and their role in the prevention of surgical wound infection, *Adv Surg* 27:43–58, 1994.

Stein PD, et al: Antithrombotic therapy in patients with mechanical and biologic prosthetic heart valves, *Chest* 108(suppl 4):371S–378S, 1995.

Stoelting RK: *Pharmacology and physiology in anesthetic practice,* ed 2, Philadelphia, 1991, JB Lippincott.

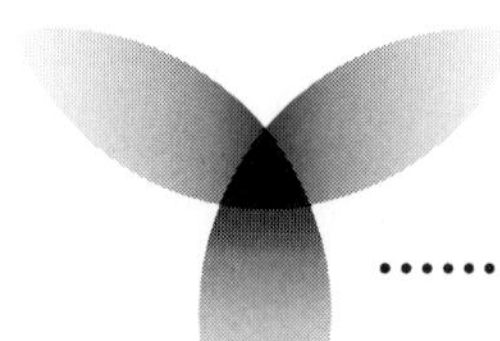

Chapter 27

Prevention of Venous Thromboembolism

Daniel M. Becker, MD, MPH

Deep venous thrombosis (DVT) and pulmonary embolism (PE), manifestations of a single entity, venous thromboembolism (VTE), are major complications of surgery and trauma. A variety of effective prophylactic agents are available, and surveyed surgeons agree that prophylaxis is indicated. Yet, most patients in acute care hospitals in the United States who are at significant risk for VTE do not receive proper preventive care. This chapter will review the risks and benefits of various prophylactic regimens and summarize how and when anticoagulant and mechanical devices can be used safely and effectively to reduce hospital morbidity and mortality.

Because there are widely available objective tests for the presence of acute VTE, a common and, to some extent, predictable postoperative event, studies of different prophylactic regimens have lent themselves to randomized and controlled methods. Thus, estimates of effectiveness generally rest on solid scientific evidence. Currently available and useful types of prophylaxis are listed in Table 27-1. In addition to agents that prevent clot formation through direct effects on clotting factors, several mechanical devices are available that either augment venous flow (graded elastic compression stockings, intermittent pneumatic compression boots) or interrupt flow to prevent embolization (vena cava filters). While various anticoagulant and mechanical methods have been shown to prevent DVT, the available studies are generally too small to demonstrate significant reductions in postoperative PE. Presumably, PE and PE death are prevented if DVT is prevented.

Several well-studied anticoagulants will not be discussed in any detail in this chapter. Aspirin would be an ideal prophylactic agent, if only it worked. While there

Table 27-1. Types of Prophylaxis

METHOD	DESCRIPTION
Warfarin—low dose	1–2 mg daily, no monitoring
low intensity	Dose varies, INR 2.0–3.0*
Low-dose unfractionated heparin	5000 U SC BID*, no monitoring
Adjusted dose unfractionated	5000 U or more BID or TID to keep APTT* high normal
Low-molecular weight heparin	Enoxaparin 30–60 mg SC BID
Dextran 40 or 70	10 ml/kg during surgery 7.5 ml/kg postoperatively 7.5 ml/kg days 3–5
Graded elastic compression stockings	Applied from surgery to ambulation
Intermittent pneumatic compression boots	Applied from surgery to ambulation
Inferior vena cava filters	Various types depending on thrombus and anatomy

*INR; international normalized ration; see text
SC; subcutaneous injection
BID, TID; 2 or 3 times daily-dose schedule
APTT; activated partial thromboplastin time

have been a few suggestive results, the bulk of clinical evidence is not convincing that aspirin or other antiplatelets agents prevent VTE. The combination of heparin and ergotamine, while effective, has vascular complications that led to its withdrawal from the American market. It is too early to comment on the clinical utility of products still in development, such as antithrombin III. Low-molecular-weight dextran, available in molecular weights of 40,000 or 70,000 (40 or 70), is an effective prophylactic agent. It has been used more often in Europe, but associated volume expansion and osmotic diuresis can lead to congestive heart failure and renal dysfunction. Dextran 40 or 70 may be useful for patients at particular risk for bleeding with anticoagulant prophylaxis.

Risk factors for VTE are listed in Box 27-1 Virchow's triad of delayed flow, abnormal clot formation, and vessel wall injury predicts these risks and characterizes the postoperative or posttraumatic state. Surgery and trauma tend to tip the dynamic plasma equilibrium between thrombosis and thrombolysis, towards thrombosis. Venous stasis is an unavoidable feature of the perioperative state. Vessel injury is common after surgery or trauma. Despite the obvious pathophysiologic predilection to VTE in these settings, the incidence rates in certain settings are astoundingly high. Table 27-2 lists estimates of postoperative and posttrauma DVT, and for some situations, thrombosis is the norm. These estimates vary considerably from study to study, depending on the end point used for assessing DVT and methods for patient enrollment. Age, comorbidity such as cancer or congestive heart failure, duration of surgery, type of anesthesia (general vs regional), and delayed ambulation all affect

Box 27-1 Risk Factors for Postoperative Deep Venous Thrombosis (DVT)

Delayed Flow
- Bed rest and postoperative stasis
- Congestive heart failure
- Venous insufficiency
- Prior venous thrombosis
- Proximal obstruction caused by injury or mass effect

Hypercoagulability
- Lupus anticoagulant
- Protein C deficiency
- Protein S deficiency
- Factor V resistance
- Antithrombin III resistance
- Dysfibrinoginemia
- Homocystinuria
- Paroxysmal nocturnal hemoglobinuria
- Inflammatory bowel disease
- Nephrotic syndrome
- Estrogen oral contraceptives
- Postoperative or posttrauma

Vessel Injury
- Trauma
- Surgery
- Vasculitis
- Prior deep venous thrombosis

the incidence rates and need to be considered when assessing an individual's risk for postoperative DVT.

Most postoperative VTE is asymptomatic and, hence, the need for a standardized approach to prophylaxis. Waiting for the symptomatic presentation of DVT or PE may be waiting too long. Most PE deaths occur in the first 30 minutes of symptoms, and this interval is too short for any intervention, however bold. Serial surveillance of high-risk patients is feasible but expensive, and some of the easily used tests, such as impedance plethysmography and duplex ultrasonography, lack sensitivity in the postoperative setting.

GENERAL, GYNECOLOGIC, AND UROLOGIC SURGERY

Patients undergoing general, gynecologic, and urologic procedures have comparable risks for postoperative DVT. Older patients undergoing extensive cancer surgery have a much higher chance of developing DVT, and decisions about prophylaxis should take this into account. Low-dose unfractionated heparin (LDUH) is generally effective and will reduce the incidence of postoperative DVT by more than 50%

Table 27-2 Incidence of Deep Venous Thrombosis

SETTING	INCIDENCE (%)
General surgery, age <40	10–20
General surgery, malignancy or age >40	20–40
Gynecologic surgery	10–20
Gynecologic surgery for malignancy	20–40
Urologic surgery	10–20
Urologic surgery for malignancy	20–40
Hip fracture	40–60
Total hip replacement	45–60
Total knee replacement	45–70
Intracranial neurosurgery	15–25
Acute spinal cord injury	40–70

following uncomplicated abdominal and pelvic surgery. Major cancer surgery requires more aggressive prophylaxis, and adjusted low-dose unfractionated heparin (ADUH), given in sufficient dosage dose to push the activated partial thromboplastin time (APTT) into the high-normal range is more effective than LDUH. However, monitoring the effect by means of the APTT is cumbersome, and low-molecular weight heparin (LMWH) is supplanting ADUH for these high-risk patients. In addition to reducing the rate of DVT compared to LDUH, LMWH appears to reduce bleeding complications, as well.

Low-molecular weight heparin is fractionated and consists of smaller heparin fragments which have more specific factor Xa effects. It can be used without monitoring and in a fixed dosage. Currently only enoxaparin is available in the United States, and it is expensive compared to unfractionated heparin. The cost is likely to fall as other fractionated heparins are marketed, and there are some laboratory savings with LMWH which need to be factored into cost considerations.

In addition to heparin in various guises, graded elastic compression stockings (ES) and intermittent pneumatic compression boots (IPCB) are effective in this population. For low-to-moderate risk patients, ESs reduce the risk of DVT by more than 50%. Higher-risk patients may not benefit, and, not infrequently, the stockings don't fit well enough to compress calf veins, the initial site of most postoperative DVT. Intermittent pneumatic compression boots have been shown to be as effective as LDUH in moderate and high-risk populations. If bleeding from heparin is a serious concern, IPCB should be considered. Both ES and IPCB need to be applied during the operation and worn until full ambulation. This is easier said then done, and their effectiveness is limited by unavoidable breaks in routine postoperative care. While there are relatively few studies assessing the additive benefits or ES and IPCB, or ES and/or IPCB with heparin, it is likely that different modalities used concurrently increase the benefit of either alone. Therefore, for example, it would be reasonable to use IPCB and LMWH for an elderly patient with a past history of postoperative DVT undergoing curative surgery for a gastrointestinal, urologic, or gynecologic malignancy.

ORTHOPEDIC SURGERY

Elderly patients undergoing major orthopedic surgery of the hip or knee represent a large population at high risk for postoperative DVT and PE. In addition to the high rates of DVT outlined in Table 27-2, the risk of PE in patients who do not receive effective prophylaxis is approximately 5%, and the case fatality rate for such events approaches 20%. Efforts to ambulate these patients early have helped to lower the rate of thromboembolic complications, but anticoagulant prophylaxis is indicated routinely for hip fractures, hip arthroplasty, and knee arthroplasty.

While LDUH will reduce the incidence of postoperative DVT in these patients, and perhaps even reduce the PE mortality rate, there are more effective anticoagulant regimens. Adjusted low-dose unfractionated heparin works but requires APTT monitoring and dose adjustment. Low-molecular weight heparin is approximately twice as effective as LDUH, reducing the risk by 70% after hip replacement and 50% after knee replacement.

Low-intensity warfarin is also effective. The goal with this warfarin regimen is to prolong the prothrombin time (PT) so that the international normalized ratio (INR) is 2.0 to 3.0. The INR adjusts the PT result by differences in thromboplastin sensitivity to deficiencies of vitamin-K-dependent clotting cofactors. Thromboplastin is used for the PT measurement, and the international sensitivity index (ISI) rates different commercially available thromboplastins with values ranging from 1.0, the most sensitive, to over 3.0, relatively insensitive. The formula for the INR is shown in the following, and most laboratories now report PT results by the INR, as well as the PT, in seconds.

$$\text{INR} = (\text{PT patient/PT control})^{\text{ISI}}$$

Low-intensity warfarin is as effective as LMWH after hip surgery but less effective after knee replacement. Unlike LMWH, warfarin requires laboratory monitoring and dose adjustment. The costs and nuisance of laboratory testing with warfarin add to the growing popularity of LMWH. The promise of less bleeding with LMWH has not been fulfilled, and clinically significant bleeding after orthopedic surgery occurs as often with LMWH as with low-intensity warfarin, in approximately 5% of patients.

Augmenting venous flow up the lower extremity by means of ES and IPCB, reduces postoperative DVT in the orthopedic patient population. After total hip replacement the DVT, risk is reduced approximately 25% by ES and 50% by IPCB.

The type of anesthesia also appears to make a difference. The risk of DVT after repair of hip fracture or hip replacement appears to be lower after spinal anesthesia compared to general anesthesia. However, for such patients spinal anesthesia alone is not considered effective prophylaxis, and low-intensity warfarin or LMWH should also be used.

Because the risk of postoperative DVT is so high in these settings, prophylactic vena-cava filter placement may have a role for patients at particularly high risk of bleeding from anticoagulants or developing DVT despite conventional anticoagulant prophylaxis. There are no clinical trials of prophylactic filter use, and use of these devices in this manner depends on the local experience with filters and a belief that no other means of preventing fatal PE is available.

NEUROSURGERY

Patients undergoing intracranial procedures and patients with acute spinal cord injuries are both at high risk for DVT. Most thrombi start in the calf veins and are asymptomatic. After spinal cord injury, the greatest risk is in the first few weeks, with clinical DVT or PE rare after 3 months. Thus, prophylaxis should be continued for at least 3 months.

There are limited data to guide decisions about prophylaxis in this patient population. In spinal-cord-injury patients treated with ADUH or LMWH, the risk of DVT is below 10%, a clinically significant benefit compared to untreated patients in whom the risk is consistently above 50%. Because such comparisons are indirect and not the result of large controlled rials, the benefits of ADUH and LMWH are presumptive. Combination therapy using ES, IPC, and LDUH also appears effective.

In studies of prophylaxis following intracranial surgery, IPC with or without ES appears effective, as if it were LDUH. The combination of IPC and LDUH may reduce the incidence of DVT even further. Central nervous system (CNS) bleeding from LDUH prophylaxis does not seem to be an issue.

Neurosurgery or spinal-cord-injury patients at unusually high risk for DVT may benefit from elective vena-cava filter placement. The same caveats for filter use, mentioned in the discussion of orthopedic patients, applies to neurosurgery patients.

TRAUMA

The incidence of DVT after major trauma is high, but in many instances such patients have injuries that pose contraindications to anticoagulant prophylaxis. Graded elastic compression stocking, with or without IPCB, are a reasonable starting point and likely to be effective. If the risk of pulmonary embolism is high and anticoagulants contraindicated, vena cava filters may be useful.

DECISIONS TO USE DVT PROPHYLAXIS

In most instances, the use of prophylactic agents or devices to prevent postoperative DVT is routine and part of standard, postoperative care. On occasion, the decision is complicated by unusual, associated conditions that increase the risk of thrombosis or bleeding from anticoagulants. The general recommendations in this chapter provide a starting point for selecting the right agent or device for a particular setting. Medical consultation may be necessary to insure that DVT risk is addressed in a safe and effective manner.

BIBLIOGRAPHY

Anderson FA, et al: Physician practices in the prevention of thromboembolism, *Ann Intern Med* 115:591–595, 1991.

Ballew KA, Philbrick JT, Becker DM: Vena cava filter devices, *Clin Chest Med* 16:295–305, 1995.

Clagett GP, et al: Prevention of venous thromboembolism, *Chest* 108 supplement:312s–334s, 1995.
Colditz GA, Tuden RI, Oster G: Rates of venous thrombosis after general surgery: combined results of randomized clinical trials, *Lancet* 19:143–146, 1986.
Green D, et al: Deep vein thrombosis in spinal cord injury-summary and recommendations, *Chest* 102 supplement:633s–635s, 1994.
Imperiale TF, Speroff T: A meta-analysis of methods to prevent venous thromboembolism following total hip replacement, *JAMA* 271:1780–1785, 1994.
Salzman EW, Hirsh J: Prevention of venous thromboembolism. In. Colman RW, et al, editors: *Hemostasis and thrombosis: basic principles and clinical practice,* ed 3, Philadelphia, 1994, JB Lippincott.

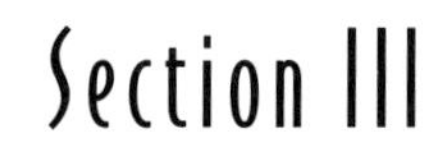

Section III

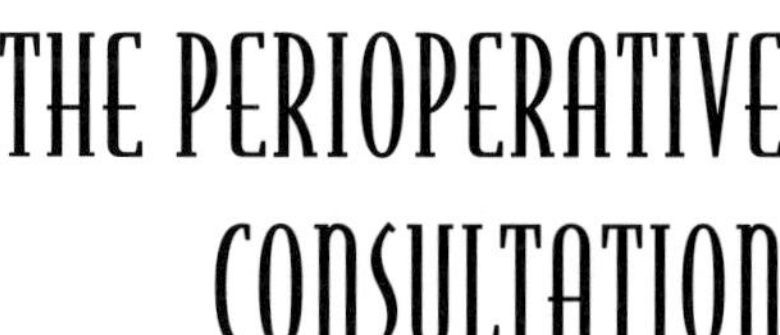

THE PERIOPERATIVE CONSULTATION

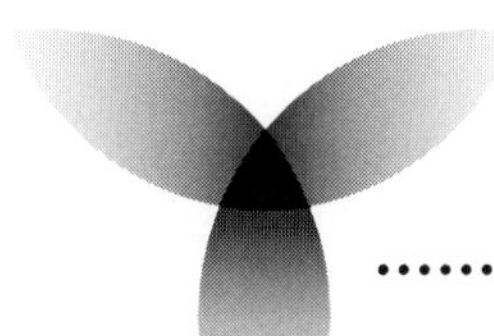

Chapter 28

An Approach to Perioperative Consultation

David J. Stone, MD

WHO? COURTESY AND COMMUNICATION
WHAT? MEDICAL CONSIDERATIONS IN THE PERIOPERATIVE PERIOD
WHEN? TIME AND TIMING
WHERE? ACCESSIBILITY AND ENVIRONMENT
HOW? RECOMMENDATIONS AND INTERVENTIONS

In journalism school, aspiring reporters are taught to seek out the who, what, when, and where of a story (personal communication, Debra Stone, M.S.J.). The perioperative consultant certainly needs to seek out and understand these elements of the "story," but the job does not end there. The consultant also contributes to the "how" of patient care, in that the recommendations and care provided by the consultant contribute to optimal care of the surgical patient in the perioperative period. The role of the consultant is to provide supplemental knowledge, judgment, and technical abilities to the care of patients when problems arise: problems requiring expertise not ordinarily possessed by the "primary care physicians" of the perioperative period, that is, the anesthesiologist and surgeon.

WHO? COURTESY AND COMMUNICATION

The first question those seeking a consultation should ask themselves is—who should be doing the consultation? Often, the surgeon and/or anesthesiologist request a consultation from a medical specialist. If there are several elements of medical care that need to be addressed, a general internist or family practitioner may provide the best consultative expertise. This may also be the case if the patient's problem cannot be easily assigned to a particular system. If the problem is clearly limited to the cardiovascular or endocrine systems, for example, medical subspecialists may be preferable, if available. In the academic medical center, one is often confined to consulting the attending physician who is "on-service," with a resultant wide variation in skills, experience, and interest in perioperative problems. In addition, students, house staff, and fellows may be expected to perform and complete these consultations before an attending physician is available. Few, if any, medical trainees, regardless of the quality of the training program, possess the expertise and experience to provide perioperative medical consultations on their own. If a consultation is being obtained as a mere formality, then the previous scenarios are acceptable. If a genuine opinion is required, it is best to seek out those individuals who can provide real help, regardless of who is actually "on-service." In private practice, those who have been shown to provide a timely, useful, and courteous service can (and will) be consulted repeatedly for this purpose.

In fact, the first element in perioperative consultation generally consists of the consultation to a surgeon from a medical practitioner, and regards the former's opinion on a potential surgical problem. This opinion includes the possible need for, type of, and urgency of surgical intervention. With experience, the medical practitioner tends to develop a favorite group of surgeons in varying surgical specialties. These will generally be individuals who can be trusted to provide an objective and thoughtful surgical opinion, rather than a sprint to the operating room schedule. The surgeon then proceeds to consult an anesthesiologist for perioperative management, including anesthesia. That interaction is not often considered a consultation, but in fact, requires an opinion based on consideration of the patient's medical status and the proposed surgery. The board certification process of the American Board of Anesthesiology has granted the status of "Consultant in Anesthesiology" to the physicians who meet the training and examination standards of that body. The considerable knowledge, experience, and skills of the anesthesiologist generally remain an underutilized resource in perioperative medicine. Anesthesiologists should also be directly available to primary care physicians for consultation on matters of perioperative care. It is important to remember "who" one is dealing with because physicians in any specialty may vary widely in knowledge, abilities, and experience. Be careful not to *in*sult, rather than *con*sult.

Another "who" element regards "who" is responsible for various aspects of care, particularly in the postoperative period. This issue is not simply a matter of medical "turf." It concerns the inadvertant neglect of some element of care. Both the medical consultant(s) and the anesthesiologist should pursue some element of postrecovery room care, even if this is only the briefest visit to the patient, accompanied by documentation in the chart. Before signing off the case, the consultant should make certain that his or her input is no longer required and that future coverage is available if the situation changes. It is especially important for medical consultants to suggest or establish routes of patient follow-up by the appropriate primary care and subspecialty physicians. This is particularly relevant because inadequate preoperative medical care often necessitates a perioperative consult in the first place.

The final element in the category of "who" involves who actually needs a consultation. Glibly put, this is what the first part of this book is about. In functional terms, it is any patient with whom the surgeon or anesthesiologist, or other involved physicians, feel uncomfortable without further opinion or investigation. Sometimes, there is a well-defined problem such as unstable chest pain, but at other times, there may only be a gut feeling that something is not quite "right" with a patient. As with appendectomies, it may be best to call for a few unneccesary consultations to ensure that needed consultations are obtained (see Chapter 47). In any case, there is no "standard of care" for consultative need. It is a matter of medical judgment that considers the patient's medical state, the expertise of the surgical team, the urgency of the planned procedure, and the quality and availability of consultative expertise.

WHAT? MEDICAL CONSIDERATION IN THE PERIOPERATIVE PERIOD

The specific details of medical care are covered throughout the various chapters of this book. This section addresses the more general principles involved. The first element is to establish what factors originally necessitated the consultation. While this procedure may seem trivial, it is one of the most frequent problems in perioperative consultation, and it comes from both sides of the consultation arena. It is vital for those seeking a consultation to clearly indicate the reason for it. A consultation asking a physician to "clear" the patient for anesthesia is not only uninformative, it is misguided because it is not the job of the consulting physician to do so. The job of the consultant is to identify what is wrong, how wrong it is, and what can be reasonably done about it in a perioperative context. While the four lines at the top of the consultation form may be adequate for purposes of communication, the whole process is usually facilitated by direct contact, either in person or by telephone. Electronic mail and telemedicine may prove to be important to this interaction in the near future. An effort should be made to provide available medical records to the consultant. Although it is often inconvenient to do so, the consultant should seek out those requesting the consultation if the tissues are not clear. While the consultant may go on to identify other issues of equal or even greater perceived importance, it is still critical and courteous to answer the original question. Courtesy and communication in the business of seeking and providing perioperative consultations cannot be overemphasized.

The perioperative consultation is unique, in that the physician may identify a number of issues, but only those relevant to the moment should be addressed preoperatively. These immediate issues must be evaluated in terms of what is to be done to the patient and the urgency of the procedure. For example, guiac positive stools should be worked-up before a lung lesion is resected but not before an open ankle fracture is repaired. The consultant should then make certain that the ball is not dropped on those issues that are delayed until the patient has recovered from surgery.

The exact nature of the written consultation may vary, depending on whether one is practicing in a teaching institution or not. Physicians should recognize that surgical communication is a bit more terse than that occurring during medical services. It is essential to make key points in a direct fashion, rather than bury them in a list of a dozen suggestions, some of which are much less important than others. The important new findings and suggestions should be clearly communicated at the beginning of the consultation form, with some designation of which are urgent, which are elective, and which are academic. Teaching is an important part of academic consultation, but crucial points should not be hidden by a slew of references and other demonstrations of great learning. Keep the consultation as simple as possible, within the requirements of completeness. Once again, direct communication is a great plus. If possible, use the chart to document, not to communicate. Certainly, the chart should not be used to communicate disagreements or criticisms. Always imagine that plaintiff's attorney reading the chart back to you 3 years later.

The consultation consists of what the consultant believes to be wrong, and what should be done about it. Tests and treatments are suggested, not ordered without discussion involving the surgeon or anesthesiologist. It is essential to ensure follow-up of all test results. It is reasonable to provide some estimate of risk, but a risk estimate alone does not constitute a consultation. In most cases, the patient is eventually going to have the operation, regardless of risk. The consultant is part of the team that is trying to reduce risk, not simply predict it. It is vital to determine whether surgery should be delayed because further tests or treatments will *actually reduce the risk of surgery*. At times, this conflicts with the need for urgent surgery and compromises must be made. Before committing one's opinion to the chart, a legal document, it may be best to first discuss matters with those requesting the consultation. This is not merely courteous. It may clarify some previously misunderstood issues, improve patient care, and reduce the risk of subsequent lawsuits.

WHEN? TIME AND TIMING

In the best of all possible worlds, patients are screened well before surgery, so that consultation can proceed at a leisurely pace in the week or two before a scheduled operation. When this scenario takes place, consultation can be delayed for the day or two that it takes to fit a patient into a busy schedule. Conversely, if the patient has traveled a great distance to arrive at the surgeon's office and subsequent preoperative screening clinic, the patient should be seen at that time, if at all possible. In today's competitive medical environment, it is best not to inconvenience patients who will return to their primary physicians with these tales. In addition, an immediate consultation allows for plenty of time to set up needed tests, additional consultations, discussions, and so forth.

Until the fairly recent advent of preoperative screening clinics, the usual preoperative consultation was requested on the evening before surgery. If possible, last minute consultations should be prevented. When preoperative consultations are called for 7 PM. The physician must determine whether the issues involved can be sorted out before a 7 AM start the next day. Sometimes, this matter can be solved by switching around the surgical schedule so that the patient's operation starts later in the day, after further tests are completed. While those requesting a "night-before-surgery" consultation can justifiably expect a response at this time, they cannot justifiably expect all the patient's medical problems to be solved before the next day's planned procedure. Cordial perioperative relations will be reinforced by a sincere attempt to avoid these last-minute consultations as well as by an attempt to do them as well as possible on the (hopefully, infrequent) occasions that they are required. Last minute consultation occur more often at the academic medical center, than at the community hospital because patients will arrive on the right before surgery with problems of which the surgical team was simply unaware. In addition, medical records may be unavailable or incomplete. The medical record problem may eventually be solved by intranetworks of clinics and hospitals maintaining updated patient records in a digitized form that is available to physicians with the proper security clearance. The successful completion of this institutional mission also requires full cooperation from laboratory, radiology, and medical records departments, as well.

Even more unfortunate and difficult are consultations that arise on the day of surgery in ambulatory surgery patients who are not hospitalized on the night before a planned procedure. The preoperative admission of patients, solely for the purpose of next-day surgery, is becoming more unusual. We have patients arrive on the day of surgery for thoracic, intracranial, and even coronary bypass surgery, at times. In theory, these patients have been screened at the aforementioned clinic for problems that need attention and might delay surgery. In fact, important problems sometimes slip through the cracks of any system. The efficiency of preoperative clinics has improved over time, and is likely to continue to do so as anesthesiologists involve themselves in this process as "perioperative physicians," who are well aware of the problems in the perioperative period. Consultations on the day of surgery are almost certain to cause some scheduling delays, particularly if the patient represents the first scheduled case of the day. It is essential to practice medicine in a responsible manner, and not cut corners simply to facilitate a busy surgical schedule. Sometimes, delays are a lesson to those involved, that they did less than a complete job in the process of evaluating the patient for surgery in the first place. Conversely, it is also essential to characterize problems as sufficiently minor so that surgery can proceed as planned, as long as postoperative attention is paid to the noted problems. These are not always easy decisions to make, because there has not been a practical textbook of perioperative medicine (until now). In fact, complex combinations of problems seem to arise in this time period which are difficult to predict and cannot be acutely solved with absolute certainty. This is probably the most important time for the consultant, anesthesiologist, and surgeon to get together and discuss the problems privately. While such a meeting is often difficult to accomplish, it is still the best way to sort out a stick issue on the day of surgery. Perhaps teleconferencing will facilitate this kind of interaction in the future.

• WHERE? ACCESSIBILITY AND ENVIRONMENT

The "where" of consultation generally involves a compromise between patient and consultant convenience. Preoperative screening clinics should have adequate examining rooms for consultants if they can find the time to visit the patient. The traditional location for perioperative consultation is the hospital room bedside, but a curtained-off area in a preoperative holding area may do as well, if necessary. Consultants should also be prepared to work in the recovery room or intensive care unit. It is courteous to introduce oneself to the charge nurse in these settings and ask if there are any special requirements in these units such as gowns or masks. In academic medical centers, a resident or fellow is often present on a full-time basis in these areas. It is worthwhile to speak to them, as well. Both of these socializing interactions will lead to a more satisfactory personal and medical experience for all involved. Actual consultation in the operating room is rare but might be required under special circumstances, especially in a small community hospital where back-up help for the anesthesia/surgery team is limited. In private practice, in a 90-bed community hospital, I was called from my office practice to the operating room on several occasions when my patients developed problems, which could not be solved by the operative team. Physicians who refer patients to surgery should feel free to put on scrubs and observe part or all of the patient's procedure. This is especially fitting if they were involved in special difficulties in preoperative management and are likely to be required for further postoperative help. The physician should not enter the operating area with an attitude of superiority because this space is the daily territory of the anesthesiologist and surgeon, who know their business. Those who enter with a respectful curiosity are obviously welcome if their presence was requested. Because things often need to be done quickly in the operating area, answers to questions may have to wait until th matter at hand is resolved. The surgeons or anesthesiologist's delayed response to a question may only represent concentration or concern, not rudeness. If special cultures of fluids or tissues are required, this may be the best way to ensure proper handling of specimens in unusual cases.

• HOW? RECOMMENDATIONS AND INTERVENTIONS

Many of the elements of "how" have been covered in the preceding sections. The consultant needs to perform an examination directed towards the problem discussed in the consultation. Yet the examination must be sufficiently broad enough to pick up details that may impact on overall perioperative or long-term care. Obviously, the consultant should not comment negatively on the care that the patient has received to date (whether at the current site or the referring hospital; praise, however, is always acceptable). The consultant should be careful in conversation to avoid statements, best discussed with the primary physicians before the patient is informed. The actual written consultation should be as brief and complete as possible, with the realization that the medical and surgical cultures have differing definitions of "brief." Direct communication, in person or by telephone, is optimal before pen is taken to chart. In the academic setting, the consulting service has the responsibility of ensuring that the patient is thoughtfully evaluated by an attending physician, even after students, residents, and fellows may have poked, prodded, and questioned the patient. It is crucial to keep feelings in mind even when stupid, careless, lazy, and uninformed care has been provided. No one likes to be told directly about these traits, but the information can be conveyed in a way that transmits the information without the pejorative connotation. Furthermore, don't tell everyone else in the vicinity (nurses, attendants, desk clerks) about what a fool Dr. X is, or what a horrible job the urology team has done in managing Joe's heart. Teaching should be done in the appropriate context, whether in an academic center or a private practice setting. Tests and further consultations should not be ordered without first discussing these matters with the referring physicians.

The consultation is just that—a recommendation, an opinion. It is not a command or a substitute for the authority of the physicians primarily responsible for the patient's care. On the other hand, it is the duty of those requesting the consultation to provide the consultant with the most complete information possible, to prepare the patient for the consultant's arrival, and to seriously consider the recommendations of the consultant, even when there are disagreements. It is also the duty of the physicians requesting the consultation to carefully consider the recommendations and then to follow them in whole, in part, or not at all, as they see fit.

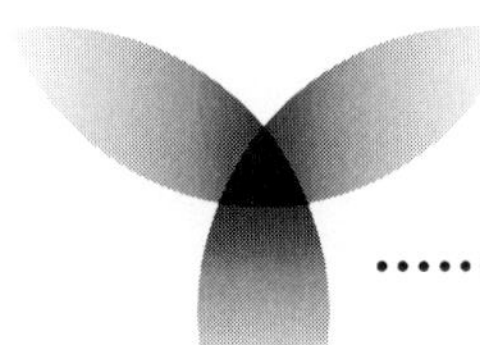

Chapter 29

Perioperative Consultation: The Viewpoint of the Internist

Daniel M. Becker, MD

THE ROLE OF THE GENERAL INTERNIST

General internists have much to contribute to patient management during the perioperative period. Several aspects of their training and clinical skill are particularly suited for perioperative care: emphasis on continuity between office practice and the hospital and, hence, availability to follow their patients through surgical illnesses; a general, yet deep, understanding of pathophysiology, which allows an integrated understanding of the clinical issues which arise both before and after surgery; experience in the role of coordinator, whether in the outpatient setting dealing with managed care, or in the hospital marshalling resources for critically ill patients; and finally, adherence to evidence-based practice, a means of clinical decision-making that takes costs, outcomes, and the quality of the available clinical evidence into account.

The important contributions of the internist are clearest when involved with their own patients in planning surgical treatment. With managed care, most patients will need a primary care physician's endorsement to proceed with surgery, and many adult patients have general internists as their primary care physicians. General internists are, thus, often involved from the beginning, both in the decision to operate and in the estimation of the risks and benefits of surgery. Their input reassures the surgeon that surgery is feasible for a particular patient and informs the anesthesiologist what specific problems may arise from induction of anesthesia through the next 48 hours of postsurgical care. The internist's presence is also reassuring to the patient who, otherwise, might not know any of the physicians involved in the operation.

What exactly should the internist do before surgery? First, assess the need for surgery and, thus, ensure that the decision to operate is validated early in the process. This assessment is based on an understanding of the underlying disease and therapeutic options. Second, assess the patient's specific risks for anesthesia and surgery. The demographic and clinical factors entering into this risk assessment are discussed later in this chapter. Third, consider the timing of surgery. Can it wait to allow medical interventions that might improve outcomes? Fourth, arrange for preoperative testing, a subject that will also be discussed further. Fifth, communicate with the surgeon and, in some instances, the anesthesiologist. While it is considered the standard of care for the referring physician and the surgeon to discuss the patient, this discussion does not routinely involve the anesthesiologist. However, for high-risk patients or patients particularly anxious about the operation, it is prudent to involve the anesthesiologist early in the planning process. Sixth, offer recommendations, both diagnostic and therapeutic, that will help guide perioperative management.

After the operation the internist continues to play an important role. Medical complications of surgery, whether routine or unexpected, frequently require internal medicine skills. Chronic problems, such as diabetes and hypertension, need to be managed perioperatively. As the patient recovers, the primary care physician, often the internist, should be available to reassure the patient and family, assist the patient in a return to normal function, reassess medication needs, complete the evaluation of any new or lingering medical problems, assess the need for rehabilitation, and arrange appropriate follow-up.

PREOPERATIVE RISK ASSESSMENT

General issues

In general, the risk of surgery escalates with age, the duration of the procedure, intraoperative blood loss, poor nutritional status, and preexisting disease that predisposes the patient to cardiac, pulmonary, renal, neurologic, nutritional, and psychiatric complications. Detailed organ and procedure-specific discussions of preoperative risk are presented elsewhere in this book.

The general internist helps to prepare the patient for surgery. It is up to the surgeon and anesthesiologist to decide what is best for the patient in the operating room. This management is influenced by the medical assessment. The internist needs to point out existing disease and fine tune chronic and acute medical problems, sometimes with constraints on time, until the time of surgery.

The process of risk assessment is not precise, and it is not possible in absolute terms to "clear" a patient for surgery. It is possible, however, to identify patients at increased risk for certain complications and, at times, reduce this risk through perioperative management. While this paradigm of risk identification and intervention is sensible, its efficacy has not been demonstrated in controlled clinical trials for any particular patient group or type of complication.

Mortality after surgery is associated with increasing age and impaired physical status, as assessed by the American Society of Anesthesiology (ASA) Physical Status Measure (Box 29-1). Average across all procedures, the young (less than 35 years old) and healthy (ASA physical status 1 or 2) are at low risk, with postoperative mortality well below 1.0%; whereas the elderly (more than 65 years old) and infirm (ASA 4 or 5) have an estimated postoperative mortality rate of up to 30%. The risk increases substantially for emergency procedures, compared to elective surgery. Across all ages, the risk of surgery is relatively flat at higher ASA scores, demonstrating that comorbid factors other than age are the relevant determinants of risk. Looking at age alone as a risk factor, those over 65 years undergoing major vascular, thoracic, or abdominal surgery face a 5% to 10% postoperative mortality rate. It is hard to decipher mortality estimates generally derived from case series which reflect selection biases, and it is likely that estimates from the literature overstate the current risk of surgery. Because the average 65 year old has a 16-year life expectancy with 9.5 years of functional independence, the risk of surgery that might extend or improve life is generally worth taking.

Cardiac Considerations

PREDICTING CARDIAC COMPLICATIONS

Common postoperative medical complications include myocardial infarction (MI), congestive heart failure (CHF), cardiac arrhythmias, pneumonia, venous thromboembolism, delirium, electrolyte imbalance, and renal failure. These occur as a function of preoperative status, type of surgery, and circumstances of surgery (elective vs emergent). Other chapters in this book deal with these specific topics, but for several reasons, cardiac risk assessment deserves further mention here. First, cardiac

Box 29-1 American Society of Anesthesiology Physical Status Scale

Class 1—No physiologic, biochemical, or psychiatric disturbance. Surgery unlikely to lead to clinically significant systemic illness.

Class 2—Mild-to-moderate systemic problems related either to the underlying surgical illness or associated pathophysiologic processes.

Class 3—Relatively severe systemic disturbance, related to surgical illness or underlying medical problems.

Class 4—Severe and life-threatening systemic disturbance, not necessarily correctable by surgery.

Class 5—Moribund patient undergoing surgery as a desperate life-saving effort.

If the surgery occurs in emergent circumstances, the suffix “E” is included in the numerical classification and physical status is presumably slightly worse.

complications are the most common cause of postoperative death, and the possibility of cardiac disease must be considered for any patient facing surgery. Second, validated cardiac-risk indices are available and demonstrate how quantitative clinical reasoning can help physicians "play the odds" and win. Third, hypertension is a common finding in patients facing surgery, and its contribution to postoperative morbidity and mortality, as well as its management, are commonly part of the general internist's consultative task. Fourth, the process of identifying adult patients at high risk of cardiac complications usually begins with the internist.

Patients with known cardiac problems who undergo surgery are at increased risk for postoperative MI, CHF, and death. Attaching a number to this risk is difficult, because definitions of cardiac disease vary from study to study, but there is, at least, a three-fold increased risk for cardiac complications after surgery for patients with known cardiac disease. Goldman et al. (see references at end of the chapter) quantified the contributions of various cardiac and noncardiac conditions to the probability of life-threatening and fatal postoperative cardiac complications. The oft-quoted Goldman criteria for cardiac risk are shown in Tables 29-1 and 29-2. In the original study, patients with more than 13 points had at least a 13% chance of life-threatening or fatal postoperative cardiac event. The independent risk factors identified in Goldman's study were not surprising, but other common cardiac problems, such as angina or history of CHF were conspicuously absent. Other studies have shown that recent MI (within 6 months), unstable angina, or any history of CHF increase the possibility of severe, postoperative cardiac complications. Predictions using the Goldman criteria, or for that matter, any prognostic index, should be considered estimates of risk, rather than precise measures. The predictive value of any statistical model will vary with the underlying risk of the patient or population to which it is applied. The Goldman criteria, as well as other cardiac findings from the history or physical examination, are best noted and remarked on by the internist who has an integrative role in assessing cardiac, as well as other risk factors. Combining the Goldman criteria with the ASA classification provides a sensitive means of identifying patients at high risk of poor outcome, cardiac or otherwise.

It should be pointed out that risk estimates derived from published prognostic indices are unlikely to be as precise in day-to-day practice as in their original cohorts. The estimate of risk is only the beginning of perioperative management, which should then proceed to identify exactly what is wrong, and what can then be done to reduce perioperative cardiac and medical complications.

Perioperative management must take coronary artery disease into account. Details of preoperative testing and perioperative management of patients with known or suspected coronary artery disease are discussed elsewhere by Drs. Stone and Dent. Recent MI raises the risk of perioperative reinfarction, and is an important consideration when assessing a patient with coronary disease. The more recent the infarction, the greater the risk of reinfarction during or soon after surgery. The perioperative reinfarction rate within 6 months of a previous MI is probably less than 10% and overall mortality after surgery less than 15%. The mortality for perioperative reinfarction during this 6 months convalescent phase is high, perhaps 50%. These estimates of the reinfarction rate used to be higher, and it is possible that preoperative

Table 29-1. Cardiac Risk Assessment

RISK FACTOR	RELATIVE POINTS
Age >70	5
MI within 6 months	10
S3 gallup	11
Significant aortic stenosis	3
Arrhythmia or PACs on EKG	7
>5 PVCs/minute on EKG	7
Any of the following:	3
pO_2 <60 or pCO_2 >50	
k <3.0, HCO_3 <20	
BUN >50, Cr >3.0	
Chronic liver disease	
AST (SGOT) increased	
Bedridden for noncardiac cause	
Intraperitoneal, thoracic, or aortic surgery	3
Emergency surgery	4
	Total 53

identification of high-risk patients allows more intensive hemodynamic monitoring, which then reduces perioperative ischemia. The risk of reinfarction and fatal cardiac complications drops sharply beyond 6 months, and until recently, it has been thought to be worth waiting this long to schedule surgery after MI. However, the current ability of cardiologists to stratify postinfarction risk allows earlier surgery in selected patients who have undergone appropriate study.

HYPERTENSION

Because approximately 10% of the adult population has hypertension, the general internist is frequently consulted to recommend treatment for elevated blood pressure before surgery and control of hypertension perioperatively. Fortunately, for the millions of patients with borderline, mild, and moderate hypertension (all with diastolic pressure less than 110 mm Hg), there is little evidence that slightly elevated preoperative blood pressure increases the risk of postoperative complications. Poorly controlled hypertensive patients have greater, relative intraoperative drops and postoperative elevations in their blood pressure, reflecting the autoregulation defect characteristic of hypertension. The clinical consequences of the exaggerated response to anesthetic induction and recovery are uncertain.

For patients with diastolic pressures greater than 110 mm Hg, expert opinion suggests a greater risk of myocardial ischemia associated with intraoperative hypotension and postoperative hypertension. However, it is not clear that MI, CHF, or stroke after surgery are more common in this group of patients. It is important to consider the end-organ consequences of hypertension and to manage expectantly hypertensive cardiovascular disease, cerebrovascular disease, and renal disease.

Table 29-2. Prognosis Based on Cardiac Risk Assessment

POINT TOTAL	CARDIAC COMPLICATION	CARDIAC DEATH
0–5	0.7%	0.2%
6–12	5.0%	2.0%
13–25	11.0%	2.0%
>26	22.0%	56.0%

From Goldman L, et al: Multifactorial index of cardiac risk in non-cardiac surgical procedures, *N Engl J Med* 297:845, 1977.

Hypertensive medications should generally be continued throughout the perioperative period. If sympatholytic medications, especially β-blockers and clonidine, are discontinued abruptly just before surgery, rebound hypertensive crises can occur. This phenomenon is dose-dependent and occurs at moderate and high-dose ranges. Parenteral formulations of β-blockers and transdermal formulations of clonidine are available.

• EVALUATION OF THE HEALTHY PATIENT BEFORE SURGERY

Routine Testing Before Surgery

PRINCIPLES OF TESTING

Box 29-2 presents a paradigm for test interpretation, comparing results of a test to actual presence of disease as determined by a "gold" or criterion standard of diagnosis. Note that a sensitive test is positive in the presence of disease, and a specific test is negative in the absence of disease. Rarely is any test 100% sensitive or specific, and, thus, we have to consider whether a positive result is a true or false-positive and a negative result is a true or false-negative. Applying a test result to the patient who was tested relies on the concept of predictive value. Sensitivity and specificity refer to the proportion of diseased or normal subjects with positive or negative results. Predictive value refers to the proportion of test positive or negative subjects who are diseased or normal. As shown in Box 29-2, the denominator used for positive or negative predictive value calculations, that is, the numbers of test positive or negative subjects, varies with the prevalence of disease in the population or the pretest probability of disease for the individual patient.

EXAMPLES OF PREOPERATIVE TESTING

Examples of some common preoperative tests illustrate the limitations of screening tests for asymptomatic patients facing surgery. Box 29-3 shows what happens when the limitations of chest radiograph interpretation are combined with preoperative screening. Chest radiographs are often ordered before surgery. Their interpretation varies with the observer, and, thus, their sensitivity and specificity are well below 100% for most common cardiopulmonary conditions.

Box 29-2 Operating Characteristics of Tests

CRITERION STANDARD FOR DIAGNOSIS

Test Result		Positive	Negative
	Positive	A	B
	Negative	C	D

A = true-positive; B = false-positive;
C = false-negative; D = true-negative.
Sensitivity = A/A+C, positive in disease
Specificity = D/B+D, negative when disease absent
Positive-Predictive Value = A/A+B among patients with positive tests, proportion with disease
Negative-Predictive Value = D/C+D among patients with negative tests, proportion without disease

Assuming relatively high sensitivity and specificity, as for the radiographic diagnoses of chronic obstructive pulmonary disease (COPD), in a low-prevalence population or for an individual unlikely to have COPD, the positive-predictive value of a positive radiograph (what proportion of patients in this population with this reading actually have COPD?) is low. Even when there are unexpected positive findings on a preoperative chest radiograph, these results rarely affect operative management. With the exception of intrathoracic procedures, or for patients with known cardiopulmonary disease, routine preoperative chest radiographs contribute little to patient management.

Preoperative clotting studies, activated partial thromboplastin time (APTT) and prothrombin time (PT) may also be routinely ordered in an effort to identify patients at increased risk for perioperative bleeding complications. However, the PT adds little to the APTT in terms of screening for clotting factor deficiency (factor VII deficiency, a rare disorder, might be detected by PT and not APTT), and the APTT is neither sensitive nor specific as a test for perioperative bleeding. Inordinate bleeding in this setting is usually not caused by coagulation defects. In a low-risk population, the positive-predictive value of a prolonged APTT is less than 10%. Generally, the history (abnormal bleeding after prior operations, dental surgery, or menstruation; liver disease; poor nutrition) and the examination (petechiae, stigmata of liver failure, ecchymoses) can accurately identify patients at risk for bleeding complications.

In contrast to the examples cited previously, the preoperative electrocardiogram (ECG) is generally more useful. The incidence of abnormal findings increases steadily with aging. Silent MI is common, accounts for more than 25% of all infarcts, and can be detected by routine ECG. However, even for older men who are at particular risk for silent infarction, the 6-month incidence of clinically inevident ECG-only infarction is less than 0.5%; thus, repeating the ECG over a short interval, simply for preoperative reassurance, is not justified.

Box 29-3 Low Positive-Predictive Value for Preoperative Chest X-Ray

Assume low prevalence of asymptomatic chronic obstructive lung disease (COPD) in the patient population to be screened—5%

Assume relative high sensitivity and specificity for interpretation of COPD on chest radiograph: 90% and 90%

		COPD	
		Positive	Negative
Test Result	Positive	A	B
	Negative	C	D

Positive-predictive value = 45/90 = 50%

Negative-predictive value = 855/860 = 99%

Only one-half of the patients with "COPD" on chest radiograph actually have COPD.

In addition to its utility in identifying silent infarction, ECGs serve also to document sinus rhythm (nonsinus rhythm and premature beats are risk factors on the Goldman cardiac index), identify cardiac end-organ damage from systemic diseases, monitor cardiac effects and toxicity from various medications, and establish a baseline for patients at risk for perioperative ischemia.

Most hospitals recommend routine, preoperative ECGs for men over age 40 and women over age 50. The ages for these recommendations vary somewhat. While this recommendation is sensible for the reasons listed earlier, it will also lead to increased testing and monitoring for clinically unimportant ECG findings. The full cost implications of ECG screenings are not known.

In addition to the examples discussed previously, other screening tests sometimes ordered routinely are complete blood count (CBC), chemistry panel, urinalysis, syphilis serology, pregnancy testing, pulmonary function tests including arterial blood gas analysis, and human immunodeficiency virus (HIV) serology. Aside from the CBC, renal function indices, and basic electrolytes, the clinical utility of these tests is hard to justify, except on a case-by-case basis. Routine HIV screening is ethically and epidemiologically questionable, especially when current occupational health standards mandate universal precautions.

Despite the high costs and limited clinical utility associated with routine preoperative testing, the practice of ordering multiple tests before surgery persists. Whether this is simply defensive medicine, a convenient time for gaining laboratory reassurance, or habit is not clear.

History and Physical Examination

The initial "test" in assessing the risks and benefits of a procedure and then planning postoperative care, involves the history and physical examination performed by the primary care physician or internist consultant. Generally, this evaluation will identify patients at increased risk for anesthesia and surgery, as well as those likely to have abnormal and clinically meaningful screening laboratory results. These evaluations may serve the patient and physician in other ways by creating an opportunity to: (1) review old and current problems and medications; (2) obtain routine tests that serve the dual purposes of preoperative screening and monitoring of chronic conditions or medication side effects; (3) confirm the need for surgery and clarify for the patient and family what the experience will be like; and (4) identify specific concerns of the patient and family that may need to be reviewed by the anesthesiologist or surgeon.

The physicians performing these preoperative evaluations are obliged to provide recommendations in a timely and organized manner. Personal communication, in addition to a written report, is necessary to convey concerns that are likely to change management, either surgical, anesthetic, or postoperative.

BIBLIOGRAPHY

Buxbaum JL, Schwartz AJ: Perianesthetic considerations for the elderly patient, *Surg Clin North Am* 74:41–58, 1994.

Djokovic JL, Hedley-White J: Prediction of outcome of surgery and anesthesia in patients over 80, *JAMA* 242:2301–2306, 1979.

Goldman L, Caldera DL: Risks of general anesthesia and elective operation in the hypertensive patient, *Anesthesiology* 50:285–292, 1979.

Goldman L, et al: Multifactorial index of cardiac risk in non-cardiac surgical procedures, *N Engl J Med* 297:845–850, 1977.

Kaplan EB, et al: The usefulness of preoperative laboratory screening, *JAMA* 253:3576–3581, 1985.

Mangano DT, Goldman L: Preoperative assessment of patients with known or suspected coronary disease, *N Engl J Med* 333:1750–1756, 1995.

Prys-Roberts C: Hypertension and anesthesia—fifty years on. *Anesthesiology* 50:281–282, 1979.

Ziffren SE: Comparison of mortality rates for various surgical operations according to age groups, 1951–1977, *J Am Geriatr Soc* 27:433–438, 1979.

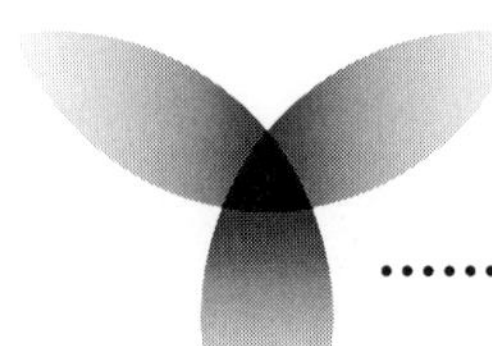

Chapter 30

Preoperative Evaluation Clinic and Preoperative Screening Tests

Donald D. Mathes, MD

PREOPERATIVE EVALUATION CLINIC

The preoperative evaluation clinic has been in a state of evolution over the past 10 years. In the late 1980s and early 1990s, many surgeons, anesthesiologists, and hospital administrators questioned the need for having a preoperative evaluation clinic. They saw the preoperative clinic as an unnecessary inconvenience for the surgical patient, an additional cost for the hospital to provide a facility and support staff, and a burden to the anesthesiology staff to provide personnel for the clinic. Clearly, their concerns have been proved wrong. The preoperative evaluation clinic is now playing a vital part in the perioperative management of the surgical patient.

Advantages of the Preoperative Evaluation Clinic

Today, at most institutions, 70% to 80% of surgical patients are arriving the day of surgery. Insurance companies or managed care groups will no longer pay for patients to be admitted the day before surgery. Furthermore, patients with complex medical problems are now arriving the day of surgery. This group includes patients scheduled for major open heart or vascular surgery.

The preoperative evaluation clinic allows appropriate evaluation of these complex medical patients in an unhurried manner. The clinic also allows the perioperative physician to obtain appropriate medical consults or risk stratification tests in advance, without delaying or cancelling surgery.

The preoperative evaluation clinic has reduced the turnover time between surgical patients, allowing the operating room to be used efficiently with fewer staff. No longer does the anesthesiologist need to do a history and physical on the patient immediately before surgery or answer multiple questions from an anxious patient. Before surgery, the anesthesiologist already knows the patient history and physical status, as well as the results of any consultations or laboratory work performed. Fischer found an 87.9% decrease in day-of-surgery cancellations in the year after starting a preoperative evaluation clinic.

Another clear advantage of the preoperative evaluation clinic is the dramatic reduction in unnecessary laboratory work and the assurance that appropriate laboratory work has been completed. Before the development of the preoperative clinic, many surgeons ordered excessive laboratory tests to try to foresee any concerns the anesthesiologist might have that would delay surgery. Not only did the excessive laboratory work increase costs, it often led to further inappropriate investigation for false-positive laboratory abnormalities. At Stanford University, the number of preoperative laboratory tests performed decreased 55.1% after the formation of a preoperative evaluation clinic.

Lastly, the preoperative clinic reduces the anxiety level of the patient. The value of reducing patient anxiety level with advanced preoperative evaluation is clearly established. Furthermore, patient education is improved greatly on such issues as what medications to take before surgery and when not to eat or drink before surgery. The patient's preoperative education leads to further reduction in delays or cancellation of surgery.

Hence, the establishment of a preoperative evaluation clinic is justified for multiple reasons. The clinic allows more efficient use of expensive operating room time, reduction in laboratory tests, appropriate medical consultation without cancellation or delay of surgery, decreased patient anxiety, improved patient education, and patient satisfaction with anesthesia care. Furthermore, in a managed-care environment, the hospital and managed-care group can justify the expense of staffing a preoperative clinic by total reduction in costs from improved efficiency of the operating room and a decrease in laboratory work expenses. At our institution, we have justified being reimbursed from the insurance company for patients' visits to our preoperative evaluation clinic by showing the overall cost saving to the patient and insurance company.

Infrastructure of the Preoperative Evaluation Clinic

For most preoperative evaluation clinics, the number of patients seen per day has greatly increased over the past 5 years. Furthermore, the patients evaluated in the preoperative clinic have continued to have both more complex medical problems and to be undergoing more major surgeries. The preoperative clinic has had to evolve to have multiple support personnel, to allow maximal efficiency for the anesthesiologist to spend time directly evaluating patients.

The Wake Forest University Preoperative Evaluation Clinic represents a good model of the evolution of the preoperative evaluation clinic and will be used as a model in this chapter. Each preoperative evaluation structure will vary, depending on how many patients are seen per day and the complexity of the patients. At Wake Forest University Preoperative Evaluation Clinic, an average of 40 to 70 patients are seen per day. The clinic has one to two nursing aides to take vital signs, direct patients into their rooms, and obtain medical records. One to two receptionists work to register and schedule appointments and to obtain faxed copies of key medical records such as prior electrocardiogram (ECG) or lab work from other hospitals and physicians. Two to three nurses work to further educate patients about fasting and medication instructions and where to arrive for surgery. Both a phlebotomist and ECG technician are available in the clinic for laboratory and ECG work. In a smaller clinic, both ECG and blood work can be done by nursing staff. Lastly, physician assistants or nurse practitioners can be used to assist the anesthesiologist in obtaining a history and physical before evaluating the patient. This infrastructure allows the clinic to run in an efficient manner for the anesthesiologist.

Preoperative Evaluation Flow Pattern

At Wake Forest University, the following flow pattern of patient care has been developed to maximize both direct patient contact and efficiency for the anesthesiology staff. This subsection is written in hopes of helping other practice groups to improve or set up their own preoperative evaluation clinics.

Initially, before the clinic opens, all the scheduled patients' old charts are reviewed, documenting prior anesthetics, medical problems, and important tests such as cardiac catheterization or recent laboratory work. Also, all ECGs and labs from the day before are reviewed. Upon arrival, the patient fills out an anesthesia questionnaire (Figure 30-1). Upon completion of the questionnaire, the patient's vital signs and weight are obtained. Any patient undergoing cardiac or vascular surgeries has blood pressure readings taken in both arms. The patient is then directed into an examining room.

While waiting for an anesthesiologist, the patient watches a video containing general information on anesthesia, including such issues as fasting status and risks of anesthesia. The video has reduced the number of questions asked by patients to the anesthesiologist and has given the patients a better sense of satisfaction and understanding about their upcoming anesthetics.

The anesthesiologist then goes over the questionnaire sheet with the patient addressing further any positive finding. Also, the old chart review sheet is incorporated into the questionnaire. The physical examination is performed, focusing on airway, lungs, heart, and other pertinent parts of the physical examination such as documentation of a neuropathy.

At the end of the examination, the anesthesiologist discusses the type of anesthesia and postoperative pain control options available, along with risks of anesthesia.

**THE NORTH CAROLINA
BAPTIST HOSPITALS, INCORPORATED
OUTPATIENT AND SAME-DAY ANESTHESIA QUESTIONNAIRE**

FOR PATIENT TO COMPLETE:
Name of Person Completing Form: ____________________
Relationship to Patient if not Patient: ____________________
Patient's Telephone Number: ____________________

Family Physician: ____________________
City: ____________________
Phone Number: ____________________

List Your Medicines: (Include eye drops, birth control pills, aspirin-like medicine and patches) ____________________

List any allergy to food, medicine or latex: ____________________

If you presently have, or have had any of the following medical conditions, please check "yes" in the appropriate space. Check "no" for negative answers. Circle all that apply.

	Yes	No
Heart Surgery/Treadmill/Cardiac Cath		
Heart Murmur		
Mitral Valve Prolapse/ECHO Diagnosis		
Skipped Heartbeat - Palpitations		
Angina (Chest Pain)		
Heart Attack		
Heart Failure		
High Blood Pressure		
Low Blood Pressure		
Stroke - TIA		
Pacemaker/Battery Checkdate:		
Born with Heart Disease		
Blood Clots or Phlebitis		
Rheumatic Fever		
Recent Cold/Cough/Flu/Fever		
Asthma		
Pneumonia within past 6 months		
Bronchitis within past month		
Emphysema/Shortness of Breath		
Use Tobacco Products/Smoke/Chew/Dip		
Tuberculosis/Brown Lung		
Born with Lung Disease		
Sinus Problems		
Kidney Stones		
Kidney Failure/Dialysis		
Bladder/Kidney Infections		
Brain/Spine/Nerve Disease		
Back Pain or Back Surgery		
Seizures or Epilepsy or Convulsions		
Depression/Panic Attack/Anxiety		
Headaches: Tension/Migraine		
Head Injury/Concussion		

Nurse Only
Age ________ WT. ________ HT. ________
BP ________ HR ________

Exposure to Communicable Disease within the last 21 days? Yes ☐ No ☐

Doctor Comments Only
H&P Present: Yes No
Old Chart Present? Yes No
Surgery ____________________
Surgeon ____________________
Operating Room: OPS SDS Date ________
Allergy comment: ____________________
Medication comment: ____________________

Continued on back: Please complete other side

	Yes	No
Hepatitis (Yellow Jaundice)		
Recent Vomiting or Diarrhea		
Hiatal Hernia/Ulcers/Heartburn		
Reflux (Choke in sleep)		
Diabetes: Usual Glucose Readings ( )		
Thyroid Problem or Goiter		
Steroid Use (Cortisone, Prednisone)		
Alcohol Use - How much per day/week		
Non-Prescribed Drug Use Dependence-DeTox		
Women: Could you be pregnant, or have you missed a recent menstrual cycle?		
Loose Teeth/Dentures/Crowns		
Dental Caps/Bridgework/Chipped Teeth		
Contact Lenses/Glasses		
Hearing Problems		
Glaucoma		
Blood or Sickle Cell Disease		
Easy Bleeding		
Chemo or Radiation Therapy		
Anemia/Low Iron		
Rheumatoid or Osteo Arthritis		
Blood Transfusion		
Muscle Weakness		
Low Blood Sugar		
Donated Blood for your surgery?		
Cancer Diagnosed		
Have you ever had surgery?		
Hospitalized for reasons other than surgery?		
Have you or a close relative had problems with anesthesia?		
Malignant Hyperthermia		
FOR PARENTS OF CHILDREN TO FILL IN:		
Premature Delivery		
Problems in Nursery		
Breath-Holding (Apnea)		
Crib or Sudden Infant Death in family		
Problems "Keeping up" physically		
Developmental Delay		
Croup/Frequent Bronchitis		
Child's Preferred or Nickname:		

DOCTOR ONLY

Physical Exam

Airway: Class 1 2 3 4

Neck: From/Limited

Heart: Rhythm: Regular Irregular

Extra Sounds

Lungs: Normal Sounds

Rhonchi Wheezing

Rales

Prolonged Expiratory Time

Carotid Bruits R L

ASA Class
1 2 3 4 5 E

Other Findings

Date

Signature M.D.

Signature P.A.

Attending Anesthesiologist

Figure 30-1
The patient fills out an anesthesia questionnaire like this upon arrival at the preoperative evaluation clinic.

The patient's preference for the type of anesthetic is documented, and the anesthesia consent form is signed (Figure 30-2). Instructions on fasting status and what medication to take the day of surgery are then discussed by the anesthesiologist. The anesthesiologist then orders any laboratory work. The 12-lead ECG is done in the examination room by an ECG technician. All laboratory work is obtained in a central location in the preoperative clinic by a phlebotomist. Finally, nurses review with the patients all anesthesia instructions including fasting status, what medication to take the morning of surgery, time of arrival, and where to arrive the day of surgery before discharging the patient. The total average time of a patient's visit is 40 to 60 minutes (Figure 30-3).

PREOPERATIVE SCREENING TESTS

The goal of preoperative tests is to detect abnormalities that may change anesthetic management and improve the perioperative outcome of the patient. The second goal of preoperative tests is to be cost-efficient by decreasing perioperative morbidity and medical costs. A third controversial goal of preoperative tests is to screen for general medical problems that may have significance in improving long-term health care, but have no bearing on perioperative care. This last goal should be determined by the philosophy of each anesthesia group and should be based on the patient-population group seen and quality of general medical care. At Wake Forest Medical Center, our department philosophy is not to actively do general medical screening unless the patient's history and physical examination reveals a potential problem. Instead, we focus on laboratory tests which have a direct bearing on the perioperative period only.

Many authors have concluded that indiscriminate preoperative laboratory screening is ineffective and an unnecessary additional expense to the medical system. Furthermore, indiscriminate preoperative screening can do more harm secondary to further evaluation of false-positive tests and lead to unnecessary delays in surgery.

Multiple studies on routine preoperative screening have found 1% to 2% of tests to be significantly abnormal. There is little evidence, however, that these abnormalities have any effect on anesthetic or surgical management. Furthermore, it is unclear if these abnormal findings improved actual patient perioperative or long-term outcome. It is hard to justify the cost of preoperative labs when even the abnormalities that are found are likely to have no bearing on anesthetic or surgical management or overall outcome. In preoperative tests obtained, but not indicated by history or physical examination, Kaplan et al. found only 0.22% of the actual abnormalities might have influenced perioperative management. In addition, of the 0.22% of abnormalities potentially influencing perioperative care, none was acted upon, and actual anesthetic and surgical management remained unchanged (Figure 30-4). Turnbull and Buck found only 4 of 5003 preoperative screening tests in healthy patients could have benefited the perioperative patient.

Although indiscriminate preoperative laboratory screening is clearly not indicated, the perioperative physician must be careful not to become nihilistic and not obtain preoperative screening tests, which, in fact, may improve perioperative management

NORTH CAROLINA BAPTIST HOSPITAL
WINSTON-SALEM, NORTH CAROLINA

ANESTHESIA CONSENT FORM

I understand that in addition to the risks of surgery, anesthesia carries its own risks, but I request the use of anesthetics for my own protection and pain relief. I realize that the type and form of anesthesia may have to be changed before or during surgery, possibly without explanation to me. Such changes would be made for my protection and benefit.

A doctor from the Anesthesia Department has explained to me that there may be complications resulting from the use of any anesthetic, and I understand that these complications may include AMONG OTHERS the following:

1. Nausea and vomiting
2. Headache
3. Back pain
4. Damage to blood vessels
5. Dental damage
6. Damage to eyes, nose, or skin
7. Sore throat
8. Vocal cord injury
9. Windpipe injury
10. Respiratory problems
11. Drug reactions
12. Infection
13. Nerve injury
14. Esophageal laceration
15. Paralysis
16. Brain damage
17. Heart damage
18. Death
19. Damage to baby if you are pregnant

I understand that medical care is not an exact science and that no guarantee is made as to the outcome of the administration of anesthesia. I have been given an explanation of the proposed plan of anesthesia and have been given an opportunity to ask questions about it as well as alternative forms of anesthesia. I have been given an explanation of the procedures and techniques to be used, as well as the risks and hazards involved, and I believe that I have sufficient information to give this informed consent.

I certify that this form has been fully explained to me, that I have read it or have had it read to me, and that I understand its contents.

Patient or person authorized to consent for patient ______________________ Date and Time ______________________

I have discussed the contents of this form with the patient, as well as the risks, hazards, and potential complications of anesthesia, in addition to the alternatives to anesthesia.

Physicians Signature ______________________ Date and Time ______________________

Figure 30-2
The patient signs the anesthesia consent form after discussing anesthesia and postoperative pain control options and risks with the anesthesiologist.

and outcome and be cost-efficient in lowering total medical costs by lowering perioperative morbidity.

The determination of what preoperative laboratory tests to obtain should be based on history, physical examination, gender, age, type of surgery, sensitivity and specificity of the test, and the prevalence of the abnormality sought. Furthermore,

Preoperative Clinic Flow Pattern

Old charts and laboratory and EKGs from the day before reviewed before clinic opens

↓

Patient fills out anesthesia questionnaire

↓

Vital signs obtained

↓

Patient placed in examination room and preoperative videos reviewed

↓

Anesthesiologist reviews questionnaire and performs physical exam

↓

Types and risk of anesthesia discussed

↓

Anesthesia consent obtained

↓

Further instruction on NPO status and preoperative medications discussed

↓

Labs ordered and obtained within the clinic

↓

Nurses provide further patient education

↓

Patient discharged

Figure 30-3
Preoperative screening flow chart.

positive abnormalities must have direct bearing in improving anesthetic and surgical management.

The prevalence of the abnormality sought based on history and physical examination is the key determination of what appropriate preoperative laboratory tests to perform. Those tests with a high sensitivity and specificity, but a low prevalence of

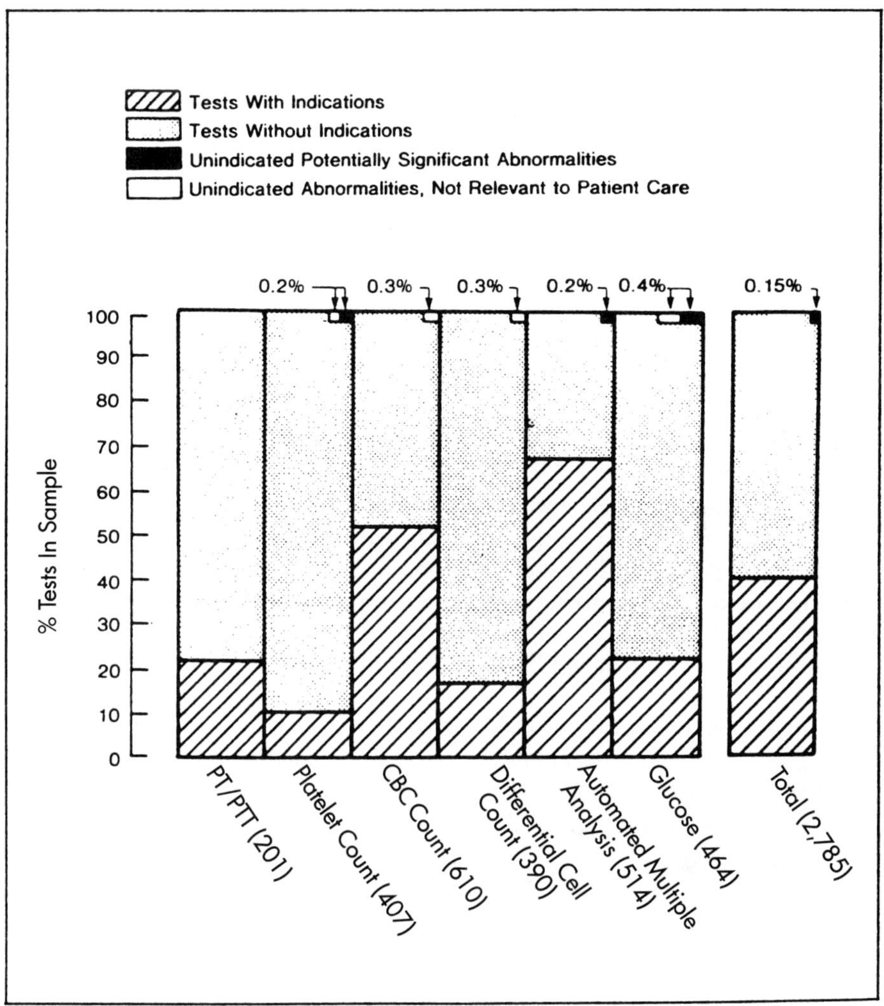

Figure 30-4
Proportions of indicated and unindicated preoperative tests, drawn to scale. Numbers in parentheses represent sample sizes used. PT/PTT indicates prothrombin time/partial thromboplastin time; CBC, complete blood cell. Automated multiple analysis is six factor. (Used with permission from Kaplan EB, et al.: The usefulness of preoperative laboratory screening, *JAMA* 253: 3578, 1985.)

abnormalities sought, will likely not be beneficial because of a low positive-predictive value. The positive-predictive value is the probability of a positive finding actually revealing an abnormality. The positive-predictive value is normally what is most important to the physician when ordering a preoperative test.

A good illustration of the importance of the positive-predictive value is assessing the value of a screening prothrombin time (PT) and partial thromboplastin time

(PTT) for predicting the risk of postoperative hemorrhage in children undergoing tonsillectomy. Manning et al. studied 994 children undergoing tonsillectomy and/ or adenoidectomy, whose PT and PTT were screened. They found a sensitivity of only 5.5%, a specificity of 94.2%, and a positive-predictive value of only 3.4% (Table 30-1).

This example reinforces the importance of there being a reasonable prevalence of disease before a test can be useful. Even with a high specificity, if the prevalence of disease is low, there will be a great increase in the number of false-positives compared to true-positives, thus, making the positive-predictive value of the test low.

Hemoglobin and Hematocrit

Traditionally, hemoglobins less than 10 gm/dl were considered too low for elective surgery. However, most perioperative physicians now realize that most chronic anemias are well-tolerated for asymptomatic patients undergoing minor-to-moderate surgery. Currently, no data have shown improved perioperative outcome from correction of mild-to-moderate anemia. Ranstron found no difference in perioperative complications between 145 surgical patients with a hemoglobin less than 10 gm/dl and a control group of 412 patients with normal hemoglobin levels. The National Institute of Health (NIH) Consensus Conference on perioperative red cell transfusion concluded that transfusion indications for surgery should often be lower than a hemoglobin of 10 gm/dl and be patient-dependent.

The incidence of undiagnosed anemia greatly varies in different studies from 0.5% to 5%, but the highest incidence of anemia appears to be in infants under 12 months, in teenage girls, in young women, and in elderly men. Thus, for general medical screening, these high-risk groups of patients should undergo hemoglobin screening. However, it is unlikely that the discovery of mild-to-moderate anemia for an asymptomatic individual without significant medical problems improves perioperative outcome in surgery, without potential for major blood loss. Clearly, all patients undergoing surgery in which a type and screen is needed should have a preoperative hematocrit checked.

For the pediatric population, obtaining a preoperative hemoglobin or hematocrit in infants less than 1 year old, perhaps can be justified as a public health concern. The prevalence of iron deficiency anemia is highest in this subgroup. Studies by Oski in 1993 and Lozoff et al. in 1987 showed infants with iron deficiency anemia had delayed neurologic development. Most pediatricians now screen infants for anemia within the first year; hence, repeating a preoperative hematocrit is unnecessary. However, if we see an infant with poor general medical care with no prior hematocrit screening, we routinely check a hematocrit and inform the parents of our reasons for obtaining the hematocrit. If we discover a child to be anemic, then we refer that child to the family pediatrician or to a pediatrician in our own institution.

A second group of infants who warrant routine preoperative hemoglobin or hematocrit screening are premature infants of less than 60 weeks postconceptional age. Hemoglobin values of less than 10 gm/dl in this subgroup of infants have a higher incidence of postoperative apnea. Depending on the critical nature of surgery, the perioperative physician may elect to postpone surgery until the anemia has been corrected.

Table 30-1. Assessment of Preoperative Coagulation Screening for Tonsillectomy and Adenoidectomy

PT/PTT	BLEED	NO BLEED
Abnormal	2	56
PT/PTT Normal	34	902

$$\text{Sensitivity} = \frac{\text{true } (+)}{\text{true } (+) + \text{false } (-)} = \frac{2}{2 + 34} = 5.6\%$$

$$\text{Specificity} = \frac{\text{true } (-)}{\text{true } (-) + \text{false } (+)} = \frac{902}{902 + 56} = 94.2\%$$

$$\text{Positive predictive value} = \frac{\text{true } (+)}{\text{true } (+) + \text{false } (+)} = \frac{2}{2 + 56} = 3.4\%$$

(Adapted with permission obtained from Manning, et al: An assessment of preoperative coagulation screening for tonsillectomy and adenoidectomy, *Int J Pediatr Otorhinolaryngol* 13:241, 1987.)

A third group, in whom hematocrit levels routinely have been obtained, consists of children undergoing tonsillectomy or adenoidectomy or both. We now do not routinely check hematocrits for these patients. Nigan et al. found a less than 1% incidence of anemia in children undergoing tonsillectomy. The low incidence of anemia combined with a 2% to 5% rate of postoperative hemorrhage after a tonsillectomy, does not justify a routine screening hematocrit. Furthermore, if postoperative hemorrhage occurred, the decision for transfusing a child would not be based on the preoperative hematocrit, but on the hemodynamic status of the child. However, patients at risk of a blood dyscrasia, such as sickle cell anemia, routinely have a screening hematocrit and sickle cell preparation if no prior screening has been done. Also a screening hematocrit is done if a clinically suspicious anemia is found on history or physical examination.

Complete Blood Count

Rarely is a complete blood count (CBC) indicated over a screening hematocrit or hemoglobin. At our institution a CBC is 3 times as expensive as a hematocrit and rarely provides any additional useful information. Turnbull et al. found that only 0.02% of preoperative patients had a low white blood cell count (WBC) and 0.04% of preoperative patients had a clinically nonsignificant thrombocytopenia. A few indications for ordering a CBC include known bone marrow dysfunction, hypersplenism, and recent chemotherapy. Another indication would be to confirm heavy alcohol abuse by looking for an elevated mean corpuscular volume (MCV), commonly associated with alcohol abuse. Lastly, in the perioperative setting, a differential WBC is rarely useful. At our institution, a CBC with a differential count is almost twice as expensive as a normal CBC and 5 times more expensive than a hematocrit.

PT, PTT, and Bleeding Time

Coagulation tests are useful as screening tests in those patients with risk factors for coagulopathy, as determined by the history and physical examination. However, a screening PT, PTT, and bleeding time have no value for screening asymptomatic patients without risk factors for bleeding abnormalities. Suchman et al. found, in patients without a risk factor for a coagulopathy, a 33% sensitivity and 84% specificity for a screening PTT but a positive-predictive value for intraoperative or postoperative hemorrhage of only 2.6%. The reason for the low positive-predictive value of the PTT was because of the low prevalence of actual bleeding abnormalities in asymptomatic patients and, hence, a high number of false-positive tests despite an 84% specificity.

Manning et al. found the PT or PTT ineffective in screening for hemorrhage from tonsillectomy or adenoidectomy surgeries. The risk of hemorrhage is estimated to be 2% to 5% from a tonsillectomy, but Manning found the positive-predictive value of an abnormal PT or PTT to be 3.4% for hemorrhage (see Table 30-1), thus, making the preoperative screening PT or PTT to be of no predictive value for hemorrhage.

Screening bleeding time in patients without risk factors is also of little to no value. Barber et al. found a 1.5% incidence of abnormal bleeding times in patients without risk factors and only 0.1% of significant elevation of bleeding times. Furthermore, Barber et al. could not find a direct correlation between intraoperative hemorrhage and an abnormal bleeding time.

Hence, the previously mentioned authors, along with several other authors, have concluded that asymptomatic patients without risk factors for bleeding abnormalities should not be screened for a coagulopathy with either PT, PTT, or bleeding time. However, patients with risk factors, including liver disease, malnourishment, malabsorption, a family history of bleeding disorders, or significant bleeding with prior operations or dental work should be screened with coagulation studies because of the increased positive-predictive value of an abnormal finding.

Chemistries

Routine preoperative screening of biochemical panels of 6 to 20 tests in asymptomatic patients is unnecessary, costly, and can lead to unnecessary further testing or future medical legal liability for ignoring abnormalities not relevant to perioperative care. Instead, the perioperative physician should order specific biochemical tests as directed by the history, physical examination, and type of surgery. Most biochemistry normal values are set within 95% confidence intervals, meaning 5% of the normal population will have abnormal values. For a 12-biochemical panel, the chance of the entire panel being normal in a normal patient is only 0.95^{12} which equals 54%. Hence, 46% of normal patients will have at least one abnormality on a 12-biochemistry panel.

ELECTROLYTES

In healthy patients, there is no need to check sodium, potassium, bicarbonate, chloride, or magnesium levels. The incidence of significant abnormalities in healthy patients is small, and there is no evidence that mild abnormalities affect perioperative outcome. However, again, electrolytes should be ordered only if warranted by history and physical examination. An example of this would be a patient presenting with oat-cell carcinoma of the lung for a lobectomy. Because of the increased incidence of a syndrome of inappropriate secretion of antidiuretic hormone (SIADH) paraneoplastic syndrome, sodium should be checked to rule out significant hyponatremia. Of the electrolytes, the perioperative physician is most interested in potassium and magnesium because of abnormal levels being associated with arrhythmias.

POTASSIUM

Potassium only needs to be checked when the prevalence of potassium abnormalities is increased, the patient has a history of serious arrhythmias, or the patient is on digoxin. Vitez et al. found few perioperative problems with chronic hypokalemia with K^+ above 2.5 mEq/l in patients not on digoxin or with a history of significant arrhythmias (Box 30-1).

MAGNESIUM

This electrolyte is not normally screened with many biochemical profiles. However, hypomagnesemia often is associated with hypokalemia. Hence, magnesium should be screened for in patients with hypokalemia or a recent history of arrhythmias.

GLUCOSE

A 2% to 5% incidence of fasting, elevated glucoses above 120 mg/dl is found in patients without a history of diabetes mellitus. Velanovich found that almost 25% of patients over age 60 have glucoses over 120 mg/dl. The prevalence of hyperglycemia is relatively common in certain subgroups of patients and, perhaps, justifies routine screening of glucose. However, few of these abnormalities, as Blery et al. stated, were deemed clinically significant enough to pursue.

No evidence exists to support the theory that tight control of glucoses in the operating room improves perioperative outcome for most surgeries. However, in open heart and intracranial surgeries, maintaining control of glucose levels to below 200 to 250 mg/dl has shown to improve outcome. Thus, for these surgeries, preoperative screening of glucose should be done. Furthermore, in patients with increased prevalence of hyperglycemia, such as in the morbidly obese or elderly, a glucose should be screened before for any moderate-to-major stressful surgery. This is because

Box 30-1 Indications for Potassium Screening

1. Potassium wasting diuretics
2. Digoxin
3. Known renal dysfunction
4. History of serious arrhythmias
5. History of other potassium wasting drugs such as amphotericin or *cis*-platinum
6. ± New diagnosis of moderate to severe hypertension (screening for hyperaldosteronism causing hypokalemia)

of the increased risk of significant hyperglycemia postoperatively from the stress of surgery in an undiagnosed diabetic. Other indications for glucose screening are patients on systemic steroids undergoing moderate-to-major surgery. In addition, patients with soft tissue infections should have their glucose levels screened because of the increased prevalence of hyperglycemia and evidence that tight control of glucose improves tissue healing (Box 30-2).

CREATININE

Creatinine is a better marker of actual glomerular filtration rate than blood urea nitrogen. Creatinine does not begin to elevate until there is a 50% loss of renal function. The creatinine is dependent on such factors as muscle mass, making it often an inaccurate test in the elderly with low muscle mass. Kaplan et al. found the prevalence of renal insufficiency among asymptomatic patients with no history of renal disease is only 0.2%. Furthermore, mild-to-moderate elevations of creatinine likely have minimal input on perioperative outcome for most surgeries. The avoidance of long-acting neuromuscular relaxants excreted renally, could arguably be a reason to screen for renal insufficiency. However, today for most shorter surgeries requiring muscle relaxants, anesthesiologists are using vecuronium, rocuronium, *cis*-atracurium, or atracurium in which moderate renal insufficiency has little effect. For longer surgery, the longer-acting neuromuscular relaxant should be titrated to effect, only with a neuromuscular monitor. However, there are particular indications when checking a screening creatinine is beneficial because of either the increased prevalence of renal dysfunction or the increased risk of postoperative renal dysfunction (Box 30-3).

Liver Enzymes

Schemel found the likelihood of finding elevated liver enzymes in the asymptomatic surgical patient to be 1 in 700 and the risk of developing jaundice to be 1 in 2540. It remains unclear if knowledge of liver-enzyme elevations changes perioperative outcome. When Schemel's study was conducted in the early 1970s, halothane was the major volatile agent used, and the etiology of halothane hepatitis was not clear. Hence, Schemel recommended that all preoperative patients undergo liver enzyme screening.

Today, since halothane is used rarely and the incidence of significant liver enzyme elevation in asymptomatic patients is low, liver enzyme screening normally is not indicated. However, a screening SGOT is indicated in the following patients: (1) patients undergoing upper abdominal surgery, in which surgery traction can cause liver ischemia; (2) patients at increased risk of hepatitis; and (3) patients with history

Box 30-2 Indications for Glucose Screening

1. Surgery involving intracranial or cardiac bypass
2. Obese patients undergoing moderate-to major-surgery
3. Elderly >60 undergoing moderate-to major-surgery
4. Surgery for ongoing soft tissue infection
5. Patients on systemic steroids undergoing moderate-to-major surgery

Box 30-3 Indications for Obtaining Screening Creatinine

1. Operations at risk of perioperative renal ischemia such as cross-clamping the aorta or bypass surgery.
2. Diseases with increased prevalence of renal dysfunction such as diabetes mellitus or moderate-to-severe hypertension.
3. Recent use of renal toxic drugs such as IV contrast dye, aminoglycosides, recent new use of angiotensin converting enzyme inhibitor without a creatinine being checked.

of liver-toxin exposure, such as alcohol abuse. An SGOT greater than 2 times the normal value, warrants further investigation with full liver enzymes, bilirubin and hepatitis panel, and possible medical consultation.

In conclusion, indiscriminate ordering of biochemistry panels with 6 to 20 tests should not be done for preoperative testing. Instead, specific biochemistry labs, such as potassium, creatinine, SGOT and glucose, should be ordered based on the history, physical examination, and type of surgery.

Value of Repeat Laboratory Tests

Macpherson et al. found that normal results from laboratory tests performed within the preceding year (although the majority of tests were within 4 months), showed an extremely low probability of changing significantly when repeated. However, 17% of patients with previous abnormal tests were found to have significant changes on preoperative tests, likely to affect perioperative management. Therefore, this author does not repeat normal laboratory values obtained within the past 6 to 12 months if there is no change in history or physical examination; but, this author does repeat tests if previous abnormalities were present or there is a change in history or physical examination which would increase the likelihood of a significant change in the test results.

Urine Analysis

Lawrence et al. concluded that routine urinalysis in asymptomatic patients should not be obtained preoperatively for most surgeries. The incidence of wound infection from asymptomatic bacteriuria in clean, nonprosthetic wound surgeries is low, and the cost of treating a wound infection caused by asymptomatic bacteriuria is 500-fold less than the cost of routine urine analysis. Clearly, patients with symptoms compatible with an active urinary tract infection should have a urinalysis performed preoperatively and be treated to prevent active inflammation of the genitourinary tract increasing the risk of hematogenous seeding of bacteria.

Operations involving the genitourinary tract likely warrant a screening urinary analysis because of the increased risk of infection from direct manipulation of the urinary tract. Performing screening urinary analysis in patients undergoing foreign body placement, such as hip arthroplasty, remains unclear. Glynn and Sheenan found no increased risk of infection in patients with untreated asymptomatic bacteriuria undergoing hip or knee arthroplasty. However, all these patients were treated with appropriate antibiotics when the urine cultures returned positive postoperatively. In asymptomatic bacteriuria, 80% of the organisms are *E. coli.* Any patient undergoing foreign body placement routinely gets a first-generation cephalosporin in which *E. coli* has a 90% sensitivity. The first-generation cephalosporins, such as cefazolin, are excreted in the urine at high levels above the needed killing concentration for a urinary tract infection. This greatly reduces the number of patients with continued asymptomatic bacteriuria in the postoperative period and may be one of the reasons why there is no evidence of asymptomatic bacteriuria increasing the rate of postoperative infection with foreign body placement.

Lastly, a screening urine analysis may be useful when screening for glucose and protein in the urine. However, direct screening by measuring glucose and creatinine as indicated by history and physical examination is a better screening tool for diabetes and renal dysfunction. In conclusion, a preoperative urine analysis should only be obtained for the majority of surgeries when the history indicates an increased likelihood of a urinary tract abnormality.

Electrocardiography

The University Hospital Consortium found the majority of academic institutions obtain a 12-lead ECG preoperatively on all males at least 40 years of age and women at least 50 years of age. Roizen, along with several authors, recommend this current guideline for ordering ECG. This recommendation was based on studies using a heterogeneous general medical population and did not focus on any specific subgroups of patients or types of surgery. Currently, the faculty at Wake Forest University has taken a different approach to ordering preoperative ECGs based on age, cardiac risk factors and types of surgery to reduce the number of unnecessary ECGs.

VALUE OF ECG SCREENING WITHOUT RISK FACTORS

The incidence of significant ECG abnormalities in apparently healthy, middle-aged men is low. Sox et al. in a review analysis of the literature found the prevalence of Q waves to be 0.014, the prevalence of T-wave inversion to be 0.033 to 0.074, and the prevalence of ST-segment abnormalities to be 0.009 to 0.02 in apparently healthy, middle-aged men. These studies on ECG abnormalities included asymptomatic men with risk factors for coronary artery disease (CAD). The actual incidence of significant abnormalities in middle age men without cardiac risk factors has not been examined in large numbers but is likely to be even lower.

Based on Framingham risk score, the annual incidence of CAD in men with no cardiovascular risk factors is 1.4 per 1000 at age 40 and 7.4 per 1000 at age 60. In the asymptomatic patient with underlying CAD, the ECG by itself is imprecise and will miss a large percentage of actual patients with CAD. Uusitupa et al. in a large autopsy study on transmural infarcts found the sensitivity of Q waves with an ECG to be only between 33% to 62%. In other words, the ECG had a high false-negative rate for diagnosing significant CAD causing a transmural infarct.

Furthermore, it is unclear if the detection of a significant ECG abnormality in the preoperative period in an asymtomatic patient without risk factors will improve patient perioperative outcome or long-term survival. Cohn et al. found that in 32% of normal coronary arteriograms, the patient's ECG had significant Q waves, ST-segment abnormalities, or T-wave changes. The annual mortality rate in apparently healthy men with Q waves, ST-segment abnormalities, or T-wave inversions is less than 1%, and there is little evidence supporting the argument that the early detection of these ECG abnormalities changes overall patient survival.

A second reason to obtain a preoperative ECG is to evaluate for arrhythmias, such as atrial fibrillation, AV block, and ventricular ectopy. The incidence of arrhythmias increases in the elderly and in those with cardiac risk factors. However, in the asymptomatic patient without cardiac risk factors who is under 60 years of age, the incidence of undiagnosed significant arrhythmias is low. Furthermore, careful physical examination should disclose the majority of arrhythmias such as ectopy or atrial fibrillation. Lastly, ECG monitoring in the operating room should disclose any missed arrhythmias. Although the diagnosing of an arrhythmia before induction could lead to postponement of surgery, the percentage of asymptomatic patients without cardiac risk factors, who are under 60 years, and in whom cardiac examination did not note an abnormality is, likely, minuscule.

A third reason for obtaining an ECG is to have a baseline ECG for comparison with intraoperative or postoperative questionable ECG abnormalities. No study has been done looking at the value of baseline ECG in the perioperative period. For patients arriving in the emergency room with chest pain, a baseline prior ECG was found to have little significance in deciding admission to the hospital. Certainly, a baseline ECG may be helpful in determining ECG changes during major intracavitary or vascular surgery in which there is a higher incidence of ECG changes and myocardial ischemia. In the asymptomatic patient who is under 60 years and not undergoing major surgery, the incidence of significant ECG abnormalities intraoperatively, and postoperatively, is low. Furthermore, the value of the baseline ECG in these patients when ECG abnormalities are noted intraoperatively and postoperatively has not been proved.

Gold et al. studied the usefulness of preoperative ECGs in 751 consecutive adults undergoing ambulatory surgery. They found 12 adverse cardiovascular events in which the preoperative ECG may have been useful in 6 of these 12 patients. Five of the six patients in whom the ECG may have been useful were older than 60, and none of the patients with cardiovascular events was American Society of Anesthesiology Class I (ASA I). Gold et al. concluded the preoperative ECG was of limited or no value in the relatively healthy ambulatory-surgery patients younger than 60 without other medical illnesses.

Callaghan et al. examined 90 preoperative ECGs in patients older than 50 without cardiac-risk factors. Only 6 were abnormal (7%), and all 6 abnormal ECGs were in patients over age 60. Callaghan et al. concluded that the routine preoperative ECG in all patients over 50 without cardiac disease or risk factors, be changed to all patients 60 years or older (Table 30-2).

If the low percentage of significant ECG abnormalities found in asymptomatic patients without cardiac-risk factors changed anesthetic management, then the preoperative ECG in this subgroup might still be a useful test. However, Rabkin and Horne reported that the detection of new ECG abnormalities did not change anesthetic management, except in 2 of 812 cases.

Table 30-2. The Incidence of ECG Abnormalities in Patients With or Without Risk of Cardiac Disease in Different Age Groups, Number (%)

	NO CARDIAC DISEASE OR RISK FACTORS			CARDIAC DISEASE OR RISK FACTORS		
AGE (YEARS)	NUMBER	ECG PERFORMED	ECG ABNORMAL	NUMBER	ECG PERFORMED	ECG ABNORMAL
0–29	55	15	0	0	—	—
30–39	28	3	0	6	2	0
40–49	43	23	0	6	5	0
50–59	42	30	0	25	23	9(39%)
60–69	42	31	2(6%)	26	25	14(56%)
70–79	21	19	2(11%)	36	33	22(67%)
80+	11	10	2(20%)	13	11	6(54%)
Total	242	131	6	112	99	51

(Used with permission from Callaghan LC, et al: Utilization of the preoperative ECG, *Anaesthesia* 50:490, 1995.)

In conclusion, a preoperative ECG should be ordered if the finding of abnormalities will change perioperative management and improve patients' overall outcome. Secondly, the ECG should be ordered only if there is a reasonable positive-predictive value of the test. For there to be a reasonable positive-predictive value, requires both a reasonable prevalence of CAD in the subgroup of patients and a low false-positive value of ECG abnormalities. The subgroup of patients aged 40 to 60, who are asymptomatic without cardiac-risk factors, has a low prevalence of significant CAD, a low positive-predictive valve, and a high false-positive rate for ECG abnormalities. Electrocardiogram abnormalities in this subgroup may lead to unnecessary, further noninvasive or invasive cardiac testing before surgery. All these reasons combined, make the routine ordering of the ECG for nonmajor surgeries in asymptomatic patients 40 to 60 years old without risk factors for CAD, an unnecessary cost. In asymptomatic patients 60 or older without cardiac-risk factors, a preoperative ECG should be obtained, secondary to a higher prevalence of undiagnosed CAD. Again, no large study has been done to verify this hypothesis and this recommendation may change as studies are done on preoperative ECG in asymptomatic patients older than 60.

VALUE OF ECG SCREENING WITH CARDIAC-RISK FACTORS

Although not proved directly in the perioperative setting, the ECG is likely justified in men older than 40 or women older than 50 with cardiac risk factors or even in younger patients with multiple risk factors. The prevalence of significant CAD is higher with an increased incidence of true-positive abnormalities. These patients are likely to have a higher incidence of intraoperative and postoperative abnormalities for whom a baseline ECG could perhaps avoid an unnecessary cardiac workup. An example would be a 44-year-old male with a history of hypertension found to have left ventricular hypertrophy with an ST-strain pattern. If baseline ECG had not noted this, these abnormalities could be confused with myocardial ischemia intraoperatively and lead to an unnecessary cardiology consultation postoperatively.

Hence, the decision to order a preoperative ECG should be based on the combination of age, cardiac-risk factors, and type of surgery. Rigid guidelines that base the decision to order an ECG on age alone cause unnecessary ECG testing and elevate costs with no benefit to the patient (Table 30-3).

VALUE OF REPEAT ECG SCREENING

Rabkin and Horne found no benefit in repeating a preoperative ECG within 2 years of an initial ECG in patients younger than 60, in whom the ECG showed no abnormalities. In general, this author agrees with Rabkin and Horne's conclusion on not reordering previous normal or nonsignificant ECG abnormalities within 2 years of surgery. However, in patients with a high risk of CAD, such as stable angina and diabetes mellitus, this author will want a 12-lead ECG done within a 2- to 3-month period because of a higher likelihood of significant changes.

Chest Radiography

Multiple studies have shown a high incidence of chest radiographic abnormalities in the subgroup of patients with risk factors for cardiopulmonary disease, and in the elderly who are older than 70. The majority of abnormalities consist of chronic obstructive lung changes or cardiomegaly. Many of the authors of these studies concluded by recommending routine preoperative chest radiography in the previous subgroup of patients. However, one significant problem with these authors' conclusions is the lack of evidence that the actual preoperative chest radiography had any influence in improving perioperative management or outcome.

The landmark study on the efficacy of preoperative chest radiography was performed by the Royal College of Radiologists in 1979. In this study, 10,619 patients undergoing nonacute, noncardiopulmonary surgery were studied. The preoperative chest radiograph did not influence the decision to operate or the choice of anesthetic. Furthermore, the preoperative chest radiograph was of little value as a baseline to compare to patients with postoperative pulmonary problems. Lastly, 25.7% of those patients with preoperative radiographs proceeded to surgery without knowing the radiologist's report; 25% of these patients' subsequent radiologic reports had significant abnormalities. In this study, no evidence was obtained that a preoperative

Table 30-3. Indications for Preoperative ECG for Non-Major Surgery

	M	F
≥40 without risk factors	No	No
≥50 without risk factors	No	No
≥60 without risk factors	Yes	Yes
≥40 with risk factors	Yes	±
≥50 with risk factors	Yes	Yes
<40 with significant risk factors	Yes	Yes

chest radiograph, even in the high-risk patient, changed perioperative management, improved perioperative outcome, or predicted postoperative cardiopulmonary complications.

Excluding intrathoracic surgery, this author does not recommend a routine, preoperative screening chest radiograph in any population subgroup. However, a preoperative chest radiograph should be obtained when the chest radiograph will answer a particular question which will directly influence perioperative management. A few examples of when a preoperative chest radiograph would be helpful are the following:

1. Ruling out a possible pneumonia in a patient with severe chronic obstructive pulmonary lung disease and a productive cough in which physical examination is limited because of distant breath sounds.
2. Examining for cardiomegaly in a patient with a questionable history of congestive heart failure. If cardiomegaly is present, then the perioperative physician obtains echocardiography to assess left ventricular function.
3. Obtaining a chest radiograph for evidence of metastatic disease for a scheduled tumor resection. Finding of metastatic disease on chest radiograph would lead to cancellation of the surgery.

In conclusion, this author agrees with the concluding statement from the Royal College of Radiologists, "It is advisable, on financial and ethical grounds, that the preoperative chest radiography service should in the future be used selectively only in circumstances where the clinical history or signs place the patient at very high risk of postoperative pulmonary complication and where it is considered the investigation will provide important additional information."

• SUMMARY

The ordering of preoperative screening tests should be based primarily on history, physical examination combined with the age, gender, and type of surgery. Furthermore, the tests ordered should have a reasonable positive-predictive value for any positive finding to be useful. The positive-predictive value of a test can only be significant if there is a reasonable prevalence of disease. The prevalence of disease can greatly be increased by subgrouping patients by history, physical examination, age and gender in which the prevalence of the abnormality sought is increased. Lastly, the goal of preoperative screening tests should be not just to find an abnormality but to find an abnormality whose discovery will change and improve perioperative management and outcome and lower medical costs because of decreased patient morbidity.

BIBLIOGRAPHY

Barber A, et al: The bleeding time as a preoperative screening test, *Am J Med* 78:761–764, 1985.

Blery C, et al: Evaluation of a protocol for selective ordering of preoperative tests, *Lancet* 1:139, 1986.

Callaghan LC, Edwards ND, Reilly CS: Utilization of the preoperative ECG, *Anaesthesia* 50:488–490, 1995.

Cohn PF, et al: A quantitative clinical index for the diagnosis of symptomatic coronary-artery disease, *N Engl J Med* 286:901–907, 1972.

Fischer SP: Development and effectiveness of an anesthesia preoperative evaluation clinic in a teaching hospital, *Anesthesiology* 85:196–206, 1996.

Glynn MK, Sheehan JM: The significance of asymptomatic bacteriuria in patients undergoing hip/knee arthroplasty, *Clin Ortho Related Res* 185:151–154, 1984.

Gold BS, et al: The utility of preoperative electrocardiograms in the ambulatory surgical patient, *Arch Intern Med* 152:301–305, 1992.

Goldberger AL, O'Konski M: Utility of the routine electrocardiogram before surgery and on general hospital admission, *Ann Intern Med* 105:552–557, 1986.

Kaplan EB, et al: The usefulness of preoperative laboratory screening, *JAMA* 253:3576–3581, 1985.

Lawrence VA, Gafri A, Gross M: The unproven utility of the preoperative urinalysis: economic evaluation, *J Clin Epidemiol* 42:1185–1192, 1989.

Leigh JM, Walker J, Janaganatham P: Effect of preoperative anaesthetic visit on anxiety, *Br Med J* 2:987–989, 1977.

Lozoff B, et al: Iron deficiency anemia and iron therapy effects on infant developmental test performance, *Pediatrics* 79:981–995, 1987.

Macpherson DS, Snow R, Lofgren RP: Preoperative screening: value of previous tests, *Ann Intern Med* 113:969–973, 1990.

Manning SC, et al: An assessment of preoperative coagulation screening for tonsillectomy and adenoidectomy, *Int J Pediatr Otorhinolaryngol* 13:237–244, 1987.

National Study by the Royal College of Radiologists: Preoperative chest radiology, *Lancet* 2:83–86, 1979.

Nigam A, Ahmed K, Drake-Lee AB: The value of preoperative estimation of haemoglobin in children undergoing tonsillectomy, *Clin Otolaryngol* 15:549–551, 1990.

Oski FA: Iron deficiency in infancy and childhood, *N Engl J Med* 329:190–193, 1993.

Rabkin SW, Horne JM: Preoperative electrocardiography effect of new abnormalities on clinical decisions, *Can Med Assoc J* 128:146–147, 1983.

Rabkin SW, Horne JM: Preoperative electrocardiography: its cost-effectiveness in detecting abnormalities when a previous tracing exists, *Can Med Assoc J* 121:301–305, 1979.

Rawstron RE: Anaemia and surgery: a retrospective clinical study, *Aust N Z Surg* 39:425–432, 1970.

Schemel WH: Unexpected hepatic dysfunction found by multiple laboratory screening, *Anesth Analg* 55:810–812, 1974.

Sox HC, Garber AM, Littenberg B: The resting electrocardiogram as a screening test, *Ann Intern Med* 111:489–502, 1989.

Suchman AL, Mushlin AI: How well does the activated partial thromboplastin time predict postoperative hemorrhage? *JAMA* 256:750–753, 1986.

Turnbull JM, Buck C: The value of preoperative screening investigations in otherwise healthy individuals, *Arch Intern Med* 147:1101–1105, 1987.

Uusitupa M, et al: Sensitivity and specificity of Minnesota Code Q-AS abnormalities in the diagnosis of myocardial infarction verified at autopsy, *Am Heart J* 106:753–757, 1980.

Vitez TS, et al: Chronic hypokalemia and intraoperative dysrhythmias, *Anesthesiology* 63:130, 1985.

Welborn LG, et al: Anemia and postoperative apnea in former preterm infants, *Anesthesiology* 74:1003–1006, 1991.

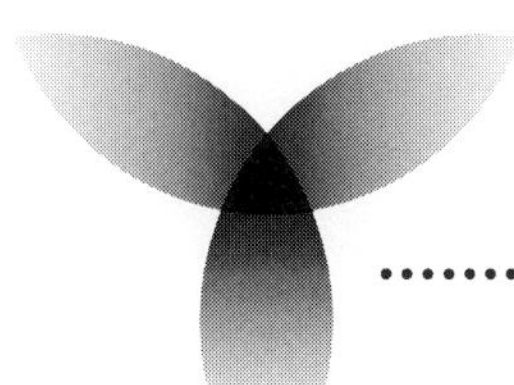

Section IV

SPECIAL SURGICAL CONSIDERATIONS

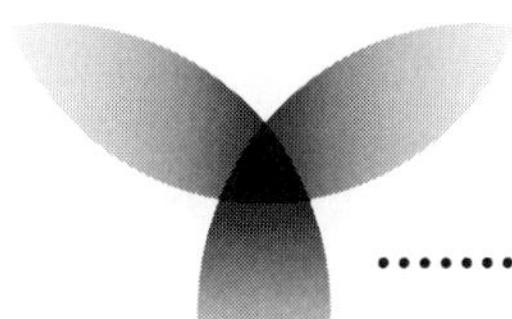

Chapter 31

Laparoscopic Surgery

David L. Bogdonoff, MD, Bruce Schirmer, MD

Despite the use of laparoscopic techniques in gynecology since 1967, it took the report of the first successful laparoscopic cholecystectomy in France in 1988 to transform the face of modern surgery. Today, the minimally invasive laparoscopic approach is the standard of care for removal of the gallbladder. The availability of such minimally invasive procedures altered many surgical decisions as operative procedures are considered earlier in the course of treatment. The dramatic decrease in postoperative morbidity following minimally invasive procedures has shortened both hospital stays and recuperative times.

The explosion of laparoscopic surgery was made possible by innovations in video and mechanical technology. Surgical telescopes have been greatly improved, and the miniaturization of the attached television cameras has allowed improved flexibility in manipulating the scope. All participants in the procedure can observe and thereby, more easily assist the operating surgeon in the performance of more and more complex undertakings. New mechanical staplers and retractors have facilitated operations on the gastrointestinal tract. Expanding balloons inserted through trocars create a space outside the peritoneal cavity allowing the use of laparoscopic techniques for preperitoneal inguinal hernia repair. Newer diagnostic and therapeutic tools for intraoperative use, such as ultrasound probes and the harmonic scalpel, hold great promise for further advances in the field.

The number of procedures now undertaken totally by the minimally invasive approach, or partially assisted with the aid of laparoscopy, has continued to increase steadily. Videotelescopic surgery has additionally revolutionized some thoracic procedures, discussed in a separate chapter. Despite the apparent advantages of these minimally invasive approaches, consultants must be aware that the anesthetic management and surgical interventions still represent a significant intraoperative physiologic hurdle for some patients, even if their postoperative course may be easier to manage. All abdominal procedures, whether laparoscopic or otherwise, will result in some postoperative respiratory and gastrointestinal dysfunction, in addition to variable amounts of pain.

• SURGICAL PROCEDURE

The principal differences between laparoscopic procedures and their open counterparts involve patient positioning and the creation of a pneumoperitoneum. Both of these will have significant hemodynamic and respiratory effects and actually will dictate whether the procedure is feasible for an individual patient.

The majority of patients will require general anesthesia for laparoscopy. While a regional anesthetic approach eliminates somatic pain from penetration of the abdominal wall, abdominal distention and visceral retraction may produce visceral discomfort carried by sympathetic and parasympathetic fibers far outside the reach of practical conduction anesthesia. In addition, because of the use of carbon dioxide as the most common gaseous agent to create the pneumoperitoneum, the absorption of this gas produces a concentration gradient of carbolic acid at the peritoneal surface, which is highly irritating. Occasionally, highly motivated patients may tolerate laparoscopy with epidural anesthesia and intravenous sedation of a heavy nature. Though less common, extraperitoneal approaches can be well adapted to regional techniques.

Following the induction of general anesthesia, it is imperative that the anesthesiologist decompress the stomach with either an orogastric or nasogastric tube. A distended stomach is at risk of perforation during entry of the peritoneal cavity. Similarly, the bladder must be emptied with a Foley catheter.

The surgery begins with the establishment of a pneumoperitoneum. This is usually accomplished by puncturing the abdominal wall with a Verres needle which allows the insufflation of carbon dioxide. The needle is usually placed in the midline, infraumbilically with the patient in the Trendelenberg position, to minimize damage to intraabdominal organs. Care is taken to ensure that the tip of the needle is free within the peritoneal space and not in a hollow viscus or within the abdominal wall. Carbon dioxide is insufflated until the abdomen is tense. A trocar is placed through the site formerly occupied by the initial Verres needle, and the surgical telescope is advanced into the peritoneal cavity. Additional trocars are then placed under direct vision afforded by the telescope. If the patient has had previous abdominal surgery and the surgeon is concerned about adhesions, a trocar is placed under direct vision following a miniaparotomy incision.

Carbon dioxide is chosen almost uniformly as the insufflating gas. In the past, other gases were used under either experimental or routine conditions. Carbon dioxide is highly soluble and, therefore, poses the least danger in a case of inadvertent entry into the circulation in the form of a gas embolus. Additionally, it does not support combustion, which is important, given the extensive use of cautery during surgery. Nitrous oxide, often used in the early days of laparoscopy, supported combustion even in the absence of oxygen and, therefore, proved to be unacceptable. Helium is effective but is expensive and, because of its low solubility, more dangerous in the rare case of air embolism. Compressed air also supports combustion and is no longer utilized. The use of carbon dioxide as the insufflating gas, as will be discussed later, represents a physiologic load for the lungs because its systemic absorption from the peritoneal space will only add to the burden of elimination of this metabolically produced waste gas.

It is the insufflation of gas under pressure into the abdominal cavity that produces the important physiologic stresses of this surgery. The insufflation of gas is controlled by a mechanical insufflator that has a pressure-limiting function, and this must be set at a reasonable level. Insufficient insufflation pressure will result in an inadequate amount of pneumoperitoneum and impair the visualization necessary for the conduct of the surgery. Excessive pressure will result in difficulties in circulation and ventilation, which will be discussed later. The usual pressure is near 15 to 18 cm H_2O.

CIRCULATORY CHANGES DURING LAPAROSCOPY

The pressure created in the abdominal cavity may have profound effects on the circulation. Insufflated gas at low pressure decreases mesenteric venous capacity by compressing the veins within the gut. This results in an initial increase in preload to the heart and, perhaps, a rise in the central venous pressure (CVP). It would take a much larger pressure to completely compress the inferior vena cava; this is unlikely with modern insufflators, which accurately control insufflation pressures. There is, however, some degree of added resistance in the inferior vena cava (IVC). This is reflected as an increase in femoral venous pressure and decreased flow, when measured. Patient position during surgery is still the most significant variable affecting venous return.

The increase in abdominal pressure also increases the resistance to arterial flow, but this is not the only explanation for the significant increases in afterload that are observed. Neurohumoral reflexes, resulting from the stretching of the abdominal wall, and perhaps, from hypercarbia if ventilation is impaired or improperly managed, will lead to sympathetic nervous system stimulation. As with conventional laparotomy, increased levels of catecholamines, vasopressin, and cortisol have been measured and the renin-angiotensin and prostaglandin systems are implicated, as well. A much deeper level of anesthesia may be necessary to block these responses which, if unsuppressed, may lead to hypertension and further increased afterload capable of significantly stressing the compromised myocardium. However, deeper levels of anesthesia and the attendant cardiovascular depression have their own negative impact on a compromised patient. Extremes of positioning, such as steep Trendelenberg or reverse Trendelenberg, will only serve to accentuate these hemodynamically stressful changes.

The actual observed responses to laparoscopy depend on the underlying physical status of the patient. It is difficult to determine the individual effects of induced pneumoperitoneum as it occurs in the presence or multiple, interrelated variables such as the intravascular volume status of the patient, surgical conditions, ventilatory techniques, volume of carbon dioxide absorbed systemically, choice of anesthetic agent, patient position, and differences in the insufflating pressure itself. The healthy cardiovascular system is resilient in the face of the preload and afterload changes associated with laparoscopy. Nevertheless, numerous physiologic changes are readily demonstrable. In the supine patient, an initial increase in CVP and blood pressure, and an increase in cardiac output is observed at low insufflating pressures. As the insufflating pressure increases, cardiac output decreases. Increases in filling pressures are misleading as intrathoracic or more specifically intrapleural pressure is also increased. Thus, net transmural pressures in the heart are actually unchanged. In fact, in healthy patients, transesophageal echocardiographic studies do not reveal any changes in end-systolic or diastolic volumes of the heart, despite increases in filling pressures. Hypertension is commonly observed because of increased afterload from both the mechanical compression of abdominal vessels by the induced pneumoperitoneum, and direct hemodynamic effects of the neurohumoral responses to surgery and elevated carbon dioxide tensions. The sympathetic nervous system stimulation also produces some degree of venoconstriction in peripheral capacitance vessels, and tends to counteract preload decreases from mild IVC compression, secondary to the pneumoperitoneum. While the resulting hypertension is usually not dangerous to the healthy patient whose heart can still eject against the additional resistance, its treatment is often undertaken with deepening of the inhalation anesthetic. This tends to decrease sympathetic nervous system stimulation resulting from the procedure, while simultaneously serving to vasodilate and, thus, directly treat the hypertension. Vasodilation decreases afterload and enhances the return of cardiac output back towards normal levels. Narcotics may supplement the anesthetic but often are not effective in lowering the blood pressure. Hypertension usually resolves when the abdomen is deflated, and may be followed by prolonged periods of hypotension if excessive amounts of long-acting antihypertensive drugs have been used intraoperatively.

Laparoscopic cholecystectomy and other upper abdominal procedures require the use of steep (up to 30°) reverse Trendelenberg. This represents a significant impediment to normal venous return, already somewhat impaired by the pneumoperitoneum. A hypovolemic patient will become severely unstable following insufflation and head-up positioning. The decrease in venous return lowers filling pressures, and the subsequent drop in cardiac output may approach 50%, even in the healthy individual. The anesthetized state is also associated with decreased cardiac output, regardless of technique, and interferes with the body's ability to adapt to these changes.

It is the case of the patient with significant cardiovascular disease which presents the greatest physiologic challenge to the consultant, surgeon, and anesthesiologist. There is an increasing trend to propose minimally invasive approaches for these patients who, in fact, are the subset least equipped physiologically to tolerate them. Certain patients simply will not tolerate the accompanying hemodynamic compromise and will require an open-surgical procedure, despite concerns about increased postoperative morbidity. Fortunately, there are only a few patients who meet these criteria, but they may often be difficult to identify preoperatively. Often, a procedure will be attempted laparoscopically regardless of these concerns, with utilization of careful monitoring and with a low threshold for conversion to an open technique.

Patients with poor myocardial function may deteriorate from the increases in afterload accompanying abdominal insufflation. These patients are often on afterload-reducing medications, such as vasodilators, to enhance their cardiac output and decrease susceptibility to congestive failure. Such patients are recognized preoperatively by a history of severely limited exercise tolerance and echocardiographic evidence of significant wall motion abnormalities with significantly reduced ejection fraction. The patient with myocardium at risk from ischemic coronary disease is also problematic because the increase in afterload will significantly raise the myocardial oxygen requirements and enhance the likelihood of ischemic dysfunction or infarction. Cardiac risk factors for many of these patients are often well-known or are suspected on the basis of preoperative evaluations, as discussed in previous chapters. Unsuspected myocardial ischemia is, occasionally, encountered intraoperatively and the anesthetic plan must include a strategy for its detection and treatment. As the degree of hemodynamic compromise relates directly to insufflation pressure and patient positioning, it may be difficult to truly eliminate all adverse effects presented by laparoscopic interventions. Often, surgical techniques can be altered, such as lowering insufflation pressure, using a less steep, reverse Trendelenberg position, and using additional operating ports in the abdominal wall to compensate for advantages lost to the former concessions. The proficiency of the surgeon also is a factor, because it will directly determine the chance for success under the less-than-ideal conditions mandated by the decreased tolerance of the high-risk patient. Another surgical alternative that may be adopted in the face of a patient at high risk for cardiovascular compromise is the use of a gasless laparoscopic approach by the surgeon. For certain procedures this is an option, based upon the skill and experience of the surgical team with such an approach.

The use of invasive hemodynamic monitoring is essential in patients with severe cardiovascular disease, except for the rare exceptionally short procedures, such as a biopsy or diagnostic examination. Invasive arterial pressure and myocardial ischemia monitoring with ST-segment analysis are an absolute minimum, pulmonary artery catheters or transesophageal echocardiography may be added, at the discretion of the anesthesia team. An anesthetic should be chosen to provide an adequate level of analgesia without undue myocardial depression. It is particularly important to modulate any increases in preload to the heart, which may result when forward flow is impaired from the compromised ventricle by the presence of increased afterload. To this effect, short-acting, afterload-reducing drugs, such as nitroprusside, are effective at enhancing or attempting to normalize cardiac output. Nitroglycerin may be helpful by increasing coronary blood flow and, perhaps, contributing to afterload reduction. Beta blockers are considered only if undesirable tachycardia is an issue because contractility must be maintained as near to normal as is possible. If difficulties with cardiac performance arise, an important maneuver is to lower the insufflation pressure as much as possible. The surgeon may be able to perform the operation with a lesser degree of abdominal distention to lessen the physiologic impasse to the compromised patient. Similarly, extremes of position may be modified. At times, despite all efforts, conversion to an open technique may be necessary. Patients and families should, of course, always be informed of such possibilities, preoperatively.

• RESPIRATORY SYSTEM CHANGES DURING LAPAROSCOPY

Because of unusual patient positioning and insufflation of the peritoneal cavity, laparoscopic surgery produces profound changes in the respiratory system. Carbon dioxide absorption from the peritoneal cavity into the blood stream may increase the effective carbon dioxide production (VCO_2) by 20% to 30% and easily produce hypercarbia. In addition, increases in abdominal pressure, secondary to insufflation of the peritoneal cavity, lead to a decrease in the efficiency of ventilation and impaired ability to handle the increased carbon dioxide load. Both of these factors require discussion.

Induction of general anesthesia is followed by a well-documented decrease in functional residual capacity (FRC). There are numerous factors contributing to this volume loss including cephalad shift of the diaphragm, loss of inspiratory muscle tone, and changes in intrathoracic blood volume. These changes are even more significant in the obese patient in whom the weight of the abdominal contents leads to even more cephalad shift of the diaphragm. Insufflation of the peritoneal cavity will further aggravate this problem by the direct pressure exerted on the diaphragm by the insufflating gas. In a sense, the normal patient becomes more like an obese one. The net result of this lower FRC will be a tendency toward atelectasis and an increase in the magnitude of ventilation-perfusion (V/Q) mismatching, largely in the form of low V/Q areas, that is, with low ventilation relative to perfusion. While severe hypoxemia will rarely occur, there will clearly be an increase in the alveolar to arterial oxygen tension gradient.

There is a significant decrease in compliance of the respiratory system during laparoscopy. Studies have shown that the decreased compliance is caused by changes in both the chest wall and the lungs. When the abdomen is distended, the result is increased stiffness of the entire chest wall (comprising rib cage, diaphragm, and abdominal wall and contents). This leads to increases in intrathoracic pressure, which diminish venous return and cardiac output. The cephalad movement of the diaphragm decreases FRC and explains some of the observed decreased lung compliance, as well. Increases in lung resistance caused by reduced lung volumes produce increased airway pressures with the potential for further aggravation of V/Q mismatching by overdistending some lung areas. This same overdistention may also lead to rupture of bullae, with resultant pneumothorax in at-risk patients with emphysematous pulmonary changes.

Patient positioning will also significantly affect the mechanics of the respiratory system. The Trendelenberg position is characterized by additional upward pressure on the diaphragm by the abdominal contents. The reverse Trendelenberg position is actually helpful in this regard because it tends to offset the adverse effect of increased intraabdominal pressure on the cephalad translation of the diaphragm. However, the reverse Trendelenberg position does not completely correct the problem because of its adverse hemodynamic effects. Decreases in cardiac output lead to a decrease in mixed-venous oxygen saturation, which is not well tolerated in the presence of pulmonary shunting, or more specifically, increased venous admixture, already so prevalent in the anesthetized patient.

Most patients will not be significantly impaired by these alterations to the respiratory system. However, obese patients and those with obstructive pulmonary disease may be at far greater risk. Obese patients may not tolerate the additional decreases in FRC and compliance imposed on the already significant decreases associated with induction of anesthesia. Patients with obstructive disease or emphysema usually have inefficiencies in ventilatory function, which are intensified by the pneumoperitoneum. These patients may develop severe difficulties with carbon dioxide elimination.

Carbon dioxide is absorbed from the peritoneal cavity during laparoscopy. The exact amount absorbed is variable, but may be significant. As much as a 30% increase in carbon dioxide delivery to the lungs has been measured, necessitating a similar increase in minute ventilation. Volumes of carbon dioxide were shown to increase from approximately 150 ml/min to 200 ml/min in one study. It is the elimination of this additional metabolic gas load that is often the most problematic task during the conduct of the anesthetic. Studies of arterial carbon dioxide tension, following peritoneal insufflation with gases other than carbon dioxide, have usually demonstrated levels closer to normal, thereby implicating carbon dioxide absorption as a significant factor in the increase. As discussed earlier, carbon dioxide, nevertheless, remains the insufflating gas of choice because other gases have distinct disadvantages.

Early studies of anesthesia for laparoscopic procedures demonstrated significant hypercarbia in spontaneously ventilating patients. Such management without controlled ventilation is no longer considered acceptable. Most healthy patients are effectively and safely managed by a reasonable increase in minute ventilation of 10% to 15% and do not suffer significant hypercarbia. However, normocarbia is not always ensured by this management approach and hypercarbia may be difficult to detect because of unnoticed increases in end-tidal-to-arterial carbon dioxide gradients, resulting from reduced cardiac output and/or V/Q mismatching, which leads to falsely low carbon dioxide readings. As a result of this process, patients with pulmonary disease or significant cardiac disease are at additional risk of developing hypercarbia. Low preoperative levels of forced expiratory volume in 1 second (FEV_1) and vital capacity and high ASA physical status scores have been identified as risk factors for the development of intraoperative hypercarbia. Studies have shown hypercarbia refractory to increases of minute ventilation of up to 2 times baseline levels. End-tidal-to-arterial carbon dioxide gradients are unreliable and variable, and detection of the presence or absence of hypercarbia will require actual serial measurement of arterial blood gases. Therefore, in patients with significant cardiopulmonary disease, it is mandatory to monitor intraoperative arterial blood gases during the laparoscopic procedure to prevent potentially dangerous undetected arterial hypercarbia.

There are two complications of insufflation that have profound influence on the respiratory system, either by directly affecting its function or by overwhelming its capabilities. On occasion, persistent pleuroperitoneal communications may be present and lead directly to pneumothorax upon peritoneal insufflation. Surgical trauma to the diaphragm may also result in such a situation. As this is functionally a tension pneumothorax and carries with it all of the associated adverse hemodynamic and respiratory effects, the procedure will almost certainly not be able to be accomplished without opening the abdomen. Emergent, intraoperative tube thoracostomy may also be required to decompress the pleural space. Tension pneumothorax may be identified by its late, severe hemodynamic sequelae but may be detected earlier by a sudden rise in inspiratory plateau pressure caused by lung collapse and the accompanying decrease in lung compliance.

Insufflated gas commonly escapes outside the peritoneal cavity and, in fact, usually does not enter the pleural space. Most commonly, the gas will track up into the mediastinum and then into the neck. Similarly, the gas may escape from trocar sites into abdominal subcutaneous tissues with potential spread into the groins or chest wall. Use of minimally invasive techniques with insufflation outside of the peritoneal cavity, such as in the preperitoneal space for inguinal hernia repair, places the patient at even greater risk from extensive, subcutaneous emphysema of carbon dioxide gas. In fact, there is much more extensive spread of gas and a much larger quantity of carbon dioxide absorbed systematically with such techniques, even though the initial operative space is much smaller.

While not causing any adverse hemodynamic or respiratory system effects directly, such extensive spread of carbon dioxide may result in a highly significant increase in the systemic absorption of carbon dioxide. Occasionally, it is necessary to convert to an open technique, even in healthy patients in such situations because of the inability to adequately excrete this significant carbon dioxide load. Arterial pH monitoring is mandatory to determine when such carbon dioxide loads are reaching dangerous levels.

Rarely, subcutaneous emphysema will significantly affect the submucosal spaces in the pharyngeal tissues and place the patient at risk for upper airway compromise. Subcutaneous emphysema is not uncommon in the skin of the neck, and when this is noticed, one must rule out the presence of airway involvement before extubation. Also, one must remember that when extensive subcutaneous gas is present, there is a significant demand being placed on the respiratory system for carbon dioxide excretion, and the patient can be expected to be tachypneic and, thus, dynamically worsen any upper airway obstruction. There will be a reduced margin of safety from any potential airway obstruction with the need for high minute ventilation in the early postoperative period.

Certain adjustments in surgical technique may increase the patient's ability to tolerate laparoscopy. Minimal uses of adverse positioning may be helpful. An obese patient may well tolerate the reverse Trendelenberg position needed for upper abdominal surgery but not do well with head-down positioning used in laparoscopically assisted vaginal hysterectomy. Use of some of the newer abdominal wall retracting devices may allow creation of an adequate pneumoperitoneum, without increased intraabdominal pressure. Similarly, such devices can provide adequate abdominal wall lifting in many cases, allowing surgeon to perform gasless laparoscopy. Once again, in the high-risk patient, the probability of complications and their resultant adverse effects will be lessened by the use of the minimum necessary insufflating pressure.

COMPLICATIONS

Laparoscopic surgery may result in a number of complications. The extensive alterations in normal physiology, which result from peritoneal insufflation and patient positioning, may lead to cardiac complications in a patient at risk. Patients with pulmonary disease are also at risk for postoperative events, as will be discussed in the following section. There are additional complications directly related to the surgical procedure which should be mentioned. Damage to various structures with the Verres needle or a trocar occurs in 0.1% to 1.0% of cases. Reports exist documenting that virtually all intraabdominal structures have been injured at some time. Perforations or injury to the bowel, bladder, liver, spleen, omentum, and major vessels have been reported. The latter can be life-threatening if not detected immediately. Late herniation of the abdominal contents through a previous abdominal wall trocar site can result in the need for additional surgery.

One of the most feared complications of laparoscopy is intravascular entry of gas, or gas embolism. Penetration of a major vessel during insufflation, particularly with a Verres needle, can lead to the immediately life-threatening complication of venous gas embolism. The solubility of carbon dioxide is high, and there are multiple mechanisms for carriage of carbon dioxide gas within the red blood cells. This certainly represents an advantage if gas is absorbed in large quantities, especially when compared to embolization of nitrogen-containing room air, such as that entrained during a sitting craniotomy, for example. Still, rapid entry of gas poses a major risk to the patient. Flow rates should be kept low (about 1 l/min) until it has been established that the needle or trocar is correctly placed. Reports of cardiovascular collapse and arrest have been attributed to gas embolism. Suspicion of this complication follows the detection of hypotension, tachycardia, dysrhythmias, ECG evidence of right ventricular strain, mill wheel murmur, increases in filling pressures, if measured, and alteration in capnographic tracings. Interestingly, a biphasic pattern would be present on the capnograph with an initial rise in end-tidal carbon dioxide from the embolism, followed by a decrease secondary to diminished cardiac output. Treatment requires the immediate deflation of the peritoneal cavity, cessation of nitrous oxide administration, placement in a head-down and left-lateral decubitus position, and hemodynamic support until recovery ensues. Reports of successful gas aspiration from the right side of the heart, using existing central venous catheters, exist. Patients have also been salvaged using cardiopulmonary bypass. Unfortunately, however, this rare event (estimated 0.1% incidence) is often fatal.

The creation of increased intraabdominal pressure may predispose to gastric regurgitation with the risk of pulmonary aspiration. The use of nitrous oxide can result in bowel distention, which may hamper the surgical procedure if significant amounts of intraluminal gas are present. The use of nitrous oxide is somewhat controversial for other reasons. Nitrous oxide will diffuse into the peritoneal cavity as it will into any closed, gas-containing space. There is a risk of explosion if three events occur simultaneously: bowel injury with leakage of methane or other flammable gas from the gut, use of cautery, and concentrations of diffused nitrous oxide into the peritoneal space. Despite this theoretical risk, the authors routinely use nitrous oxide unless directly contraindicated by the presence of significant intraluminal air.

Other surgical complications such as injury to adjacent structures, that is, the bile duct, or bleeding and infection may occur, but are not unique to laparoscopic techniques. Significant morbidity may result from such injuries, particularly if they go unrecognized during the procedure. The anesthesiologist must also be prepared for sudden, significant, and unexpected intraabdominal hemorrhage which during a laparoscopic procedure poses a much greater likelihood of imminent hypovolemic shock to the patient. This is because control of hemorrhage may be difficult to impossible using a laparoscopic approach, and, if this is truly the case, considerable delay may result before arrest of the hemorrhage can be accomplished through creation of an emergent celiotomy. Rapid infusion of crystalloid and, if available, blood products may be suddenly required in such situations.

POSTOPERATIVE CONSIDERATIONS

Pain after laparoscopy is significantly less than that following any comparable open procedure. Nevertheless, postoperative pain is variable and unpredictable. Somatic abdominal wall pain, the predominant complaint following open procedures, is present but is less severe and is readily controlled with a small dose of systemic narcotic. There is a tendency to treat this pain solely with nonsteroidal medications and local anesthetics placed at the time of wound closure. Ketorolac can be given systematically during the procedure and is effective at reducing analgesic requirements. While no definitive data exist, one must consider the potential side effects on platelets. The ability to control bleeding laparoscopically is reduced, compared to that possible with direct hands-on surgery. One may choose to withhold nonsteroidal agents until the end of the procedure when bleeding has ceased. It still takes a highly motivated patient with a high pain threshold to completely avoid narcotics in the postoperative period. The use of narcotics is best kept to a minimum for those patients expected to be discharged following minor laparoscopic cases. The combination of narcotics and motion (necessary for ambulating) is a great stimulus for debilitating nausea and vomiting.

Following major laparoscopic operations such as cholecystectomy, visceral discomfort is more difficult to treat and is an unpredictable variable. This pain revolves around the amount of retained gas in the peritoneal cavity and irritation of the parietal peritoneal surfaces. Interestingly, carbon dioxide leads to more discomfort than nitrous oxide when used as the insufflating gas because of the irritation of the carbolic acid formed at the parietal peritoneum upon absorption of carbon dioxide. There is significant interpatient variability and, in fact, intrapatient variability when compared to previous experiences with similar procedures. Pain is commonly experienced in the shoulders and is attributable to diaphragmatic irritation by the retained gas. Four fifths of cholecystectomy patients have neck and shoulder pain 24 hours following surgery; fully one half of patients still complain at 48 hours. Occasionally, discomfort may persist for days.

Various maneuvers have been used to treat postoperative pain. Nonsteroidals are effective as previously mentioned. Local anesthetics injected into fallopian tubes, the rectus sheath, trocar wounds, and even as irrigant solutions placed into the peritoneal cavity and onto diaphragmatic surfaces, are relatively effective for the duration of the drugs' action. Efforts have even been made to warm the insufflated carbon dioxide gas in an attempt to eliminate hypothermia and the contributions made by this gas to postoperative pain.

Postoperative nausea and vomiting are a significant problem following any intraabdominal procedure, and laparoscopic procedures are no exception. The incidence ranges from 40% to 75%. Narcotics clearly increase the incidence while propofol used as an induction agent may decrease the frequency. Prophylactic use of ondansetron is helpful, although routine use may represent an unnecessary expense. Etiologies of nausea are multiple and include side effects from anesthetic drugs (especially narcotics) and manipulation of intraabdominal viscera and the ileus which results. Routine drainage of the stomach will decrease the unpleasantness of nausea at the expense of considerable discomfort associated with the tube itself. At a minimum, the stomach should always be aspirated at the end of the procedure. A tube is always present, having been used earlier in the surgery.

One of the main advantages of minimally invasive surgery is in the recovery phase, with the expectation of reduced pulmonary morbidity. Abdominal surgery, particularly of the upper abdomen, produces profound effects on postoperative pulmonary function. A restrictive pattern of breathing is noted with significant reductions in forced vital capacity and FEV_1, largely caused by decreased inspiratory capacity. There is a diminution of the diaphragmatic contribution to breathing and a tendency toward hypoxemia. There is a simultaneous decrease in lung defense mechanisms, with alterations in mucociliary flow. Postoperative pain is partially responsible for these abnormalities, although effective epidural analgesia only partially restores lung volumes. Reflex inhibition of diaphragmatic function presumably results from nociceptive activation of visceral or somatic afferents. While numerous studies have shown much improvement in these abnormal values following laparoscopic approaches to comparable open procedures, the unfortunate reality is that significant alterations, nevertheless, occur. There is still a 20% to 40% decrease in vital capacity after laparoscopic cholecystectomy. This is one half of the decrease following open cholecystectomy. Fortunately, it also resolves in one half the time, usually over the first 2 or 3 days. Values of forced expiratory flows dropped by 25% versus 50% in the open surgical counterparts, but slight abnormalities were still noted after 72 hours in some studies.

Reductions in the previously mentioned lung volumes result in decreases in functional residual capacity (FRC); this leads to atelectasis and hypoxemia. Smaller reductions in FRC are noted after laparoscopic surgery, but there is significant variability between patients. Larger decreases in FRC may be seen the groups of patients who are smokers, are obese, elderly, or have underlying pulmonary disease.

Reflex inhibition of the diaphragm, though less in magnitude following laparoscopic procedures, is qualitatively similar to that seen following open operations. The postoperative time course for these changes is also similar to those following other abdominal procedures; initial near-normal tidal breathing in the immediate postoperative course is followed by decreased abdominal contributions after a few hours. These abnormalities will be well tolerated in younger, healthier patients and may have significant morbid effects on those more compromised patients. It is important to ensure that aggressive breathing exercises and pulmonary toilet are performed, despite the current thrusts toward early discharge of patients from the hospital. Pulmonary complications of atelectasis, hypoxia, and, possibly, pneumonia may still develop a few days postoperatively, even after a patient is sent home if ambulatory activity is not resumed.

BIBLIOGRAPHY

Couture JG, et al: Diaphragmatic and abdominal muscle activity after endoscopic cholecystectomy, *Anesth Analg* 78:733–739, 1994.

Cunningham AJ, McCoy D: Anesthetic implications of laparoscopic surgery. *Advances in anesthesia*, vol 11, St. Louis, 1994, Mosby-Year Book.

Dhoste K, et al: Haemodynamic and ventilatory changes during laparoscopic cholecystectomy in elderly ASA III patients, *Can J Anaesth* 43:783–788, 1996.

Iwasaka H, Yamamoto H, Taniguchi K: Respiratory mechanics and arterial blood gases during and after laparoscopic cholecystectomy, *Can J Anaesth* 43:129–133, 1996.

Mullet CE, et al: Pulmonary CO_2 elimination during surgical procedures useing intra- or extraperitoneal CO_2 insufflation, *Anesth Analg* 76:622–626, 1993.

Wahba RWM, Tessler MJ, Kleiman SJ: Acute ventilatory complications during laparoscopic upper abdominal surgery, *Can J Anaesth* 43:77–83, 1996.

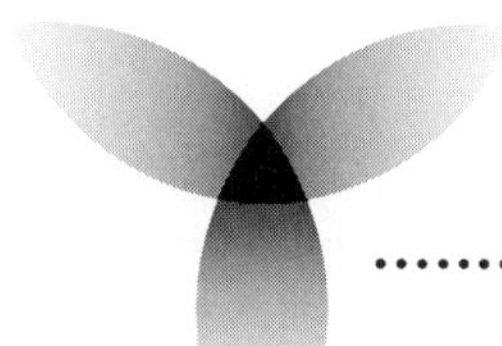

Chapter 32

Major Vascular Surgery

David L. Bogdonoff, MD, Mark E. Lovelock, MBBS, FRACS

Vascular surgery is an evolving discipline with significant complexity and patient acuity. It represents a subspecialty area within general surgery and claims some neuro- and cardiovascular surgeons (intracranial, cardiac, and thoracic vascular procedures will not be discussed here). The incidence and severity of concomitant medical diseases are high and contribute significantly to intra- and postoperative morbidity and mortality in vascular surgical patients. Perhaps in no other surgical discipline are the preoperative assessment and optimization of the patient so important. The role of the medical consultant is integral to this process and continues after surgery with the need for sophisticated intensive care and cardiopulmonary monitoring.

The urgency and timing of vascular procedures ranges from the immediate life-threatening repair of a ruptured abdominal aortic aneurysm to the purely elective endarterectomy for asymptomatic carotid stenosis or aortoiliac bypass grafting for chronic claudication. The opportunity for careful preoperative assessment and planning will, therefore, also vary between the two extremes, as well. The implications of a surgical intervention derive from the underlying medical comorbidity and from the effects of temporary or permanent cessation of blood flow in the vascular beds supplied by vessels in the surgical field. Major central nervous system (CNS), renal, and gastrointestinal complications may result, requiring expensive and demanding medical care, and producing significant morbidity and mortality. Interruption of flow to lower extremity nerve and muscle tissue, though less essential to the survival of the organism, may, nevertheless, result in major patient morbidity and necessitate prolonged rehabilitative care and permanent alterations in lifestyle.

Following general comments common to all vascular surgical patients, three major categories of vascular procedures will each be considered sequentially. The physiologic ramifications of the different procedures are sufficiently different as to drastically alter the approaches to care of the same patient being considered for different procedures.

PREOPERATIVE ASSESSMENT

The risk of complications in any given vascular surgery patient is approximately 30%. Such risks will only increase as the population ages and as more complicated surgical procedures are performed. Successes are commonplace given the increasing sophistication of pre-, intra- and postoperative care. These successes are not inexpensive; rather, they consume an inordinately large portion of financial and human resources. The challenge, therefore, remains to attempt to risk-stratify the vascular patient to determine which patient will benefit from the most aggressive evaluation and care and which patient will do fine with somewhat less attention.

Vascular surgery patients are burdened by the effects on other organ systems of the same etiologic factors that have led to their vascular disease. Hypertension, diabetes, and tobacco abuse are the major culprits and lead to significant cardiopulmonary comorbidity. Chronologic age itself is a risk factor because the elderly patient will have a higher likelihood of having a concomitant disease and, in fact, will respond less well to the stresses of surgery. Vascular patients seem to have a greater physiologic age than chronologic age because of their various comorbid medical conditions. Cardiac disease is responsible for the majority of intra- and postoperative morbidity and mortality in this patient group and rightly deserves the attention it receives in the hierarchy of preoperative assessment.

Cardiac Evaluation

Significant coronary artery disease has a high prevalence in patients with both atherosclerotic occlusive disease and aneurysmal disease. Between 50% and 70% of patients presenting for vascular surgery will be found to have significant coronary artery disease. At least one third will have evidence of previous myocardial infarction and a smaller fraction will have active angina at the time of presentation. Severity of disease is often masked by diabetes, given its high association with silent ischemia, and by physical inactivity. This inactivity comes from the infirmities of increasing age and from the limitations to activity resulting from symptomatic peripheral vascular disease.

Cardiac evaluation has been well covered in its own previous chapters but will be briefly discussed in this setting. Two questions must be addressed initially. What is the level of ventricular function, and how much myocardium is at risk for infarction caused by ischemia? These two questions are entertained by some of the criteria contained in various, multifunctional cardiac-risk indices, initially and subsequently championed by Goldman. Ultimately, however, these questions and the results of risk stratification must be integrated, along with a determination of the severity of the proposed surgical procedure and the expected physiologic implications of the intra- and postoperative events. For example, the Goldman index has been shown to *under*estimate the degree of cardiac risk for aortic aneurysm patients. Most likely, this is because of the high degree of physiologic stress represented by the procedure, compared with other surgical interventions.

There has been much debate in the literature concerning the use of preoperative percutaneous transluminal coronary angioplasty (PTCA) or coronary artery bypass grafting (CABG) in the vascular surgical population. No consensus has been achieved and each approach has its advocates. Many of the studies have involved aortic surgical patients because these are clearly the highest-risk vascular surgical group. Significant coronary artery lesions as documented by angiography are found in almost 30% of even asymptomatic patients presenting for abdominal aortic aneurysm surgery. Enough cases have been done to date to show that when the mortality rates for CABG and subsequent postCABG aneurysm rupture are combined, there is no overall reduction in mortality from that of aneurysm surgery performed without the benefit of the preoperative coronary revascularization. Some have chosen to do both CABG and aneurysm repair simultaneously. The major risk is rupture of the aortic aneurysm postCABG caused by increased collagenase activity. The size of the aneurysm will need to be considered. The largest (>9cm) aneurysms will require repair preCABG or during CABG, while smaller aneurysms may allow temporization and be repaired at a later date. The use of PTCA in this situation, when feasible, should not place the patient at increased risk from peri-procedure aneurysm rupture and may be advantageous. Because of the considerable postPTCA restenosis rate, surgical intervention should be undertaken between 3 days and 3 months following angioplasty.

Pulmonary Considerations

The pulmonary implications of the heavy tobacco use in this patient population are obvious. Whenever possible, cessation of smoking should be encouraged and optimization of respiratory symptomatology should be accomplished. When problematic, the underlying pulmonary status will alter the anesthetic management of the patient, depending on the site of surgery. For example, one might consider regional anesthesia for those vascular procedures not requiring an abdominal incision. Similarly, pain management schemes may be altered toward the same goals of avoidance of perioperative pulmonary complications. Epidural pain analgesia is being used more commonly for aortic cases with great success. Additionally, surgeons may wish to alter techniques, such as with the use of a retroperitoneal approach to the aorta, the transabdominal approach is the one with the greatest challenge.

Diabetes

As discussed previously, there is no single best approach to diabetic management. As with pulmonary disease, the type of vascular procedure may well determine the diabetes management schema. For example, the major stress and prolonged fasting which follows abdominal aortic surgery will preclude a simpler approach that may be taken in a peripheral vascular case which permits the early resumption of dietary intake. Carotid surgery with its known potential risk for intraoperative cerebral ischemia requires the most stringent control because of the possibility of neural injury aggravation in the presence of hyperglycemia.

Hypertension

Blood pressure management in the vascular patient needs to be managed with potentially conflicting goals. Hypotension must be avoided because of its potential adverse effects on vascular beds distal to coexisting uncorrected arterial stenoses, particularly in the myocardium. Hypertension, though less worrisome preoperatively, will be a considerable risk factor in the postoperative period with the presence of new arterial suture lines.

SURGICAL PROCEDURES

Carotid Endarterectomy

Carotid endarterectomy is a serious undertaking because of the significant potential for cardiac and, particularly, neurologic morbidity. The latter is responsible for most of the anxiety of the referring physician, patient, and surgeon even though cardiac morbidity is responsible for the majority of the actual risks from the procedure. Nevertheless, the procedure produces a relatively minor physiologic impasse, as far as the surgical wound and postoperative recovery period is concerned.

RELEVANT ANATOMY

The carotid artery is superficial in the neck. Structures that must be sacrificed to gain access are crossing veins, minor neck muscles, superficial cervical nerves innervating skin over the neck and chin, and small branches of the ansa cervicalis, which innervate the strap muscles. Significant structures that are nearby and at risk of injury include the hypoglossal nerve and the vagus nerve, including its laryngeal branches. The surgical procedure takes place adjacent to the airway that is susceptible to obstruction from a postoperative hematoma resulting from arterial suture-line bleeding.

INTRAOPERATIVE PHYSIOLOGY

The superficial nature of the procedure means that so-called "third space" losses of fluid are minimal. This is occasionally problematic for the inattentive anesthesiologist who is used to much larger fluid losses in almost all other surgical procedures. Care must be taken to avoid fluid overload, particularly in the patient with impaired contractility who is at risk for congestive failure or when the surgeon plans to use a platelet-inactivating (and volume-expanding) agent such as Dextran postoperatively.

During the endarterectomy, flow through the common, external, and internal carotid arteries will be interrupted. Even if shunting is to be performed, 3 or 4 minutes of cessation of flow are to be expected. Patient tolerance of this brief, yet significant, lack of flow is determined by multiple variables, some of which are unknown preoperatively and intraoperatively. A patient with a severe stenosis may, in fact, not have much flow to lose from cross-clamping, while the patient being operated on for a symptomatic ulcerated plaque would have essentially normal baseline internal carotid blood flow. The anatomic completeness of the Circle of Willis and the extent of any simultaneous stenosis in the contralateral carotid system are the predominant factors affecting the patient's ability to tolerate the procedure from the viewpoint of neurologic survival. Intracranial atherosclerotic lesions in distal vessels can be problematic. A lack of normal cerebral autoregulation can also be problematic, such as would be present in areas of brain suffering from recent stroke, reversible ischemic neurologic deficit (RIND), or transient ischemic attack (TIA). While a recent permanent ischemic insult used to represent an absolute contraindication to endarterectomy, it has evolved currently to become only a relative contraindication.

The debate over the use of intraoperative shunts to reestablish internal carotid arterial blood flow during the endarterectomy has continued for the last 3 decades since the development of the surgical procedure. Various determinants have been used in the decision-making process, including the degree of contralateral occlusion on arteriography, estimation of the degree of backbleeding from the cranium or the measurements of the pressure driving that flow, and determinations of neurologic function as assessed by any of a variety of neurologic function monitors. There has been no correlation between stump pressure, electroencephalogram transcranial doppler, or angiography and the need for shunting. The only correlation between clamping of the carotid and neurologic function has been in the awake patient. One can find a report in the literature to support virtually any opinion. Hence, no universally applicable algorithm can be developed at this time. Furthermore, while shunting may elegantly permit both the normalization of cerebral blood flow and the avoidance of compensatory maneuvers necessary to counteract the occlusion, it is not always universally successful. If suboptimally performed, shunting may not result in adequate flow if technical problems such as kinking or tip obstruction occur. Additionally, placement of a shunt may, in fact, result in distal embolization or irreparable damage to the internal carotid artery.

In the absence of shunting, efforts are made to increase flow to the areas theoretically placed at risk by the temporary arterial occlusion. Characteristically, these efforts represent measures to increase blood pressure (usually by approximately 20%) to enhance the potential for blood flow through collateral vessels. Blood pressure can be increased by a decrease in the concentration of a volatile anesthetic or with the infusion of a vasopressor. There is a debate in the anesthetic literature concerning the risks involved in either approach. A patient with significant cardiac risk factors may not tolerate these interventions well, and one must take care to monitor closely for myocardial ischemia. The choice of anesthetic agent may have an impact, at least on a theoretical level. Studies have shown that some anesthetic agents allow the CNS to tolerate a lower total blood flow than other agents. Clinical studies of carotid endarterectomy patients, however, were unable to show any outcome differences between the agents. The manipulation of carbon dioxide tension is another available modality, although there are theoretical advantages to both hyper- and hypocarbia, depending on the actual intracranial anatomy and physiology at the time of cross clamping. Generally, the patient is kept normocarbic unless there is identifiable evidence of cerebral ischemia, in which case, an intentional change in ventilation may be considered. The latter is, in fact, clinically a rare event. This is, perhaps, largely because of the current lack of highly effective neurologic monitoring.

While details of neurologic monitoring techniques are outside the scope of this chapter, a brief discussion of their use is relevant. The explosion of computer technology in the last decade has resulted in a proliferation of available devices, although verification of their usefulness has yet to be established. The gold standard for monitoring (in the anesthetized patient) is the continual presence of a neurologist assessing the output from real-time, multichannel electroencephalogram (EEG). Standard, multiple-lead systems are used, just as in the EEG laboratory. The actual presence of the neurologist in the operating room can be avoided by sophisticated telemetric networks, but real-time assessment is still necessary to provide the necessary relevant feedback to the operating surgeon. The complexity and expense of formal EEG techniques is such that it is the rare center that can provide this level of service. Additionally, it is difficult, if not impossible, to claim that such sophisticated and labor-intensive monitoring actually leads to better operative results. Computerized analysis of EEG signals from a reduced number of leads is cheaper, more user-friendly, and has found its way into many operating rooms. Compressed spectral array, density spectral array, and other similar compression and presentation schemes are in widespread use. One looks for alterations in electrical activity following carotid occlusion and, presumably, uses the information to make decisions on shunting or physiologic manipulations during the endarterectomy. There is little evidence for the efficacy of these practices. However, it may be suggested that some form of monitoring should be the standard of care.

Somatosensory evoked potentials are also now more readily available and have been proposed for intraoperative cerebral monitoring. While less prone to artifact from electrosurgic units than other techniques, they are flawed by their significant sensitivity to almost all general anesthetic drugs.

One must remember that perhaps the best neurologic monitor is the physical examination. To this end, many surgical teams perform carotid endarterectomy under superficial and deep cervical plexus block, with the awake patient providing the ultimate in neurologic feedback. Regional techniques, seemingly elegant because of their avoidance of general anesthesia, have not been shown to be any safer in terms of cardiac risk. It is critical that the anesthesia team not oversedate the patient into a state of disorientation which can result in confusion regarding the cause of the neurologic changes. Nevertheless, a regional technique remains another option to be considered by the patient and the surgical team.

Intraoperative hemodynamic changes are to be expected. Dissection of the carotid sinus is necessary and intraoperative manipulation of this structure can be expected to cause severe bradycardia. Injection of the carotid sinus or the nerve innervating the sinus with local anesthesia will alleviate the bradycardia. Alternatively, the anesthesiologist can administer an anticholinergic drug such as atropine; but, this is potentially troublesome because it may lead to tachycardia and an adverse myocardial oxygen supply/demand ratio. Some surgeons will choose to permanently denervate the sinus.

POSTOPERATIVE MANAGEMENT AND COMPLICATIONS

Postoperative blood pressure changes are common and potentially problematic. Patients may be hypotensive, presumably because of the activity of an intact carotid sinus being exposed to higher blood pressure after endarterectomy has removed previously obstructive atherosclerotic plaque. One half of all patients will remain normotensive and not require intervention. The majority of patients, however, will need treatment for hypertension. Even though many patients are hypertensive preoperatively and, hence, will be hypertensive in the postoperative period, surgical stress and the potential for carotid-sinus damage lead to an even higher incidence of blood pressure elevation.

The incidence of hypo- and hypertension in different studies is likely explained, in great part, by differing treatment of the carotid sinus by individual surgeons. When the carotid sinus is intentionally denervated, the incidence of hypertension is increased. Studies showing high levels of activity in carotid sinus baroreceptor nerves in hypotensive patients confirm these suspicions.

Hypertension and hypotension have both been shown to increase perioperative morbidity, independent from other surgical variables. While hypotension may obviously lead to regional or global perfusion deficits, hypertension is particularly dangerous in the patient with previous stroke. Recovering areas of brain tissue may not have intact autoregulation and they are susceptible to hemorrhage from the higher local blood pressures which follow endarterectomy and uncontrolled hypertension. The choice of antihypertensive regimens must involve a consideration of any underlying ventricular dysfunction or coronary insufficiency.

The carotid body chemoreceptor is often denervated by endarterectomy, but this is usually of no clinical significance. Bilateral loss of carotid chemoreceptor activity will result in an absence of hypoxic ventilatory drive. The need for such respiratory drive is clinically rare, except in severe pulmonary disease. The common use of oximetry essentially makes this a moot point.

Cardiac morbidity is a major concern in the postoperative period. Hemodynamic disturbances, particularly hypertension, are commonplace as previously mentioned. The awake patient, particularly when cold and shivering, has a higher myocardial oxygen demand and, likely, a higher cardiac risk than the closely monitored and hemodynamically manipulated intraoperative patient. Careful monitoring for ischemia is crucial. A patient at exceptionally high risk may well benefit from intensive care monitoring for 2 days or longer. Most patients, however, will only require a day in an intensive care unit (ICU) or step-down unit. Patient care beds equipped with electrocardiographic telemetry may be an acceptable alternative to an ICU bed. Care must be taken to avoid fluid overload in the patient with poor myocardial function.

Neurologic complications are an obvious concern. Surveillance for such problems begins immediately following the procedure. An anesthetic technique is usually chosen to accomplish the desired goal of early restoration of consciousness after skin closure. An assessment of neurologic function is made at this point in the operating room. In the past, evidence of new neurologic dysfunction would be an indication for reexploration, to rule out occlusion of the carotid artery. Today, this possibility remains in the differential diagnosis for new neurologic abnormalities; but, noninvasive studies, that is, duplex scanning, would usually be invoked to determine that flow was present in the operated artery. An intraoperative embolic event or injury from ischemia during cross-clamping is the usual cause of new deficits. Swelling of a previously ischemic area of the brain, caused by new perfusion pressure, may also contribute to neurologic dysfunction. Swelling usually resolves in the postoperative period.

New neurologic deficits may arise in the postoperative period, even when the patient awakens from surgery with a normal examination. Embolic debris, in the form of platelet-fibrin complexes, may form on the rough surface of the endarterectomized vessel. For this reason, some surgeons will choose not to reverse anticoagulation initially, and will place the patient on an antiplatelet medical regimen. Virtually all patients receive aspirin pre- and postoperatively. While clearly addressing the potential for neurologic risk, these practices create a new risk of bleeding.

The risk of bleeding is of significant concern after any vascular procedure with arterial suture lines. The length of the suture line directly correlates with this risk, as does the use of anticoagulation regimens. The skin closure creates a closed space. Any bleeding which is not removed by the surgical drain is left to create an expanding mass. The patient must be closely observed for any evidence of bleeding for two reasons. An expanding hematoma will compress the trachea or upper airway, and may compress the carotid artery as well and lead to thrombosis. Airway obstruction is insidious and must be taken seriously. A patient who is noticed to have minimal symptoms of stridor or dyspnea from blood in the neck may go on to airway obstruction in a short period of time. Confusion or anxiety may often be the first sign of an expanding hematoma. At this point, intubation may be impossible, even by the most skilled anesthesiologist, because of the severe distortion of anatomy caused by bleeding into the cervical tissues. Treatment must be instituted immediately. Ideally, the patient should be intubated and taken back to the operating room for reexploration. Equipment for the performance of a surgical airway must be at hand. Opening of the wound to allow egress of accumulated blood may temporize the situation, but one must be prepared to place a sterile finger over an arterial bleeding site to avoid major blood loss. The previous use of a regional anesthetic technique, or the placement of local anesthesia into the wound during closure, may permit reexploration of a wound in the awake patient. This could lessen the risk associated with a failed intubation scenario in such a patient.

Peripheral Vascular Surgery

Peripheral vascular surgery is usually performed to ameliorate the effects from atherosclerotic lesions resulting in distal ischemia. Occasionally, these procedures are necessary for aneurysmal disease of the femoral or popliteal vessels. While the manifestations of peripheral vascular disease are rarely life-threatening, quality-of-life issues are serious, as are the risks to the heart during and after proposed surgical interventions.

RELEVANT ANATOMY

Peripheral arteries are either superficial or can be reached by the retraction of leg and thigh muscles. Muscles rarely need to be divided; although, at times, such approaches are chosen. Adjacent structures are the accompanying veins and nerves, but careful surgical dissection usually avoids any injury to these structures. The major risk of structural damage from peripheral vascular surgery comes from the unavoidable interruption of small collateral vessels which are sacrificed during the surgical dissection. These vessels often represent a significant contribution to tissue blood flow distal to a stenotic or obstructed artery. Loss of these collaterals and any subsequent failure of the operative procedure (or a subsequent occlusion of the bypass graft) will render the extremity more ischemic than before the procedure. It is for this latter reason that many vascular surgeons will choose not to operate on peripheral vessels solely for symptoms of claudication; they will only proceed surgically in the face of threatened tissue or limb loss.

INTRAOPERATIVE PHYSIOLOGY

As with carotid surgery, peripheral vascular procedures do not create large surgical wounds which will result in significant postoperative third-space fluid losses or respiratory embarrassment from alterations in pulmonary function. However, the wounds are larger and their significant lengths do produce a slightly greater physiologic stress postoperatively.

Intraoperative occlusion of femoral or distal arteries obviously does not carry with it the significance of carotid artery occlusion or occlusion of an artery supplying a major intraabdominal organ. Chronic stenosis results in extensive collateralization of blood flow, which is also somewhat protective. Nerve and muscle tissue will tolerate at least 4 hours of total ischemia. Time factors are rarely relevant, except when vascular occlusion occurred preoperatively and the surgical procedure is being done emergently for that reason. Hemodynamic effects on the myocardium from such distal clamping of vessels would be expected to be insignificant except for only the most compromised of hearts.

Intraoperative monitoring of distal perfusion may take many forms. Simple clinical observation of the extremity after revascularization with palpation of pulses is universal. Pulse volume recording is easily performed with the use of a sterile blood pressure cuff. Intraoperative arteriography and Doppler insonation are heavily used. More sophisticated Doppler ultrasound and spectral analysis are used by some surgeons.

POSTOPERATIVE MANAGEMENT AND COMPLICATIONS

Meticulous management of blood pressure, blood sugar, and myocardial oxygenation requirements is the order for the peripheral vascular surgical patient as well. To these basic tenets, one must add meticulous wound and tissue care. Peripheral tissues are highly susceptible to even the most trivial of injuries because of their reduced blood supply. Total amelioration of all distal blood flow does not occur, even with successful peripheral vascular procedures, because of the highly diffuse nature of vascular disease. Serial assessments of the quality of peripheral perfusion and, specifically, pulse presence, quality, and, perhaps, pressure measurement, is performed to increase the likelihood of early detection of any postoperative technical failures of graft function. This will involve checking for the continued presence of distal pulses as well as an assessment of their quality, perhaps with actual pressure measurements. Early detection and reoperation are paramount in any attempt to salvage a failed graft.

Though rarely problematic in the patient with chronic peripheral ischemia, revascularization of a severely ischemic extremity may produce two important complications that may threaten both the extremity and the entire patient. Tissues rendered acutely ischemic and then revascularized within a timeframe still consistent with viability of the tissue, may suffer significant swelling. Muscles contained within tight fascial compartments (much like the brain within the skull) may suffer from secondary vascular insufficiency as tissue tensions rise to a point above that of perfusion pressure. Diagnosis of this problem, known as "compartment syndrome," is usually made purely on a clinical basis. There is pain and palpably tense tissue compartments. There may be diminution of peripheral pulses. Pain is aggravated by passive motion of a distal joint that stretches a muscle within the involved compartment. Peripheral neurologic changes are often present in the distribution of nerves running through the involved compartment. All of these clinical signs may be muddied in the vascular patient. Sensation may not be a reliable sign because it may have been lost during the acute ischemic event and, therefore, not be present at the beginning of the procedure. Similarly, a change in pulses may not be helpful unless good pulses are restored and subsequently found to be diminished and, even so, is a relatively insensitive sign. In these situations a high index of suspicion is essential and must be supplemented with a meticulous physical examination. Compartment pressures may be measured with a needle and a manometer or transducer when quantitative measurements are necessary. Pressures above 30 mm Hg necessitate surgical fasciotomy. There must be a low threshold to perform this procedure, as failure to act in time jeopardizes the extremity and the patient.

Fasciotomy may be performed prophylactically to open tissue compartments at the time of revascularization when tissue ischemia is known to have been severe. More often, however, extremities are watched postreperfusion for evidence of compartment syndrome in an attempt to avoid the unnecessary injury to tissues which may accompany fasciotomy. Whenever possible, fasciotomy is performed with a limited skin incision overlying a more extensive slit of the fascial bands above and below the incision site. Extensive skin incision may be necessary at times of severe muscle swelling, and may even need to be supplemented with fibular resection and opening of deeper compartments. Fortunately, this latter procedure is rare.

If revascularization occurs too late, nonviable muscle may place the patient at significant risk from the systemic release of tissue-breakdown products. Rhabdomyolysis results in systemic myoglobin circulation which may lead to renal shutdown and an obvious increase in potential overall morbidity and mortality. Early diagnosis follows a high index of suspicion. The presence of myoglobin in urine is detectable by the laboratory and is quantifiable. More simply, the diagnosis is made by a urine dipstick test, positive for guaiac or benzidine pigments in the absence of red cells on the microscopic urinalysis. Early intervention with osmotic and loop diuretics and urinary alkalinization may be useful. Consideration of emergent amputation must also be undertaken immediately. The severity of this last intervention is significant. It is a difficult decision to make, albeit a necessary one. Theoretically, amputation should be performed, rather than revascularization, when tissue damage is felt to be irreversible. However, it is reasonable to attempt to save tissue as long as caregivers are observant for complications that may threaten the patient as a whole. Disseminated intravascular coagulation from the systemic dissemination of other tissue products represents another potential life-threatening threat to the patient.

Bleeding from anastomoses is an obvious complication and must be cared for urgently. Because most wounds are superficial, bleeding is usually detected as soaking through wound dressings. Loss of distal perfusion caused by acute compression of arteries by contained blood is another urgent presentation. It requires reexploration and, potentially, revascularization or thrombectomy of a graft. Though distal tissues will be more forgiving in the short-term than the CNS, as in the case of a similar post-carotid complication, the potential threat to long-term outcomes is no less significant.

Abdominal Aortic Surgery

Intraabdominal aortic surgery represents the largest and physiologically most profound extrathoracic vascular surgical intervention. Access to the major intraabdominal vessels requires an extensive laparotomy and has profound effects on the blood flow to major organ systems. It may produce a particularly large stress on the cardiovascular system, which is often compromised and at significant risk. Other coexisting diseases are similarly problematic because this surgical intervention may aggravate preexisting cardiopulmonary and renal dysfunction and contribute to perioperative morbidity and mortality.

Atherosclerotic lesions account for the bulk of aortoiliac pathology and are responsible for both stenotic and aneurysmal diseases. Plaque formation either leads to gradual obliteration of the vessel lumen by the continued accumulation of atherosclerotic material or leads to degeneration of the underlying media layer with resultant vessel dilation. The latter process is aggravated by an increase in wall tension that causes a decrease in local nutritional blood supply and further arterial wall degeneration and dilation. Decisions concerning surgical intervention will vary, depending on the presence of either stenotic or aneurysmal lesions. Decisions will vary as well with factors that take into account the severity of coexisting diseases.

RELEVANT ANATOMY

Exposure of the aorta requires extensive manipulation and dissection of multiple structures and carries a significant potential for temporary or permanent damage. An extensive vertical incision is usually used, although other surgical approaches are possible, depending on the vascular anatomy. The small bowel must be mobilized laterally and the retroperitoneal portion of the duodenum must be dissected free from the aorta. Multiple lymphatic channels lie anterior to the aorta and must be divided, though this is rarely of significance. The aorta is also surrounded by a dense network of autonomic nerves, particularly those involving the sympathetic nervous system. Despite being aware of the importance of these nerves, particularly for male sexual function, some of them must be cut to gain adequate exposure. Surgeons do make efforts to avoid them (especially over the proximal left iliac artery), if at all possible, and techniques have evolved that have lessened this problem.

Other concerns with aortic exposure involve the potential for damage to other vascular structures. The left renal vein crosses the aorta, usually at the most proximal point of dissection and may be damaged or need to be sacrificed. This is usually tolerated fairly well by the kidney, as long as the vein is divided to the right of the gonadal and adrenal veins which allow alternate routes for renal venous outflow. The inferior mesenteric artery comes off the abdominal aorta in a location frequently involved with the surgical intervention. Sacrifice of this vessel is common and is usually well tolerated. Often, the vascular pathology within the aorta has already occluded this colonic artery. Nevertheless, devascularization of the colon may result, and will mandate that the surgeon verify adequacy of the sigmoid colon blood supply intraoperatively. The ureters are located near the iliac vessels and are at risk from injury, particularly during emergent surgical exposure. For aortofemoral grafting, the dissection around the ureters will also be relevant because graft placement can lead to an obstruction of urine flow.

INTRAOPERATIVE PHYSIOLOGY

There may be profound hemodynamic changes with aortic crossclamping. A much better understanding of this physiology has been achieved recently. Much of the credit goes to Simon Gelman, and this work has been well reviewed elsewhere. It is important, however, to make a distinction between aneurysmal disease and aortoiliac occlusive disease when one considers the potential consequences of aortic cross-clamping. Patients with stenotic disease already have significant obstruction to aortic flow and are less effected by the application of a totally occlusive vascular clamp. Additionally, chronic occlusive disease has usually led to the development of extensive arterial collaterals that render the tissues (pelvic and lower extremity musculature) more resistant to the loss of aortic flow occurring during cross-clamping. Therefore, despite the need for aortic cross-clamping during repair of aortoiliac occlusive disease, the physiologic implications are much less than in the patient with aneurysmal disease undergoing the comparable surgical procedure, and the patient is likely to be at considerably less risk.

The aneurysm patient does not have collateral vessels of significance and will be significantly stressed by the placement of the aortic cross-clamp. Distal tissues will be rendered acutely ischemic, and proximal afterload will be significantly increased. The response to cross-clamping is determined almost entirely by the ability of the cardiovascular system to respond to the resulting stresses. It is for this reason that a thorough preoperative evaluation of the cardiac status of the patient must be performed and optimization of cardiac function accomplished.

Aortic cross-clamping just below the level of the renal vessels causes an increase in afterload to the heart and in proximally measured systemic blood pressure. This change is caused by the mechanical effects of the clamp, as well as an increase in the systemic levels of circulating vasoconstricting substances, which result from the physiologic response to the surgical interventions. Loss of stimulation of aortic wall endothelial pressure sensors contributes to ever-increasing levels of sympathetic nervous system stimulation. Epinephrine, norepinephrine, and angiotensin have been clearly implicated, but other substances are also involved. Still, one third to one half of the observed hypertension is not caused by these factors but, rather, to observed increases in preload.

There is a simultaneous increase in preload to the heart, the reasons for which are not intuitively obvious. Decreased flow in the venous system below the level of clamping leads to a decrease in intramural venous pressure and a subsequent decrease in venous compliance. Passive recoil of these venous systems occurs, with consequent emptying and displacement of much of the contained blood back to the heart. The nature of the circulation is such that this blood is then redistributed predominantly to the upper body.

Cardiac output generally falls because of a decrease in stroke volume accompanying the increase in afterload. The increases in both preload and afterload result in an increase in myocardial contractility and a need for an increase in coronary flow. The ability to tolerate these profound physiologic changes depends on the adequacy of coronary flow reserves. Patients with severe coronary artery disease will, hence, be at significant risk for the development of intraoperative myocardial ischemia. A normal heart will not have a problem tolerating these changes and will not require an alteration in anesthetic management. On the other extreme, the compromised myocardium must be closely monitored for the development of ischemia; therapeutic interventions to counteract these adverse effects must be close at hand. Unfortunately, vascular patients are often ravaged by coronary vascular disease as well and fall into the latter category of patients with a compromised myocardium.

Nitroglycerin infusion is a useful adjunct in the care of the aneurysm patient. Its ability to augment venous capacitance serves to ameliorate the potential increases in preload. The effect of increasing coronary flow is also obviously desirable. The potential for some arterial vasodilation may exist as well, although any antihypertensive effect likely comes predominantly from a reduction in the preload's contribution to hypertension. Even in those patients without coronary artery disease the use of nitroglycerin to increase blood capacitance just before unclamping is often helpful.

Nitroprusside is commonly used intraoperatively, but, in our opinion, it should be avoided. While effective at decreasing afterload, it is less effective in accomplishing the goal of preload reduction and is devoid of salutary effects on coronary flow. In theory, coronary vasodilation from nitroprusside could lead to coronary steal. Additionally, the most significant effect of afterload reduction with this drug is a decrease in perfusion pressure below the level of aortic clamping. The result is a potential decrease in organ blood flow from collaterals. The low pressure that exists in these distal vascular beds following cross-clamping produces a situation in which organ flow is pressure-dependent and, thus, susceptible to the adverse effects of any further decrease in pressure resulting from nitroprusside.

Unclamping of the aorta is also associated with profound and potentially adverse hemodynamic effects. Hypotension invariably occurs but may be offset by a number of pharmacologic interventions, as well as by maneuvers designed to counteract the etiologic factors in the blood pressure drop. Reactive hyperemia produces arterial vasodilation and can be corrected with a small bolus of a vasoconstricting drug, such as phenylephrine or dopamine. The earlier decrease in venous capacitance will be eliminated by the return of flow to the lower extremities and blood volume will have to be expanded to refill this new void. This expansion of the total body blood capacitance at the time of unclamping represents the largest contribution to potential instability and must be properly managed by the anesthesia team. Elevation of the legs may help augment venous return. Judicious volume loading, possibly facilitated by the use of additional nitroglycerine just before unclamping, is effective toward this goal. Reduction or termination of nitroglycerin will pharmacologically counter the anatomic and physiologic increase in blood capacitance. Prophylactic use of bicarbonate, or an increase in ventilation, may be considered in an attempt to deal with the expected small acid load from the transiently ischemic distal tissues. A decrease in the level of inhalational anesthetic before unclamping is an elegantly simple and highly effective technique.

A significant drop in blood pressure at this time can be dangerous to the compromised myocardium, as well as to other organ systems if it is prolonged. Perhaps the best technique for avoidance of significant hypotension is the gradual unclamping of the aorta, conceivably with reperfusion of only one extremity at a time. Physiologic changes then occur more slowly and with less severe fluctuations from normal levels. Close communication between the surgeon and the anesthesiologist will obviously be critical at this juncture. This is most important because manual control of the graft by the surgeon's fingers will allow control over this potentially unstable situation, by controlling changes in afterload and blood flow to the extremities.

Careful observation of the distal extremities must be made to assure that adequate perfusion exists. Concomitant peripheral vascular occlusive disease in the lower extremities and the significant potential for embolization of atherosclerotic material from the aorta greatly increase the risk for distal ischemia. Similarly, adequacy of perfusion of the abdominal viscera must be verified.

Intraoperative hemorrhage is often significant. Modern techniques of cell salvage have allowed the retransfusion of much of this shed blood and have, therefore, greatly decreased blood-bank usage. Preoperative autologous donation can be used to advantage when elective procedures are being considered. Anesthetic techniques must be planned and equipment must be available to deal with this potential for massive and sudden blood loss. Hemodilution may be considered as a means to reduce the later need for transfusion of banked blood but may not be well tolerated in sicker patients.

Renal protection is paramount during aortic surgery. The threat of perioperative renal failure is real and contributes greatly to morbidity and mortality in this patient population. Abnormalities of renal function may occur intraoperatively and result predominantly from alterations of intrarenal blood flow. Total renal blood flow diminishes by 40%, initially, and does not return to baseline after clamps are released. There is a mechanical change in renal blood flow brought about by aortic cross-clamping even when occlusion occurs below the renal arteries. Humoral changes resulting from the profound stimulation of the sympathetic nervous system have significant effects on the kidney. Other substances, including prostaglandins, are involved as well. A redistribution of flow from cortex to medulla is noted.

The hallmark of renal protection is maintenance of renal blood flow intraoperatively, as well as postoperatively. This predominantly involves optimization of volume status and cardiac output. Intrarenal blood flow redistribution patterns can be partially reversed with the use of mannitol; this drug has been shown to be helpful in prospective studies. Whether the beneficial effects of mannitol resulted from intrarenal flow distribution back to the renal cortex, or simply from its advantageous effects on total body volume status is unclear. Many practitioners also consider the use of loop diuretics routinely. These drugs block active, energy-requiring, sodium reuptake and have the theoretical potential for increasing the kidney's tolerance for ischemia. Again, this may be a real effect or may simply produce more urine output that leads one to believe the kidneys are working better.

POSTOPERATIVE MANAGEMENT AND COMPLICATIONS

Hypertension and coronary insufficiency are the two major pitfalls to avoid in the postoperative period and hemodynamic management must be precise. High blood pressure is the rule rather than the exception. It is usually present preoperatively and is aggravated by the response to the surgery, as previously mentioned, and by postoperative pain and relative hypothermia. Cardiac morbidity is a major concern but one which is managed with conventional regimens.

Surgical exposure of the abdominal aorta, having required a formal laparotomy, brings to bear all of the postoperative concerns of an upper abdominal incision as discussed elsewhere. The abdominal viscera need to be mobilized, and the necessary dissection and retraction lead to postoperative ileus, with the potential for abdominal distention and further pulmonary compromise. Fluid requirements are large and continue for several hours because of ongoing third-space losses. Nasogastric decompression is essential because of the expected ileus, and to alleviate its potential contribution to abdominal distention.

Pain control is critical because of the large incision and the usual pulmonary comorbidity. Aggressive pain management techniques should be used but are controversial for a number of reasons. Epidural techniques are the gold standard for pain control but require the placement of a catheter into a patient who will require heparinization. Thus, the catheter introduces a potential for peridural bleeding with permanent neurologic damage. Added to this is the threat of paralysis from abdominal aortic clamping itself which, though rare (about 1 in 200 to 500), may well occur. Peripheral vasodilation, from the use of epidural local anesthetics intraoperatively, would carry the same risk for decreased distal-tissue perfusion which occurs with nitroprusside during crossclamping. Postoperative use of local anesthetics also carries the potential for complicating fluid management by causing peripheral venodilation. These concerns aside, more and more practitioners are using epidural techniques. There are no published large series to attest to the safety of these techniques, and more time will be necessary before a definitive answer exists. Active trials studying these issues are underway at present.

Measures that can be taken to maximize the safety of epidural pain-management techniques will require close communication between surgeon and anesthesiologist. There must be agreement between all parties involved concerning the potential for cancellation of the surgery in the event of a complicated, bloody epidural puncture. Heparin use can be minimized intraoperatively and corrected early. The use of local anesthetic can be minimized or discontinued intermittently to permit adequate neurologic assessment.

Even with meticulous and effective pain control, there will be significant pulmonary changes postoperatively, analogous to the significant decreases seen with thoracic surgical procedures. One half of all patients can be found to have evidence of atelectasis or pneumonia. Patients with significant preexisting pulmonary compromise may require prolonged mechanical ventilatory assistance. Postoperative reductions in lung volumes and forced expiratory flow rates will take several days to resolve, even without being further aggravated by any additional abdominal distention from ileus or intraabdominal bleeding. Patients requiring large numbers of transfusions and excessive amounts of volume resuscitation will suffer higher degrees of pulmonary difficulty in the postoperative period. Any patient experiencing perioperative shock and hypotension is also at risk for development of adult respiratory distress syndrome (ARDS).

Preoperative measures can have a great impact on postoperative care; hence, treatment should begin with preoperative optimization of pulmonary function with patient education, cessation of smoking, and consideration of the use of antibiotics and bronchodilators. Continuation of these prophylactic measures into the postoperative period is then complemented with judicious analgesia, coughing and deep breathing exercises, and early mobilization. The last is extremely important and may be combined with early physical therapy aimed at rehabilitation.

Intraabdominal bleeding is one of the most serious postoperative problems and may be difficult to diagnose at times. Bleeding is often occult and not visible on dressings or in surgical drains. Significant blood loss may occur before the patient presents with profound hypotension and shock. Serial hematocrits and a close watch of intravascular volume status are mandatory. The latter is particularly problematic in the face of ongoing third-space losses, warming of the cold postoperative patient, epidural pain-management techniques, and the almost obligatory use of antihypertensive regimens. Again, a high index of suspicion and compulsive monitoring is necessary.

Treatment of bleeding must involve a search for etiologies while resuscitative measures are ongoing. Technical factors are commonly involved, but one must rule out contributory medical factors. Residual heparin effects are not unusual. Thrombocytopenia and prolongation of clotting times requiring blood component therapy are common when bleeding occurs to any significant degree. Inadequate levels of clotting factors and platelets may lead to the bleeding, or may result from the bleeding while they are consumed in the body's attempts to seal holes in open vessels.

Renal failure is not uncommon because of the significant intraoperative stress to the kidneys. The threat of renal failure may further complicate fluid management. Care must be taken to avoid overload, particularly in the days following surgery. Nonoliguric renal failure may occur with the risk for electrolyte disturbances without fluid overload and mislead the less vigilant caregivers. Patients taking prostaglanding inhibitors, and those exposed to a dye load from angiographic interventions pre- and intraoperatively, may be at higher risk for perioperative renal dysfunction. One must also be cognizant of the potential for ureteric obstruction from an aortofemoral graft, causing oliguria.

The left colon is especially susceptible to ischemia from sacrifice of the inferior mesenteric artery or of branches of the internal iliac arteries. It is to be hoped that such ischemia is noted intraoperatively and followed by corrective measures. However, subtle colonic ischemia may be present in the postoperative period (even up to a month postoperatively), as well. Pain and ileus are common findings but may be missed in the postoperative period when such events are not uncommon. Guaiac-positive stools and rectal bleeding may well be the only signs and symptoms. Peritonitis and sepsis may follow a delayed diagnosis and are extremely serious, especially in a case involving synthetic graft material. Treatment is immediate surgical excision, often requiring colostomy and takedown at a much later date.

Bowel obstruction can occur in the early or late postoperative period, as it can after any intraabdominal procedure. The duodenum is specifically at risk after aortic surgery because of its mobilization intraoperatively and its proximity to the aortic suture line. The proximal aortic anastomosis is performed at the infrarenal level and lies directly posterior to the fourth portion of the duodenum. There is little, if any, tissue interposed between these structures, and the duodenum is at risk for erosion because of friction from the pulsatile anastomosis. Such a problem is dangerous and it may lead to nonhealing of the proximal anastomosis, as well as to infection of the foreign graft material by endogenous gut flora. The presence of any upper intestinal bleeding must immediately lead to a search for a potential life-threatening aorto-duodenal fistula, a complication which occurs months to years after aortic surgery.

BIBLIOGRAPHY

Ernst CB, Stanley JC, editors: *Current therapy in vascular surgery,* ed 3, St. Louis, 1995, Mosby-Year Book.

Fleisher LA, Eagle KA: Screening for cardiac disease in patients having noncardiac surgery, *Ann Intern Med* 124:767–772, 1996.

Gelman S: The pathophysiology of aortic cross-clamping and unclamping, *Anesthesiology* 82:1026–1060, 1995.

Haimovici H, editor: *Haimovici's vascular surgery: principles and techniques*, Cambridge, MA, 1996, Blackwell Science.

Mangano DT, Goldman L: Preoperative assessment of patients with known or suspected coronary disease, *N Engl J Med* 333:1750–1756, 1995.

Rutherford RB, editor: *Vascular surgery,* ed 4, Philadelphia, 1995, WB Saunders.

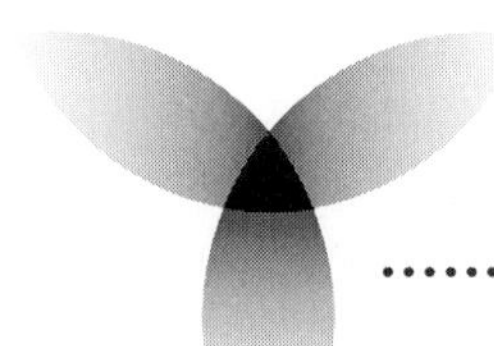

Chapter 33

Trauma and Emergency Surgery

Jeffrey S. Young, MD, David L. Bogdonoff, MD

Care of the trauma patient is often fraught with danger and uncertainty. Trauma results in a myriad of injuries and a variety of presentations, which can tax the skills and resources of all perioperative care providers. A major problem, especially in blunt trauma, is that a single, obvious injury often overshadows less obvious problems. For example, the open femur fracture or massive scalp laceration may, in less experienced centers, take center stage and delay the initiation of careful airway management and vigorous resuscitation. Thus, while the physicians caring for traumatized patients must be compulsive in their search for and treatment of all major injuries, they must remain vigilant in their attention to the current status of the patient. Additionally, efforts must be made simultaneously to obtain information about underlying medical conditions which may further complicate the perioperative care of the trauma patient. This latter issue is important because knowledge of coexisting medical conditions is paramount. The urgent care of the trauma patient often dictates that there will be little or no time for a careful preoperative assessment.

• SURGICAL PROCEDURES

A variety of surgical procedures, involving different surgical services, may be performed on a trauma patient. Often, trauma care may involve resuscitation and observation without a definitive operative intervention. Virtually all surgical subspecialties may become involved in these efforts, usually after major organ system injuries are treated or ruled out by the general surgical team. At times, a cardiac or neurosurgical problem will require the initial life-saving intervention. Surgical subspecialties such as orthopedics, urology, plastic and reconstructive surgery, otolaryngology, ophthalmology, and oral surgery will play important roles in the final outcomes and successful recovery of these patients. Thus, their intervention must be carefully coordinated with other resuscitative efforts. The trauma team must have a designated leader who will coordinate the overall care of the patient and be responsible for determining the appropriateness of the planned interventions by the consulting services.

INITIAL CARE

The purpose of a trauma team in a trauma center should be to: resuscitate, diagnose, intervene, and resuscitate. These functions usually occur simultaneously.

Airway, Breathing, and Circulation

The ABCs of resuscitation form the basis of the initial care of the traumatized patient. An adequate airway and the presence of effective ventilation are, of course, primary and essential prerequisites. However, it is surprising how often assessments of these functions differ among practitioners. A stable airway may deteriorate and adequate initial ventilation may become more labored as the traumatic disease processes continue or as the patient undergoes diagnostic and therapeutic procedures.

Personal opinion dictates that an intubated patient is a safe patient. Often, in emergency departments, personnel are unwilling to perform intubation in patients who can still grunt. We feel this is a dangerous policy. Patients who cannot follow commands, especially if extremely agitated, can be difficult to manage, even if they are still ventilating adequately. If these patients are expected to undergo multiple radiologic tests which require sequestration in rooms with poor monitoring equipment, disaster may ensue. We recommend that patients who cannot follow simple commands and those who are combative are better served by calm, elective intubation rather than emergent intubation in the radiology suite. This intubation should be performed by those personnel most experienced and qualified in endotracheal or nasotracheal techniques. Short-acting paralytics are recommended, initially, to allow resumption of spontaneous respirations if the airway cannot be secured, and to allow gross follow-up neurologic examination. Airway management should be performed by the most skilled personnel available and should be undertaken with the knowledge that the neck may be unstable as will be discussed below.

No critically injured patient should be moved from the emergency department until adequate venous access has been obtained. Exceptions would be those patients whose immediate transfer to the operating room is anticipated and when an operating room is available. Intravenous lines should be of adequate size and placement should be secure. Electrocardiographic and pulse oximetry monitoring is also considered essential. If the patient does not have a secure airway, equipment and medications for emergent airway control should be immediately available at all times.

Hypotensive or otherwise hemodynamically unstable patients should not, under any circumstances, be left unaccompanied at any time. Vigorous resuscitation and diagnostic measures should be ongoing in these patients. In our opinion, all hemodynamically unstable patients should be intubated. This removes one variable from the diagnostic equation and will enable maximum oxygen delivery for the degree of circulation present. Additionally, it will prevent aspiration, which is very common in these patients.

Spinal Considerations

There is no more dangerous position for a patient with suspected spinal injuries than with the head affixed to a spine board and the unsecured extremities and torso flailing wildly. A calm, well-organized intubation is far preferable to a drawn-out battle with a delirious or combative patient. We assume that the spine is broken in all cases of blunt trauma and in select cases of injury. Attempts to completely assess the spine during the initial evaluation of the trauma patient are misguided and ineffective. Controversy exists over the need for the lateral cervical spine film in the secondary survey. We have found, as have others, that up to 80% of these films are totally inadequate to evaluate the lateral cervical spine. Furthermore, an adequate film will rule out only approximately 85% of cervical spine injuries. Thus, the spine should be kept immobilized. The spine can be cleared clinically if the patient has a normal mental status, no distracting injuries, and the absence of pain and tenderness of the cervical spine. The advantage to obtaining a lateral c-spine film early, is that serious unstable injuries can be diagnosed immediately and safer stabilization can be applied. The only real disadvantage is the cost of wasted films. At our institution, the portable lateral c-spine costs $140. Elimination of the portable lateral c-spine has saved $140,000 in patient charges. Our recommendation is that if the patient is adequately immobilized and there are no focal motor deficits, all spine films should be performed after life-threatening conditions are ruled out. The films can then be performed in the radiology suite under optimal conditions.

All patients with focal motor deficits, and who are being taken directly to the operating room, do have a portable lateral spine film performed. The argument that a lateral c-spine film be performed before intubation is attempted, in my mind is specious. Spine films may miss the presence of ligamentous injuries and odontoid or compression/burst-type fractures. Thus, the anesthesiologist must always assume the cervical spine is unstable and use appropriate precautions when performing intubation, regardless of any radiographic findings.

In the operating room, positioning for thoracotomy or laparotomy must be performed by log rolling the patient. The backboard may be removed while the back is inspected for other injuries. Spinal precautions should otherwise be continued.

Occult Thoracic and Abdominal Injuries

One of the great dangers of perioperative care of the trauma patient is an incomplete trauma workup. An example follows:

A 45-year-old male, intoxicated, unrestrained driver is posted for open reduction and internal fixation of a left midshaft femur fracture. The patient has been evaluated by orthopedics and the emergency room physician. Circumstances of the accident are unknown to these physicians. The patient is writhing in agony from his femur fracture and seemingly has no other complaints. A chest film reveals broken ribs 7, 8, and 9 on the left. Pelvis radiograph is negative. Hematocrit is 38%; urine has 50 rbc/hpf. The patient has no cervical collar in place because he "didn't complain of neck pain" and is not on a backboard. Blood pressure is 105/60 and pulse rate 120 beats per minute. On induction of anesthesia the patient's blood pressure drops to 95 systolic, oxygen saturation drops to 80% and the pulse increase to 125 bpm. These improve with 2 liters of crystalloid and are attributed to the blood loss from the femur fracture. After the patient is placed on the fracture table and the operation begun, the blood pressure drops to 60 systolic, pulse rate 145 bpm, and oxygen saturation to 80%. Two units of packed cells are given with some improvement. An arterial blood gas is obtained which reveals: pH 7.19, pCO_2 45, pO_2 87 on 100% FIO_2, base excess –10, bicarbonate 15. The patient begins to have ventricular arrhythmias and increased hypothermia, as well as continued hemodynamic instability. A cardiac arrest occurs 60 minutes into the case and the patient can not be resuscitated. Autopsy reveals a large splenic laceration with 3 liters of hemoperitoneum.

Prevention of such a scenario requires a basic understanding of the essentials of the workup of the trauma patient and the indications for certain tests and studies. One does not need to be an expert in traumatology to recognize the errors made in this case presentation. A high level of suspicion and a comfortable level of paranoia will suffice. Knowledge of the mechanism of injury for an accident helps the clinician predict the probable organs involved and the risks of associated injuries. Generally, ejection from a vehicle and autopedestrian mechanisms have the highest risk of injury. Unrestrained victims also should raise concern. The speed and direction of collisions can aid in the expectations of various abdominal, thoracic, and neurologic injuries.

Any obtunded patient should be assumed to have a closed head injury. Hence, mental status changes must not be simply attributed to intoxication until pathologic intracranial injury has been ruled out with cranial computed tomography.

For patients with thoracic and abdominal injuries, a chest and pelvic film, urinalysis, and basic laboratory tests should be performed. These should include complete blood count, electrolytes, and, possibly, arterial blood gases. Rib fractures, pneumothorax, hemothorax, and mediastinal abnormalities all warrant further diagnostic intervention. Lower rib fractures mandate an abdominal evaluation. Diagnostic peritoneal lavage, abdominal computed tomography, and/or ultrasound examination should be performed depending on institutional preferences. While this may seem like overkill, ignoring the previously listed physical and radiograph findings can result in a poor outcome from a failed diagnosis.

A general surgical consultation should be obtained before specialty surgeons (orthopedics, otolaryngology, etc.) become involved in the care of patients with serious mechanisms of injury or abnormal physical findings, radiographs, and severe laboratory irregularities. The patient must be protected at all times from overly eager orthopedic interventions when a complete workup has not yet been performed.

Once diagnostic interventions are completed and therapeutic interventions are undertaken, all parties caring for the patient must remain vigilant and suspicious for the presence of a missed underlying problem. Prophylactic and expectant management schemes may be invoked which help eliminate or reduce some of these concerns.

All pneumothoraces seen on routine chest films should be treated with tube thoracostomy, even if small and stable. Any episodes of hypotension should be assumed to be caused by occult internal bleeding and NOT simply from oozing from the orthopedic procedure. An unstable patient should have the operation IMMEDIATELY terminated and resuscitation performed, especially in the face of severe acidosis, hypothermia, and ventricular arrhythmias.

EMERGENCY "BAIL-OUT"

One of the great advances in the treatment of the critically injured multiple trauma patient in the past decade has been the widespread recognition of the need to terminate operative and diagnostic procedures in the face of physiologic collapse. This is most often performed by "packing" of the abdominal, and even the thoracic, cavities followed by immediate termination of the procedure, and rapid transfer to an intensive care unit for rewarming, fluid and blood product administration, and correction of severe electrolyte and coagulation disturbances. To proceed with surgery in the event of severe hypothermia, coagulopathy, acidosis, and cardiac dysrhythmias is to risk an intraoperative death. Naturally, there are cases in which termination of the procedure is not possible. However, with increasing use of these "bail-out" procedures, it has been found that even continued severe venous bleeding can almost always be temporized with abdominal packing and that, to an extent, arterial bleeding can be managed similarly. In these situations, bowel injuries can be stapled proximally and distally and left *in situ* without consequence. That is because reoperation will be performed usually within 48 hours.

Close cooperation between the anesthesiologist and surgeon are essential for optimal outcome. Often, the surgeon is preoccupied with the problems at hand and will not be cognizant of the physiologic changes that are occurring. It is the responsibility of the anesthesia team to keep the surgeon constantly aware of the patient's condition. In addition, it is the surgeon's responsibility to inform anesthesia of the estimated length of operation, when large amounts of blood loss are expected, and if obvious coagulopathic oozing is present in the surgical field.

Patient warming devices such as heating blankets, humidifiers, and forced air warmers can decrease hypothermia. High-flow fluid warming and infusion devices are also essential. The cascade of bleeding–inadequate blood replacement–bleeding-hypothermia-coagulopathy can be avoided with close communication and meticulous anesthetic management. Injuries often associated with this cascade are massive liver lacerations, pelvic fractures, pelvic gunshot wounds, and retroperitoneal injuries. The large fluid and blood requirements for these situations must be anticipated, and arrangements with the blood bank made before excessive blood loss is encountered. The surgeon should immediately inform the anesthesia team of the presence of any active bleeding or of the intention to enter a large retroperitoneal hematoma. Furthermore, whenever possible, the surgical team should be prepared to wait to begin until the patient is adequately prepared and blood and blood products are present in the operating room. A good guideline for these severe injuries is the ability to give "10 units of blood in 10 minutes" if necessary. To accomplish this, large IV access, high-flow blood warmers, and adequate monitoring are needed, as well as the availability of the blood and blood products themselves.

POSTOPERATIVE CARE: ONGOING RESUSCITATION AND CRITICAL CARE

After transfer to the intensive care unit (ICU), the anesthesia team should remain with the patient for a short period of time. This ensures that optimum resuscitative care continues until the critical care team is prepared to assume total care of the patient. It is also prudent to be certain that immediate return to the operating room will not be necessary. Occasionally, continued bleeding is still present and difficult management decisions will face the trauma team at this juncture. Aggressive correction of hypothermia and persistent coagulation abnormalities must be undertaken immediately.

Resuscitation of the trauma patient should be ongoing and should not terminate upon arrival to the ICU. Although the endpoints of adequate resuscitation are controversial, we follow some simple guidelines. In the absence of continued bleeding, acidosis should be corrected. We find that serum lactate is a good indication of adequate perfusion and its presence should be determined at several times during the initial and subsequent phases of resuscitation. Arterial blood pH and base deficit should also be examined, though they tend to parallel serum lactate levels in the absence of diabetic ketoacidosis or respiratory insufficiency. Continued acidosis, or increasing acidosis after initially normal values, should prompt immediate therapy and a search for any correctable underlying problems.

We feel that in elderly patients and in those patients with severe multiple system injuries and evidence of continued inadequate perfusion (as demonstrated by lactic acidosis), a pulmonary artery catheter should be placed to help guide therapy. Inadequate cardiac performance can be treated with optimization of preload, and vasopressors can be added as needed. Urine output should be followed closely and there should be a low threshold for initiating low-dose dopamine therapy. Frequent reassessments of the patient's perfusion status through repeated physiologic measurements and laboratory determinations of arterial pH, base deficit, and lactate are warranted.

It has been shown that persistent lactic acidosis in the early posttrauma period inevitably leads to respiratory complications, as well as multiple system organ failure. This is especially true of the elderly population in whom inadequate cardiac reserve may not be able to meet the demands of injury and lead to severe hypoperfusion, despite adequate blood pressure.

Adequate sedation and analgesia must be maintained in an effort to minimize the stress response and any potential adverse effects on hemodynamics and cardiac performance. A high degree of compulsiveness and aggressiveness are necessary to ensure optimal outcomes in these patients.

EMERGENCY GENERAL SURGERY

Contrary to what the general surgeon may say in the middle of the night, few general surgical emergencies require IMMEDIATE operative intervention. While occasional emergencies (such as exsanguinating hemorrhage from a disrupted vascular graft) do occur, almost all other cases result from pathology which has been present for hours or days, with the patient being slowly debilitated by the process. Therefore, there is almost always time for a prompt, yet careful, examination of the patient's fluid and cardiac status, as well as renal function. If possible, rapid institution of invasive monitoring followed by directed fluid resuscitation, antibiotics, and vasopressors may make the subsequent operation safer and the postoperative course less rocky. Conversely, in the young patient showing the signs of sepsis without severe physiologic derangement, immediate operation to remove the source of sepsis is the most prudent action. Close communication and cooperation between surgeon and anesthesiologist are, once again, imperative. Surgery should be delayed only long enough to permit adequate resuscitation of vital signs and organ perfusion without waiting too long, which may worsen the septic process.

INTRAOPERATIVE COURSE

Operating for 5 hours on a septic, elderly patient is not likely to lead to a good outcome. There are many options in emergency general surgery, which should allow most operations to be completed in no more than 3 hours. The anesthesia team must inform the surgeons constantly of the patient's condition so that the proper operative strategy can be chosen. Eradication of the septic focus and thorough irrigation should be adequate to immediately treat most septic problems in the abdomen. In many cases, reoperation may be necessary, but the removal of the offending organ should allow improvement in the patient's condition and allow definitive operation at a later date.

No proven antiseptic therapies are currently available outside of antibiotics. Thus, none is recommended. Lack of urine output, hypotension refractory to fluid administration and vasopressors, and a worsening of respiratory function should all prompt rapid termination of the procedure after the essential basic lifesaving components of the operation are completed.

FINAL RECOMMENDATIONS

Optimal outcome for injured and septic patients requires close communication and exchange of information between the anesthesia and surgery teams. Trust is also a vital component of this relationship. The surgical team must trust the anesthesiologists to adequately follow the procedure and provide fluids, blood, and drugs necessary to resuscitate the patient. The anesthesia team should expect the surgeons to provide information about the course of the operation and to be open to suggestions regarding any potential delay of the procedure to permit placement of adequate monitoring devices and continue resuscitation. A decision to terminate a procedure, should it become necessary, must be made jointly by all members of the care team.

A final word should be said about transfer of critically ill patients. Many surgeons, possibly because of the surgical ego, may resist transfer of patients to tertiary care facilities, even though operative care of these patients may be well beyond the primary hospital's capabilities. It is a responsibility of the anesthesia team to ensure the safe care of the patient. This may entail expeditious transfer to another facility. Furthermore, it is important for any hospital to decide on criteria for patient transfer so that delay is minimized and survival optimized.

• SUGGESTED ALGORITHMS FOR TRAUMA MANAGEMENT

See Appendixes 1–4.

BIBLIOGRAPHY

Eddy VA, Key SP, Morris JA Jr: Abdominal compartment syndrome: etiology, detection, and management, *J Tenn Med Assoc* 87:55–57, 1994.

Hoyt DB, et al: Death in the operating room: an analysis of a multi-center experience, *J Trauma* 37:426–432, 1994.

Lewis FR: Initial assessment and resuscitation, *Emerg Med Clin Amer* 2:733–748, 1984.

Morris JA Jr, et al: The staged celiotomy for trauma. Issues in unpacking and reconstruction, *Ann Surg* 217:576–584, 1993.

Rutherford EJ, et al: Base deficit stratifies mortality and determines therapy, *J Trauma* 33:417–423, 1992.

Appendix 1

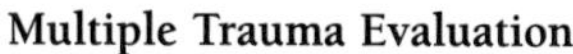

Multiple Trauma Evaluation

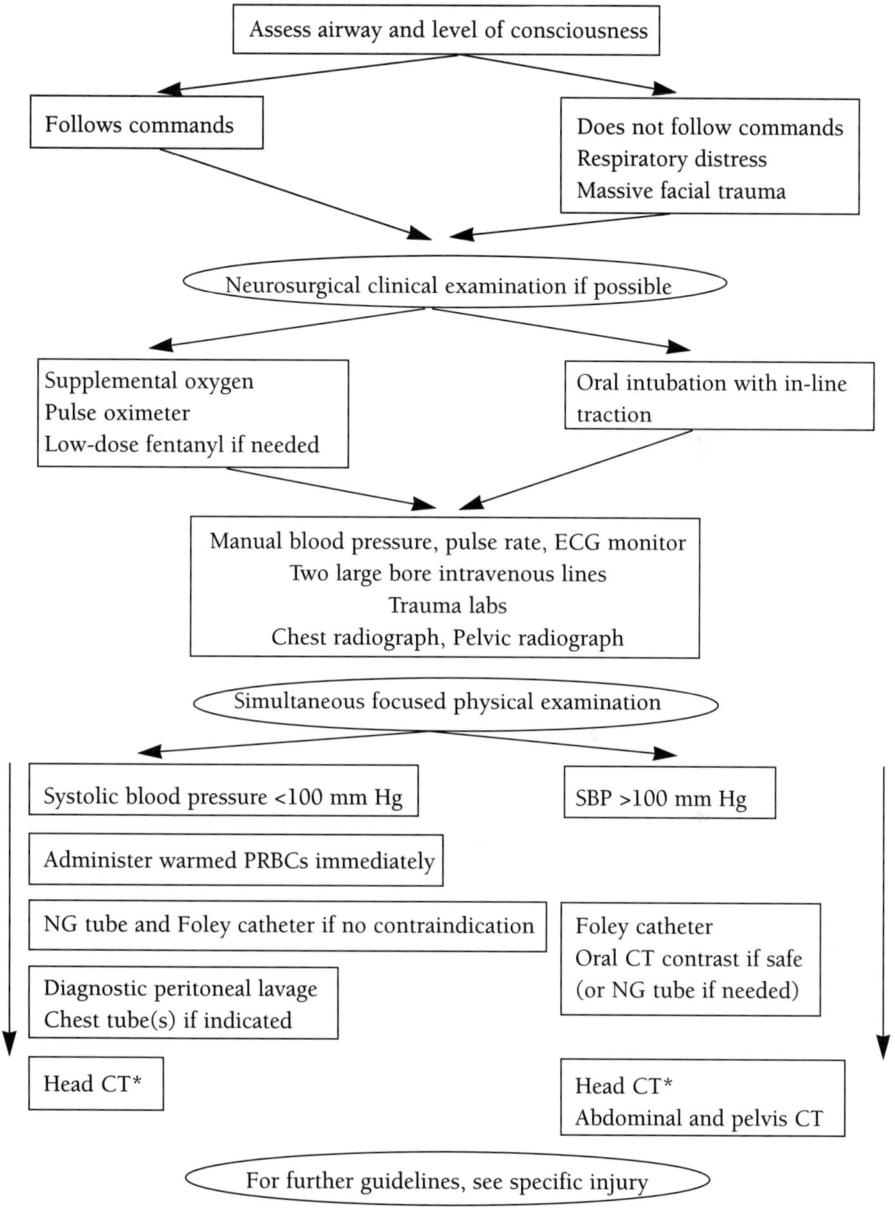

Assess airway and level of consciousness

Follows commands

Does not follow commands
Respiratory distress
Massive facial trauma

Neurosurgical clinical examination if possible

Supplemental oxygen
Pulse oximeter
Low-dose fentanyl if needed

Oral intubation with in-line traction

Manual blood pressure, pulse rate, ECG monitor
Two large bore intravenous lines
Trauma labs
Chest radiograph, Pelvic radiograph

Simultaneous focused physical examination

Systolic blood pressure <100 mm Hg

Administer warmed PRBCs immediately

NG tube and Foley catheter if no contraindication

Diagnostic peritoneal lavage
Chest tube(s) if indicated

Head CT*

SBP >100 mm Hg

Foley catheter
Oral CT contrast if safe
(or NG tube if needed)

Head CT*
Abdominal and pelvis CT

For further guidelines, see specific injury

* Many of the aspects of this guideline will occur simultaneously. Head CT will always be performed before abdominal CT in the stable patient. In the unstable patient with a positive DPL, the patient with focal neurologic signs, whose blood pressure can be maintained with fluid and blood administration, should undergo a quick head CT before laparotomy. Sedation should be withheld in all cases until the neurosurgery resident can examine the patient, if possible. If any question about neuro or airway status exists, the patient MUST have the airway controlled.

Appendix 2

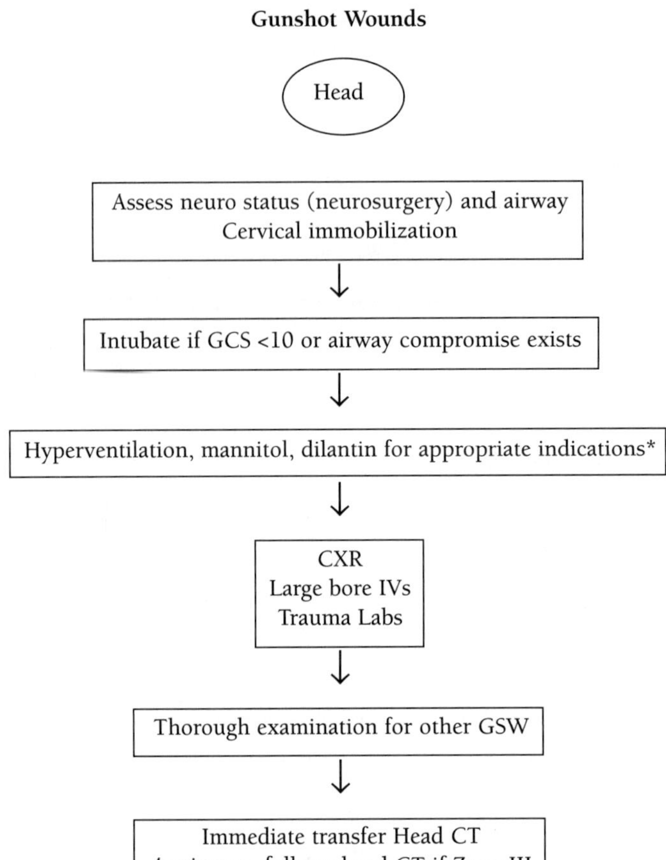

* Hyperventilation (pCO_2 <25 mm Hg) and mannitol should only be used if signs of significant intracranial hypertension or herniation are present. The need for Dilantin will be assessed by the neurosurgery team.

Appendix 3

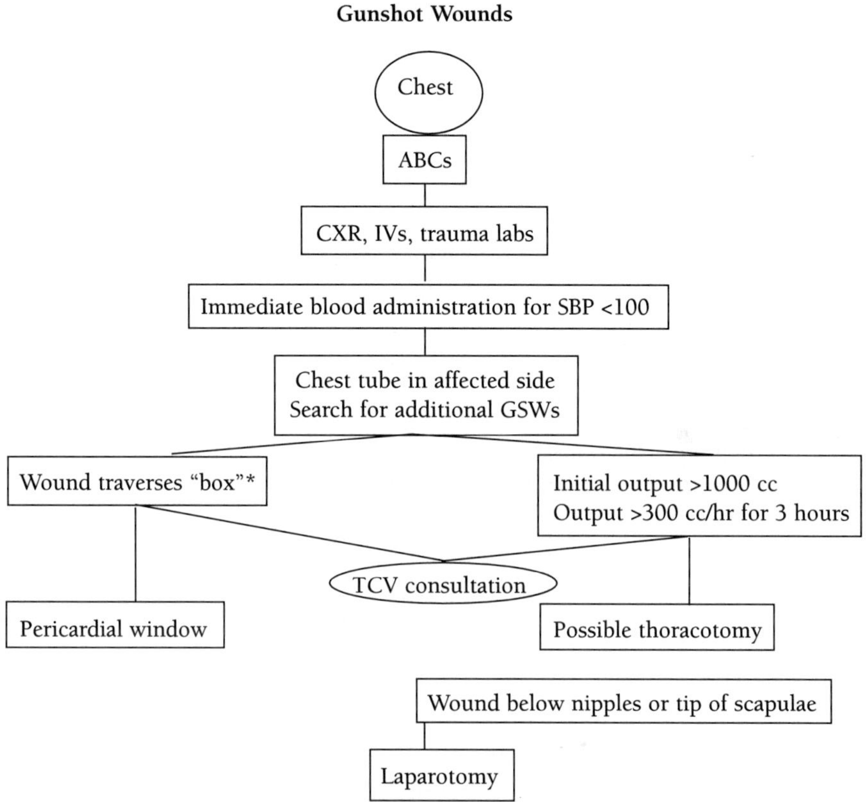

* "Box" refers to area between nipples, below the thoracic inlet, and above the xiphoid.

Appendix 4

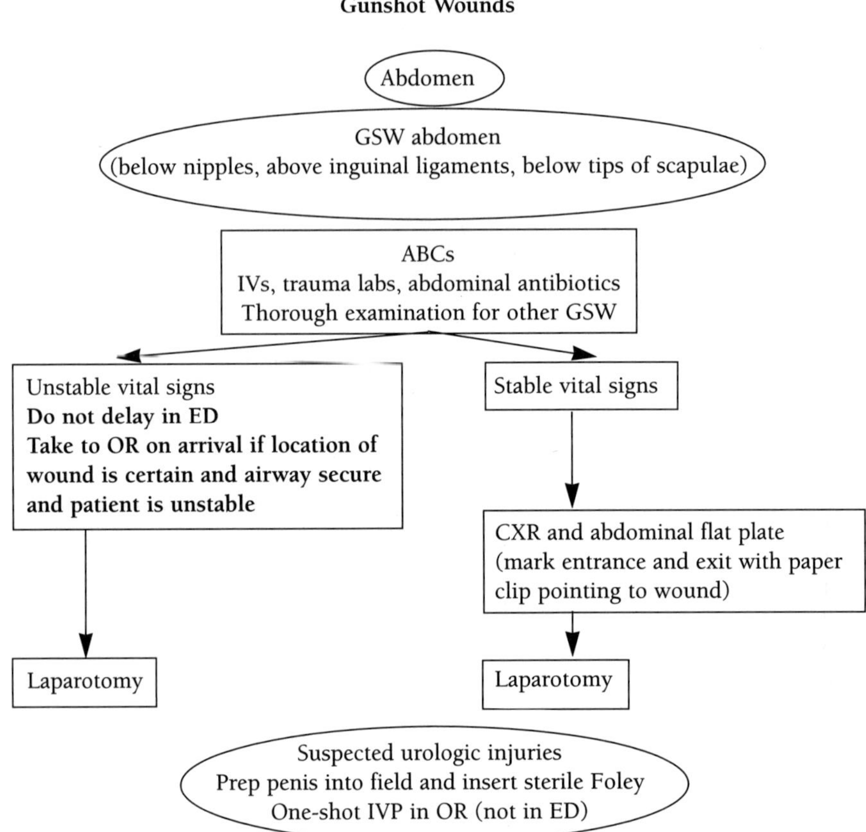

Safest place for patient with abdominal gunshot wound is in the OR, NOT the ED.

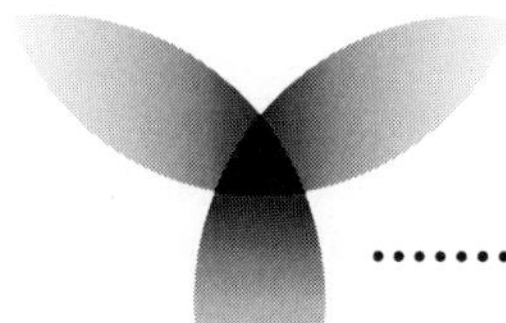

Chapter 34

Thoracic Surgery

David L. Bogdonoff, MD, John A. Kern, MD

Thoracic surgery is a discipline intimately involved with vital organs and their life support functions. As such, these organs are the primary focus of thoracic surgical procedures or are significantly effected by their proximity to the operative field. Cardiac surgery and procedures using cardiopulmonary bypass are usually not included in discussions of thoracic surgery and are discussed elsewhere. In the field of thoracic surgery, even the least invasive interventions, such as mediastinoscopy or bronchoscopy, may have may profound physiologic effects, with life-threatening implications. Major operative interventions require meticulous pre-, intra-, and, particularly, postoperative care by all parties involved.

The domain of thoracic surgery, like many others, remains dynamic. Video-assisted, minimally invasive thoracic surgery has evolved and become a common undertaking, having revolutionized the diagnostic and therapeutic possibilities for a number of different medical conditions. The techniques of esophageal resection and antireflux surgery have undergone less in the way of change, though their relative indications continue to be debated along with the choice of which procedure is best to perform. Pulmonary resection for malignancy has become more commonplace with the continued improvements and successes of preoperative radiation and chemotherapeutic regimens. Surgical treatment for nonmalignant end-stage lung diseases has entered the therapeutic arena with the advent of lung volume reduction surgery and transplantation.

Evaluation of the thoracic surgical patient is rarely straightforward. Coexisting diseases are the rule, rather than the exception. Heavy smoking and alcoholism are not infrequent and concomitant coronary artery disease is highly prevalent. Restrictive, obstructive, and reactive airway diseases are concerns central to the entire process and so their treatment must be optimized before surgery. Decisions regarding the feasibility of pulmonary resection must be made on the basis of preoperative information, with an understanding of the intra- and postoperative effects of the proposed reductions in total lung mass.

SURGICAL PROCEDURES

The thoracic surgeon uses a number of operative approaches depending on the surgical goals. Each approach has its own unique physiologic implications, in addition to those common to all procedures in the chest.

Mediastinoscopy

Diagnostic procedures involving the mediastinum are needed to determine resectability of lung cancers and to obtain diagnoses of certain mediastinal masses and mediastinal adenopathy. A small suprasternal incision permits access to the anterior and middle mediastinum for the probing mediastinoscope. Highly relevant to this procedure are questions concerning the clinical manifestations resulting from the masses. Proximity to the tracheobronchial tree, pulmonary arteries and veins, and the superior vena cava may allow abnormal tissue to have profound effects. While signs and symptoms from metastatic lymph nodes are uncommon, large masses may have profound physiologic implications. A careful history must search for any symptoms related to airway compression such as dyspnea with exertion, wheezing, or new onset of stridor. Symptoms relating to positional changes, such as lightheadedness, syncope, or dyspnea are particularly ominous. Signs of superior vena caval obstruction are also of major concern. Even asymptomatic patients may be at risk because of the alterations in physiology which result during anesthesia and surgery. Computed tomography (CT) or magnetic resonance imaging (MRI) scans, inspiratory and expiratory flow volume loops from pulmonary function tests, and echocardiography are effective in ruling out subclinical impingement on vital organs.

Induction of general anesthesia results in changes in intrathoracic volumes and pressure dynamics and may result in airway obstruction or circulatory collapse. Use of paralytic drugs, inhibition of spontaneous ventilation with need for positive airway pressure, and changes in positioning all contribute to potential adverse reactions. Though rare, cardiovascular collapse may be difficult to treat. It may require that the patient be rolled to a lateral decubitus position, seated upright, or even turned prone. Loss of the airway, resulting from intrathoracic tracheal or bronchial collapse, may be similarly difficult to treat, and may require rigid bronchoscopy as a lifesaving maneuver. Avoidance of general anesthesia, or careful inhalational induction in a spontaneously breathing patient, is necessary for the known symptomatic patient. Surgery under local anesthesia, percutaneous needle biopsy, or other noninvasive diagnostic approaches should be considered, if at all possible.

The physical introduction of the mediastinoscope into the mediastinum also has profound implications. The trachea and mainstem bronchi are subject to compression, with resultant airway obstruction or damage by perforation. Inadvertent biopsy of a pulmonary artery mistaken for a lymph node is a recognized possibility. It is the reason why the patient must always be prepared for the possibility of massive bleeding requiring transfusion. In such a situation, conservative measures of holding pressure may be effective, but median sternotomy or thoracotomy is usually necessary. Compression of the inominate artery by the rigid scope, with loss of blood flow to the right carotid artery, presents a risk of stroke to the patient with cerebrovascular disease. Monitoring for the loss of pulses in the right arm is a necessary component of the patient's anesthetic management.

In the absence of anesthetic or surgical complications, mediastinoscopy is often helpful diagnostically, and is well-tolerated postoperatively by the patient. Pain is minimal and the surgical wound is small and resistant to infectious complications. Patients are usually discharged within 24 hours. Previous mediastinoscopy results in scarring of tissue planes and represents a relative contraindication to a subsequent identical procedure.

Anterior Thoracotomy

For the patient with contraindications to mediastinoscopy (significant cerebrovascular disease, known significant symptoms relating to a mediastinal mass, or previous mediastinoscopy) and for patients with predominantly aortopulmonary window adenopathy, a left anterior thoracotomy is chosen for the diagnostic intervention. This small left anterior thoracotomy, known as a Chamberlain procedure, carries a smaller risk for surgical misadventures, though its anesthetic risks are equal. Postoperative pain is significantly greater than with mediastinoscopy but is still limited, considering the significant pain associated with the alternative of a formal lateral thoracotomy. In addition, because the pleura is usually entered and the lung can be injured, a chest tube may be required postoperatively.

Thoracoscopy

Minimally invasive surgical techniques initially developed for laparoscopy have been applied in the thorax as well. Thoracoscopic talc pleurodesis, undertaken for spontaneous or persistent pneumothorax, is one of the simplest endoscopic procedures. Nevertheless, it represents an improvement over previous "blinded" techniques in that it allows diagnostic visualization of the pleural space and lung and the possibility for detection and treatment of underlying blebs or large air leaks, which previously would have resulted in a failed pleurodesis. Familiarity and experience with thoracoscopic techniques have led to an increase in the magnitude and complexity of these procedures. In addition to blebectomy, actual wedge resections of lung tissue can be accomplished, and lung biopsies are often performed in this manner. Removal of some pleural lesions is possible, as well. Access to intrathoracic, retropleural structures is possible and esophageal myotomy and thoracic sympathectomy are prime examples of procedures well suited to these thoracoscopic techniques.

As in laparoscopy, adequate visualization requires that air be present to permit manipulation of the scope in a free space. While the abdominal wall is expandable, the chest wall is not. Therefore, the ipsilateral lung must be collapsed. Insufflation of air (carbon dioxide) under pressure into the pleural space is equivalent to a tension pneumothorax and can result in significant untoward hemodynamic sequelae. It is safest to passively collapse the lung without external pressure whenever possible. This, of course, requires mechanical separation of the lungs, usually accomplished with a double-lumen endotracheal tube. As will be discussed, single lung ventilation requires significant technical expertise on the part of the anesthetic team. Additionally, single lung ventilation represents the most significant physiological impasse to the patient and greatly complicates the anesthetic management of the case.

Thoracotomy

Formal thoracotomy is a significant undertaking and produces a major surgical wound. The standard posterolateral thoracotomy is one of the most painful incisions in surgery. Ribs are frequently removed or purposely fractured during spreading. Multiple layers of muscle must be incised. Most thoracic surgeons now attempt to enter the chest with muscle-sparing incisions, without complete division of the serratus anterior and latisimus dorsi muscles. Such attempts may be rewarded by some diminution in postoperative pain and morbidity (although recent studies fail to prove this). Nevertheless, thoracotomy produces an extremely painful incision and results in significant decreases in postoperative respiratory function in a patient group ill-prepared to deal with such consequences. Decreased vital capacity is significant. It may drop by 25% to 50% over the first 24 hours postoperatively, even with excellent pain management. Ability to cough is also impaired and tracheobronchial toilet becomes problematic. Expiratory reserve volumes have been found to decrease up to 60% following thoracotomy. Pulmonary compliance and functional residual capacity are reduced as well, dropping by one third. These volumes would be further reduced by any concomitant resection of lung tissue. As will be discussed, the use of a variety of pain management regimes will significantly decrease pain and enhance the patient's participation in coughing and deep breathing exercises. It will not, however, eliminate all the adverse sequelae of this major surgery.

Chest tubes are usually required, except in the case of pneumonectomy where they are omitted. Following pneumonectomy it is desirable to have the pleural space fill with fluid and no attempt is made to drain it. For patients with chest tubes, proper care and understanding of the function of these tubes is essential because mismanagement can lead to tension pneumothorax or infection. The presence of a chest tube additionally contributes to postoperative discomfort, often in a different dermatome from the thoracotomy incision.

Pulmonary resections performed through formal thoracotomy will have profound effects on postoperative pulmonary function, simply from the reduction in total lung mass, separate from the obligatory and unavoidable adverse effects on the remaining lung tissue. Pneumonectomy obviously leaves no lung mass on the operative side, although lobectomy may produce similar short-term effects in the early postoperative period. One must ensure that patients undergoing a planned lobectomy can tolerate pneumonectomy because they may, in fact, require such a procedure or suffer the same consequences physiologically. The remaining ipsilateral lung tissue after lobectomy is atelectatic and invariably injured by intraoperative surgical manipulation. Optimal pain management and pulmonary toilet are essential to prevent lobar collapse and pneumonia in the remaining lobe.

Following pneumonectomy, the mainstem bronchial suture line is at risk of rupture or air leak from positive-pressure ventilation; hence, attempts are made to extubate as early as possible. The empty hemithorax fills with fluid over the next several days to weeks and is at risk for infection with empyema formation if there is contamination from the bronchial stump. If this occurs, prompt drainage of the empyema and further surgical intervention is needed. Air leaks following lobectomy and wedge resection are not unusual. They are rarely unable to be controlled with chest tube suction unless the patient is difficult to ventilate and requires high ventilator pressure settings. Early extubation, resulting from effective anesthetic and pain management techniques, in patients with adequate pulmonary function in the remaining lung tissue serves to minimize problems from persistent air leaks.

Median Sternotomy

Sternotomy is most commonly used for cardiac surgery but does provide access to the mediastinum for cases involving anterior mediastinal masses. It also permits access to both hemithoraces for the occasional case requiring bilateral resections of lung tissue, such as for pulmonary metastases. Recently, lung volume reduction or "lung shaving" operations have been performed for the treatment of end-stage lung disease from emphysema. This operation is usually accomplished through a sternotomy incision. Surgical staplers are used to reduce lung volume by the resection of small strips of lung tissue with the use of xenografts of pleura or pericardium to seal the edges. The resultant reduction of lung volumes ameliorates dyspneic symptomatology, possibly by producing an elevation of the diaphragm back to a more normal domed configuration and away from its previous flattened and dysfunctional position. It may also obliterate areas of severe ventilation/perfusion mismatch. These cases require meticulous attention to postoperative pain control and respiratory therapeutics. These cases are particularly problematic because of massive air leaks, even in the absence of positive pressure ventilation. Physical therapists, respiratory therapists, pulmonologists, and nurses who are familiar with this procedure are required before the hospital undertakes the care of these most difficult patients.

Esophageal Resection

Classical esophageal resections are performed through a right or left thoracotomy, depending on the level of the lesion. Left thoracotomy is used for lower esophageal lesions and any work near the diaphragm. Right thoracotomy permits access to the middle and upper esophagus. Resection for cancer is often accomplished through a right thoracotomy and then reconstructed through laparotomy and mobilization of the stomach into the chest or, more frequently, the neck. Thoracic surgeons are divided on their thoughts concerning the proper procedure for cancer resection. Recently, more surgeons have advocated a blinded, blunt, transdiaphragmatic resection of the esophagus through a laparotomy incision, with subsequent cervical-esophageal anastomosis to the mobilized stomach. While elegant in its avoidance of thoracotomy, the procedure may result in damage to adjacent vital structures. It certainly causes transient major hemodynamic consequences, especially during dissection behind the heart.

Esophageal myotomy for achalasia and some antireflux procedures are performed through left thoracotomy. The former undertaking is now being done more commonly through a thoracoscopic approach. The latter is being displaced by an increasing tendency towards transabdominal and laparoscopic repair, not to mention increasingly effective nonoperative medical therapy.

PREOPERATIVE CONSIDERATIONS

The surgeon and consultant must have a good understanding of the underlying condition of the patient before surgery. Optimization of treatable disease is integral to the workup and preoperative preparation. Nowhere else is this more crucial than in the evaluation leading up to surgery for pulmonary resection. Most patients already have significant lung disease for which thoracotomy, even without resection, likely represents a significant risk. There is clear evidence that morbidity and mortality can be reduced with proper preoperative intervention.

Wheezing can result from asthma or chronic obstructive pulmonary disease (COPD). Responsiveness to bronchodilators should be sought with screening studies and treatment initiated or optimized. The treatment of reactive airway disease must continue right up to the time of surgery, with additional prophylactic measures strongly considered in the operating room or surgical holding area before anesthetic induction. Patients with severe asthma may benefit from perioperative steroids. These must be started at least an hour before airway manipulation (intubation) to be most effective. Bronchitic patients should make extra efforts to clear any airway secretions preoperatively. A course of antibiotics should be considered for any patient with a suspicion of harboring an underlying bacterial infection. Preoperative instructions relating to the proper performance of deep breathing and coughing exercises and demonstrations of planned postoperative respiratory therapy maneuvers are helpful and worth any extra time and effort.

All of these attempts are even more important when considering that intubation, with resultant stimulation of tracheal, and particularly carinal mechanoreceptors, is one of the most potent inducers of bronchospasm. Patients with reactive airway disease must be at their best before anesthetic induction.

Acute illnesses should always be allowed to run their course. Unless absolutely necessary, surgery must be delayed until the patient has recovered, with regard to pulmonary symptomatology, recognizing that there will always be underlying disease present.

Smoking is clearly a major perioperative risk factor, not to mention it being the most common etiologic factor leading to the need for thoracic surgery in the first place. Smoking produces a multitude of adverse effects and each sequela requires a variable amount of time of abstinence before any improvement in seen. Carbon monoxide levels are maintained at a few percent in the chronic smoker and have the obvious effects of decreasing oxygen-carrying capacity and oxygen unloading at the tissue level. These levels drop off rapidly with cessation of smoking and are at normally nominal levels within 24 to 48 hours. This shows that there is some benefit to cessation of tobacco use, even if only for a brief period of time preoperatively.

Chronic smoking leads to hypertrophy of mucous secreting cells, a decrease in mucociliary transport, mucosal edema, and irritability of the airways. These profound effects demonstrably lead to an increase in postoperative morbidity in all surgical patients. The effects are, unfortunately, not readily reversible and one must wait a minimum of 4 to 6 weeks to see improvements after tobacco use has ceased. A decrease in volume of secretions will be apparent by this time and mucociliary transport will have rebounded as well. Perhaps the most notable effect will be a significant decrease in airway reactivity. Two or three months are needed to demonstrate an improvement in lung volumes by pulmonary function testing; but this should be expected eventually. While most conditions requiring thoracic surgical intervention will not permit a delay of this duration, whenever possible in a patient who is truly motivated to quit smoking, measurable benefits will be achieved by any smoke-free interval, even if for only a few days.

EVALUATION FOR LUNG RESECTION

In determining the suitability of the patient for lung resection, one starts with an evaluation of the extent of reversible disease as previously discussed. After the evaluation, a determination must be made concerning how much lung tissue, if any, can be removed without placing the patient at risk of dying or being made a pulmonary cripple. Finally, a prediction of the potential need for prolonged postoperative ventilatory support is made.

The evaluation for potential resectability of the abnormal lung involves up to three states, progressing from simple, noninvasive tests to sophisticated and invasive studies. Successive stages of investigation are only undertaken if previous steps are suggestive of inoperability.

Spirometric measurements taken from standard pulmonary function tests (PFTs) are the first steps in this assessment of resectability. An arterial blood gas measurement accompanies the initial PFTs. The following four results have been identified as major risk factors for pulmonary resection and each is highly correlated with an increased risk of postoperative complications and death:

1. Forced expiratory volume in 1 second (FEV_1) <50% predicted or specifically <2 l/sec.
2. Maximum voluntary ventilation (MVV) <50% predicted.
3. Residual volume (RV)/Total lung capacity (TLC) >50%.
4. pCO_2 >46 mm Hg on room air blood gas.

Absence of any of these high-risk results on screening tests serves as the endpoint for the workup preceding pulmonary resection. A positive result will require additional evaluation. This is often a worthwhile undertaking because many patients have special considerations, which may invalidate an initial stage screening test. An obvious example would be a patient with atelectatic lung distal to an obstructing carcinoma. Decreased lung volumes on screening spirometry would result in a drastic miscalculation of anticipated residual lung volumes following resection, because removal of any atelectatic lung would fail to produce an adverse effect of further diminishing the measured spirometric values. Determinations of the relative individual contributions of each lung will thus be necessary in the second stage of evaluation.

Ventilation-perfusion scanning is used to identify the percentage of function attributable to each lung or lung lobe. Xenon or technetium radioisotopes are most commonly used. The derived estimate of the relative contribution from the diseased lung segments permits a calculation of expected lung volumes following the anticipated resection. A predicted post-resection FEV_1 less than 0.8 l/sec is considered to represent an unacceptably high risk for postoperative respiratory failure. Some have suggested using the value of FEV_1 of less than 30% of predicted, rather than the specific value of 0.8 l/sec. This is because the latter would not take into account actual size or age of the patient. Values above this level, needless to say, do not guarantee success, but values below are associated with dismal results.

The third stage of evaluation, if necessary, proceeds only if the previous studies still suggest inoperability. This stage involves invasive studies using temporary occlusion of the bronchi or pulmonary arteries supplying the affected lung segments. Bronchoscopically directed bronchial balloon occlusion with repeat measurements of lung volumes can be performed but is really rare in clinical practice. Rather, temporary occlusion of the branch of the pulmonary artery supplying the lung to be resected is the procedure most often performed during this final stage of evaluation. This isolates all pulmonary blood flow to the normal or unoperated lung that would be present following resection. Measurements of pulmonary artery pressure are made and values above 35 mm Hg will suggest an inability of the patient to tolerate resection. Additionally, arterial blood gas documentation of hypoxemia (pO_2 <45 mm Hg) or hypercarbia (pCO_2 >60 mm Hg) will preclude resection. The latter measurements cannot be simulated and must actually be determined with the blood flow diverted.

Some researchers have used invasive measurements of pulmonary vascular resistance during exercise. Levels above 190 dynes sec/cm^5 depict an inability of the remaining lung to compensate for the increase in pulmonary blood flow post-resection. Measurements of maximal oxygen consumption with exercise have similarly been suggested as being predictive of ability to tolerate resection. Maximal levels of oxygen consumption below 1 l/min are ominous, with higher levels being more consistent with survival. On a weight basis, these critical values have been reported as below 15 ml/kg/min or above 20 ml/kg/min. The actual significance of the suggestions of these researchers is yet to be tested in prospective trials. It is interesting to note, however, that these latter tests seem to bring the sophisticated levels of preoperative testing full circle, back to the beginning basics of history and physical examination. The old-time thoracic surgeons used to do well without even the simplest PFT by going for a walk with the patient in the stairwell. Those patients not able to maintain a decent pace for a couple of flights of stairs were not deemed to be operable candidates. This test is still found to be accurate. All of the sophisticated measurements may well serve only to confirm the assessments and suspicions of the insightful clinician.

INTRAOPERATIVE CONCERNS

The anesthesiologist will need to accomplish several goals, many of which are unique in the thoracic surgical patient. The choices to be made begin with a decision concerning the potential need for separation of the lungs. Patient positioning is often a bit of a challenge. Intraoperative management will require extreme vigilance for hemodynamic and ventilatory disturbances, many of which will be difficult to manage. Ultimately, the ability to deal with these disturbances in physiology may well determine whether or not the procedure may be accomplished at all.

Separation of the Lungs

There are both absolute and relative indications for separation of the lungs during thoracic procedures (Box 34-1). Even when not absolutely indicated physiologically, surgical preference often represents a strong indication for intraoperative lung separation. Obvious indications include cases of lung abscess in which spillage of pus to the opposite lung could result in disaster. A massive bronchopleural fistula will cause a huge air leak during positive pressure ventilation and may well necessitate ventilation of each lung individually, in an effort to prevent most of the delivered tidal volume from being lost through the fistulous tract. Significant bleeding from one lung may require separation of individual lungs. Bleeding from the upper operated lung, positioned above the normal lung in the decubitus position, will lead to obstruction of the bronchi in the unaffected dependent lung below. Collapse of the operated lung is helpful to the surgeon. Not only will it increase the space available for performing the procedure within the confines of the chest, but it will decrease the motion associated with ventilation. Surgery can still be done in the absence of these conveniences but is less efficient and, at times, can lead to excessive manipulation of the operated lung with resultant micro- or macroatelectasis. In the case of the thoracic vascular surgical patient requiring intraoperative anticoagulation, the latter goals of having the lung collapsed and out of the surgical field result is an

Box 34-1 Indications for Separation of the Lungs

ABSOLUTE	RELATIVE
Infection (lung abscess)	Lung resection
Bleeding	Thoracoscopy
Massive air leak	Esophageal resection
Lung collapse during heparinization	
Bronchoalveolar lavage	

absolute indication for lung separation. A heparinized lung is highly susceptible to pulmonary hemorrhage, resulting from even minor degrees of surgical manipulation.

Separation of lungs is accomplished with use of a double-lumen endotracheal tube or with use of a bronchial blocking device placed through or along the side of a conventional endotracheal tube. Modern improvements made to the original double-lumen tube designs have resulted in available products that are safe and effective for most scenarios requiring lung separation. The tubes allow either lung to be ventilated individually, or for both to be inflated simultaneously. Larger and more compliant balloon cuffs minimize damage to bronchial mucosa and tube construction with D-shaped cross sections allow larger lumens for both air movement and the important function of allowing passage of a suction catheter to remove blood and secretions. This latter need represents a shortcoming of bronchial blockade techniques, which do not provide a means to suction secretions or blood, or even allow additional egress of air, necessitated by further subsequent collapse of the operated lung. Additionally, as the use of bronchoscopically aided placement becomes the standard of care, and with the increasing use of scopes for therapeutic and diagnostic maneuvers, the ability to gain access to the operated lung represents another argument favoring the use of a double lumen tube.

In most situations, a left-sided double lumen tube is chosen. There is a larger margin of error for placement of a left-sided tube. Malposition of a tube is possible when the endobronchial component is placed too far into the mainstem bronchus and, thereby, obstructs a segmental bronchus to a lung segment. Additionally, the tube may not be inserted far enough, thereby failing to actually separate the two lungs, or to result in partial obstruction of the contralateral side by a herniating balloon cuff. Finally, it is possible for the endobronchial tube to go down the wrong side altogether. The margin of safety for the first two malpositions is significantly larger with the use of a left-sided tube. Initial placement is more successful, and it is less prone to intraoperative movement, which is not at all uncommon during positioning and operative manipulation of the lungs. A right-sided tube also presents some challenge associated with ventilation of the right upper lobe. The right upper lobe bronchus takes off immediately after the carinal bifurcation of the trachea (with some anatomic variability being fairly common) and, thus, is easily obstructed by the occluding bronchial cuff.

There is some room for preference of the anesthesiologist in choice of tube or lung separation technique. In fact, at times, the best technique is the one with which the anesthesia staff has the most experience. There are some clear cases where choices are made by the anatomy, pathology, or surgical approach. Left endobronchial lesions will preclude use of a left-sided tube. Procedures that involve resection and reanastomosis of a section of a mainstem bronchus will eliminate the use of an endobronchial device or tube on that side, unless plans are made which will include intraoperative repositioning of the device.

Single Lung Ventilation

The challenge of single lung ventilation is to maintain oxygenation and carbon dioxide elimination. While there is no ventilation of the operated lung, perfusion is still ongoing, except to the extent that it is diminished by hypoxic pulmonary vasoconstriction and the mechanical factors of surgical compression and gravity. Use of the lateral decubitus position is helpful in this regard, because gravity tends to increase perfusion to the dependent, ventilated lung. Because of the persistence of flow to the nonventilated lung, hypoxia is a significant problem, use of 100% oxygen is frequently required, despite any theoretical concerns about absorption atelectasis. Tidal volumes are usually decreased slightly in an effort to avoid high mean airway pressures, which have the adverse effect of increasing pulmonary vascular resistance and diverting blood flow to the upper, nonventilated lung. Higher respiratory rates are, therefore, necessitated to maintain normocarbia.

Not infrequently, hypoxia results and necessitates an alteration in technique for the anesthesiologist. There are algorithms that may be followed and much of this discussion is beyond this chapter's intent. Briefly, one may attempt to increase oxygen delivery to the nonventilated lung with either intermittent inflation or CPAP or an increase in ventilation to the dependent lung in such a manner as to not divert blood flow away from that functioning lung unit. Dependent lung positive end-expiratory pressure (PEEP) should be instituted only after nondependent lung CPAP is started, again in an effort not to nullify any potential gains by a resultant diversion of blood flow to the nonventilated lung. Actual surgical ligation or compression of the pulmonary artery will dramatically improve oxygenation, if such maneuvers are possible.

Drugs and anesthetic techniques that blunt hypoxic pulmonary vasoconstriction must be considered. While anesthetic potent agents have some definite adverse effects in this regard, they are, nevertheless, frequently used to advantage because they allow the use of nearly 100% oxygen for ventilation. Use of antihypertensives, such as nipride and nitroglycerin, may prove troublesome and may well not be tolerated.

There must be a low threshold for suctioning and for rechecking the position of the double lumen tube. The bronchi of the dependent lung are vulnerable to blockade by any secretions or blood from the nondependent lung or by malposition of balloon cuffs. Change of position and surgical manipulation of the lung result in significant shifts of the mediastinum, and the bronchi may actually move over the relatively fixed, secured endobronchial tube.

POSTOPERATIVE CARE

Postoperative care of the thoracic surgical patient requires the continuation of all pertinent pre- and intraoperative therapeutic measures. It also involves close monitoring of fluid administration and vital signs, as well as a high vigilance for the development of postoperative complications. There are a myriad of potential complications in the postoperative period. Those unique to thoracic surgery and of life-threatening significance will be discussed.

An important part of care involves the use of chest tubes. While a comprehensive discussion of chest tube physiology and management is outside the scope of this discussion, a brief review is useful and essential. The purpose of chest tubes is to ensure drainage of the pleural space (or mediastinum) of air, blood, or fluid until a pleural symphysis is achieved after approximately 2 or 3 days. Modern-day chest tubes are usually connected to self-contained, commercially available units. Such units are based on the old three-bottle collection system, which is actually three separate containers (or bottles) in one unit. The part of the unit that the tube from the patient directly drains into is called the drainage collection chamber and is simply a graduated chamber, which allows accurate measurement of how much fluid is being drained from the chest. The next chamber in the unit is the water seal. When filled to the proper level with water, this chamber effectively seals off the system from the atmosphere and prevents air from being sucked back into the chest tube (and pleural space) during periods of negative intrathoracic pressure. When this chamber is filled properly, the entire system may be disconnected from wall suction (as is necessary for patient transport) with no adverse effects to the patient. This chamber will not function if the unit is not upright because the water level may not appropriately cover the tube connecting this chamber to the drainage chamber in continuity with the pleural space. The third chamber is the suction control chamber. This final chamber determines how much negative pressure is applied to the system and, hence, the pleural space; it is regulated by the height of the water level in the chamber. The tubing from the vacuum suction is connected to this chamber and suction applied only until bubbles start to appear in the water column. Higher levels of applied vacuum only lead to more active bubbling and do not result in a higher level of suction being applied to the pleural space. The standard amount of suction for an adult patient is 20 cm of water.

The tubes leading to the Pleurovac unit from the vacuum source and from the patient **must never be clamped** or kinked. Clamping of the chest tube coming from the patient can prevent evacuation of leaking air (from pulmonary staple lines after a lung resection, for example), which can rapidly lead to a tension pneumothorax. To transport a patient who has a chest tube connected to a Pleurovac unit, make sure the water seal chamber is appropriately filled and is upright, and simply disconnect the unit from the wall suction source. Never clamp the tubes. The decision as to when chest tubes are to be removed should always be made by the operating surgeon. Generally, the tubes are removed once it has been documented that air leaks are gone and significant drainage of blood and fluid is no longer anticipated.

POSTOPERATIVE COMPLICATIONS

Numerous complications may occur following thoracic surgical procedures. Respiratory complications are the most frequent and may be of a severe nature. Other rare but life-threatening conditions may occur and vigilance along with a high index of suspicion are necessary attributes for the postoperative caregivers. Cardiac herniation with hemodynamic collapse, major hemorrhage from a slipped ligature, bronchial disruption, pulmonary edema, paradoxical embolism, and serious cardiac arrhythmias are all possible. Troublesome though nonlife-threatening problems include neural injuries to the phrenic, vagus, or recurrent laryngeal nerves and airway injuries to the vocal cords, larynx, or trachea resulting from double-lumen tube interventions. In addition, severe pain is the rule and must be managed effectively.

Respiratory Failure

With appropriate preoperative evaluation, respiratory failure following thoracic surgical procedures, in particular pulmonary resections, should be minimized. Nevertheless, occasional high-risk patients, either by the nature of their disease or through intraoperative events, will be encountered whose postoperative pulmonary management is not straightforward. An acute awareness of subtle changes in oxygenation and ventilation or of altered pain management or mental status is essential to avoid a downward pulmonary spiral leading to prolonged respiratory failure.

Careful intra- and postoperative fluid management is critical in patients undergoing a lung resection. Any extra volume through unnecessary intravenous fluid administration can rapidly lead to pulmonary edema in the nonoperated lung. In addition, lengthy lobectomy procedures during which the remaining ipsilateral lobe was collapsed during single-lung ventilation can render that lobe very sensitive to volume overload and severe reexpansion pulmonary edema. Intravenous fluids should be maintained at one-half to two-thirds maintenance levels for this reason. Furthermore, more patients are undergoing lung resections for malignancy after undergoing preoperative chemo- and radiotherapy. While no scientific data exist, it appears these patients may be even more susceptible to postoperative pulmonary edema, perhaps because of direct pulmonary toxicity of the preoperative regimen, or to altered lymphatic and mucociliary clearance of parenchymal fluid and endobronchial secretions within the irradiated lung.

Postoperative respiratory failure is almost always reversible and should be treated aggressively. If need be, mechanical ventilation should be reinstituted. Bronchoscopy should be used to clear the tracheobronchial tree and help reexpand areas of lobar collapse. Appropriate antibiotics should be used to help clear any developing pneumonia. Careful diuresis should be carried out and, if cardiac function is in doubt, pulmonary artery catheterization should be considered for optimal management. One must be very careful when floating a pulmonary-artery catheter following lobectomy or pneumonectomy because of to the presence of fresh vascular staple or suture lines. If the patient is severely debilitated, thought must be given to performing a tracheostomy for prolonged ventilatory support, while concomitant medical conditions are corrected and nutritional status is improved.

Reexpansion Pulmonary Edema

Patients presenting with large pleural effusions and complete lung collapse also seem particularly prone to reexpansion pulmonary edema. If the pleural effusion (at times, 6 liters or more) is drained off all at once, the underlying lung rapidly reexpands and is suddenly reperfused. This rapid reperfusion leads to endothelial injury and a profound capillary leak. Pulmonary edema in such instances can be so severe that it requires intubation and mechanical ventilation. Large long-standing pleural effusions should probably be drained slowly, one liter at a time over several hours.

Cardiac Herniation

The pericardium is often entered intraoperatively, especially for control and ligation of major pulmonary veins. Additionally, pericardium may be resected because of its involvement by contiguous tumor. A large pericardial defect may remain, through which the myocardium can herniate. Mechanical herniation causes blockage of venous return and a near total cessation of cardiac output. Herniation usually follows a change in patient position, such as a turn to the lateral decubitus position, but it could involve a change in the level of suction in a chest tube as well. Treatment involves a return to the prior position or a turn to the contralateral side immediately. If the original position is unknown, the patient is placed with the nonoperated side down. Treatment is surgical and involves emergency thoracotomy in the ICU or a return to the operating room. Obviously, this problem is best treated by surgical maneuvers which prevent the condition from occurring in the first place. Closure of the pericardial defect with autologous tissue or bovine pericardial grafts is the technique of choice during the primary procedure.

Somewhat analogous to cardiac herniation is torsion of a pulmonary lobe following resection of the other lobe or lobes on that side. Torsion is rarely possible when the lobe is fully inflated but may occur in an atelectatic lobe. Torsion blocks blood flow to the involved segments and will require surgical correction. A double lumen tube must be in place to deal with reexpansion pulmonary edema and bleeding from the involved lung with release of torsion and to help with expansion of the atelectatic lung.

Major Hemorrhage

Ligatures are placed around major pulmonary vessels during pulmonary resections. Slippage of a ligature is fortunately rare, because of the low pressures in the pulmonary vasculature. Slippage may be caused by poor intraoperative surgical technique or, more likely, movement and traction caused by deep breathing and coughing in the postoperative period. The large pleural space will do little to retard bleeding before massive amounts of blood loss have occurred. Close monitoring of vital signs and chest tube drainage are, therefore, essential after pulmonary resection. In the case of pneumonectomy, in which no chest tubes are left in place, one must be extra aware of the possibility of postoperative hemorrhage. Any hemodynamic instability or fall in hematocrit must be evaluated with a chest radiograph. If the pleural space has filled too quickly with fluid one must assume it is blood, and prompt reexploration should be considered.

More common than massive bleeding is bleeding of a persistent nature from raw pleural surfaces. Such bleeding may be difficult to control intraoperatively; patients are often closed with the hope that such bleeding will stop. Following pneumonectomy there is a higher risk of bleeding because there will be no remaining lung tissue to be inflated against the raw pleural surfaces. Other causes of bleeding can be from the bronchial and intercostal arteries.

Significant bleeding must be suspected in the case of an instability of vital signs. A lack of chest tube drainage does not rule out blood loss. Chest tubes can be easily blocked by blood clots and blood can pool in areas not drained by the specific chest tube. Furthermore, chest tubes are not placed following pneumonectomy. Chest radiographs may reveal accumulation of fluid in the chest and suggest bleeding in the presence of unstable vital signs and dropping hematocrit. Treatment is obviously surgical in a severe case but can represent a difficult clinical decision in the face of slow, indolent bleeding post thoracotomy.

Bronchial Disruption and Pneumothorax

Acute bronchial disruption is a life-threatening complication following major pulmonary resection. It is caused by a technical failure of the bronchial suture or staple line. Massive air leak from the chest tube is seen and is followed by hypoxia and hypercarbia as ventilation becomes ineffectual secondary to excessive loss of tidal volume through the bronchopleural fistula. Chest tube suction should be discontinued, with the tube left to underwater seal only. Clamping of the tube must not be done because it would result in a tension pneumothorax. Reintubation with a double lumen tube may be necessary before return to the operating room for definitive closure.

Pneumothorax and lung collapse can occur because of a malfunction of chest tube drainage. Clogging with blood or simple mechanical kinking are potential causes of chest tube occlusion. A lack of adequate chest tube drainage may result in pneumothorax or tension pneumothorax. Additionally, one must be cognizant of the fact that the contralateral, nonoperated hemithorax is at risk for developing pneumothorax, either from intraoperative injury of its mediastinal pleura or from high airway pressures necessitated during reexpansion of the operated lung.

Arrhythmias

Arrhythmias are not uncommonly seen after thoracic surgical procedures and are most common with pulmonary resections. As many as 20% of patients undergoing lobectomy or pneumonectomy may develop postoperative arrhythmias. Rarely are these disturbances life-threatening. Atrial fibrillation is the most commonly occurring arrhythmia. Treatment of atrial arrhythmias in this setting consists of rate control followed by attempts at medical, or if necessary for hemodynamic stability, electrical cardioversion. Besides treatment with digoxin, rate control is best achieved with the administration of the calcium channel blocker diltiazem. Beta blockade will often be contraindicated in these patients, many of whom already have significant reactive airway disease.

PAIN MANAGEMENT

The thoracotomy wound is one of the most painful surgical incisions. Not only is good pain control important for patient satisfaction, it is essential to minimize postoperative pulmonary complications in this high-risk group. Pain comes from a variety of sources, the most important of which is the incision. Respiratory motion stretches the wound and produces an increase in painful stimulation. The patient will attempt to minimize this discomfort by splinting and actively exhaling, thereby, minimizing the amount and duration of motion. Coughing, with its need for a large volume inspiration and forceful exhalation, is also actively avoided by the patient. The net result of such abnormal respiratory patterns will be a loss of lung volumes of a restrictive nature, retention of secretions, airway closure, and atelectasis.

The severe pain of the thoracotomy wound crosses at least seven somatic dermatomes, as well as being transmitted by afferents of the vagus nerve. Soft tissue, muscle, and bone pain are accompanied by visceral pain from the lungs and mediastinal structures. The former nociceptive signals pass through the intercostal nerves and are sensed as intense, localized pain in the wound itself. Diaphragmatic irritation may lead to shoulder or scapular referred pain, while pain from visceral discomfort traveling over the more vague vagal afferents is sensed as intense and deep, and is difficult to localize. Treatment of pain must not involve maneuvers that will interrupt all function of the mixed motor and sensory nerves involved in its transmission. For example, blockade of the phrenic nerve would paralyze the diaphragm and vagal blockade would eliminate important cough reflexes and lead to tachycardia.

Narcotics have traditionally been the mainstay of pain treatment. Adequate analgesia is indicated by a decrease in splinting and active exhalation. These drugs obviously carry the important side effect of causing central respiratory depression. Some aggravation of hypercarbia is expected and unavoidable. The use of patient-controlled analgesia (PCA) infusion pumps has minimized complications with narcotics. That is because periods of oversedation and inadequate pain control can be avoided with the narrow therapeutic window of narcotics being more easily maintained. Some patients do not do well with PCA because of their inability to properly use the devices. Regardless, narcotics themselves may be inadequate for pain relief in one-fifth of thoracotomy patients.

A variety of other pain control modalities have been brought to bear on postthoracotomy pain. Intercostal or paravertebral blocks using local anesthetic drugs can be performed intraoperatively by surgeons, or postoperatively by any caregivers. Continuous methods using indwelling catheters are possible, as well. Complications such as pneumothorax are usually negated by the presence of chest tubes on the operated side. Vascular uptake of local anesthetics is often rapid. Care must be taken to observe for signs of local anesthetic toxicity and to ensure that treatment for such complications is immediately available. While not treating deep-seated visceral pain, these blocks are effective in decreasing narcotic requirements and improving pulmonary function.

Interpleural analgesia is a variant of intercostal blockade. Local anesthetics placed within the pleural cavity will diffuse through the parietal pleura and block intercostal nerves. The spread of drug within the pleural space is greatly affected by gravity so patients must be placed supine to permit drug to reach the desired posterior aspects of the intercostal nerves. Problems also derive from loss of drug out through chest tube drains, which must necessarily be clamped for at least 10 minutes after drug instillation. Such clamping would be impossible in the presence of large air leaks. Significant bleeding or actual adhesions obliterating the pleural space would also result in a failure of this technique. Once again, toxicity from local anesthetics is a risk. Despite the fallbacks of interpleural analgesia, there are times when this proves to be simple and elegant and is fairly effective at alleviating somatic pain from thoracotomy.

Cryoanalgesia is practiced by some surgeons. At the completion of surgery, a cryo-probe is used to create a long-lasting, but hopefully temporary, neuropraxia of intercostal nerves. The probe must be placed directly on the nerve; this will require a small amount of additional dissection. Chest tubes should then be placed through dermatomes rendered insensate by the cryo blockade. Somatic pain control is effective but lasts longer than does the significant postoperative pain. Further disadvantages of this technique are the potential for permanent numbness or intercostal muscle paralysis, and some reports of troublesome dysesthesias.

Perispinal opiates are evolving into the standard of care for postthoracotomy pain control. There are a wealth of opioid receptors in the substantia gelatinosa of the dorsal horn of the spinal cord and nociceptive stimulation can be effectively modulated at this level with the use of narcotics. Analgesia obtained by this route is predictable, prolonged, and devoid of effects on the sympathetic nervous system. Furthermore, blockade of other sensations, such as proprioception and temperature, does not occur and the important motor functions necessary for active respiration and ambulation are not blocked. Studies have shown that effective peridural opioid therapy increases forced vital capacity, expiratory reserve volumes, and patient compliance and tolerance of respiratory therapy maneuvers.

Opiates can be given intrathecally or epidurally and from caudal, lumbar, or thoracic sites. Drug effects and side effects differ considerably on the basis of differences in lipid solubility. While details are clearly outside the scope of this discussion, some generalizations are important to understand.

The intrathecal route is used sparingly because it requires repeat dural punctures. There are significant risks to long-term use of indwelling catheters in the subarachnoid space, which are not as high with similarly placed epidural catheters. Morphine is relatively hydrophilic and spreads significantly within the thecal sac. Therefore, it is effective for thoracic pain even when given by lumbar dural puncture. Analgesia is profound and lasts 18 to 24 hours. However, the excellent spread offered by this lipophobic drug is responsible for its high incidence of side effects. Rostral spread to the central nervous system is responsible for late respiratory depression in a small percentage of patients. This risk is significantly reduced with epidural administration and with other drugs. It represents another reason for the relatively infrequent use of intrathecal opioids in thoracotomy patients.

Epidural administration, thus, has become the route of choice for most practitioners. Catheters can be placed and used for up to 5 days with a low incidence of infectious complications. Analgesia is effectively delivered from both lumbar and thoracic routes. The former is associated with a lower risk of neural damage because the spinal cord ends at the level of the first lumbar vertebra. Lumbar administration of morphine, the least lipophilic drug, has an onset within 60 minutes and lasts also for 18 to 24 hours. Lumbar administration of lipophilic drugs, such as fentanyl, is characterized by an onset within 10 to 20 minutes and less tendency to spread rostrally to thoracic levels because of the rapid binding of drug to neural tissues. Fentanyl must be administered in a large volume of diluent to physically force its rostral spread, or it must be given at the thoracic level through a highly placed epidural catheter. Most studies suggest that either route is effective and neither has been definitively shown to be more effective. Thoracic placement has the advantage of being at the level of the desired analgesic effects, is more amenable to use with a constant infusion to maintain analgesia, and can be combined with diluted local anesthetic solutions to add to potential pain control.

Side effects from epidural narcotics are significant but are usually less morbid than those from systemically administered drugs. Delayed respiratory depression is the most feared complication, particularly in the thoracic surgical patient. The incidence is only approximately 0.09%, and its onset is slow and readily detected with monitoring of level of consciousness and respiratory rate. Nausea and vomiting also result from rostral spread of drug to the chemoreceptor trigger zone, near the fourth ventricle in the brain. Pruritis is common and probably mediated at the spinal level. Urinary retention is similarly common and likely results from a resulting imbalance in innervation of the bladder musculature. The latter is often not observed because of the frequent use of indwelling urinary catheters in the thoracic-surgical patient population. Other side effects are readily treated with narcotic antagonists and without reversal of analgesia if used in small doses.

Respiratory depression can be monitored by floor nurses taking frequent vital signs at least twice per hour. Because onset is slow, adequate time for treatment is afforded. Any patient with increasing somnolence deserves particular attention as does one with diminishing respiratory effort and rate. Additional teams of observers or intensive care are not mandated solely because of the use of epidural narcotics. Narcotic antagonists should be readily available for the treatment of delayed respiratory depression. A separate infusion at a low rate can be started or drug can simply be added to maintenance intravenous solutions. Bolus doses must be carefully titrated to avoid rapidly reversing all analgesic effects, but this is rarely a problem because the respiratory depressant effects are readily reversible with only small doses of antagonists.

The use of dilute local anesthetic solutions may add to analgesia when given at the thoracic level. While administration of local anesthetic and lipophilic narcotics through thoracic epidural catheters has become relatively common, there is little formal evidence that it is better than epidural narcotic alone. Future studies will need to be performed and analyzed. Sympathetic fibers are blocked with the use of low concentrations of local anesthetics and, therefore, some degree of sympathectomy is unavoidable. Motor blockade is usually avoidable and, thus, cough effectiveness is often not further impaired.

Fluid management must be meticulous and undertaken with full knowledge of whether local anesthetics are being used and whether any sympathetic blockade has resulted. Vasodilation and, particularly, venodilation are the result of sympathetic blockade and will increase intravascular fluid needs. Cessation of epidural sympathetic blockade will be accompanied by a return to basal vascular tone, a decrease in blood capacitance, and a resultant potential for fluid overload. The thoracic surgical patient is already at significant risk for the ravages of overhydration and this risk can be compounded by inattention to this detail. Communication between pain management, surgeon, and consultant teams is imperative.

BIBLIOGRAPHY

Baue AE, et al: *Glenn's thoracic and cardiovascular surgery,* ed 6, Stamford, Conn., 1996, Appleton & Lange.

Elefteriades JA, Geha AS, Cohen LS: *House officer guide to ICU care: fundamentals of management of the heart and lungs*, New York, 1994, Raven Press.

Pearson FG, et al: *Thoroacic surgery*, New York, 1995, Churchill Livingstone.

Sabiston DC Jr, Spencer FC: *Gibbons's surgery of the chest*, Philadelphia, 1983, WB Saunders.

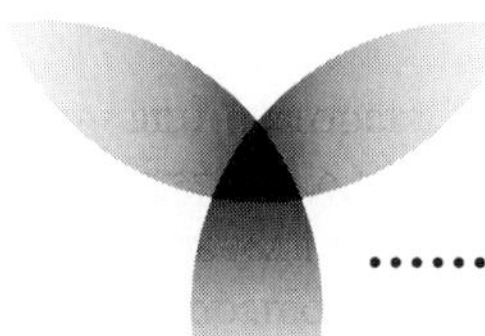

Chapter 35

Cardiopulmonary Bypass

David J. Di Benedetto, MD, George S. Leisure, MD, Curtis G. Tribble, MD

The pursuit of artificial oxygenation and perfusion traces its origins back to the 19th century when physiologists developed the earliest oxygenators and pumps. As early as the 1880s, work by von Frey and Gruber resulted in the first rudimentary heart-lung machine. Despite these developments, it was not until the discovery of heparin by McLean in 1916 that the science of perfusion could begin to advance because heparin allows for the exposure of blood to foreign surfaces without the formation of a clot. In 1934 DeBakey described the use of the roller pump, and by 1950, the use of bubble oxygenators became possible with the development of defoaming agents. The accomplishments of these early pioneers culminated in the first successful clinical application of cardiopulmonary bypass (CPB) when it was used during the repair of an atrial septal defect (ASD) in a young woman by Dr J.H. Gibbon Jr in 1953. Since that time the use of extracorporeal circulation has become commonplace. Cardiopulmonary bypass now makes possible the routine surgical repair of diseases which once were associated with significant morbidity and mortality. Yet, despite the great advances in the science of perfusion that have continually improved its safety, the use of CPB is not without risk. Significant sequelae still remain a concern, resulting in up to 30% of the postoperative morbidity occurring in these patients. This chapter will examine the perioperative issues and concerns facing the patient preparing to undergo CPB.

• INDICATIONS FOR CARDIOPULMONARY BYPASS (CPB)

Since its first successful clinical application in 1953, the utility of CPB has grown. It is estimated that over 250,000 surgical procedures using extracorporeal circulation are performed each year. Today, CPB is essential, not only for cardiac surgery, but for a wide variety of noncardiac procedures, as well (Box 35-1).

• PREOPERATIVE EVALUATION

Patients undergoing surgery in which CPB is to be used often have a multitude of medical problems in addition to the underlying cardiac pathology. Both cardiac and noncardiac diseases have an impact on perioperative morbidity and mortality. Higgins et al. found that chronic pulmonary disease, anemia, renal impairment, and, to a lesser extent, diabetes mellitus, obesity, and cerebrovascular disease were significant predictors of postoperative morbidity and mortality, in addition to the traditionally accepted cardiac risk factors. Thus, it is essential that both the cardiac status as well as coexisting conditions be assessed and treated preoperatively, so as to optimize outcome.

Cardiac Evaluation

The cardiac risk factors associated with increased perioperative morbidity and mortality have been well defined. Left ventricular (LV) dysfunction, emergency surgery, advanced age, female gender, history of prior coronary artery bypass grafting (CABG), and presence of left main coronary disease have been shown to influence perioperative risk in most studies. The presence of LV dysfunction is the most important of these risk factors for two reasons. First, it is the only predictive factor mentioned that can be improved by preoperative management. Second, studies have shown that in patients with severely depressed LV function (i.e., ejection fraction <20%), none of the traditional risk factors are significant. Urgency of surgery becomes the only predictor of operative mortality. Thus, it is important to accurately assess and maximize LV function preoperatively.

In patients ready to undergo a surgical procedure using CPB, an evaluation of LV function should be performed. This should begin with the cardiac history, physical

Box 35-1 Indications for CPB

Cardiac procedures
- Coronary artery bypass grafting (CABG)
- Valvular repairs/replacements
- Congenital heart anomaly repairs
- Heart transplantation

Noncardiac procedures
- Ascending aortic surgery
- Single lung transplantation (CPB standby)
- Double lung transplantation
- Pulmonary embolectomy
- Complex neurologic procedures (e.g., highly selected cases of basilar-tip aneurysm surgery)
- Treatment for severe hypothermia

examination, and electrocardiogram (ECG). Contrast ventriculography and echocardiography are also likely to be included. If LV dysfunction is discovered, attempts should be made to improve ventricular performance preoperatively through the appropriate use of medications to reduce afterload, improve contractility, and control ventricular rate. In the patient with severely depressed LV function, intensive therapy with intravenous inotropic medications, and use of an intraaortic balloon pump, may decrease perioperative morbidity and mortality. In addition, a critical consideration in the patient with depressed LV function is whether or not the function can be improved by the surgical intervention.

Neurologic Evaluation

There exists the potential for postoperative neurologic dysfunction in patients undergoing CPB, especially for those with preexisting cerebrovascular disease. Recent studies have found the incidence of cerebrovascular accident (CVA) to be 2% to 5%. When studies have tested for more subtle neuropsychiatric dysfunction, the incidence of immediate postoperative deficits has been found to be as high as 80%, with up to 50% showing some subtle, residual deterioration 6 months later. Fortunately, the majority of these patients normalize within the first year. It is, therefore, important to evaluate carefully the patient's neurologic status to differentiate preoperative from postoperative deficits, to identify patients at higher risk for postoperative neurologic impairment, and to provide the patient with an accurate assessment of perioperative risk, as well.

Of special interest is the patient in whom significant cerebrovascular disease exists (i.e., carotid stenosis >70% and/or symptomatic disease). It is estimated that the incidence of carotid stenosis in patients undergoing CABG is 40%. Furthermore, the incidence of having a CVA is 17 times greater in patients with symptomatic carotid disease, as compared to patients free of carotid stenosis. A greater incidence of hypoperfusion and embolization from vascular disease in the ascending aorta and carotid arteries is thought to be the etiology responsible for this increase in risk. Two questions commonly arise in the preoperative evaluation of these patients. First, can the risk of postoperative neurologic deficit be reduced? Second, should the patient undergo a combined carotid endarterectomy (CEA)/CABG or staged procedure?

Interventions that have been made to reduce the incidence of postoperative deficits in high-risk patients have been met with limited success. It has been shown that by paying meticulous attention to aortic cross clamping, by using a membrane oxygenator and appropriate arterial filters, and by limiting bypass time, the risk for embolization is reduced. Obviously, these techniques benefit all patients undergoing CPB. The use of drugs such as barbiturates, steroids, prostacyclines, calcium-channel blockers, and N-methyl-D-asparate (NMDA) antagonists have been studied for possible cerebroprotective effects; but have either shown little benefit or are still under investigation. Other than the surgical maneuvers and methods mentioned earlier, protecting high-risk patients often centers around attempts to ensure adequate cerebral perfusion pressures. Traditionally, this has meant using higher perfusion pressures during CPB. The validity of this approach has been questioned in a recent study by Johnsson et al., which found preservation of cerebral blood flow down to bypass pressures of 50 mm Hg in patients with severe bilateral carotid disease. As this and other studies suggest, embolization from the aorta and heart is the main source of neurologic morbidity in these patients, rather than the carotid disease. Consequently, surgical and bypass techniques to minimize embolization are the key to reducing postoperative neurologic morbidity and mortality.

Whether the patient should undergo a staged or combined CEA/CABG procedure has been long debated. If the cerebral blood flow in patients with significant carotid disease is preserved down to the lower limits of autoregulation as the previous study suggests, then the criteria for performing a combined approach should not be based on the flow-limiting influence of the carotid stenosis. Combined CEA/CABG has a 17% major morbidity/mortality, so it should be reserved for those who are unstable from both a neurologic and cardiac standpoint.

Renal Evaluation

Preoperative renal insufficiency has been shown to be a significant predictor of postoperative mortality. In the study by Higgins et al., a creatinine level over 1.8 mg/dl was found to be second in importance only to urgency of surgery, in predicting postoperative morbidity and mortality. Deterioration of renal function is also more likely in these patients, possibly because of the decrease in renal perfusion, loss of pulsatile blood flow, and hemoglobinuria that can occur during CPB. Additionally, these patients have a greater incidence of anemia, diabetes, cerebrovascular disease, all of which are significant risk factors for postoperative morbidity and mortality. Attempts should be made to improve renal function, maintain adequate volume status, avoid nephrotoxic insults, and correct anemia and electrolyte abnormalities before surgery.

Medications

Specific recommendations regarding the management of the patient's routine medications are covered elsewhere in this book. In general, medications should be continued up until the night before surgery. Each medication should be well documented, and the anesthesiologist should be prepared to treat the potential toxicities and adverse drug interactions of these drugs with anesthetics. Prior exposure to aprotinin and protamine should be noted because the risk for anaphylaxis is increased with reexposure.

Cardiovascular drugs should be continued up until the time of surgery. Premature discontinuation of these drugs may precipitate rebound tachycardia, hypertension, and tachyarrhythmias, thus, placing the patient at an increased risk for myocardial ischemia. These medications are unlikely to interact adversely with anesthetics, and they may provide greater intraoperative hemodynamic stability. Heparin infusions may be discontinued 6 hours before surgery to minimize the risk of hemorrhage and hematoma formation during the prebypass period. However, patients who experience angina after discontinuation of the infusion should be immediately reheparinized and the infusion continued until the time of CPB.

PHYSIOLOGY OF CARDIOPULMONARY BYPASS

Cardiopulmonary bypass transfers the functions of gas exchange, circulation, and thermoregulation from the patient to the CPB machine, thus, allowing the performance of complex surgical procedures. The basic machine consists of a pump, an oxygenator, a heat exchanger, a cardiotomy reservoir, arterial and venous cannulas, filters, and interconnecting tubing (Figure 35-1). During CPB, blood bypasses the heart and lungs and drains by gravity from the venous cannula to the venous reservoir. The venous blood is then oxygented, temperature adjusted, filtered, and pumped at arterial pressure into either the aorta or femoral artery. The goal is to provide the respiratory and perfusion needs while minimizing the impact of CPB on the patient. Despite the advances in perfusion science that have occurred, extracorporeal circulation imposes a unique set of physiologic alterations on the patient.

Circulatory Changes

With the initiation of CPB, blood pressure typically decreases because of the decrease in viscosity that occurs when the patient's blood is mixed with the priming solution used in the bypass circuit. Other possible mechanisms include the dilution of catecholamines and the transient hypoxemia that occurs with the abrupt decrease in oxygen-carrying capacity, related to the dilutional effect of the priming solution. After this initial decrease in blood pressures, systemic vascular resistance (SVR) and systemic pressure increase. Several factors are thought to be responsible for this rise in blood pressure, including increases in viscosity caused by hypothermia, and decreased vascular cross-sectional area, secondary to increasing catecholamine levels, hypothermia-induced vasoconstriction, and, possibly, microvasculature closure related to the use of nonpulsatile perfusion during CPB. Finally, as the patient is rewarmed and the aortic cross clamp is removed before separation from CPB, SVR and systemic pressures typically decrease. This is thought to occur because of vasodilation induced by rewarming, as well as the release of vasodilating metabolites such as adenosine. As these hemodynamic changes occur, interventions are made to maintain systemic pressures within a predetermined range (usually 50 mm Hg

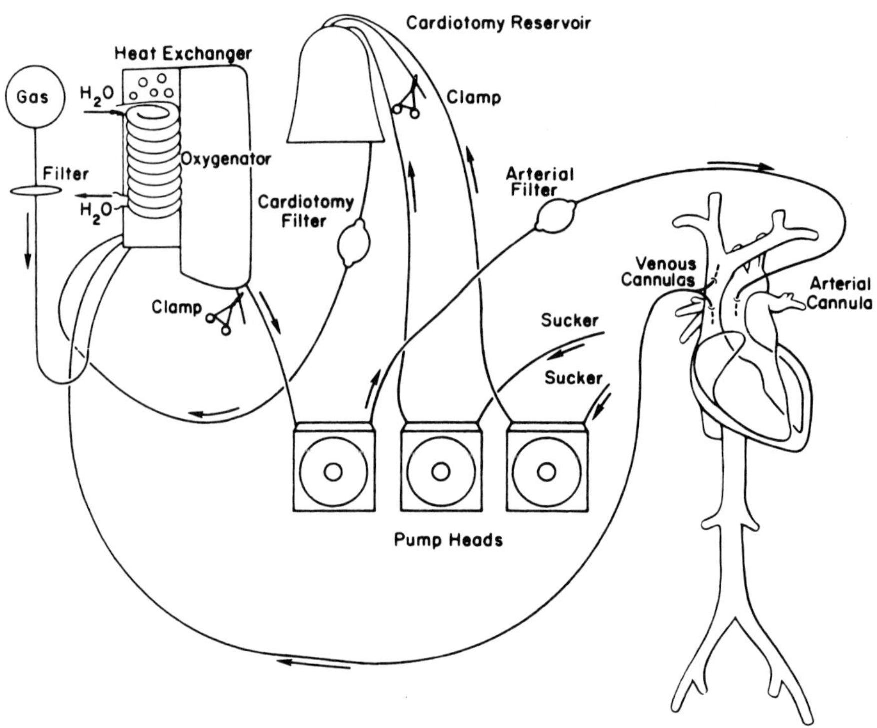

Figure 35-1
A schematic drawing of the extracorporeal circuit.

to 80 mm Hg). Increases in pressure during CPB are first treated with additional anesthetics to ensure an adequate depth of anesthesia, followed by the use of sodium nitroprusside or α-1 receptor-blocking agents such as phentolamine, if needed. Decreases in pressure are best treated by first ensuring adequate intravascular volume, followed by the use of α agonists such phenylephrine.

Ultimately, the goal of systemic pressure manipulation is to ensure adequate end-organ perfusion. We know that this goal is not always achieved, because patients continue to experience renal, neurologic, pulmonary, and cardiac dysfunction postoperatively that is, in part, caused by our inability to reproduce exactly normal circulatory physiology during CPB. To monitor for end-organ hypoperfusion, we ideally would obtain measurements of tissue-oxygen tensions. Unfortunately, this is currently not possible and, instead, estimates of global-tissue perfusion and oxygen supply are used. Of the indices of global-tissue perfusion currently used, determination of oxygen consumption is the most sensitive indicator. Using the Fick Principle, global-oxygen consumption can be determined by first measuring arterial and venous PO_2, hemoglobin concentrations, and perfusion flow rates. Measured venous PO_2 can also be used as an indicator of global perfusion but is a less accurate index because the arterial-venous shunting that occurs during CPB may yield normal venous PO_2 measurements, despite ongoing tissue hypoperfusion. Lactate and base excess levels are also used as indicators of the adequacy of end-organ perfusion but are fairly insensitive markers and, therefore, of limited use. Urine output has long been used as an indicator of tissue perfusion and volume status for all types of surgical procedures. Unfortunately, it is an inaccurate index during CPB because hypothermia-induced diuresis, and the frequent use of osmotic diuretics in the pump-priming solution influence urine production.

In an attempt to ensure adequate end-organ perfusion, flow rates are set to maintain a cardiac index over 1.9 $l/min/m^2$, which is thought to represent the level below which, the risk for tissue hypoperfusion is increased. The mean arterial pressure (MAP) necessary to maintain adequate perfusion is more controversial. Studies have demonstrated that autoregulatory mechanisms remain intact during CPB as long as α-stat pH management of arterial blood gases is used (see following). As a result, MAP is usually maintained above 50 mm Hg. The validity of this practice has been challenged by several studies which have shown preservation of cerebral blood flow at MAP as low as 30 mm Hg. Given the fact that many of these studies excluded patients with untreated hypertension, diabetes mellitus, and cerebrovascular disease, it would seem prudent to maintain MAP above 50 mm Hg in the adult population.

Hypothermia

Most procedures performed using CPB use hypothermia as a means to decrease the metabolic activities of vital organs such as the heart and brain, thus, providing protection against ischemic damage. It has been shown that a 10°C reduction in body temperature results in a 50% reduction in overall oxygen consumption. With this beneficial decrease in metabolism, several other physiologic changes also occur.

Hypothermia increases blood viscosity, potentially causing an impairment in tissue perfusion. It is estimated that a 30% increase in blood viscosity accompanies a 10°C reduction in body temperature. Under these conditions, a state of hyperviscosity is produced, possibly resulting in sludging, tissue hypoperfusion, and end-organ damage. These problems are overcome by simultaneously decreasing blood viscosity through hemodilution.

Tissue oxygenation also may be altered as hypothermia induces a leftward shift in the oxygen-hemoglobin dissociation curve. As a result of the increased affinity of hemoglobin for oxygen, oxygen transfer to tissues may be impaired. This detrimental effect is offset by the 25% increase in dissolved oxygen and 50% reduction in oxygen consumption that occurs with a 10°C decrease in body temperature.

Acid-base physiology is also altered by hypothermia. The solubility of both oxygen and carbon dioxide are increased by hypothermia, resulting in a reduction in their partial pressures. This effect is more apparent for carbon dioxide given its high solubility, and results in an elevation in the pH of blood as the patient is cooled. This alteration in blood pH has lead to the development of two acid-base management strategies during CPB. The first, known as pH-stat, strives to maintain a pH of 7.4 during CPB by adding carbon dioxide to the oxygenator, thereby, increasing the partial pressure of this gas to its normal range (i.e., 40 mm Hg). Proponents of this strategy cite the cerebral vasodilatory effects of carbon dioxide and the possible protection this may provide against the reduction in cerebral blood flow induced by hypothermia. The second and most commonly used technique, know as α-stat, maintains a pH of 7.4 and a $PaCO_2$ of 40 mm Hg when the blood gas is warmed to 37°C before analysis. Proponents cite the maintenance of the intracellular hydroxide ion: hydrogen ion ratio under this strategy. This, in turn, maintains the dissociation state of the imidazole group on histidine, which has been shown to be necessary for optimal enzyme function. Unlike pH-stat which produces pressure-passive cerebral blood flow, α-stat has been shown to preserve cerebral autoregulation. Furthermore, α-stat has been shown to improve myocardial contractility and metabolic profiles as compared to pH-stat management. Despite these facts, no study has yet to show improved outcome when using α-stat, rather than pH-stat management.

Hemodilution

Hemodilution is used to prevent the end-organ damage and pulmonary congestion that once occurred when pumps were primed with blood, resulting in states of hyperviscosity and volume overload. The need for blood transfusions may also be decreased by the use of hemodilution. However, hemodilution also causes a reduction in the concentration of other blood components, possibly resulting in adverse consequences. For example, colloid-oncotic pressures are decreased primarily because of the dilution of albumin, resulting in increased tissue edema. Impaired coagulation may also result from the dilution of platelets and coagulation factors.

PATHOPHYSIOLOGY OF CARDIOPULMONARY BYPASS

Myocardial Ischemia and Preservation

Myocardial preservation during CPB is of paramount importance. Alterations in perfusion that occur during CPB place the myocardium at risk for both ischemic damage and reperfusion injury. With the onset of CPB and aortic cross clamping, blood flow to the myocardium is minimal and ischemia results. Metabolic changes occur, resulting in a shift from aerobic to anaerobic metabolism and the accumulation of lactate and hydrogen ions. Myocardial energy stores are rapidly depleted, adenosine levels rise, and calcium homeostasis is impaired. If allowed to progress, cellular swelling, membrane disruption, and cytolysis will occur. When coronary flow is restored early, cellular changes are fully reversible and rapid recovery occurs. Immediate recovery may not result if the duration of ischemia is prolonged, but, instead, takes hours to days to occur. Myocardial compliance and the ejection fraction are reduced during this period, resulting in so-called "stunned" myocardium.

Myocardial reperfusion injury occurs when previously ischemic myocardial tissue is reperfused, such as what occurs at the end of CPB. Reperfusion injury is characterized by mitochondrial dysfunction, which results in impaired oxygen utilization. Etiologic factors include the inhibition of ATP production by the rapid influx of calcium ions which occurs with reperfusion, and the release of proteolytic enzymes and free radicals, which occurs from reperfusion activation of neutrophils.

Intraoperative myocardial preservation attempts to minimize the ischemic and reperfusion damage that occurs during CPB. Preservation is achieved by decreasing metabolic demands through the use of hypothermia, hyperkalemic cardiac arrest, and the prevention of ventricular distention and edema formation by venting the LV and the use of mannitol. Under conditions of hypothermia and cardiac arrest, oxygen comsumption is only 5% of that at baseline. Despite this reduction in metabolic demand and the intermittent infusion of oxygenated cardioplegia, damage caused by ischemia and reperfusion can still result.

Hematologic Abnormalities

Exposure of the patient's blood to CPB causes significant destruction of both cellular and plasma components. Hemolysis can result when red blood cells (RBC) are exposed to foreign surfaces and sheer stresses, which are present during the passage through the oxygenator and pump. Cardiopulmonary bypass also leads to increased RBC fragility, resulting in decreased RBC lifespan and delayed hemolysis. As a result of these processes, free hemoglobin is generated. When the amount of free hemoglobin exceeds binding and removal by haptoglobin and the reticuloendothelial system, hemoglobinuria results and acute tubular necrosis can occur.

Platelet dysfunction and thrombocytopenia are common complications of CPB. Thrombocytopenia results from several factors that include hemodilution, platelet activation, and destruction in the cardiotomy suction systems and blood filters, hepatic sequestration induced by protamine administration, and the destruction that occurs at blood-gas interfaces when a bubble oxygenator is used. The etiology of platelet dysfunction is also multifactorial. Exposure to the artificial surfaces of the CPB circuit causes platelet adhesion and activation, resulting in the major source of dysfunction. Hypothermia can also result in platelet dysfunction. Of these two factors, platelet dysfunction is the more significant contributor to postoperative hemorrhage. As a result, platelet counts do not usually correlate with the degree of postoperative hemorrhage.

Cardiopulmonary bypass also results in alterations in the coagulation and fibrinolytic systems. Hemodilution secondary to the pump prime, RBC transfusion, and cell washing can reduce coagulation factor levels. A consumptive coagulopathy may also result from extensive fibrinolysis. Fibrinolysis appears to occur commonly during CPB, and likely results from both increased plasmin activation and decreased plasmin-inhibitor activity. The use of hetastarch has also been shown to exacerbate the coagulopathy.

Immunologic Abnormalities

Leukocyte function is altered by exposure to CPB, as well. With the onset of CPB, white-blood-cell counts decrease primarily because of the margination and aggregation of neutrophils in the pulmonary and cardiac microcirculations. Subsequently, a leukocytosis occurs and persists for up to a week postoperatively. Leukocyte activation also appears to occur during CPB, resulting in tissue damage secondary to the release of lytic enzymes and free radicals. This activation has been shown to contribute to the pulmonary dysfunction that can occur after CPB.

Complement activation also occurs during CPB and appears to be a key stimulus for the leukocyte aggregation which occurs in the pulmonary and cardiac vasculature.

The complement system consists of at least 20 proteins which interact with one another. During CPB, several factors lead to abnormal complement activation. Antibody molecules tend to denature during CPB, resulting in aggregates which become potent stimultors for complement activation. Heparin-protamine complexes also have been shown to activate the complement cascade. When unrestrained, complement activation produces widespread inflammation, tissue damage, and, possibly, reduces the immunologic competence of the patient.

Neuroendocrine Response

Studies have shown that catecholamine, vasopressin, and renin levels are elevated in excess of that seen in nonCPB procedures. Catecholamine and vasopressin increases result from the stimulation of aortic and carotid sinus baroreceptors, which repond to the low-pulse pressures occurring with nonpulsatile CPB. Hypothermia also is a potent stimulus for catecholamine release. Decreased MAP experienced by the kidneys during bypass stimulates renin release, resulting in increased levels of angiotensin II and aldosterone. By increasing the levels of catecholamines, vasopressin, and angiotensin II, the neuroendocrine response to CPB results in vasocostriction. If perfusion flow rates are held constant in this setting, systemic pressures will rise. As a result, blood flow is redistributed to organs most sensitive to elevations in perfusion pressure (i.e., brain, heart, kidneys). Occasionally, organ hypoperfusion results from an excessive vasoconstrictor response, necessitating the reduction of vascular tone through the use of volatile anesthetics or other vasodilating drugs.

Clinical Problems in Establishing and Weaning From CPB

Despite the safety of CPB, there are potential problems that may happen during the establishment of or weaning from CPB. Misplacement of arterial or venous cannulae can have catastrophic consequences. For example, if the arterial or "return" cannula is placed within the arterial wall and not in the true lumen, aortic dissection may ensue. A misdirected arterial cannula can be placed into the left carotid artery, leading to possible arterial rupture or cerebral edema. Massive gas embolization with disastrous consequences can also occur with inattention to the oxygenator-reservoir level. Air can be pumped from an empty reservoir leading to possible stroke, myocardial infarction, or death. Pump failure, oxygen supply failure, and a clotted CPB circuit caused by inadequate systemic heparinization are other rare, but serious, complications.

Weaning from CPB involves a complex process whereby the mechanical work needed to pump blood is transferred from the CPB pump back to the patient's heart. Weaning begins with rewarming of the patient, and resumption of normal sinus rhythm. Spontaneous ventricular fibrillation that is difficult to convert during rewarming, may be caused by inadequate rewarming, air in the coronary arteries, or poor myocardial preservation. Subsequently, the heart is allowed to fill by restricting the venous return. Right-atrial pressure rises with the increased resistance of the venous line. As a result, some blood will begin to flow into the right ventricle instead of draining fully into the pump. As preload rises, the cardiac output will increase, and the heart will eject blood more forcefully as it fills and enlarges. The patient needs to be warm and in optimal metabolic and hemodynamic condition, with appropriate inotropic support instituted and the heart, great vessels, and grafts properly de-aired. Once these conditions are met, arterial inflow is stopped, and CPB is terminated.

The most common cause of cardiovascular insufficiency during weaning is left or right ventricular failure which can be caused by a myriad of factors including ongoing ischemia, graft or valve failure, incomplete myocardial preservation during CPB, increased myocardial oxygen demand, protamine reaction, inadequate oxygenation, and inadequate or excessive preload. The following risk factors have been associated with difficulty weaning from CPB: prolonged CPB duration, incomplete myocardial preservation, preoperative ejection fraction less than 40%, inadequate surgical repair such as in diabetic patients with severe distal disease, and evolving myocardial infarction or ongoing ischemia in the pre-CPB period. To avoid right ventricular failure, pulmonary hypertension must be minimized by correcting acidosis, and avoiding hypoxia and hypercarbia. In addition, drugs such as milrinone, isoproterenol, and nitroglycerin may ameliorate pulmonary hypertension. In the future, inhaled nitric oxide may prove the best treatment for pulmonary hypertension.

POSTOPERATIVE CONCERNS

While many of the postoperative concerns are similar to those facing other postsurgical intensive care unit (ICU) patients who have not undergone CPB, others are unique to this patient population. The successful outcome of the surgical procedure, performed with the use of extracorporeal circulation, depends greatly on the management of these problems in the immediate postoperative period.

Cardiovascular Function

The stress on the cardiovascular system continues into the postoperative period, frequently resulting in rapid hemodynamic fluctuations. Hypotension is a common postoperative complication, resulting from either a reduction in cardiac output, a decrease in SVR, or both. When a reduction in cardiac output occurs, a decrease in preload, secondary to hypovolemia, may be responsible. Other causes of reduced cardiac output include ischemia and infarction, acidosis, electrolyte imbalances, tamponade, dysrhythmias, and myocardial failure caused by increased afterload. When a pulmonary artery catheter is present, the diagnosis of a low-cardiac output state can be quickly made by use of thermodilutional measurements.

Decreases in SVR most commonly result from rewarming-induced vasodilation, but also can result from drug reactions and the presence of vasodilating drugs such as nitroglycerin and α-1 receptor antagonists commonly used in the management of these patients. Correction of the underlying cause for hypotension must occur quickly, because prolonged myocardial and systemic hypoperfusion will exacerbate the hemodynamic instability of the patient.

Myocardial ischemia and infarction can also occur postoperatively, resulting in reduced LV function, right ventricular failure, dysrhythmias, and death. Factors predisposing to ischemia and infarction include incomplete revascularization because of distal coronary vascular disease, preexisting ventricular dysfunction, vein graft closure, internal mammary artery vasospasm, and commonly, intracoronary air. Increased myocardial oxygen consumption because of hypertension can also lead to ischemia, and is frequently caused by inadequate postoperative analgesia, vasoconstriction induced by residual hypothermia, or the presence of hypertensive disease. Rapid diagnosis and treatment of the underlying cause for ischemia is essential. To prevent clinical deterioration of the patient, prompt insertion of an intraaortic balloon pump should be considered, in addition to increased inotropic support and calcium administration.

Pulmonary Function

Modern CPB techniques have virtually eliminated the development of postperfusion lung syndrome. However, postoperative pulmonary dysfunction still occurs. While the dysfunction appears to be maximal 24 hours after the completion of the surgery, many of the derangements take weeks to resolve. Furthermore, preexisting pulmonary disease is clearly associated with more severe postoperative pulmonary dysfunction.

Respiratory function is impaired after CPB for multiple reasons. Vital capacity, total lung capacity, inspiratory capacity, and functional residual capacity are all decreased postoperatively for up to 2 weeks. Total lung capacity may be decreased by 25% postoperatively. As a result, the work of breathing required for spontaneous ventilation is increased. At the same time, respiratory drive can be depressed by the narcotics and sedatives commonly used in these patients, thus, blunting the response to hypoxia and hypercapnia. Intrapulmonary shunting also frequently occurs because of the decrease in total lung compliance and functional residual capacity, as well as the inhibition of hypoxic pulmonary vasoconstriction by the use of vasodilating drugs such as nitroglycerine or, more commonly, nitroprusside. Ventilation can also be impaired, secondary to residual neuromuscular blockade.

Atelectasis is almost universally present, commonly resulting from small airway closure associated with decreased functional residual capacity and inadequate lung reexpansion after CPB. Other factors that can result in atelectasis include a decrease in surfactant production, a decrease in the clearance of secretions, and the presence of pleural effusions that frequently occur in patients exposed to CPB.

Pulmonary vascular resistance is increased after CPB and is related to the absence of pulmonary circulation, the aggregation of platelets and leukocytes in the pulmonary vasculature, and the release of vasoactive substances by leukocytes and the pulmonary endothelium that occurs during CPB. Pulmonary hypertension can occur postoperatively, and usually occurs in those patients with elevated pulmonary artery pressures preoperatively. When severe, weaning patients from the ventilator or from CPB can become difficult.

All of these factors must be considered when attempting to provide the proper respiratory support for these patients. Ventilators should administer appropriate tidal volumes (10–15 ml/kg) and reexpansion maneuvers, such as sustained inspiration (30cm H_2O held for 10 seconds) should be used to prevent and treat atelectasis. An assessment of the patient's ability to support ventilation after extubation needs to made and is accomplished by gradually shifting the work of breathing from the ventilator to the patient while monitoring key parameters such as respiratory rate, minute ventilation, and tidal volumes. Arterial blood gases can be analyzed to ensure adequate gas exchange and to guard against acidosis as the patient is weaned from the ventilator, and as inspired concentrations of oxygen are decreased. Residual neuromuscular blockade should be reversed if needed. Once hemodynamic stability, hemostasis, adequate rewarming, and recovery from anesthesia have occurred, the patient should be weaned rapidly. Thereafter, it is important to minimize the deleterious effects on gas exchange, work of breathing, and risk of pneumonia that result from the postoperative pulmonary derangements through the use of incentive spirometry, early ambulation, and appropriate use of analgesics.

Hemostasis

Bleeding is a common postoperative complication. Suture or cannulae site bleeding can result in profound hemorrhage, instability, and even tamponade. Prompt surgical intervention is required should this occur. Massive chest tube drainage is indicative of surgical bleeding and the need for reexploration.

More commonly, postoperative bleeding occurs because of the hemostatic abnormalities induced by CPB. Inadequate heparin reversal, platelet dysfunction, ongoing fibrinolysis, hypothermia, and the reduction in coagulation factors all can cause postoperative bleeding. Management should be directed at the diagnosis and treatment of the underlying aberration, rather than empiric treatment for all possible etiologic factors. A reasonable approach would be to first check an activated clotting time (ACT) and administer additional protamine if indicated. If bleeding persists despite normalization of the ACT, a coagulation profile should be checked; it should include a platelet count, prothrombin time, partial thromboplastin time, fibrinogen, and fibrin-split products level. Given the high incidence of platelet dysfunction after CPB, a platelet transfusion is often administered. Further therapy should then be guided by the results of laboratory analysis, and may include the administration of fresh frozen plasma, cryoprecipitate, additional platelets, and desmopression (DDAVP). Importantly, many patients will stop bleeding if their temperatures can be maintained at 37°C or warmer. Nitroglycerin is a platelet inhibitor and bleeding may be decreased if this drug can be discontinued.

Antifibrinolytic agents also are used when bleeding is thought to be secondary to primary fibrinolysis. Epsilon-aminocaproic acid (amicar) and transexamic acid are synthetic drugs which both prevent fibrinolysis by inhibiting plasminogen activation. Aprotinin is a naturally occurring polypeptide that also inhibits plasminogen activation. Additionally, it is reported to preserve platelet function when given intraoperatively. All of these drugs have been shown to decrease blood loss when given intraoperatively and postoperatively. Premature graft closure, the questionable ability of these drugs to reduce banked RBC usage, and in the case of aprotinin, cost and possibility of anaphylaxis limits the routine use of these drugs. These drugs are often reserved for patients expected to have potentially significant bleeding associated with complex surgical procedures such as repeat CABGs, multiple valve replacements, and, especially, with surgery for aortic dissection.

BIBLIOGRAPHY

Aladj LJ, et al: Cerebral blood flow autoregulation is preserved during CPB in isoflurane-anesthetized patients, *Anesth Analg* 72:48–52, 1991.

Christakis GT, et al: Coronary artery bypass grafting In patients with poor ventricular function, *J Thoracic Cardiovasc Surg* 103:1083–1092, 1992.

Dietrich W, et al: High-dose aprotinin in cardiac surgery: three year experience in 1784 patients, *J Cardiothorac Vasc Anesth* 6:324, 1992.

Estafanous FG, Barash PG, Reeves JG: *Cardiac anesthesia, principles and clinical practice*, 1994, JB Lippincott.

Guidman DR, et al: *Perioperative medicine,* ed 2, 1994, Mcgraw-Hill Inc.

Hall TS: The pathophsiology Of cardiopulmonary bypass, the risks and benefits of hemodilution, *Chest* 107:1125–1133, 1995.

Hardy JF, Desroches J: Natural and synthetic antifibrinolytics in cardiac surgery, *Can J Anaesth* 39:353, 1992.

Hertzner NR, et al: Staging for simultaneous coronary and carotid disease: a study including prospective randomization, *J Vasc Surg* 9:455–463, 1989.

Higgins TL, et al: Stratification of morbidity and mortality outcome by preoperative risk factors in coronary artery bypass patients, *JAMA* 267:2344–2348, 1992.

Johnsson P, et al: Cardiopulmonary perfusion and cerebral blood flow In bilateral carotid artery disease, *Ann Thorac Surg* 51:579–584, 1991.

Kay PH: *Techniques in extracorporeal bypass*, ed 3, 1992, Butterworth-Heinemann LTD.

Lake C: *Cardiovascular anesthesia,* New York, 1985, Springer-Verlag.

Shaw PJ, et al: Early intellectual dysfunction following coronary bypass surgery, *Q J Med* 58:59–68, 1986.

Shaw PJ, et al: Long-term intellectual dysfunction following coronary artery bypass surgery, *Q J Med* 62:259–268, 1987.

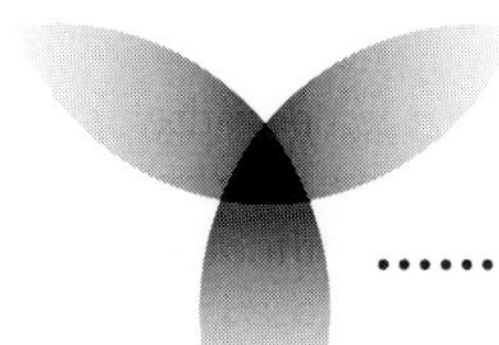

Chapter 36

Major Hepatobiliary Surgery

David L. Bogdonoff, MD, Burkhard F. Spiekermann, MD,
Timothy L. Pruett, MD

Surgical procedures involving the liver run the full spectrum—from a simple diagnostic tissue biopsy to hepatic transplantation. The liver may be functionally and anatomically normal or may be extensively altered by the ravages of acute and chronic diseases. Alterations in normal hepatic function and anatomy will have profound effects on the ability to successfully accomplish the surgical goals. In addition to the physiologic abnormalities secondary to the liver disease, coexisting medical disorders may complicate a planned surgical intervention.

Liver surgery has become more common because surgical care and technique have become more sophisticated. For example, in the last 15 years, liver transplantation has evolved from a radical procedure performed by maverick surgeons to a routine procedure recognized as an integral form of therapy for a wide spectrum of liver diseases. With the increasing complexity of both the surgical undertakings and the severity of underlying diseases, there is a crucial need for the early involvement of medical consultants and anesthesiologists in the perioperative period.

HEPATIC ANATOMY AND PHYSIOLOGY

The liver is the largest gland in the body, weighing approximately 1.5 kg and comprising 2% of total body weight. It is divided into two lobes along a line from the gall bladder bed to the vena cava. Each lobe has its own branch of the hepatic artery, portal vein, and bile duct. The left lobe is further divided into two sections, separated by the ligamentum teres. An anatomic division of the liver into eight segments (based upon the distribution of portal blood vessels) can be defined, but this anatomy is highly complex and its useful application during resectional procedures requires the knowledge and skills of an experienced hepatic surgeon.

Liver blood supply derives from contributions made by both the portal vein and the hepatic artery. Total blood flow approaches 100 ml/min/100 g tissue and represents fully 25% of the total cardiac output. The hepatic artery contributes approximately 25% of total flow but, because of the higher oxygen content of its arterial blood, provides almost one half of the oxygen supply to the liver. Portal venous inflow supplies 75% of the liver blood flow and the other one half of the liver's oxygen needs. In addition, the portal vein provides nutrients and other substances from the gastrointestinal tract, as well as unknown trophic factors, and is essential for normal liver functioning.

Control of liver blood flow involves a semireciprocity of blood flow between its two supplying vascular beds. During a reduction of portal (or splanchnic) flow, local release of adenosine in the liver results in hepatic arteriolar dilation and a resultant increase in hepatic arterial flow. This compensation for diminished portal flow protects the oxygen supply to the liver. A reciprocal increase in portal flow to the liver in a setting of decreased hepatic arterial inflow, however, is not possible. Portal flow is regulated at its arteriolar level in the gut and spleen and, therefore, is not affected by local changes in the liver.

The highly vascular liver can act as a blood reservoir in hemodynamically stressful situations, such as hemorrhage. The sympathetic nervous system controls resistances in the hepatic veins, and with sympathetic activation, the normal liver can reduce its blood capacitance and "squeeze" out a unit (approximately 500 cc) of blood.

PREOPERATIVE EVALUATION

A thorough preoperative assessment of the patient undergoing liver surgery is necessary to evaluate the extent of any underlying liver disease and its effects on metabolic and physiologic functional reserves, as well as the presence of any associated anatomic alterations. The extent of these abnormalities will determine the feasibility of any proposed surgery.

The etiology of the liver disease often allows one to predict the underlying physiologic derangement, particularly early in the course of disease. Liver diseases are generally divided into parenchymal disorders (acute and chronic viral hepatitides, cirrhosis with or without portal hypertension) and cholestatic disorders (cholestasis and biliary obstruction).

The preoperative evaluation also includes a careful search for underlying and coexisting medical conditions; attempts will be made to optimize the care of these disorders.

Some surgical interventions on the liver will be carried out on an organ with only minor physiologic and anatomic abnormalities. For example, a blunt trauma patient with a hepatic laceration or the rare individual with a liver abscess or cyst will usually have normal liver function and normal underlying medical physiology. Patients presenting for liver resection for malignant disease will often have normal underlying liver function but may be suffering from cirrhosis, a condition that may significantly affect the successful outcome of the procedure. Occasionally, surgical interventions are carried out in patients suffering from acute hepatitis. Surgery may have profound implications on the course of the disease, regardless of whether or not the liver is the focus of the procedure. Patients undergoing transplantation or portal decompressive procedures usually have extensive underlying liver disease and multisystem organ involvement. Therefore, their management will be complex and difficult.

Parenchymal Diseases

The most common causes of parenchymal liver disease are the viral hepatitides and alcohol. Other drugs, toxins, and chemicals, as well as inborn errors of metabolism (Wilson's disease, hemochromatosis, and α_1-antitrypsin deficiency) make up the remainder of the causes.

The usual result of *long-standing* parenchymal disease of the liver is cirrhosis, with or without accompanying portal hypertension. *Acute* parenchymal disorders do not result in the physiologic alterations associated with cirrhosis but, nevertheless, carry their own risks because a surgical and anesthetic intervention may aggravate the disease process and lead to perioperative hepatic decompensation. Only emergent surgical procedures should be performed on patients with acute hepatitis. *Chronic* disorders, if early in their course, generally have little overall effect on the liver, and are of much less perioperative significance (because of the large hepatic reserve). Longstanding chronic diseases will eventually progress to cirrhosis, which will have a profound impact on other organ systems.

CIRCULATORY CHANGES IN CIRRHOSIS

Cirrhotic patients are characterized by a hyperdynamic cardiovascular state. A high cardiac output and a low systemic vascular resistance are the rule. Cardiac filling pressures are usually normal, despite an increase in circulating blood volume. As blood flows are increased above normal, and without any increase in oxygen consumption, there is a resultant oversupply of oxygen to the tissues and mixed-venous oxygen tensions are high.

The cause of this vasodilated state is multifactorial but not well understood. Animal research suggests that increased glucagon levels may be responsible for roughly 40% of these effects. Ferritin, vasoactive intestinal peptide, and increased nitric oxide levels may also play a role. Cirrhotics have an increased level of circulating catecholamines. End-organ responsiveness to these substances is reduced, possibly because of the effects of glucagon.

Cardiac function is ordinarily maintained until late in the course of cirrhosis. In the late stage, a cardiomyopathy may develop, but clinical effects are possibly offset by the inotropic actions of the increased catechol levels. Interestingly, alcoholics typically either develop cardiomyopathy or cirrhosis, and the two conditions rarely coexist. Similarly, the cirrhotic state seems to be somewhat protective for cardiovascular disease, because the incidence of coronary disease in these patients is statistically less than would be expected. Deterioration of cardiac function late in the course of cirrhosis is accompanied by a decrease in stroke volume and an increase in heart rate. Tense ascites can result in decreased cardiac output by mechanically decreasing transmural cardiac filling pressures and shifting ventricular pressure-volume relationships.

Total renal blood flow is often normal in cirrhotic patients, but its distribution can be altered; decreased renal cortical blood flow develops early on, caused by afferent arteriolar vasoconstriction. An increase in renal vascular resistance may occur, despite the significant vasodilation present in other vascular beds. The abnormal humoral milieu and the high levels of catechols may be responsible.

The hepatic circulation is characterized by decreased portal vein flow to the liver, despite an overall increase in both total portal blood flow and portal venous pressure. Hepatic sinusoidal resistance increases secondary to parenchymal scarring, and results in significant impairment to normal portal flow to the liver. This increase in portal resistance was formerly thought to explain portal hypertension but does not explain the observed increase in total portal flow. The currently popular "forward" theory of portal hypertension suggests that certain factors, such as glucagon, lead to vasodilation and the formation or dilation of arteriovenous fistulae. This results in an overall increase in portal blood flow, much of which drains through portosystemic venous collaterals and not through the liver. Hepatic arterial flow and oxygen supply to the liver are not affected by the cirrhotic process and are usually maintained at normal levels.

PULMONARY FUNCTION IN CIRRHOSIS

A multitude of factors may contribute to arterial hypoxemia in cirrhotic patients. The result is that up to 25% of patients will have a p_aO_2 of less than 70 mm Hg and some may have a p_aO_2 less than 50 mm Hg. The patient may complain of dyspnea, orthopnea, and reduced exercise tolerance. Signs on physical examination may include clubbing, cyanosis, and a worsening of oxygenation when assuming the standing position (orthodeoxia). The last is in stark contrast to other pulmonary conditions, in which oxygenation actually improves in the upright position. Patients with severe pulmonary abnormalities secondary to cirrhosis are said to have the *hepatopulmonary syndrome*. Patients without obvious pulmonary disease, however, may well have subclinical pulmonary disorders which warrant attention.

Ascites may result in an elevation of the diaphragm and an increase in closing volume, with a tendency towards atelectasis. Pulmonary volumes may be reduced by pleural effusions, which often accompany ascites. Increased extracellular fluid volume, characteristic of chronic liver disease, may result in a decreased pulmonary diffusing capacity. Anatomic portopulmonary venous shunts may be present and result in direct passage of deoxygenated portal venous blood into the pulmonary veins. Pulmonary spider angiomata may cause shunting of blood past pulmonary capillaries, directly into the pulmonary venous system. A rightward shift of the oxyhemoglobin saturation curve is often encountered, secondary to a red blood cell content of 2,3-diphosphoglycerate (and, therefore, a reduced affinity for oxygen).

Despite the factors mentioned, the bulk of hypoxemia in liver disease results from the effects of the hyperdynamic, vasodilated circulatory state which characterizes cirrhosis. Blood flow through the pulmonary capillaries occurs at a rapid rate, and through an abnormally dilated vessel, so that there is actual flow of deoxygenated blood through the lung without an opportunity to become saturated with oxygen. This results in pulmonary shunting, which is partially overcome by the administration of supplemental oxygen. Furthermore, vasodilation impairs hypoxic pulmonary vasoconstriction; thus, any minor underlying pulmonary abnormalities, such as atelectasis, will have an exaggerated effect on oxygenation.

Despite the high incidence of pulmonary disorders, the administration of supplemental oxygen allows most patients to tolerate anesthesia and surgery without ventilatory difficulties. Postoperative care, however, requires close attention to prevent hypoxemia.

RENAL FUNCTION IN CIRRHOSIS

Renal dysfunction and electrolyte abnormalities are common in cirrhotics. Renal failure develops in over one half of dying cirrhotics. The etiology of renal impairment is multifactorial. It is incompletely understood, but its pathogenesis is secondary to hemodynamic, neural, and hormonal interactions, both endogenous and exogenous to the kidneys. The result is profound sodium retention and the production of dilute urine.

Ascites and edema are associated with renal functional abnormalities. Various theories suggest that either the renal abnormality leads to ascites or vice versa, with the formation of ascites leading to renal malfunction. The "revised underfill theory" suggests that peripheral vasodilation is perceived by the kidney as a decreased effective intravascular volume, leading to a feedback response of renal sodium and water retention. This response may also be triggered by the high levels of circulating catecholamines in the cirrhotic patient. Retention of salt and water, in combination with a decreased plasma oncotic pressure, aggravates ascites and edema. As a result, low urinary sodium levels are common in the cirrhotic patient.

Renal prostaglandins play a role in counteracting the abnormalities leading to functional renal impairment. Renal decompensation often occurs late in the course of cirrhosis, particularly during periods of stress, such as with a variceal hemorrhage. Abnormalities in renal blood flow develop, characterized by a decrease in total flow, particularly flow to the renal cortex. This leads to progressive oliguric renal failure, termed the "hepatorenal" syndrome. It is difficult to differentiate the hepatorenal syndrome from prerenal azotemia and acute tubular necrosis. Hepatorenal syndrome is a functional, rather than a pathologic disorder. A kidney affected as such will function normally following successful treatment of the underlying liver disease.

Treatment of the late abnormalities of renal dysfunction is supportive. Early in the course, however, drug therapy and water restriction will improve the functional abnormalities. Spironolactone is effective in blocking the high levels of aldosterone which are present in the cirrhotic patient, thereby, decreasing Na^+ and water reabsorption. Spironolactone may be combined with a loop diuretic. Sodium and potassium ion concentrations need to be monitored when instituting diuretic therapy, because rapid electrolyte changes may contribute to the development of hepatic encephalopathy.

HEMATOLOGIC AND COAGULATION ABNORMALITIES IN CIRRHOSIS

Blood abnormalities are common and relate mostly to underlying vitamin deficiencies and malnutrition. Alcoholics may also suffer from alcohol-induced bone marrow suppression. Hypersplenism secondary to portal hypertension may lead to hemolysis, thrombocytopenia, and leukopenia. Albumin levels are often decreased, owing to the decreased synthetic mass of the liver, which leads to a decrease in plasma oncotic pressure. Coagulation abnormalities are one of the hallmarks of cirrhosis. They contribute to morbidity and mortality and have profound effects on the perioperative management of these patients.

The liver is responsible for the synthesis of all coagulation factors, except for Factor VIII. As a result, diminished levels of clotting factors will be present in the later stages of cirrhosis when functioning hepatic cell mass and reserve synthetic capacity is reduced. In addition to decreased factor synthesis, there is reduced activity of the decarboxylation functions which are integral to the proper synthesis of the vitamin K–dependent Factors (II, VII, IX, X). Interestingly, fibrinogen and Factor-VIII levels are increased, as are the levels of other "acute-phase reactants." In severe cirrhosis, fibrinogen synthesis in the liver may be abnormal, resulting in dysfibrinogenemia, which further contributes to coagulation inefficiencies.

The clearance and breakdown of activated coagulation factors is also decreased in patients with cirrhosis, potentially causing fibrinolysis. Increased levels of tissue-plasminogen activator are encountered and lead to high levels of plasmin in the blood. Additionally, decreased hepatic synthesis of plasmin inhibitors such as α_2-antiplasmin contribute to this fibrinolytic tendency. Fibrinolysis may be difficult to discern from disseminated intravascular coagulation.

Laboratory studies to assess the coagulation status include a platelet count, prothrombin time (PT) and activated partial thromboplastin time (aPTT). Because platelet function is generally normal in liver disease, measurement of platelet numbers is sufficient and a bleeding time is not indicated. The PT is the most sensitive measurement of clotting function in the liver-disease patient, because it only involves factors synthesized by the liver. In fact, the PT is a good indicator of overall synthetic liver function in the absence of active bleeding. A prolongation of the PT suggests that hepatic functional reserve has been exceeded and that the patient has significant underlying liver disease.

METABOLIC ABNORMALITIES IN CIRRHOSIS

The liver is responsible for gluconeogenesis. Gluconeogenesis is not deficient until late in the course of cirrhosis, although it is often impaired in acute, fulminant liver failure resulting in hypoglycemia. Increased glucagon and growth hormone levels may explain the glucose intolerance which is occasionally observed in cirrhotics.

The metabolism of xenobiotics (drugs) may be altered because of abnormalities in both liver function and liver blood flow. An increase in acid glycoproteins and acute-phase reactants may change the volume of distribution of some drugs. Decreased albumin levels will increase the free fraction of other drugs. The alterations in protein binding, extracellular fluid volumes, and metabolism of drugs lead to unpredictability in the dosing of medications in the perioperative period. In addition to pharmacokinetic changes, pharmacodynamic changes will influence the response to medications, as discussed further on.

ENCEPHALOPATHY IN CIRRHOSIS

The pathogenesis of hepatic encephalopathy involves insufficient hepatic elimination of ammonia and other nitrogenous compounds caused by the loss of hepatic functional mass and the presence of portosystemic venous-collateral flow, which allows, gut-venous drainage to bypass the liver. The serum level of ammonia does not correlate with the severity of encephalopathy and, therefore, cannot be the sole factor. Other molecules such as mercaptans, short-chain fatty acids, and false neurotransmitters (octopamines) may contribute.

An increased sensitivity of the central nervous system (CNS) to nitrogenous compounds is present in the cirrhotic patient. Increased levels of the inhibitory neurotransmitter gamma aminobutyric acid (GABA) in the CNS system may contribute to the pathogenesis of hepatic encephalopathy. Interestingly, flumazenil, a benzodiazepine-receptor antagonist, may reverse symptoms seen with the early stages of hepatic encephalopathic coma. As benzodiazepines increase CNS levels of GABA, the partial reversal of hepatic coma with benzodiazepine antagonists solidifies the suggestion that GABA is a contributor in the pathogenesis of hepatic encephalopathy.

The early symptoms of hepatic encephalopathy include subtle personality changes or alterations in speech, often noted first by a family member. Confusion may progress along a spectrum of symptoms, culminating in unresponsiveness and hepatic coma (Table 36-1). Various neurologic findings may be present. Periods of stress and, particularly, gastrointestinal hemorrhage are likely to aggravate any preexisting subclinical encephalopathy.

In fulminant hepatic failure, CNS involvement may progress to cerebral edema. Brain swelling and intracranial hypertension are the terminal events for many patients dying of acute liver failure. Chronic liver disease rarely causes increased intracranial pressure.

Treatment of hepatic encephalopathy is supportive and involves the administration of lactulose to enhance ammonia elimination and neomycin to block bacterial

Table 36-1. Hepatic Encephalopathy/Coma

LEVEL	SYMPTOMS	INTELLECTUAL FUNCTION	NEUROLOGIC FINDINGS
0	Normal	Normal	None
1	Personality changes	Forgetful, inattentive	Slight tremor, poor coordination
2	Lethargy, inappropriateness	Disoriented	Asterixis, abnormal reflexes
3	Somnolent but arousable, confusion	Unable to communicate	Asterixis, abnormal reflexes
4	Unarousable	None	Babinski, decerebration

formation of toxins. There may be a role for dopamine agonists and L-dopa to counteract effects of false neurotransmitters. Encephalopathy can be aggravated by aggressive treatment of electrolyte abnormalities and correction of pH.

As hepatic encephalopathy progresses, it is important to consider the issue of airway protection. The patient's loss of the ability to protect the airway often occurs insidiously. This is dangerous, especially in the face of a high concomitant risk of vomiting, such as with the presence of esophageal and gastric variceal bleeding, and/or the delayed gastric emptying, which is characteristic of cirrhosis.

PORTAL HYPERTENSION

Continued attempts at regeneration and scarring which occur in response to chronic parenchymal injury, lead to a progressive increase in sinusoidal resistance to blood flow. This increased resistance may contribute to portal hypertension, or may be occurring in parallel with other changes that lead to the increased portal blood flow seen in cirrhosis. Regardless of the causation, portal hypertension has potentially grave consequences.

Normal portal pressures are 5 to 10 mm Hg (7–10 cmH_2O). Portal hypertension may be defined by a portal pressure either 5 mm Hg above that in the inferior vena cava pressure or any reading above 22 mm Hg. This chronically elevated pressure contributes to both portosystemic collateralization of venous drainage and to hypersplenism. The latter has already been mentioned as a contributory factor in thrombocytopenia.

Portosystemic collaterals allow portal venous blood to bypass the liver and, because of that bypass, may ultimately contribute to encephalopathy. Similarly, those same collaterals in the pulmonary system, though rare, may contribute to hypoxemia. The major risk of this neovascularity, however, is that of upper gastrointestinal hemorrhage. Esophageal and gastric varices can be large and fragile; they may lead to profound, potentially life-threatening hemorrhage. Bleeding from these venous collaterals is commonly the precipitating event in the ultimate deterioration of the end-stage cirrhotic patient. Medical and surgical interventions, in attempts to control variceal bleeding, will often need to be undertaken with little time for stabilization of the patient, let alone time for detailed preoperative evaluation and optimization.

Cholestatic Diseases

Cholestatic diseases are characterized by a reduction in the hepatic secretion of bilirubin, cholesterol, and bile acids. Most causes of cholestasis that require a surgical intervention are related to extrahepatic biliary obstruction. Presenting symptoms may be pain, infection, or pruritis, jaundice and malabsorption. Persistent obstruction of the biliary tree over time, will eventually lead to liver damage and cirrhosis. Other medical conditions may cause a decrease in bile secretion and progressive liver dysfunction but are rarely amenable to easy surgical interventions. Primary biliary cirrhosis begins as a periportal process and, ultimately, progresses to a cirrhotic process. Primary sclerosing cholangitis consists of scarring and fibrosis of extrahepatic bile ducts and, possibly, intrahepatic bile ducts. The latter are not amenable to surgical (nontransplant) treatments and will, in the end, lead to a cirrhotic picture.

Early in the course of cholestatic diseases, abnormalities are related to the accumulation of bilirubin and the effects of the absence of normal bile secretion. Elevated bilirubin levels, in either a conjugated or unconjugated form, can be toxic to various enzyme systems and can lead to organ dysfunction. Only late in the course of these diseases does the clinical picture fuse with that of parenchymal disorders, because cirrhosis is the final common pathway for nearly all chronic liver diseases.

CARDIOVASCULAR FUNCTION

There is some evidence that high bilirubin levels impair myocardial contractility. It may also blunt the response to catecholamines, perhaps by a mechanism of interference with receptor binding. Hyperdynamic circulatory changes also characterize the cholestatic patient, though to a lesser degree than with cirrhotic patients. It is known that patients with biliary obstruction tend to develop hypotension with minimal blood or fluid loss. This may result from a decreased sensitivity to catecholamines and an inability to mobilize fluids from the splanchnic vascular bed as a compensatory response.

RENAL FUNCTION

High levels of bilirubin or bile salts have been suggested to be toxic to the kidneys. It is now believed that coexisting conditions present in biliary obstruction are the etiologic factors in associated renal dysfunction. Hypotension secondary to a stressed cardiovascular system and endotoxemia from sepsis are etiologic factors leading to perioperative acute tubular necrosis (ATN) in these patients. Close observation and meticulous fluid management are required in patients undergoing procedures for biliary obstruction, in an effort to prevent the development or aggravation of renal dysfunction.

BLOOD COAGULATION

Bile is a necessary substance for the enteric absorption of fats and, hence, the fat-soluble vitamins A, D, E, and K. Vitamin K is required for decarboxylation of coagulation

Factors II, VII, IX, and X. Prolongation of the PT is characteristic and is often responsive to treatment with parenteral vitamin-K supplements. Failure to respond to vitamin K is ominous and suggests a deterioration of liver function from significant parenchymal involvement.

SURGICAL PROCEDURES

Anesthetic Implications for Liver Surgery

It is important for the anesthesiologist to be aware of the extent of the liver disease. It has long been recognized that patients with end-stage liver disease present a challenge for the anesthesia/surgery team. Therefore, prognostic tools to predict risks of procedures on these patients have been sought. Depending upon the duration of the procedure, the amount of blood loss, and the severity of the insult upon metabolic and physiologic functions, the risk of an operative procedure will vary. As centers have increased their surgical and anesthetic expertise for patients with marginal liver function (often through experiences with liver transplantation), traditional guidelines have been modified. Many tests have been proposed to assess liver reserve before an operation: indocyanine green clearance, aminopyrine breath test, lidocaine metabolism (MEGX), and galactose elimination. While these tests assess different components of liver function, none has been proved to be consistently reliable in the prediction of either perioperative morbidity or mortality. Table 36-2 shows the risk assessment for portasystemic shunting procedures which was originally devised by Child and modified by Pugh this has been one of the most commonly used schemes.

Using Pugh's modification, those patients who score 5 to 6 (Child's A) are considered good anesthetic and surgical risks; patients with 7 to 9 points (Child's B) are at intermediate risk. Those with 10 to 15 points (Child's C) are poor operative risks. In certain cases, there may be a benefit from the delay of a surgical procedure so that a patient's overall condition may improve. Clearly, all preoperative assessments of anesthetic and surgical risks have to account for changes in hepatic mass (i.e., after resection) or significant changes in hepatic blood flow (hemodynamic changes with anesthetic agents, surgical bleeding, portasystemic shunting), which will affect the ability of the liver to function.

Significant alterations in both pharmacokinetics and pharmacodynamics should be expected when administering drugs; they should be carefully titrated to their desired therapeutic end points. Alterations in pharmacokinetics are numerous and involve altered volumes of distributions and clearances. Protein binding is significantly different from that in normal patients, but generalizations concerning the effects of such changes are not possible. For example, while albumin levels are generally decreased and, therefore, result in higher free levels of drugs, which bind to this protein, acute-phase reactant proteins and acid glycoproteins are increased in cirrhosis and will, therefore, lead to decreased blood concentrations of drugs with affinities for this latter group of carrier proteins. Increases in volumes of distribution are common but are not necessarily applicable across even the same class of drugs. An example is the increased volume of distribution measured for the neuromuscular

Table 36-2. Risk Assessment for Liver Surgery Patients (see text for details)

CLINICAL AND BIOCHEMICAL MEASUREMENT	POINTS SCORED FOR INCREASING ABNORMALITIES		
	1	2	3
Encephalopathy (grade)	None	1 and 2	3 and 4
Bilirubin (mg/dl)	<1.5	1.5–2.3	>2.3
Albumin (gm/dl)	3.5	2.8–3.5	<2.8
Prothrombin time (sec greater than control)	1–4	4–6	>6

blocking agent pancuronium and the findings of unaltered distribution volume in cirrhotics for the closely related drug vecuronium. Without such detailed studies for each specific drug, it is difficult to accurately predict the specific alterations in pharmacokinetics or pharmacodynamics.

Intraoperative bleeding is common and should be anticipated. Preparations must be made to permit the rapid administration of blood products and other fluids through large-bore intravenous lines. The potential for metabolic derangement, particularly with respect to blood pH, K^+, Ca^{++}, and glucose, requires frequent intraoperative blood sampling. Appropriate vascular access for blood sampling is thus, necessary, most commonly in the form of an indwelling arterial catheter.

All anesthetics will affect liver blood flow and hepatic oxygen supply. While much attention has been paid to their effects (particularly from the inhalational agent halothane, which is well known for its hepatotoxicity), the effects of other interventions are much more clinically significant. The stress of laparotomy, placement of retractors and abdominal packs, and decreases in blood pressure or cardiac output accompanying hypovolemia will all decrease hepatic blood flow to a much greater extent than will the effects of anesthesia. Liver blood flow is directly proportional to blood pressure and cardiac output. Hence, attempts should be made to keep these variables at normal levels. Hyperventilation resulting in respiratory alkalosis can cause hepatic arterial vasoconstriction and should be avoided if not otherwise indicated.

As mentioned previously, all anesthetics may decrease liver blood flow. However, techniques can be adopted that minimize such effects. Isoflurane and fentanyl have been studied extensively. Both maintain the hepatic oxygen supply-demand ratio. Fentanyl preserves blood pressure and cardiac output, keeping portal flow and hepatic oxygen supply unaffected. Isoflurane causes a slight decrease in blood pressure and total hepatic flow but produces a parallel decrease in both splanchnic and hepatic oxygen consumption, maintaining a favorable hepatic oxygen supply-to-demand ratio.

Meticulous anesthetic technique and resuscitative efforts to minimize hemodynamic instabilities will be particularly important for any patient with an ailing liver, whether compromised by acute or chronic stressors. Even a functionally normal liver (when subjected to profound hypotension with a decreased blood and oxygen supply during hepatic trauma or resection) may be at risk for irreversible hepatocyte damage and the potential for hepatic failure.

SURGICAL PROCEDURES

Liver Biopsy

A liver biopsy is frequently required for diagnostic and staging purposes. Percutaneous needle biopsy of the liver is fraught with the potential for insidious bleeding, especially in the scarred, cirrhotic liver. Open liver biopsy requires a general anesthetic. Today, liver biopsies are performed laparoscopically, more and more commonly in the outpatient clinic setting. Bleeding can be controlled with conventional electrocautery or with an argon electron beam coagulator. Minimal insufflating pressures are used to decrease the potential for adverse hemodynamic sequelae (see Chapter 31 on laparoscopy). Platelets and fresh frozen plasma are indicated if the platelet count or coagulation studies are abnormal to minimize the potential for bleeding. Patients who are at increased risk of bleeding require an extended period of postbiopsy observation before discharge. Despite the significant potential risks, laparascopic liver biopsy seems to be a safe procedure. If the etiology of the liver disease is in doubt, serious consideration should be given to performing a liver biopsy before one considers a more invasive procedure, especially if the possibility of acute viral hepatitis is present.

Hepatic Trauma

Most cases of hepatic trauma occur in patients without underlying liver disease. Anesthetic efforts are directed towards resuscitation from hypovolemia and attempts to maximize liver oxygen delivery. Early in the surgical treatment for liver trauma, surgical packs will be placed into the abdomen to tamponade bleeding from the liver and other organs. Such actions may result in near total cessation of blood flow to the liver, causing a functionally anhepatic condition. This means that citrate metabolism will be impaired and the patient will be at risk of developing hypocalcemia, secondary to the exogenous administration of citrate in blood products. Even without the decreases in liver blood flow, decreased liver function may result secondary to hypothermia, so commonly encountered in the trauma victim.

Surgeons may use the *Pringle* maneuver in an attempt to transiently control hepatic bleeding. This involves the temporary clamping of the portal triad containing the hepatic artery and portal vein. The normal liver can tolerate an ischemic time of 60 minutes without major damage. Intermittent flow may be considered if this maneuver needs to be continued for longer periods. On rare occasions, a surgeon may consider hepatic artery ligation in an effort to control hemorrhage. Such a scenario should prompt the anesthesiologist to ensure adequate hepatic oxygen supply by efforts directed toward maximizing portal blood flow and oxygen content. This involves efforts to minimize sympathetic nervous system stimulation to avoid sympathetically mediated vasoconstriction, to maintain a high hematocrit, and to normalize the blood pressure and cardiac output. Persistent uncontrolled bleeding will likely result in a surgical "bail out" with the placement of packs around bleeding sites and a rapid, temporary abdominal wound closure followed by transfer to an intensive care unit for ongoing resuscitation.

Hepatic Resection

Most hepatic resections in this country are performed for malignant disease. Metastases from colonic carcinoma are the most common treatable malignant lesions excised, although various hepatic primary tumors may be resectable. Hepatic trauma with resultant necrotic tissue, hepatic cysts, and granulomas may require resectional treatment, as well.

Removal of up to 80% of the liver is tolerated without significant morbidity as long as the underlying liver is normal and not subjected to prolonged intraoperative ischemia. Regeneration of liver tissue resulting from hypertrophy of the remaining healthy tissue is relatively rapid but will not occur in a diseased, cirrhotic liver. Therefore, the extent of any underlying cirrhosis will determine the capacity of the liver for regrowth and the underlying pathology dictates how much liver tissue can, ultimately, be removed.

Hepatic resections can be subsegmental (wedge) or segmental. Major segmental resection usually requires an anatomic dissection with division of the major branches of the portal vein, hepatic artery, and bile duct to the involved segments. Multiple segments can be excised together, as in a right or left hepatic lobectomy or an extended left or right trisegmentectomy. Couinaud's eight hepatic segments (based on portal anatomy) can also form the anatomic basis for resection; they are particularly useful for the excision of the gall bladder fossa or limited resections on patients at risk for postoperative liver failure.

The major intraoperative threat associated with liver resection results from the potential for massive hemorrhage. Anesthetic preparations must include large-bore venous access and invasive intravascular monitors. Surgical techniques vary, but all require strict attention to hemostatic efforts. Particularly effective are efforts to compress or ligate vessels within the substance of the remaining liver, or temporary clamping of the portal triad outside the liver (Pringle maneuver). Hemostatic adjuncts such as gelfoam, micronized collagen, thrombin spray, and fibrin glue may be used following control of the major bleeding sites. An aggressive technique has recently become more popular which involves total vascular isolation of the liver. Despite clamping of inflow vessels, retrograde bleeding from the vena cava still occurs from the cut surface of the liver because of the lack of valves in the hepatic veins and sinusoids. Total vascular isolation involves clamping of the vena cava above and below the liver to stop this retrograde venous bleeding. The result is a loss of venous return to the heart from both the splanchnic vascular bed and the systemic circulation below the diaphragm. The associated decrease in preload is not well tolerated. It will require extensive volume administration by the anesthesia team or the utilization of veno-venous bypass techniques, as with liver transplantation. Release of the clamps following completion of the resection is associated with a sudden increase in preload of approximately 2 liters, secondary to the return of massive amounts of blood previously trapped in the venous capacitance beds behind the occluding clamps. Management of these cases is difficult and should be left to experienced teams. Close communication between surgical and anesthesia teams is essential. Preoperative screening of patients, in an effort to exclude those with poor cardiovascular reserve who may not tolerate significant adverse hemodynamic swings, is essential. Even when not clamped, the vena cava is sbject to compression by mechanical retractors, surgeons' hands, and mobilization of the liver, thereby impairing venous return and causing hypotension.

A rare but serious potential complication that can occur during hepatic resection is that of massive air embolism from an opening in the hepatic veins, particularly during a period of hypovolemia with low central venous pressure. The anesthesiologist must be aware of this possibility in the differential diagnosis of hypotension.

Support of the patient undergoing extensive hepatic resection also includes maintenance of glucose and calcium homeostasis and replacement of clotting factors and blood. Since the production of albumin will be impaired for days postoperatively, albumin is the colloid of choice if fresh frozen plasma is not required. Clotting factors are consumed at a rapid rate in the body's attempts to stop bleeding from the extensive surgical field. Synthesis will be similarly impaired by resection of hepatic synthetic mass. Aggressive efforts must be made to maintain normal body temperature. Heat loss during laparotomy is considerable and hypothermia will impair platelet function and clotting, not to mention the potentially adverse effects of hypothermia on wound healing and infection.

Portal Decompressive Procedures

Manifestations of portal hypertension, which may prompt a surgical intervention, include bleeding esophagogastric varices, intractable ascites, and hypersplenism. Portosystemic collaterals, which develop with long-standing portal hypertension, include the coronary vein, hemorrhoidal veins, paraumbilical veins, retroperitoneal veins of Retzius, and the veins of Sappey. The coronary vein drains into a network of esophageal veins, which may dilate to potentially enormous sizes in the patient with portal hypertension. Erosion of such an esophageal varix may lead to exsanguinating hemorrhage or clinical deterioration eventually culminating in the death of the cirrhotic patient.

The prophylaxis and acute management of the patient with esophageal varices has changed a great deal over the last 2 decades. Sclerosis of esophageal varices is performed as a prophylactic procedure in cirrhotic patients. This has led to a decrease in the incidence of fatal variceal hemorrhage. Transesophageal sclerotherapy is also used in the face of ongoing hemorrhage. Interventional radiographic efforts at embolization of the coronary vein are available in some centers. While effective in preventing and treating hemorrhage, sclerosing procedures do not, however, alter the course of the cirrhotic disease. Other conservative, nonoperative measures include balloon tamponade with a Sengstaken-Blakemore (or the more modern Minnesota) tube, in combination with medical therapy. Vasopressin is effective at reducing portal pressure but is associated with coronary vasospasm and may increase the likelihood of cardiovascular morbidity, especially in the patient with coexisting coronary artery disease. Somatostatin also decreases portal blood flow and pressure, presumably by blocking the effects of glucagon and by decreasing intestinal activity and, hence, mesenteric inflow. The beta-blocker propranolol is well known for its effects of decreasing portal venous inflow and portal pressure. Chronic propranolol use is associated with a reduction in the incidence of variceal bleeding. Subsequent withdrawal, however, may increase the likelihood of bleeding. Nitroglycerin may be beneficial secondary to its venodilating properties, although it must be used with caution in the hypovolemic patient.

Another nonsurgical option is *transjugular intrahepatic portosystemic shunting* (TIPS) performed by interventional radiologists. This procedure involves the creation of a portosystemic shunt through the substance to the liver from the hepatic vein to the portal vein. It uses an angioplasty balloon and a wire mesh stent. The portal vein is not injured along its intrabdominal length and the abdomen is not entered surgically: both important factors if a liver transplant will be considered at a later stage. Management of these patients usually includes a general anesthetic. These critically ill patients will benefit from the care provided by an anesthesiologist.

If medical and nonoperative measures are ineffective, surgery may be required to alleviate portal hypertension or control variceal bleeding. Direct ligation of a bleeding esophageal varix is rarely performed. Direct approaches to gastric varices are seldom effective in the absence of other measures. Devascularization procedures of the esophagus and stomach (Sigura procedures) have been described, although they are rarely considered by American surgeons. The most common surgical interventions involve the decompression of the portal vein into the systemic circulation by the creation of an anatomic shunt.

Portosystemic shunts are classified as "selective" and "nonselective." The type of shunt will affect the hepatic blood supply. Nonselective or "total" shunts divert all splanchnic blood flow away from the liver. They are associated with a high incidence of hepatic encephalopathy, even in patients with reasonable hepatic reserve. Side-to-side portocaval shunts may behave functionally as total shunts; the degree of portal flow to the liver will be determined by the vascular resistance in the hepatic sinusoids and portosystemic collateral vessels, and by the actual level of portal pressure elevation. A selective shunt does not deprive the liver of portal inflow, because only the splenic and coronary veins are diverted. The latter veins are the source of the venous inflow into gastric and esophageal varices. Encephalopathy is less likely with selective shunting because portal flow to the liver is not dramatically altered. With time, however, the pattern of flow through a selective shunt may change and may approximate the flow pattern of a nonselective shunt. The choice of shunt is made with consideration of the urgency of the operation and individual patient anatomy and physiology.

Management of the patient requiring a shunting procedure is supportive and involves a continuation of any ongoing resuscitative efforts. Replacement of blood products takes center stage with attention directed towards correction of coagulation disturbances. Efforts to lower portal pressure by pharmacologic means may decrease intraoperative blood loss. Anesthesia is helpful in this regard because all general anesthetic agents have a tendency to decrease splanchnic blood flow and portal pressure.

Liver Transplantation

The patient undergoing liver transplantation is generally in a severely debilitated condition. Many recipients are gravely ill with multiple organ system failures. Conditions previously considered to represent absolute contraindications to surgery have today become only relative contraindications; in some cases they are considered only minor inconveniences. Extremes of age, significant concomitant disease, previous portocaval surgery, and viral hepatitis are among the factors that no longer preclude surgery. However, with the increasing success rates of liver transplantation and the growing shortage of donor organs, there is a movement to transplant the healthier or acutely ill patient, in light of their increased likelihood of a successful long-term outcome.

Preparations for liver transplantation remain a significant undertaking for the consultant hepatologists, their medical colleagues, and for the surgical team consisting of surgeons, anesthesiologists, and intensivists. The operation is probably the most technically demanding procedure in modern surgical practice. It is performed on patients with often severely dysfunctional, nonhepatic organ systems. Renal failure, encephalopathy with possible intracranial hypertension, primary or secondary pulmonary diseases, and major coagulopathies are the predominant problems that need to be addressed by the team. The operation is associated with a high potential for blood loss and involves interruption of major veins supplying all infradiaphragmatic structures of the body. Extracorporeal circulation may be used and preparations must be made to deal with the likelihood of major hemodynamic alterations and instability during the procedure. Metabolic perturbations and worsening coagulation disturbances only add to the challenge. While more and more surgical teams have become adept at the surgical challenge, no center is immune to the occasional transplant case that "goes bad."

If renal function is impaired in the recipient, preoperative potassium and fluid balance deserves special attention. It is important for the consultant nephrologist to recognize that the intraoperative period may be characterized by the administration of large volumes of banked blood, which is often high in potassium. Intraoperative metabolic acidosis may further contribute to hyperkalemia. Oliguria and decreased renal potassium excretion occurs even in patients with near normal renal function. This mandates that potassium needs to be maintained in the low-normal range immediately before surgery. Preoperative dialysis may be required to keep potassium levels low, even if these efforts may temporarily aggravate hepatic encephalopathy.

Coagulation disturbances are the norm in this patient population. The aggressive administration of fresh frozen plasma is rarely effective and can result in fluid overload. Unless thrombocytopenia is so severe that it represents a threat of intracranial hemorrhage, efforts to increase the platelet count are best left for the late intraoperative period, once surgical hemostasis is achieved. Electrolyte disturbances are best treated gradually, because aggressive correction (other than severe hyperkalemia) may result in untoward consequences including CNS damage. Magesium levels are often low and replacement has been shown to positively influence postoperative recovery.

Reversible cardiopulmonary disturbances need to be addressed. Active respiratory infections may represent a contraindication to transplantation. Postoperative immunosuppression and the true nature of any acute lung disorder must be discerned. Chronic conditions such as pleural effusions may be treated pre- or intraoperatively. Patients with hepatopulmonary syndrome respond well to higher oxygen levels, as described earlier. Irreversible pulmonary hypertension represents a major risk to the patient and may preclude surgery. A thorough cardiac evaluation is needed to ensure the patient will tolerate the intraoperative hemodynamic challenges represented by this procedure.

Psychological and social situations need to be considered as well, including the assurance that an alcoholic patient will not return to drinking. Social support services must be in place to enable adequate compliance with follow-up medical care, including immunosuppressive regimens vital to survival of the allografted organ.

Although only occasionally encountered, acute fulminant hepatitis may result in progressive neurologic deterioration, characterized by cerebral edema and intracranial hypertension. Consultation with the neurosurgical service for placement of an intracranial pressure monitor in the preoperative period may be required. Irreversible neurologic damage must be ruled out before a patient is considered for transplantation.

Intraoperative management mandates peripheral and central large-bore vascular access permitting volume administration of up to several hundred milliliters per minute. This also requires the ability to warm cold fluids and blood at a rapid rate. Sophisticated equipment (and possibly other technicians to operate the equipment) must be used, further complicating the management of these cases. Access to the central circulation in the severely coagulopathic patient is a challenge in itself.

Removal of the liver often involves interruption of all the venous drainage from the lower body and from the splanchnic circulation. Systemic and portal veno-venous bypass (performed without anticoagulation) may be used to lessen the hemodynamic effects from caval and portal venous clamping. This necessitates more equipment and a dedicated perfusionist or other technician. While the extracorporeal bypass decreases the hemodynamic perturbations, and possibly lessens intraoperative bleeding, it is associated with complications related to placement of the cannulae, heat loss, and the potential for air and thrombotic emboli. Management of the transplant without veno-venous bypass is performed at many centers. It may require volume loading and the sudden administration of up to 2 liters of fluid before cross clamping the major vessels to compensate for the sudden decrease in preload. This additional fluid may further stress the cardiovascular system when clamps are released and large volumes are returned from previously obstructed capacitance vessels. An experienced team is needed to care for these unique intraoperative events.

The intraoperative management of coagulation and platelet deficiencies present preoperatively are further complicated by excessive blood loss. A high potential for fibrinolysis is perhaps the most difficult aspect of managing the coagulation status of these patients. The prophylactic or expectant administration of ε-aminocaproic acid, tranexamic acid, or aprotinin may need to be considered.

Peritoneovenous Shunting

Peritoneovenous shunting is occasionally used to treat intractable ascites which does not respond to diuretics and sodium restriction, and for patients who are not candidates for TIPS or transplantation. There are two types of shunts, LeVeen and Denver. These devices are placed into the peritoneal cavity and allow the passage of ascitic fluid through tubing connected with a one-way, low-pressure valve to the venous circulation, usually through the internal jugular vein. The Denver shunt has a pumping chamber to permit active flushing in the hopes of decreasing the likelihood of shunt occlusion.

Local anesthesia with sedation and monitoring by the anesthesia team is usually the preferred approach to these ill patients. Systemic fluid overload is a major risk caused by translocation of ascitic fluid from an extra- to an intravascular location. Removal of some ascitic fluid before opening the shunt, and meticulous fluid management postoperatively, will diminish the severity of this problem. Infection in the peritoneal cavity can lead to systemic septicemia.

A severe coagulopathy may be initiated by soluble collagen procoagulants from the peritoneal cavity which set off a disseminated intravascular coagulation-type situation. Removal of ascitic fluid and its replacement with saline into the peritoneal cavity before shunt opening will decrease the risk of coagulopathy. Treatment involves immediate surgical ligation of the shunt and possible treatment with clotting factor replacement, platelets, and perhaps an antifibrinolytic agent such as ε-aminocaproic acid.

POSTOPERATIVE CARE

The postoperative course of patients after hepatic surgery can range from the uncomplicated to the very complex, mostly dependent upon the degree of perioperative hepatic dysfunction and the extent of the surgical procedure. Besides the postoperative complications discussed in Chapters 41 and 43, an increased postoperative morbidity rate following hepatic surgery can be anticipated in regards to hepatic failure, persistent coagulopathy, and major bleeding, renal dysfunction, infection, and wound healing.

Hepatic Failure

Postoperative hepatic failure after major liver surgery is more frequent than after other surgical interventions, even in patients with normal preoperative hepatic function. Prolonged intraoperative hepatic ischemia from surgical manipulation or systemic hypotension and resection of large parts of functional hepatic tissue, may lead to transient or irreversible hepatic failure. Patients with diminished hepatic reserve preoperatively are at even greater risk of developing postoperative hepatic failure. Treatment is supportive, just as in the nonsurgical patient.

Even in the absence of outright hepatic failure, a limitation in hepatic functional reserve may be apparent and result in mild jaundice and drug accumulation. The latter is potentially problematic, particularly with regard to the accumulation of hepatically metabolized analgesics, resulting in insidious oversedation and respiratory insufficiency. Patients with cirrhosis often develop postoperative hepatic encephalopathy.

Coagulopathy and Major Bleeding

Persistent coagulation defects, secondary to compromised hepatic synthetic function, may be the cause of early or late postoperative bleeding. Alternatively, continued oozing of blood from the surgical field may result in further consumption of the already limited coagulation factors and platelets. Large amounts of blood, plasma, and platelet transfusions may be required in the early postoperative period. This necessitates adequate vascular access and the availability of a fluid-warming device to avoid transfusion-associated hypothermia, which may further compromise blood coagulation. There should be a low threshold for surgical reexploration and evacuation of accumulated blood. Breakdown products from blood have anticoagulant effects and will contribute to ongoing bleeding. Accumulated blood is also a major risk factor for intraabdominal infection.

Renal Dysfunction

Postoperative acute renal failure is not uncommon in the patient with liver disease. The differential diagnosis includes the same causes as in other surgical patients. Prerenal causes of renal failure need to be addressed and treated aggressively. In patients with poor liver function or hepatic failure, the hepatorenal syndrome has to be considered as a cause of renal dysfunction. Ensurance of adequate intravascular volume is paramount. The medical treatment for renal failure includes dopamine, diuretics, and hemodialysis. Early involvement of the nephrologist in the care of the patient with renal compromise will aid in accurate diagnosis and optimal treatment.

Infection

Patients with extensive hepatic disease have a decreased resistance to infection. However, there is little evidence to suggest that the surgical infection rate is higher than in other patient groups. An exception is the patient who underwent liver transplantation in whom immunosuppressive therapy will increase the likelihood of infections.

WOUND HEALING

Problems with wound healing secondary to decreased protein synthesis, anemia, and poor nutritional status in the patient with decreased hepatic function can be anticipated. If ascites is present, mechanical stress may also interfere with abdominal wound healing. Meticulous surgical wound closure is essential. Optimal wound dressing care and prophylactic antibiotics will improve wound healing and decrease the incidence of wound infection.

Pain Control

Postoperative pain control in patients undergoing major hepatic surgery has to be tailored to the remaining metabolic function of the liver. Because most analgesics are hepatically metabolized, drug accumulation is possible and adjustments in drug dosage are required. Patients with underlying liver dysfunction often have subclinical encephalopathy and have low analgesic requirements. On one end of the spectrum is the ill liver transplant recipient whose analgesic requirements are initially satisfied with only diphenhydramine. Nonsteroidal analgesics may be contraindicated in patients with renal dysfunction or ongoing coagulation defects. The latter may also make continuous postoperative epidural analgesia an undesirable or impossible option for pain control.

BIBLIOGRAPHY

Brown BB Jr: *Anesthesia in hepatic and biliary tract disease,* Philadelphia, 1988, FA Davis.

Carton EG, et al: Perioperative care of the liver transplant patient: part 1, *Anesth Analg* 78:120–133, 1994.

Carton EG, et al: Perioperative care of the liver transplant patient: part 2, *Anesth Analg* 78:382–399, 1994.

Emond JC, et al: Surgical and anesthetic management of patients undergoing major hepatectomy using total vascular exclusion, *Liver Transplantation and Surgery* 2:91–98, 1996.

Quan D, Wall WJ: The safety of continuous hepatic inflow occlusion during major liver resection, *Liver Transplant Surg* 2:99–104, 1996.

Sherlock S, Dooley J: *Diseases of the liver and biliary system,* ed 9, London, 1993, Blackwell Scientific.

Strunin L, Thomson S, editors: The liver and anaesthesia, *Baillieres Clin Anaesth* 6:697–956, 1992.

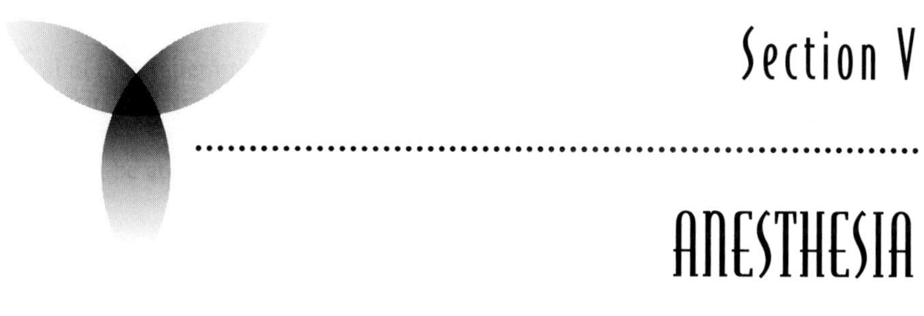

Section V

ANESTHESIA

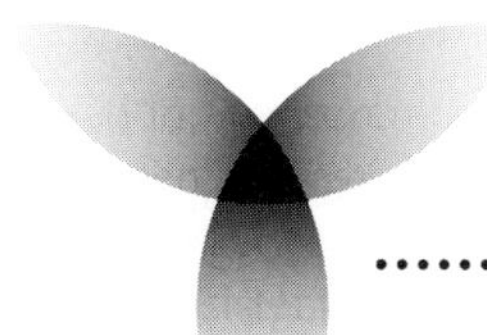

Chapter 37

Airway Management and the Induction of Anesthesia

David J. Stone, MD, Thomas J. Gal, MD

• PREOPERATIVE ISSUES

Considerations in airway management are important in determining the precise mode of inducing anesthesia. Thus, the topics of equipment, airway evaluation, and induction of general anesthesia are clinically inseparable and must be considered together.

To an anesthesiologist the "airway" refers to the entire channel for gas flow between the lips and the alveoli. Maintaining the airway refers to the task of ensuring the patency throughout this channel. This is often synonymous with endotracheal intubation, but other means may be used to maintain the airway. Airway obstruction at any level obviously leads to hypoxemia and hypercarbia if not corrected. The anesthesiologist is the medical specialist best suited to providing a patent airway, unless a surgical airway is required. This chapter is intended as a basic introduction to airway management for the nonanesthesiologist. Those interested in a more extensive general review of airway management are referred to the chapter in Miller's *Anesthesia*, a major textbook in the field. A complete monograph published on the subject by Benumof also provides extensive information. (See Bibliography at the end of the chapter).

Equipment for Airway Management

An oxygen source and capability for suction must be available for any elective attempt at airway management. These may not be present if an airway must be managed in an urgent/emergent nonoperating-room situation. An anesthesia face mask of appropriate size attached to a ventilating bag is required to provide gas flows by positive-pressure ventilation. The use of a tight-fitting anesthesia mask will improve inspired oxygen concentration during spontaneous ventilation, compared to face tents, and allows controlled ventilation. Currently, these masks are often made of clear plastic so the patient can be more easily observed for cyanosis and vomiting. In addition, the clear masks are relatively odorless and less intimidating to the patient than the old, black rubber reusables.

One potential source of confusion arises from the fact that the small mechanical devices used to aid airway patency are referred to as "airways." In the operating room, oral airways are frequently used to preserve a conduit of gas flow dorsad to a potentially obstructing tongue. The insertion of these airways is a noxious stimulus that can provoke gagging, coughing, vomiting, laryngospasm, and bronchospasm in the inadequately anesthetized patient. Care must be taken during insertion to assure that the airway tip is behind the tongue, and not simply pushing the tongue backwards into the oropharynx. Nasal airways or trumpets are softer and less stimulating devices placed through the nares down into the oropharynx to provide a patent gas column. These are useful in patients emerging from anesthesia or when the airway is inadequate with an oral airway alone. However, extensive hemorrhage can occur when nasal airways are jammed into an unprepared nose and, occasionally, even after careful preparation and insertion. Preparation consists of a vasoconstrictor (phenylephrine nose drops) and lubricant/anesthetic (usually, viscous lidocaine jelly). Neither oral nor nasal airways guarantee airway patency. It is helpful for the nonanesthesiologist to have some understanding of the use of these devices because they may be used in an emergency situation until intubation is accomplished or if intubation is impossible.

The basic requirements for endotracheal intubation include endotracheal tubes of appropriate size (includes smaller than predicted size), syringes to inflate the endotracheal tube cuff, and a laryngoscope. Intubation is performed to provide leak-free ventilation with a controlled F_IO_2, for simple airway maintenance and protection, or toilet. For surgery, intubation may be required because of patient position, length of the procedure, or the location and nature of the planned surgery. Today's endotracheal tubes are manufactured of polyvinylchloride and have high-volume, low-pressure cuffs designed to minimize tracheal injury during prolonged intubation. Before use, the tube is inspected for obvious flaws, including lack of patency, and the cuff is tested with an attached syringe for leaks or aberrant inflation. Once the tube is intratracheal, a seal can generally be achieved with approximately 4 to 8 ml air. Intratracheal location is best confirmed by the persistent presence of exhaled carbon dioxide on a capnograph. The valve into which the syringe is inserted is referred to as the pilot valve and is designed to prevent backleak of airflow from an inflated cuff. During long-term intubations, leaks may occur in this valve or, more commonly, in the plastic housing that contains the valve mechanism. The palpable tension of the little balloon next to the valve gives some idea of the pressure within the cuff but is not a quantitative measurement of cuff pressure. Clinically, an endotracheal tube that has migrated partway out of the glottis is a much more common source of cuff leak or inability to provide leak-free ventilation than actual physical disruption of the cuff/

valve mechanism. In the operating room, endotracheal tubes (ETTs) of 7-mm internal diameter (ID) are usually used in adult females and 8-mm ID tubes in males. Depending on manufacturer, the external diameter of the tube will be approximately 3 mm greater than the internal one. It is actually the outer diameter that primarily determines what size ETT should and can be used. If prolonged intubation is anticipated, a 7.5-mm ID ETT can be placed in females to facilitate bronchoscopy. The problem with larger diameter tubes is that they may be more likely to produce laryngeal damage during relatively long periods of intubation, that is, more than 48 hours. For those interested in the issue of prolonged intubation as may occur in the intensive care unit (ICU), several sources are provided in the bibliography.

While a vast number of laryngoscope blade designs have been manufactured, the curved Macintosh and the straight Miller blades are, by far, the most commonly used. The laryngoscope blade is designed to lever the tongue mass into the subglottic space and, thereby, open an illuminated pathway to a glottis whose exposure is facilitated by proper head and neck positioning (viz infra). The laryngoscope is held in the left hand, and the endotracheal tube inserted with the right. While so-called "left-handed" laryngoscopes are manufactured (so-called because these are actually held in the right hand, like a left-handed baseball glove), they are rarely seen because most left-handed laryngoscopists are perfectly happy to perform the task of laryngoscopy with their dominant hand. The laryngoscope blade is carefully inserted into the mouth and passed down the right side of the tongue. The Miller blade is used to actually lift the epiglottis while the Macintosh blade is inserted into the vallecula between the tongue base and epiglottis. While the blade opposes the tongue surface, the entire laryngoscope is gently, but firmly, lifted in a 45° angle away from the vertical. The laryngoscope should not be levered using the blade/handle attachment as a fulcrum because this will tend to break incisors and is not as effective in exposing the glottis as a true lifting motion.

Other commonly used airway devices include stylets, bougies, tube changers, fiberoptic bronchoscopes, and the laryngeal mask airway. Stylets are rigid insertions which should not protrude past the ETT tip. They are used to maintain the ETT tip in a fixed, predictable location and aid glottic entry when visualization is incomplete or poor, or simply to quicken the intubation process when this is an issue, as in an emergent or full-stomach situation. Stylets are also manufactured with lights on the tip to provide a guide for blind intubation as the path of the light is followed through the skin of the upper neck. The gum elastic bougie is a moderately flexible stylet-type device that is longer than the aforementioned conventional stylet. It is used as a blindly-inserted conduit into the glottis when little or none of the laryngeal structures can be visualized during laryngoscopy. It can also be used as a tube-changer, although it is a bit short. Devices are now produced expressly for this purpose. Formal tube changers are manufactured with thick, rigid plastic walls, well-marked with distances from both ends. They are sufficiently long so that even when the indwelling tube is removed, there is still some length of tube changer accessible to the operator. These maneuvers are no guarantee that the first tube can be replaced and alternative airway measures should be considered, including the high-pressure insufflation of oxygen through the hollow tube changer.

Fiberoptic technology is now used to facilitate oral and nasal intubations in both conscious and anesthetized patients. The fiberoptic bronchoscope allows visualization of the glottis when this cannot be achieved by more conventional means. Examples include patients whose necks cannot be moved, or when there is severe distortion of anatomy as may occur in rheumatoid arthritis or acromegaly. Training in this modality is relatively new so that the anesthesiologist trained more than a decade ago may not possess this skill. Furthermore, the equipment is expensive and fragile and may not be universally available.

The laryngeal mask airway (LMA) is an ingenious device that lies somewhere between face-mask ventilation and endotracheal intubation. The airway consists of a small mask-type device attached to a large tube that can be connected to airway tubing. The miniature face mask is inserted down to the laryngeal level and has an inflatable rim that provides some degree of seal, so that positive-pressure ventilation can be provided if high pressures are not required. The LMA may be inserted under general anesthesia, usually without muscle relaxants, and is nearly as stimulating as an oral airway. The LMA does not protect the airway against aspiration, and is not as reliable an airway as an ETT. However, it is well suited for many kinds of procedures and can also be inserted under emergency circumstances when the anesthesiologist can neither intubate nor ventilate by face mask.

Extreme measures that may be required if the patient can be neither ventilated nor intubated include cricothyrotomy, tracheostomy, and translaryngeal jet ventilation. In the last case, an intravenous catheter is inserted into the cricotyhroid membrane and attached to a high-pressure oxygen source to provide oxygenation and, at times, ventilation.

Airway Evaluation

This constitutes the most important component of the anesthesiologist's selective physical examination and an important part of the perioperative history, as well. The patient should be asked about difficulties with airway management during previous anesthetics or intubations for respiratory failure. Other historic components include radiation therapy or airway trauma, long-term intubations and the presence of a variety of diseases that may interfere with airway management. These include congenital, infectious, metabolic, neoplastic, and inflammatory diseases and are listed in detail in anesthesia texts. Old anesthetic records should be reviewed, as available. In some cases, the patient will have more complete information such as a Medic Alert (Medic Alert Foundation, Turlock, CA) bracelet for this purpose.

The physical examination evaluates those anatomic features that may interfere with mask ventilation, laryngoscopy, and/or endotracheal intubation. Basic physical attributes are first noticed such as obesity, short or thick neck, scars on the neck, and obvious problems such as neck collars and halo devices. The laryngoscopic view of the glottis involves alignment of the oral, pharyngeal, and laryngeal axes. This is done by slight flexion at the lower cervical spine, extension at the atlanto-occipital and atlantoaxial joints, and wide opening of the mouth. Therefore, the examination includes an evaluation of adequate mouth opening while viewing the mouth and oropharynx for tongue size relative to the oral cavity and obvious signs of pathology or dental problems, because chipped or fractured teeth are the most common complication of direct laryngoscopy. This is followed by full-neck extension, if permitted by concomitant pathology, with attention to extension at the upper cervical levels, and the distance this extension creates between the mandible and the thyroid cartilage. Because the laryngoscope displaces the tongue muscle into the floor of the mouth, it is also important to evaluate the distance between the hyoid bone and the mandible in the midline. A large tongue, combined with a small mandibulohyoid distance, are likely to impair one's attempts to view the glottic aperture. While an obvious problem, such as a cervical spine fracture, renders airway management difficult, a combination of mild defects in mouth opening, neck movement, and mandibulo-hyoid space can also result in difficulties. Other problems, such as lingual tonsils or tracheal stenosis, may be hard to predict. Finally, some patients present airway management difficulties that can not be explained by obvious anatomic derangements, even in retrospect. Today's anesthesiologist should be prepared to deal with both the predicted and unanticipated difficult airway. On rare occasions, laboratory measures such as magnetic resonance imaging (MRI), flow-volume loops, and other radiographic tests may be used preoperatively.

• AIRWAY MANAGEMENT AND THE INDUCTION OF ANESTHESIA

These two elements are inextricably intertwined because one's predicted ability to manage the airway determines the mode of anesthesia induction. In the majority of cases, the airway is judged to be manageable and the patient is anesthetized with an intravenous anesthetic, mask ventilation is established, and laryngoscopy and intubation facilitated with a muscle relaxant. If there a risk of aspiration, the relaxant is administered with the intravenous anesthetic while dorsal pressure is maintained over the cricoid cartilage to occlude the esophagus (Sellick maneuver). If difficulties with mask ventilation occur, there are a number of options which include use of oral and/or nasal airways and two-handed mask ventilation with anterior mandibular displacement. An attempt at intubation without or (usually) with muscle relaxant, may be made. If unsuccessful, it may be necessary for the patient to wake up or to attempt ventilation with a laryngeal mask airway. If mask ventilation is adequate but intubation can not be accomplished, the patient's head position is reexamined, a different laryngoscope blade may be tried, and a more experienced operator may attempt the procedure. Digital manipulation of the larynx in a backwards, upwards, and/or rightwards direction may improve visualization. A smaller ETT should be tried if the tube will not pass down through the larynx or if blind measures are unsuccessful. Actual intubation may be facilitated by the use of a stylet, an elastic gum bougie, or a lighted ("lite-wand") stylet. Other possible measures include the traditional blind nasal approach, fiberoptic techniques, retrograde techniques over a translaryngeal guide, or using the laryngeal mask airway (LMA) as an intubation guide. If the procedure is elective, it may be best to stop attempts at intubation and manage the airway by mask or LMA until consciousness and muscle strength are restored. This is because further attempts can cause edema, bleeding, and trauma, which can result in complete upper airway obstruction.

If neither mask ventilation nor intubation can be accomplished, the aforementioned translaryngeal jet ventilation or a surgical airway will be required, unless the patient resumes spontaneous ventilation with an acceptably well-maintained airway. In our opinion, this is the main reason that succinylcholine is still used. It is the only relaxant with a duration of action so short that spontaneous ventilation will return before cerebral hypoxia ensues if the patient has been adequately denitrogenated ("preoxygenated") before the induction of anesthesia. Succinylcholine is metabolized by plasma pseudocholinesterase. Duration of action will be somewhat prolonged if the level of the enzyme is reduced or extremely prolonged if a genetically abnormal form of the enzyme is present. Serious problems may occur with the use of succinylcholine, including severe hyperkalemia in the presence of a variety of medical problems (spinal-cord injury, stroke, burns, other neuromuscular disease; see an anesthesia text for complete list) and the production of malignant hyperthermia. Succinylcholine is the only depolarizing relaxant commonly used in North America. All the other neuromuscular blockers are nondepolarizing agents, which act primarily by blocking the postjunctional nicotinic acetylcholine receptor. To facilitate intubation, a large dose of these agents is used so that spontaneous or pharmacologic reversal of the blockade is generally impossible for at least 20 to 30 minutes after administration. Pharmacologic reversal with an inhibitor of cholinesterase (neostigmine or edrophonium) is not effective until the block has receded to the point where at least one "twitch" can be produced by the clinical nerve stimulators commonly used in the operating room. For this reason, nondepolarizing relaxants should not be administered until mask ventilation is proven, or one has confidence that the airway does not present severe difficulties. This latter judgment is one that requires a fair amount of clinical experience and should not be taken lightly by any physician involved in airway management.

When the anesthesiologist judges that the airway cannot be safely managed in the anesthetized state, intubation can be accomplished while the patient is conscious. While this is frequently referred to as "awake" intubation, the patient almost always receives some degree of sedation unless life-threatening airway compromise is present. Just as importantly, local anesthesia is also applied topically and, at times, in specific nerve blocks to improve patient comfort and intubating conditions. Physicians and surgeons should not be outraged that their patient is being intubated "awake"; instead, they should be grateful that a caring and insightful anesthesia clinician has attempted to avoid a potentially life-threatening situation. Preparation for conscious intubation may include administration of an anticholinergic drying agent to improve visualization and diminish dilution of topical anesthetics with saliva. Anticholinergics are not restricted to conscious intubations and are also useful in patients who are smokers, who have airway hyperreactivity and/or copious secretions, and in any situation in which decrease in secretions is judged to be clinically desirable. Topical anesthetics (usually lidocaine) can be applied by nebulization, direct spray, gargling of viscous preparations, application of lidocaine gels, and through a translaryngeal approach as well. The glossopharyngeal and/or the superior laryngeal nerves can be specifically blocked if so chosen. Sedation may be accomplished by the judicious administration of narcotic, benzodiazepine, butyrophenone, or diphenhydramine. These are titrated in small, incremental doses because patient response is variable in terms of both consciousness and respiratory depressant effects.

After the chosen sedative and local anesthetics are administered, the actual intubation can proceed in a variety of ways. Blind nasal intubation was heavily relied on in the past, but has been replaced to a large extent by fiberoptic techniques. The nasal approach avoids the discomfort of direct laryngoscopy and affords a straighter route to the glottis than the oral approach. The nasal approach requires vasoconstriction as well as analgesia, as noted. Blind techniques may stir up bleeding and edema that make a subsequent fiberoptic approach more difficult. Direct oral laryngoscopy, as generally used in the anesthetized patient, may also be used. While some clinicians may take an "awake look" to see if the glottis is visible, and then administer anesthesia and relaxants, we believe that if the glottis is visualized by this technique, the endotracheal tube should be inserted after proper topicalization. The view may worsen in the anesthetized, paralyzed patient because the larynx tends to move cephalad and anteriorly, compared to the awake state. Basically, all the techniques used in the anesthetized patient may be used in the conscious patient. Success with conscious intubation requires thorough explanation to the patient, adequate topical anesthesia after administration of an anticholinergic drying agent, and patience with sedation so that neither under- nor oversedation results. In most cases, the ETT can be safely placed without undue discomfort to the patient.

POSTOPERATIVE CARE AND AIRWAY MANAGEMENT OUTSIDE THE OPERATING ROOM

The most careful intraoperative management can be undone by a casual approach to wake-up and extubation. Care must be taken, particularly in patients who presented difficulties in ventilation or intubation during the induction process. However, any extubation can be further complicated by laryngospasm, soft-tissue airway obstruction, laryngeal edema, or aspiration. This also applies to extubation after longer-term ICU intubations, although they are much more prone to structural complications such as laryngeal or tracheal stenosis. Laryngospasm and soft-tissue obstruction may be generally avoided by extubating the patient who is sufficiently awake to follow verbal commands and who has adequate return of neuromuscular function. Laryngospasm is treated with gentle, sustained positive pressure, low doses of succinylcholine, and reintubation, if necessary. Adequate muscle strength can be demonstrated by sustained tetanus with an anesthesia nerve stimulator, or, clinically, by the ability to hold the head up or stick the tongue out of the mouth for 5 seconds. Airway maintenance maneuvers such as mechanical airways and proper positioning are helpful if there is soft-tissue obstruction, although additional cholinesterase inhibitor and even reintubation may be required. Laryngeal edema is unlikely in adults who have no premorbid condition, appropriate-sized ETTs, and atraumatic intubations and who have undergone surgery remote from the neck. However, it may occur in any patient especially those who have had neck surgery, because extremes in neck positioning are often required for exposure. Glottic edema is manifested as stridor (inspiratory wheezing can be heard over the trachea) and is treated with heated, humidified oxygen which may be supplemented by nebulized epinephrine and intravenous steroids. Once again, reintubation may be required if the airway cannot be maintained and if the patient's general clinical condition, oxygenation, or ventilation deteriorates.

In cases in which there is particular concern about extubation, the ETT is not removed until the patient is fully awake and consistently responsive to verbal stimuli. These cases might include difficult intubations, patients who have had their mouths wired shut or cervical spines fused and those with upper-airway pathology /surgery. Patients in the ICU who have failed prior extubations because of apparent upper-airway obstruction would fall into this category. Skilled clinicians with the proper airway equipment should be present at bedside. In selected cases, this will include preparation for surgical airway intervention, as well. A tube changer may be inserted into the trachea before the old tube is removed over the changer, which is left in place. A hollow tube changer can also be used for jet ventilation, as well as maintaining the trail to the glottis. Most patients tolerate the small tube changer without too much difficulty, but care must be taken to avoid stimulating carinal contact. The changer can then be removed when the patient is judged to have passed the test of extubation.

Acute management of the airway outside the operating room is subject to several important disadvantages relative to usual elective operative airway management. These problems include possible lack of basic equipment, usual lack of more sophisticated equipment, lack of experienced help, and a critically ill patient. The actual approach to the airway is dictated by the experience of the practitioner, the availability of equipment, and the urgency and exact nature of the patient's medical/ surgical problem. While the patient in full-blown cardiopulmonary arrest requires no supplement to simple laryngoscopy and intubation, other patients may be best handled with topical anesthesia alone. The use of muscle relaxants outside the operating room is a calculated risk, and we would encourage the nonanesthesiologist not to use these drugs without extensive clinical experience. The reviews listed in the bibliography provide approaches to a variety of problems encountered. In general, it is usually best to start off with a conservative approach of topicalization, later supplemented by intravenous adjuncts, anesthetics, and muscle relaxants only as absolutely required. In addition to airway difficulties, these patients may have unstable cardiovascular systems, which will respond poorly to negative inotropes, vasodilators, drugs that diminish sympathetic outflow, and even the institution of positive-pressure ventilation. These situations can represent extreme airway difficulties and, as a rule, are not the place for the beginner to acquire experience in airway management.

The patient requiring long-term intubation has come to receive more attention in recent years (see bibliography). Issues include oral versus nasal locations, cuff leak, ETT size, tube changes, laryngotracheal injury, and timing of tracheostomy. Nasal ETTs were frequently used in the past and have the advantages of potential placement without a laryngoscope. Although they appear to provide greater stability and patient comfort, the frequent association of maxillary sinusitis with nasotracheal intubation has made the latter undesirable for intubations lasting more than a day or two. While less-experienced clinicians are quick to diagnose a ruptured ETT cuff when leak-free ventilation cannot be provided, other explanations are actually more likely. Most common is an ETT tip that is positioned nearly out of the larynx but leaks in the pilot balloon/valve system are also more common than actual disruption of the cuff. Structural problems such as tracheomalacia or tracheoesophageal fistula are more serious causes for ongoing cuff leak, unremediable by what normally is adequate cuff inflation. Endotracheal tube size is important because a tube that is too small may result in cuff leaks or requirement for cuff hyperinflation to produce a seal. The latter will overcome the normally low tracheal-wall pressure applied by the modern ETT cuff producing ischemia, malacia, and, eventually, stenosis at the site. The 7.0-ID ETT, usually used in females, makes diagnostic/therapeutic bronchoscopy in the ICU somewhat difficult. However, larger tubes may predispose to laryngeal damage in the smaller female glottic inlet. We have reached a local compromise by inserting 7.5-ID ETTs in women, so that bronchoscopy can be accomplished and the potentially more damaging 8.0-ETT can be avoided. Tube size may be raised as an issue during weaning because smaller tubes increase the work of breathing. While the patient ready to be weaned can generally do so with a 7.0-ETT, a small amount of pressure support (5–10 cm H_2O) can be applied to obviate this issue. Finally, smaller tubes may limit exhalation in patients with airway obstruction and predispose them to dynamic hyperinflation during mechanical ventilation. This can generally be overcome by lengthening expiratory times and shortening inspiratory times as well, if necessary. Endotracheal tubes may need to be changed for a variety of reasons including nasal-to-oral positioning, true cuff leak, or ETT size. These "simple" tube changes can be challenging and are best accomplished by a consultant anesthesiologist. At this time, tracheostomy should also be considered as an option. In past years, patients often received tracheostomy after a short period. Patients now more commonly remain intubated for 10 to 14 days before tracheostomy is performed. In brief, the tracheostomy trades off the laryngeal complications of intubation for the stomal complications of tracheostomy. The tracheostomy does provide a more comfortable, secure route for long-term ventilation, and facilitates nursing care and ambulation. It also may be required because of complicating upper-airway obstruction. It is important to remember that a reliable tracheocutaneous tract does not form for a week after tracheostomy and that tracheostomy changes in that first week are best handled by those who are capable of airway management. They should probably be done over a changer stylet if necessary.

BIBLIOGRAPHY

Benumof J: *Airway management*, Philadelphia, 1996, Mosby.

Bogdonoff DL, Stone DJ: Emergency management of the airway outside the operating room, *Can J Anaesth* 39:1069, 1992.

Dorsch JA, Dorsch SE: *Understanding anesthesia equipment-construction, care, and complications*, Baltimore, 1994, Williams & Wilkins, (good source on airway equipment).

Leisure GS, Stone DJ, Spiekermann BF, et al: Airway management of the chronically intubated patient, *Respir Care* 40:644, 1995.

Spiekermann BF, et al: Nonsurgical airway management: general considerations and specific considerations in patients with coexisting disease, *Respir Care* 40:1, 1995.
Stone DJ, Bogdonoff DL: Airway considerations in the management of patients requiring long-term intubation, *Anesth Analg* 74:276, 1992.
Stone DJ, Gal TJ: Airway Management. In Miller RD, editor; *Anesthesia*, ed 4, New York, 1994, Churchill Livingstone.

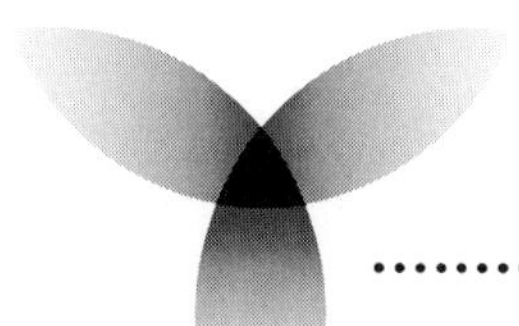

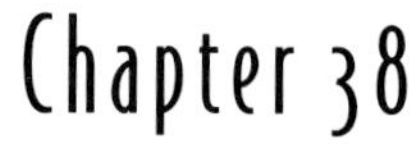

Chapter 38

Monitoring

Burkhard F. Spiekermann, MD, Robert C. Li, MD

One of the primary functions of the anesthesiologist in the operating room is to monitor and document changes of a multitude of patient parameters. In fact, patient monitoring occupies more than one half of the anesthesiologist's time while in the operating room. As such, monitoring can be regarded as an integral part of patient care and advances in monitoring technology over the last decade have made a significant contribution towards decreasing perioperative morbidity.

The choice of monitoring is governed by the status of the patient and by the type of operation performed. This chapter will discuss the principles of monitoring, the current basic monitoring standards, and the selection of monitors for specific cases. We attempted to functionally group the monitoring requirements for patients with or without specific organ diseases, while taking into consideration the invasiveness of the planned surgical procedure.

In addition to monitoring the patient, continuous monitoring of the anesthesia machine is required to prevent adverse anesthetic events related to equipment malfunction. Modern anesthesia equipment is designed with many fail-safe devices and built-in alarm systems to minimize the potential for such events. Monitoring of anesthesia equipment function will not be discussed in this chapter.

THE PRINCIPLES OF MONITORING

Every monitoring technique underlies the same principle: continuous and repeated observations of specific patient parameters to identify trends and prevent untoward events. This implies that the value of a monitor depends on how accurately it will predict an adverse event, and how early it will display the trend towards an adverse event to allow adequate time to intervene. Pulse oximetry, for example, accurately displays a decrease in oxygen saturation with a short lag time and is a much better monitor of hypoxia than visually inspecting the patient for cyanosis. Monitoring for hypoxia through signs of cyanosis will give the anesthesiologist a late warning signal and will allow little time to correct the problem of oxygen delivery. In spite of the often stated cliché "there is no better monitor than the vigilant anesthesiologist," new advances in monitoring technology, when applied knowingly, may help anticipate untoward events early, and allow prompt therapeutic intervention before permanent damage to the patient occurs. Although this sounds logical, data for improved outcome with sophisticated monitoring technology is lacking. This is one reason why, with the exception of basic monitoring as specified by the American Society of Anesthesiologists (ASA), monitoring practice varies among different practitioners. A well-meant suggestion in the preoperative consultation form by the cardiologist, such as "use Swan Ganz catheter" is, therefore, not appropriate and may only have legal implications if such suggestions are not followed and an adverse event occurs. In addition, invasive monitors may be the cause of morbidity and mortality. Their inherent dangers should always be weighed against their potential benefits.

THE AMERICAN SOCIETY OF ANESTHESIOLOGISTS' MONITORING STANDARDS

In 1986 the ASA adopted a set of standards for basic monitoring of oxygenation, ventilation, circulation, and body temperature, which was amended in 1992 to include a recommendation for capnometry (Box 38-1). These standards were adapted from similar standards introduced by the Harvard Medical School in 1986 and apply to all anesthesia care provided, including conscious sedation, regional anesthesia, and general anesthesia. Standard I requires the continuous presence of qualified anesthesia personnel in the anesthetizing location. Standard II defines monitoring requirements

Box 38-1 American Society of Anesthesiologists' Standards for Intraoperative Monitoring

These standards apply to all anesthesia care, although, in emergency circumstances, appropriate life-support measures take precedence. These standards may be exceeded at any time based on the judgment of the responsible anesthesiologist. They are intended to encourage quality patient care, but observing them cannot guarantee any specific patient outcome. They are subject to revision from time to time, as warranted by the evolution of technology and practice. This set of standards addresses only the issue of basic intraoperative monitoring, which is one component of anesthesia care. In certain rare or unusual situations, (1) some of these methods of monitoring may be clinically impractical, and (2) appropriate use of the described monitoring may fail to detect untoward clinical developments. Brief interruptions of continual monitoring may be unavoidable. Under extenuating circumstances, the responsible anesthesiologist may waive the requirements marked with an asterisk (*); it is recommended, that when this is done, it should be so stated (including the reasons) in a note in the patient's medical record. These standards are not intended for application to the care of the obstetrical patient in labor or in the conduct of pain management.

STANDARD I

Qualified anesthesia personnel shall be present in the room throughout the conduct of all general anesthetics, regional anesthetics, and monitored anesthesia care.

Objective:

Because of rapid changes in patient status during anesthesia, qualified anesthesia personnel shall be continuously present to monitor the patient and provide anesthesia care. In the event there is a direct known hazard, e.g., radiation, to the anesthesia personnel which might require intermittent remote observation of the patient, some provision for monitoring the patient must be made. In the event that an emergency requires the temporary absence of the person primarily responsible for the anesthetic, the best judgment of the anesthesiologist will be exercised in comparing the emergency with the anesthetized patient's condition, and in the selection of the person left responsible for the anesthetic during the temporary absence.

STANDARD II

During all anesthetics, the patient's oxygenation, ventilation, circulation, and temperature shall be continually evaluated.

Oxygenation

Objective:

To ensure adequate oxygenation concentration in the inspired gas and the blood during all anesthetics.

Methods:

1. Inspired gas: During every administration of general anesthesia using an anesthesia machine, the concentration of oxygen in the patient's breathing system shall be measured by an oxygen analyzer with a low oxygen concentration-limit alarm in use.*
2. Blood oxygenation: During all anesthetics, a quantitative method of assessing oxygenation such as pulse oximetry shall be employed.* Adequate illumination and exposure of the patient is necessary to assess color.* *(continued on p. 658)*

Box 38-1 American Society of Anesthesiologists' Standards for Intraoperative Monitoring *(Continued)*

Ventilation

Objective:
To ensure adequate ventilation of the patient during all anesthetics.

Methods:
1. Every patient receiving general anesthesia shall have the adequacy of ventilation continually evaluated. While qualitative clinical signs such as chest excursion, observation of the reservoir breathing bag, and auscultation of breath sounds may be adequate, quantitative monitoring of the CO_2 content and/or volume of expired gas is encouraged.
2. When an endotracheal tube is inserted, its correct positioning in the trachea must be verified by clinical assessment and by identification of carbon dioxide in the expired gas.* End-tidal CO_2 analysis, in use from the time of endotracheal tube placement is strongly encouraged.
3. When ventilation is controlled by a mechanical ventilator, there shall be in continuous use a device that is capable of detecting disconnection of components of the breathing system. The device must give an audible signal when its alarm threshold is exceeded.
4. During regional anesthesia and monitored anesthesia care, the adequacy of ventilation shall be evaluated, at least, by continual observation of qualitative clinical signs.

Circulation

Objective:
To ensure the adequacy of the patient's circulatory function during all anesthetics.

Methods:
1. Every patient receiving anesthesia shall have the electrocardiogram continuously displayed from the beginning of anesthesia until preparing to leave the anesthetizing location.*
2. Every patient receiving anesthesia shall have arterial blood pressure and heart rate determined and evaluated at least every 5 minutes.*
3. Every patient receiving general anesthesia shall have, in addition to the above, circulatory function continually evaluated by at least one of the following: palpation of pulse, auscultation of heart sounds, monitoring of a tracing of intraarterial pressure, ultrasound peripheral pulse monitoring, or pulse plethysmography or oximetry.

Body Temperature

Objective:
To aid in the maintenance of appropriate body temperature during all anesthetics.

Methods:
There shall be readily available a means to continuously measure the patient's temperature. When changes in body temperature are intended, anticipated, or suspected, the temperature shall be measured.

related to oxygenation, ventilation, circulation, and temperature. The rationale behind adopting uniform, basic monitoring standards stems from analysis of data in which patient mortality and morbidity was judged to be preventable in more than 30% of all cases with improved monitors. Approximately 80% of those preventable incidents were associated with adverse respiratory events, for example, undetected esophageal intubations, or an undetected disconnection within the breathing circuit. Reflecting this preponderance of adverse outcomes related to respiratory events, is the ASA's suggestion to include pulse oximetry, as a monitor in all anesthetics, and capnometry whenever general anesthesia is administered.

MONITORING OF THE PATIENT WITHOUT MAJOR ORGAN DISEASE

Healthy patients undergoing minimal-to-moderate invasive surgery generally will not require invasive monitoring. Basic monitoring techniques congruent with the ASA standards are almost always sufficient. This includes continuous electrocardiography, noninvasive blood-pressure monitoring, pulse oximetry, capnography, and temperature monitoring. Monitoring that can be performed without any devices on every patient includes direct inspection of the patient for changes in color, skin turgor, signs of movement or perspiration (which may indicate inadequate anesthetic depth), and symmetrical chest excursions. Observing the surgical field for tissue color and the amount of blood loss may also give valuable information regarding the adequacy of peripheral perfusion.

Electrocardiography

Electrocardiographic (ECG) monitoring in the form of a continuous visual display of the ECG on a screen informs about (1) heart rate, (2) cardiac dysrhythmias, (3) myocardial ischemia (4) conduction defects, and (5) electrolyte abnormalities. A five-lead system consisting of leads I, II, III, aVF, and lead V5 is used for every anesthetic at our institution. Lead II is sensitive for detecting cardiac dysrhythmias, because it most prominently depicts the P wave. Lead V5 is the single best lead in detecting myocardial ischemia and, when combined with lead II, detects 80% of all ischemic events. If the patient is at increased risk for myocardial ischemia, lead V4 may be monitored, as well. The combination of lead II, V4, and V5 was shown to have a 96% sensitivity for detecting ischemic events.

Noninvasive Blood Pressure Monitoring

Automated blood pressure monitoring in the anesthetized patient is routinely performed with an oscillometric device such as the Dinamapp (Critikon, Tampa, FL). Oscillometric systems measure and display systolic, diastolic, and mean arterial pressure. The system is accurate even in small children, provided that a properly sized blood pressure cuff is applied. The width of the cuff should be approximately 40% of the arm circumference. At times, in the very small neonate, only mean arterial pressure may be displayed: Low blood pressure values in the small child cause low amplitude deflections. Therefore, the monitor algorithm is unable to assess systolic and diastolic values accurately.

Pulse Oximetry

Pulse oximetry allows continuous noninvasive monitoring of arterial hemoglobin oxygen saturation and provides an early warning sign of hypoxia. The pulse oximeter is usually applied to the finger or the earlobe of the patient. A diode emits light at a wavelength of 660 nm and 940 nm (reflecting the absorption spectrum of oxy- and deoxyhemoglobin). A photodetector receives the light signals and electronically calculates the amount of light absorbed, which is (according to the Lambert Beer law) directly related to the amount of saturated and unsaturated hemoglobin. There is a 10- to 15-second delay in the response time of the pulse oximeter and the device is inaccurate at low oxygen saturation values.

Pulse oximetry depends on pulsatile flow. Extreme hypotension, cardiopulmonary bypass, peripheral vasoconstriction, or any other situation that compromises pulsatile flow to the periphery interferes with proper pulse-oximetry function. Similarly, patient movement causes monitor malfunction.

Dyshemoglobinemias will cause inaccuracy of the pulse oximeter reading. Carboxyhemoglobin has similar absorption characteristics to oxyhemoglobin and will give falsely elevated values. Methemoglobinemia will cause a pulse oximetry reading approximately 85%. Ambient light, nail polish, and intravenously injected dyes will cause spurious readings. Intravenous methylene blue, for example, decreases oximetry readings to 65% for approximately 1 to 2 minutes after injection.

Capnography and Respiratory Gas Analysis

Capnography monitors and continuously displays carbon dioxide (CO_2) concentrations in the inspired and expired gases of the patient. Capnography has become a routine monitor in most operating rooms. The most commonly used technology uses infrared spectroscopy to determine CO_2 concentration in the gas mixture. Other systems use mass spectrometry or Raman spectroscopy, a laser-based system. In addition to CO_2 analysis, these systems also will calculate and display the in- and expired concentrations of anesthetic gases, oxygen, and nitrogen. Infrared devices, however, cannot register nonpolar molecules and, therefore, will not directly measure nitrogen and oxygen.

Capnography is used to confirm proper endotracheal intubation. Even though the presence or absence of CO_2 in the exhaled gas does not absolutely confirm endotracheal or esophageal intubation, capnography is a sensitive monitor for proper tube placement, when used in conjunction with other clinical parameters (i.e., bilateral breath sounds over both lung fields).

The shape of the capnogram (Figure 38-1) and analysis of its four phases will help identify different potential patient and anesthesia-machine problems. Elevations in the inspiratory baseline (Segment A-B) is caused by rebreathing of CO_2 from either incompetent unidirectional valves in the breathing circuit or an exhausted CO_2 absorber. A delayed expiratory upstroke (Segment B-C) is consistent with unequal alveolar emptying, as for example in patients with chronic obstructive pulmonary disease. Dips in the expiratory plateau (Segment C-D) may indicate spontaneous respiratory efforts, whereas a delayed inspiratory downstroke (Segment D-E), may be caused by an incompetent inspiratory valve within the circle breathing system.

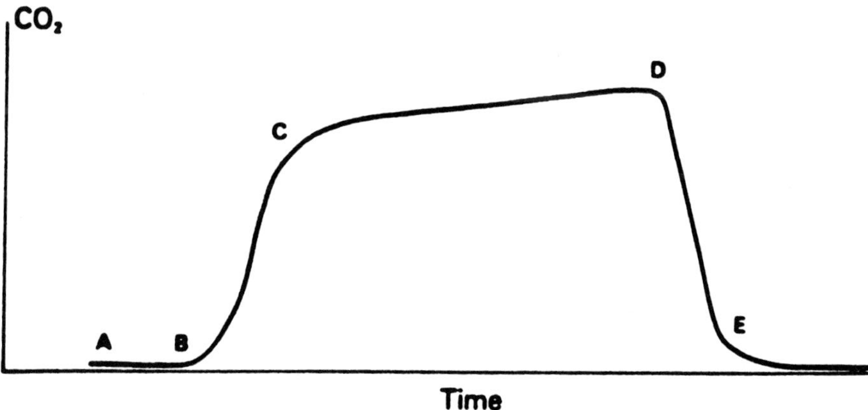

Figure 38-1
The shape of a normal capnogram. See text for details. (Reprinted with permission from Cohen N, Schwartz D: Monitoring the airway and pulmonary function. In Benumof JP, editor: *Airway management: principles and practice*, St. Louis, 1996, Mosby–Year Book, Inc.)

Causes of a decrease in expired CO_2 without changes in minute ventilation include decreased cardiac output or cardiac arrest (i.e., decreased or no pulmonary blood flow and CO_2 delivery), hypotension, a pulmonary embolus or decreased CO_2 production (i.e., hypothermia, neuromuscular blockade.) The causes of increases in expired CO_2 include increased endogenous CO_2 production as with malignant hyperthermia or a febrile illness. The release of a vascular clamp or an orthopedic tourniquet will also temporarily increase expired CO_2, secondary to the CO_2 load from the ischemic tissue. Carbon dioxide insufflation and absorption during laparoscopic procedures will cause an exogenous CO_2 load and will be reflected by an increase in exhaled CO_2.

Temperature Monitoring

Except during short procedures the patient's temperature should be monitored. Mild, unintentional hypothermia, that is, a decrease in body-core temperature by 1 to 3°C, is common during general anesthesia: Heat redistribution from the central to the peripheral compartment (secondary to anesthesia-induced vasodilation), and subsequent heat loss to the cold, operating room environment contribute to this temperature drop. In addition, hypothalamic temperature regulation is altered in the anesthetized patient. Hypothermia is responsible for postoperative patient discomfort and delayed awakening. Shivering increases oxygen consumption by 400%. It has been shown that in patients with poor myocardial reserve, hypothermia correlates with the incidence of perioperative myocardial ischemia. Other problems related to hypothermia include increased systemic vascular resistance, platelet dysfunction, a left-shift of the oxygen-hemoglobin dissociation curve, and impaired drug metabolism and clearance. Excessive decreases in temperature should be recognized and avoided. At times, however, mild-to-moderate hypothermia is used intentionally, as with intracranial vascular operations in which it has been shown to be protective against the effects of cerebral ischemia. Again, accurate temperature monitoring is required to allow adequate patient cooling. A rise in body temperature during the perioperative period should also be noted, because it may indicate sepsis, excessive peripheral warming (common in small children), or malignant hyperthermia.

Esophageal temperature monitors (incorporated into esophageal stethoscopes), placed in the lower third of the esophagus, are most commonly used to monitor the patient's temperature, since they are inexpensive, minimally invasive, and accurately reflect core temperature. Tympanic membrane sensors reflect brain temperature, but their placement is associated with a risk of tympanic membrane rupture and bleeding in the external auditory canal. Skin, rectal, and axillary probes do not accurately correlate with core temperature. If the patient has a pulmonary artery catheter, the thermistor on the catheter also measures core temperature.

Monitoring of Neuromuscular Blockade

Monitoring of neuromuscular function is required if neuromuscular blockers are used during the operation to monitor adequate intraoperative muscle relaxation and recovery of neuromuscular function postoperatively. Electrodes are typically placed over the ulnar or facial nerve, and the response to an electrical stimulus from the nerve stimulator is assessed by evaluating contraction of the adductor pollicis and orbicularis oris muscle, respectively. The degree of neuromuscular blockade is assessed by delivering a supramaximal stimulus (50 mA) to the nerve and evaluating muscle contraction in response to this stimulus. The most commonly used patterns of electrical stimulation are the "Train of Four (TOF)," "Tetanic Stimulation," "Posttetanic Potentiation," and "Double Burst Stimulation (DBS)." Tactile and visual evaluation of the motor response is normally used to quantify the degree of neuromuscular blockade, although electromyography can be used for a more accurate quantitative measure. The motor response not only depends on the degree of neuromuscular blockade, but is determined by the type of neuromuscular blockers used. Depolarizing (i.e., succinylcholine) and nondepolarizing neuromuscular blockers have a different effect on the pattern of neuromuscular response. In addition, different muscle groups have different sensitivity to neuromuscular blockade. For example, the orbicularis oris muscle, for example, is more resistant to neuromuscular blockade than the adductor pollicis. Diaphragmatic and laryngeal muscle function also recovers sooner from neuromuscular blockade than does the adductor pollicis.

TRAIN OF FOUR

Train-of-four stimulation consists of four supramaximal stimuli delivered to the nerve at a frequency of 2 Hz. In the presence of a nondepolarizing neuromuscular blocker, a decrease in the motor response (twitch) is present between each consecutive twitch. The ratio of the fourth response to the first response (TOF ratio) determines the degree of blockade (Figure 38-2). Surgical relaxation is present when only one to two twitches are present. (80%–90% block) If the TOF ratio is greater than 0.7, respiratory muscle strength is usually not compromised. If succinylcholine is used

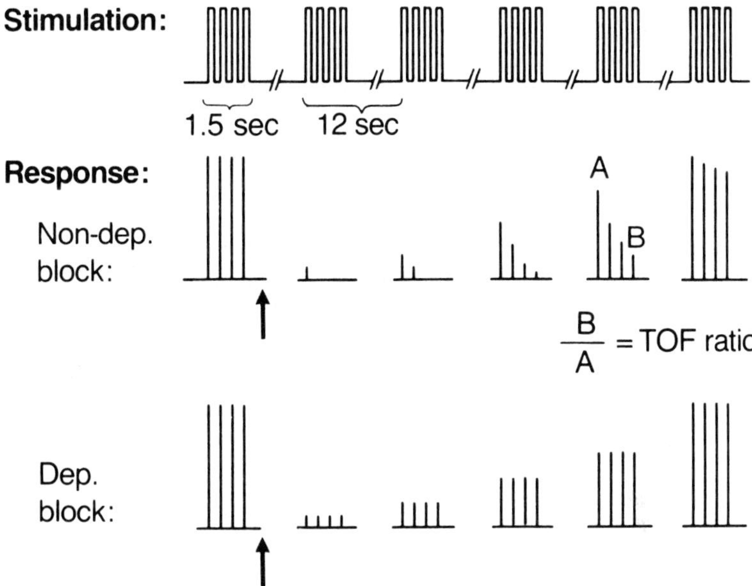

Figure 38-2
Monitoring of neuromuscular blockade in the presence of nondepolarizing and depolarizing neuromuscular blockers. TOF, train of four. See text for details. (Reprinted with permission from Viby-Mogensen J: Neuromuscular monitoring. In Miller R, editor: *Anesthesia,* ed 4, New York, 1995, Churchill Livingstone.)

for neuromuscular blockade, the TOF ratio remains 1.0, but the height of all four twitches is depressed according to the amount of neuromuscular blockade present (Figure 38-2).

TETANUS

Tetanic stimulation consists of a 50-Hz supramaximal stimulus applied for 5 seconds. In the absence of neuromuscular blockade, a sustained contraction is elicited. In the presence of nondepolarizing blockers, the contractile muscle force will fade depending on the degree of blockade. Succinylcholine will not produce a fade but will cause a constant but overall decreased response to tetanic stimulation.

POSTTETANIC POTENTIATION

Tetanic stimulation augments the neuromuscular response to an immediately following stimulus in the presence of nondepolarizing blockade (probably as a result of increased calcium release within the myocytes). The number of twitches recorded after a tetanic stimulus correlate with the depth of block. A posttetanic count of less than 10 (at a 1-Hz frequency) correlates with good surgical relaxation, while a count of at least 15 predicts easy reversibility of neuromuscular blockade.

DOUBLE-BURST STIMULATION

Double-burst stimulation consists of the application of three short bursts of supramaximal stimulation followed after a 750-msec pause by 2 ($DBS_{3,2}$) or 3 ($DBS_{3,3}$) additional stimuli. In the presence of nondepolarizing blockade, a fade in the second set of stimuli is appreciated. It has been shown that DBS is more sensitive in detecting residual neuromuscular blockade than TOF stimulation.

Urine Output

If the procedure is expected to take more than 3 hours, an indwelling urinary catheter should be placed for two reasons: to avoid urinary retention and bladder distension, and to monitor urine output. Urine output serves as an excellent gauge for assessment of intravascular volume. In general, if urinary output is at least 0.5 to 1 ml/kg/hr, intravascular volume and perioperative fluid administration is adequate.

MONITORING OF THE PATIENT WITH CARDIOVASCULAR DISEASE

The prevalence of cardiovascular disease in patients requiring surgical procedures is high. The spectrum is wide, ranging from patients with well-controlled hypertension without end-organ involvement to poorly controlled hypertensives with ventricular hypertrophy. Ischemic heart disease with and without preserved myocardial function is common, as are valvular diseases, cardiac conduction abnormalities, arrhythmias, and congenital cardiac defects. Again, the monitoring requirements depend on the degree of pathology and the invasiveness of the procedure. For example, a patient with stable angina undergoing a cataract extraction under local anesthesia most likely will not benefit from a pulmonary artery catheter, whereas a patient with hypertension undergoing a liver resection deserves an arterial and central venous catheter; a child undergoing repair of a complex, congenital cardiac lesion will benefit from transesophageal echocardiography (TEE). This section will discuss the principles and indications for invasive arterial, central venous and pulmonary artery–pressure monitoring, ECG monitoring for myocardial ischemia, and the indications for perioperative TEE.

Invasive Cardiovascular Pressure Monitoring

Measurement of pressure waves requires a system that converts the dynamic forces generated in the heart and distributed through the arterio-venous circulation, into an electronic signal that can be displayed on a monitor. The basic components of this kind of system are an intravascular catheter, a coupling system (i.e., tubing and stopcocks), a transducer (which converts mechanical energy into electrical energy), and a display unit. The natural frequency, (i.e., the frequency of the pressure oscillations at which the system responds with the maximum output amplitude), and the damping coefficient, (measure of the friction to oscillations within the system), determine the response of the pressure measurement system. Multiple factors, including the length and compliance of the tubing, the presence of small air bubbles within the system, and the size of the intravascular catheter used, influence these characteristics and may, therefore, interfere with the accuracy of invasive pressure monitoring.

Most transducers are based on the principle that electrical resistance changes when mechanical pressure is applied to a resistive element. The element is commonly a small silicone diaphragm with resistors engraved into it (Wheatstone's bridge). The diaphragm moves as a result of pressure of the arterial pressure waveform. This causes a change in resistance, proportional to the amount of movement, which is then electronically translated and displayed as a pressure-wave form.

Invasive arterial blood pressure (BP) monitoring is the gold standard for BP monitoring: Accurate, beat-to-beat measurement of systolic, diastolic, and calculated mean arterial pressure is the most common reason for placement of an arterial catheter. However, pressure-waveform analysis gives additional valuable information, in regard to cardiovascular performance that is often not well appreciated.

The contour of the arterial pulse form relates to myocardial contractility. A quick upstroke represents good myocardial contractility, whereas a poorly contracting heart will generate a delayed upstroke. Arrhythmias and their hemodynamic consequences are easily recognized by waveform analysis. Cyclic ventilatory changes reflect the intravascular volume status of the patient. Analysis of the systolic pressure variation (SPV), which is the difference between the maximal and minimal values of the systolic BP during one respiratory cycle, is indicative (and potentially more sensitive than central venous-pressure monitoring) of hypo- or hypervolemia. During mechanical ventilation, SPV is approximately 8 to 10 mm Hg, reflecting the effects of a positive-pressure breath on (1) decreasing venous return resulting in a decrease in preload, and (2) increasing right ventricular afterload with shifting of the ventricular septum towards the left ventricle and impeding ventricular filling. Observing SPV during a respiratory cycle, using the systolic pressure during a period of apnea as the reference value, the delta-up segment is the difference between the maximal systolic pressure and the apneic reference, while the delta-down value reflects the difference between the apneic reference and the minimum value (Figure 38-3). Delta-down values correlate well with the degree of hypovolemia; delta-up values are most prominent during hypervolemia. Myocardial contractily also influences SPV and a patient in congestive heart failure totally lose the delta-down segment with a relative prominence of the delta-up segment. It should also be kept in mind that arterial pressure tracings differ when moving distally along the arterial tree (Figure 38-4): Peripherally systolic pressures are higher, mean and diastolic pressures are lower, and the waveform displays a greater amplitude.

The radial artery is the most commonly cannulated vessel. Patients who are severely vasoconstricted (shock, cold) may have a low radial-artery pressure that does not accurately reflect the true central-aortic pressure. Cannulation of the femoral or brachial artery may be more useful and technically easier. Also, radial-arterial pressure is frequently significantly less than central-aortic pressure after cardiopulmonary bypass.

The indications for placing an arterial catheter include major surgical procedures with large fluid shifts (i.e., massive trauma, thoracic surgery, abdominal aneurysms, burns), intracranial and cardiac procedures, or operations requiring hypotensive

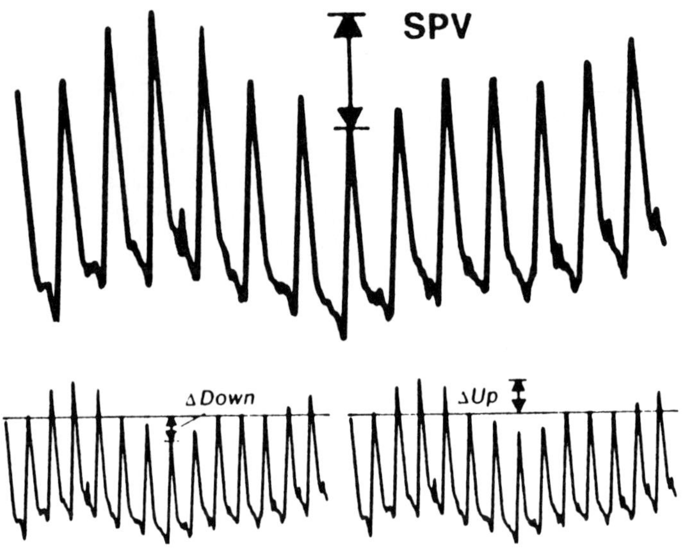

Figure 38-3
Systolic pressure wave form (SPV) variations of the arterial wave form with positive-pressure ventilation. See text for detail.

techniques. Patients with unstable cardiovascular disease, dysrhythmias, or severe pulmonary disease, as well as patients requiring frequent blood sampling or patients in whom noninvasive BP monitoring is technically impossible (i.e., morbid obesity, burns) also require invasive BP monitoring. This list is by no means inclusive.

Contraindications to placing an arterial catheter include a local infection at the insertion site, a proximal vascular obstruction, Raynaud's syndrome and severe peripheral vascular disease. A coagulopathy is only a relative contraindication, but sites where manual compression can easily be performed (in case of a hematoma formation) should be selected. Complications are rare and include infection, bleeding, thrombosis or emboli with distal ischemia, skin necrosis, hematoma, neurologic injury, and pseudoaneurysm formation.

By far, the most common reason for inserting a central venous-pressure (CVP) catheter is to guide fluid administration and to assess the patient's volume status. It has to be kept in mind, however, that the numeric value of the CVP is influenced by factors other than intravascular volume, including (1) right atrial compliance, (2) right ventricular afterload, (3) pleural pressures, and (4) peripheral venoconstriction. Since CVP monitors measure right ventricular filling pressures, they indirectly assess intravascular volume status and right cardiac performance. If left ventricular function is good and the ejection fraction is greater than 50%, CVP monitoring also will indirectly reflect left ventricular preload. Furthermore, analysis of the right atrial wave form (a, c, v waves and X, Y descents) is useful in diagnosing pathologic conditions (Figure 38-5). The a wave corresponds to atrial contraction and follows

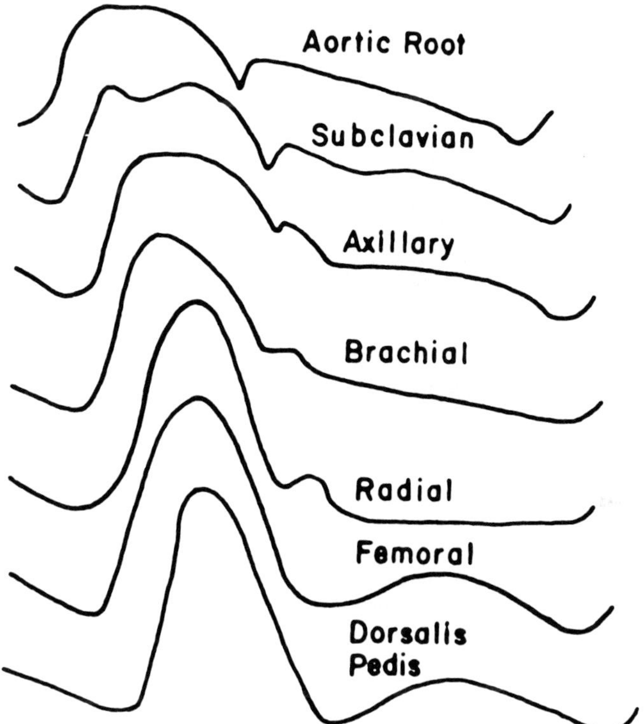

Figure 38-4
Invasive arterial blood pressure monitoring. As the arterial wave form travels distally, systolic blood pressure increases while mean pressure decreases. (Reprinted with permission from Bedford R, Shah N: Blood pressure monitoring, invasive and noninvasive. In Blitt C, Hines R, editors: *Monitoring in anesthesia and critical care medicine,* ed 3, New York, 1995, Churchill Livingstone.)

the P wave on the ECG. The c wave is produced by closure and upward movement of the tricuspid valve into the right atrium. During ventricular systole the tricuspid valve moves toward the right ventricle producing the atrial X descent. The v wave reflects passive atrial filling and the Y descent is the result of opening of the tricuspid valve and blood flow from the atrium into the ventricle. Cannon a waves are the result of atrial contraction against a closed tricuspid valve (nodal rhythm, AV dissociation). Cannon v waves can occur with tricuspid regurgitation, right ventricular failure, or a noncompliant right ventricle.

Percutaneous central venous access is established in the operating room most commonly through cannulation of the right internal jugular vein. External jugular, subclavian, femoral, and antecubital veins are other sites that lend themselves to central venous cannulation. Each site has its own advantages and disadvantages, which will not be discussed here.

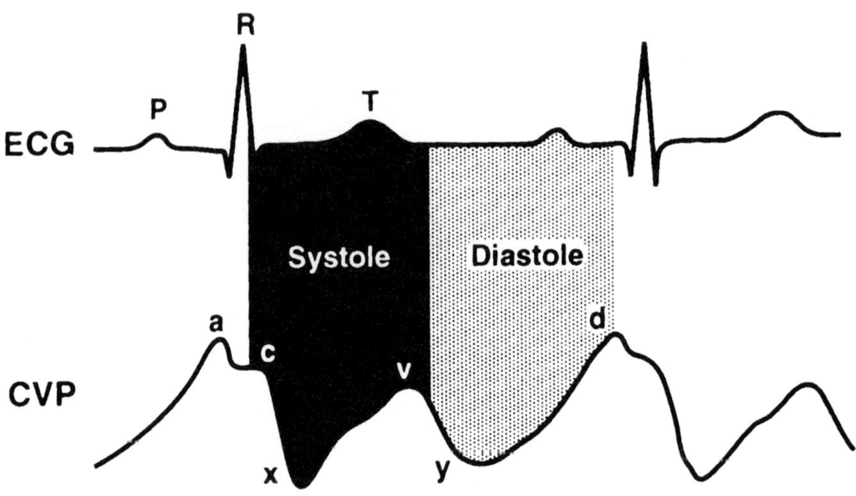

Figure 38-5
Normal CVP tracing with corresponding ECG tracing. See text for detail. (Reprinted with permission from Miller R, Stoelting RK, editors: *Basics of anesthesia,* ed 3, New York, 1995, Churchill Livingstone.)

Other than the previously mentioned, indications for establishing central venous access are the ability to administer drugs centrally and the ability to rapidly give large amounts of fluids. Surgical procedures with high risk for venous air embolism (to aspirate intracardiac air through a multi-orifice CVP catheter), patients requiring frequent blood sampling where an arterial line is not indicated or contraindicated, chronic drug administration, and inadequate peripheral access are other common reasons for placing CVP catheters.

Complications are related to accidental injury of structures adjacent to the vein that is chosen for access. They include arterial puncture with potentially life-threatening hemorrhage and hematomas (i.e., airway compromise if the carotid artery is punctured), hemothorax, pneumothorax, hydrothorax, chylothorax pericardial effusion and tamponade, embolism from entrained air or catheter fragments, and various nerve injuries (brachial plexus, stellate ganglion, phrenic nerve, femoral nerve, median nerve).

The balloon flotation pulmonary artery catheter (PAC) was introduced in 1970 and since then has been modified to become an important tool for assessing and treating critically ill patients. Modern PACs allow the measurement of other clinical parameters besides central venous, pulmonary artery (PA), and pulmonary artery occlusion pressures (PAOP). Continuous cardiac output catheters continually calculate and display cardiac output. Fiberoptic catheters display mixed venous-oxygen saturation "on line." Catheters are manufactured with pacing capabilities and sophisticated monitor electronics allow instant calculations of cardiac indices, systemic and pulmonary vascular resistance, and shunt fractions. Ideally, monitoring data derived from PACs are superior to clinical parameters in the cardiovascular assessment of a patient. A recent task force of the American Society of Anesthesiologists has concluded that the knowledge of such data may reduce the incidence of perioperative complications. However, it has been repeatedly shown that data obtained from the PAC are frequently misinterpreted and result in incorrect therapeutic decisions. The effectiveness of PACs to reduce perioperative morbidity and mortality remains largely unproved. Because the invasiveness of the procedure carries its own substantial risk, PAC monitoring can only be recommended in the critically ill patient undergoing major surgical procedures.

The principle behind the PAC catheter rests on the assumption, that when the pulmonary artery is occluded by inflating the distal balloon, the tip of the catheter measures the PAOP, which under ideal circumstances reflects left atrial pressure, left ventricular end-diastolic pressure (LVEDP), and, ultimately, left ventricular end-diastolic volume (LVEDV). In patients with reduced left ventricular function, PAOP provides a better measure of volume status than CVP. However, PAOP can wrongly over- or underestimate estimate LVEDV, as summarized in Box 38-2. Cardiac output measurements are based on thermodilution techniques and accuracy depends on technical aspects when performing the measurement, as well as certain pathologic conditions of the patient. (i.e., intracardiac shunts).

Besides assessing cardiac indices, changes in PA pressures and PAOP, PACs may also be used as monitors for cardiac ischemia. Myocardial ischemia decreases ventricular compliance which should result in increased LVEDP/PAOP. Similar to a CVP tracing for the right ventricle, the PAOP tracing can be further analyzed and subendocardial ischemia may manifest itself as V waves on the tracing. However, clinical studies found PAC pressure analysis to be unreliable and not as sensitive as noninvasive ECG ST-segment analysis as markers for cardiac ischemia.

In general, a PAC is indicated for major surgical procedures with massive fluid shifts in patients with coronary artery disease, patients with a recent myocardial infarction, unstable angina, or poor left ventricular function (with a history of congestive heart failure). Patients with multiple organ failure, massive trauma, high positive end expiratory pressure (PEEP) requirements, patients on inotropes or an intraaortic balloon pump, or patients undergoing operations that involve cross clamping of the aorta, coronary artery bypass, or liver transplantations may also

Box 38-2 Factors That Cause a Discrepancy in Pulmonary Artery Occlusion Pressure (PAOP) and Left Ventricular End Diastolic Pressure (LVEDP)

PAOP > LVEDP
- Mitral stenosis
- Left atrial myxoma
- Pulmonary venous obstruction
- Elevated pulmonary alveolar pressure

PAOP < LVEDP
- Decreased left ventricular compliance
- Aortic insufficiency

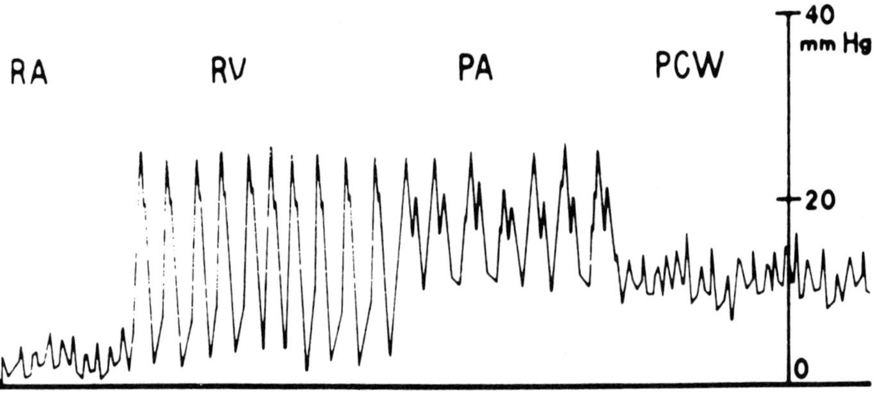

Figure 38-6
The normal pressure tracing as a pulmonary artery catheter is advanced from the right atrium (*RA*) to the right ventricle (*RV*) into the pulmonary artery (*PA*) and into the wedge position (*PCW*). (Reprinted with permission from Hines R, Barash P: Pulmonary artery catheterization. In Blitt CR, editors: *Monitoring in anesthesia and critical care medicine,* ed 3, New York, 1995, Churchill Livingstone.)

benefit from a PAC. The list of indications is not inclusive and varies within different institutions and between practitioners.

Placement of a PAC requires central venous cannulation. The right internal jugular vein or right subclavian vein are most commonly used. The PAC is advanced through an introducer, with the balloon inflated, while continuously monitoring the ECG for arrhythmias and the PAC pressure tracing for a "step-up" in the diastolic pressure, indicating PA placement (Figure 38-6). Once the catheter is in the wedge position, the balloon is deflated and return of the PA tracing verified. Permanent wedging may cause pulmonary artery rupture. Dysrhythmias are common with PAC placement, while a transient right-bundle branch block is observed less frequently.

Absolute contraindications to placing a PAC include tricuspid or pulmonic stenosis, a right atrial or ventricular mass, and tetralogy of Fallot (where it may precipitate infundibular spasms). Relative contraindications include severe dysrhythmias, a left-bundle branch block (where it may precipitate complete heart block), and newly inserted pacer wires (where wire dislodgment is possible).

Complications are either related to the central cannulation, as discussed in the section on central venous pressure (CVP) monitoring, or they are caused by the PAC itself. This includes complete heart block in patients with a preexisting left-bundle branch block, severe dysrhythmias, endobronchial hemorrhage, pulmonary infarction, catheter knotting, valvular damage, thrombus formation, thrombocytopenia, and infection. The authors are personally aware of a case of pulmonary artery rupture leading to the death of a patient. Because of the severity of such a potential complication, the risks should always be weighed against the benefits when inserting a PAC, and the patient should be made aware of such risks.

Automated ST-Segment Analysis

Most modern ECG monitors have computerized ST-segment analysis. These monitors trend and display ST-segment changes in specific leads and will facilitate the detection of ischemic ST-T wave changes. Although the various systems differ in technology, they perform the same basic functions. A baseline template is formed by sampling a number of ECG complexes. Subsequent beats are compared to the template and ST-segments are analyzed. In some systems, the current complex can be superimposed on the template for direct comparison to evaluate for significant changes. ST deviation from the isoelectric point are displayed numerically as well as trended. Any major ST-segment deviation from the baseline will cause the monitor to alarm. However, artifacts may lead to invalid conclusions, and in spite of the widespread use of ST-segment analysis, there are only limited data as to their ability to modify the outcome from perioperative ischemic events. As already mentioned, observing leads II, V4, and V5 will have the highest sensitivity in detecting myocardial ischemia. If a patient has known ischemic heart disease and cardiac catheterization data suggest specific areas of myocardium at heightened risk, the choice of leads to be monitored can be guided by their coronary anatomy.

Transesophageal Echocardiography

Transesophageal echocardiography was introduced in the perioperative care setting in the 1980s. Modern transducers and color Doppler imaging permit both surgeon and anesthesiologist to evaluate overall ventricular function, diagnose myocardial ischemia, assess valvular function, confirm the adequacy of repair of congenital cardiac lesions and diagnose traumatic injuries to the heart and great vessels. Transesophageal echocardiography is a powerful and relatively noninvasive monitor which requires expertise, often only provided by an experienced echocardiographer. Similar to misinterpretation of PAC information, the inaccurate interpretation of TEE data by inexperienced practitioners may lead to fatal therapeutic decisions. Box 38-3 summarizes the current indications for perioperative TEE in which it is most likely to improve clinical outcome. Transesophageal echocardiography is probably not indicated for uncomplicated coronary artery bypass grafting in patients with preserved ventricular function.

MONITORING OF THE PATIENT WITH PULMONARY DISEASE

Pulse oximetry and capnography provide the mainstay of respiratory monitoring. However, patients with substantial pulmonary disease or patients undergoing operations which will severely compromise pulmonary function (i.e., thoracotomies) often will benefit from additional monitors. Monitors that assess pulmonary compliance, inspiratory and expiratory flow dynamics, and direct blood gas analysis with an indwelling arterial catheter, will provide information regarding baseline pulmonary function. In addition, the effects of anesthesia, surgery, and positioning, as well as the effects of therapeutic interventions can be assessed.

Box 38-3 Indications for Perioperative Transesophageal Echocardiography

- Intraoperative evaluation of acute, persistent, and life-threatening hemodynamic disturbances in which ventricular function and its determinants are uncertain and have not responded to treatment
- Intraoperative use in valve repair
- Intraoperative use in congenital heart surgery for most lesions requiring cardiopulmonary bypass
- Intraoperative use in repair of hypertrophic obstructive cardiomyopathy
- Intraoperative use for endocarditis when preoperative testing was inadequate or extension of infection to perivalvular tissue is suspected
- Perioperative use in unstable patients with suspected thoracic aortic aneurysms, dissection, or disruption who need to be evaluated quickly
- Intraoperative assessment of aortic valve function in repair of aortic dissections with possible aortic valve involvement
- Intraoperative evaluation of pericardial window procedures
- Use in intensive care unit for unstable patients with unexplained hemodynamic disturbances, suspected valve disease, or thromboembolic problems (if other tests or monitoring techniques have not confirmed the diagnosis or patients are too unstable to undergo other tests)

Modified and reprinted with permission from The American Society of Anesthesiology, Park Ridge, IL.

Airway Pressure Monitoring

Aneuroid gauges to monitor airway pressure (Paw) are present in most anesthesia machines and give reliable qualitative information regarding peak and plateau airway pressure. Since anesthesia machines also measure delivered tidal volumes, pulmonary compliance (C), that is, the change in lung volume (VT) over the change in pulmonary pressure, can be calculated.

Dynamic compliance equals VT/peak airway pressure. Dynamic compliance decreases with endotracheal tube obstruction from a mucus plug or kink, or endobronchial movement of the endotracheal tube. Static compliance equals VT/plateau airway pressure. A decrease in static compliance is associated with an increase in small airway resistance, as in asthma or pulmonary edema. Changes in peak and plateau airway pressure will alert the anesthesiologist to changes in pulmonary compliance.

Pressure–Volume and Flow–Volume Loops

Some respiratory gas monitors have a built-in, pressure-based flow sensor and are capable of graphically displaying flow-volume and pressure-volume loops of each single breath. (Capnomac Ultima, Datex Inc., Helsinki, Finland) This monitor will allow the determination of compliance and flow resistance and will calculate such variables automatically. Figure 38-7 illustrates a flow-volume loop of a patient with a fixed large airway obstruction causing in- and expiratory flow compromise (A), with a variable extrathoracic obstruction causing inspiratory flow limitations (B), with a

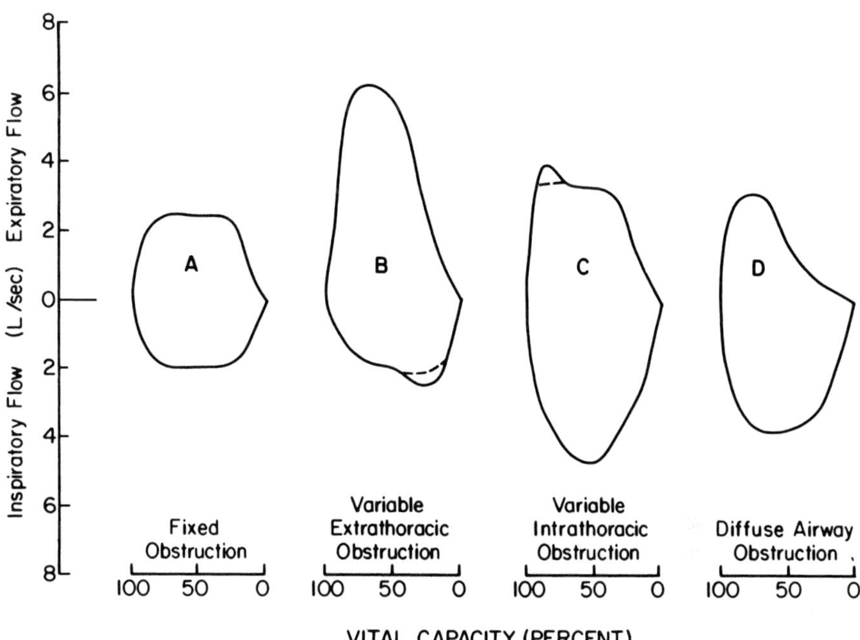

Figure 38-7
Flow-volume loops. The shape of the flow-volume loop will vary with the site of the airway obstruction. See text for detail. (Reprinted with permission from Gal TJ: Pulmonary function testing. In Miller R, editor: *Anesthesia,* ed 4, New York, 1995, Churchill Livingstone.)

variable intrathoracic obstruction and expiratory flow limitations (C), and with a flow-volume loop of a patient with diffuse airway obstruction (D). Patients undergoing surgery for lung tumors and lung transplantation are routinely monitored with this type of capnograph at the University of Virginia.

Arterial Blood Gas Analysis

The gold standard for assessing arterial oxygenation and ventilation is still arterial blood gas (ABG) analysis. Artertial blood gas monitoring is invasive and requires an indwelling arterial catheter. Transcutaneous, noninvasive monitors for PO_2 (PtO_2) and PCO_2 ($PtCO_2$) are available but are not commonly used, except in the premature infant. In the adult they are of limited accuracy, especially in patients undergoing general anesthesia. In addition, they have problems with electrode maintenance and calibration. There is also a potential for skin burns at application sites.

The placement and the potential complications associated with arterial catheters have already been discussed. A small sample of arterial blood (as little as 0.1 ml) is aspirated into a heparinized syringe (with all the air bubbles eliminated), and then immediately placed on ice and sent to the ABG analyzer. Electrodes measure PO_2, PCO_2, and pH. The HCO_3^- concentration is a calculated value.

Alternatively, continuous monitoring of PO_2, PCO_2, and pH with a small sensor that can be passed through an arterial cannula is possible. Recently developed optodes allow accurate on-line measurements of ABG values. Unlike the Clark and Severinhaus electrodes which calculate PO_2 and PCO_2 by the amount of electrical current passing through the respective polarographic cell, optodes use the phenomenon of photoluminescense quenching to calculate gas tensions and pH. Continuous ABG monitoring may facilitate rapid diagnosis and treatment of cardiorespiratory and metabolic derangements. They may be especially useful and more economic during operations in which frequent ABG analysis is necessary.

Besides the adequacy of arterial oxygenation and ventilation, additional information that can be easily derived from ABG analysis includes the alveolar-to-arterial oxygen gradient (A-a gradient) and the amount of dead space ventilation (V_D).

A-A GRADIENT

The A-a gradient is equal to P_AO_2 (alveolar oxygen tension) minus P_aO_2 (arterial oxygen tension). It is a reflection of venous admixture, and in normal individuals is between 5 to 10 mm Hg when breathing room air. This corresponds to normal right-to left-shunting through bronchial, pleural, and Thesbesian veins. To calculate the A-a gradient, alveolar oxygen tension needs to be calculated first:

$$P_AO_2 = (P_B - P_{H_2O}) \times F_IO_2 - P_aCO_2/0.8$$

P_B = barometric pressure, mm Hg

P_{H_2O} = partial pressure of water vapor, 47 mm Hg at 37°C

F_IO_2 = inspired concentration of oxygen

P_aCO_2 = arterial partial pressure of carbon dioxide, mm Hg

0.8 = respiratory quotient

If the P_aO_2 is at least 150 mm Hg, the amount of shunting can roughly be estimated to be 1% of the cardiac output for every 20 mm Hg of A-a gradient. For P_aO_2 levels below 150 mm Hg the amount of shunting will be underestimated with this formula.

DEAD SPACE VENTILATION

Under normal conditions the amount of physiologic V_D is less than 30% of the tidal volume (V_T). An increase V_D is reflected by an increase in the difference in end-tidal CO_2 (P_ECO_2) and P_aCO_2. This relationship is expressed in the following equation:

$$V_D/V_T = (P_ECO_2 - P_aCO_2)/P_aCO_2$$

ABG analysis in combination with capnography will allow for quick calculations of V_D.

• MONITORING THE PATIENT WITH SPECIFIC NEUROLOGIC DISEASE

Patients undergoing intra- and extracranial vascular procedures (i.e., aneurysm clipping, resections of an arteriovenous malformation [AVM], carotid endarterectomy), craniotomies for tumor removal, or extensive surgery around the spinal cord are at heightened risk for perioperative central nervous system (CNS) ischemia. Ideally, the goal of neuroanesthesia monitoring is to assess the adequacy of oxygen delivery to the neurons at risk. Today, this can only be done indirectly by assessing global or regional cerebral blood flow (CBF) and oxygenation, and by monitoring the functional integrity of specific neuronal pathways.

Intracranial Pressure Monitoring

Increased intracranial pressure (ICP) may cause cerebral ischemia since it lowers cerebral perfusion pressure (CPP, which equals the difference between mean arterial pressure and ICP.) An increase in ICP may also precipitate cerebral herniation and cerebral edema. Increased ICP is defined as sustained elevations of ICP over 15 mm Hg. Besides the absolute value derived from the ICP monitor, different types of waveforms can be diagnosed and are associated with characteristic events:

A-waves: sustained waves (6–10 mm Hg), every 5 to 20 minutes. Life-threatening, representing cerebral vasodilation secondary to decreased CPP.

B-waves: small, brief waves (10–20 mm Hg), every 30 to 120 seconds. Because of fluctuations in cerebral blood volume in patients with poor cerebral compliance.

C-waves: small oscillations (0–10 mm Hg), reflecting changes in systemic arterial pressure.

Intracranial pressure monitoring is routinely used in patients in the neurointensive care unit who are at risk for increased ICP. Commonly, ICP monitors are placed just before skin closure in the neurosurgical patient, prone to develop postoperative cerebral edema, to guide and facilitate care. At our institution, intraoperative ICP monitoring is reserved only for patients who are at extreme risk for ICP increases during the surgical procedure (i.e., patients with hepatic encephalopathy undergoing liver transplantation) or who present to the operating room with an ICP monitor in place. (i.e., head trauma patients.)

Intracranial pressure monitors are placed either in the cranium or in the lumbar subarachnoid space, measuring lumbar cerebrospinal fluid pressure (CSFP). Lumbar CSFP assumes a free communication between spinal and intracranial CSF. With obstructive hydrocephalus, for example, CSFP will not reflect ICP. Figure 38-8 illustrates monitors placed at the skull, which include epidural transducers, ventriculostomies, subdural bolts, and subdural/intraparenchymal catheters.

CNS Ischemia Monitoring

Carotid endarterectomy is a classic example of how a neurosurgical procedure is directly responsible for potentially causing severe limitations in CBF. When the internal carotid artery is clamped, blood flow to the respective cerebral hemisphere depends entirely on collateral flow, primarily through the circle of Willis.

ELECTROENCEPHALOGRAPHY

Computerized electroencephalogram (EEG) monitoring system which analyze and display data in a variety of forms (power spectrum analysis, compressed spectral array, aperiodic analysis, bispectral analysis) are electrophysiologic monitors of cerebral

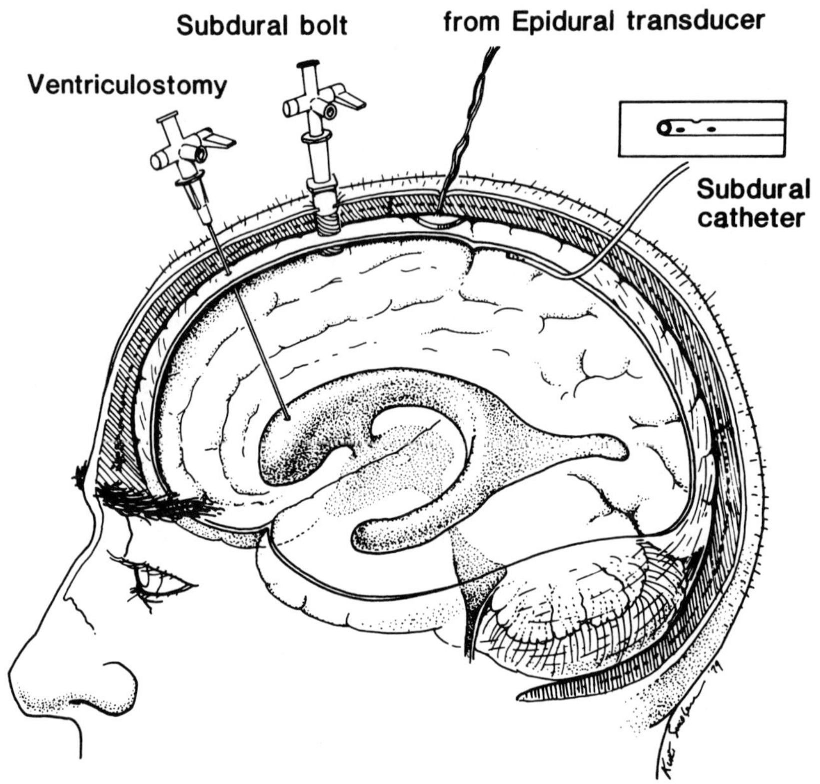

Figure 38-8
Various monitoring devices to monitor intracranial pressure. (Reprinted with permission from Shapiro H, Drummond J: Neurosurgical anesthesia. In Miller RD, editor: *Anesthesia,* ed 4, New York, 1995, Churchill Livingstone.)

ischemia. Changes in frequency and amplitude, and the development of interhemispheric assymetry of the EEG are predictive of ischemic changes. However, a multitude of other factors affect the EEG and its sensitivity and specificity as an ischemia monitor; thus, its value is questionable. For example, a decrease in amplitude and frequency, which can accompany cerebral ischemia, is also seen with commonly used anesthetic agents.

SENSORY EVOKED POTENTIAL (SEP) MONITORING

A SEP is the response of the CNS to a peripherally applied stimulus and, therefore, reflects the integrity of a neuronal pathway. A peripheral nerve is stimulated and electrodes along the sensory pathway record the CNS response up to the sensory cortex.

Somatosensory EPs (SSEP), brain stem auditory EPs (BAEP), and visual EPs are used to monitor the integrity of the posterior column/sensory pathway, and cranial nerve VII and II, respectively. As with EEG, their statistical power is far from perfect and anesthetic agents alter the response. Extensive spine surgery (i.e., Harrington rod placement) is often monitored with SSEP.

Motor evoked potentials (MEPs) are infrequently used to assess the integrity of the motor pathway. They are even more affected than SEPs by parameters that do not reflect CNS ischemia. Like EEG and EPs, MEPs are electrophysiologic monitors of ischemia.

TRANSCRANIAL DOPPLER (TCD) MONITORING

TCD measures CBF velocity (cm/sec) by isolation of the middle cerebral artery. It has been shown to be useful in the detection of vasospasm after subarachnoid hemorrhage, as a monitor during carotid endarterectomy, and for the diagnosis of brain death. It can also detect cerebral emboli.

JUGULAR VENOUS OXYGEN SATURATION ($SJVO_2$)

$SjVO_2$ monitors are percutaneously inserted through the internal jugular vein into the jugular venous bulb. Oximetric technology allows continuous monitoring of cerebral venous oxygen saturation. Normal $SjVO_2$ values are 60% to 70%. A decrease in venous saturation correlates with increased brain oxygen extraction in the presence of decreased oxygen supply. However, since the jugular venous blood represents global hemispheric blood flow, $SjVO_2$ cannot predict the adequacy of regional CBF.

CEREBRAL OXIMETRY AND NEAR INFRARED SPECTROSCOPY

Monitors using optical spectroscopy, applied noninvasively over brain regions at risk for ischemia, are available to predict regional CBF and cellular ischemia. Similar to pulse oximetry, these monitors can detect oxyhemoglobin and the redox state of mitochondrial cytochrome a, a3 in the neuronal cell population. A decrease in the oxydative state of cytochrome a, a3 correlates with cellular ischemia. More experience with this kind of monitor is needed, before its routine use can be advocated. However, its noninvasive technology and selectivity for small regions within the CNS make it a potentially attractive monitor for cerebral ischemia.

Monitors for Venous Air Embolism

Venous air embolism (VAE) is a well-known complication of craniotomies performed in the sitting position and, if large, may cause fatal cardiovascular collapse. Precordial doppler ultrasonography is the most practical VAE monitor and should be used during all sitting craniotomies. A doppler probe placed over the right second intercostal space can detect amounts as small as 0.25 ml of entrained air. Expired gas analysis is also a sensitive monitor. A decrease in end-tidal CO_2 with a concomitant increase in nitrogen is a characteristic finding of a VAE. Echocardiography is probably the most sensitive of all VAE monitors and the only monitor that will detect paradoxic emboli. However, echocardiography requires special training, is expensive, and currently requires constant visual attention to detect intracardiac air.

• SUMMARY

Perioperative care of the patient with and without coexisting medical problems involves monitoring of physiologic parameters to assess the patient's responses and to guide further medical interventions. Basic monitoring standards have been developed by the American Society of Anesthesiologists, which should be followed whenever anesthesia care is assumed. Despite the multitude of monitoring technology available, it should be stressed that monitors themselves do not cure patients. Even the most accurate monitor is only as good as the physician who knows how to interpret the derived data and who makes the appropriate therapeutic decisions.

BIBLIOGRAPHY

Blitt, CD, Hines, RL, editors: *Monitoring in anesthesia and critical care medicine*, ed 3, New York 1995, Churchill Livingstone.

Dorsch, JA, Dorsch, SE: *Understanding anesthesia equipment*, ed 3, Baltimore, 1993, Williams & Wilkins.

Lake CL, editor: *Clinical monitoring for anesthesia and critical care*, ed 2, Philadelphia, 1994, WB Saunders.

Royston D, Feeley TW, editors: Monitoring in anesthesiology: current standards and newer techniques, *Int Anesthesiol Clin* (Nr 3). Boston, 1993, Little Brown.

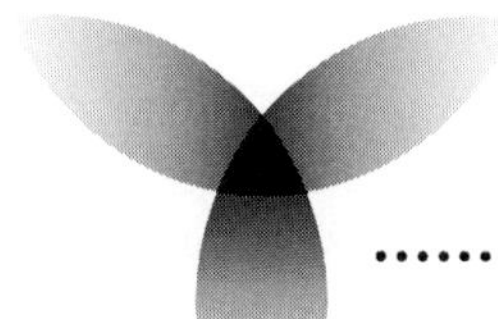

Chapter 39

General Anesthesia

Burkhard F. Spiekermann, MD

It is impossible to discuss all aspects associated with the perioperative care of the patient undergoing a surgical procedure under general anesthesia (GA) in one book chapter. Following a brief discussion defining the term and describing the theories regarding the mechanism of GA, this section will primarily focus on the major intra- and postoperative physiologic alterations and complications associated with it. Many of the principles touched upon are covered in more depth in other relevant chapters, and no attempt is made to discuss the technical aspects surrounding the administration of GA.

DEFINITION

General anesthesia, as the patient understands it, is "getting put to sleep." However, the actual state of anesthesia is certainly distinct from the "sleep" the patient experiences under GA. General anesthesia is better defined as a state of a "carefully induced reversible coma," producing immobility to noxious stimuli, hypnosis (loss of consciousness), amnesia (absence of recall), and analgesia (reduced or loss of pain perception). In clinical practice this is accomplished with a variety of drugs, most commonly a combination of inhaled and intravenous anesthetics ("balanced anesthesia"). As of yet, there is no direct monitor that allows us to assess the depth of anesthesia and the anesthesiologist has to primarily rely on observing quantifiable patient parameters such as blood pressure, heart rate, pattern of respiration, and patient movement. Different electrophysiologic monitoring techniques have been evaluated in their capacities to monitor anesthetic depth (as discussed in the chapter on monitoring) with widely variable results. The fact that anesthetic depth is difficult to measure objectively, and the fact that the anesthesiologist uses a diverse group of anesthetic drugs with different mechanisms of action (that are only partly understood), constitutes a large part of the problem defining the term *GA*.

THEORIES OF ANESTHESIA

For a long a time a "unitary theory" of anesthesia was favored by most researchers, that is, a common pathway of action of all anesthetic agents (inhalational and intravenous) to produce the anesthetic state. The addition of new classes of anesthetic agents and recent investigations have challenged this view. Currently, it is more likely that different classes of anesthetic agents act at different sites to produce different neuropharmacologic events. The effects may be combined to work in an additive or synergistic fashion to generate clinical anesthesia.

Inhalational Anesthesia

Classically, the term *GA* was synonymous with the term *inhalational anesthesia*. Most older theories on the mechanisms and actions of anesthetics are, therefore, related to inhalational anesthetics. Because all inhalational anesthetics are lipid-soluble, the focus of research early on was on the lipid bilayer of the cell membrane as the target of anesthetic action. Near the year 1900 Meyer and Overton suggested that anesthetic potency is directly related to lipid solubility ("Mayer-Overton rule"). The "critical volume hypothesis" proposes that a defined number of anesthetic molecules need to be disolved within the lipid membrane of neuronal cells, altering their normal function, before anesthesia is induced. In the most simple terms, the minimum alveolar concentration (MAC, which is the concentration of anesthetic gas in the alveoli at which 50% of the patients will not move on skin incision), at a steady-state level (i.e., after equilibration of the anesthetic gas between alveolus, blood, and tissue), would reflect the amount of anesthetic gas dissolved in the neuronal membrane within the central nervous system (CNS), which is equal to this "critical volume." Although the concept was appealing, many experimental data disagree with both the Meyer-Overtone rule and the critical volume hypothesis. It is far from certain whether the lipid bilayer is the sole site of action, or whether specific receptor proteins are mediating anesthetic action. It also appears that amnesia is produced by a different mechanism at a different site within the CNS than the suppression of movement to noxious stimuli (i.e., the definition of MAC). Current theories suggest that inhalational anesthetics may produce hypnosis and amnesia through interactions through a $GABA_A$ receptor-mediated pathway in the hippocampus (similar to the actions of benzodiazepines and barbiturates), whereas the inhibition of movement and, possibly, analgesic effects may be mediated by inhibition of excitatory synaptic transmisson of spinal-cord neurons.

Intravenous Anesthesia

A diverse group of intravenous (IV) anesthetic agents all seem to have a common feature that may explain their anesthetic action. Many aspects of the anesthetic properties of IV anesthetics appear to result from enhancement of the inhibitory action of the GABA receptor on neuronal transmission within the CNS. These include the short-acting barbiturates (thiopental, methohexital), benzodiazepines (midazolam), etomidate, propofol, and the steroid anesthetics alphalaxalone and pregnanalone. The phencyclidine derivative ketamine is a notable exception.

Except for ketamine, IV anesthetic agents do not have analgesic effects and opioids are typically administered in conjunction with these agents to prevent either voluntary movement or cardiovascular responses to profoundly painful stimuli.

In summary, it appears that, even though the exact mechanism and site of action most likely is different for various anesthetic agents and for the various aspects that constitute clinical anesthesia, the underlying principle of all anesthetics is that they cause a disruption of normal synaptic communication between neuronal cells within the CNS.

• WHEN TO USE GENERAL ANESTHESIA

It is not uncommon that a patient will say during the preoperative visit, "My doctor told me that I am too sick to go to sleep," or that a consultant will write in the patient record "patient cleared for surgery under spinal." There is a common misconception among nonanesthetists that GA is not as safe as alternative techniques of anesthetic care, that is, regional anesthesia or monitored anesthesia care (MAC). However, there are no clearly supportive data that suggest that the choice of anesthetic technique affects overall morbidity and mortality. Outcome is determined by how a specific technique is implemented. Certain operations can only be performed under GA (sometimes in combination with regional anesthesia). Examples include most thoracic procedures, cardiac, and intracranial operations. Besides the constraints related to the operation, the next variable that should determine which technique is chosen is the preference of the patient (once surgical requirements and alternative anesthetic techniques with their possible risks and benefits have been explained to him/her.) The preference of the surgical team as to the anesthetic technique should also be considered, if possible. A factor that comes to no surprise is that the patient will receive better care if the anesthesiologist is using an anesthetic technique with which he/she is familiar and comfortable. Avoiding GA because the "patient is too sick" in favor of a complicated regional technique that the anesthesiologist has only read about will not improve patient care.

There are, however, situations in which the avoidance of GA is advantageous. For example, regional anesthesia may be preferred over GA in a patient with a full stomach or a difficult airway if it can be performed in a safe way. Outpatient surgery that lends itself to MAC or peripheral nerve blocks (i.e., carpal tunnel release, opthalmologic procedures) usually is associated with a shorter recovery-room stay and faster discharge. Whatever the final decision regarding the anesthetic plan may be, this plan should be mutually agreed upon by the patient and the anesthesiologist. "Talking a patient into" an anesthetic technique that he or she does not want is never appropriate.

PREOPERATIVE EVALUATION

The preoperative evaluation serves at least two important functions. First, allows the anesthesiologist to gather all the information necessary through a goal-oriented history and physical examination to formulate an anesthetic plan. Second, just as importantly, it allows the patient to ask any questions related to his/her perioperative care and to hopefully alleviate anxieties and fears regarding the pending operation. Studies have documented that an appropriately informative preoperative visit by an anesthetist is more effective than pharmacologic measures to alleviate the fear and anxiety patients experience before an operation. In addition, premedications or specific consultations may be ordered during a preoperative visit, if necessary. As mentioned, the preoperative evaluation should be goal-oriented. A chart review will reveal pertinent information, especially if the patient has had previous operations and the anesthetic records are available. The history and physical examination should focus on a review of major organ systems, since the anesthetic plan will be influenced by the patient's cardiopulmonary and other organ function, and since GA and surgery have a potentially negative impact on already compromised organ function. The goal of such a review is to assess the overall physiologic reserve of the patient. This reserve will determine the anesthetic plan and the drugs selected to induce and maintain GA. For example, a patient with poor ventricular function and an ejection fraction of 20% will not tolerate the cardiac depressant effects of inhalational anesthetics. Thus, the anesthetist may chose a primarily narcotic-based anesthetic technique. Conversely, a patient with a history of severe asthma may benefit from the bronchodilator effects of inhalational anesthetic agents.

Perhaps unique to an anesthetic preoperative examination, as compared to the preperative assessment by other medical teams, is the focus on examination of the airway. The ability to open the mouth, neck mobility, and other anatomic features related to the oropharynx, will impact on airway management plans and endotracheal intubation, as discussed in Chapter 37. Box 39-1 summarizes a general outline of a goal-oriented preoperative visit.

At the end of the preoperative assessment, it is costumary, that the anesthesiologist classifies the patient within the "American Society of Anesthesiologists (ASA) Physical Status Classification." (Table 39-1). The American Society of Anesthesiologists developed this five-category classification to facilitate statistic analysis of outcome data within one hospital and between different institutions. The ASA physical status

Box 39-1 Outline for a Goal Oriented Preoperative Visit

1. What are the problems that brought you to the hospital, and why do you need surgery?
2. Have you previously been under the care of a physician, or are you currently seeing a physician for other unrelated medical problems?
3. Previous operations/anesthetics and potential problems associated with such?
4. Family history of anesthesia-related complications?
5. Current medications?
6. History of allergic reactions?
7. Tobacco, alcohol, or other drug use?
8. How far can you walk; what makes you stop?
9. Review of organ systems:
   cardiovascular
   pulmonary
   CNS
   hepatorenal
   musculoskeletal
   endocrine
   coagulation
10. Physical examination:
    vital signs and weight
    airway
    cardiopulmonary
    gross neurologic exam

assignment also provides the anesthesiologist with a quick summary of the patient's overall physical condition. Even though there is a correlation between the ASA physical status and perioperative morbidity and mortality, the ASA physical status was not designed as a tool for patient risk stratification and should not be used as such. Patients who are ASA physical-status I and II are not immune from anesthetic-related deaths!

• INTRAOPERATIVE COURSE

In the adult patient, anesthetic induction is most commonly performed intravenously. The short-acting barbiturate thiopental is largely replaced by propofol for the routine IV induction. Propofol has a faster recovery profile, may potentially have an antiemetic action, and, possibly, has less of a myocardial depressant effect than thiopental. Other IV induction agents may be selected for specific clinical situations as discussed in Chapter 26.

After induction, anesthesia is usually maintained using a combination of IV anesthetic agents (primarily narcotic or hypnotic agents like morphine, fentanyl, sufentanil, propofol, benzodiazepines), a potent, inhaled anesthetics (which is delivered through an agent-specific, calibrated, and easily controllable vaporizer) with nitrous

Table 39-1. The ASA Physical Status Classification

STATUS	DESCRIPTION
Class 1	Healthy patient.
Class 2	Mild-to-moderate systemic disease.
Class 3	Severe, but not incapacitating, systemic disease.
Class 4	Severe, life-threatening systemic disease.
Class 5	Moribund patient who is not expected to live longer than 24 hours with or without surgery.
Emergency (E)	Any patient who needs an emergency operation. E is added to the ASA status classification.

oxide (N_2O) and neuromuscular-blocking drugs. The goal of this "balanced anesthetic technique" is to (1) meet the criteria of general anesthesia as defined earlier, (2) modify the stress response to surgery and provide hemodynamic stability, (3) modify hemodynamic parameters as required for specific surgical procedures, (4) select specific drugs to minimize the negative impact anesthetic agents may have on compromised organ systems, and (5) titrate drugs to facilitate a safe emergence and a smooth transition to postoperative recovery. Since most of those goals vary for different operations and different patients, a thorough knowledge of pharmacokinetic and pharmacodynamic principles and side-effect profiles of the many drugs used by the anesthesiologist is mandatory. Only if the physiologic changes associated with the administration of GA are appreciated, is it possible to tailor an anesthetic to the specific needs of the patient and the operation. Anticipation of the change of intensity of the surgical stimulus throughout the anesthetic course is imperative, so one can adjust the depth of anesthesia to meet the anesthetic goals. As already mentioned, the many anesthetic agents, when used in the hands of a skillful anesthesiologist, makes GA generally a safe anesthetic option, even in the sickest patient.

Providing a smooth emergence from a general anesthetic is a "skill" that requires sound knowledge of the pharmacology of the anesthetic agents used, in addition to an ability to predict how certain patients will behave. This skill develops with practice and experience. The principle goal of the immediate emergence phase is to have the patient recovered from GA with regard to his/her overall physiologic functions. Other goals are (1) recovery of protective airway reflexes, (2) permitting extubation of the trachea if an endotracheal tube was used, and (3) restoration of normal hemodynamic parameters. The challenge for the anesthesiologist is to allow recovery as fast as possible without compromising operating conditions during the last minutes of surgery and without denying the patient an adequate amount of pain medication for the immediate postoperative period. Recovery from inhalational anesthetics is primarily a function of the blood and lipid solubility of the anesthetic gas chosen, the patient's cardiac output, the effective alveolar ventilation, and the fresh gas flow of the anesthesia circuit. "MAC awake," the minimum alveolar concentration at which 50% of patients respond to a verbal stimulus, is approximately 30% of MAC. Intravenous anesthetic recovery is related to the drug's half-life and clearance. Neuromuscular blockade needs to be fully reversed before extubation. This can be documented with a peripheral nerve stimulator or, in the responsive patient, with the patient's ability to lift his/her head against gravity for at least 5 seconds. Provisions should be made early during recovery to facilitate a safe transfer to the postanesthesia care unit (PACU). This includes a transport stretcher with an oxygen delivery system and a transportable monitoring device. Most newer hospitals have interchangeable modular monitors that allow continuous cardiopulmonary monitoring from the operating room to the PACU. This especially facilitates transport of sick patients in whom even short periods of absent monioring may be detrimental.

INTRAOPERATIVE PHYSIOLOGIC CHANGES AND COMPLICATIONS DURING GA

GA affects every organ system, either because of the direct pharmacologic action of the particular anesthetic agents, as a result of the hemodynamic alterations associated with GA, or as a result of a combination of both factors. I will limit my comments mostly to physiologic alterations seen in the healthy patient, since more specific information regarding the effects of GA on patients with organ dysfunction is also discussed in other chapters in this book.

Cardiovascular Changes and Complications

General anesthetics cause cardiovascular alterations secondary to their direct and indirect action on arteriolar and venous vascular tone, their effects on myocardial contractility, on myocardial innervation (through alterations of the autonomic nervous system), and on the cardiac conduction system. The magnitude of these effects depends on the patient's underlying intrinsic or pharmacologically altered sympathetic tone, and are potentiated in the patient with cardiovascular disease (i.e., ischemic or valvular heart disease or hypertension), the patient on medication affecting the cardiovascular system (i.e., β-blockers, calcium channel blockers), and the hypovolemic patient. They are also potentiated by the effects of positive-pressure ventilation (i.e., decreased venous return) and intraoperative patient positioning (i.e., Trendelenburg, reverse Trendelenburg, prone, lithotomy, lateral, sitting).

INHALATIONAL ANESTHETICS

All inhalational anesthetics (N_2O, halothane, enflurane, isoflurane, sevoflurane, desflurane) are myocardial depressants and produce a dose-dependent reduction in cardiac output and stroke volume. Of the potent anesthetics, enflurane and halothane cause the greatest depression of stroke volume; it is possible to cause cardiovascular collapse with high concentrations of these vapors, easily. Except for N_2O, all inhalational anesthetics will cause a dose-dependent decrease in arterial blood pressure, either because of decreased myocardial contractility (halothane) or peripheral vasodilation with a decrease in systemic vascular resistance (isoflurane) or both (enflurane). The heart rate is unchanged by halothane, minimally increased by N_2O, but tachycardia may be associated with isoflurane, sevoflurane, and desflurane (in the last especially, if the dose is rapidly increased). An overdose of inhalational anesthetics may be associated with severe bradycardia. Halothane is arrhythmogenic because it sensitizes the myocardium to intrinsic and extrinsic catecholamines. Therefore, ventricular tachyarrythmias may be more common than with other inhalational anesthetic agents. Isoflurane is a coronary vasodilator and has been implicated in causing coronary steal precipitating myocardial ischemia in patients with steal-prone coronary anatomy. However, most recent studies refute this concept. For all the reasons discussed, inhalational anesthesia is generally avoided as the sole anesthetic agent in patients with poor cardiac reserve and GA is maintained with IV anesthetics, with or without a low concentration of volatile agents.

IV ANESTHETICS

Intravenous agents most commonly used for the maintainance of anesthesia include propofol and opiods. Less commonly, barbiturates (thiopental), ketamine, benzodiazepines or etomidate may be used. Propofol may cause arterial hypotension because of arterial and venous vasodilitation; also, it has a mild, direct-negative inotropic effect. Bolus injections compare less favorably to a continuous infusion in this regard. High-dose opioids are frequently used as the sole anesthetic in patients with poor cardiac function because of their negligable effects on the cardiovascular system. Bradycardia is common with rapid administration of high doses; large bolus doses of morphine may cause hypotension secondary to histamine release. Thiopental reduces arterial and venous tone and is a myocardial depressant. Hypotension may develop from a decrease in preload, myocardial depression, and a decrease in systemic vascular resistance (SVR). Compensatory tachycardia usually occurs. Ketamine interferes with the reuptake of catecholamines and will cause an increase in heart rate, blood pressure, and SVR. However, it has a direct, negative-inotropic effect on the myocardium. Midazolam, a short-acting benzodiazepine, produces only small hemodynamic effects if given alone in low doses. Its principal effect is related to a small decrease in SVR which translates into a clinically insignificant decrease in arterial blood pressure. When combined with narcotics it may cause a more profound decrease in sympathetic tone and SVR. Etomidate has a neutral cardiovascular profile, and may be desirable in the patient with poor cardiac reserve. Its inhibitory effect on steroidegenesis may contraindicate a continuous infusion.

Respiratory Changes and Complications

All anesthetic agents produce a dose-dependent depressant effect on ventilation. Respiratory function is also compromised during GA because of altered pulmonary mechanics which are introduced with the use of anesthetics, neuromuscular blockers, surgical positioning of the patient, and the site of surgery itself (i.e., the use of retractors, or abdominal or thoracic incisions). For example, the functional residual capacity (FRC) may decrease by 15% to 20% just with induction of GA. This is discussed in more detail in other chapters. Mucociliary clearance is decreased significantly during and after GA, because of a direct drug effect and because of the dryness and coldness of the gas mixture inhaled. In addition to the patient's underlying baseline pulmonary function, other variables which compound the effects of GA are duration of surgery greater than 2 to 3 hours, advanced age, obesity, and a history of smoking. Complications that may contribute to impaired respiratory function with GA include upper airway obstruction and/or laryngospasm, secondary to premature extubation, bronchospasm, cardiogenic and noncardiogenic pulmonary edema, aspiration pneumonitis, or pulmonary emboli. Many of the respiratory alterations persist into the recovery period (as discussed in Chapter B.2) and necessitate attention to prevent more serious complications from prolonged hypoxia and hypercarbia. Before a patient is scheduled for surgery, especially under GA, all reversible factors that may worsen pulmonary function should be addressed. This includes treatment of pulmonary infections, reversible elements of bronchospasm, and the negative effects of smoking.

INHALATIONAL ANESTHETICS

The depressant effects of all the inhalational anesthetics on ventilation is dose-dependent. They are related to the depressant effect on the medullary respiratory center and, perhaps, to a smaller degree, on the diaphragmatic and intercostal musculature. Inhalational anesthetics generate a respiratory pattern consisting of a rapid, respiratory rate and small tidal volumes with an overall decrease in minute ventilation. This results in an increase in $PaCO_2$, which is most prominent with the administration of enflurane (approximately 60 mm Hg at 1 MAC enflurane). Inhalational anesthetics also attenuate the ventilatory response to carbon dioxide (which in the healthy awake patient is an increase in minute ventilation of 1 to 3 l/min for every mm Hg increase in $PaCO_2$) and, at 1 MAC concentration, abolish the hypoxic ventilatory response. Surgical stimulation counteracts some of these effects, but the respiratory depressant effects may necessitate controlled positive-pressure ventilation in the patient with underlying pulmonary disease or in the patient who does not tolerate even a small increase in $PaCO_2$. Hypoxic pulmonary vasoconstriction, the protective reflex that attempts to maintain V/Q matching in response to alveolar hypoxia, is inhibited by all inhalational anesthetics. However, a number of studies have suggested that this property is of no significant clinical consequence. A desirable property of an inhalational anesthetic agent is its bronchodilator effect. Some clinicians believe (although scientific data are lacking) that the use of inhalational anesthetics may be preferred over predominantly IV anesthetic agents in the patient with reactive airway disease.

IV ANESTHETICS

All IV anesthetic agents depress the central ventilatory regulatory mechanism and, at higher doses, will cause apnea. Ketamine at low concentration has classically been thought to cause only modest or no ventilatory depression. However, ketamine will not guarantee adequate air exchange during anesthesia, especially if used at higher doses or in combination with other drugs. In addition to the effects on the respiratory control center, large doses of the synthetic opiods (fentanyl, sufentanil), because they are commonly used for induction and anesthetic maintainance during cardiac surgery, may cause chestwall muscle rigidity in the absence of neuromuscular blockade, which may make mask ventilation difficult or impossible. Most clinicians pretreat with an adequate dose of a neuromuscular blocker before the administration of large doses of fentanyl or sufentanil.

In summary, GA and surgery affect the respiratory system at many levels, and many of the effects seen persist into the postoperative period. Hypercarbia will undoubtedly develop in the spontaneously ventilating patient under GA and controlled ventilation needs to be instituted if normocarbia or hypocarbia is desired. In the healthy patient, intraoperative hypoxemia during spontaneous ventilation is prevented by increasing the inspired FIO_2; it usually will not occur. Today, intra- and postoperative respiratory monitoring in the form of pulse oximetry and capnometry are considered the standard of care. By providing early indicators of dysfunction, they have decreased the incidence of perioperative morbidity from adverse respiratory events.

Hepatic Changes and Complications

Even in healthy patients without preexisting liver disease, perioperative hepatic dysfunction after GA does occur. This may be as a result of the direct effects of anesthetic agents on hepatocytes, secondary to the hemodynamic effects of anesthetics that may alter hepatic blood flow and, probably most importantly, secondary to the direct surgical effects on hepatic perfusion and hepatocyte injury. Postoperative hepatic dysfunction is more common if the surgical site is close to the liver, possibly because of decreased blood flow from retractor pressure and visceral manipulation. Generally, perioperative hepatic dysfunction in the healthy patient is mild and of little clinical significance, often only detected with laboratory tests. Concerns related to the patient with preexisting liver disease are discussed in Chapter 21.

INHALATIONAL ANESTHETICS

All potent inhalational anesthetics decrease portal venous hepatic blood flow and, except for isoflurane and sevoflurane, also decrease hepatic artery flow. However, unless excessive hypotension ensues, oxygen delivery to hepatocytes is not compromised. In addition, inhalational anesthetics decrease the hepatic oxygen requirement, therefore, maintaining a favorable supply and demand ratio. Direct hepatocellular toxicity from inhalational anesthetics was first described with halothane. This so-called "halothane hepatitis" is an immune-mediated process, where one of the halothane metabolites (trifluoroacetate) acts as a hapten when bound to hepatocytes, triggering an autoimmune response that may cause fulminant hepatic failure. Halothane hepatitis is rare (1 in 35,000 halothane anesthetics) and is seen more commonly in obese women in their 40s with previous exposure to halothane. Such immunologically triggered hepatitis has since been described with every potent inhalational anesthetic, although with even lower incidence. The avoidance of halothane, in favor of another potent vapor in a patient with a suspected history of halothane hepatitis, will decrease but not eliminate the potential problem, because trifluoroacetate is a metabolic by-product of all inhalational anesthetics; even a small concentration of trifluoroacetate may initiate an immulogic response. Nitrous oxide does not seem to be associated with hepatic toxicity.

IV ANESTHETICS

Intravenous anesthetic agents seem to have little effect on perioperative hepatic function. Opioids can precipitate sphincter of Oddi spasm in 3% of patients, which is of theoretical concern during biliary surgery. Intravenous naloxone or glucagon readily reverse these effects and the routine avoidance of narcotics for hepatobiliary surgery is not indicated.

In summary, transient postoperative hepatic dysfunction is relatively common, but seems to be related more to the type of surgery than to GA. Hepatic complications directly related to GA are rare and should be a diagnosis of exclusion.

Renal Changes and Complications

Anesthetic affect renal function either directly, through alterations in renal vascular tone and glomerular filtration rate or direct toxic effects, or indirectly through their effect on cardiovascular parameters (i.e., decreased cardiac output causing decreased renal perfusion). All inhalational anesthetics, when metabolized, will release inorganic fluoride, which may cause dose-dependent tubular nephrotoxicity manifested by an inability to concentrate urine. Since all agents used today are scarcely metabolized, this is not clinically significant. A theoretical exception may be sevoflurane. (In addition to hepatic metabolism, sevoflurane is also degraded in carbon dioxide absorbers to nephrotoxic byproducts.) Therefore, the use of sevoflurane in patients with preexisting renal disease is probably not indicated. As with perioperative liver dysfunction, surgical factors, blood transfusions, and other nonanesthesia-related conditions predominantly will influence perioperative renal function. Unless GA causes prolonged periods of hypotension with poor renal perfusion, postoperative renal dysfunction in the healthy patient secondary to GA is rare.

Central Nervous System Changes and Complications

General anesthesia implies an alteration in mental status and as such, GA produces a profound reversible change in mental function. In addition, anesthetics affect cerebral blood flow (CBF), cerebral oxygen consumption ($CMRO_2$), and cerebrospinal fluid dynamics. An altered mental state after GA is common in the immediate postoperative period, especially in the elderly population. It is argued by some that regional anesthesia in the elderly avoids this potential problem, presuming that perioperative sedation is minimal. Prolonged mental status changes after GA, however, should not be attributed to the effects of anesthesia, unless other etiologies have been thoroughly ruled out.

INHALATIONAL ANESTHETICS

All inhalational anesthetics decrease $CMRO_2$ to a variable extent, while CBF is increased because of their direct cerebral vasodilator effects. Since in the awake patient, CBF is coupled to $CMRO_2$, inhalational agents are said to be "uncouplers." In patients with poor intracranial compliance, this increase in CBF may cause an unacceptable rise in intracanial pressure (ICP).

IV ANESTHETICS

With the exception of ketamine (a direct cerebral vasodilator), all IV anesthetic agents cause a decrease in CBF and $CMRO_2$. For this reason thiopental, propofol, or etomidate infusions may be used (instead of inhalational anesthesics) in patients with increased ICP.

Endocrine Changes and Complications

General anesthesia in itself does not produce significant effects on hormone secretion. However, surgery will induce a "fight or flight" hormonal response in many patients. "Stress free anesthesia" may be possible with regional anesthetics that completely abolish afferent input from the surgical site, but GA with low narcotic doses only attenuates the body's endocrine response to surgery.

Surgery induces an increase in catecholamine levels (epinephrine and norepinephrine). Inhalational anesthetics, as well as high-dose opioids, blunt this response. The hypothalamic-pituitary-adrenal axis, the predominant regulator of the stress response, is triggered by surgical stress, resulting in elevated perioperative cortisol levels. Etomidate is the only anesthetic that will significantly decrease cortisol synthesis, not by inhibiting the neurohumoral axis, but by inhibiting the adrenocortical enzymes 11-β and 17-α hydroxylase. Adrenocortical hypofunction is a relative contraindication to the use of etomidate, unless hormone supplementation is part of the perioperative care. The adrenocortical response to surgery is only partially blunted with GA and its effect is very short-lived. Surgery induces the release of ADH (antidiuretic hormone), which may be a reason for decreased perioperative urine output. Adequate depth of anesthesia will prevent the rise in serum-ADH levels and higher doses of opioids seem to be more efficacious than inhalational anesthetics in this regard. Antidiuretic-hormone levels may remain elevated for up to 4 days postoperatively. Insulin levels also increase perioperatively, but because of the increased levels of cortisol, epinephrine, and glucagon, hyperglycemia is common during the surgical period.

In summary, surgical stimulation induces endocrine responses which persist in the postoperative period. The hormonal changes are proportional to the amount of stress and trauma secondary to the surgery. Increased catecholamines and adrenocortical hormones are the most prominent changes seen and, although it attenuates it, GA does not eliminate the body's stress response.

SUMMARY

General anesthesia is probably the most widely used anesthetic technique. Many times, it is the only option in providing care for patients undergoing surgery. Although regional techniques and MAC have established themselves as excellent and, in specific situations, superior modes of anesthesia, GA should not be withheld as an option for anesthetic care for fear of the patient being "too sick." As discussed in this chapter, the multitude of anesthetic agents available, in combination with a thorough knowledge of their pharmacologic and physiologic effects, makes GA a safe technique. In addition, regional anesthetics and MAC cases may need to be urgently converted to GA because of patient discomfort or anesthetic or surgical complications. Avoiding GA for the wrong reasons in a situation like this will stress the patient (and the anesthesiologist) much more than a carefully planned general anesthetic, which was initiated in a controlled fashion.

BIBLIOGRAPHY

Copp MV, Feneck RO: Cardiovascular function and the safety of anesthesia. In Taylor TH, Major E, editors; *Hazards and complications of anaesthesia*, ed 2, New York, 1993, Churchill Livingstone.

Selsby DS, Jones JG: Respiratory function and the safety of anaesthesia. In Taylor TH, Major E, editors: *Hazards and complications of anaesthesia*, ed 2, New York, 1993, Churchill Livingstone.

Stevens WC, Kingston HGG: Inhalation anesthesia. In Barash PC, Cullen BF, Stoelting RK, editors: *Clinical anesthesia*, ed 2, Philadelphia, 1995, JB Lippincott.

Willenkin RL, Polk SL: Management of general anesthesia. In Miller RD, editor; *Anesthesia*, ed 4, New York, 1995, Churchill Livingstone.

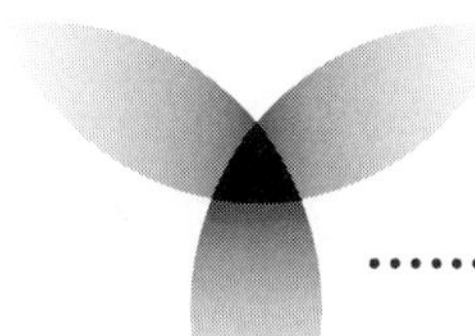

Chapter 40

Regional Anesthesia

Burkhard F. Spiekermann, MD, David M. Sibell, MD,
Cosmo DiFazio, MD

Carl Köller, an Austrian ophthalmologist, who in 1884 applied topical cocaine to the cornea of his patients before eye surgery, is generally recognized as the person who introduced regional anesthesia into the clinical arena. Systemic regional anesthesia was introduced in 1899 by August Bier who performed the first spinal anesthetic. Regional anesthesia is now a standard alternative, or an adjunct, to general anesthesia (GA) for a wide variety of surgical procedures. Today, virtually every part of the body can be anesthetized with specific nerve blocks. After a brief discussion on the mechanism of action, pharmacology, and potential side effects of local anesthetics, this chapter will focus on the principles, indications, contraindications, and complications of epidural and spinal anesthesia, as well as the most frequently used peripheral nerve blocks for intraoperative anesthesia. It is beyond the scope of this chapter to address the technical aspects of administering regional anesthesia or to cover the vast variety of techniques available for peripheral neuronal blockade.

• MECHANISM OF ACTION OF LOCAL ANESTHETICS

All excitable cells maintain a negative *resting membrane potential* of –60 to –70 mV, generated by active and passive diffusion of ions. The sodium-potassium pump is primarily responsible for the maintenance of this trans-membrane gradient by actively transporting sodium out of and potassium into the cell. Chemical, mechanical, or electrical excitation of a neuron will cause an opening of the membrane sodium channels and a sudden influx of sodium ions intracellularly, resulting in membrane depolarization following achievement of a certain critical threshold potential (+35 mV). The depolarization (action potential) is propagated along the nerve axon and reaches and excites other neurons through chemical synaptic transmission of the electrical impulse.

Local anesthetics (LAs) enter the sodium channel from the axoplasmic side of the cell membrane, reversibly bind to the sodium channel, and prevent subsequent sodium-channel activation and membrane depolarization. Local anesthetics do not change the resting membrane potential or the threshold potential but prevent achievement of the threshold level. This effectively and reversibly blocks neuronal conduction.

All LAs contain a lipophilic (usually a benzene ring) and a hydrophilic moiety (usually a tertiary amine) connected either through an amide or an ester linkage. This linkage classifies LAs either as amino*esters* (benzocaine, tetracaine, procaine, chloroprocaine, cocaine) or amino*amides* (lidocaine, bupivacaine, ropivacaine). Local anesthetic are relatively poorly water-soluble weak bases and are marketed as positively charged salt preparations.

The *potency* of LAs is directly proportional to their lipid solubility. The *onset of action* depends on the local anesthetic pKa and is related to the amount of unionized drug available to cross the axonal membrane and bind to the sodium channel. This is the reason why alkalization of commercially available lidocaine with sodium bicarbonate (1 meq for each 10 ml of lidocaine solution) will speed up the onset of lidocaine blockade. The *duration of action* is related to the amount of protein- and lipid-binding, regional-tissue blood flow, and the addition of epinephrine to the LA. Metabolism of LAs is minimally important in their termination of LA action. Once absorbed from the site of action into the general circulation, drug clearance is effected by metabolism. Esters are metabolized by plasma cholinesterases, and amides are hepatically degraded by dealkylation and/or amide hydrolysis.

• SIDE EFFECTS AND TOXICITY OF LOCAL ANESTHETICS

Systemic side effects and toxic reactions of local anesthetic agents are principally related to their effects on sodium channel blockade in tissues and organ systems other than the spinal cord and peripheral nerves. Toxicity is directly related to the dose, the route of administration, and the type of local anesthetic. In general, toxicity is proportional to anesthetic potency. Toxic reactions can be avoided by slow, incremental administration, repeated aspirations between injections, and adherence to the guidelines for maximum safe dosages. Table 40-1 summarizes the safe dosages of the more popular local anesthetic agents in use.

Cardiovascular Side Effects

Local anesthetics decrease myocardial automaticity and reduce the refractory period, which may result in severe cardiac arrhythmias, such as ventricular fibrillation and heart block, when accidentally administered intravascularly at high doses. At high doses they also have negative inotropic effects and cause decreased myocardial contractility. With the exception of cocaine, higher doses of local anesthetics cause smooth muscle relaxation and arteriolar dilatation. This may accentuate hypotension caused by local anesthetic-induced myocardial depression.

At high blood levels, *bupivacaine* is especially cardiotoxic, probably because of it's high affinity and binding properties to the sodium channel. Predisposing factors accentuating this toxicity include pregnancy, hypoxemia, and respiratory acidosis. There are many case reports in the literature of fatal cardiovascular collapse, secondary to unintentional intravascular bupivacaine injections. Resuscitation is difficult and often will not respond to the usual pharmacologic measures. *Ropivacaine*, a new LA chemically similar to bupivacaine, but with a much lower cardiovascular-toxicity profile, will most likely replace bupivacaine for some anesthetic procedures.

Cerebral Side Effects

Increasing plasma concentrations of local anesthetics will cause signs and symptoms of central nervous system irritation which may eventually progress to tonic-clonic seizures. Early symptoms of increasing LA concentrations include circumoral numbness, tinnitus, blurred vision, and slurred speech. Seizures, which occur at high drug concentrations, may be followed by apnea and may be lethal without intervention. Hyperventilation with 100% oxygen will ensure adequate oxygenation and will decrease cerebral blood flow, thereby decreasing the amount of LA delivered to the brain. If mask ventilation is impossible, succinylcholine should be administered and the trachea intubated. Small doses (1–2 mg/kg) of sodium thiopental or midazolam (1–2 mg) will raise the seizure threshold and will frequently terminate the seizure.

Allergic Reactions

Many patients report to be allergic to LAs; however, true allergic reactions to amide LAs are rare. Often, the patients believes to be an allergic reaction are actually systemic effects felt from accidental intravascular administration of small amounts of LA secondary to the systemic absorption of epinephrine. Ester-type LAs, which are metabolized to paraaminobenzoic acid (PABA), are more likely to produce true allergic reactions. If a true allergy to ester-type LAs is present, local anesthetic neural blockade can be produced by the use of LA amides, provided PABA is not present as a preservative in the LA solution.

Table 40-1. Safe Dosages of Local Anesthetic Agents

DOSE (MG/KG)	PERIPHERAL BLOCKS	CENTRAL +EPI	BLOCKS –EPI	INTERCOSTAL BLOCKS +EPI
Chloroprocaine	N/A	20	25	N/A
Lidocaine	14	7	9	6
Bupivacaine	5	2	2	2
Tetracaine	N/A	2	2	N/A

The safe total doses of the most commonly used local anesthetics for neuraxial and regional anesthesia. N/A = nonapplicable, +epi = 5 mcg/ml epinephrine added to the local anesthetic, –epi = epinephrine-free solution.

NEURAXIAL ANESTHESIA–EPIDURAL AND SPINAL ANESTHESIA

Principles of Neuraxial Anesthesia

The spinal cord travels within the spinal canal and extends in the adult patient from the foramen magnum to the L1 lumbar vertebra. It is surrounded by the meninges, the pia mater, arachnoid, and dura mater. Below L1, the spinal cord splits into terminal branches, the cauda equina, which is suspended in cerobrospinal fluid CSF. The dura is a dense, watertight connective tissue that protects the spinal cord and prevents leakage of CSF. The dura is a continuum of the intracranial dura and extends as far as the S1 sacral vertebra. The spinal nerves (mixed motor, sensory, and autonomic nerves) exit the vertebral foramina at the level of the corresponding vertebral body.

Spinal anesthesia, or subarachnoid blockade, involves deposition of a local anesthetic *subdurally* into the subarachnoid space and is performed similarly to a lumbar puncture. To avoid the possibility of direct injury to the spinal cord, a subarachnoid block is usually performed by entering the spinal canal at the L3/L4 or L4/L5 vertebral level. The LA mixes with the CSF and directly bathes the spinal nerves, causing blockade of motor, sensory, and autonomic fibers. The extent of spread of the LA depends primarily on (1) the baricity of the LA solution (hyperbaric solutions are used most commonly, which tend to travel to dependent areas in the CSF), (2) patient positioning after injection (a slight Trendelenburg position facilitates a cephalad spread of the blockade), and (3) the amount of LA injected. Motor, sensory, and autonomic fibers have different sensitivities to LA blockade, autonomic fibers being more sensitive than the others. *Differential neuronal blockade* is the reason why autonomic blockade typically precedes and exceeds motor and sensory blockade.

Even though it is possible to insert a subarachnoid catheter and perform a *continuous spinal anesthetic*, subarachnoid blockade is usually performed as a *"single shot,"* that is, the LA is injected as a single dose and the needle withdrawn. Subarachnoid blockade is technically easier than epidural blockade, has an almost immediate onset of action, and blocks lower sacral segments more reliably than epidural blockade. The cephalad spread of the block, however, is not as predictable as with epidural blockade, which more likely, may cause profound hypotension from extensive autonomic blockade or inadequate block at higher abdominal levels. Another disadvantage of single-shot spinal anesthesia is that redosing with LA is impossible. If the surgical procedure exceeds the expected length and the block wears off, conversion to a general anesthetic may be necessary. The most commonly used LA agents for spinal anesthesia are lidocaine (for short procedures), bupivacaine (for procedures lasting 1 to 2 hours), and tetracaine (for long procedures).

Surgeries that lend themselves to spinal anesthesia include many urologic procedures (ureteroscopy, cystoscopy, transurethral prostatectomy), orthopedic surgery (knee- and hip-replacement surgery), peripheral vascular surgery, perineal surgery (hemorrhoids, rectal fissures), and gynecologic surgery (vaginal hysterectomy, cervical cerclage).

Epidural anesthesia involves placing the LA into the epidural space, which is a potential space between the ligamentum flavum posteriorly, and the dura mater anteriorly. The epidural space is located with a specially designed epidural needle. The technical aspects of epidural anesthesia require considerably more expertise and will be more time-consuming than spinal anesthesia. Once the epidural space is located, a small catheter is placed through the epidural needle and the epidural needle is removed. The catheter allows repeated injections of LA and can remain in place for the first postoperative days and used for continuous epidural analgesia.

Unlike spinal anesthesia, epidural anesthesia can be performed at various lumbar and thoracic levels. It allows *segmental blockade* of the spinal nerves upon leaving the spinal cord through the spinal foramina. For example, a thoracic epidural catheter can provide anesthesia and postoperative analgesia for an open cholecystectomy, while leaving sensation and motor function to the lower extremities intact. More and more commonly, combined epidural and general anesthesia is used for invasive and painful operations like thoracotomines. This approach provides a lighter plain of GA intraoperatively and excellent, postoperative thoracic epidural analgesia.

Unlike spinal anesthesia, incremental administration of LA into the epidural space allows a more controlled distribution of neuronal blockade, especially in the cephalad direction. This may be especially important in a patient who will not tolerate excessive sympathetic blockade and hypotension, such as the patient with aortic stenosis. Because LA seems to spread preferentially upwards in the epidural space, it is sometimes difficult with epidural anesthesia to produce a dense block in the perineal region. Spinal anesthesia (a so-called “saddle block”) may be selected if perineal anesthesia is required.

Another advantage of epidural blockade is that epidural anesthesia can be maintained as long or as short as needed. For shorter cases, a shorter-acting drug like lidocaine may be chosen. If the procedure is expected to take longer, bupivacaine may be the drug of choice. In either case, if the block starts to recede, redosing through the epidural catheter is always possible, no matter what type of LA is chosen. Since the total LA requirement for epidural anesthesia is much higher than required for spinal anesthesia, there is a larger potential for toxic blood levels of LA (from accidental intravascular injections or excessive redosing through the catheter).

In general, the same surgical procedures that lend themselves to spinal anesthesia can also be performed under epidural anesthesia.

The Rationale for Using Neuraxial Anesthesia

One obvious reason for the administration of neuraxial anesthesia (NA) instead of GA is patient preference. Many patients are afraid of "going to sleep" and may be less anxious having the surgical procedure performed under NA. Another common reason for NA is that epidural *anesthesia* during surgery can easily be converted to epidural *analgesia* for superior, continuous postoperative pain control, as discussed in Chapter 42. General anesthesia has significant intraoperative and postoperative physiologic effects (see Chapter 42) which may be avoidable or less severe with NA. There are many recent studies that address the potential benefits of NA over GA, primarily regarding the neuroendocrine stress response to surgery, cardiopulmonary morbidity, perioperative blood loss, and the frequency of thromboembolic complications.

NA AND THE STRESS RESPONSE

Surgical stimulation increases the plasma concentrations of cortisol, insulin, renin, angiotensin, aldosterone, growth hormone, and circulating catecholamines. This stress response may be detrimental in patients with cardiovascular disease who may not be able to respond to the increasing circulatory and metabolic demands. There is a considerable amount of discussion as to whether attenuation of this stress response translates into reduced perioperative morbidity. General anesthesia, with the possible exception of high-dose opioid anesthesia, does not effectively blunt the body's generalized "fight and flight" response. However, most surgically induced endocrine and metabolic changes are effectively blocked by afferent blockade of nociceptive input, as produced by adequate spinal or epidural anesthesia. These effects are seen primarily during regional anesthesia for lower-extremity procedures; neuraxial anesthesia only *attenuates* the rise in circulating mediators when surgery includes upper abdominal or thoracic procedures.

NA AND BLOOD LOSS

Studies have shown that intraoperative blood loss is decreased by 25% to 40% during hip and knee replacement surgery, as well as retropubic and transurethral prostatectomies when performed under NA, as compared to GA. However, abdominal surgery performed under NA is not associated with a similar decrease in blood loss. The diminished blood loss with NA may be caused by the decrease in blood pressure that occurs, secondary to the regional blockade-induced sympathectomy, and may be similar to GA when blood pressure is pharmacologically maintained at levels similar to the NA group.

NA AND THROMBOEMBOLIC COMPLICATIONS

Thromboembolic complications (deep venous thrombosis and pulmonary embolism) are decreased by 40% to 60% when hip and knee arthroplasties and retropubic prostatectomies are performed with NA, compared to GA. Peripheral vascular surgery (e.g., femoral-popliteal bypass grafting) with NA also had a lower incidence of early graft stenosis, requiring fewer repeat operations during the first postoperative month than patients who had the operation under GA. It is believed that the sympathectomy produced by NA promotes lower-extremity blood flow, and that adequate afferent blockade by NA prevents the hypercoagulable state induced by surgical stress. It has been shown that an increase of the plasminogen activator Inhibitor-1 (PAI-1) during the perioperative period is directly related to the incidence of postoperative thromboembolic events. Unlike GA, NA prevents such an increase.

NA and Cardiovascular Function

The extent of the cardiovascular changes associated with NA are primarily depended on the extent of sympathetic blockade produced by NA, the baseline blood volume (preload), and the underlying cardiac function. In general, the more extensive the neuraxial blockade, the more likely there will be a decrease in preload, afterload, and blood pressure. Capacitance and resistance vessels of all vascular beds dilate below the level of the sympathetic blockade, which may only partially be compensated for by the vasoconstricted state of the vasculature above the level of the sympathetic block.

A reduction in pre- and afterload may be beneficial in patients with poor ventricular function and angina because of decreased myocardial oxygen demand. However, oxygen supply may also be jeopardized, if an excessive decrease in diastolic blood pressure reduces coronary perfusion pressure. Improvements of regional wall-motion abnormalities of the myocardium with thoracic epidural anesthesia have been documented in patients with ischemic heart disease. It is thought that thoracic sympathetic blockade will cause coronary vasodilatation and improve subendocardial blood flow. If volume loading and vasopressor therapy is necessary to avoid severe hypotension, the benefits of improved myocardial oxygen supply during thoracic epidural anesthesia will be offset. Thoracic (T1–T4) anesthesia will also block cardioaccelerator fibers, sometimes resulting in profound bradycardia unresponsive to atropine therapy. Mild-to-moderate bradycardia may be beneficial, improving the myocardial oxygen-supply balance. Bradycardia resulting in hypotension, conversely, will decrease oxygen supply to the myocardium.

Earlier studies suggested a decrease in perioperative cardiac morbidity in patients undergoing major abdominal or thoracic procedures with a combination of GA and epidural anesthesia and postoperative epidural analgesia for pain control, when compared to patients who had the operation performed under GA with postoperative IV analgesia. These results have been challenged because recent studies suggest there is no difference in perioperative cardiac complications.

NA and Pulmonary Function

Unlike GA, lumbar and low-thoracic epidural anesthesia have only minimal effects on pulmonary parameters. Avoiding the negative effects of GA and airway manipulation in patients with pulmonary disease, especially chronic obstructive pulmonary disease (COPD) and asthma, may, therefore, be advantageous. More effective postoperative pain control with continuous epidural analgesia, will improve respiratory dynamics and restoration of functional residual capacity (FRC), decrease atelectasis, and, hopefully, decrease the possibility of postoperative pulmonary infections.

Mid- and high-thoracic anesthesia may decrease vital capacity, total lung capacity, and forced expiratory volume in 1 second (FEV_1). Patients with obstructive airway disease, who depend on muscle function for expiration, may have even more difficulty with expiration when effective thoracic anesthesia causes motor blockade of the internal intercostal muscles.

NA and Gastrointestinal Function

Sympathetic outflow to the gut (T5–L1) decreases peristalsis, increases sphincter tone, and counteracts vagal action. With a sympathectomy from NA, vagal tone predominates, resulting in increased peristalsis. It seems that postoperative gastric emptying and bowel activity is unaffected by NA, and NA is associated with a lower incidence of postoperative ileus, when compared to general anesthesia.

In summary, despite the potential benefit of NA over GA, convincing evidence from well-designed studies regarding the superiority of NA is still lacking. Critically ill patients, in whom the benefits of NA may be most beneficial, are often too sick for NA and require intraoperative intensive care, which entails controlled ventilation and full pharmacologic support, including the administration of IV or inhaled anesthetic agents.

Patient Evaluation

Patients scheduled to have an operation under epidural or spinal anesthesia should be evaluated just as carefully as patients receiving GA as outlined in Chapter 39. Information regarding the patient's cardiovascular status will reveal whether precipitous or excessive sympathetic blockade may be detrimental, which would favor the choice of epidural over spinal anesthesia. Patients who are taking antihypertensives or adrenergic blockers may have a more exaggerated physiologic response to epidural and spinal blockade. An examination of the patient's back is necessary to rule out any anatomic abnormalities, skin breakdown, or infection at the site of entry.

Laboratory studies should include a coagulation profile in patients at risk for coagulopathies, such as the patient who is taking anticoagulants preoperatively or the alcoholic patient or patients who give a history of easy bleeding (i.e., when brushing the teeth). Coagulation defects are considered a contraindication to NA, as discussed further on.

During the preoperative visit, the advantages and disadvantages of regional anesthesia should be explained to the patient. The technical procedure of neuraxial blockade need to be discussed, because patient cooperation when performing the block is necessary. Patients should to be told that they will be aware of the operating room environment during surgery. Because many patients will find remaining awake during surgery of concern, they should be reassured that supplemental IV sedation can be administered if needed, or that conversion to a general anesthetic is always possible. It should also be explained that in the small chance NA is not completely successful, GA may be necessary as a backup option. As is the case with the patient undergoing GA, preoperative medication depends on the anxiety level of the patient. Excessive premedication needs to be avoided, however, since it makes cooperation during neuraxial blockade and evaluation of the adequacy of the block difficult.

Contraindications

There are only a few absolute contraindications for NA. Patient refusal is an obvious reason not to perform spinal or epidural anesthesia and a patient should never be talked into a specific anesthetic technique. Uncorrected coagulation defects, from either systemic disease or therapeutic anticoagulation, are another absolute contraindication because they increase the risk of epidural hematoma formation from accidental vascular puncture. Severe hypovolemia, bacteremia, and skin infection at the site of injection are other absolute contraindications. Patients with increased intracranial pressure should also not have spinal or epidural anesthesia, because CSF leakage from the spinal canal may increase the risk of cerebral herniation.

Relative contraindications include peripheral neuropathies, demyelinating neurologic disorders like multiple sclerosis, cardiac lesions like aortic stenosis or asymmetric septal hypertrophy (where excessive pre- and afterload reduction may be detrimental), emotional instability, and mini-dose heparin therapy. Therapy with antiplatelet drugs, like aspirin, are not a contraindication to neuraxial blockade.

Complications

Major complications from spinal and epidural blockade are rare and are related to neurologic injuries secondary to infection or mechanical trauma. Minor complications usually consist of transient hypotension, high-spinal blockade, postdural puncture headache, and back pain.

Hypotension

Hypotension during spinal and epidural anesthesia results from decreased cardiac output secondary to decreased venous return caused by venous pooling. The amount of venous pooling is directly related to the degree of sympathetic blockade. The overall physiologic condition of the patient determines whether the degree of hypotension should be treated or will be tolerated by the patient. Pregnant patients, for example, should not be left hypotensive (systolic blood pressure less than 100 mm Hg) for a prolonged time, otherwise, uterine blood flow and fetal oxygenation will be compromised. Hypotension from neuraxial anesthesia can be attenuated by giving the patient a fluid bolus (500–1000 ml) before the procedure. Incrementally administered epidural blockade is less likely to cause hypotension than spinal anesthesia. If hypotension occurs, administration of fluids, leg elevation, and small doses of vasopressor (ephedrine 5–10 mg IV) are usually sufficient to treat the episode. Repeated episodes of hypotension after the block may be treated with the intramuscular injection of 25 to 50 mg of ephedrine.

High-Spinal Anesthesia

High-spinal anesthesia from excessive cephalad spread of LA can occur in any patient but is most frequently seen in the parturient. With high-thoracic and lower-cervical blockade, severe hypotension with profound bradycardia and respiratory compromise are likely. If hypotension is so extreme that brainstem perfusion is compromised, the patient will become unresponsive. Treatment consists of circulatory and respiratory support. Left-uterine displacement, aggressive administration of fluids, leg elevation, and the administration of direct acting vasopressors such as epinephrine are required to stabilize the blood pressure. Atropine may not be adequate to treat bradycardia caused by blockade of the cardiac accelerator fibers. Oxygen therapy by mask may be sufficient. However, inadequate ventilation secondary to brainstem anesthesia requires the induction of general anesthesia and endotracheal intubation. The extensive spread is usually short lived and respiratory function will return to normal fairly quickly.

BACK PAIN

Back pain after epidural and spinal anesthesia may be secondary to local tissue irritation, small hematomas, reflex skeletal muscle spasm or secondary to the surgical position. Back pain after NA is not very common and some studies suggest that patients who have had general anesthesia have the same incidence of back pain as patients after NA.

If back pain does occur, a careful examination of the back and a neurological exam should be performed to rule out the more serious problem of an epidural hematoma or infection/epidural abscess. Reassurance, rest, locally applied heat and nonsteroidal analgesics are usually sufficient treatment.

POSTDURAL PUNCTURE HEADACHE

Postdural puncture headache (PDPH or spinal headache) is most likely related to the persistent leaking of cerebrospinal fluid (CSF) through the dural hole, causing a lowering of CSF pressure within the spinal canal. This results in downward traction on the structures of the CNS and it's blood vessels, causing a headache similar to an acute vascular cluster headache. Postdural puncture headache is probably the most common complication after spinal and epidural (with accidental dural puncture) anesthesia. The incidence of PDPH is related to gender (females > males), age (younger > older), and pregnancy status (more likely during pregnancy) of the patient. The size and type of the needle used for the dural puncture is also important in predicting the frequency of a PDPH. (Larger cutting needles cause a much higher incidence of PDPH.) To minimize the frequency of PDPH, a small noncutting spinal needle (24–27 gauge with a Whitacre or Sprotte needle) should be used in the younger patient population.

The classic feature of a PDPH is its postural component. Postdural puncture headache is typically relieved when assuming the supine position, and made worse when sitting or standing erect. If a postural association is absent, other etiologies for the cause of the headache are likely.

Once the diagnosis of PDPH is made, the initial treatment consists of hydration, oral analgesics, and bedrest. Nearly all PDPHs resolve over the first 24 hours, and no further therapy is needed. Persistent, debilitating headaches can be treated with IV-caffeine benzoate (500 mg) or an epidural blood patch.

Caffeine is a potent vasoconstrictor, and may attenuate the vascular component of the headache. It may also increase production of CSF. The epidural blood patch involves the sterile injection of 15 to 20 mL of the patient's own blood through an epidural needle in the patient's epidural space. Formation of a blood clot probably seals the epidural tear and prevents further leakage of CSF. Ninety-five percent of patients have complete relief if an epidural blood patch is performed 24 hours after the onset of a PDPH. A second blood patch increases the success rate to 99%.

URINARY RETENTION

Blocking the S2 to S4 sacral nerve roots will cause a loss of bladder tone and inhibition of the voiding reflex. Overdistension of the bladder is possible and voiding may, at times, be a problem, even when the block has resolved. This problem is more common in males than females. To avoid bladder distension, an indwelling urinary catheter should be inserted for prolonged surgical procedures. If postoperative voiding is a problem and the bladder seems to be distended (which is often associated with hypertension and tachycardia), "in and out" catheterization may be required.

NAUSEA

Nausea during NA may often be the first sign of impending hypotension. The initial step in treating nausea is to rule out significant hypotension, administer oxygen, and treat low blood pressure, if present.

Nausea can also result from unopposed vagal activity secondary to a sympathetic block, causing increased peristalsis. Atropine (0.2–0.4 mg IV) may help in this situation.

VASCULAR INJURY

Trauma to the epidural venous plexus can occur from spinal and epidural anesthesia. Persistent bleeding from traumatized vessels may cause an epidural hematoma, which, if not surgically decompressed, may cause permanent nerve injury and paraplegia. Any motor or sensory function that does not resolve after NA, suggests the possibility of an epidural hematoma and should be aggressively investigated. Contrast enhanced computerized tomography (CT) or magnetic resonance imaging (MRI) will reliably diagnose an epidural hematoma and imaging studies cannot be delayed.

The risk for epidural hematoma formation is higher in patients who are on anticoagulants or who are thrombocytopenic preoperatively. NA should be avoided in this group of patients. Patients who had a traumatic epidural or spinal anesthetic (i.e., grossly bloody when inserting the needle) and require intraoperative anticoagulation (for example abdominal aortic aneurysm surgery) should probably have their surgical procedure delayed for 24 hrs, if possible. In patients undergoing these type of operations, the risk/benefit ratio of NA needs to be carefully evaluated and discussed with the surgical team as part of planning the anesthetic procedure.

Aspirin or other nonsteroidal analgesic interfering with platelet function are not a contraindication for NA. Neuraxial anesthesia with the use of subcutaneous minidose heparin, or with the use the newer, low-molecular weight heparins is controversial, especially if the patient is also taking aspirin.

NERVE INJURY

Injury to the spinal cord can be caused by direct trauma to the spinal nerves from the needle or chemical irritation of the spinal cord from the LA solution. Permanent nerve injury after NA is rare, estimated to be less than 1:10,000.

Nerve injury from mechanical trauma can be prevented by performing spinal anesthesia below the L2 lumbar level in the adult, because the spinal cord ends at L1 to L2. Local anesthetic should never be injected when persistent paraesthesias are elicited with needle placement. This usually indicates placement of the needle in the nerve bundle. Injection at this point may cause permanent nerve disruption.

Chemical nerve injury is possible from high local concentrations of the LA itself, the preservative solution in the LA, or inadvertent injection of other drugs into the CSF or the epidural space. Inadvertent subarachnoid injection of 2-chloroprocaine has been associated with the cauda equina syndrome, and is attributed to the low pH and the preservative sodium bisulfite. 2-chloroprocaine has since been reformulated and now contains sodium-EDTA as a preservative. Recently, subarachnoid hyperbaric 5% lidocaine in 7.5% dextrose, injected through microcatheters for a continuous spinal anesthetic, has been implicated in causing a cauda equina syndrome. It is probably wise to avoid repeated subarachnoid injections of any LA for a "failed spinal" to prevent a high concentration of LA. Solutions containing preservatives should not be administered into the CSF. Diluting the LA with 2 to 3 ml of CSF, simply by aspirating through the spinal needle before its subarachnoid injection, may also help prevent deposition of concentrated LA solution close to the spinal cord.

MENINGITIS AND EPIDURAL ABSCESS

Chemical or infectious meningitis is rare after NA when careful aseptic technique is maintained during the procedure. Seeding of the CSF in a patient with an infection is only of theoretical concern and has never been shown to be a clinical problem. This includes patients with human immunodeficiency virus (HIV), who will not increase their likelihood of CNS-HIV symptoms after NA. However, patients with septicemia who are not receiving antibiotics or are refractory to antibiotic therapy are unlikely candidates for NA. The possibility of infectious meningitis should be considered in any patient who develops meningeal signs after NA.

The formation of an epidural abscess is rare and, potentially, catastrophic. It has been reported in septic patients receiving epidural anesthesia. Diagnosis and therapy include a careful examination of the back, CT or MRI, IV antibiotic therapy, and emergent decompressive surgery.

SYSTEMIC TOXICITY FROM ABSORBED LA

Because of the small amount of LA required for spinal anesthesia, systemic reactions are unlikely, even if inadvertently injected intravascularly. Epidural anesthesia, however, requires larger total dosages of LA, which even if not injected intravascularly, may cause toxic blood concentrations when large dosages are administered. The blood and tissue concentration of LA are determined by the total dosage administered, the rate of absorption from the epidural space, tissue redistribution, metabolism, and excretion. To avoid complications from systemic LA toxicity, incremental administration of LA, the adherence to safe maximal dosages, the avoidance of excessive redosing, and the addition of epinephrine when applicable to the LA to decrease systemic absorption, should be used.

• PERIPHERAL NERVE BLOCKADE

Principles of Peripheral Nerve Blockade

Peripheral nerve blocks involve deposition of local anesthetic agents in close proximity to certain nerves or nerve plexi. Unlike with neuraxial anesthesia, specific limbs or smaller anatomic structures can be selectively anesthetized. Sympathetic blockade, with its associated side effects, is generally not encountered. Peripheral nerve blocks alone, or in combination with GA, may provide superior, intraoperative physiologic and surgical conditions, and better postoperative analgesia with faster postoperative recovery times. This section addresses the more commonly used plexus- and peripheral-nerve blocks. Again, technical details will not be discussed and the reader is referred to the bibliography at the end of the chapter.

Patient Evaluation and Selection

The indications for neuraxial regional anesthesia have already been outlined, and they apply similarly to peripheral regional anesthesia. As with NA, one of the few absolute contraindications to peripheral nerve blockade anesthesia is patient refusal. Frequently, a patient who bluntly refuses to consider a regional anesthetic does so out of misconceptions and misinformation. At institutions where regional anesthesia is a priority and patient education is done properly, patient refusal is not much of an issue. Ideally, the anesthesiologist has an opportunity to meet with the patient before the immediate preoperative period, to discuss anesthetic options with the patient in a more relaxed atmosphere. In many ambulatory settings, this is not possible, and every effort must be made to give the patient balanced information by other means. This is the beginning of a successful perioperative anesthetic care system, of which the intraoperative anesthetic is only a part.

The anesthesiologist must consider the postoperative plans for the patient by the surgeon, and the social setting for an ambulatory patient. A prolonged femoral nerve block, for instance, may prevent a patient from ambulating, and result in an unplanned admission. A patient with a long drive home must be counseled regarding the use of postoperative analgesic medications to avoid the sudden onset of uncontrollable pain as a block recedes. These considerations underline the need for communication between the health care practitioners within the perioperative care system.

Complications

There are potential complications associated with peripheral regional anesthesia. Some of those common to all peripheral regional anesthetics are intraneural injection, local anesthetic toxicity (both systemic and local), intravascular or neuraxial injection, bleeding, infection, and pain at the injection site, as discussed earlier. The subject of intraneural injection deserves special mention in regard to plexus anesthesia. Intraneural injections can result in devastating postoperative neuropathies or plexopathies. The only indicator for an intraneural injection is the intense, crampy burning the patient experiences upon injection from the increased hydrostatic pressure within the fascicles or perineurium. In the anesthetized patient, this crucial feedback is eliminated. Therefore, there is a measurable hazard in performing a general anesthetic before block placement. In the appropriately counseled patient, minimal premedication should result in a tolerable block placement.

Cervical Plexus Block

The cervical plexus is derived from the cervical nerve roots from C_1 to C_5 and is responsible for the sensory innervation of the area from the occiput to the scapula, posteriorly and to the neck and proximal shoulder girdle, anteriorly. It also serves as the motor innervation to the diaphragm and several intrinsic cervical muscles. Although less commonly anesthetized than the brachial and lumbar plexi, regional anesthesia of the cervical plexus does have a potentially significant role to play in patient care.

The most common application of deep and superficial plexus block is for carotid artery surgery. Many practitioners believe it less likely to cause major pulmonary and hemodynamic alterations than GA in patients undergoing carotid endarterectomy. One significant advantage of regional anesthesia for carotid procedures is that patient response during carotid cross clamping has been shown to be the most sensitive and specific indicator of intraoperative neurologic ischemia. Because intraluminal carotid shunting is associated with a significant risk of embolization itself, selectively shunting patients who show temporary deficits upon cross clamping has established benefits. There are several large studies in the surgical and anesthetic literature, demonstrating the safety and efficacy of cervical plexus anesthesia for carotid surgery. In addition to medical benefits, one study has shown a significant reduction in intensive-care-unit stay (a 2-day reduction in hospital stay) and significant savings in total hospitalization cost.

For successful regional anesthesia for carotid surgery, several considerations must apply. The patient must be able to follow commands and lie still for what may be prolonged periods of time. He/she must have sufficient cognitive reserve to avoid significant disinhibition caused by sedative medications, if these are to be used. In addition, even candidates who meet these criteria may fail to tolerate lying still for a prolonged procedure. Considering the difficulty of emergent, intraoperative airway management of a potentially unstable patient who has an open, sterile wound, it is prudent to weigh these considerations heavily.

Cervical plexus anesthesia may also be used in thyroid and parathyroid surgery, but one must consider the potentially uncomfortable position of extreme cervical neck extension, as preferred by some surgeons. Tracheal manipulation may also cause significant airway compromise in a prolonged case.

One hypothetical risk of cervical plexus anesthesia is blockade of the phrenic nerves. There is a high incidence of phrenic nerve paresis or paralysis with these procedures. This may potentially result in significant respiratory distress in patients with preexisting severe pulmonary disease who rely heavily on diaphragmatic contribution for adequate gas exchange.

Upper Extremity Blocks

The brachial plexus involves the C_5 to T_1 nerve roots and can be anesthetized with a range of approaches, from the proximal (interscalene) technique to distal peripheral nerve blocks, and local field infiltration for minor procedures. The anesthesiologist must decide between these blocks based on anatomic location of surgery, operator experience, and postoperative goals, among other priorities. The interscalene approach to the brachial plexus is probably the most commonly used block for shoulder surgery; the axillary is used, for distal upper-extremity procedures. Many anesthesiologists prefer the supraclavicular and infraclavicular approaches for the placement of catheters for postoperative regional analgesia, although this practice has yet to be thoroughly evaluated in the anesthetic literature. Peripheral nerve blocks, typically performed at the level of the elbow, wrist, or digits, may be used as the primary anesthetic or to supplement a partially effective plexus anesthetic.

Outcome analysis in brachial plexus anesthesia, principally interscalene blocks for shoulder procedures, indicates significantly reduced pain scores on the operative day and postoperative day 1. Sleep is improved on the first postoperative night, as well, likely because of better analgesia. Of consummate importance, however, is the equivalent usage of oral analgesics between the block and general anesthesia groups in these studies. This consistent finding indicates that unless a continuous technique is used, the block will terminate and require the need for continuous postoperative analgesia in these patients.

Typically, the principal difference between postoperative analgesia requirements in general and regional anesthesia patients occurs in the postanesthesia care unit (PACU). General-anesthesia patients ordinarily require upwards of 15 to 30 mg of intravenous morphine (or its equivalent) to control their pain, whether they had intraarticular and subcutaneous infiltration of their wounds with local anesthetics or not. This commonly results in sedation and/or nausea, incompatible with discharge home. The patients with regional anesthesia are frequently able to take oral medications soon after reaching the PACU and do well with the early initiation and maintenance of oral or parenteral nonsteroidal antiinflammatory drugs, and oral narcotic/acetaminophen preparations. Attempts to use medications only "as needed" can result in the onset of significant shoulder pain when the outpatient is at home, or worse, en route. Oral medications are rarely sufficient to control this runaway pain, and emergency room visits are common in this group. A well-integrated system of optimal preoperative counseling and postoperative analgesia techniques is necessary to allow these patients maximum benefit from the block.

One commonly held belief is that regional anesthesia significantly prolongs perioperative time, when compared to a general anesthetic. In fact, a retrospective analysis of several perioperative-time increments in outpatient shoulder surgery showed several advantages to interscalene anesthesia, when compared to GA. The average preoperative time, in one such study, was 11 minutes longer in the block group, but positioning, "wake up," and room-turnover times were all significantly reduced in the block group because of improved patient consciousness and participation in positioning. This led to a 9-minute reduction in the "anesthesia-dependent" portion of the perioperative time, and was also associated with a 30-minute reduction in PACU time. Add to this the 8.1% incidence of unplanned admission in the GA group, and there are several potent indicators of improved perioperative efficiency, which strongly suggest that cost savings attributable to the inclusion of regional anesthesia is possible.

Although there are several demonstrated advantages to performing brachial plexus anesthesia for upper-extremity procedures, these techniques are still uncommon at many institutions. One major deterrent is the incomplete training of the practitioners, and the perception that patients will refuse the procedure is another. However, as a part of a properly constructed system, patient acceptance of this type of anesthesia can be high.

Aside from the aforementioned risks of any regional anesthetic, an interscalene block carries a nearly 100% incidence of ipsilateral phrenic nerve paresis or paralysis. Generally, this is not a major issue, but as with cervical plexus anesthesia, it must be considered in preparing the patient. Furthermore, there are scattered reports of high-spinal or epidural blockade because of inappropriately placed interscalene blocks.

Lower Extremity Blocks

Before considering peripheral regional anesthesia in the lower extremity, the anesthesiologist must understand the complex anatomy of the lumbosacral plexus. Compromised of the T_{12} to S_4 spinal nerve roots, the lumbosacral plexus is responsible for the sensory and motor innervation of the lower extremity and distal pelvis. For the sake of this discussion, the branches innervating the lower abdomen and pelvis will not be reviewed.

The femoral nerve is responsible for the sensory and motor innervation for the vastus muscle groups and the anterior thigh. The saphenous nerve is the only branch of the femoral nerve to occur reliably distal to the knee, and it is responsible for innervating part of the medial leg and foot. The obturator nerve is formed from the branches of L_{2-4}, and innervates the adductor muscle groups, as well as a variable patch of skin on the medial thigh. The lateral femoral cutaneous nerve is comprised of L_{2-3}, and provides sensory innervation to the lateral thigh. It is particularly important in mediating tourniquet pain.

The sciatic nerve is the largest peripheral nerve in the body and results from input from L_4 to S_3 spinal nerve roots. It and its branches comprise the mixed innervation of the entire posterior thigh and the leg distal to the knee, with the exception of the saphenous nerve.

There are several approaches to lower-extremity regional anesthesia, from posterior lumbar plexus blockade, to the simpler and better tolerated three-in-one and fascia-iliaca compartment approaches. Raj has demonstrated a supine approach to both the femoral and sciatic nerves. The peripheral nerves may be approached in the pelvis, popliteal fossa, and ankle; local infiltration or field blocks may result in satisfactory anesthesia for minor procedures.

Given the compact nature and multitude of approaches to the brachial plexus, and the ease of neuraxial anesthesia, many practitioners would choose to stop considering extremity regional anesthesia beyond this. Unfortunately, because of these concerns, the literature on outcomes in lumbosacral-plexus anesthesia is limited. What does exist points toward data similar to that reviewed in the section on brachial-plexus anesthesia.

Most of this literature investigates the use of either femoral nerve, three-in-one (femoral, lateral femoral cutaneous, and obturator nerves), or fascia-iliaca compartment block for femur or knee procedures. Typically, these procedures are combined with another type of anesthetic, either sciatic nerve block or general anesthesia for surgery, with the possibility of a femoral sheath catheter left for postoperative analgesia in knee procedures. Generally, patients receiving bolus techniques show improved postoperative analgesia for 12 to 24 hours postoperatively. Patients with catheters inserted in the fascia-iliaca or femoral-sheath compartments can derive effective postoperative analgesia for several days, and are spared the contralateral extremity effects associated with epidural analgesia. Moreover, they are not at increased risk of developing urinary retention, requiring bladder catheterization, as are some patients who receive epidural analgesia.

As with any regional anesthetic, there are concerns regarding needle placement. Fortunately, the femoral nerve is not comprised of a compact collection of neurons, as are the branches of the brachial plexus. Rather, the nerve is composed of several loose strands, which are less prone to damage by a needle. The nerve is, however, lateral to the femoral artery, and arterial complications are the predominant complication of this block. These range from uncontrollable bleeding if the artery is punctured proximal to the inguinal ligament (where it can not be tamponaded), to transient postoperative pain and/or femoral nerve palsy caused by hematoma formation. The use of a blunt-tipped needle allows access to the fascia iliaca sheath in a fashion less likely to cause neural or vascular trauma, and also allows the introduction of a catheter for postoperative analgesia.

The sciatic nerve is more like the branches of the brachial plexus in its construction, and is more prone to needle-related injury than the femoral nerve. Although it is partially responsible for innervation of the knee, it does not appear to be necessary for postoperative analgesia, even in total-knee-arthroplasty patients requiring continuous passive motion. Many practitioners report the successful use of a single sciatic nerve block, and placement of a femoral-sheath or fascia-iliaca-compartment catheter for intraoperative management, with the catheter alone used for postoperative analgesia.

SUMMARY

Many times, regional anesthesia is an attractive alternative or supplement to GA and an excellent choice for postoperative analgesia. However, it requires sound knowledge of the technical aspects, the physiologic implications, side effects, and potential complications associated with the various techniques. Perhaps even more so than with GA, an informed and cooperative patient is necessary. Otherwise, regional anesthesia will become frustrating and undesirable for patients, surgeons, and anesthesiologists. Lastly, a clear picture regarding the extent of the surgery is essential. Misunderstanding may lead to insufficient blockade and may require urgent conversion to a general anesthetic, which could have been avoided by better communication with the surgical team.

BIBLIOGRAPHY

Cousins MJ, Bridenbough PO: *Neuroblockade in clinical anesthesia and management of pain*, ed 2, Philadelphia, 1992, JB Lippincott.

Greene NM: *Physiology of spinal anesthesia*, ed 4, Baltimore, 1993, Williams & Wilkins.

Katz J: *Atlas of regional anesthesia*, ed 2, 1994, Appleton & Lange.

Raj PP: *Practical management of pain*, ed 2, Philadelphia, 1992, Mosby–Year Book.

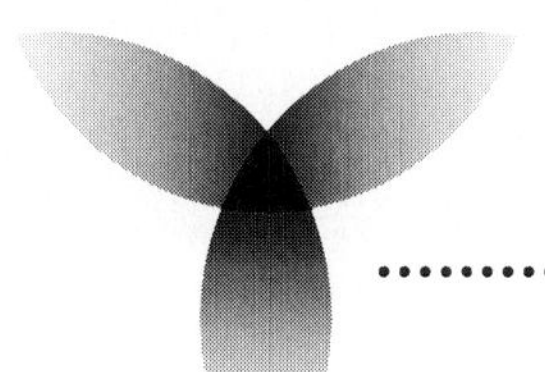

Section VI

POSTOPERATIVE CARE

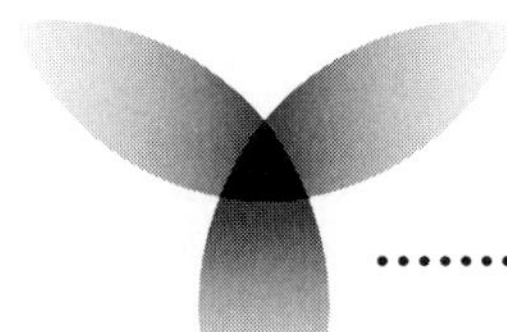

Chapter 41

Postanesthesia Care

George S. Leisure, MD

Recovery from either general or regional anesthesia can impose a significant physiologic stress on many patients. In fact, before the advent of dedicated recovery rooms, many early postoperative deaths occurred immediately following anesthesia and surgery. Some of these deaths were preventable, and this fact has led to the development of the modern postanesthesia care unit (PACU). Although the period of emergence from anesthesia is associated with a relatively high incidence of potentially life-threatening circulatory and respiratory events, such problems should be preventable or treatable by an experienced recovery room staff.

• TRANSFER TO THE POSTANESTHETIC CARE UNIT

Ideally, following an uncomplicated, elective procedure, the patient should be extubated in the operating room. This facilitates the immediate assessment of neurologic and respiratory function. In addition, if reintubation is necessary, it can be accomplished in the best setting possible. However, patients may have to remain intubated if their preoperative medical conditions prevent early postoperative extubation. Furthermore, patients with inadequate blood gas values, elevated intracranial pressure (ICP), hemodynamic instability, or patients who are hypothermic may also have to remain intubated. If there is any question as to whether or not the patient will tolerate extubation, he or she should remain intubated.

Supplemental oxygen is usually administered during transport because as many as 30% to 50% of patients will develop transient hypoxemia with saturations below 90% while breathing room air during transport. Patients with significant underlying pulmonary dysfunction may do best being transported in the head-up position, while those at high-risk for upper-airway bleeding or vomiting may do best in the lateral position. In the PACU, a full report is made to the staff assuming care of the patient. This report should include a pertinent past medical history, a review of all preoperative and intraoperative medications, a history of allergies, and the patient's intraoperative course including blood loss, fluid administration, urine output, and any special events or complications that may have occurred. The clinician must remain with the patient until the patient's condition is stable and patient care responsibilities are transferred to the appropriate PACU personnel.

RESPIRATORY COMPLICATIONS

Respiratory complications are the most common complication in the PACU, and they are usually related to airway obstruction, hypoventilation, or hypoxemia.

Airway Obstruction

The most common cause of airway obstruction in the unconscious patient is the tongue falling backward against the posterior pharynx, which occludes the airway. This condition is manifested by absence of breath sounds, intercostal and suprasternal retractions, and paradoxical chest movement. Under normal conditions, the abdomen and chest should rise together during inspiration. However, if the airway is obstructed, the chest descends as the abdomen rises during inspiration giving this paradoxical rocking motion of the chest. Airway obstruction caused by the tongue usually responds to administration of 100% oxygen by mask with neck extension, accompanied by a jaw-thrust. Insertion of a nasal and/or oral airway may also be necessary.

Laryngospasm is another important cause of airway obstruction. Spasm of the vocal cords may occur during emergence from anesthesia or shortly after extubation, and may be precipitated by blood or secretions in the airway. Simple airway measures such as those outlined earlier should be instituted, as well as suctioning of the oropharynx. Refractory laryngospasm may need to be treated with a small dose of succinylcholine (10–20 mg) and temporary bag-mask ventilation with 100% oxygen. Reintubation may also be necessary to secure the airway.

Other causes of airway obstruction include swelling of the tongue. This condition may result from veinous outflow obstruction, particularly in patients operated on in the prone position for protracted periods or in those positioned with extreme neck flexion. The oral airway, if left in place for the duration of the operation, may also interfere with proper veinous drainage of the tongue. Time should be permitted before extubation to allow the edema to subside. Upper airway obstruction can also occur in patients with a history of obstructive sleep apnea caused by enlarged anatomic structures. Remnants of a surgical throat packing must always be considered as a possible cause of airway obstruction.

Expanding wound hematomas must always be considered as a possible cause of airway obstruction after surgery involving the thyroid, the carotid artery, or a neck dissection. Despite the distorted airway anatomy, endotracheal intubation may still be possible. Reopening of the wound may be necessary to relieve the airway compression. A cricothyrotomy may also be necessary should reintubation prove impossible, even with reopening of the wound.

Airway obstruction can also occur because of glottic or subglottic edema. Glottic edema can result from surgery involving this area, trauma caused by intubation, or toxic or allergic reactions. Inspiratory stridor is the hallmark of this condition. The obstruction is worsened during inspiration when the extrathoracic tracheal wall is pulled inward by the negative pressure in the airway. It is important to remember that a decrease in stridor may not represent clinical improvement but rather, less air movement. Subglottic edema is more common in children because of the rigid, cricoid cartilage being the narrowest region of the pediatric airway. Treatment of these conditions includes administration of humidified oxygen, inhalation of racemic epinephrine, and intravenous dexamethasone.

Bilateral vocal cord paralysis must also be considered as a possible cause of airway obstruction, especially if the procedure involved the area of the recurrent laryngeal nerves. Unilateral vocal cord paralysis should not result in complete airway obstruction.

Bronchospasm

True bronchospasm and airway hyperreactivity can occur, but the clinician must be aware that not all wheezing is caused by bronchospasm. For example, airway obstruction may present as inspiratory wheezing. In this case, extrathoracic obstruction is worsened by the negative pressure of inspiration, which tends to bring laryngeal surfaces closer together. Wheezing can also occur with pulmonary edema either from a cardiogenic (high-pulmonary venous pressures) or noncardiogenic (increased permeability) cause. Cardiogenic causes are unlikely in the absence of underlying cardiac dysfunction. Special causes of noncardiogenic pulmonary edema in the neurosurgical patient include edema resulting from venous air embolism and neurogenic pulmonary edema. Neurogenic pulmonary edema is thought to be caused by a high catecholamine state and may be associated with acute rises in ICP. Other causes of noncardiogenic pulmonary edema include pulmonary aspiration, allergic reactions to drugs or transfusion components, sepsis, and postobstructive pulmonary edema. Pulmonary edema can mimic bronchospasm because the small airways are mechanically compressed by peribronchial edema. In addition, wheezing can occur from obstruction of the endotracheal tube by mucus, a clot, a foreign body, a kinked endotracheal tube, an overinflated cuff, or by a biting patient. Pneumothorax and endobronchial intubation must also be considered in the differential diagnosis of wheezing.

Once bronchospasm has been properly identified and other causes of bronchospasm have been ruled out, appropriate pharmacologic treatment should be instituted. Treatment includes humidified 100% oxygen and the following drugs as clinically indicated:

1. Inhaled β-2-agonists: nebulized metaproterenol (0.2–0.3 ml in 2 ml normal saline) or isoethrine (0.5 ml in 2 ml normal saline).
2. Anticholinergics: glycopyrrolate 0.4 to 1 mg intravenous (IV) or nebulized glycopyrrolate 0.4 to 1 mg in 2 ml normal saline. This agent will decrease secretion volume without increasing viscocity.
3. Corticosteroids: Hydrocortisone 2 to 3 mg/kg IV or equivalent dose of another preparation. These agents are not useful for acute bronchospasm because they may require 4 to 6 hours to show a clinical effect.
4. In the intubated patient, lidocaine 1 to 1.5 mg/kg IV or fentanyl 1 to 2 mcg/kg may decrease reactivity to the endotracheal tube. In cases of severe bronchospasm, deeper anesthesia may be required. The inhaled agents can be used to treat severe refractory bronchospasm. Isoflurane, enflurane, and halothane are nearly equally potent bronchodilators, so the choice of drug should be made for other considerations.
5. Parenteral β-2-agonists: Terbutaline 0.25 mg subcutaneous.
6. Intravenous β-2-agonists: isopreterenol or epinephrine. Infusions should start at 0.5 mcg/min and titrate. As with parenteral β-2 agonists, tachyarrhythmias and myocardial ischemia are possible so careful monitoring is important.

Hypoventilation

Hypoventilation is common following general anesthesia and is usually of little clinical significance. However, hypoventilation can become significant when the $PaCO_2$ rises above 60 mm Hg, resulting in profound somnolence, airway obstruction, and weakness. As the respiratory acidosis progresses, tachycardia, cardiac irritability, and circulatory depression can ensue.

Hypoventilation, with resultant hypercarbia, occurs because of a variety of different causes. Any neurosurgical procedure that leads to injury of the central respiratory centers may lead to hypoventilation, with subsequent hypoxemia and hypercarbia. The control of respiration involves pathways within the reticular formation of the medulla and the ventrolateral portions of the spinothalamic tract of the cervical cord, as well as two pontine areas, the apneustic and pneumotactic centers. In addition, patients with a history of sleep apnea may manifest disturbances of central control of respiration; close observation in the immediate postoperative period is imperative. Clearly, residual depressant effects of anesthetic agents is the most common cause of hypoventilation in the PACU. In fact, some patients may be particularly prone to the respiratory depressant effects of the potent inhalational agents, narcotics, benzodiazepines, and barbiturates. Naloxone in dosages of 20 to 40 mcg can be carefully administered to reverse narcotic-induced respiratory depression. However, renarcotization must be closely watched for, as well as the possible development of hypertension, dysrhythmias, and even pulmonary edema from naloxone. Flumazenil may be useful in reversing the effects of benzodiazepines if these agents are thought to be contributing significantly to hypoventilation.

Postoperative hypoventilation can occur secondary to residual neuromuscular blockade. This may be from incomplete reversal of neuromuscular blocking agents because of inadequate pharmacologic reversal or extreme sensitivity to the relaxants. In either case, the trachea should remain intubated until the patient demonstrates adequate muscle strength by being able to stick out the tongue or sustain a headlift for at least 5 seconds. Myasthenia gravis and the Eaton-Lambert Syndrome, as well as other neuromuscular diseases, may cause extreme sensitivity to muscle relaxants, and the possibility of a pseudocholinesterase deficiency should be considered after a prolonged neuromuscular blockade from succinylcholine. Other causes of weakness may also need to be considered such as preexisting myopathies, hypermagnesemia, or hypercalcemia. Hypercarbia should also be ruled out as a cause of muscle weakness. A blood gas determination or the use of end-tidal gas monitoring may be helpful in this case.

Hypoxemia

As with hypoventilation, mild hypoxemia is relatively common after general anesthesia. Fortunately, the routine use of the pulse oximeter in the PACU allows early detection and treatment. Hypoxemia in the recovery room usually results from increased intrapulmonary shunting caused by a decreased functional residual capacity, hypoventilation, or, sometimes, both. Hypoxemia must be suspected in any patient with unexplained agitation, cardiac irritability, obtundation, or bradycardia.

Many patients come to surgery with underlying pulmonary dysfunction such as chronic bronchitis and chronic obstructive pulmonary disease (COPD). These patients may be particularly susceptible to postoperative hypoxemia. In healthy patients undergoing surgical procedures not involving the abdomen or thorax, lung volumes may be reduced by one half for approximately 4 hours after general anesthesia. As a result, V/Q mismatching may be exacerbated, especially in patients with already-diminished pulmonary reserves. In this group of patients, resting hypercarbia (P_aCO_2 >45 mm Hg) noted on a preoperative arterial blood gas may be a good indicator for the development of postoperative pulmonary problems. Other possible causes of hypoxemia include pulmonary edema caused by cardiogenic or noncardiogenic factors and pulmonary embolization. The possibility of a pneumothorax must always be considered, especially following any retroperitoneal or intraabdominal procedure in which the diaphragm may have been penetrated, and following central line placements, rib fractures, and upper-extremity regional anesthesia.

As the etiology of hypoxemia is being evaluated and treated, the FiO_2 should be increased either through nasal prongs, face mask, or endotracheal intubation, as clinically indicated. In the intubated patient, positive end-expiratory airway pressure (PEEP) may be used in the mechanically ventilated patient or continuous positive airway pressure (CPAP) may be used in the spontaneously breathing patient to improve oxygenation. Continuous positive airway pressure can also be applied by mask in the unintubated patient. However, gastric distension and pulmonary aspiration are possible consequences, so CPAP should only be used in the fully awake patient.

• CARDIOVASCULAR COMPLICATIONS

Hypertension

Hypertension is a common occurrence in the PACU. The most common causes include untreated or poorly treated preoperative hypertension, pain, bladder distension, and discomfort associated with the presence of the endotracheal tube. In addition, causes such as hypoxemia, hypercarbia, and metabolic acidosis should be sought and treated. Mild hypertension rarely requires treatment.

Severe hypertension can precipitate cerebral hemorrhage, myocardial ischemia, heart failure, and postoperative bleeding. In patients with raised ICP, hypertension must be treated to a degree that lowers ICP without causing further cerebral ischemia by decreasing cerebral perfusion pressure (CPP). Before instituting pharmacologic treatment, the clinician should rule out other causes of hypertension such as pain, shivering, bladder distension, hypothermia causing peripheral vasoconstriction, hypercapnia, hypoxia, or residual vasopressor effects. A serious cause of hypertension in the neurosurgical patient is the "Cushing reflex," which involves extreme blood pressure elevations, along with bradycardia and an increase in ICP. This may signal the possibility of brain-stem herniation and demands immediate surgical attention. Treating the hypertension pharmacologically in these patients may actually be detrimental because it may decrease CPP. Again, the accuracy of the blood pressure determination must be assured. For example, an invasive blood pressure measurement, with the transducer placed below the left atrium, will falsely elevate the reading. Once the clinician has confirmed the diagnosis of hypertension and determined its etiology, treatment is started with a variety of pharmacologic agents, based on specific, clinical considerations.

Alpha- and β-blockers can be used successfully to lower blood pressure. Propranolol in 0.5-mg increments or metoprolol in 5-mg increments can be administered intravenously and titrated to effect. Labetolol, a combined α- and β-blocker may be the best choice because of its rapid onset, usually less than 5 minutes. It reduces blood pressure by decreasing cardiac output and systemic vascular resistance. The β_1 effect of the drug allows preservation and, possibly, reduction of myocardial oxygen consumption by preventing any reflex tachycardia. The α_1 effect causes a reduction in afterload, thus, diminishing myocardial wall tension. These drugs are limited by their relatively prolonged half-life, as well as their potential for causing bronchoconstriction and cardiac depression. Esmolol, an intravenous, short-acting, cardioselective β-blocker, may be a desirable agent in cases in which fast dissipation is advantageous. This drug has a rapid onset and is metabolized primarily by esterases in the erythrocyte cytosol. It is rapidly eliminated, even in patients with impaired renal or hepatic function. The clinician must be aware that the administration of β-blockers can blunt the normal hemodynamic response to acute postoperative blood loss.

Direct-acting vasodilators, such as sodium nitroprusside (SNP), are often used postoperatively to control hypertension. Sodium nitroprusside is potent, acts rapidly, and has a short elimination half-life upon termination of the infusion. The dose of this drug is in the range of 0.5 mcg/kg/min to 5 mcg/kg/min. Its mechanism of action is primarily through arteriolar dilation mediated by nitric oxide. Because of it's potency, SNP should only be used when an arterial line is in place. Elderly and hypovolemic patients may be sensitive to the hypotensive effects of this drug. In addition, SNP impairs hypoxic pulmonary vasoconstriction and inhibits platelet aggregation. SNP can cause cyanide toxicity, so doses should be kept below 8 mcg/kg/min. Cyanide, a breakdown product of SNP, is toxic because it interferes with tissue-oxygen utilization by blocking the action of cytochrome oxidase. Tachyphylaxis is often the first sign of toxicity. Other manifestations of toxicity are metabolic acidosis, hypotension, and an increased, mixed venous-oxygen saturation. Treatment of SNP toxicity includes discontinuation of the drug, hemodynamic support, and IV administration of sodium nitrite, 5 mg/kg, followed by IV sodium thiosulfate, 150 mg/kg, in cases of severe toxicity.

Rebound hypertension and reflex tachycardia can be a problem following the use of SNP because SNP-induced hypotension increases renin excretion, which stimulates the production of angiotensin I and the potent vasoconstrictor angiotensin II. This rebound effect can be limited by slowly tapering the SNP infusion, as well as by adding a β-blocking agent or angiotensin-converting enzyme (ACE) inhibitor. In addition, SNP should be used with extreme caution in those at risk for intracranial hypertension. Sodium nitroprusside can cause a rise in ICP, especially in those in whom intracranial compliance is decreased. Although SNP decreases cerebral blood flow (CBF), it may increase cerebral blood volume and, hence, ICP by dilating cerebral capacitance vessels.

Nitroglycerin (at a dose of 0.25–10 mcg/kg/min IV) can also be used for blood pressure control. It offers the advantages of a short plasma half-life (2 minutes) as well as a more favorable distribution of coronary blood flow than SNP in patients with coronary artery disease. It acts by dilating capacitance vessels, rather than resistance vessels, thus, decreasing venous return, stroke volume, and cardiac output. Nitroglycerin is less predictable than SNP in its antihypertensive effect and may not achieve the desired blood pressure reduction, especially in younger patients. The drug may increase ICP by the same mechanism as SNP, but it produces no toxic metabolites nor rebound hypertension when discontinued.

Trimethaphan, a ganglionic blocker with a short plasma half-life of 1 to 2 minutes, causes relaxation of both capacitance and resistance vessels. It is rapidly inactivated by plasma cholinesterase, then renally excreted. Unlike nitroglycerin and SNP, trimethaphan rarely raises ICP, because the ganglionic blockade usually spares the cerebral circulation. Trimethaphan can cause histamine release, bronchospasm, tachyphylaxis, and fixed, dilated pupils, which may confuse the neurologic examination postoperatively. The infusion is begun at 1 mg/min and titrated to effect. Other drugs such as hydralazine, in doses of 5 to 20 mg doses IV, and nifedipine 10 to 20 mg sublingually, can be used to treat postoperative hypertension. However, they may be more difficult to titrate to effect and also may increase ICP. Enalaprilate 1.25 to 2.5 mg IV can also be used, and it has little effect on CBF.

Hypotension

The most common cause of postoperative hypotension is hypovolemia. Other causes of hypotension include the persistent effect of anesthetic agents or antihypertensives, adrenal or thyroid failure, peripheral vasodilation from rewarming of a hypothermic patient, cardiac tamponade, or tension pneumothorax related to central-venous catheter insertion, sepsis, anaphylaxis, profound myocardial damage, hypoxia, and hypocalcemia.

Many methods exist to gauge the adequacy of intravascular volume. The clinical assessment begins with a review of the patient's preoperative history and intraoperative course, with special emphasis on medications and fluids received, as well as blood lost. Before continuing with evaluation or treatment, the clinician must be sure that the diagnosis of hypotension is real and not an artifact from an erroneous measurement. Oliguria, supine hypotension, tachycardia, and significant variation in pulse pressure with positive-pressure ventilation, all support the diagnosis of hypovolemia. The development of lactic acidosis may indicate severe hypovolemia with systemic hypoperfusion. The clinician must be aware that normotension may represent relative hypotension in the chronically hypertensive patient. Patients with autonomic dysfunction, such as those with long-standing diabetes mellitus, or patients on antihypertensive therapy, may not exhibit the expected cardiovascular response to hypovolemia. In addition, they may be more subject to hypotension caused by failure of the compensatory baroreceptor responses.

Treatment is directed at correcting the underlying cause of hypotension. In some instances, a central venous-pressure or pulmonary-artery catheter may be required to diagnose the etiology and appropriately treat the hypotension. Transthoracic or transesophageal echocardiography may also be a useful diagnostic tool. In the case of hypovolemia, a fluid challenge with an isotonic crystalloid or colloid solution, or blood, is used to replace volume as clinically indicated. The legs may be raised in the acute setting to provide autotransfusion of volume into the central circulation. The Trendelenburg position is generally contraindicated in the patient at risk for increased ICP, because it may actually decrease CPP. In addition, this position has not been shown to be effective in raising the central circulating blood volume. A vasopressor such as ephedrine (5–10 mg IV) or phenylephrine (25–50 mcg IV) may be judiciously used as a temporizing measure to increase blood pressure, but it should not replace adequate volume resuscitation.

Arrhythmias

Arrhythmias are a common postoperative occurrence, and may be caused by hypoxemia, hypercarbia, acid-base disturbances, hypokalemia from diuretic therapy, myocardial ischemia, pain, stress, cranial nerve injuries, and hypothermia. The clinician should investigate and treat underlying causes of the arrhythmia, if possible, and ensure that the disturbance does not represent a serious threat to the patient.

Premature atrial contractions (PACs) are not usually a serious rhythm disturbance, and rarely necessitate treatment. Premature ventricular contractions (PVCs) may be benign, although the common causes mentioned previously should be ruled out. Polymorphic, multifocal PVCs should be aggressively investigated because they are often a sign of significant myocardial ischemia. Frequent PVCs that cause hemodynamic compromise should also be treated. If a central venous catheter is in place, its position should be checked because PVCs may result from the catheter irritating the endocardium. Treatment includes the correction of underlying abnormalities as well as lidocaine, 1.5 mg/kg bolus IV, followed by an infusion of 1 to 4 mg/min. Lidocaine may cause significant sedation.

Sinus bradycardia can result from residual β-blockade, administration of narcotics and cholinesterase inhibitors, as well as underlying sinus-node dysfunction, especially in the elderly population. An ominous cause of bradycardia is the Cushing reflex. This reflex was described in 1901 by Harvey Cushing. The classic triad involves bradycardia, which is often irregular, systemic hypertension, and raised ICP. The reflex is caused by compression of the blood supply to the medulla. This results in an increased catecholamine release from the brainstem in an attempt to restore CBF. As systemic blood pressure increases, the arterial baroreceptors cause a reflex bradycardia.

Supraventricular tachyarrhythmias (SVTs) can occur. Therefore, it is important to distinguish from atrial fibrillation, atrial flutter, sinus tachycardia, and ventricular tachycardia, all of which may require different treatment approaches and have different etiologies. Supraventricular tachyarrhythmia can be treated with a β-blocker such as esmolol (0.5 mg/kg IV), adenosine (6 mg IV), verapamil (5 mg IV), as well as carotid sinus massage. Diltiazem has also proved to be useful for rate control (0.25 mg/kg IV followed by 0.35 mg/kg IV, if needed). Cardioversion can be used, if necessary, in the unstable patient.

Atrial fibrillation is characterized by fragmented and disorganized atrial electrical activity, and is often caused by disease processes that produce stretching of the atria. Treatment includes controlling the heart rate by cardioversion or drug administration. If the patient is hemodynamically unstable, cardioversion should be used, beginning with 50 watts (joules) and ensuring synchronization of the defibrillator to avoid initiating ventricular fibrillation. Drug therapy includes digoxin (0.125–0.25 mg IV every 15 minutes to a total dosage of 1 mg), verapamil, diltiazem, or β-adrenergic blocking agents.

Myocardial Ischemia

The detection and treatment of myocardial ischemia in the PACU may be of extreme importance because perioperative myocardial infarctions have a higher mortality rate than those occurring in other settings. Myocardial ischemia may be diagnosed by electrocardiogram (ECG) with new ST-segment depression or elevation, T-wave inversion, the appearance of new Q waves, or certain arrhythmias. It must be kept in mind, however, that T-wave changes found in the PACU may not reflect myocardial ischemia. Surgery in close proximity to the stellate ganglia may alter their autonomic output; this may cause the observed ECG phenomena. In addition, stress, cold, electrolyte abnormalities, raised ICP, temperature, and drug effects can alter the ECG nonspecifically.

The complaint of substernal chest pain in the patient sufficiently awake to relay this information, or a rise in pulmonary artery diatolic blood pressure if a pulmonary-artery catheter is in place may also be suggestive of ischemia. If ischemia is suspected from the ECG-monitor display, a 12-lead ECG must be obtained and compared to the preoperative study. Transesophageal echocardiography in the anesthetized patient or transthoracic echocardiography in the awake patient may be used as a more sensitive tool to confirm the diagnosis of ischemia by demonstrating diagnostic focal wall motion and wall-thickening abnormalities. As with the ECG, comparison with a preoperative study may be helpful.

Treatment of ischemia involves adjusting the delicate balance between myocardial oxygen demand and supply. Supply can be improved by administering oxygen to the patient and maintaining an adequate circulating blood volume, thus, ensuring adequate oxygen-carrying capacity. Intravenous nitroglycerin begun at 0.25 mcg/kg/min may provide coronary artery vasodilation. In addition, treatment of hypotension will ensure an adequate coronary perfusion pressure.

Demand can be decreased by carefully reducing preload, afterload, and heart rate without inducing hypotension. Nitroglycerin, again, may be helpful in reducing preload, and SNP or hydralazine can reduce afterload. Heart rate can be reduced with β-blockade. However, because cardiac output is the product of stroke volume and heart rate, beta blockade can profoundly depress cardiac output. Consequently, a short-acting drug such as esmolol is helpful to determine the cardiovascular response to β-blockade. If favorable, longer-acting drugs can be used. It may be wise to consult a cardiologist to aid in the postoperative care of a patient with suspected or active myocardial ischemia.

HYPERTHERMIA

Hyperthermia is a relatively uncommon problem in the recovery room. It may be seen in patients, especially small children, who have been in a warm operating room covered with drapes for a long period of time. The clinician should investigate whether a fever existed preoperatively. Malignant hyperthermia must be ruled out because this may present in the recovery room. In addition to fever, these patients may exhibit unexplained tachycardia, hypotension, and an increased carbon dioxide production. An arterial blood gas usually shows a mixed respiratory and metabolic acidosis. The administration of phenothiazines such as chlorpromazine, or butyrophenones such as droperidol and haloperidol, can cause malignant neuroleptic syndrome. Anticholinergic agents, especially the tertiary amines such as atropine, can cross into the central nervous system (CNS) and cause toxicity manifested by fever, flushing, delerium, and anhydrosis. Treatment consists of the administration of physostigmine, 1 to 4 mg IV. Meperidine, in combination with monoamine oxidase inhibitors, may cause hyperpyrexia with seizures and death. Neurogenic hyperthermia may be associated with brainstem or hypothalamic damage, or with blood in the ventricles or in the subarachnoid space. It can occur after resection of a large pituitary tumor or craniopharyngioma. Finally, other medical conditions that can cause fever include atelectasis, aspiration pneumonia or other infections, thyroid storm, and a pheochromocytoma.

Fever should be treated to improve patient comfort, as well as to avoid an increase in carbon dioxide production. In addition, fever can cloud the patient's mental status and interfere with the neurologic examination. Acetaminophen can be administered per os (PO) or per rectum (PR) at a dose of 650 to 1000 mg. In children, a dosage of 10 to 15 mg/kg is suggested. Uncovering the patient and the use of cooling blankets may also be helpful.

HYPOTHERMIA

Hypothermia is a common finding postoperatively because of heat loss from convection, conduction, and radiation, as well as infusion of cold intravenous solutions. In addition, compensatory thermoregulatory mechanisms initiated by the hypothalamus are suppressed during general anesthesia. Moderate hypothermia may also be used intentionally in the neurosurgical patient to protect the brain from ischemic injury. Severe hypothermia can predispose to ventricular arrhythmias, and even mild hypothermia can prolong emergence from general anesthesia. Shivering can increase oxygen consumption by as much as 400%, possibly placing the patient with coronary artery disease at risk for myocardial ischemia. The hypothermic patient can be warmed with warming lights, a warming blanket, covering the head, and warmed intravenous fluids.

OLIGURIA

Postoperative oliguria is most frequently caused by hypovolemia. First, obstructive causes like a kinked Foley catheter or urinary retention should be ruled out before a fluid challenge is given to optimize the patient's intravascular volume and to prevent prerenal causes of acute tubular necrosis. The use of diuretics to increase urine output in the face of hypovolemia is dangerous, and may actually precipitate further renal damage. If the etiology of oliguria is unclear, appropriate laboratory studies should be performed (urine sodium, urine creatinine, urine osmolarity, urine specific gravity, and serum sodium and creatinine). The measurement of central venous pressures may be indicated if oliguria persists.

NAUSEA AND VOMITING

Nausea and vomiting are relatively common following general anesthesia and often do not require pharmacologic interventions. However, nausea and vomiting should be treated promptly in some patients because they may cause an increase in systemic blood pressure and ICP. Refractory nausea and vomiting may also be caused by intracranial pathology with an increase in ICP. The possibility of acute hydrocephalus, cerebral edema, or intracranial hematoma formation should always be kept in mind.

Commonly used drugs to treat nausea and vomiting include droperidol (Inapsine), 0.625 mg to 2.5 mg IV, promethazine (Phenergan), 12.5 mg to 25 mg IV or IM, prochlorperazine (Compazine), 5 to 10 mg IV or intramuscularly (IM), and metoclopramide (Reglan), 10 mg IV. All of these agents are dopamine antagonists and may cause dystonic reactions or exacerbations of Parkinson's disease. Dystonic reactions may be treated with diphenhydramine (Benadryl), 25 to 100 mg IV or IM or benztropine (Cogentin), 1 to 2 mg IV. The new serotonin-antagonist ondansetron has also been used successfully in doses of 4 mg IV in adults, or 0.15 mg/kg IV in children. In some studies it has been shown to be more effective in preventing and treating nausea and vomiting than both droperidol and metoclopramide.

DELAYED EMERGENCE

The rapidity of emergence from an inhalational agent is directly proportional to the alveolar ventilation and indirectly proportional to the blood solubility of the agent. As the duration of anesthesia increases, other factors become important such as total tissue uptake, and the average concentration of the agent used. Consequently, a prolonged deep anesthetic with a relatively soluble agent, such as halothane, may result in a slower emergence.

Emergence from intravenous anesthetics is dependant on the pharmacokinetics of the medications used. Recovery from the effects of most of these agents is dependant on redistribution. However, as the doses increase, the termination of the effects becomes increasingly dependant on the elimination half-life of the drug. Consequently, renal and hepatic disease, along with advanced age, can lead to a delayed emergence.

The most common cause of delayed emergence is residual anesthetic drug effect caused by either absolute or relative drug overdose. In addition, anesthetic effects can be potentiated by prior drug ingestion such as alcohol. Causes such as hypoxemia, hypercarbia, hypotension, hypoglycemia, sepsis, acid-base, and electrolyte disturbances must all be considered. Hypothermia can also greatly potentiate the effect of anesthetic agents. Finally, stroke can lead to persistent obtundation and must be considered.

DISCHARGE CRITERIA

To be suitable for discharge from the PACU, patients must meet a variety of criteria to ensure their continued safety. They must be easily arousable with verbal stimuli, fully oriented, and able to maintain and protect the airway. Patients should exhibit hemodynamic stability and have no obvious surgical complications, such as bleeding. Patients should also be reasonably warm and comfortable with minimal nausea and vomiting. They should be observed for respiratory depression for at least 30 minutes following the last dose of parenteral narcotic. In addition, those recovering from spinal or epidural anesthesia should exhibit signs of resolution of both motor and sensory blockade.

BIBLIOGRAPHY

Alon E, Himmelseher S: Ondansetron in the treatment of postoperative vomiting: a randomized, double-blind comparison with droperidol and metoclopramide, *Anesth Analg* 75:561, 1992.

Breslow MJ, et al: Changes in T-wave morphology following anesthesia and surgery: a common recovery room phenomenon, *Anesthesiology* 64:398, 1986.

Craig DB: Postoperative recovery of pulmonary function, *Anesth Analg* 60:46, 1981.

Rinde-Hoffman D, Glasser SP, Arnett DK: Update on nitrate therapy, *J Clin Pharmacol Ther* 31:697, 1991.

Stoelting RK, Dierdorf SF, McCammon RL: *Anesthesia and coexisting disease*, ed 3, New York, 1993, Churchill Livingstone.

Stone DJ: Recovery room care. In Sperry RJ, Stirt JA, Stone DJ, editors: *Manual of Neuroanesthesia:* Philadelphia, 1989, BC Decker.

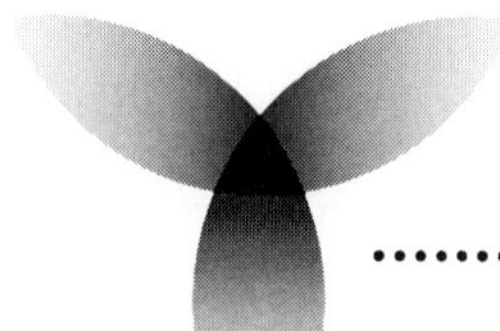

Chapter 42

Acute Postoperative Pain Management

Jerry A. Hall, MD, Burkhard F. Spiekermann, MD

Pain is a subjective experience that varies tremendously from one patient to another. The International Association for the Study of Pain defines pain as "an unpleasant sensory and emotional experience associated with actual or potential tissue damage, or described in terms of such damage." Acute postoperative pain management has evolved over the years from the traditional intramuscular (IM) injection of opioids to include many, often very specialized, treatment modalities. Effective postoperative pain control is now being recognized as an essential aspect of perioperative surgical care. Many hospitals have a postoperative pain management service, usually organized by the anesthesiology department, to continue intraoperative pain management into the postoperative period. The concept of preemptive analgesia establishes that effective postoperative pain control starts preoperatively and, during that time, there it requires a joint effort by surgeons and anesthesiologists.

After a brief introduction to the physiology of nociception and the organism's response to pain, this chapter will give an overview of the many contemporary management options for postoperative pain control, including the various pharmacologic agents available and their routes of administration. Chronic pain management will not be discussed.

• PHYSIOLOGY OF NOCICEPTION

Acute postoperative pain is caused by the noxious stimulus of surgical tissue injury. The initial step in the neuronal pain pathway is initiated by perturbations of cutaneous, deep or visceral nociceptors, that is, receptors that respond to painful stimuli. Most nociceptors are free nerve endings, which respond to chemical, thermal, and mechanical tissue destruction. The chemical mediators of pain include a long list of neuropeptides (e.g., substance P, somatostatin, calcitonin gene-related peptide [CGRP], leukotrienes, histamine, serotonin, bradykinin) and excitatory amino acids (e.g., glutamate). Sensory impulses travel through the axons of the afferent neurons (A-δ and C fibers) and enter the spinal cord through the dorsal horn, where the axons synapse with second-order neurons, primarily in lamina I and V of the dorsal horn. *Wide dynamic range* (WDR) neurons in lamina V are important in modulating the pain response and are thought to be responsible for the "wind-up" phenomenon (i.e., an augmentation of the neuronal response that results from repetitive application of the same stimulus and which results in increased pain sensation). The axons of most second-order neurons cross the midline and travel on the contralateral side of the spinal cord in the *medial (paleo-)* and *lateral (neo-) spinothalamic tracts*, where they synapse primarily in the *medial* and *posterolateral thalamic nuclei*, respectively. The neospinothalamic tract is responsible for transmitting the discriminatory aspects of pain, whereas the paleospinothalamic tract mediates the autonomic and emotional aspects of pain. Third-order neurons send fibers from the thalamus to the *somatosensory cortex*. Figure 42-1 is a schematic presentation of the pain pathways described.

In addition to these "classic" pain pathways there are many alternate and collateral pathways, as well as highly active segmental and suprasegmental reflex responses. Anxiety and emotional stress associated with pain will activate hypothalamic centers and may trigger additional sympathetic and neuroendocrine responses in the patient experiencing pain. Inhibitory and excitatory modulation of the neuronal pain response occurs at various peripheral and cortical levels in the nervous system. Inhibitory modulation at the level of the nociceptor, in the spinal cord and supraspinally, is the goal of all postoperative pain management.

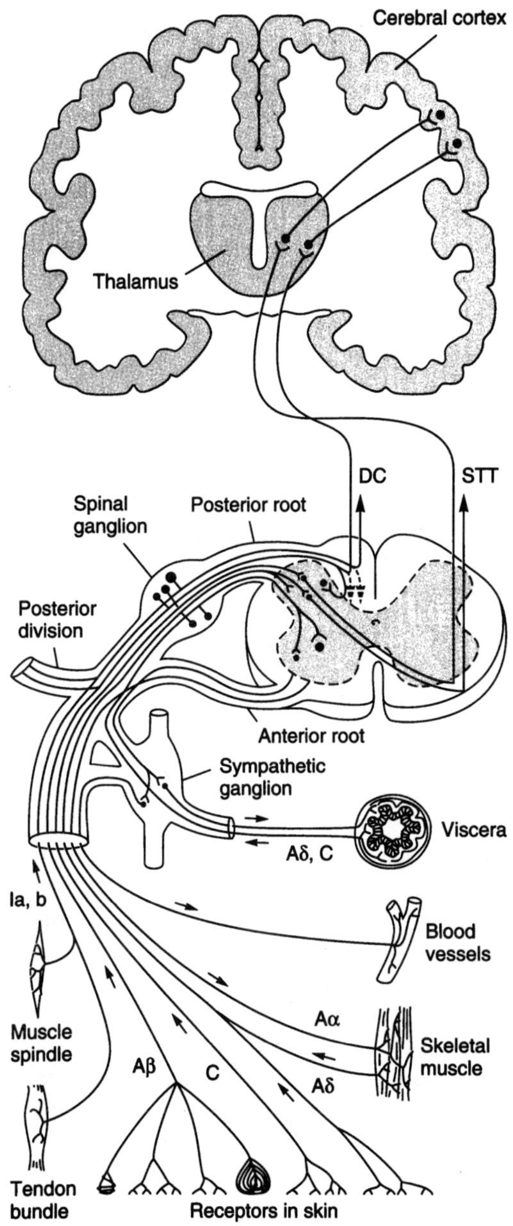

Figure 42-1
Diagram of the primary pain pathways. DC, dorsal column; STT, spinothalamic tract. See text for details.

Aside from effective analgesia, the most important factors modifying postoperative pain are related to the site, nature, and duration of the surgery, the physiologic and psychologic condition of the patient, his or her preoperative physical and emotional preparation, the presence of any surgical complications, and the quality of anesthetic management and postoperative care. It is, therefore, not surprising that the most effective postoperative pain management begins in the preoperative period.

PHYSIOLOGIC RESPONSES TO PAIN

Aside from the adverse psychologic and emotional trauma caused by acute and prolonged pain, the body's physiologic "stress response" to postoperative pain includes all organ systems, contributes to postoperative morbidity and mortality, and may be responsible for a prolonged hospital stay. This implies that aggressive postoperative pain management is not only compassionate, but is an integral element in facilitating and expediting postoperative recovery.

The magnitude of the body's stress response is related to the invasiveness of the operative procedure and is most pronounced after thoracic and major abdominal operations. With currently available techniques in pain management, major reductions in this stress response and its associated adverse side effects are possible.

Endocrine and Metabolic Effects

Heightened sympathetic tone and hypothalamic activation caused by pain stimulates adrenal catecholamine release and the secretion of catabolic hormones (cortisol, growth hormone, glucagon). This causes a state of negative nitrogen balance with glucose intolerance) and lipid and protein breakdown. Increased release of antidiuretic hormone, renin, angiotensin, and aldosterone results in sodium and water retention, which leads to an increase in extracellular fluid.

Cardiovascular Effects

Sympathetic stimulation from pain causes hypertension, tachycardia, an increase in systemic vascular resistance, and cardiac stroke volume. The end result is an increase in myocardial work, which leads to increased myocardial oxygen consumption. Patients with coronary artery disease may not be able to meet such an increase in oxygen demand, which places them at heightened risk for myocardial ischemia.

Respiratory Effects

In addition to the adverse effects of general anesthesia and surgery (as discussed in other previous chapters) on the respiratory system, pain from upper-abdominal and thoracic incisions will cause splinting and poor respiratory efforts, which further compromises adequate pulmonary function. Pain during respiration may result in reduced tidal volumes, ineffective ventilation, and hypercarbia. Atelectasis may be responsible for hypoxemia. Poor pulmonary toilet caused by ineffective coughing and clearing of secretions may lead to postoperative pulmonary infections.

Gastrointestinal Effects

Increased sympathetic discharge from inadequately treated pain increases gastrointestinal sphincter tone and relaxes intestinal smooth muscles. This leads to postoperative ileus and bowel distension. Abdominal distension not only increases the patient's misery but will elevate the diaphragm and contribute further to poor pulmonary mechanics. Postoperative nausea and vomiting are common and may be a direct result of nociceptive input from visceral and abdominal receptors. Hypersecretion of gastric acid may lead to stress ulceration.

Genitourinary Effects

Pain causes ureteral and bladder hypomobility, which leads to urinary retention. Urinary retention itself can be very painful and unpleasant to the patient, often necessitating ureteral catheterization.

Hematologic Effects

Pain interferes with patient movement and bed rest promotes venous thromboembolism. Stress also induces a hypercoagulable state because of an increase in specific coagulation factors, platelet aggregation, and a decrease in fibrinolysis. All these factors may lead to a higher incidence of pulmonary embolism.

Immunologic Effects

The stress response may induce neutropenia and depress reticular, endothelial system function, which increase the risk of postoperative infection.

THE ACUTE PAIN SERVICE

With the increasing complexity and invasiveness of postoperative pain management, many institutions have developed postoperative pain management services, which make comprehensive pain management available to all patients in the hospital. Typically, the Acute Pain Service (APS) is a branch of the anesthesia department and is designed to provide continuous postoperative pain care as an extension of intraoperative pain management. Anesthesiologists with postgraduate training in pain management frequently get involved preoperatively, or at least early during the intraoperative period, to guarantee a smooth transition toward effective postoperative analgesia. At our hospital a dedicated APS team is available on a 24-hour basis to assist with postoperative pain issues. For the APS to function effectively, 24-hour coverage and a short response time are essential. To alleviate the surgeon's reluctance to relinquish part of his or her control over postoperative patient care (i.e., pain management), close cooperation with the surgical team is necessary and should include a detailed discussion of the postoperative pain management plans. Similarly, nurses taking care of the postoperative patient need to be educated in regard to the expectations, limitations, and potential dangers of some of the more interventional types of pain control. To avoid the dangers of duplicating orders for pain medication, *all* pain-related therapeutic interventions should be cleared by the APS. Protocols need to be instituted which specifically outline postoperative pain care. A well-functioning APS has a significant impact on the quality of postoperative patient care. It is our experience that the acceptance by and enthusiasm of patients, surgeons, nurses, and other health care providers has grown steadily over the last years.

THE CONCEPT OF PREEMPTIVE ANALGESIA

Although clinical evidence is not conclusive, there is a substantial amount of experimental evidence showing that the administration of effective intravenous (IV) or regional analgesia *before* surgical trauma decreases postoperative pain. It is thought that preemptive analgesia prevents the development of "wind up," that is, the hyperexcitable state of central neurons after exposure to repetitive noxious afferent input. Preemptive analgesia may decrease postoperative analgesic requirements, prevent the development of phantom limb pain associated with limb amputations, and prevent persistant neuropathic pain states induced by surgical trauma. Early consultation with the pain specialists is important to properly plan for adequate preemptive techniques.

PHARMACOLOGIC AGENTS FOR MANAGEMENT OF POSTOPERATIVE PAIN

There are a number of classes of pharmacologic agents that are appropriate for treating postoperative pain. Traditionally, focus has centered around the use of opioid analgesics. Alternatively, nonopioid analgesics, such as nonsteroidal antiinflammatory agents, acetaminophen, and tramadol, as well as the judicious use of local anesthetics, may provide satisfactory postoperative analgesia.

Opioid Analgesics

Opioid analgesics bind specific receptor sites in the central nervous system (primarily located in the substantia gelatinosa of the dorsal horn of the spinal cord) to inhibit the presynaptic release of neurotransmitters that facilitate nociception. Opioids may be given orally, intramuscularly, intravenously, transmucosally (nasal, oral and rectal), transcutaneously, and through the central neuraxis (epidural and spinal administration). Optimal use of these agents for postoperative pain is frequently limited by unfounded fears and misconceptions regarding the relationship between their use and the development of tolerance, dependence, and addiction.

Tolerance is defined as a decrease in drug effect with repeated administration. The rate of tolerance development depends on several factors, including the dose administered (higher doses promote faster tolerance development), interdose interval (frequent dosing promotes tolerance development), and environmental factors, such as the situation in which the drug is administered. Clinically significant tolerance may develop in the postoperative period, leading to increased demand (and need) for analgesics.

Dependence is a state produced by repeated administration of a drug and is not limited to opioids. It is expressed as an abstinence syndrome, precipitated by cessation of the drug or administration of a reversal agent. The abstinence syndrome associated with opioid use is characterized by lacrimation, rhinorrhea, yawning, and sweating in its early stages, followed by weakness, chills, gooseflesh, nausea and vomiting, muscle aches, involuntary movements, hyperpnea, hyperthermia, and hypertension. These later signs may last for 7 to 10 days. While physical and psychologic dependence on analgesic medications may develop in the postoperative period, it is unusual to see classic withdrawal symptoms. Most patients will spontaneously wean their use of these medications as their postoperative pain decreases.

Addiction is a psychiatric disorder characterized by drug-seeking behavior which places a person at economic, social, or physical risk. It is exceedingly rare to see true drug addiction develop in the course of treatment of routine postoperative pain. It is more common to see the phenomenon called "pseudo-addiction." That is when fear of producing dependence or addiction leads to inadequate prescription of analgesics, which, in turn, leads to increasing patient demands for more analgesics. When this phenomenon is recognized, and adequate analgesia is prescribed, demands for analgesia subside.

Animal studies have suggested that the δ-opioid receptor is most likely responsible for the phenomena of tolerance and dependence associated with opioid administration. There may also be involvement of excitatory amino-acid receptor systems and neuropeptides, such as cholecystokinin. These findings suggest that it may be possible in the future to develop analgesics with greatly attenuated tolerance and dependence properties, while still retaining analgesic efficacy.

The opioid analgesics may be divided into three major classes: opioid agonists for mild-moderate pain, opioid agonists for moderate-severe pain, and opioid agonist-antagonists.

Opioid Agonists for Mild-Moderate Pain

Codeine is a semisynthetic derivative of morphine, formed by methylation of the -OH group on the third carbon of the phenol ring of morphine. Codeine is a prodrug and requires hepatic-enzyme demethylation to morphine for analgesic effect. This conversion is mediated by a subset of the cytochrome P-450 system known as CYP2D6. It is now known that 7% to 10% of the caucasian population has reduced or absent activity of this enzyme system, this absence may account for side effects of profound nausea with the use of codeine. Codeine is available as the pure drug in liquid and solid forms, as well as in combination with acetaminophen as Tylenol #3 or #4. It is dosed on a 4 to 6 hourly schedule.

Hydrocodone is also a synthetic derivative of morphine. Again, it is a prodrug and must be metabolized to an active form before it is effective. It is available only in fixed combinations with acetaminophen (Vicodin, Lortab, Lorcet, Lorcet Plus, Hydrocet, Norcet, and others), or with aspirin (Lortab ASA). This drug is dosed on a 6-hourly schedule.

Oxycodone is another a synthetic derivative of morphine. It is more potent than the other opioids in the mild-moderate class and approximately 7 to 8 times greater in potency than codeine. It is available in pure form (Roxicodone) or in fixed combination with acetaminophen (Percocet, Tylox) or aspirin (Percodan). The somewhat short duration of action requires 4-hourly dosing. There is a controlled-release form of oxycodone (Oxycontin) for long-term analgesic use in special situations. Because of the long duration of action, the routine use of oxycontin for intraoperative pain control is not warranted.

Propoxyphene is a derivative of methadone that is one half to two thirds as potent as codeine. Several studies have unsuccessfully attempted to show that propoxyphene is superior to placebo. Equianalgesic studies have shown propoxyphene to be equivalent in analgesic effect to 600 mg aspirin. Propoxyphene is only available in fixed combinations with aspirin (Darvon) or acetaminophen (Darvocet). Propoxyphene and its metabolite, norpropoxyphene, can accumulate with chronic dosing and may lead to central nervous system (CNS) excitability, confusion, and cardiac toxicity.

This drug has a short duration of action and needs to be dosed every 4 hours. For all of these reasons, propoxyphene is not usually recommended as a primary agent for postoperative analgesia.

Opioid Agonists for Moderate-Severe Pain

Morphine is the prototype opioid for moderate-to-severe pain. Morphine is a naturally occurring product of the opium poppy and is extracted from unripened seeds of the plant. The extract contains several other alkaloids, and morphine must be separated from these. Morphine is usually the initial choice for postoperative analgesia because of its low cost, variety of administration routes, and clinical efficacy. Its duration of action is dependent on the route of administration, with epidural and spinal effects ranging from 12 to 24 hours, compared to IV effects lasting approximately 1 hour. Controlled-release (MS Contin) or sustained-release (Oramorph) preparations of morphine have consistently been shown to be inappropriate for postoperative routine analgesia.

Methadone is a synthetic narcotic, first produced by German chemists during World War II. It has a plasma half-life of 18 to 24 hours, but its clinically useful duration of action is only 6 to 8 hours. Methadone is of equal potency compared to morphine, however, because of its long half-life, it must be titrated slowly and carefully to prevent unintentional overdose from accumulation. Therefore, it is of very limited use in the postoperative setting.

Meperidine (Demerol) has long been used for postoperative analgesia. It is a synthetic opioid originally synthesized for its atropine-like effects. It is structurally dissimilar to other opioids, although it exhibits many of the same effects. Meperidine is available in both oral and parenteral forms, although the oral bioavailability is less than one-half that of the parenteral form. Its duration of action, again, depends on the route of administration, ranging from 1 to 2 hours for IV administration, to approximately 12 hours for epidural administration. Repeated dosing with meperidine leads to accumulation of the metabolite, normeperidine, which has a 12 to 15 hour half-life. It is capable of causing CNS excitation, which can be intense enough to generate seizure activity. This effect may be mediated through dopamine receptors, and is not reversible by opioid antagonists.

Oxymorphone is a synthetic morphine derivative with high potency. It is available in parenteral form (Numorphan) and as a rectal suppository. It is approximately 10 times more potent than morphine. The duration of action of an IM dose is approximately 4 hours, while that of an IV dose is approximately 1 hour.

Hydromorphone (Dilaudid) is another synthetic morphine derivative, with a potency approximately 7 times greater than that of morphine. It is available in both oral and parenteral forms, and the oral bioavailability is approximately one fifth that of the parenteral form. Its duration of action ranges from 30 to 60 minutes for IV administration, to 4 to 5 hours with oral administration.

Fentanyl is a synthetic opioid derived from meperidine. It is approximately 80 to 100 times as potent as morphine and traditionally has been infrequently used outside of the operating room. Fentanyl is becoming more prominent now outside the operating room environment as a component of epidural analgesic infusions for postoperative pain and in IV PCA infusions. It is only available in parenteral form, either injectable (Sublimaze) or transdermal (Duragesic). The IV duration of action is approximately 20 minutes, while that of epidural administration is approximately 1 to 2 hours. Transdermal administration results in highly variable plasma levels, requiring 8 to 12 hours to reach peak plasma levels, with potential residual effects lasting up to 17 hours from the cutaneous reservoir *after* the patch is removed. This makes Duragesic an unwieldy and potentially dangerous form of analgesia; use for postoperative analgesia is not recommended.

Agonist-Antagonist Opioid Analgesics

Most drugs in the agonist-antagonist class of agents act as agonists at the kappa opioid receptor and antagonists at the mu opioid receptor. Interest in these agents for postoperative analgesia comes from their ability to achieve analgesia without μ-related side effects, such as respiratory depression, somnolence, and nausea/vomiting. While this profile is attractive, most of these agents exhibit a ceiling effect for analgesia, above which, further dosing does not increase analgesia. These opioids are most commonly used in the obstetric suite and as supplementary analgesics with epidural analgesia techniques. These agents should be used with caution in patients on chronic opioid regimens, because they have the potential to precipitate opioid withdrawal.

Pentazocine (Talwin) was the first agent in this class of drugs, representing an attempt to produce a synthetic analgesic compound with little abuse potential. It is nearly as potent as codeine. It is associated with dysphoric effects, which limit its clinical usefulness. The duration of action after oral administration is approximately 2 to 3 hours.

Dezocine (Dalgan) is an agonist-antagonist with potency and duration of action similar to morphine. It is available only in IV form and has a duration of action of approximately 1 hour. Above a dose of 30 mg/70kg, it does not exhibit further analgesia nor does it produce progressive respiratory depression.

Nalbuphine (Nubain) is an agonist-antagonist opioid with higher antagonistic potency at mu receptors than pentazocine and less propensity for dysphoria. It is available only in parenteral form, and typically lasts 3 to 6 hours after parenteral administration. Doses below 160 mg per 24 hours rarely result in dysphoric side effects.

Butorphanol (Stadol) is similar to pentazocine in effect. Like pentazocine, it can increase pulmonary artery pressure and cardiac work in analgesic doses. Its duration of action is approximately 3 to 4 hours. Butorphanol has recently become available in a nasal transmucosal form, which appears to have rapid onset, short duration of action, and moderately high abuse potential.

Table 42-1 lists approximate relative potencies of various opioid agents.

Nonopioid Analgesics

Nonsteroidal antiinlammatory agents (NSAIAs). Possibly, the most frequently used NSAIA in the perioperative period is ketorolac (Toradol). It is the only parenteral NSAIA available, and a 30-mg intramuscular (IM) dose is reported to be equianalgesic to 10 mg of IM morphine. Controversy surrounding the use of this agent in the postoperative period centers around its effects on platelet function and renal function.

Table 42-1. Relative Potencies of Opioid Analgesics

DRUG	EPIDURAL DOSE (MG)	INTRAVENOUS DOSE (MG)	ORAL DOSE (MG)	DURATION OF ACTION (HR) E/I/O		
				E	I	O
Morphine	1*	10*	30	12–24	1–2	2–4
Methadone	—	10	20	—	4–6	6–8
Meperidine	10*	100*	300	4–12	1	3
Oxymorphone	—	1	—	—	1–2	—
Hydromorphone	0.15*	1.5*	7.5	2–4	1–2	4
Fentanyl	1 mcg/kg*	0.1*	—	1–2	1	—
Codeine	—	—	90–180	—	—	3–4
Hydrocodone	—	—	180	—	—	4–6
Oxycodone	—	—	30	—	—	4
Propoxyphene	—	—	180–360	—	—	4–6

* The epidural-intravenous equivalencies are estimates based on clinical practice. There are currently no studies comparing doses for clinical effect.

Because of the ability of ketorolac (and other NSAIAs) to block the function of cyclooxygenase, and, thus, interfere with production of prostaglandins and thromboxanes (specifically thromboxane A_2), which are active in hemostasis, there is a theoretical concern that use of ketorolac in the postoperative period may lead to an increase in surgical and gastrointestinal (GI) bleeding. Multiple studies have shown that this effect does not translate into clinically significant bleeding. However, ketorolac should be used cautiously in patients who will be receiving other anticoagulants, such as heparin, warfarin, and low-molecular weight fractionated heparins, such as enoxaparin. The combined effects of these agents may well lead to a greatly enhanced propensity for spontaneous bleeding in the postoperative period.

The renal effects of NSAIAs are negligible in normovolemic patients. However, in patients with congestive heart failure, hepatic cirrhosis with ascites, chronic renal disease, or hypovolemia, they can reduce renal blood flow and glomerular filtration rate, and precipitate acute renal failure. These effects are presumed to be caused by the loss of vasodilatory prostaglandins which regulate renal response to norepinephrine and angiotensin II. In addition, NSAIAs reduce the prostaglandin-induced inhibition of the action of antidiuretic hormone and the reabsorption of chloride, thus, leading to sodium and water retention. This sodium and water retention may exaggerate retention normally associated with the stress response to surgery. The combined effects of acute renal failure and sodium and water retention can result in morbidity by causing total body fluid overload, congestive heart failure, or pulmonary edema in the postoperative period.

While these potential complications of NSAIA therapy are serious, in the majority of postoperative patients, their effect is small. Clinical experience suggests that those patients most at risk for complications of NSAIA therapy in the postoperative period are those with preexisting renal, cardiac, or hematologic disease; those patients requiring anticoagulation; patients needing excessively negative fluid balance (e.g., thoracotomies, pneumonectomies); and those at risk for GI bleeding (e.g., coagulopathic patients, trauma patients, and those with anticipated prolonged postoperative fasting period).

Acetaminophen

Acetaminophen can be a useful postoperative adjunct in patients able to take oral medications. Studies suggest that acetaminophen is synergistic in effect with many of the less potent opioids, and may well have additive analgesic effects when used with more potent opioids. Attention must be given to the total dose of acetaminophen per 24 hours when using fixed combination preparations. Increasing the dose of these medications may result in toxic levels of acetaminophen and subsequent hepatic damage. When titrating less potent opioids to analgesic effect, using a pure preparation, such as codeine or oxycodone, in conjunction with regularly dosed acetaminophen as a separate drug, will decrease the potential for toxicity.

Tramadol

This drug is the most recent analgesic released in the United States, although it has been used for many years in Europe. Pharmacologically, tramadol is quite distinct in its mechanisms of action from the pure opioid and nonopioid analgesics discussed earlier. Tramadol possesses both catecholamine-reuptake-inhibition properties, as well as agonist activity at mu-1 receptors. Thus, some of its actions resemble those of antidepressants, especially the selective-serotonin-reuptake inhibitors, while others resemble the effects of mild opioid agonists. Potency studies have determined the analgesic effect of tramadol to be equivalent to that achievable with oral meperidine or codeine.

Tramadol has been marketed as an analgesic for mild-to-moderate pain. While a parenteral form exists, it has not been approved in the United States, therefore, dosing is limited to those patients able to take oral medications. A typical dosing regimen begins at 50 mg bid, followed by increases to qid dosing as tolerated. The maximum recommended dose of tramadol is 100 mg qid, although studies from Europe have examined doses as high as 100 mg q4h without demonstration of adverse effects.

The primary side effects of tramadol include GI upset, dizziness, agitation, increased sweating, and decreased libido. These side effects tend to appear early in treatment, and regress over the first week of therapy. It is not unusual to see temporary recurrence of side effects with dosage increase. These effects can be minimized by starting therapy with 25 mg bid, and advancing to the maximum dosage over 1 to 2 weeks.

Local Anesthetics

Local anesthetics are being used in increasingly inventive ways as adjuncts or primary means for postoperative analgesia. They are administered through wound infiltration, peripheral nerve blocks, field blocks, in intraarticular injections, and in the epidural and subarachnoid spaces to block nociceptive input from A-δ and C fibers. While there are several different local anesthetics available, the ones primarily used for postoperative analgesia are lidocaine and bupivacaine.

Lidocaine is the prototype amide local anesthetic. Lidocaine contains a methyl-substituted benzene ring connected to an ethyl-substituted tertiary amine through an amide linkage. The duration of action of lidocaine depends on the location of injection, with drug given by IV injection being cleared most rapidly, and epidural injection most slowly. The typical duration of action of lidocaine injected for peripheral nerve blockade or field block is 75 to 90 minutes. This can be significantly prolonged to 90 to 180 minutes with the addition of epinephrine, but injecting such solutions subcutaneously can lead to tissue necrosis. Epidural injection typically lasts 80 to 120 minutes and can safely be prolonged with the addition of epinephrine to 120 to 180 minutes.

Local injection, field blocks and peripheral nerve injections are usually performed with 1% to 1.5% lidocaine solution, while epidural blockade is performed with 2% solutions. Injection of lidocaine in the subarachnoid space is not generally useful for postoperative pain control, because it predictably results in profound motor paralysis, as well as analgesia. For the same reason, lidocaine is not normally used for continuous epidural analgesia, either.

Bupivacaine is a long-acting amide local anesthetic, which has some advantages over lidocaine for postoperative analgesia. It has a longer duration of action without the addition of epinephrine, thus, achieving prolonged analgesia without tissue-bloodlow compromise. It is also possible to reliably achieve analgesia with dilute concentrations of the drug (0.125% or less) without causing motor blockade. It may also exhibit less tachyphylaxis in conditions of continuous infusion.

All local anesthetics have the potential for adverse cardiovascular and CNS side effects with IV injection or rapid vascular uptake. Blockade of the cardiac conduction system can lead to asystole with accompanying hypotension and circulatory arrest, while local anesthetic effects on the CNS can lead to confusion, lethargy, and seizures. Care must be taken when injecting these medications to avoid intravascular injections, and to avoid giving toxic doses of drug. The maximum dose of lidocaine per injection is 5 mg/kg without epinephrine and 7 mg/kg with epinephrine, while the maximum dose for of bupivacaine is 3 mg/kg.

ROUTES OF ADMINISTRATION FOR POSTOPERATIVE ANALGESIA

There are many potential means of delivering analgesia in the postoperative period. The choice depends on factors such as patient or surgeon preference, location of surgery, extent of surgery, length of expected NPO status, and others. This section will begin with a discussion of routes of administration of the medications discussed previously, and follow with a discussion of nerve block options for pain control. Specific concerns related to epidural and subarachnoid injection of local anesthetics are further discussed in Chapter 4.

Oral Administration

The routes of administration available for opioid and nonopioid analgesics are multiple, and include oral, intramuscular, subcutaneous, intravenous and neuraxial (epidural or spinal administration). Oral medication is appropriate for those patients who have not had abdominal or other major surgery and is frequently used for patients who have had regional anesthetics for their surgical procedures. The major disadvantage of using oral analgesics is manifested in the patient with nausea and vomiting, who will not likely be able to absorb enough medication in a reliable fashion to attain adequate pain control.

Intramuscular Injection

Intramuscular injections have been the standard in postoperative analgesia for many years. Reasons for this include ease of administration, slow rise in blood levels with supposedly less potential for respiratory depression from opioids, and no need for sophisticated delivery systems. However, there are several disadvantages to this form of administration. First, injection into muscles is painful. There is risk of tissue damage. Many opioid preparations lead to formation of scar tissue in muscle, and it is not uncommon for injections to be given repeatedly in the same area, which may increase this risk. There are also reports of nerve damage, mainly arising from gluteal injections with unintentional injection into the sciatic nerve; there are similar reports from injections into or near the radial nerve in the upper arm. As with oral administration, absorption is slow, and it may be 30 to 60 minutes or longer before a patient benefits from the injection. A major disadvantage of IM injections today is the nursing time required for their use: nurses must respond to the patient's request for medication, check orders for dose and frequency, obtain keys for getting the medication, draw up the medication, verify the dose, route and frequency again, and then administer the medication to the patient. In many cases, this leads to a unacceptable delay in provision of analgesic medication.

Intravenous Administration

The intravenous method of administering analgesics overcomes many of the disadvantages of oral or IM dosing. Medication can be given through intermittent IV boluses (with the same disadvantages as with intermittent IM dosing), or, as is more commonly done today, through *patient-controlled analgesia* (PCA) systems. The theory of PCA is simple; the patient is given a means by which to give a small IV dose of medication whenever (s)he hurts. The parameters of dose, dose interval, and total hourly dose are programmed as specified by the physician caring for the patient. This method allows the patient to achieve a more uniform level of pain relief than can be obtained with intermittant boluses.

Figure 42-2 points out several important features of PCA versus intermittent dosing regimen. First, intermittent dosing of large boluses rapidly achieves therapeutic blood levels, as demonstrated by the rapid rise into the analgesic zone. However, there is usually significant overshoot with this method of management, with the patient spending a significant amount of time above the analgesic zone, at levels where side effects predominate over analgesia. Also, there is a substantial period of time where the blood level is subtherapeutic before the next dose is given; the patient is usually uncomfortable during this time. Patient-controlled anesthesia dosing eliminates this problem by giving smaller doses closer together, with the patient in effect "cycling" between the boundaries of the analgesic zone, without over- or under-shooting into the side effect or subtherapeutic zones, respectively.

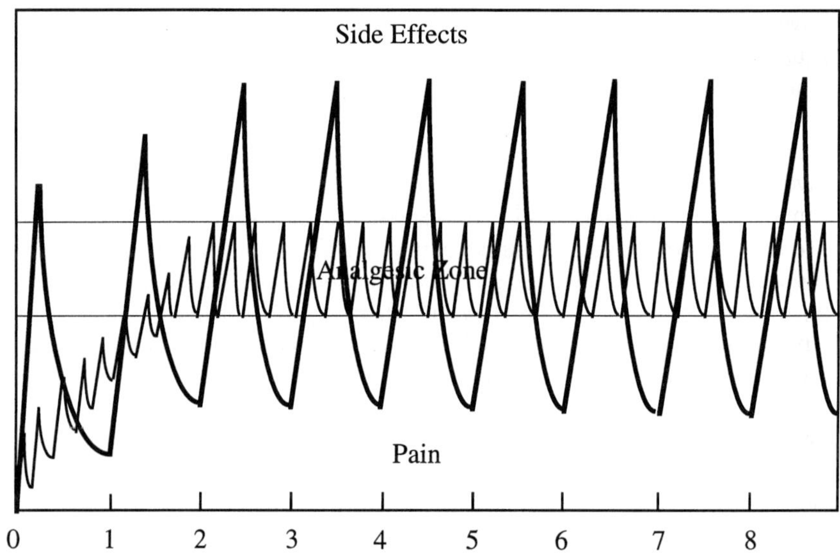

Figure 42-2
Analgesic drug concentration when administered intravenously as a continuous infusion or intermittent boluses (bold). Therapeutic levels are more easily achieved with a continuous infusion. See text for details.

It is also apparent from Figure 42-2 that it is impossible to achieve rapid therapeutic blood levels of opioid with PCA dosing alone. Rather, a patient should be given small, frequent boluses (e.g., 2 mg every 1 to 2 minutes) until satisfactory analgesia is achieved, and *then* be connected to the PCA system. In this manner, there will be rapid establishment of analgesia, with minimal side effects and minimal complaints of breakthrough pain.

A unique phenomenon is often seen with PCA dosing. When patients sleep, they are not able to push the button for further doses of analgesia. Having other members of the medical care team (or, in some cases, the family) push the button while the patient is sleeping defeats the inherent safety features of the system. This problem can be overcome by using a basal infusion of opioid along with intermittent PCA dosing. The usual starting range in an opioid-naive individual is 0.5 to 1 mg/hr of morphine for a basal dose, with 1 to 2 mg every 6 to 10 minutes PCA dose. Thus, the patient still receives analgesia while sleeping, and is able to self-administer doses for breakthrough pain, but the total opioid dose per hour can still be controlled by the medical staff. This practical technique for providing analgesia represents optimum use of the IV route of administration.

Some physicians fear use of basal opioid infusions, because they believe their use will lead to opioid overdose, serious respiratory depression, and even death. Such concerns are valid, although the actual incidence of such occurences is exceedingly low. Most reported instances in which basal opioid infusions have caused problems involve human error in programming the pump, pump malfunction, and failure to adequately monitor the patient. Human error and pump malfunction can be reduced, but not prevented, by applying protocols for programming infusions and regular equipment checks. However, there is no excuse for failure to monitor a patient's respiratory rate and level of consciousness, along with other vital signs in the postoperative period. A review of the most serious adverse events implicates this failure as a primary contributor to morbidity.

Neuraxial opioids are gaining in popularity because of their potential for profound analgesia with an extremely low opioid dose, the safety of continuous infusion, and the long duration of action. Indeed, epidural and spinal administration of morphine can give sustained analgesia for 12 to 24 hours following major surgical procedures. Side effects of this route of administration include the usual opioid side effects of sedation, nausea/vomiting, pruritus, and respiratory depression. The last must be monitored closely while the patient is receiving neuraxial opioids, because the onset of respiratory depression may be 18 to 24 hours after the initial administration of the drug.

Peripheral Nerve Blocks for Postoperative Analgesia

Peripheral nerve blocks may be very efficacious in surgery affecting the upper and lower extremities. They can be used for both anesthesia and analgesia, and may offer increased safety in critically ill patients. Care must be taken to ensure that there is a plan for pain management after the block wears off, because few blocks last longer than the expected postoperative pain course. At our hospital, ambulatory surgery patients are instructed to begin taking their routinely-prescribed analgesics as soon as they arrive home, while inpatients are started on alternative medications as soon as they begin to experience discomfort. In this manner, the patient can avoid the development of disconcerting breakthrough pain.

UPPER EXTREMITY BLOCKS

Analgesia of the upper extremity most commonly involves blockade of the brachial plexus in the neck, the supraclavicular fossa or the axilla, or the individual peripheral nerves more distally in the arm. *Interscalene block* is frequently used for shoulder procedures, either as the sole anesthetic, or more commonly, in conjunction with light general anesthesia. Use of a long-acting local anesthetic, such as bupivacaine with epinephrine, will not only decrease anesthetic requirements during surgery but is capable of giving 12 to 24 hours of postoperative analgesia. There is controversy in the anesthesia literature as to whether these blocks should be performed with the patient awake or under general anesthesia. As with any nerve block procedure, there is an undefined risk of neurologic injury. It is possible that this risk may be increased by performing the block in a sedated or insensate patient, and many practitioners of regional anesthesia feel these blocks should be done before instituting general anesthesia.

Supraclavicular brachial plexus block may be useful for procedures centered around the elbow. The interscalene approach may fail to cover the lower extent of the joint, and the axillary approach may fail to cover the upper end. This procedure may be associated with increased risk of morbidity in inexperienced hands, the most feared complication being pneumothorax.

Axillary blockade of the brachial plexus is frequently used for surgeries on the forearm and hand. With use of a catheter technique for continuous local anesthetic infusion, the effects of the blockade can be prolonged into the postoperative period. This allows increased blood flow to an extremity, with its attendant improved wound healing, crucial in digit reimplantation surgery and nerve and blood vessel reconstructive surgery.

Distal blockade of the major nerves of the brachial plexus is rarely done for postoperative analgesia because the blocks last only as long as the local anesthetic. It is difficult to repeat these blocks indefinitely because the site becomes tender and inflamed. The reader is referred to standard texts of regional anesthesia for descriptions of performing these blocks.

LOWER EXTREMITY BLOCKS

Lower extremity nerve blocks have not found a significant place in the modern postoperative analgesic armamentarium, primarily because of lack of familiarity with how to perform them, and the relatively long period of time necessary for them to become effective. While education in regional anesthesia can address the former, the latter issue is less concerning if one is using the block primarily for postoperative analgesia. The block can be performed shortly before induction, and by the time the case has finished, analgesia will have been achieved.

Blockade of the *sciatic nerve* will result in analgesia of the posterior thigh and the entire leg below the knee, with the exception of the medial calf. Femoral nerve blockade will provide pain relief in the anterior thigh and medial calf. Obturator nerve block is necessary to provide analgesia of the medial thigh, while blockade of the lateral femoral cutaneous nerve is necessary for pain relief in the lateral thigh. This is important to remember when using peripheral nerve blockade for analgesia after knee arthroscopy or arthroplasty. Many patients will experience pain in the medial knee if the obturator nerve is not adequately blocked. The so-called "3-in-1" technique attempts to provide blockade of all three major nerve trunks of the lower extremity through one needle entry site. The technique may be useful for postoperative analgesia, especially in outpatient surgery.

Other Therapeutic Options

There are several analgesic adjuncts which may have some utility in the postoperative period. *Transcutaneous electrical nerve stimulation (TENS)* applies a low-voltage electrical current between two electrodes placed on the skin, thus, stimulating the underlying nerve fibers. Theoretically, this electrical stimulation excites larger diameter A-beta fibers in peripheral nerves preferentially to A-δ and C-fibers, and, thus, contributes a greater degree of input to the nociceptive processing centers in the dorsal horn of the spinal cord. This increased "noise" then obscures the pain signals carried by the A-delta and C-fibers. Studies of the use of TENS in postoperative patients generally show low efficacy, but this may be a useful adjunct in certain situations.

Massage therapy has been studied for its ability to raise the pain perception threshold in the postoperative period. A small study at our hospital looking at the effect of postoperative massage on analgesic requirements for cancer patients undergoing both curative and palliative surgery, suggested that massage may be able to significantly decrease the need for narcotic pain medications, thereby decreasing sedation and other drug side effects in the postoperative period and increasing patient well-being.

Formal *pyschologic intervention* in the form of relaxation therapy, supportive counseling, and behavioral interventions may be useful in some instances. Many patients have significant anxiety about experiencing pain, and even if they receive adequate analgesia, may continue to demand pain medications because of a fear of hurting. Clinical psychologists, working together with the rest of the patient care team, are an indispensable resource at our institution. They help redirect patients' expectations and can serve as arbiters between patients and care teams with patients who may be felt to have unreasonable demands for postoperative analgesia.

SUMMARY

Optimal pain control is an integral part of the postoperative patient's recovery. Specialized techniques are available to provide analgesia, even for the most invasive types of surgical interventions. The safe administration of such techniques requires knowledge of their side effects and their potential complications. Plans for adequate postoperative analgesia should be drawn preoperatively. Early consultation with a pain management specialist will facilitate such planning.

BIBLIOGRAPHY

Bonica, JJ: *The management of pain*, ed 2, Philadelphia, 1990, Lea & Febiger.

Cousins, MJ, Bridenbough, PO: *Neural blockade in clinical anesthesia and management of pain*, ed 2, Philadelphia, 1988, JB Lippincott.

Raj, PR: *Practical management of pain*, ed 2, St. Louis, 1992, Mosby–Year Book.

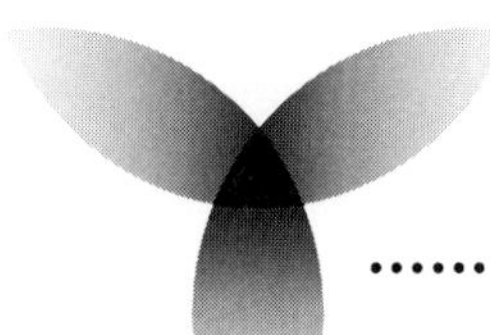

Chapter 43

Routine and Specialized Postoperative Care

Cassandra Kennedy, MD, Alan T. Lefor, MD

The care required by a patient in the postoperative period depends on a number of factors including the patient's preoperative status, the nature of the operation, and the continuing physiologic insults suffered by a patient secondary to the disease process and surgery (e.g., a patient with a pancreatic abscess and continued retroperitoneal necrosis/inflammation). Providing care in the immediate postoperative period is usually the responsibility of the surgical service, but it is incumbent upon the surgeons to pay close attention to the anesthesiologists involved in the intraoperative care, to learn as much as they can about the physiologic responses demonstrated by the patient during the stress of surgery. The dependence of excellent patient care on close cooperation between surgeons, anesthesiologists, and nursing staff in the postoperative period cannot be overstated.

Postoperative care for the surgical patient begins when the operation ends and continues until the patient has returned back to the baseline level of function. This can be broken down into the immediate postoperative period or postanesthetic phase; an intermediate phase, which encompasses the continued hospital stay; and a convalescent phase, during which the patient recuperates (usually at home). Our concern in this chapter is primarily during the immediate and intermediate postoperative periods, because this is the time frame when complications are most likely to be noted; however, with the continually increasing popularity of outpatient surgery (even if only with payers), close surveillance of patients and potential complications in all clinical settings is required.

IMMEDIATE POSTOPERATIVE CARE: INTENSIVE CARE UNIT (ICU)

The care of the postoperative patient in the intensive care unit (ICU) is well discussed elsewhere in this text. Here, we will discuss two issues of great importance to the surgeon: indications for ICU monitoring and transport to the ICU.

Surgical Indications for ICU monitoring

The decision to provide immediate postoperative care in the ICU is usually made jointly by the surgeon and anesthesiologist either before, during, or at the end of a procedure. There are a wide variety of factors that contribute to this decision, including specific institutional policies. For example, in many tertiary care hospitals the need for continued postoperative mechanical ventilation requires an ICU bed. However, in other institutions, there are "step-down" units, which allow ventilators and, therefore, may be appropriate for such patients.

Some of the specific indications for postoperative monitoring in an ICU include the need for ventilatory support or invasive monitoring. Patients with severe comorbid diseases (such as a patient with coronary artery disease 1 month after myocardial infarction who requires a bowel resection for cancer) are usually monitored in the ICU postoperatively. Similarly, patients receiving large amounts of intraoperative intravenous (IV) fluid who are expected to undergo major postoperative fluid shifts may require ICU monitoring.

In institutions that allow direct transfer of patients from the operating room (OR) to the ICU, the nursing staff has usually received in-service training to acquaint them with early postoperative assessment and care. The care rendered in the ICUs is usually of the same high caliber as that in the postanesthesia care unit (PACU), making such immediate transfer to the ICU logical and in the best interest of patient and staff.

Transportation of the Postoperative Patient

The decision to provide ICU care to the postoperative patient is effected by immediate bed availability and other logistic factors. Transportation of the patient to the ICU from the OR requires some planning and a great deal of cooperation between the surgical service, anesthesiologist, and nursing staff. Particular attention must be paid to management of ventilation, vascular access, and hemodynamic monitoring during transport. Institutional factors such as elevator availability and the clearing of hallways must also be taken into account. Safe transport of a patient will require at least three people: anesthesiologist, surgeon, and a nurse or technician. Those personnel assisting in such transport should be senior level residents or attending physicians who are well versed in the management of emergencies that could occur during transit. In ideal circumstances, there is another person to take care of the vascular access and hemodynamic monitoring lines and still another person to walk ahead of the transport team, clearing any obstructions in the hallways.

POSTOPERATIVE CARE

While details of care in the PACU are discussed elsewhere in this text, there are some issues of this care of significant concern to the operating surgeon which will be discussed here. Once surgery has ended, most patients are taken to the recovery area with a physician in attendance during transport. This is a critical time for observing the patient because the majority of early morbidity and mortality in the postoperative setting (secondary to acute pulmonary, cardiovascular, and fluid derangements) can potentially be identified and treated early by an alert staff. Most patients are initially monitored in the PACU and then transferred to an inpatient floor or an outpatient surgery recovery unit if the patient is to go home. A small percentage of patients are transferred directly from the OR to the ICU (see earlier).

Once the patient has recovered sufficiently to leave the PACU or ICU, the patient is usually transferred for routine "floor care." During this phase of recovery, the daily care is almost always under the direct supervision of the treating surgical service. There are a number of significant issues of concern to the surgeon at this time, as well as required vigilance for early postoperative difficulties.

Patient Monitoring

Vital signs, including pulse, blood pressure, and respiratory rate, are checked and recorded at least every 15 minutes for the first hour, and then, every 30 minutes thereafter if the patient remains stable in the PACU. Continuous electrocardiographic monitoring is recommended in the PACU for the first hour; if any abnormalities are noted, monitoring should be continued. Any such prolonged monitoring should ideally occur on a telemetry floor, and if severe electrocardiogram (ECG) changes are noted, ICU admission is warranted. Suspicion of serious ECG changes leads the PACU nurse to contact a physician (anesthesiologist or surgeon) and obtain a 12-lead ECG. Pulse oximetry should also be monitored continuously in the somnolent postoperative patient to ensure adequate oxygenation. Supplemental oxygen is initially administered and then reduced to room air while keeping the oxygen saturation level above the usual threshold of 94%. After major operations, patients are often hypothermic; the core temperature is checked on arrival to the PACU and warming begins immediately, if needed. Warming lights, hyperthermia blankets, and, particularly, forced-air devices may be used.

Consideration of fluid and electrolyte balance begins before surgery and continues until the patient is discharged. It is important to recognize any potential for fluid derangements which began in the preoperative period, for example, a patient who is hypovolemic secondary to an oral preoperative bowel preparation, or a patient who is hypervolemic secondary to not receiving dialysis because of a clotted arterio-venous fistula. The anesthesiologist should have titrated the amount of intraoperative fluid needed based on vital signs and urine output. This treatment is continued in the PACU, based on the fluid status of the patient during the operation, the type of operation, and any concomitant disease processes that may affect ongoing fluid needs. If there is a concern about fluid balance, careful monitoring of urine output with a urinary catheter and urimeter to keep urine output greater than 0.5 to 1 cc/kg/hr is recommended. Invasive monitoring of central venous or pulmonary artery pressure may also be helpful if the patient's fluid status remains in doubt. Often, these invasive monitoring devices are placed in the OR and may be used postoperatively until no longer needed.

Assessing Stability of the Patient Postoperatively

The PACU staff monitors the postoperative patient until stable, usually for approximately 1 hour. During this time, the patient awakens from the effects of anesthesia and becomes more responsive. Vital signs should normalize and the immediate nursing demands decrease. At this point, a patient whose discharge is planned for the same day can be transported to a less intensive recovery situation where vital signs are monitored every 30 minutes, pain is controlled, spontaneous urination is achieved, and the patient is able to tolerate a liquid diet before discharge home. Patients who are to be admitted postoperatively can be transported to the floor, where for the next 3 hours vital signs will be checked every 30 minutes; if vitals have normalized, the patient can then be monitored less frequently, usually every 4 hours. The nurse should be given parameters of vital signs for which the physician will be notified. For a normal adult, we typically choose to be notified if respiratory rate is between 14 and 34, pulse is between 60 and 120, systolic blood pressure is between 90/50 and 160/90, and temperature is above 38.5°C. The nurse should also be instructed to check the bandage for excessive drainage and to notify the physician if it becomes saturated. All drains are monitored by the nursing staff and parameters of output given for notification of the responsible physician (e.g., chest tube output >200 mls/hr after heart surgery).

The patient is examined by the physician postoperatively and every day thereafter, until discharge; progress notes document each examination and evaluation. During these examinations, the trends of vital signs are evaluated, as well as the breakdown of fluid intake and output. The patient's overall demeanor should be noted, including adequacy of pain control and appropriateness of response. An examination of the surgical wound site, drains, lung, heart, abdomen, and extremities should take place and be documented.

Fluid and Electrolyte Therapy

Maintaining homeostasis in the postoperative period requires meticulous attention to detail in the administration of fluid and electrolyte therapy. Proper administration of fluids and electrolytes in the postoperative period depends on five factors:

1. Preexisting medical conditions (e.g., congestive heart failure, renal failure, hepatic failure).

2. Maintenance fluid requirements.
3. Fluid and electrolyte deficits present preoperatively.
4. Fluids and electrolytes administered intraoperatively.
5. Consideration of ongoing fluid and electrolyte losses in a particular patient (e.g., gastrointestinal fistula, nasogastric tube, etc.).

MAINTENANCE FLUID REQUIREMENTS

The basis of all fluid and electrolyte therapy is the detailed knowledge of baseline fluid requirements, which may be calculated in a number of ways. In the average 70 kg adult, maintenance requirements are most easily estimated at 2400 ml daily. This value is based on daily water losses. In 24 hours, the average patient loses 1500 ml of water in urine, 250 mls in the gastrointestinal (GI) tract, 600 ml by insensible loss (75% through skin and 25% through lungs) for a total daily water loss of 2350 ml. In children, one estimates maintenance requirements based on body weight. Using body weight, one gives 100 ml/kg/day for the first 10 kg, plus 50 ml/kg/day for the next 10 kg, plus 20 ml/kg/day for each kg above 20 kg. Note that using this method, the daily fluid requirement for a 70 kg person is calculated at 2500 ml, close to the 2400 ml estimate used previously. In children, one can alternatively calculate fluid requirements based on body surface area using 1500 ml/m^2/day.

Maintenance electrolyte requirements are somewhat more variable than fluid requirements, but as a general rule, the average 70 kg person requires roughly 40 to 60 mEq K^+ daily and 90 to 120 mEq Na^+ daily. Calculations of baseline fluid requirements must be tempered by coexisting medical conditions such as congestive heart failure, renal failure, or hepatic failure.

The electrolyte content of commonly used parenteral fluids is shown in Table 43-1. Using the fluid and electrolyte estimates stated previously, it is easy to determine that the daily maintenance requirements for fluids and electrolytes are met by administration of D_5 0.25NS + 20 mEq K^+/l at 100 ml/hr. This will provide 2400 ml fluid, 125 g dextrose, 50 mEq K^+ and 95 mEq Na^+ daily. The use of fluids containing more electrolytes is not needed to meet maintenance requirements.

PREOPERATIVE DEFICITS

In most cases, surgery is performed electively on patients with normal fluid and electrolyte status. In fact, significant attention is paid to this aspect of the preoperative status during the preanesthesia evaluation. However, in patients brought urgently or emergently to the OR, significant fluid and electrolyte deficits may be present. The planning of postoperative fluid and electrolyte therapy demands attention to preoperative electrolyte abnormalities, such as hypokalemia or hypocalcemia. Patients who present with massive fluid losses from GI hemorrhage or prolonged emesis and diarrhea, may have continued fluid deficits.

INTRAOPERATIVE FLUID AND ELECTROLYTE ADMINISTRATION

In most patients, fluids given during surgery are sufficient to meet physiologic needs. Most patients with normal renal function lose this extra fluid over the first few days postoperatively in the urine. It is important to determine what fluids were

Table 43-1. Composition of Commonly Used Parenteral Fluids

SOLUTION	NA+	K+	CL−	CA++	HCO3−
Extracellular fluid	142	4	103		27
LR	130	4	109	3	28
NS	154		154		
0.5NS	77		77		
0.25NS	38		38		

Adapted from Gomella LG and Lefor AT: *Surgery on call,* Norwalk, CT, 1996, Appleton & Lange, p. 339.

administered during the operation. This should be accurately recorded in the operative note to allow anyone involved in the care of the patient to easily determine what was given. Intraoperative urine output must be evaluated as a guide to overall fluid balance. The patient who remains oliguric at the end of a large surgical procedure most likely has continued fluid deficits or catheter dysfunction, which must be corrected in the postoperative period.

ONGOING LOSSES

Fluid and electrolyte therapy in the postoperative period must take into account any ongoing fluid and electrolyte losses. Careful monitoring of fluid losses is essential to properly follow fluid balance. This may require continuous monitoring of urine output (urinary catheter), nasogastric tube losses, drain output, fistula output, and the quantitation of postoperative bleeding. Ongoing third-space losses are not unusual following major surgical procedures and are often difficult to measure. Estimates of such anticipated losses may require the insight of experienced practitioners. The average fluid and electrolyte content for a variety of bodily fluids is shown in Table 43-2.

The type of fluid administered is guided by the source of the ongoing losses. Patients with bleeding are replaced with isotonic fluids or blood products depending on their hematocrits. Fluid deficits in patients with large nasogastric tube outputs are replaced using $D_5$0.5NS + 20 mEq K^+/l on a cc for cc basis because this most closely approximates the electrolyte content of gastric fluid (see Table 43-1). Large diarrhea outputs require repletion using D_5LR + 15 mEq K^+/l, while biliary and pancreatic drainage (e.g., from a fistula or postoperative drain) require D_5LR containing additional HCO_3^-. Ongoing third-space losses should be replaced with an isotonic fluid such as LR, Normosol R or Plasmalyte-A.

COMPLICATIONS

There are a number of potential complications associated with fluid and electrolyte therapy. Infusion-related phlebitis occurs in approximately 70% of patients with IV catheters. Catheter-related infection is also a frequent occurrence, which may manifest itself as a local process or even as systemic septicemia, requiring removal of the line and parenteral antibiotic administration. Fluid administration is frequently complicated by electrolyte disturbances. This can be avoided by careful monitoring of serum electrolyte levels and careful adjustment of electrolyte concentration in

Table 43-2. Composition and Daily Production of Body Fluids

FLUID	VOLUME (CC)/DAY	NA^+	K^+	HCO_3^-	CL^-
Sweat	variable	50	40	0	40
Saliva	1500	10	26	50	15
Stomach	1500	60	10		100
Duodenum	300–2000	140	5	10	90
Pancreas	100–800	140	5	115	75
Ileum	2000–3000	140	5	30	100
Bile	50–800	140	5	30	100
Diarrhea	variable	50	35	45	40

Adapted from Gomella LG and Lefor AT: *Surgery on call*, Norwalk, CT, 1996, Appleton & Lange, p. 337.

administered fluids. A common mistake is the replacement of third-space losses with a hypotonic fluid, resulting in hyponatremia, particularly at a time when the normal kidney is actively holding on to free water. Acute electrolyte deficiencies are repleted with boluses of electrolytes, rather than by adding the electrolytes to large volumes of IV fluid to be given over a long period of time. Fluid overload and pulmonary edema are also common complications which can be avoided by careful monitoring of intake and output as well as clinical status.

Antibiotic Therapy in the Postoperative Period

The administration of antibiotics in the postoperative period depends a great deal on what antibiotic therapy was given preoperatively, if any, as well as the intraoperative findings which may alter the indications for antibiotic administration. The number and diversity of antibiotics are ever-expanding, making it increasingly difficult to base decisions on sound data. Because the treatment of infectious problems is common in surgical practice, it must be remembered that antibiotic therapy is often used as an adjunct to surgical therapy (incision and drainage, debridement, etc.). The use of antibiotics in the surgical patient is divided into three categories: prophylaxis, empiric therapy and directed therapy.

PROPHYLACTIC ANTIBIOTICS

The administration of prophylactic antibiotics is indicated for patients undergoing clean contaminated operations (e.g., biliary tract surgery, bowel resection, etc.). Some authors suggest the benefit of prophylactic antibiotics in clean cases in which a subsequent infection would be catastrophic, such as neurosurgical procedures and certain vascular operations. Their administration is also accepted in procedures that include foreign-body implantation, such as artificial joints or hernia repair with mesh.

Data regarding the efficacy of agents given for prophylaxis was obtained in patients undergoing biliary and upper GI surgery, using first-generation cephalosporin drugs. A key principle in the use of prophylactic antibiotics is that they must be administered before the skin is incised to be beneficial, because they are most effective in preventing bacterial infection when they are at peak levels in the tissue before bacterial contamination. Most often, they are ordered to be administered "on call" to the OR, but may have to be given upon the patient's arrival in the OR, because that is when IV access may be initiated. Adequate communication between surgeon and anesthesiologist is essential to assure timely administration of antibiotic therapy.

In upper GI and biliary procedures, the pathogens likely to be encountered are *Enterobacteriaceae* and other gram-positive cocci, making a first-generation cephalosporin a likely drug choice. Cefazolin is commonly used in this situation. In colonic surgery, the presence of anaerobes requires additional coverage for which second-generation cephalosporins are commonly used. The use of third-generation cephalosporins has not been associated with improved results and is generally not indicated in prophylaxis. The duration of antibiotic administration is also a controversial issue, and current recommendations suggest that one dose preoperatively and two doses postoperatively should suffice. There are no data suggesting that administration beyond 24 hours is of any benefit. Recent data also suggest that intraoperative dosing, in an effort to maintain tissue levels, should be performed in extended procedures (longer than 3 hours) or in those procedures with excessive blood loss (greater than 1500 ml).

EMPIRIC ANTIBIOTIC THERAPY

In many cases, antibiotic administration must be initiated based on a patient's clinical course in the absence of specific microbiologic data. Often, this situation is encountered in the absence of a proven site of infection. Thus, the empiric therapy of antibiotics must include a careful search for septic foci and a predefined (at least in the mind of the ordering physician) time limit on the course of empiric antibiotic therapy. Careful selection of agent(s) involves knowledge of patterns of pathogen activity in a specific institution, as well as known spectrum of activity of the agent(s) selected. Most hospital laboratories track the incidence of various bacteria in culture specimens, as well as their susceptibilities. This information is invaluable for the clinician faced with an empiric decision. The use of broad-spectrum single agents is becoming more common than the use of combination regimens for a variety of reasons, including ease of administration (with concomitant lower costs) and somewhat diminished toxicities (e.g., nephrotoxicity associated with aminoglycoside agents).

DIRECTED ANTIBIOTIC THERAPY

Directed antibiotic therapy is that given after specific pathogens have been identified, based on their individual sensitivity patterns. There are only guidelines available for prescribing directed antibiotic therapy because there are no solid data on which to base these decisions. It is believed that treatment of both aerobic and anaerobic components of infections in sites likely to harbor both types of organisms is important because of pathogenic synergy between aerobic and anaerobic organisms. Antimicrobial agents with specific activity against culture-documented organisms should be administered with an attempt to minimize toxicity. Broad-spectrum agents may be appropriate in this role, as long as they have activity against the organisms present.

GENERAL PRINCIPLES OF ANTIBIOTIC THERAPY

Antimicrobial agents are divided into a number of groups, based on structure or spectrum of activity. These include β-lactams (e.g., penicillins, cephalosporins, monobactams, and carbapenems), quinolones, aminoglycosides, antianaerobes, macrolides, tetracyclines, glycopeptides, sulfa drugs, and antifungal drugs. There are a number of reference works published annually, detailing the dose and spectrum of activity of these agents, which should be referred to before writing orders for these ever-changing classes of drugs. The general objective is to achieve high tissue levels of drug; it is usually believed that the level should exceed the minimum inhibitory concentration (MIC) for a given drug against a specific organism. This may be achievable with oral drugs in some situations; however, in severe infections commonly encountered by the surgeon, it is usually necessary to parenterally administer these drugs.

The initial choice of drug should be based on organisms expected to be involved. Patients must be regularly reevaluated for response to the selected antibiotics. There are a number of explanations for the patient who fails to improve, including inadequate surgical procedure (debridement, incision, and drainage, etc.), complication of a surgical procedure (anastomotic failure, etc.), development of a superinfection, development of resistant organisms, inadequate antibiotic dose, or incorrect choice of antibiotics.

The length of time antibiotics are used is highly controversial. In the patient whose clinical status is stable and whose white blood count has returned to normal, there is a scant likelihood of further infectious problems. In general, antibiotics are continued until the patient is clinically stable and afebrile for 48 hours. New infections usually require the initiation of new antibiotic therapy, and are best evaluated after stopping the initial therapy.

Respiratory Care

Patients in the PACU are usually given supplemental oxygen and monitored continuously with pulse oximetry. Once sedation diminishes, the patient is encouraged to frequently breathe deeply and cough. During this time, the patient should be weaned off oxygen as tolerated, while maintaining oxygen saturation above 94%. It is important to be cognizant of the decreased respiratory drive which occurs when a sedated patient falls asleep. Satisfactory saturation values may become unacceptable as consciousness is lost. Patients unable to tolerate decreased oxygen support should continue to receive oxygen and have routine pulse oximetry readings to ensure adequate oxygen saturation. These patients should have early mobilization, starting with turning side-to-side, progressing to moving the patient into a chair, and finally ambulation. Patients should also be instructed to frequently use an incentive spirometer. Lung auscultation should be performed routinely, and a chest radiograph obtained if abnormalities are noted on physical examination. Chest physiotherapy and bronchodilators may be given to patients with atelectasis, volume loss, chronic obstructive pulmonary disease (COPD), or asthma. Diuretics may be required in patients with signs of fluid overload.

Early postoperative respiratory failure is most likely caused by a mechanical problem and occurs in patients with marginal preoperative pulmonary function who undergo a thoracic or upper abdominal operation. Adequate analgesia is required to decrease pain and respiratory splinting so the patient can breathe as deeply as possible and minimize atelectasis. Lung volumes decrease significantly following thoracic and upper abdominal surgery, and even optimal epidural analgesia will not prevent these changes totally. The patient needs to be kept in a euvolemic state to avoid dry secretions associated with hypovolemia, and pulmonary fluid overload associated with hypervolemia.

Late postoperative respiratory failure is often associated with a new event such as pulmonary embolism, vomiting with aspiration, oversedation, or abdominal distension. This failure usually occurs more than 48 hours after the operation and is heralded by tachypnea, low tidal volume, and an arterial blood gas with a PCO_2 greater than 45 mm Hg or a PO_2 less than 60 mm Hg. These patients usually require immediate intubation and ventilation. A postintubation chest radiograph is required to check endotracheal tube positioning, as well as to evaluate the existence of any pulmonary problems which may have caused the patient's respiratory collapse (e.g., pneumonia, pneumothorax, large effusion, or atelectasis). Further studies should then be obtained to diagnose the cause of the respiratory decompensation.

Wound Care and Wound Complications

WOUND CARE

Sterile dressings are applied to primarily closed wounds and are usually left in place for 48 hours if they remain clean and dry. These dressings provide a protective barrier and allow epithelial cells to migrate and seal off the deeper structures from the external environment. If the dressings become wet or the patient develops a temperature above 38.5°C, the dressings are removed and direct wound inspection is performed. In the first 48 hours, aseptic technique is used when inspecting any wound and a new sterile dressing applied; after 48 hours, if the wound is dry, a dressing is no longer required.

Skin sutures and staples may be removed on postoperative day 6 and replaced with skin tapes. Sutures may be removed earlier on the face (by the fourth postoperative day), and later on the extremities or over a joint (usually by the fourteenth postoperative day). Patients with decreased wound healing potential (e.g., elderly, malnourished, diabetic, or patients on corticosteroids) should have their sutures left in place longer, with frequent inspection to make sure there are no signs of infection. Wound infection is commonly noted after the fourth postoperative day, when the wound becomes erythematous, edematous, tender, and, occasionally, may break down with purulent drainage. If this occurs, the wound needs to be opened and wet-to-dry dressings are applied to the wound twice daily or more often, depending on the degree of contamination. Necrotic tissue may need to be debrided. Fascial integrity of abdominal closures must be assured in the case of abdominal wound infections.

An open wound can continue to undergo dressing changes, allowing the wound to close slowly, that is, by secondary intention. However, once a wound has undergone packing and no longer appears infected, it can be approximated with skin tapes for a delayed primary closure. After an open wound is approximated, it must be reexamined to make sure healing is progressing without further signs of infection.

WOUND COMPLICATIONS

Optimal wound healing occurs when the incised tissue beds are reapproximated and collagen is allowed to bridge this space. The process is delayed when blood, serous fluid, or infection occurs within the wound. Wound hematoma most often occurs immediately postoperatively and is caused by imperfect hemostasis at the time of operation. Patients with coagulopathies, or those receiving anticoagulants, are at greater risk for wound hematomas. The wound appears discolored and elevated and is tender; occasionally bleeding can be seen from between the cut surface of the wound. Small hematomas may be left alone to resorb, with a slightly higher risk of wound infection. Large hematomas or those located in an anatomically dangerous area (e.g., a hematoma of the neck with potential for compression of the trachea and upper airway) should be taken back to the OR for evacuation, assuring adequate hemostasis and meticulous reclosure of the wound.

A seroma is a fluid collection within a wound. The fluid typically collects underneath a wound because of the disruption of lymphatic drainage at the time of surgery. If lymphatic disruption is anticipated (e.g., lymph node dissection, mastectomy, underneath rotated skin flaps, etc.), drains are placed. Seromas delay wound healing by keeping the adjacent tissue from forming the collagen crosslinks which are necessary for wound contraction. Small seromas will usually resolve without specific therapy. Larger seromas are evacuated by sterile needle aspiration, followed by placement of a compressive dressing; this procedure may have to be repeated. Occasionally, a sclerosant solution (tetracycline had been used for this in the past but is no longer available) is placed into a drained seroma that has recurred. The risk of draining and sclerosing a seroma includes the possibility of introducing bacteria into the wound and causing a subsequent wound infection.

Wound dehiscence is a breakdown of the fascial layer in an incision, while evisceration is the breakdown of all layers of an abdominal wound with extrusion of abdominal viscera. Dehiscence occurs in 1% to 3% of abdominal operations and is more common in patients over 60 years of age. Increased risk of dehiscence is also seen in patients who have diabetes mellitus, uremia, cancer, obesity, malnutrition, jaundice, COPD, steroid dependence, sepsis, or who are immunocompromised from medications or disease. Wounds which have been closed inadequately or are subjected to increased intraabdominal pressure from ascites, dilated bowel, vomiting, coughing, or COPD are also more likely to break down. If these factors are present at the original surgery, meticulous closure of the fascia and use of retention sutures is prudent. Presentation of dehiscence usually occurs on the fifth to eighth postoperative day and is heralded by serosanguinous drainage from the incision. This fluid should be examined and cultured. Wound dehiscence without evisceration is usually electively repaired with reclosure of the fascia. If the skin remains intact with evidence of partial disruption, the patient is closely followed because a ventral hernia often results. An abdominal binder is worn and skin staples left in place for at least 2 weeks, to decrease the risk of complete dehiscence with evisceration. If the wound is also noted to be infected, appropriate antibiotics are started, wet-to-dry dressing changes are initiated 2 to 4 times a day, and surgical repair delayed until after the infection has cleared. This process may take as long as 6 months or more.

In cases of evisceration, the bowel is kept clean and covered with moist towels and the patient urgently returned to the OR for repair. Antibiotics covering gram-positive organisms are given preoperatively. In the OR, the eviscerated bowel is irrigated with copious amounts of normal saline. The fascia is meticulously repaired and retention sutures placed. Evisceration is associated with a 10% mortality rate caused, in part, by the patient's overall general health and associated abdominal infections. Incisional hernias occur in 20% of patients with dehiscence or evisceration, and are more prevalent if a wound infection is also present.

Drains

Drains are typically placed in the sterile intraoperative environment and are used to prevent or treat the unwanted accumulation of fluid. This creates a tract from the sterile intracavitary environment to the skin surface and is a potential site of contamination and infection because organisms can use the drain as a portal of entry. Drains should be brought out through a separate skin incision to reduce the incidence of herniation; that way, if a deep infection does occur, the surgical wound does not become involved. The handling of drains in the postoperative period should include aseptic technique at the skin surface, with sterile dressings replaced whenever the dressing becomes saturated, or every 24 hours, when the skin surface at the drain site is examined. The drain output should also be recorded daily, and the characteristics of that output documented (i.e., serosanguinous, purulent, bilious, etc.). Once the drain has served its purpose and there is less than 20 ml of drainage per day, it is usually removed.

There are a variety of types of drains; the use of a specific type of drain is both surgeon- and situation-dependent. Open drains, such as soft latex or Penrose drains, are often placed for dependent drainage and to form a tract. They should be sutured to the skin with a safety pin placed on the end, so that it does not become lost within the cavity it is draining. These drains may be advanced slowly or pulled out after a tract has formed. If left in place too long, the drains may eventually act to plug the tract, instead of draining it. Closed drainage systems are often used because they minimize external environmental contact. Closed drainage systems may be placed to gravity (e.g., a biliary t-tube or suprapubic urostomy tube) or suction. These drains function best when the fluid is thin, and drains easily. One of the main complications is plugging with clot or cellular debris, which renders the drain nonfunctional. Rigid drains run the risk of erosion into adjacent structures and must be monitored closely.

Sump drains are best used when large amounts of fluid are to be drained, or if the draining fluid is thick and likely to clog other drains. Sump drains have an airflow port that permits air from the outside to be sucked in, thus, decompressing the drain and preventing its collapse. Some of these drains also come with an irrigation port, which is useful when the material being drained is thick or particulate in nature (e.g., pancreatic abscess). The main channel of these drains can be placed on intermittent or continuous suction. Once drainage has decreased or stopped, these drains are usually gradually advanced out, or removed and replaced with progressively smaller catheters until the drain tract is closed.

Pain Management: Surgical Considerations

Postoperative pain is dependent upon the type of operation, duration of surgery, amount of tissue trauma, extent of retraction, and patient threshold. Severe pain is more common following intrathoracic, intraabdominal, and major bone and joint procedures, than after head, neck, breast, or superficial extremity surgery. Adequate pain control can be achieved by a variety of medications given by various routes, and patient education before surgery is helpful in alleviating fear and anxiety, both of which contribute to postoperative pain.

Pain is transmitted through somatic pathways and also splanchnic afferent fibers to the central nervous system (CNS). Spinal cord, brainstem, and cortical responses are then initiated. Spinal responses result in skeletal muscle spasm, vasospasm, and postoperative GI ileus through stimulation of neurons in the anterior horn. Brainstem responses result in tachypnea, tachycardia, hypertension, and alterations in endocrine function. Cortical responses control psychologic changes including fear, anxiety, and apprehension. Voluntary movement is also controlled by the cortex, and patients typically minimize pain by shallow breathing and decreased voluntary activity. This contributes to the risk of postoperative complications (e.g., atelectasis, pneumonia, deep venous thrombosis, pulmonary embolism, or decubitus ulcers), as well as prolonging hospitalization. Optimum pain control decreases the discomfort to a tolerable level and enables the patient to be alert and cooperative. Thus, the patient is able to more completely participate in the recovery process (which is an active process for the patient!). More evidence continues to show that adequate pain management will improve surgical recovery, and may even shorten hospital stays.

Management of postoperative pain begins by including the patient in the planning process. This gives the patient a sense of control, often relieving anxiety. Standard analgesic medications include opiates, nonsteroidal antiinflammatory drugs, and other adjuvants such as phenothiazine derivatives; they can be given intravenously, intramuscularly, or orally. The route of delivery is not as important as is the assurance of adequate doses and proper dosing intervals. Nursing staffs must have the time to carefully monitor the patient's pain levels and provide appropriate therapy in a timely fashion. Patient controlled analgesia (PCA) systems place the analgesic administration in the patient's hands with safety checks and preset limits to ensure safety.

All analgesic medications have side effects, which must be monitored. It is important to be cognizant of these potentially troublesome effects and make efforts to counteract them without compromising patient comfort. Opiates can cause constipation, nausea, vomiting, pruritis, sedation, and decreased respiratory drive. Nonsteroidal antiinflammatory drugs (NSAIDs) have analgesic and antiinflammatory effects. Ketorolac is a NSAID, which may be given parenterally (30 mg given intramuscularly has the same amount of analgesic effect as 10 mg of morphine), and is devoid of the sedative actions and respiratory depression usually accompanying opiate administration. Synergism between the NSAIDs and narcotics will permit prescribing lower doses of each. Complications of NSAIDs include GI ulceration, impaired platelet function, and potential renal impairment.

Epidural analgesia with opiates and/or local anesthetics produces segmental analgesia without causing CNS depression. Pain relief is often more profound than that from systemic administration of analgesics and is particularly desirable in high-risk patients undergoing extensive abdominal or thoracic surgery. Patients with epidural catheters tend to be more alert and have better respiratory and GI function. Common side effects include pruritis, nausea, and urinary retention. Fluid management must also be watched closely, particularly during discontinuation of an epidural local anesthetic infusion; the loss of any sympathectomy will result in a relative increase in intravascular volume. This may occur concomitantly with the mobilization of third-space fluids and place a sick patient at further risk of pulmonary edema. An experienced pain management team is needed to properly care for these patients.

Postoperative Fever: Evaluation and Therapy

Postoperative fever is common and is best evaluated in light of the timing subsequent to the surgical procedure. This is because certain causes of postoperative fever most commonly occur at characteristic times postoperatively. It is important to remember that over 40% of all postoperative fevers resolve spontaneously without any particular cause ever being identified.

The causes of postoperative fever include: atelectasis, urinary tract infection, wound infection, thrombophlebitis, and drug reaction. These are commonly remembered using the “5 Ws” mnemonic: **W**ind (atelectasis), **W**ater (urinary tract infection), **W**ound (wound infection), **W**alking (thrombophlebitis), and **W**onder drug (drug reaction). Identification of a fever pattern is also helpful; fevers that “spike” are commonly associated with closed space infections such as abscesses. Some patients have fevers preoperatively, which are caused by something totally unrelated to surgery.

Fevers caused by atelectasis commonly occur in the first 12 to 48 hours postoperatively, and rarely exceed 39°C. By 48 hours postoperatively, fevers caused by atelectasis commonly have associated changes which are visible on chest radiograph. Physical examination may show decreased breath sounds in patients with fevers caused by atelectasis. Fever from atelectasis is usually treated with aggressive chest physiotherapy and/or incentive spirometry. Other causes of early postoperative fever (12 to 36 hours) include metabolic abnormalities, thyroid storm, adrenocortical insufficiency, transfusion reaction, or early wound infection with streptococcus or clostridium species.

Urinary tract infection-associated fever ordinarily does not occur until more than 48 hours postoperatively, and is usually associated with an indwelling urinary catheter. These patients will typically have complaints of dysuria, and urinalysis will show the typical findings of white blood cells and, possibly, organisms in the urine. A urine sample should be obtained, using sterile technique, and sent for culture. Patients with a positive urinalysis are usually begun on oral antibiotics pending culture results.

Wound infections can cause postoperative fever, but rarely do so before the fifth postoperative day. The exception to this is early, postoperative wound infection caused by clostridium or streptococcus which, if not recognized and treated immediately, may lead to a fatal outcome. These wounds usually have watery drainage that looks like “dirty water.” An immediate gram stain should be obtained and the patient brought to the OR for debridement if this is suspected. Most wound infections occur later in the postoperative course and present with a tender, erythematous wound with purulent drainage. Opening these wounds at bedside is possible and allowing secondary closure usually suffices (see "Wound Care" earlier).

Drug reactions and thrombophlebitis can occur at any time in the postoperative course. Thrombophlebitis tends to occur later in the course but can occur early if associated with an IV catheter which has been indwelling for a prolonged period of time.

Other causes of fever include severe CNS lesions, postpericardiotomy syndrome, anastomotic leak (usually 7–10 days postoperatively with associated peritonitis), acalculous cholecystitis, connective tissue diseases, endocarditis, and paraneoplastic syndrome.

The usual evaluation of postoperative fever is to obtain wound cultures (if indicated), urinary cultures, blood cultures, sputum culture (if indicated), and a complete blood count with differential. A chest radiograph may be indicated, as well as a computed tomographic (CT) scan of the abdomen if intraabdominal abscess is suspected. Therapy is dependent upon the underlying cause. The use of antipyretics remains an individual matter, with many surgeons avoiding their use, except in the case of systemic reaction to fever. That is because antipyretics only treat the symptom and not the cause of the fever. Treatment of fever should be more aggressive in sicker patients who may not tolerate the increased demands posed by the hypermetabolism and stress of fever.

Nutritional Considerations in the Postoperative Period

The decision to provide nutritional supplementation in the postoperative period is made after consideration of many factors. Unfortunately, the use of nutritional support is based largely on empirical knowledge and habit, rather than on convincing data from prospective randomized controlled trials. Clearly, patients who cannot tolerate regular oral feedings will eventually die in the absence of nutritional support. However, the optimal timing to begin providing nutritional support to the postoperative patient is unknown. Some authors recommend beginning nutritional support after just 5 days of caloric starvation, while others wait as long as 21 days before beginning nutritional support. The most recent guidelines from the American Society of Parenteral and Enteral Nutrition (ASPEN) state "patients should be considered malnourished or at risk of developing malnutrition if they have inadequate nutrient intake for 7 days or more, or if they have a weight loss of 10% or more of their preillness body weight."

Once the decision to provide nutritional support has been made, there are a number of steps that must be undertaken to initiate this therapy in a logical and safe manner. The first step is a careful assessment of nutritional status which begins with a careful history. Nutritional assessment is difficult to quantitate, and a variety of parameters have been used. Acute malnutrition is starvation, which occurs during catabolic stress, while chronic malnutrition (marasmus) is characterized by growth retardation and wasting of muscle and subcutaneous fat while maintaining an appetite. These two nutritional insults are often superimposed in the surgical population. While quantitation of nutritional status is important, the parameters used are often less than reliable. Anthropometric measurements have been used (triceps skin fold, etc.), but the interobserver variability diminishes their reliability. Serum protein levels have also been used (prealbumin, transferrin, albumin) although levels reflect hydration status as well as metabolic response to injury (i.e., acute-phase response), and may be of little value. The most useful parameter is nitrogen balance, with a negative nitrogen balance indicating insufficient protein replacement to meet skeletal muscle loss.

Nutritional requirements are calculated based on baseline energy expenditures and increased losses caused by existing disease states. Caloric requirements may be calculated in a number of ways. The Harris-Benedict equation is one of the most popular, and takes into account a number of factors, including activity level and severity of injury (Box 43-1).

Having assessed the patient's nutritional status and needs, one must then select a route for nutritional support with enteral nutrition and parenteral nutrition as the two available choices. In almost all cases, the maxim "If the gut works, use it" is applicable. Thus, patients who will tolerate enteral feedings should be supplemented through the GI tract. Consideration of this factor may lead to the placement of a jejunostomy catheter during an abdominal operation or radiographically assisted passage of a duodenal feeding tube. Enteral feedings are usually avoided in patients with high-GI obstruction, high-output fistulas, or short-gut syndrome. Some recent animal studies have demonstrated the importance of integrity of the GI tract in preventing bacterial translocation. Enteral nutrition has been shown to preserve gut morphology and, thus, may have an important role in preventing septicemia, although this has not been proven in humans.

ENTERAL NUTRITIONAL SUPPORT

Enteral feedings may be administered by a variety of methods including nasogastric, gastric, or jejunal catheters. Enteral nutrition is best tolerated when instilled into the stomach. There are fewer problems with feeding volumes and osmolarity because the stomach serves as the GI tract's guardian against hyperosmolarity. Aspiration secondary to enteral feeding is a significant cause of morbidity and must be closely guarded against by monitoring of residual volumes and appropriate patient positioning. The ideal time to initiate enteral feedings requires careful patient assessment. The use of bowel sounds as a single criterion is not appropriate because the presence of bowel sounds does not necessarily correlate with the presence of prograde GI motility.

Box 43-1 The Harris-Benedict Equation

Calculation of caloric requirements (kcal/day) adjusted for activity level and injury factors.

Men: [66 + (13.75 x wgt) + (5.0 x hgt) – (6.76 x age)] x A x I

Women: [655 + (9.56 x wgt) + (1.85 x hgt) – (4.68 x age)] x A x I

wgt in kgs, hgt in cms, age in years, **A** = activity factor (range from 1.1 for a paralyzed patient to 1.5 for normal activity), **I** = injury factor (range from 1.1 for minor surgery, 1.3 for major surgery, to 1.95 for >40% BSA burn)

Patients in whom jejunal feeding tubes have been placed may tolerate initiation of feedings in the PACU.

Enteral feeding products are classified by nutritional components and osmolarity. Proteins are intact, partially digested, or fully digested into crystalline amino acids. Carbohydrate sources are categorized as intact complex starches, glucose polymers, or simple disaccharides. Fats are usually supplied as long-chain fatty acids. Medium-chain triglycerides (MCT) are supplied in some products but cannot be used as the sole source of fats because they do not contain essential fatty acids. Low osmolarity formulations usually contain approximately 1 kcal/ml and require approximately 2000 ml/day to meet minimum dietary requirements. In patients requiring volume restriction, high osmolarity formulas may be appropriate, which provide up to 2 kcal/ml, meeting requirements with 1500 ml/day or less. While enteral feedings typically are associated with fewer complications than parenteral feedings, the complications of diarrhea, constipation, aspiration, and drug interactions can be significant.

PARENTERAL NUTRITIONAL SUPPORT

Parenteral nutrition is most often provided through a central venous catheter because the osmolarity of solutions needed to provide total nutritional needs is too high to be given in a peripheral vein. While peripheral parenteral nutrition (PPN) remains an option, there are relatively few patients who will benefit from the provision of calories peripherally. Because patients who receive PPN must also receive some other form of nutritional support to meet the remainder of their needs, most can receive all of their nutritional needs by other means, thus, obviating the need for PPN. The details of prescribing total parenteral nutrition are well delineated in many sources and will not be expounded upon here. The solutions used are generally over 1900 mosm/ml and contain at least 1 kcal/ml so that the usual infusion of 2000 to 2500 ml/day provides 2000 to 2500 kcal/day. Most hospitals now use a single infusion bag containing all components for a 24-hour period. This bag typically contains amino acids (10%, 1000 ml), dextrose (50%, 500 ml), and fat emulsion (20%, 500 ml) for a total volume of 2000 ml. Electrolytes, trace elements, and vitamins are added in appropriate amounts (see Table 43-2). The exact amounts of all additives must be adapted to the individual nutritional and electrolyte requirements of each patient. Total parenteral nutrition is generally started at a low rate (25–50 ml/hr) and gradually increased to the rate needed to meet requirements. Laboratory studies are followed closely until a “recipe” is settled upon which maintains the patient’s needs; studies are then obtained less often. Total parenteral nutrition may usually be stopped whenever indicated without a weaning process. Complications of total parenteral nutrition include mechanical complications associated with the catheter, infectious complications, hyperglycemia, refeeding syndrome, electrolyte abnormalities, acid-base disturbances, impaired liver function, prerenal azotemia, bleeding diatheses, and overfeeding.

Nutritional support must be modified for patients with certain preexisting medical conditions such as hepatic failure, chronic renal failure, cardiac failure, or pulmonary dysfunction. Patients with cardiac failure require limitation of total fluid administration. Patients with diabetes mellitus usually require increased calories from fats to limit carbohydrate administration. Patients with hepatic dysfunction may benefit from increased administration of branched-chain amino acids (leucine, valine, isoleucine) and reduced amounts of aromatic amino acids (e.g., phenylalanine). Patients with renal failure require limited protein administration, and generally do not receive potassium or magnesium as part of the total parenteral nutrition prescription. Since carbohydrate metabolism results in a higher production of carbon dioxide, patients with impaired ventilatory reserve (e.g., COPD) may decompensate from hypercarbia. This is usually treated by increasing the supply of calories from fat (lower R value) to limit carbohydrate administration with its higher relative production of carbon dioxide.

Assessment of Return of Gastrointestinal Tract Motility

The majority of operations have no effect on GI motility and patients may resume a diet when mental status returns to normal. Laparotomy and other operations which violate the peritoneal cavity have the potential to cause a cessation of GI peristalsis (i.e., GI ileus). Return of peristaltic activity typically occurs in the small intestine within 24 hours (peristaltic activity in the small bowel often persists throughout the procedure), in the stomach between 24 and 48 hours, and is followed by the right colon in 48 hours, and, finally, the left colon after 72 hours. The typically coordinated propulsive action between the stomach and small intestine remains disorganized after upper GI surgery for 3 to 4 days. Nasogastric tubes are seldom indicated in patients following routine lower GI surgery. Patients with upper GI or esophageal surgery should have a nasogastric tube placed to low-intermittent suction during this period. Once bowel function has resumed, heralded by bowel sounds and flatulence, the nasogastric tube may be removed, although the patient is not fed for another 24 hours. If the patient tolerates nasogastric tube removal, an oral intake may be resumed in gradual steps.

Occasionally, a patient develops a prolonged ileus; this may be secondary to pain, opiate administration, electrolyte changes, pancreatitis, preoperative peritonitis, or a postoperative bowel obstruction. Patients with prolonged ileus require careful monitoring and represent difficult management issues. Once the medical causes of GI ileus have been ruled out, the possibility of a mechanical obstruction may become more significant. Immediate postoperative bowel obstruction is a rare event and can be secondary to adhesions, internal herniation, or inflammation. Treatment is initiated with gastric decompression and expectant observation. If resolution does not occur, or if the patient develops signs of bowel ischemia, laparotomy is indicated.

Delirium Tremens

The risk of delirium tremens occurs in any patient with a long-standing history of alcohol consumption who suddenly stops drinking. Contributing factors include hypomagnesemia, hypokalemia, alkalosis, and nutritional deficiencies. Alcohol withdrawal symptoms occur because of excessive sympathetic nervous system activity. Signs and symptoms include hyperthermia, diaphoresis, tachycardia, hypertension, anxiety, arousal, agitation, nausea, vomiting, sleeplessness, hyperreflexia, tinnitus, and generalized tonic-clonic seizures. Symptoms usually start 6 to 8 hours after cessation of alcohol intake and last approximately 72 hours. Delirium tremens is associated with a 9% to 15% mortality rate, and, thus, prevention is of paramount importance.

Patients at risk should be given thiamine 100 mg, folate 1 mg, a multivitamin ampule, and magnesium sulfate 2 g added to the first bag of IV fluids each day. Patients are then placed on a tapering dose of benzodiazepines. We use diazepam (Valium) for patients without liver disease and lorazepam (Ativan) for patients with liver disease because of the shorter half-life and renal elimination of lorazepam. On the first day, diazepam is started at 10 to 20 mg IV/po every 4 hours and a 5 to 10 mg IV bolus is given every 5 to 10 minutes as needed for agitation, up to a total of 40 mg/hr. On the second day, diazepam is decreased to 5 to 10 mg every 6 hours, and on the third day it is further decreased to 5 to 10 mg po every 8 hours. Diazepam should be withheld if sedation is noted. Ativan is also given on a daily tapered scale starting with 2 to 4 mg po every 4 hours and 2 to 4 mg IV every 5 to 10 minutes, if needed for agitation, up to 12 mg/hr. On the second day, the dose is decreased to 2 to 4 mg po every 6 hours and on the third day the patient is given 2 to 4 mg po every 8 hours. Antiadrenergic therapy is also required in the early withdrawal phase to control heart rate and blood pressure. Metoprolol 100 mg po qid is given for a heart rate greater than 80. Metoprolol 50 mg po qid is given for a heart rate between 50 to 80/min. Clonidine may be substituted for metoprolol at a dose of 0.2 mg po q12 hours. Haldol may be given for hallucinations refractory to sedation in the presence of adequately treated autonomic and neuromuscular symptoms.

Seizures in the alcoholic patient suggest withdrawal and may be precipitated by hypoglycemia, hypomagnesemia, and respiratory alkalosis. These are usually generalized tonic-clonic seizures characterized by the absence of an aura, focal onset, a significant postictal state (more than 30 minutes), and agitation or aggression. Initial treatment starts with IV fluid of 5% dextrose and saline, thiamine 100 mg, 25 g of dextrose, and 1.2 mg of naloxone IV. Diazepam is then given at 2 to 4 mg/min, up to 20 mg; if seizures persist, a diazepam infusion may be started. Phenytoin should be started with a loading dose (13 to 18 mg/kg) and delivered at 50 mg/min. Seizures persisting may indicate *status epilepticus* and if these last more than 60 minutes, irreversible brain damage may occur. Intubation is used to secure an airway and supplemental oxygen is given. If there is no response to phenytoin or diazepam, phenobarbital is started at 25 to 50 mg/min after a loading dose of 7 to 20 mg/kg; diazepam is discontinued because of potential incompatibilities between the two drugs. The patient at this point should be transferred to the ICU for continuous monitoring. A complete neurologic examination and computed tomography scan of the brain is required as part of the complete workup of a seizure, even when delirium tremens is suspected as the etiology.

BIBLIOGRAPHY

Dyer CB, Ashton CM, Teasdale TA: Postoperative delirium: a review of 80 primary data collection studies, *Arch Intern Med* 155:461–465, 1995.

Galandiuk S, Fazio VW: Postoperative irrigation suction drainage after pelvic colonic surgery: a prospective randomized trial, *Dis Colon Rectum* 34:223–228, 1991.

Hall JC, et al: Incentive spirometry versus routine chest physiotherapy for prevention of pulmonary complications after abdominal surgery, *Lancet* 337:953–956, 1991.

Koretz RL: Nutritional supplementation in the ICU: how critical is nutrition for the critically ill? *Am J Respir Crit Care Med* 151:570–573, 1995.

Levine R, Alvarez FG: Intravenous fluid therapy, *Hospital Physician* November 1994, pp 21–37.

Levy E, et al: Septic necrosis of the midline wound in postoperative peritonitis, *Ann Surg* 207:470–479, 1988.

Ng SKC, et al: Alcohol consumption and withdrawal in new-onset seizures, *N Engl J Med* 319:666, 1988.

O'Hanlon-Nichols T: Commonly asked questions about wound healing, Am J Nurs 95:22–24, 1995.

Ready LB, the Task Force on Pain Management: Practice guidelines for acute pain management in the perioperative setting, *Anesthesiology* 82:1071–1081, 1995.

Swoboda SM, et al: Does intraoperative blood loss affect antibiotic serum and tissue concentrations? *Arch Surg* 131:1165–1172, 1996.

van Heurn LWE, Brink PRG: Prospective randomized trial of high versus low vacuum drainage after axillary lymphadenectomy, *Br J Surg* 82:931–932, 1995.

Wolff BG, et al: Elective colon and rectal surgery without nasogastric decompression: a prospective, randomized trial, *Ann Surg* 209:670–673, 1989.

Woods JH, et al: Postoperative ileus: a colonic problem? *Surgery* 84:527–533, 1978.

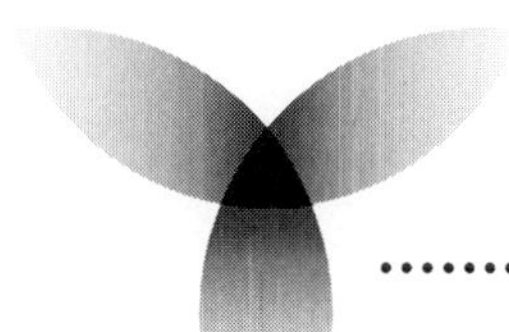

Chapter 44

Perioperative Medicine and Intensive Care

Charles G. Durbin, MD, David J. Stone, MD

Currently, there are a large number of texts on the practice of critical care medicine and the "how-to" aspects of critical care practice. Some of these are listed in the bibliography at the end of this chapter. Rather than attempt to cover the entire field in a brief space, this chapter will cover some less-frequently addressed aspects of critical care medicine as they specifically relate to the perioperative period. These issues are political, administrative, economic, and legal in addition to strictly medical concerns. Who belongs in the intensive care unit (ICU), what the ICU has to offer these patients, and how long patients should be kept in the special care unit will be discussed in this chapter. The issues of shared responsibility and decision making, relationships with allied health professionals and other physicians, and resource allocation (triage decisions) make the ICU a unique and stressful environment for physicians as well as patients.

CRITICAL CARE MEDICINE IN THE PERIOPERATIVE PERIOD

In the operating room (OR), cardiovascular, respiratory and other functions are monitored and managed meticulously by an anesthetist who is continuously present. In fact, much of what is done in the OR, especially if the patient is sick or the operation complex, is similar to what is done in the ICU. The primary goal in both environments is the maintenance and, if necessary, restoration of basic physiologic functions. In the OR, physiologic functions are influenced by the presence of anesthetic agents, as well. The closure of the incision does not necessarily signal the end of problems. For this reason, the postanesthesia care unit (PACU), or recovery room, was developed to deal with airway, respiratory, cardiovascular, and other problems immediately after surgery. While the most important effects of the anesthesia agents per se are usually limited to the immediate postoperative period, the patient's underlying medical problems are often worsened by the operation. Recovery from anesthesia and surgical trespass extends beyond the brief recovery room stay.

The modern ICU evolved mainly from two sources, the PACU and the respiratory care unit, which was originally organized to care for patients with neuromuscular respiratory failure from poliomyelitis. The basic function of the ICU is to continue the intensive nursing care available in the PACU while providing advanced airway management, mechanical ventilation skills, and immediate resuscitation for as long as they are required. This basic service level has been augmented in many ways in some ICUs including special considerations in patients with neurologic, cardiac, and infectious disease problems as well as in transplant and trauma patients. The presence of the nurse in close proximity allows continuous or near-continuous monitoring of noninvasive measures such as electrocardiogram (ECG), automated blood pressure by oscillometry, and pulse oximetry. It also allows the safe use of invasive monitors, such as arterial and pulmonary artery catheters, and the administration of potent cardiovascular pharmacologic agents. Most importantly, the nurse serves as an on-site monitor and advocate of overall patient status. Currently, many ICUs have a physician in the ICU or immediately available to respond to urgent or emergent problems so that needed care will not be delayed while bedside nurses are locating physicians. The ICU consequently represents an unrivaled resource in terms of medical and nursing care, combined with the ability to use potent and invasive medical measures to patients whose chances of survival would be considerably diminished in the absence of such care. The actual and potential harm that can and does occur in the critical care unit makes the unit a high medical-legal risk.

The cost of critical care is also high, perhaps accounting for 20% of the total hospital budget. In the United States, approximately 1% of gross domestic product is spent on critical care; in 1994, this was estimated to be approximately 100 billion dollars. In times of diminishing economic support, careful resource management is essential for hospital survival. Appropriate, cost-effective ICU care can improve the hospital's financial viability.

• INTENSIVE CARE UNIT (ICU) ORGANIZATION

As mentioned previously, the first ICUs were respiratory care units, dealing with a single patient group with similar problems. This allowed specialized equipment and patient care expertise to be concentrated in a single location for efficiency and safety. Today, specialized ICUs catering to specific patient groups with similar clinical needs are the rule. Individual ICUs for patients following acute myocardial infarction, coronary care unit (CCU), after cardiac or transplant surgery, with neurologic diseases, after major trauma, or of a particular age (neonatal and pediatric) are common in most larger hospitals. However, general medical, surgical and combined medical-surgical ICUs, providing basic and specialized critical care for a larger range of patients and clinical problems, are common in many hospitals. The organization, administration and staffing of the ICU depends on which patients it serves and what services it supplies.

Medical direction, required for special care units (including the PACU), is usually provided by a specialist physician with interest and experience in critical care medicine (CCM). Subspecialty certification in critical care medicine is offered by the American Board of Anesthesiology, the American College of Surgeons, the American Board of Internal Medicine, and the American Academy of Pediatrics. Additional certification opportunity will soon be available for diplomates of other specialties. The medical director is responsible for the appropriateness of admission and discharge of patients, assuring availability of physician coverage, and the overall quality of care provided in the unit. This usually means developing policies and procedures for ICU functions that are then approved though the hospital physician governing body. The way in which medical care is provided will vary, depending upon unit organization and institutional politics.

The medical coverage of CCUs follows one of two basic models: "closed" or "open." In a closed unit, all primary medical decisions are made by a unit-based, dedicated critical care physician. Patients may actually be transferred to the CCM physician's service when they enter the unit. On unit discharge, patients may stay on the intensivist's service or revert to the hospital admitting physician. This model is most common in medical ICUs, CCUs, and some surgical subspecialty units. Specialty consultations are initiated by the CCM service attending, and all patient care communications are directed through the intensivist.

The other basic model for ICU medical care is the "open" model. Most common in surgical and mixed medical-surgical ICUs, this model identifies the admitting attending as the primary coordinator of critical-care decision making. Often, a unit-based or CCM consultant attending physician actively collaborates to enhance the care process. However, final patient management decisions rest with the primary attending physician. Many units exhibit characteristics of both models. For instance, in an "open" general surgical ICU, following major urologic surgery, patients may be entirely managed by the unit-based surgical intensivist (often, an anesthesiologist) while patients on the trauma service may be primarily managed by the trauma surgeon with consultation from the intensivist.

Understanding the medical organization of a unit is important when turning over postoperative care after providing anesthesia to patients in the OR. If the patient will not require continued intubation following surgery and anesthesia, extubation in the OR or PACU may be appropriate if the unit is an open unit in which the surgical attending directs care, or a closed unit without an anesthesiologist intensivist. Under these circumstances, direct physician-to-physician communication of the intraoperative events and anesthetic concerns should be reported to the unit or surgical attending physician at the end of the procedure, or on transfer to the unit after recovery in the PACU. Patients can be transported anesthetized and recovered in the

ICU, if the immediate postoperative recovery period is managed by an anesthesiologist or anesthesiology intensivist, or if postoperative airway support and mechanical ventilation are planned. Local politics and unit organization will determine these issues.

Nursing care in ICUs is usually specialized, as well. Nurses may obtain specialty certification as Critical Care Registered Nurses (CCRN) from the American Association of Critical Care Nurses. To achieve this recognition requires extensive critical care experience, continued education, and successful completion of a certification examination. Intensive-care unit nursing care may be provided by registered nurses or practical nurses (LPNs). Nurse-to-patient ratios vary according to policy and intensity of care needs. Ratios of 1:2 are the usual average in most ICUs; however, for the most ill patients, ratios of greater than 1:1 are occasionally needed.

Because airway care or mechanical ventilation are needed in the majority of ICU patients, respiratory therapists are often a part of the ICU staffing mix. In some units they provide all needed ventilator care; in others this is a shared service with nurses. In addition, respiratory therapists may provide bronchodilator treatments, endotracheal intubation, weaning and extubation, chest physical therapy, and other technical services such as physiologic monitoring, invasive-line insertion and maintenance, determination of cardiac output, 12-lead ECG recording, and some laboratory services (e.g., arterial blood gas analysis). Therapists may be unit-based or have the responsibility of assessing and treating patients as they progress through the hospital system. Other specialized personnel may provide additional patient services such as line dressing teams, nutritional support teams, clinical pharmacists, and clinical laboratory services. Unit and institutional policy will determine what services will be provided by which groups. Understanding how these services work and interact is important when delivering or seeing a patient in the perioperative period in an ICU.

INTENSIVE CARE UNIT ADMISSIONS

In the perioperative period, intensive-care unit admissions are either planned or unplanned. Planned admissions are done so on the basis of patient factors or the type of operation. A large number of surgical procedures produce sufficient physiologic trespass so that the need for intensive care is readily predictable. These needs include continued airway management with or without mechanical ventilation, potential for specific complications, monitoring for cardiac ischemia or hemodynamic instability, and a demand for frequent attention and care that simply cannot be provided outside an ICU. These include cases requiring cardiopulmonary bypass, major vascular and thoracic procedures, severe multiple trauma, and liver transplants. Other cases may receive intensive care mainly for neurologic monitoring, such as after intracranial vascular surgery or craniotomy for brain tumor, especially involving the posterior fossa. The location of postoperative care for a variety of procedures may vary from institution to institution. These include kidney transplants, carotid endarterectomies, selected cervical spine procedures, and major head and neck operations. The choice of locale may depend on institutional philosophy, nursing availability on regular units, and the availability of special "step-down" units that can provide an intermediate level of nursing care and monitoring. Procedures that may result in a need for intensive care include major urologic, gynecologic, and general surgery procedures. The actual need for an ICU bed may depend on the course of the operation (e.g., degree of blood loss and anticipated large fluid shifts). Other urgent general surgery cases may need postoperative intensive care and include operations for GI bleeding, ischemic bowel, and perforated viscus. In these cases, the decision to request an ICU bed may only be finalized in the recovery room when the patient demonstrates the need for continued intensive nursing and medical care. While these admissions may not strictly be planned, they are not unplanned in the sense that a possible need for ICU care was anticipated in view of the magnitude of the surgery.

Patient issues may also determine a need for planned, postoperative ICU placement. The most obvious of these includes those patients already in the ICU who come to the OR for a procedure during that period of time when ICU care is still necessary. Often, these procedures involve establishment of long-term airway (tracheostomy) and feeding (gastro- or jejeunostomy) conduits, which will facilitate eventual ICU discharge. In some institutions, these procedures are performed in the ICU but other surgeons feel that equipment and conditions are optimized in the OR environment. This is especially important if all does not go well with the procedure. Even a "simple" tracheostomy can result in severe, acute life-threatening complications such as loss of the airway, tracheostomy tube misplacement, and tension pneumothorax. Patients from burn units also may require frequent visits to the OR for debridement and grafting procedures.

Other planned admissions may well be on the basis of clinical judgment and cover a wide variety of clinical problems. These can be approached by system: Box 44-1 provides a listing of some of the possible reasons for anticipated ICU admission.

Unplanned admissions, by definition, arise from unanticipated problems or complications which occur in the operative or recovery period. Analysis by continuous quality improvement (CQI) programs has revealed that these unplanned admissions fall into two basic categories. The first consists of unplanned admissions as a result of preoperative misjudgment, that is, in retrospect, it became evident that the admission should have been planned. The other category includes admissions which truly could not have been anticipated preoperatively.

Anesthetic problems which may result in a need for an ICU bed include aspiration of gastric contents, upper airway problems, cardiac arrest, prolonged paralysis, malignant hyperthermia or neuroleptic malignant syndrome, or an episode of hypoxemia or hypotension that is so severe that reawakening has been delayed. A large variety of problems may cause delayed emergence from anesthesia, and ICU care may be required if these do not resolve during a reasonable period of time in the recovery room. Analysis by our CQI program has indicated that respiratory failure, including pulmonary edema caused by fluid overload, comprises a significant proportion of these cases. (personal communication, TA Yemen, MD) Other problems which may partly be related to the anesthetic include myocardial ischemia/infarction, congestive heart failure, stroke, and acute renal failure. A very common scenario involves the patient with mild ST-T wave changes who is otherwise stable and

Box 44-1 Reasons for Anticipating Postoperative Admission to an ICU

1. Cardiovascular
   a. Severe myocardial dysfunction caused by myocardial, valvular, congenital, or pericardial disease
   b. High risk of myocardial ischemia/infarction—unstable angina, recent myocardial infarction in high-risk or unstratified patient (may go to CCU or postcardiac surgery unit)
2. Respiratory
   a. Severe preoperative compromise of lung volumes—incapacitating restrictive-lung disease, chest wall deformities, extreme obesity, chest wall trauma, incipient respiratory failure
   b. Preoperative ventilatory failure—especially if complicated by neuromuscular weakness and procedure that involves thorax or upper abdomen
   c. Special difficult airway considerations
3. Neuromuscular
   a. Severe neuromuscular disease likely to result in a need for postoperative airway maintenance/protection and/or mechanical ventilation
   b. Monitoring and care for decreased mental status, increased intracranial pressure, epilepsy
4. Endocrine
   a. Presence of endocrine emergency such as diabetic ketoacidosis, thyroid storm or myxedema coma, adrenal insufficiency with shock, pituitary apoplexy
   b. Endocrinopathy that may produce hemodynamic instability—pheochromocytoma, carcinoid
5. Renal
   a. Gross fluid overload with pulmonary edema, metabolic disturbances requiring intensive therapy such as hyperkalemia, acidosis judged to be too severe to be treated on the ward
6. Infectious Disease
   a. Fulminant septic shock—may also *result* from surgery such as perforated viscus, mesenteric ischemia
   b. Isolation—patient requiring isolation may receive closer attention in ICU isolation area than in floor area where near constant supervision is impossible

usually asymptomatic, but who may require some further degree of cardiac intervention and monitoring while the process is evaluated for genuine myocardial ischemia/infarction vs nonspecific changes as a result of surgery, hypothermia, electrolyte shifts, etc. Perioperative myocardial infarction carries a significant risk of death. If myocardial infarction is being "ruled out" by drawing cardiac enzymes, it does not seem logical to follow a patient in an unmonitored bed on the floor where detection and treatment of a malignant dysrrhythmia could be delayed.

Unanticipated surgical problems which result in a need for ICU admission involve technical complications, as well as unexpected findings and difficulties which arise in the course of an operation. These include unanticipated severity of hemorrhage with subsequent need for massive fluid and blood product replacement, possibly further complicated by coagulopathy; entry into a structure such as a major blood vessel or viscus that was inadvertent and resulted in severe, prolonged hypotension; or discovery that a more extensive or different procedure than originally planned was required. An example of the last would be the discovery of a large amount of infarcted bowel in an elderly patient suspected of a relatively mild problem, such as appendicitis.

INTENSIVE CARE UNIT DISCHARGES

Criteria for ICU discharge will vary among circumstances, depending on the availability of various support modalities outside the unit. For example, can patients be mechanically ventilated outside an ICU? This may be safe in the tracheotomized but not for the intubated patient, in view of the difficulties involved in replacing the respective airway devices if dislodged. In many instances, the patient must be weaned from mechanical ventilation, but the presence of a tracheostomy for airway maintenance, protection, and pulmonary toilet is perfectly acceptable on the regular floor. While central venous catheters are allowed, usually arterial and pulmonary artery catheters are not permitted outside the ICU. Patients must be hemodynamically stable and off pressor and inotropic support. Most other functions such as enteral nutrition, multiple intravenous infusions, pleural drainage, basic respiratory care, etc. can be provided outside the ICU if the nursing and respiratory care staff has the quality and quantity of workers to do so. However, discharge from the ICU must be undertaken with the realization that there is some risk involved in leaving the haven of intensive care, and that some individuals may soon return to the unit because discharge was predictably or unpredictably premature.

Patients who return unexpectedly to the ICU may represent premature discharge (early triage), worsening of the same problem for which the patient was originally admitted to the ICU, or development of a new problem. Mortality is lowest with a new problem, similar to that of the "new" problem on a first ICU admission. Return for worsening of the same problem carries the highest mortality. This is probably because the original problem is now chronic, and unlikely to improve significantly in the short run. Respiratory problems are a common cause of ICU readmission, occurring in between 45% and 65% of these patients.

OUTCOME FROM CRITICAL CARE

Patient outcome for CCU treatment is influenced by many factors. The severity of the underlying disease and reason for ICU admission are extremely important in determining patient survival. The quality and appropriateness of treatment should play a part in outcome. Quality of care in an ICU is often assessed by crude mortality rate. Because critically ill patients are cared for in the ICU, mortality of ICU patients will be high, even with the best quality care. To estimate and improve quality, it is important to know what the expected mortality of a group of critically ill patients is likely to be, and compare this to the actual mortality. Several acuity-adjusted outcome (mortality) systems have been developed. One of the best known ICU mortality-predictive systems is the APACHE System (Acute Physiology and Chronic Health Evaluation). The APACHE II score is based on the patient's age, presence of chronic disease, area from where the patient is admitted, and a weighted score based on the worst deviation from normal of 17 physiologic measures during the first 24 hours in the ICU. This system has been validated in many different ICUs and between different countries. It predicts approximately 90% of the outcome of critically ill patients (alive or dead at hospital discharge). Differences between predicted and actual outcome in an individual ICU can be used as a measure of quality of lack of quality relative to the "average" ICU outcome, represented in the original APACHE II data set.

A newer version of this system, APACHE III, is a commercial product with a larger set of diagnosis-specific outcome predictions with a slightly different physiologic data set. Outcomes can be compared between similar institutions, units within the same region, or with the entire database. Periodic updating and calibrating with current data makes the comparisons more useful over time. Similar to APACHE II, slightly more than 90% of the patient outcome is determined by the status of the patient on ICU admission during the first 24 hours of treatment. A significant improvement in the APACHE III system is the daily prediction of the probability of death in each individual patient. This prediction is based on algorithms relating to expected physiologic improvements over time and the development of organ system failures. Patients who have less than a 10% chance of needing ICU resources are also identified with the APACHE III system. These patients are only being monitored and can often be cared for in a less intensive (and expensive) hospital location with no significant risk of poor outcome.

Other models predicting ICU patient mortality include the Mortality Prediction Model (MPM II), the Simplified Acute Physiology Score (SAPS I and II), the Trauma Score, the Pediatric Risk of Mortality (PRISM) system, and Project Impact, a growing ICU database sponsored by the Society of Critical Care Medicine. These can also be used to stratify patients according to risk of death and identify quality concerns when applied across units. Other quality measures include monitoring the frequency of complications of critical care treatment. The incidence of unplanned patient extubation, invasive-line removal, pneumothorax drug central-line insertion, cardiac arrest, incorrect drug or drug dosage, unexpected return to the OR, nosocomial infection rate, need for reintubation after elective extubation, pressure ulcer rate, and death, or return to the ICU after discharge have been used to identify quality issues in the ICU.

By identifying ICUs with better acuity-adjusted outcomes than predicted, organizational and care delivery methods which may contribute to this improvement have been identified. From the original APACHE study of 13 ICUs, the best units had a patient-centered culture, strong medical and nursing leadership, effective communication and coordination, and an open, collaborative approach to solving problems and resolving conflict. In a study of pediatric ICUs, the presence of a certified intensivist as Unit Director and a senior physician decision-maker in the unit, correlated with the best patient outcome. Other studies have confirmed the contribution of an intensivist as unit medical director to improved outcome. The complexity and differences of ICU organization, missions, resources, and patient populations make generalities relating to different management strategies difficult to conclude in the current critical care environment. The best ICUs are concerned about the quality of patient care delivered, attempt to measure quality, and change operations when opportunities to improve are identified.

Patients undergoing surgical procedures experience a lower acuity-adjusted mortality than medical patients admitted to an ICU with similar physiologic derangements. This is most likely because of the acute, reversible, physiologic abnormalities induced by anesthesia and surgery. Surgical patients experience more pain in the ICU than medical patients and are often inadequately treated with analgesics. The advent of novel pain-relief strategies (i.e., epidural analgesia, patient-controlled analgesia) has positively impacted critically ill surgical patients, and probably has reduced perioperative complications and mortality.

Patients are admitted to an ICU for active treatment (such as mechanical ventilation, vasoactive drug infusions, airway protection) or for "monitoring." Patients being monitored have a low frequency (generally less than 10% chance of needing active treatment) and experience a relatively low mortality, usually less than 5%. Between 20% to 40% of ICU admissions to surgical ICUs are for monitoring. The amount of active treatment a patient is receiving can be quantitated in several ways. The Therapeutic Intervention Scoring System (TISS) point total is a commonly used method, which reflects this quantity and correlates well with ICU costs. The system's points do not correlate with severity of illness because they are determined by local physician- and nursing-treatment practices.

Although not possible to test in a randomized fashion, the survival of patients requiring life support technologies is undoubtedly improved from ICU care. Patients who are unstable and moderately ill, seem to benefit most from ICU care. The fact that ICU admission earlier in the course of critical illness is associated with lower mortality, suggests the benefit of critical care units. An experienced staff with technical expertise, a strong multidisciplinary team, and active medical involvement in unit management are necessary to provide maximum patient benefit and reduce risk.

• CONSULTING IN THE ICU

While some physicians may provide "primary care" in the ICU or act as the unit medical director, the majority will see patients residing in an ICU during a preoperative evaluation before surgery and anesthesia, or as a consultant about specific medical issues. The preoperative evaluation of the ICU patient is often complicated by the active treatment the patient is receiving. If the patient is receiving mechanical ventilation, sedative drugs or neuromuscular blocking agents may be in use. Verbal communication is often impossible. Families are often distressed or not available, and information transfer about the planned procedure and medical problems is difficult. The intensive care physician and other caregivers are often the primary source of medical information needed by the consultant. Care priorities in the ICU and the OR are similar. However, because ICU care is often segmented and provided by a team rather than a single individual, all members of the team may need to be involved in relating relevant information to the anesthesiologist who is seeing the patient preoperatively.

The nurse will provide the current vital signs and describe any continuous infusions that are in use and any recent changes. The respiratory therapist will relate the current mode of ventilation, inspired oxygen, amount and character of sputum, and any airway difficulties. Psychosocial issues, including any advanced directives, are usually known to the nurse. The preoperative chart review is usually daunting task. Intensive care unit charts are often voluminous and are organized to suit the needs of the particular unit. Previous anesthetic records and other important sources of information are frequently removed when the chart is "thinned." Old charts are often hidden in the unit. It is necessary to ask for the entire chart when consulting or evaluating an ICU patient for anesthesia. Digitization of medical records may eventually provide a particular boon when it comes to practical utilization of the ICU chart.

Transfer of an unstable ICU patient to the OR can also be a difficult task. Maintenance of needed continuous pharmacologic infusions, mechanical ventilation, and the equipment needed for any unexpected emergency should be guaranteed. This may mean that a physician (the intensivist or the anesthesiologist) must accompany the patient to the OR from the ICU. Simplification of infusion lines and choosing monitoring equipment used in the OR for transport should be considered.

Anesthesiologists are, occasionally, requested to provide services or consultation in the ICU. Tracheal intubation or changing an endotracheal tube after cuff failure is a common request. Routine airway equipment may be available. However, specialized equipment (such as a gum bougie or a lighted stylette) is unlikely to be present in the ICU. Routine anesthetic drugs such as 4% topical lidocaine or pentothal are also difficult to obtain quickly in many ICUs. Bringing the necessary equipment will facilitate efficient service provision.

Anesthetics may be requested for brief surgical or medical procedures performed in the ICU. Local customs and availability of resources lead to several routine procedures being performed in the ICU, rather than the OR or other specialized area. Patient factors and stability may, at times, lead to unusual requests for anesthetic services, as well. Unintubated patients will benefit from an anesthesiologist providing airway management and sedation during endoscopy, tracheostomy, percutaneous feeding-tube placement, and other procedures performed in the ICU. Conscious sedation for radiographic studies is another area for which anesthetic skills may be needed and requested. For the anesthesiologist providing these skills and services, inadequate equipment and untrained support personnel provide a significant challenge to quality and safe care.

General anesthesia may be therapeutic and life-saving in several conditions. *Status asthmaticus* unresponsive to conventional intensive treatment may improve with deep inhalation anesthesia. The use of general anesthesia in *status epilepticus* has also been reported. Safe treatment may require transport of the patient to the OR where anesthetic machines and waste gas scavenging can be provided. Provision of general inhalation anesthesia in the ICU is possible with advanced planning and negotiation. The strangeness of the environment and lack of usual support systems makes a "dry run" a useful, preparatory exercise.

Treatment of malignant hyperthermia (MH) begins in the OR and continues into the ICU. Prescription of dantrolene and support of the hyperthermic patient is the domain of the anesthesiologist. Complications of MH, including disseminated intravascular coagulation, cardiac failure, and renal failure, should be collaboratively managed with the intensivist or appropriate organ-system specialist. The use of dantrolene in support of patients with the neuroleptic malignant syndrome or heat stroke may involve anesthesiology consultation.

Consultations can be advisory or for direct management. Direct communication with the requesting physician should be made to ensure the correct questions are being addressed and whether active services are requested. Maintaining good relations with other ICU caregivers when seeing patients in the ICU is essential for the best quality care.

MEDICAL LEGAL ISSUES

Modern anesthetic techniques, routine monitoring, and clinical education have all improved patient safety to the point that it is difficult to estimate the minimal contribution of OR anesthetic practices to perioperative mortality. In the ICU the situation is different. Many patients treated in an ICU do not survive. The duration of the physician contact with the patient extends for a longer period of time in the ICU than in the OR. More complications occur. Patient care is not continuously under the direct supervision of the physician. Many other individuals of various levels of training and experience provide aspects of the treatment plan. For these reasons, the potential for a malpractice action against the physician is greater in the ICU than in the OR or for the primary care physician. Wrongful death is a common allegation in ICU suits. Good communication is essential to reduce risk. Detailed, unhurried discussions with patients and their families, especially regarding risks and possible poor outcomes, are important. Many times this is not possible because the family is not available when care is given. Even with adequate discussion, what is said is often not remembered or given proper weight because the anxiety surrounding a critical illness makes retention of details poor. A detailed, complete note in the patient's chart including what was discussed and with whom is useful to refresh memories, should a question occur in the future. Further details on this issue are addressed in the Chapter 47.

BIBLIOGRAPHY

Ayers SM, et al, editors: *Textbook of critical care*, ed 3, Philadelphia, 1995, WB Saunders.

Bell RM: Is the timing of intensive care unit admission important? *Crit Care Med* 18:1303, 1990.

Civetta JM, Taylor RW, Kirby RR, editors: *Critical Care*, Hagerstown, MD, 1996, Lippincott-Raven.

Durbin CG, Kopel RF: A case-control study of patients readmitted to the intensive care unit, *Criti Care Med* 21:1547, 1993.

Leigh JM, Tytler JA: Admissions to the intensive care unit after complications of anesthetic techniques over 10 years, *Anaesthesia* 45:814, 1990.
Marino PL, editor: *The ICU book*, Philadelphia, 1991, Lea & Febiger.
Swann D, Houston P, Goldberg J: Audit of intensive care unit admissions from the operating room, *Canadian J Anaesth* 40:137, 1993.

Section VII

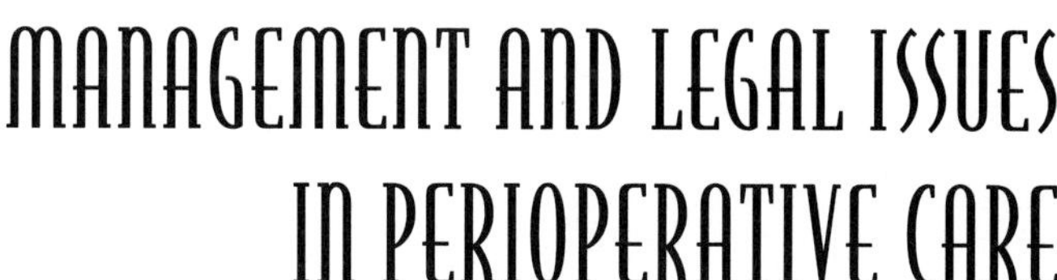

MANAGEMENT AND LEGAL ISSUES IN PERIOPERATIVE CARE

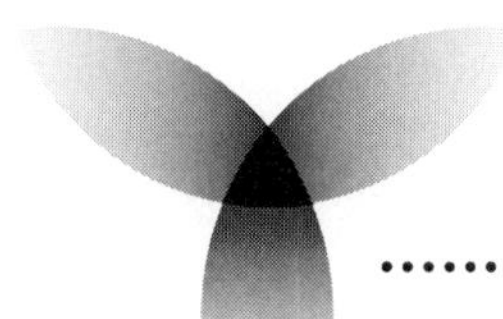

Chapter 45

Outcomes Research and Cost-Effectiveness

Jennifer E. O'Flaherty, MD, MPH

The goal of outcomes research is to fill existing gaps in medical knowledge and to direct practitioners to the best course of action for their patients. To provide quality patient care, physicians will rely more on clinical research in which outcomes of direct relevance to the patient are measured and less on personal experience and consensus opinion. Government and third-party payers are demanding independently verifiable evidence that therapy will not only be of high quality, but will actually improve patient outcome. At the same time, health care consumers are demanding greater control of their health care decisions and are requesting information on outcomes of interest to them. As the medical decision-making process and the application of medical knowledge by individual physicians are being increasingly analyzed by individual patients and society as a whole, physicians are responding by providing the evidence in question.

• THE STUDY OF OUTCOMES IN PERIOPERATIVE MEDICINE

The need for outcomes data is particularly great in perioperative medicine, a field in which patient care options are rapidly expanding and are ripe for evaluation. For example, in 1993 Warner et al.[1] published their prospective outcomes study examining major morbidity and mortality within 1 month of ambulatory surgery and anesthesia. Previous ambulatory perioperative outcomes data had been limited to the first 24 to 48 postoperative hours. Because more patients are undergoing ambulatory surgery and anesthesia, increasing numbers of patients with coexisting diseases and patients at the extremes of the age spectrum will be treated at ambulatory surgery centers. Outcomes of ambulatory surgery and anesthesia will provide useful information to physicians and patients. Warner and colleagues[1] looked at a total of 38,598 patients undergoing 45,090 consecutive anesthetics with near complete follow-up at 3 days, and again at 30 days. They found overall major morbidity (myocardial infarction, central nervous system deficit, pulmonary embolism, and respiratory failure) and mortality to be low, with only 1 in 1455 patients developing a major morbidity, and only 2 persons dying of medical conditions.

In addition to new patient care options, new medications are also frequently introduced into perioperative practice. It is no longer sufficient to demonstrate the safety and efficacy of a medication in a randomized, double-blind, placebo-controlled trial. It is now necessary to show that the new drug is either superior in action to the existing drug options, or that it is associated with significantly fewer side effects. For example, ondansetron was shown to be a safe and effective antiemetic for the treatment of postoperative nausea and vomiting in a randomized, double-blind, placebo-controlled trial in 1991 by Larijani et al.[2] Since that time, many clinical researchers have investigated whether ondansetron is superior to antiemetics already in use. In 1992, Alon and Himmelseher[3] evaluated the prophylactic antiemetic administration of ondansetron in comparison with droperidol and metoclopramide in a randomized, double-blind trial in adult patients undergoing general anesthesia for dilatation and curettage. Postoperatively, there was a statistically significant decrease in the incidence of vomiting in the ondansetron group, compared with the other two groups (incidence of vomiting was 13% with ondansetron, 45% with droperidol, and 54% with metoclopramide). In 1994, Furst and Rodarte[4] studied the prophylactic antiemetic administration of ondansetron, droperidol, metoclopramide, and placebo in children undergoing tonsillectomy under general anesthesia in a randomized double-blinded trial. They found that ondansetron reduced the incidence of postoperative vomiting from 62% to 27%, whereas droperidol and metoclopramide had no significant effect on postoperative vomiting. Similar results were obtained by Paxton et al.[5] in 1995. They compared the prophylactic antiemetic administration of ondansetron, droperidol, metoclopramide, and placebo in women undergoing laparascopic gynecologic procedures under general anesthesia in a randomized double-blinded trial. The incidence of vomiting was 18% in the ondansetron group compared with 48% in the droperidol group, 41% in the metoclopramide group, and 48% in the placebo group.

The study of outcomes allows perioperative physicians to evaluate the effect of their choice of therapeutic interventions. It has long been recognized that there are significant variations in the practice patterns of physicians. It is important to know if different practice patterns result in different patient outcomes. In 1993, Todd et al.[6] published an excellent example of this type of study. They prospectively compared three different anesthetic techniques (propofol/fentanyl, isoflurane/nitrous oxide, fentanyl/nitrous oxide) in adults undergoing elective surgical removal of a supratentorial, intracranial mass lesion. These anesthetics have distinct cerebrovascular physiologic effects *in vitro*, and in animal studies and, therefore, have theoretical differences in clinical practice. Todd et al. found few intergroup hemodynamic differences, no intergroup differences in surgical assessment of brain swelling, no clinically important intergroup differences in the mean intracranial pressure, no differences in the incidence of new postoperative deficits, and no differences in short-term outcome or length of hospital stay. There was an increased incidence of vomiting and a significantly shorter time to awakening in the fentanyl/nitrous oxide group. Todd et al. concluded that each of the three anesthetic techniques was acceptable to use in patients undergoing elective supratentorial craniotomies, although there were some differences in minor side effects. Outcomes studies help perioperative physicians choose wisely from the multitude of therapeutic options, many of which have been inadequately evaluated and have been previously recommended or rejected on theoretical grounds alone.

Outcomes research forces physicians to acknowledge that their individual biases, or even those of the "experts," can be misleading. In the late 1980s, most perioperative centers around the world incorporated pulse oximetry into their intraoperative and postoperative monitoring practices because perioperative physicians empirically believed that the power to detect subtle hypoxemia would reduce perioperative morbidity and mortality. In fact, the current American Society of Anesthesiologists' standards for basic anesthetic monitoring require that "during all anesthetics, a quantitative method of assessing oxygenation such as pulse oximetry shall be employed." Also, "during recovery from all anesthetics, a quantitative method of assessing oxygenation such as pulse oximetry shall be employed in the initial phase of recovery." However, the assumed efficacy of pulse oximetry has never been documented in a study of outcomes. In Denmark, Moller et al.[7] had the opportunity to conduct a randomized trial of pulse oximetry in 20,802 patients in the perioperative setting before there was widespread use of pulse oximetry. They examined the impact of pulse oximetry monitoring intraoperatively and postoperatively on the frequency of unanticipated perioperative events, changes in patient care, and the rate of postoperative complications. In the oximetry group, there was a 19-fold increase in the incidence of diagnosed hypoxemia in both the operating room (OR) and the postanesthesia care unit (PACU). In the OR, use of pulse oximetry was associated with a more frequent identification of hypoventilation, endobronchial intubation, and myocardial ischemia. Several changes in PACU care were observed in association with the use of pulse oximetry, including the use of higher flow rates of supplemental oxygen, longer PACU stays, a greater likelihood of receiving supplemental oxygen at discharge from the PACU, and a greater likelihood of receiving naloxone in the PACU. There was no significant difference, however, in morbiity or mortality in the monitored and unmonitored groups. Despite the increase in sensitivity for diagnosing perioperative hypoxemia and related events in the OR and in the PACU, use of pulse oximetry was associated only with a number of costly changes in patient care, but not with any ultimate effect on patient outcome.

The study of outcomes can also be used to confirm that an intervention actually has the intended effect, rather than a negative or no effect. For example, in 1973 Shapiro et al.[8] reported on the successful use of a barbiturate to reduce acutely elevated intracranial pressure in the OR. In 1974, Michenfelder[9] demonstrated that barbiturates in sufficient doses could decrease cerebral blood flow and cerebral metabolic rate, both of which significantly contribute to intracranial pressure. Because the management of increased intracranial pressure is critical in the severely brain injured patient, critical care physicians began to use barbiturate therapy to acutely and chronically control intracranial hypertension in severely brain-injured patients. In 1985, however, a well-designed, randomized, controlled trial by Ward et al.[10] demonstrated that the prophylactic use of the so-called "barbiturate coma" was not associated with an improvement in patient outcome. In fact, they found that its use was accompanied by significant side effects. Systemic hypotension occurred in 54% of the patients who received barbiturate therapy, and in only 7% of patients who did not receive barbiturates. Systemic hypotension can considerably worsen the outcome of patients with severe head injuries.

Finally, outcomes research will help perioperative physicians identify aspects of patient care, which may not be directly under the physician's control but are, nonetheless, of great importance to patients, such as ease of parking at the medical center, time spent waiting for preoperative anesthesia assessment, or the comfort of the perioperative waiting facilities. Attention to improvements in patient comfort and satisfaction will become increasingly important as competition to attract patients intensifies.

OUTCOMES RESEARCH: A NEW INVESTIGATIONAL TOOL

Outcomes research has broad applications across medicine and will become an important investigational tool in the medical field in the next decade. The success of outcomes research will depend on fundamental shifts in clinical research. The first fundamental shift involves a change in perspective to examine outcomes of interest to patients, rather than outcomes of interest to physicians. Patients have been demanding this change in perspective for decades. In 1837 Honore Daumier produced his now classic lithograph in which the physician pronounces the operation to have been a success despite the fact that the patient died (Figure 45-1). Its continued popularity is a testament to how little progress has been made in closing the gap in perspective between patients and physicians. The technical success of an intervention may be of relevance to physicians (e.g., a surgical procedure successfully removed a diseased ovary), but will be entirely irrelevant to the patient if the intervention does little to change the course of his or her disease.

Outcomes studies of relevance to patients will require new outcome measures. Conventional outcome measures tend to be biologic and physiologic measures of technical success (e.g., an improvement in hemoglobin level following preoperative treatment of anemia, documentation of a perioperative myocardial infarction, or the recording of postoperative pain-relief scores). Physicians find these measures useful because they are easy to define, quantitate, and reproduce. Patients however often have trouble interpreting these medical outcomes, and are much more interested in humanistic outcomes. From the patient's perspective it would be more important to know if an improvement in preoperative hemoglobin level would lead to a decreased risk of intraoperative blood transfusion or a swifter postoperative recovery. It would

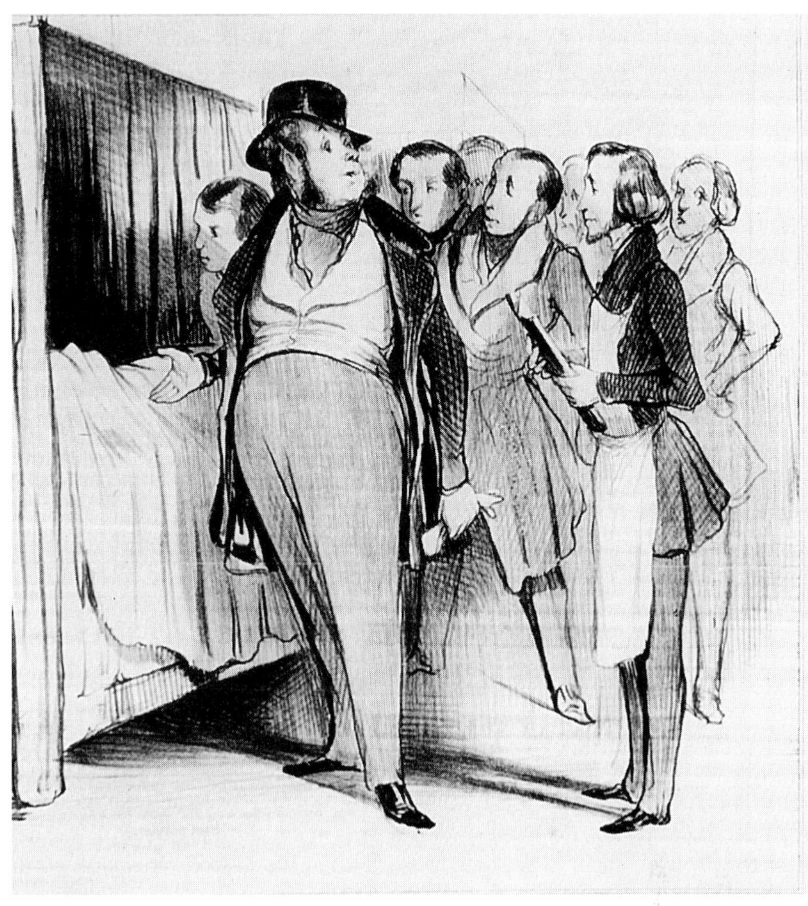

Figure 45-1

Dr. Robert Macaire's Clinic. "There you are, gentlemen, you've seen this operation, that everyone said was impossible, performed with complete success. . . .—But, Doctor, the patient's dead. . . .—What of it! She would have died anyway even without the operation." (Courtesy of the National Library of Medicine.)

be more important to know if a perioperative myocardial infarction would mean a prolonged hospital stay or any long-term functional limitations, or if an improvement in pain scores would necessarily mean an improvement in the patient's general well-being or quality of life. If a linear relationship between disease measures (e.g., a perioperative myocardial infarction) and outcome measures existed (e.g., the patient's subsequent functional status), it would be unnecessary to perform outcomes studies. This relationship however is complex rather than linear and may be affected by many different factors such as baseline health, coexisting disease, individual psychology, specific support systems, significant others, and the patient's physical environment.

New outcome measures will include measures of patient satisfaction, functional status, general well-being, quality of life, length of hospital stay, distress, ability to work, and the time it takes to get back to work. These outcomes have been referred to as "true outcomes" or patient-oriented outcomes rather than "medical outcomes" or disease-oriented outcomes. These outcomes are clearly related to end results, rather than to intermediate occurrences, such as myocardial infarction. Health care providers must become more focused on the downstream effects of the interventions they provide. Without a doubt, patient-oriented outcomes are harder to measure than disease-oriented outcomes. It is also true that several alternative outcome measures may exist for measuring patient-based outcomes. There is currently no mechanism for determining which measure would be best, and there is no overseeing body to endorse one measure over another. Much investigation and standardization will need to be done in this area. However, the use of meaningful patient outcomes will lead to relevant patient data.

Traditionally there has been an emphasis on catastrophic events in perioperative medicine. In 1858 John Snow, the noted 19th century physician, published the first study of anesthesia related deaths. Since that time, and for many reasons, anesthetic practice has become, significantly, so much safer, that death caused by anesthesia is no longer a meaningful outcome measure from the physician or the patient's point of view. Because death related to anesthesia has become such a rare event, other measures of perioperative outcome have become popular with physicians. Measures such as perioperative myocardial infarction, aspiration, or stroke, and unanticipated intensive-care unit admission have been used for many years in clinical anesthesia research to measure catastrophic perioperative events. These are all disease-oriented intermediate measures and by themselves may not be consequential to patients. Patients are interested in how these factors will affect the length of their hospital stay, the time it takes them to get back to work, their functional status, or their quality of life.

Though catastrophic events will continue to occur in the perioperative period, and must be carefully reviewed when they do occur, they now happen too rarely to remain the major focus of perioperative research. Physicians and patients are increasingly interested in the less catastrophic consequences of anesthesia because they are more likely to occur. These outcomes include postoperative nausea, dental injury, delayed awakening, and various residual discomforts such as sore throat after intubation, or back pain after regional anesthesia.

The second fundamental shift in outcomes research involves its scope. Investigators in this field will use large, linked, clinical databases. Modern computer information systems have made the collection and analysis of patient outcomes possible on a large scale. Manual systems of record keeping and information storage are being replaced with automated systems of record keeping and computer storage of information. Soon, computer-based information systems will be incorporated into all clinical practices. Information may be shared and compared between institutions on a scale, previously unthinkable. To make this sharing of information meaningful, it will be critically important to define outcome measures consistently and to require uniform collection and encoding of outcomes data. Collaborative research efforts across institutions will become more frequent and more important. Opportunities for intervention, which may not be detected on a smaller scale, may be discernible from a large central database.

The third fundamental shift in research design is the recognition that outcomes research will necessitate a multidisciplinary approach. Input from epidemiologists, biostatisticians, economists, health-science researchers, ethicists, sociologists, and health psychologists will be crucial to the success of such endeavors.

Outcomes research reflects a shift away from the classic health-care model of the individual physician providing patient care, based in large part on personal experience and expert opinion, using manual systems of record keeping and information storage. The new model is a population-based systematic approach of providing care based on evidence, then measuring outcome and providing continuous reevaluation and improvement, using computer systems for record keeping and information storage. In a medical environment in which therapeutic options are expanding rapidly, outcomes research will provide physicians with the ability to make rational, medical care choices, based on the outcomes most important to their patients.

COST-CONTAINMENT AND COST-EFFECTIVENESS

Medical care costs are increasing at a rate nearly 10% greater than inflation. Health care expenditures accounted for 14% of the gross national product (GNP) in 1992 and are projected to account for 20% of the GNP by the year 2000. As costs increase, hospital profits are steadily declining. Most of the causes of increased health care expenditures have direct significance in the perioperative arena. These include new technologies such as pulmonary artery catheters and transesophageal echocardiograms. Also included are new drugs like aprotinin, an antifibrinolytic agent used to decrease perioperative bleeding, principally in cardiac-surgery patients, and the accommodation of new circumstances, such as the need to test donor blood for HIV and hepatitis viruses, or the costs of implementing universal precautions.

Payers are searching for the optimal way to manage patients, one which results in improved patient outcomes and minimizes the cost to them. Physicians, who have always been interested in improving patient outcomes, must now also be concerned with the cost of therapy, relative to the improved outcome. Without data on outcome, payers will blindly decrease their costs. This is pure cost-containment. Cost-containment will sometimes result in the elimination of unnecessary expenses, with few consequences to physicians or patients. At other times, cost-containment might have devastating effects on the quality of patient care. Physicians can maintain their commitment to patients to provide high-quality care and, simultaneously, help decrease the overall costs of medical care, by providing therapies which are cost-effective. Physicians need not engage in blind cost-containment, but must furnish scientific evidence of effective therapies, eliminate ineffective therapies, and limit excessively expensive therapies. In the case of cost-containment, the least expensive therapy is always chosen, whereas in the case of cost-effectiveness the more expensive therapy may be chosen for sufficient reasons. More often, the least expensive option is chosen when two or more therapies are shown to result in the same patient outcome. A good example of this is preoperative testing. Traditionally, certain laboratory and diagnostic studies were routinely performed preoperatively. These usually included a complete blood count, blood chemistries, a urinalysis, and, sometimes, coagulation studies, a chest radiograph, and an electrocardiogram. Over the past decade, Roizen,[11] Apfelbaum,[12] Narr,[13] Gold,[14] Turnbull,[15] and many others have demonstrated that routine preoperative laboratory and diagnostic testing does not improve patient outcome and is very expensive. The results of these studies have led most perioperative centers to eliminate the minimum requirement for preoperative testing reulting in laboratory and diagnostic studies being ordered on an individual basis. Patient outcomes remain unchanged at a significant reduction in cost. In another example, Ledgerwood et al.[16] in 1992 examined the effects of two different anesthetic regimens on 86 morbidly obese patients undergoing gastric reservoir-reduction surgery. Baseline patient characteristics were similar in the two groups. They found that the medical outcome in patients for whom postoperative ventilation was routinely planned and arterial lines and Foley catheters were routinely inserted, was no different than the medical outcome in patients for whom postoperative ventilation was not routinely planned and arterial lines and Foley catheters were not routinely inserted. The difference however, in hospital charges for the two groups was radically different, totaling $14,524 per patient in the group in which postoperative ventilation was routinely planned and $7,580 per patient in the group in which postoperative ventilation was not routinely planned. Ledgerwood et al. concluded that gastric reservoir-reduction surgery could be performed safely, and at a significantly lower cost, without the routine use of postoperative ventilation and invasive monitoring.

Drug costs are a significant component of perioperative costs and of overall hospital costs. In 1994, Johnstone and Jozefczyk[17] demonstrated that drugs used by anesthesiologists accounted for 25% of all drug costs at their institution and 1.4% of all hospital operating expenses. Many drugs with comparable actions exist in perioperative medicine. They often vary widely in cost. In a study by Hampel et al.[18] in 1992, resident and attending anesthesiologists were unable to reliably predict which of four neuromuscular blocking agents (d-tubocurarine, pancuronium, atracurium, or vecuronium) they were using based on clinical signs. The cost to the institution per case was significantly different, however, ranging from $2.93 for pancuronium to $47.50 for atracurium. Why practitioners chose particular drugs is unknown, but it is suspected by Modell[19] and others to be related more to personal preference or convenience, rather than to specific medical indications. Hampel's[20] study suggests that it may be possible to decrease drug costs without compromising quality of care by choosing the most economical drug when there is a choice among clinically indistinguishable drugs.

Several recent studies have highlighted the fact that anesthesiologists have little knowledge about the cost of the drugs that they use routinely. In 1994, Shapiro et al.[21] surveyed the members of their department of anesthesiology at the University of California at Irvine and found that their knowledge of drug costs was limited. Faculty members were no better informed than residents, suggesting that they were unlikely to be instructing residents in this area. In 1994, Johnstone and Jozefczyk[22] surveyed members of the Department of Anesthesiology at West Virginia University and found that only 42% claimed to have a reasonable idea of the relative costs of drugs used during anesthesia. Whether drug-cost education alone will be sufficient to result in long-term cost savings is unclear. Becker,[23] Williams,[24] and Johnstone[25] have all shown that educational programs aimed at publicizing drug costs to anesthesiologists can result in significant short-term cost savings through altered drug usage patterns. Johnstone and Jozefczyk[26] noted an initial 23% reduction in anesthetic drug expenditures after their intensive cost education program. After 2 months, however, the cost education program lost its effectiveness and drug costs returned to above preeducation levels. The reasons for the long-term failure of such an education program are not fully known and have significant implications for the success of future perioperative physician education programs. Johnstone and Jozefczyk hypothesize the ultimate failure of the education program to be related to multiple causes, including a perception among physicians that the less expensive drugs were clinically inferior, that the drugs were being used increasingly by nonanesthesiologists and newer staff members who had not received the education, that drug company representatives had increased their efforts, and that there was a perceived lack of reward among the participants for saving money. Johnstone and Jozefcyk concluded that in order for there to be long-term savings from the cost-conscious use of anesthetic drugs, there would have to exist ongoing educational programs and participation incentives for perioperative physicians.

There will be times when drugs vary in their effects, as well as in their costs. Data on drug costs is equally important in these situations. Cost is now one of the variables that must be weighed when attempting to make intelligent choices among different therapies. In 1993, Wong et al.[27] compared the new nonsteroidal antiinflammatory drug ketorolac with two commonly prescribed opioid analgesics in ambulatory surgery patients. Intravenous ketorolac was associated with delayed, but otherwise equivalent, analgesic effects when compared with intravenous fentanyl. Oral ketorolac was associated with a lower incidence of nausea and somnolence and earlier return of bowel function (but no difference in analgesic effects) when compared with oral codeine and acetaminophen. Johnstone and Martinec[28] point out that the unmentioned difference in cost between the ketorolac group and the fentanyl plus codeine and acetaminophen group is more than 20-fold. This information should be available and considered when making a fully-informed choice as to which regimen to use.

The introduction of new technologies into perioperative medicine should also be accompanied by a cost analysis, in addition to outcomes data. Pulmonary artery catheters have received a lot of attention recently. Studies in perioperative and intensive-care patients by Isaacson, Pearson, Connors,[29] and others suggest that pulmonary artery catheters have not improved patient outcomes, but have significantly increased hospital costs, and have introduced the possibility of pulmonary artery catheter-related complications.

The laryngeal mask airway (LMA) is another example of a new innovation in perioperative practice. Since the introduction of LMAs into practice in the United States in 1991, multiple studies have demonstrated their safety, ease of use, low incidence of sore throat, and decreased anesthetic requirement when compared with endotracheal tubes. Joshi et al.[30] have proposed a model for studying the cost-effectiveness of airway devices to compare the costs of LMAs with those of endotracheal tubes. Macario and colleagues[31] have performed a cost analysis of LMAs in adult outpatients undergoing isoflurane–nitrous oxide–oxygen anesthetics for elective surgery. They found that the cost-effectiveness of the LMA is highly dependent upon its reuse rate. If the LMA is reused 40 times, it is the least costly airway management technique in cases lasting longer than 40 minutes.

There are already therapeutic options closed to certain patients because the tremendous cost of the therapy is unjustifiable in comparison to the small likelihood that the patient will derive any benefit. For example, lung transplants are denied to patients with a known malignancy. It is likely that in the future the number of therapeutic options will continue to expand and the ability to pay for exorbitant medical care will diminish, necessitating the further exclusion of certain patients from specific therapeutic options. This eventuality is difficult for both physicians and patients to accept. It is critically important that physicians be able to accurately assess the range of outcomes, the likelihood of each outcome, and the costs of the various alternatives. Knaus et al.,[32] in a recent article, emphasized that accurate information of this sort is likely to form the basis of many future discussions between physicians and their patients.

It is clear that changes in health care practice intended to optimize outcomes and costs are going to occur. Physicians may be entering an era when it will be necessary to justify costs for the therapies they provide and in which they will be held accountable for the costs incurred. Information on cost, cost-effectiveness, and the economic consequences of drugs and technologies relating to perioperative medicine must be included in information available to practitioners so that they can make informed choices. Economic pressure will become a powerful incentive for physicians to provide objective evidence that their practices are of high quality and, simultaneously, cost-effective.

CHALLENGES AND OPPORTUNITIES FOR PERIOPERATIVE PHYSICIANS

The study of outcomes and cost-effectiveness presents new challenges to perioperative researchers. Over the years, surgeons and anesthesiologists have taken on increased responsibility for preoperative assessment, postoperative care, intensive care, acute and chronic pain, and perioperative administration. Outcomes research and the delineation of cost-effective medical practices are additional logical areas of expansion for perioperative physicians. Perioperative physicians observe a variety of specialty practices on a daily basis and have good insight into the influence of practice patterns on disease states. Perioperative physicians are in an excellent position to reexamine the practices of individual specialties or a combination of specialties as they contribute to a patient's perioperative experience. In addition, previous experience with the administration of ORs has given perioperative physicians insights into ways to improve efficiency, quality, safety, and patient satisfaction. The current medical environment will favor those who take an activist's role in improving medical outcomes, financial outcomes, quality of care, and patient satisfaction. Perioperative physicians should be leaders in this role.

An activist approach will also highlight the perioperative physician's contribution to the health care system. The public, individual patients, administrators, and even other physicians have many misperceptions of the perioperative period. This is partly because of lack of exposure and partly because of the lack of patient-oriented outcome measures. Outcomes research is an opportunity for perioperative physicians to emphasize the breadth and integration of their medical knowledge and concern, rather than just the technical skills involved in perioperative care. Any improvements in perioperative care will be good for our image within our hospitals and with the public.

Perioperative physicians have a strong tradition in basic science research. This research has resulted in many medical advances which must be evaluated in clinical practice. Because perioperative physicians have emphasized basic science research for several decades, many academic departments will need to make changes to successfully expand into outcomes research. In particular, it will be important to have researchers trained in epidemiology and biostatistics. Many departments will choose to recruit clinicians with the skills necessary to perform outcomes studies. Others will choose to train physicians already at their institution. At some institutions, building bridges between departments may provide this expertise. Perioperative units will need to expand their computer capabilities and develop linked databases. For there to be useful sharing of information, there will need to be significant cooperation between institutions to define what information will be collected, what form the collected information will take, and how data will be stored and analyzed. As funding is shrinking, and clinical and administrative demands are growing, creativity will be necessary to accomplish these goals.

• CONCLUSION

Perioperative physicians are in a strategic position to broaden our understanding of medical outcomes. They can contribute to the delineation of the range of outcomes, the generation of outcomes data of relevance to patients, the improvement in quality of patient care, and the practice of cost-effective medicine. Although patients currently enjoy a high level of safety and satisfaction in the perioperative period, perioperative practice can be improved. Currently, outcomes data in perioperative medicine are limited. When data addressing important issues are limited, politics and anecdote often influence medical practice. If perioperative physicians want to optimize patient outcomes and remain in control of their medical practices, they must take the lead in investigating outcomes and cost-effectiveness in perioperative medicine.

REFERENCES

1. Warner MA, Shields, SE, Chute CG: Major morbidity and mortality within 1 month of ambulatory surgery and anesthesia, *JAMA* 270:1437, 1993.

2. Larijani GE, et al: Treatment of postoperative nausea and vomiting with ondansetron: a randomized, double-blind comparison with placebo, *Anesth Analg* 73:246, 1991.
3. Alon E, Himmelseher S: Ondansetron in the treatment of postoperative vomiting: a randomized, double-blind comparison with droperidol and metoclopramide, *Anesth Analg* 75:561, 1992.
4. Furst SR, Rodarte A; Prophylactic antiemetic treatment with ondansetron in children undergoing tonsillectomy, *Anesthesiology* 81:799, 1994.
5. Paxton LD, McKary AC, Mirakhur RK: Prevention of nausea and vomiting after day case gynaecologic laparoscopy: a comparison ofondansetron, droperidol, metoclopramide and placebo, *Anaesthesia* 50:403, 1995.
6. Todd MM, et al: A prospective, comparative trial of three anesthetics for elective supratentorial craniotomy, *Anesthesiology* 78:1005, 1993.
7. Moller JT, et al: Randomized evaluation of pulse oximetry in 20,802 patients: I. Design, demography, pulse oximetry failure rate, and overall complication rate, *Anesthesiology* 768:436, 1993.
8. Shapiro HM, et al: Rapid intraoperative reduction of intracranial pressure with thiopentone, *Br J Anaesth* 45:1057, 1973.
9. Michenfelder JD: The interdependency of cerebral functional and metabolic effects following massive doses of thiopental in the dog, *Anesthesiology* 41:231, 1974.
10. Ward JD, Becker DP, Miller JD: Failures of prophylactic barbiturate coma in the treatment of severe head injury, *J Neurosurg* 62:383, 1985.
11. Roizen MF, et al: The relative roles of the history and physical examination, and laboratory testing in preoperative evaluation for outpatient surgery: the "Starling" curve of preoperative laboratory testing, *Anesthesiol Clin North Am* 5:15, 1987.
12. Apfelbaum JL, et al: Do asymptomatic individuals benefit from preoperative laboratory screening? *Anesthesiology* 75:A1054, 1991.
13. Narr BJ, Hansen TR, Warner MA: Preoperative laboratory screening in healthy Mayo patients: cost-effective elimination of tests and unchanged outcomes, *Mayo Clin Proc* 66:155, 1991.
14. Gold BS, et al: The utility of preoperative lectrocardiograms in the ambulatory surgical patient, *Arch Intern Med* d152:301, 1992.
15. Turnbull Jm, Buck C: The value of preoperative screening investigations in otherwise healthy individuals, *Arch Intern Med* 147:1101, 1987.
16. Legerwood AM, et al: The influence of an anesthetic regimen on patient care, outcome, and hospital charges, *Am Surg* 58:527, 1992.
17. Johnstone RE, Jozefczyk, KG: Costs of anesthetic drugs: experiences with a cost education trial, *Anesth Analg* 78:766, 1994.
18. Hampel K, et al: Can the anesthesiologist reliably decide which muscle relaxant he is using? *Anesthesiology* 77:A941, 1992.
19. Modell JH: Must cost containment affect patient safety in anesthesia? *Am Soc Anesth Newsletter* 56:9, 1992.
20. Hampel K, et al: Can the anesthesiologist reliably decide which muscle relaxant he is using? *Anesthesiology* 77:A941, 1992.
21. Shapiro HM, et al: Rapid intraoperative reduction of intracranial pressure with thiopentone, *Br J Anaesth* 45:1057, 1973.
22. Johnstone RE, Jozefczyk, KG: Costs of anesthetic drugs: experiences with a cost education trial, *Anesth Analg* 78:766, 1994.
23. Becker KE, Carrithers JA: Cost savings in anesthesia: changing usage patterns, *Anesthesiology* 81:A1204, 1994.
24. Williams MJ, Torjman M: Anesthetic cost containment through education, *Anesthesiology* 81:A11999, 1994.
25. Johnstone RE, Martinec CL: Costs of anesthesia, *Anesth Analg* 76:840, 1993.
26. Johnstone RE, Jozefczyk, KG: Costs of anesthetic drugs: experiences with a cost education trial, *Anesth Analg* 78:766, 1994.
27. Wong HY, et al: A randomized, double-blind evaluation of ketorolac tromethamine for postoperative analgesia in ambulatory surgery patients, *Anesthesiology* 78:6, 1993.

28. Johnstone RE, Martinec CL: Anesthesia studies should include costs, *Anesthesiology* 79:195, 1993.
29. Isaacson IJ, et al: The value of pulmonary artery and central venous monitoring in patients undergoing abdominal aortic reconstructive surge, *J Vasc Surg* 12:754, 1990.
30. Joshi G, et al: A model for studying the cost-effectiveness of airway devices: laryngeal mask airway vs. tracheal tube, *Anesth Analg* 80:S219, 1995.
31. Marcario A, et al: A cost analysis of the laryngeal mask airway for elective surgery in adult outpatients, *Anesthesiology* 83:250, 1995.
32. Knaus WA, Wagner DP, Lynn J: Short-term mortality predictions for critically ill hospitalized adults: science and ethics, *Science* 254:389, 1991.

BIBLIOGRAPHY

Alon E, Himmelseher S: Ondansetron in the treatment of postoperative vomiting: a randomized, double-blind comparison with droperidol and metoclopramide, *Anesth Analg* 75:561, 1992.

Apfelbaum JL, et al: Do asymptomatic individuals benefit from preoperative laboratory screening? *Anesthesiology* 75:A1054, 1991.

Becker KE, Carrithers JA: Cost savings in anesthesia: changing usage patterns, *Anesthesiology* 81:A1204, 1994.

Connors AF, et al: The effectiveness of right heart catheterization in the initial care of critically ill patients, *JAMA* 276:889, 1996.

Furst SR, Rodarte A: Prophylactic antiemetic treatment with ondansetron in children undergoing tonsillectomy, *Anesthesiology* 81:799, 1994.

Gold BS, et al: The utility of preoperative electrocardiograms in the ambulatory surgical patient, *Arch Intern Med* 152:301, 1992.

Hampel K, et al: Can the anesthesiologist reliably decide which muscle relaxant he is using? *Anesthesiology* 77:A941, 1992.

Isaacson IJ, et al: The value of pulmonary artery and central venous monitoring in patients undergoing abdominal aortic reconstructive surgery, *J Vasc Surg* 12:754, 1990.

Johnstone RE, Jozefczyk, KG: Costs of anesthetic drugs: experiences with a cost education trial, *Anesth Analg* 78:766, 1994.

Johnstone RE, Martinec CL: Costs of anesthesia, *Anesth Analg* 76:840, 1993.

Johnstone RE, Martinec CL: Anesthesia studies should include costs, *Anesthesiology* 79:195, 1993.

Joshi G, et al: A model for studying the cost-effectiveness of airway devices: laryngeal mask airway vs. tracheal tube, *Anesth Analg* 80:S219, 1995.

Larijani GE, et al: Treatment of postoperative nausea and vomiting with ondansetron: a randomized, double-blind comparison with placebo, *Anesth Analg* 73:246, 1991.

Legerwood AM, et al: The influence of an anesthetic regimen on patient care, outcome, and hospital charges, *Am Surg* 58:527, 1992.

Macario A, et al: A cost analysis of the laryngeal mask airway for elective surgery in adult outpatients, *Anesthesiology* 83:250, 1995.

Michenfelder JD: The interdependency of cerebral functional and metabolic effects following massive doses of thiopental in the dog, *Anesthesiology* 41:231, 1974.

Modell JH: Must cost containment affect patient safety in anesthesia? *Am Soc Anesth Newsletter* 56:9, 1992.

Moller JT, et al: Randomized evaluation of pulse oximetry in 20,802 patients: I. Design, demography, pulse oximetry failure rate, and overall complication rate, *Anesthesiology* 78:436, 1993.

Moller JT, et al: Randomized evaluation of pulse oximetry in 20,802 patients: II. Perioperative events and postoperative complications, *Anesthesiology* 78:445, 1993.

Narr BJ, Hansen TR, Warner MA: Preoperative laboratory screening in healthy Mayo patients: cost-effective elimination of tests and unchanged outcomes, *Mayo Clin Proc* 66:155, 1991.

Paxton LD, McKay AC, Mirakhur RK: Prevention of nausea and vomiting after day case gynaecological laparoscopy: a comparison of ondansetron, droperidol, metoclopramide and placebo, *Anesthesia* 50:403, 1995.

Pearson KS, et al: A cost/benefit analysis of randomized invasive monitoring for patients undergoing cardiac surgery, *Anesth Analg* 69:336, 1989.

Roizen MF, et al: The relative roles of the history and physical examination, and laboratory testing in preoperative evaluation for outpatient surgery: the "Starling" curve of preoperative laboratory testing, *Anesthesiol Clin North Am* 5:15, 1987.

Shapiro HM, et al: Rapid intraoperative reduction of intracranial pressure with thiopentone, *Br J Anaesth* 45:1057, 1973.

Todd MM, et al: A prospective, comparative trial of three anesthetics for elective supratentorial craniotomy, *Anesthesiology* 78:1005, 1993.

Turnbull JM, Buck C: The value of preoperative screening investigations in otherwise healthy individuals, *Arch Intern Med* 147:1101, 1987.

Ward JD, Becker DP, Miller JD: Failure of prophylactic barbiturate coma in the treatment of severe head injury, *J Neurosurg* 62:383, 1985.

Warner MA, Shields SE, Chute CG: Major morbidity and mortality within 1 month of ambulatory surgery and anesthesia, *JAMA* 270:1437, 1993.

Williams MJ, Torjman M: Anesthetic cost containment through education, *Anesthesiology* 81:A1199, 1994.

Wong HY, et al: A randomized, double-blind evaluation of ketorolac tromethamine for postoperative analgesia in ambulatory surgery patients, *Anesthesiology* 78:6, 1993.

SUGGESTED READINGS

Becker KE: Cost containment in anesthesiology. In *1993 Annual Refresher Course Lectures*, 1993, American Society of Anesthesiologists.

Civetta JM, Kirby RR: Prediction and definition of outcome. In *Advances in Anesthesia, vol 9*, St. Louis, 1992, Mosby–Year Book, Inc.

Deutschman CS, Traber KB: Evolution of anesthesiology, *Anesthesiology* 85:1, 1996.

Eddy DM: Connecting value and costs: whom do we ask, and what do we ask them? *JAMA* 264:1737, 1990.

Knaus WA, Wagner DP, Lynn J: Short-term mortality predictions for critically ill hospitalized adults: science and ethics, *Science* 254:389, 1991.

Knill RL: Anaesthesia research: needs for the nineties, *Can J Anaesth* 39:411, 1992.

Lanier WL, Warner MA: New frontiers in anesthesia research: addressing the impact of practice patterns on outcome, health care delivery, and cost, *Anesthesiology* 78:1001, 1993.

Orkin FK, Cohen MM, Duncan PG: The quest for meaningful outcomes, *Anesthesiology* 78:417, 1993.

Tuman KJ, Ivankovich AD: High-cost, high-tech medicine: are we getting our money's worth? *J Clin Anesth* 5:168, 1992.

Snow J: *On Chloroform and Other Anaesthetics*, London, 1858, John Churchill.

Wetchler BV: Economic impact of anesthesia decision making: they pay the money, we make the choice, *J Clin Anesth* 4:20S, 1992.

White PF, Watcha MF: Are new drugs cost-effective for patients undergoing ambulatory surgery? *Anesthesiology* 78:2, 1993.

Williams MH, Blazeby JM, Eachus JI: Current challenges for outcome measurement in surgical practice, *Ann R Coll Surg Engl* 77:401, 1995.

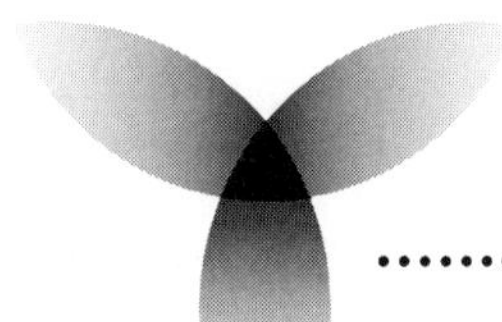

Chapter 46

Total Quality Management and Continuous Quality Improvement

Terrance Yemen, MD

Total quality management (TQM) and *continuous quality improvement (CQI)* are often confusing and threatening terms; neither should be. Total quality management and continuous quality improvement are interchangeable terms with the former primarily referring to industry-based programs and the latter to clinical or hospital settings. Used appropriately, these two terms should not threaten the clinician. Total quality management and CQI can enhance and improve the physician's function in both the hospital and office settings. Conceptually, TQM involves a common set of characteristics, starting with a council of the institution's top leadership. The council then creates training programs for personnel, mechanisms for selecting process improvements, the formation of process of improvement teams, proviso of staff support for process analysis and redesign principles, and, finally, personnel policies that motivate and support the staff as they participate in these process improvements.

Examining the principles of TQM and CQI and their application in all the separate subspecialties involved in perioperative medicine, is well beyond the scope of this chapter. The purpose of this chapter is to help explain what these principles are, how they may be used, and examine some of the problems facing the perioperative physician when using these concepts. It is my hope that this chapter will stimulate an interest in the concepts of TQM by providing a brief introduction into the reasons why such methodology is not only essential for future health care development, but how it can also be applied to subspecialties, such as anesthesiology and surgery, to improve daily performance.

Continuous quality improvement comes in a variety of forms and is used for a number of reasons. Nonetheless, such differences do not distract from the common set of characteristics and functions that all CQI programs have. These characteristics include: (1) the ability to empower commissions and managers to analyze and improve processes; (2) allowing the adoption of the norm that customer preferences are the primary determents of quality; (3) the development of a multidisciplinary approach that goes beyond conventional department lines; and (4) allowing motivation for a rational database-cooperative approach to process analysis and subsequent change.

In simple terms, the application of database management principles to the clinical administrative processes that produce patient care is what CQI is all about. It is both a management philosophy and a management method. I believe that all of us acknowledge change to be a fundamental aspect of the health care environment. Therefore, our organizational systems must have both the will and the means to master such change effectively.

Continuous quality improvement is also notable for its emphasis on avoiding personal blame. The appropriate use of CQI avoids focus on individual workmanship, negligence, or lack of interest; instead it focuses on the professional processes associated with specific outcome. The assumption is that the process needs to be changed and that the persons already involved in that process are needed to help identify how to approach the problem (or opportunity) and solve that problem.

Another fundamental principle of CQI is the decentralization of responsibility for ownership of each process into the hands of its implementers, the people most directly involved with the process. Management's role, therefore, is to encourage and support the development of process improvement teams, which may be related to a given subspecialty but which also cut across multidisciplinary lines. Thus, to be effective, management must be the model of the improvement process.

THE HISTORY OF TOTAL QUALITY MANAGEMENT

The fundamentals of TQM are based on a scientific management movement which began at the turn of this century. Traditionally, emphasis was given to the concept of "management based on facts." This meant that management was assumed to be the master of the facts. The concept assumes that it is the responsibility of management to specify one correct method of work for all people and see that they execute this method, thereby, ensuring quality. That perspective has been influenced over the past century by the recognition of the importance of the personnel actually working within the organization at nonmanagement levels. These individuals must also be involved in problem analysis and the building of quality control within the organization itself.

A traditional history of TQM involves a review of at least five key individuals. One of the first TQM pioneers was statistics expert Walter Shewhart who, while at Bell Laboratories, made multiple contributions including the control chart and "The

Plan, Do, Check, Act" (TDCA) cycle. Shewhart promoted the idea that price alone was not an indication of value, and that price without consideration of quality is meaningless. It was also Shewhart's concept that the statistical control of stable ("in control") processes was the foundation of all CQI activities. If excessive variation existed within a process, then the cause of that variation needed to be discovered and removed to provide a stable process. Determining variation and analyzing its cause(s) for removal or control, would be a primary function of TQM.

W. Edward Deming is one of the best known proponents of TQM. In the 1950s he was invited by representatives of the Japanese industry to provide conceptual methods to rebuild what was, at that time, a war-ravaged economy. It was well-known that Demings had been advocating a statistical approach to quality for sometime in the United States, but by working with the Japanese, the concepts were first implemented in industry. Although his contributions are extensive, most histories suggest that he is best known for the 14-step program developed for management to improve quality. Deming's 14-point plan includes:

1. Creating and publishing for all employees a statement of the aims and purposes of the company for which management must constantly demonstrate its commitment.
2. Learning the new philosophy from *top* management *down.*
3. Understanding the purpose of inspection, i.e., the improvement of processes and reduction of costs.
4. Ending the practice of awarding business on the basis of price tag alone.
5. Improving constantly and forever the system of reduction and service.
6. Instituting training.
7. Teaching and instituting leadership.
8. Driving out fear; creating trust; creating a climate for innovation.
9. Optimizing towards the aims and purposes of the company, using the efforts of the teams, groups, and staff.
10. Eliminating competition between the work forces.
11. a) Eliminating numeric quotas for production. Instead, learning an institute method for improvement. b) Eliminating management by objective.
12. Removing processes that rob people of the pride of workmanship.
13. Encouraging education and self-improvement for everyone.
14. Taking action to accomplish the transformation.

Deming believed that two sources of improvement can be identified in all processes. The first is the elimination of special causes of process variation; that is variation associated with specific materials, machines, or individuals. The second is the elimination of common causes of variation; those associated with the aspects with the system itself such as poor design, inadequate training, inappropriate materials, machines or working conditions. Since Deming believed that quality problems were management-controlled rather than worker-controlled, he promoted the fundamental concept that TQM must be based on a "top-down" organizational wide commitment.

Armand F. Feigenbaum and Joseph M. Juran are the two given credit for providing the theoretic constructs for TQM. The goal of quality, according to Feigenbaum, is to satisfactorily meet whatever the customer believes to be the requirements for the service or product. He noted that factors outside the organization, such as cultural attitude and technologic change, can eventually make customers dissatisfied with that which was once a satisfactory product. Hence, he stressed that continuous, quality improvement cycles are essential.

Joseph N. Juran, like Deming, was involved with Japanese industry during the 1950s. Juran's writings parallel Deming's concepts of classifying process variations. Furthermore, Juran insisted that quality goals be specific. He disagreed with vague quality statements such as "we are dedicated to improving" or "quality is job one." He insisted that specific goals should be stated. An example would be to state that the number of cancelled cases on the operating room (OR) schedule is to be reduced from 15% to 5% over a 1-year period. Juran believed in a trilogy of basic quality processes. These included quality planning, quality control, and quality improvement. Such processes must be supported by an infrastructure measuring buyer/user supply relationships, education in training, and information management. These principles rested on a foundation of customer focus.

Philip B. Crosby developed a different theoretic perspective based on changing cooperative cultures and attitudes. He emphasized the concept of "zero defects." Crosby asked two questions: What is quality? and What standards and systems are needed to achieve quality? He answered his own questions with four absolutes of quality: (1) do the right thing, the first time, (2) defect prevention is the only acceptable approach, (3) zero defects are the only performance standard, and (4) the cost of quality is the only measure of quality. His approach, like Deming's, was to implement a 14-step process, but his processes stressed changes in organizational culture and attitude. Crosby's 14-step program included:

1. Management commitment
2. Quality improvement team
3. Quality measurement
4. Cost of quality evaluation
5. Quality awareness
6. Corrective action
7. Establishing an ad hoc committee for the zero defects program
8. Supervisor training
9. Zero defects day
10. Goal setting
11. Error/cause removal
12. Recognition of success
13. Quality councils
14. Do it over again

Crosby also emphasized developing an estimate of the cost of nonconformance, or otherwise called, the cost of quality. This process identifies and assigns values to all of the unnecessary costs associated with waste and wasted effort when work is not done correctly the first time. It includes the cost of identifying errors, correcting them, and making up for the customers' dissatisfaction that subsequently resulted.

A COMPARISON OF INDUSTRIAL AND HEALTH CARE QUALITY

Quality has always been at the heart of the health services industry. The valid question is, therefore, "What is the value added by CQI?" A comparison of the industrial perspective with the health care perspective on quality reveals that the two are surprisingly similar. Both have strengths and weaknesses as outlined by Donabedian's work. The industrial model is limited however in that it: ignores the complexities of the patient-physician relationship; down-plays the knowledge, skills, and motivation of the practitioner; treats quality as free, ignoring the quality/cost trade-off; gives more attention to supportive activities and less to clinical ones; and provides less emphasis on influencing professional performance through education, retraining, supervision, encouragement, and censor. Conversely, Donabedian suggests that the professional health care model can learn the following from the industrial model:

1. Evaluation of the fundamental soundness of the healthcare quality tradition.
2. The need for even greater attention to consumer requirements, values, and expectations.
3. The need for greater attention to the science of systems and processes as a means to quality assurance.
4. The need to extend the self-motivating, self-governing tradition of physicians to other organizations.
5. The need for a greater role by management in the sharing of the goal of quality clinical care.
6. The need to develop appropriate applications of statistical control methods to monitor health care.
7. The need for greater education and training in quality monitoring and assurance for all concerned.

The application of TQM/CQI activities must take into consideration, and be modified by, a number of factors. Manufacturing processes have linear flows, repetitive cycle steps, standardized input, high analyzability and lower worker discretion. Professional services, in contrast, involve nonstandardized and variable inputs, nonrepetitive operations, unpredictable demand peaks and higher worker discretion. Despite these differences, the concepts of TQM can be applied to the clinical arena.

THE BASICS OF TQM/CQI

One of the fundamental requirements in understanding TQM or CQI is an understanding of systems. The sciences and, in this case, the science of medicine, are relevant to the knowledge of a system as a whole. The conceptualization of a system raises many questions. How can one acquire a view of the system as a whole? If we as doctors are accustomed to exploring the world in fragments, how do we connect those fragments conceptually to know which of our discoveries should be included within the system and what should be left outside? What are the different types of systems and how do they differ from one another? For example, a typical dichotomy exists between closed systems, which are self-reverential and tend towards homeostasis, such as the pituitary adrenal axis, and open systems, which are affected by nonsystem influences, such as when one resets a thermostat or when a child learns to read. How do nonlinear systems (those with feedback loops and delays) behave? When are they predictable and when are they not? When do these systems find their aims? How do people or elements communicate with each other and with the world outside their system? If a system's purpose is to meet an outside need, how does it explore and understand that need? If it understands that need, how does it translate that understanding into a co-ordinated effort to meet that need? Also, what is the relationship between the part and the whole? How does one element of a system support the performance of a system as a whole avoiding suboptimizing in favor of its own local performance (appreciating that suboptimization is a constant threat to achieving the purpose of the whole). Finally, one needs to appreciate that some systems are unsolvable. Some systems have been described as messes. A mess is a system of problems in which each problem affects every other problem. We may, therefore, adopt the illusion of solving one problem or another, when it is the nature of systems that the mess cannot be solved as a whole. Once again, the attempt to solve such problems results in suboptimization, which endangers the system as a whole.

One must also have an appreciation for the sciences of psychology in systems, which relates to four basic topics: (1) the science of group process, (2) the sciences of conflict resolution, (3) the sciences of understanding motivation, and (4) creativity.

In many complex systems our work is done by exchanges through meetings, communications, and groups of various sorts. How we react and interact within and with these groups is not a peripheral matter, but, rather, central to the functioning of human systems. In understanding such systems it is not just the elements that count but also the arrows that connect those elements, or the dynamics among the elements. Our medical departments, therefore, represent different elements, and our meetings, conversations, and communications are the arrows.

All systems experience internal and external friction. The resultant heat is wasteful and results in suboptimization. Local pride and competition thrive when co-operation would have been a more appropriate methodology. In medical care environments, the methods of handling disagreements are primitive and uninformed, in contrast to the sciences of economics, game theory, anthropology, linguistics, etc. Yet, it is key to the attainment of quality medicine that we understand how to improve the relationship between physician and patient.

Medical systems have tremendous trouble breaking from primitive assumptions concerning motivation and incentive. Little evidence supports the use of reward, punishment, and contingence pay as ways of producing continuous improvement in our systems. An argument has been made that merit pay produces defensiveness and suboptimization much more reliably than improved quality performance. In place of outmoded ideas concerning rewards and punishments as a foundation for dealing each other, one can substitute more modern concepts promoting the role of intrinsic motivations which include pride, joy, affiliation, and celebration.

Creativity involves that aspect of scientific psychology that can be applied in an effort to understand new ideas that break through the assumptions of our closed systems. It is a soft area of science that deals with the characteristics of cultures, groups, organization and thought processes which promote or hinder creative development.

An important element of TQM involves the sciences of learning, prediction, and experimentation, otherwise called the science of gaining knowledge. The sciences of learning, prediction, and experimentation are essential for promoting improvement. Deming suggests that we develop and maintain a system of cyclical, interactive investigation and learning which does its work in the real world. Keeping track of time as time passes. Deming suggests our system of learning occurs in a changing world and, therefore, it must be cyclical, because no collection of knowledge at any particular time can perfectly predict the future. We must repeatedly ask questions because the answers may, in fact, change from one period of time to another. We must repeat the cycle often enough to follow the pace of change. Learning must be interactive so that it builds on each new lesson and never assumes that there is a fixed solution.

We should be interested not only in the process of investigation but also in the process of learning. The method of gaining knowledge cannot be separated from the application of that knowledge. It is, therefore, important that we know who is gaining the knowledge, whether the knowledge will be connected to an action, and how it will be connected. Generally, we are interested in a process of learning in a real world. This is not the same as relegating learning to a laboratory or a specialized environment. To be as powerful as it can be, gainful knowledge must involve both local and general knowledge. Finally, our system for gaining knowledge must have sequential memory. Isolated snapshots in time will tell us little about the process with which we are working. In terms of prediction, it is trajectory, history, and trends that are highly informative. The simple application of such a process suggests that instead of making a list of isolated events along a pathway, we should produce graphs which track and show the trends in certain behaviors.

Total quality management/CQI requires the science of variation or statistics. Statistics which support prediction of a unknown future are different from classical statistics which focus on enumeration. This area of statistics is interested in variation stability occuring over time. Therefore, for this purpose, extremely small samples are adequate as long as they are drawn from rational and contained ample time-dependent information. In simplistic terms, we are not so much interested in what kind of product we are producing, as much as whether or not we are producing this product consistently or whether it is changing over time. Such thinking led to the use of the control chart, which is one of the most powerful practical tools developed in industry, but which can also be applied to medicine.

By recording, efficiently and informatively, the history of a process, a control chart can tell us whether a specific new event is consistent with the past history of the process, or whether the event is unexpected and new. If the event is new it is said to be attributable or of special cause. In such cases, investigating these events is very informative. If unexpected events are not observed over the history of the process, then the process or system is said to be in control, and experiencing only common causes of variation. Control charts help people to avoid tampering by using prescribed limits to guide and interpret variation. Shewhart called these controls *limits*. He suggested they be set to limit the probability that people will act on a random variation. There is considerable debate over the exact calculation of control limits, but, nevertheless, the concept of interpreting variation as a fundamental element in the science of improvement, remains valid. In dealing with variation, several challenges need to be acknowledged:

1. We need to understand the basic concepts of special cause, common cause, and tampering.
2. We need to be capable of measuring the variables of importance in real work settings as part of the whole.
3. We need to be able to display those measurements in the most informative possible formats and to avoid or reduce tampering.
4. We need to integrate all of these capabilities into the daily life of the organization rather than just to leave them to some other department, research, or otherwise.

In understanding control charts some other fundamental aspects should be appreciated. Typically, control limits indicate the amount of variation expected in a process so that a process is considered in control and stable as long as variations fall within those limits. The decision to place such boundaries, which define whether or not the system is in control, at two or three standard deviations is discretionary; but the decision should take into account the comparative cost of concluding that a process is stable when it is unstable or unstable when it is not. Wide limits predispose to the first type of error, type 1, and narrow limits predispose to the second type of error, or type 2. The control chart provides a rapid accurate assessment of the significance of the observed variation in a process or production, with variation being endemic in all systems. The value of the control chart lies not only in the novelty of the statistic principles, but also the ease and reliability from which data can be transformed into information.

The application of the control chart and other related techniques is generally known as "statistic quality control." These concepts are not new; most of statistical quality control was accomplished before and during World War II. The techniques of statistical quality control advance the quality of production systems using three types of activities: quality control, quality improvement, and quality planning. Quality control uses statistic methods, such as control charts, to maintain quality at a desired level. Quality improvement relies on a number of tools that assist workers in diagnosing or treating problems in the process of production. This allows workers to modify these processes and not just control them, thereby increasing their capabilities to elevate the level of quality that the process(es) achieve. Quality planning involves techniques whose purpose it is to design in quality by developing products superior in quality and easier to maintain and manufacture. To simplify this concept one could think in terms of intraoperative echocardiology. Quality control activities would ensure the resolution of images during intraoperative echocardiography. Quality improvement activities may seek methods to improve the resolution of the machine and its use by changing hardware or software. Quality design activities might result in rethinking of this technology to produce other machines that involve easier use, lower cost, or greater accessibility.

David Blumenthal has suggested that one can combine statistic quality control and clinical care and that the combination produces the following insights:

1. Quality must be measured to be controlled or improved.
2. Much can be learned about how to control or improve quality by studying variation in its measured levels and in the performance of the processes that produce the things we care about.
3. Control charts and other devices can greatly assist in studying variation, drawing statistically sound conclusions from them and controlling variation in cases where this will improve quality.
4. Deliberate experimentation is a powerful tool for improving the performance of processes.

TOTAL QUALITY MANAGEMENT AND PHYSICIAN DECISION MAKING

It has been suggested that there are many similarities between the problems physicians encounter and those in industries, but it is also important to appreciate the many differences. Physicians face limits in their ability to reduce uncertainty, limits which do not affect industrial workers. One irreducible source of uncertainty for physicians is the individuality of each human being, the uniqueness of that person's problem, the needs and the manner in which the person responds to given therapy. This is particularly true in situations in which patients have multiple illnesses. Complex processes do occur in industries as well, but they can be run over and over again so that their variability can be characterized. Patients however, cannot be subjected, for obvious reasons, again and again to the same surgical process, or the same medical treatment to gain better insight into the predictability of a given therapy. Additionally, one must appreciate that an industry, no matter how complex an industrial process, can theoretically be stopped, disassembled, studied, and then put back together again. The same cannot be said, under most circumstances for biologic processes, especially for human beings. Despite these differences, TQM offers a potential valuable methodology for accomplishing the tasks that enable physicians to continually improve the management of their patients.

One of the greatest difficulties in linking relating TQM with the physician is physicians' reluctance to be involved in TQM. Despite the autonomy of physicians, their key role in resource allocation within the health care system makes their active participation in and support of quality management initiatives vital to the success of these programs. The sources of this resistance seem to include, as defined by Dr. DM Berwick:

1. Physicians' general resistance to change, an attribute they share with many other professional and nonprofessional groups.
2. There is a fear that the TQM emphasis upon reducing variation in the process of care would lead to an attack on physician autonomy, including the ability to care for patients, the ability to individualize care to meet the needs of a particular patient, and the ability to innovate.

3. The fact that the early applications of TQM have been championed by administrators and used primarily to address problems perceived by physicians as the responsibility of administration. Physicians are frequently distrustful of administrators and health care organizations.
4. The strong emphasis of TQM on breaking down professional boundaries and the development of interdisciplinary teams, which many physicians find threatening to their status in health care organizations.
5. Advocates of TQM have not yet refined and developed a persuasive, theoretic empiric, or practical argument that the techniques and activities will improve the decisions individual physicians make for their patients. Therefore, one of the hurdles of TQM is to educate physicians in the processes of TQM and how it can be effectively applied to their own daily work.

If TQM is to successfully involve the physician, advocates of TQM must show the physician that these activities will improve the ability they have to care for their patients and/or reduce cost. As time and monitary resources become more scarce, physician practice priorities will be more stringent in allocating these resources. If physicians are to spend a portion of their valued time on TQM activities, then that time must be productive and results forthcoming. The real challenge for those people who believe in TQM, therefore, is to demonstrate these attributes.

• OUTCOMES RESEARCH AND CONTINUOUS QUALITY IMPROVEMENT

One of the downfalls of CQI occurs when people take a simplistic approach towards its application in health care. The danger is that emphasis upon the reduction of variation in the health care process may be viewed as an end in itself. Such efforts represent a threatening attempt to improve efficiency, without attending to the end results which are what matter most to patients and physicians.

Sheldon Greenfield has suggested that one way of avoiding this misunderstanding is by the marriage of outcomes research and CQI. He believes that because of its focus on health care outcomes that really matter, outcomes research can provide CQI with a focus on goals which are meaningful to physicians. To understand this concept, one must define and characterize three health-care delivery processes. They are efficiency, effectiveness, and quality.

Greenfield has pointed out that part of the difficulty physicians have with CQI is that they perceive the methods of CQI are most appropriate to improving efficiency, even though CQI is most interested in quality. In analyzing any patient care process, efficiency is how inexpensively, consistently, or rapidly decisions and/or actions can be carried out. It is at this point where variation can be minimized in a manufacturing sense. Effectiveness involves studying which discreet decisions work. It does not ask whether the process of care was well carried out. In simple terms then, efficiency is doing something well, and effectiveness is doing the right thing. Quality is whether the aggregate processes taken together lead to as good an outcome(s) as is scientifically possible to obtain. It is at this point where outcomes management comes in.

Quality can be related to cost. If the outcome(s) is good, can similar care be less expensive? Although a focus on any three of these elements (efficiency, effectiveness, and quality) will improve delivery of a health care process in one way or another, physicians are most interested in improving quality. In many ways, physicians are well placed to make an assessment of whether or not quality has actually been obtained, because we are the ones most closely in touch with the patient. Where outcomes research and CQI can be married, and made acceptable and relevant to physicians, is in the following areas: (1) the establishment of better measures of quality, (2) improvements in methods to ensure validity and reliability, and (3) setting priorities for improvement.

PHYSICIAN INVOLVEMENT AND ORGANIZATION-WIDE QUALITY IMPROVEMENT

One problem with focusing on specific clinical conditions is that it only serves to further the bifurcation, fragmentation, and suboptimization, which currently characterizes many health care efforts. In fact, focusing exclusively on an isolated piece of an overall puzzle of health care has been defined as committing a type 4 error, mistaking the problem for the solution.

Steven Shortell has suggested that given the growing complexity and interdependence of medical care processes and the trend to provide more care outside the hospital setting, there is a need to involve all care givers: physicians, nurses, and therapists, managers, and colleagues in quality improvement efforts. He defines a pyramid of CQI, which includes cultural, technical, strategic, and structural dimensions.

The cultural dimension refers to the organization's underlined beliefs, values, norms and behaviors which support or serve as barriers to organizational wide improvement. The technical dimension refers to the extent to which those associated with the organization have received the necessary training in CQI/TQM tools. It refers also to the quality of the organization(s) information systems, data analyses, and capabilities, etc. The strategic component refers to the extent to which organizational CQI efforts are focused on the key strategic priorities of the organization, as opposed to activities that are more peripheral. The question asked is whether or not there is a direct link between the organization's CQI efforts and what it is fundamentally trying to achieve with its plan. The structural element refers to specific coordinating committees, councils, task forces and reporting mechanisms associated with the organization(s) CQI efforts. The structural component will bring together the various cultural, technical, and strategic dimensions of the organization(s) CQI work and serves as a forum for these elements to interact.

It is Shortell's belief that all four dimensions, cultural, technical, strategic, and structural need to be in order and in place for significant organizational-wide quality improvement to occur. If the cultural component is missing CQI results will be short-lived, lacking staying power. This is also referred to as inability to hold the gain. If the technical component is missing, the result may be frustrated efforts. Many people can be motivated to work on strategically important problems, but they are frequently not supported by the necessary tools to be effective or given the appropriate time to do the work. If the strategic component is missing, the result will be isolated areas of activity occurring throughout the organization. None of these activities produces any meaningful or significant impact because the activities are not coordinated. If the structural component is missing, the organization has problems transferring learning throughout the organization and capitalizing on improved work that has been done before.

Shortell further suggests that for physicians to be successfully involved in an organization-wide quality-management plan he/she must be integrated into all four dimensions of such work. Although physicians are easily involved in the technical and structural components of such a pyramid, involving physicians in a cultural transformation, which is believed to be required for organizational CQI to work, is the greatest challenge. Traditional physician training and socialization emphasizes individual clinical responsibility. Most physicians traditionally enjoy independence status from the very organization in which they work; this does not provide the foundation for the type of interactive cross-functional teamwork, which is required for organizational CQI efforts. Undoubtedly as the health care field changes, hospital administrators and physicians will find themselves with intertwined destinies, thereby, making it easier to bridge the cultural differences. It is suggested that the use of pluralistic, segmented training, which supports the emergence of physicians who understand CQI's proviso of strong data, analytical support systems, and the support of trusting relationships, will advance the field in the desired direction.

• TQM/CQI AND ANESTHESIOLOGY

Introducing the concepts of TQM/CQI has had its difficulties in anesthesiology. In fact, little interest has been shown overall by the speciality. The popular textbooks of the field dedicate little or no space to this area of science. A recent review of the literature reveals that, although several hundred articles have appeared in the peer-reviewed medical literature concerning CQI, less than 10 of these papers directly involve the field of anesthesiology. That is not to say that anesthesiology has not been involved in CQI activities, but rather there is little evidence that TQM concepts have been incorporated in daily activities.

Traditionally most departments have taken up small CQI efforts in a response to keep hospital administrators, hospital accreditation organizations, and third-party payers happy. Such efforts usually involve measuring morbidity and mortality on an "on your honor" basis. While these efforts can, at times, provide some insight into the quality of the department as a whole, more often than not, we end up with an early morning review of why an ASA IV or V patient died within 24 hours after emergency surgery for one problem or another. These activities do little to stimulate enthusiasm for the review process, and very little learning or quality improvement occurs. In fact, a recent study showed that volunteer reporting of untoward anesthetic events seldom occurs, with the great majority of events going unreported. So what can we do?

At times, the field of anesthesia has been effective in CQI activities. For example, the closed-claims analysis of patients, who could not be intubated or effectively ventilated using a mask, was a remarkable CQI effort. This analysis measured the severity and frequency of the problem, which resulted in recommendations by an expert panel in management improvement of a difficult airway. Through the use of a flow chart, a pathway to handling patients with difficult airways was developed. These recommendations involved preventive and treatment modalities, and the whole process was given extensive exposure, both in the anesthesia literature and at major meetings. All that remains now is a review of the process once again. How well are we handling these difficult airways now? Are we doing better? Approaches like the aforementioned can be used in many other areas of perioperative medicine.

For CQI to be effective in our own departments we must avoid certain pitfalls. First, we must start to measure the quality of the work that we do. Any aspect of the care we provide can be examined, but we must first raise the question. Remember that quality cannot be improved without first defining and measuring it. Having asked the question, we must measure the event or process as accurately as possible. Reporting such events cannot be random, with some anesthesiologists reporting and others not.

To receive the co-operation of all department members, the reporting of adverse events or the like cannot result in punitive action. We are very unlikely to cooperate with any reporting system if we can be singled out and embarrassed in front of our peers or have the information used against us the next time hospital privileges are granted. Confidentiality must be maintained. Unfortunately, many teaching hospitals still have departments that take great joy in openly presenting a difficult case during a teaching round, thoroughly embarrassing and unconstructively criticizing a colleague. Such behavior does little to impart medical knowledge and residents quickly learn that it is better to hide your mistakes than learn from them. We must learn, as stated earlier in this chapter, that TQM/CQI does not seek to place individual blame but, rather, seeks to examine the process as a whole. It assumes that those directly involved in the care want the best outcome possible and are, therefore, motivated to do their best. In such an atmosphere learning and sustaining the gain may be possible.

Traditionally, anesthesia departments have tended to be insular, but one requirement of TQM is that quality improvement is most likely to occur when it involves interdisciplinary activity. Why can't many of our teaching activities involve medical specialities from other areas? Much can be learned by attending and participating in the activities of other departments. Failure to share concepts, concerns, and departmental missions with each other leads to suboptimization. The first exposure to a new surgical technique should not occur with the patient already on the table early Monday morning. An anesthetic should not be complicated by a new cardiac drug being used experimentally by the cardiologist down the hallway. We work side by side with surgical specialists each day in the OR. We must share that information which will directly or indirectly affect us.

Failure to communicate effectively distracts us from taking care of the patient as best as possible. Surgeons and anesthesiologists still struggle with the concept of suboptimization. Patients rarely want great surgery and a poor anesthetic, or vice versa. Achieving either great surgery or anesthesia, at the expense of the other, impairs patient care and leads to such unfortunate Pyrrhic victories saying as, "the operation was a success, but the patient died." The traditional concepts of communication between specialities is based on considerable confrontation and territorialism. Because communication is a key aspect of CQI, any improvement in the way we communicate with one another is likely to show an improvement in care.

As stated previously, medicine is hampered in the achievement of quality improvement because the process of patient care is not repetitive for any given patient. The ability to run and rerun a process is invaluable is studying those factors that produce variability in the process. Until recently, physicians involved in the process of perioperative medicine did not have the opportunity to study process in such a way, but the advent of computer simulators may bring change. If computer simulators can accurately reproduce rare, but dangerous, clinical situations our learning process should be enhanced. Computer simulators have been highly effective in teaching those skills that could not be taught by real life experiences alone in the airline industry. Although the data on the value of such teaching is forthcoming, there is little to suggest that the gains in anesthesia teaching will not be substantial. Improvement in teaching is fundamental to quality improvement. It is not unreasonable to challenge the traditional methods of teaching anesthesia during residency or in the area of continuing medical education, remembering that experimentation is a necessary factor in TQM.

Quality improvement occurs when we challenge the traditional. The quality of perioperative medicine will not change substantially without experimentation. Progress occurs when we challenge the current methodology of a process. New is not always better, but the challenge to the process alone gives us greater insight into the process, even if we cannot find a better process to replace the traditional one. The advent of outpatient surgery, streamlined preoperative clinics, reduction and reevaluation of preoperative bloodwork, and early extubation of postcardiopulmonary bypass patients are all examples of an effort to improve care by challenging the norm. Further improvements in care will certainly come from those unwilling to accept the present.

Lastly, CQI cannot occur without departmental and institutional support. Experimentation, reevaluation, and the measurement of quality take time and money. Governments, hospitals, and the public at large must take greater responsibility for providing the means for this support. Continuous quality improvement CQI activities will not occur if the institutes that asked for them are unwilling to give them value. Anesthesiologists, surgeons, and other specialists involved in the practice of perioperative medicine need to remain proactive in seeking such support through internal and external lobbying efforts and educating our colleagues and patients as to its benefits.

BIBLIOGRAPHY

Berwick DM: Peer review and quality management: are they compatible? *Quality Review Bulletin 16,* 12:419–420, 1990.

Blumenthal D, Scheck AC: *Improving clinical practice*, San Francisco, 1995, Jossey-Bass Publishers.

Cohen MM, Rose DK, Yee DA: Changing anesthesiologists practice patterns, *Anesthesiology* 85:260–269, 1996.

Deming WE: *Out of the crisis,* Cambridge, Mass., 1986, M.I.T. Center for Advanced Engineering Study.

Donabedian A: Criteria and standards for quality assessment and monitoring, *Quality Review Bulletin 14,* 3:99–108, 1986.

McLaughlin CP, Kaluzny AD: *Continuous quality improvement in health care*, Gaithersburg, MD, 1994, Aspen Publishers.

Posner KL, et al: Linking process and outcome of care in a continous quality improvement program for anesthesia services, *Am J Med Qual* 9:129–137, 1994.

Sanborn KV, et al: Detection of intraoperative incidents by electronic scanning of computerized anesthesia records, *Anesthesiology* 85:977–987, 1996.

Shortell S: Revisiting the garden: medicine and management in the 1990s, *Frontiers of Health Services Management 7,* 1:3–32, 1990.

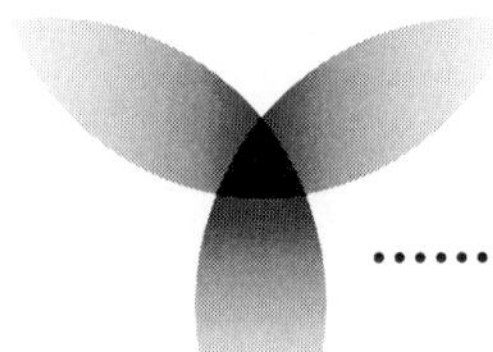

Chapter 47

Medical-Legal Risks in Perioperative Medicine

Rebecca West, JD, Frederic A. Berry, MD

HISTORIC PERSPECTIVE
ECONOMIC INCENTIVES AND LIABILITY RISKS
CONSULTING OPINIONS AND LIABILITY RISKS
LIABILITY FOR A BAD OUTCOME
ROLES AND RESPONSIBILITIES

The term *malpractice* refers to professional misconduct, defined as unreasonable lack of skill or fidelity in carrying out professional or fiduciary duties. Although the word *fiduciary* is most often associated with financial responsibilities, it actually refers to the duty of care one has when entrusted with something that belongs to another person. In the medical context it refers to the duty a physician has to a patient who has entrusted his/her medical care to a physician. The purpose of the medical malpractice lawsuit is to afford recovery for injuries suffered when physicians fail to exercise ordinary and reasonable care in the diagnosis and treatment of patients.[1] Lawsuits for patient care may also be brought on other grounds, including breach of confidentiality (in some states considered part of a medical malpractice claim, while in other states considered a separate cause of action), product liability, contract liability (failure to meet a promise or guarantee), or vicarious liability (liability for the acts of another under your supervision or control).

Negligence is the most common of the theories used to sue physicians. To succeed on under the theory of negligence, a plaintiff must establish by a preponderance of the evidence (greater than 50% likelihood) that the physician had a duty to the patient, that the physician breached that duty, and that the breach was the proximate cause of resulting injuries.

Usually, there is no dispute that a physician-patient relationship exists. When a patient accepts professional services rendered by a physician, the physician-patient relationship is established. No explicit agreement is required. In general, the relation-

[1] *Black's Law Dictionary, West Publishing Co., 5th Edition, 1979.*

ship does not exist until the physician sees the patient. However, an on-call physician who does not respond when called will likely be liable for any injury resulting to the patient who was in need of the physician's services. Moreover, if advice is given over a telephone or through other electronic means, the physician-patient relationship has most likely been established. Conversely, a relationship with the patient may not be established if the physician is simply consulted by another physician and the consulted physician never sees the patient or the patient's medical records and delivers no care or treatment.

Proving there is a breach of the applicable standard of care is a two-step process. First, the standard of care must be defined, then evidence must be defined, then evidence must be introduced to show that the physician's care fell below that standard. Competing plaintiff's and defendant's experts will assert what a reasonable physician under similar circumstances should have done for the patient. Authoritative texts and/or professional policies or standards may be used. Ultimately, it is the jury who will determine what evidence is more credible and whether a breach of the standard of care has been proven.

If a breach is found, the plaintiff must also prove that it was more likely than not that this breach caused the plaintiff's injuries. Legal causation is divided into two categories: cause-in-fact and proximate cause. Cause-in-fact merely means that injury would not have occurred "but for" the physician's negligence. Proximate cause means that the physician's negligence was a "substantial factor" in bringing about the patient's injuries. Expert testimony is again used to prove this element of negligence.

The final element of proof in the plaintiff's case is damages. Damages may include physical, financial, or emotional injury to the patient or his/her immediate family. The purpose of the damage award is to compensate the plaintiff for injury with payment of a monetary award. Punitive damages may be awarded if the facts show the negligence to be gross, or if malice, fraud, or wanton or intentional conduct is established. Punitive damages are not directly related to, or necessarily proportionate to, the injury suffered by the patient, but are intended to punish the defendant. In some states, damages have been capped in medical malpractice actions. There may be an overall cap on damages, or, more often, a cap on damages to compensate for pain and suffering, or a cap on punitive damages.

If a case proceeds to trial, a jury will decide whether the plaintiff has established all the elements of the case and what the damages are.

HISTORIC PERSPECTIVE

Before the 1950s, medical malpractice lawsuits were relatively rare. Between 1950 and 1960, they increased at a rate of 2% to 5% annually. A Congressional study reported the recent rate of annual increase in lawsuits against health care providers to be approximately 15%.[2] Another study showed that from 1981 to 1985 the

[2] *Continuing Medical Malpractice Insurance Crisis: Hearing before the Subcommittee on Health of the Community on Labor and Public Welfare, 94th Congress, 1st Session, 154, 220.*

number of medical malpractice lawsuits increased more than threefold. In 1985, the risk of being sued was 10.1 per 100 physicians, up from 3.2 per 100 physicians in 1981.[3] The risk of being sued has increased less dramatically in the 1990s, although large dollar claims have been increasing. For some specialists, the cost of insuring against malpractice claims may be as high as 25% of physician's income.[4]

Despite the growing number of claims, jury verdicts in the 1970s and 1980s favored physicians in almost 80% of cases. Many claims were settled before trial, but one third of cases filed were resolved without payment.[5] The positive trial results may have reflected a strong societal belief that physicians acted in the best interest of their patients and was evidence of the public's general trust in the medical profession. This attitude appears to be changing. Statistics show that physicians receive favorable jury verdicts in only 67% of cases, down 13% from earlier periods.

Traditionally, specialists, particularly surgeons, had a higher risk among physicians of being sued. However, as the market has increasingly shifted from fee-for-service medicine to managed care, liabilities appear to be shifting as well. A recent California study showed that between 1992 and 1995, lawsuits alleging failure to diagnose and treat were rising faster than any other category of claims. In 1995, failure to diagnose or treat claims comprised over one half of the large dollar claims, up from 34.6% in 1992. Further, indemnity payments were made on 42% of these claims, increasing from 33.5% in 1992.[6] These statistics coincide with a downturn in the number of inpatient days and the shift toward outpatient therapy.

A recent study conducted by the General Accounting Office to determine the frequency of claims further indicates that medical liability risks are shifting from the operating room to other areas of the hospital and clinic. The study showed that misdiagnosis and delay in diagnosis comprised the largest number of claims, 24.1%. Surgical complaints were the next most frequent, being alleged in 22.8% of claims. Inappropriate treatment claims followed with 16.6%. In terms of payments, failure to diagnose claims were the highest, comprising 28.5% of payments, outstripping obstetrics claims (traditionally, the highest), which comprised 26.9% of payments, and surgical claims, which comprised 21.5% of payments.[7] Still, the majority of incidents giving rise to claims, 80.5%, take place in the hospital, indicating the perioperative period remains a significant time of risk.

Changes in the economics of medicine and in medical technology may also be driving changes in risks. As more techniques are developed to minimize invasive procedures (e.g., laparoscopy, laser surgery, etc.), patients are being treated as outpatients and are being sent home with shorter hospital stays. These changes in technology, combined with managed care controls, which require approval of hospitalization,

....

[3] *Novik, Ruslan, "Medical Malpractice," st. edu/faculty/nielson/industry/med/med.htm (February 19, 1995).*

[4] *Id.*

[5] *St. Paul Insurance Company.*

[6] *Ron Neupauer, "1995 California Medical malpractice Large Loss Trend Study," Medical Underwriters of California.*

[7] *Novik, supra.*

length of stay, and diagnostic and therapeutic procedures, affect the ability of clinicians to assess a patient's condition before and after surgical procedures.

In examining changes in the liability risks of anesthesiologists, the effects of technologic changes, as well as changes in health care delivery systems, are evident. Traditionally, most claims against anesthesiologists were filed because of mortality during surgery. Today, because of changes in anesthesia practice, the risk of death has been significantly reduced. However, the overall risk of anesthesiologists has not changed. Rather, the number for claims for lack of informed consent, postoperative monitoring, and issues related to appropriate pain assessment and control have increased.[8] Communication has always been an essential risk management tool, but it generally was not considered important for the anesthesiologist who spent little time with a conscious patient. Today, however, all physicians, including anesthesiologists, are finding a need to spend more time communicating with patients and their insurers. At the same time, reimbursement is decreasing and managed care is funneling care to the least costly provider.

• Economic Incentives and Liability Risks

While the Federal government is at the center of many changes in the health care environment, the business community continues to exert a major influence. Increasing numbers of patients are being insured through managed care organizations. Concern is increasing that managed care, driven by cost containment goals, will limit or deny access to care for patients who would have benefited under a fee-for-service model.

Managed care organizations create both direct and indirect incentives to reduce the volume and levels of patient care. Under a capitated system, reimbursement increases when the physician meets targeted financial goals. Under other, less restrictive models, the incentives to limit care may not be as obvious, but they exist. For instance, as competition proliferates, a physician may be excluded from a managed care organization's provider network if the physician's utilization is higher than the managed care organization's projections, or if a physician challenges the organization's utilization review decisions too frequently or vehemently. As a result, the current health care delivery system creates incentives for a physician to think twice as to whether particular care is truly necessary. The system may inhibit care delivery, even though a physician believes the care is needed, regardless of where the patient falls in the economic projections of the managed care organization. As such, primary care physicians face increased risk of claims for failure to consult specialists, order needed diagnostic tests, or for sending a patient home too early.

Physician liability in the managed care setting arises in four contexts. First, a plaintiff may argue that managed care financial incentives create a motive for a physician to render inappropriate care. This argument may result in punitive damage awards. The second major area of risk is the failure to timely refer the patient to a specialist. Third, managed care has created a new duty for the physician to act as

[8] *Chase, Marilyn, "Health Journal," Wall Street Journal, June 24, 1996.*

an advocate on behalf of the patient. Fourth, there are issues of patient abandonment. Complaints of this type increase in situations in which the managed care organization, rather than the physician, is dictating when a patient is to be seen.

In general, liability risk for missed or delayed diagnosis, or inappropriate treatment, has rested with the physician alone. This is because federal ERISA laws have most often insulated the managed care organization from lawsuits claiming negligence.[9] However, lawyers have begun using agency theories to establish some liability on the part of the managed care organizations. The first case to establish the potential liability of an HMO arose in 1985 in California, *Wickline v. State of California.*[10] The lawsuit alleged that Medi-Cal was negligent in approving only 4 days of a requested 8-day hospital stay. The alleged premature discharge resulted in amputation of the patient's leg. The patient directed his/her anger at the managed care organization and did not sue the physician or the hospital. The jury returned a verdict in favor of the patient, but on appeal, the jury's verdict was overturned and the HMO was found not to be responsible as a matter of law. The court found that because the physician did not appeal the HMO's utilization review decision, the physician was solely responsible for the patient's injury.[11] However, the ruling left an opening in future cases for the physician to share liability with an HMO by having exhausted available appeals of the managed care organization's utilization review decision. This would effectively transfer the burden of negotiating coverage issues under the patient's insurance policy from the patient to the physician.

However, in the *Wickline* case, the physician was left solely liable for the decision to let the patient leave the hospital early and the resulting medical complication of an amputated leg. If the physician had appealed the utilization review decision of the HMO, then the issue of liability for the amputated leg could have gone to the jury for both the HMO and the physician. If the patient, chose to sue only the HMO, a jury verdict may have resulted in the HMO being solely liable. Without having fully appealed the reduced length of stay, the physician stood alone in the courtroom, leaving him solely responsible for the amputated leg, which may have been avoided by a longer hospital stay. In the words of the Court, a physician who "complies without protest with the limitations imposed by the third-party payor, when his medical judgment dictates otherwise, cannot avoid his ultimate responsibility for his patient's care."[12] *Wickline* was the first case to stand for the principle that a treating physician has a duty to appeal utilization-review decisions that are contrary to recommended treatment.

Subsequent to the *Wickline* decision was another California case, *Wilson v. Blue Cross of Southern California.*[13] In the *Wilson* case, parents sued Blue Cross alleging their son's suicide was caused by the company's utilization review decision to approve only a 10-day in-patient hospitalization stay, rather than the 3- to 4-week stay requested

[9] *29 U.S.C. 1144 (a).*

[10] *Wickline v. State of California, 192 Cal.App.3d 1630, 228 Cal.Rptr. 661 (1986).*

[11] *Id.*

[12] *Id.*

[13] *Wilson v. Blue Cross of Southern California, 222 Cal.App.3d 660, 271 Cal.Rptr. 876 (1990).*

by the boy's physician. The patient suffered from depression, drug dependence, and anorexia nervosa. Ultimately, the patient was discharged over the physician's explicit objection and committed suicide by drug overdose less than 3 weeks later. The trial court granted summary judgment in favor of Blue Cross stating that the company could not be held responsible, leaving the psychiatrist solely responsible. The trial court's decision was overturned on appeal. The appellate court cited *Wickline* stating: "[A] patient who requires treatment and who is harmed when care which should have been provided is not, should recover for the injury suffered from all those responsible for the deprivation of such care. . . ." The treating physician testified that had the patient completed his planned course of hospitalization, there was a reasonable probability that he would not have committed suicide. The appellate court remanded the case for trial by a jury. A jury, ultimately, found in favor of Blue Cross.[14] Precedent, however, was established for recovery from a managed care provider when the physician clearly objected to the utilization review decision and made attempts to appeal the decision. A physician's duty to make such appeals on behalf of the patient and to document those objections follows.

California courts were also the first to examine liability stemming from actions induced by financial incentives of a managed care provider. The premier case in this area of liability attacked the incentives given to the managed care company executives to deny coverage. In *Fox v. Health Net of California*, the estate of a breast cancer patient sued its managed care organization, Health Net, for refusal to pay for a bone marrow transplant, which the managed care organization deemed experimental.[15] Testimony at trial showed that the managed care organization had previously approved the procedure for two other women. Evidence showed the physician executive who decided to deny payment received bonuses based on denial of costly procedures. The jury concluded the managed care organization acted in bad faith, breached its contract, and committed intentional infliction of emotional distress. The jury awarded $89 million to the estate of the patient with $77 million being punitive damages.[16] The lesson to managed care companies was expensive. The case cautions against tying compensation to decisions to deny patient care.

A similar argument can be made as to why a physician under a capitated reimbursement plan sends a patient home early, fails to perform a diagnostic test, or fails to provide some other treatment. Incentives given to treating physicians can result in the same type of liability as the physician executives in the *Fox* case. The plaintiff's lawyer in the *Fox* case was the brother of the deceased patient. Since the success in the *Fox* case, his primary area of practice has become liabilities arising from managed care. A more recent case focused on the incentives to primary care providers to avoid referring a patient to a specialist. In this instance, a 33-year-old women went to her primary care physician complaining of severe stomach cramps. Despite repeated requests from the patient's husband to refer the patient to a specialist, the

[14] *Id.*

[15] *Fox v. Health Net of California, Case # 21962, Superior Court Riverside Co. Calif., January 1995.*

[16] *Id.*

primary care physician continued to follow the patient for 3 months. When the patient was finally referred to a gastroenterologist, the specialist diagnosed colon cancer within 24 hours. The patient died within 15 months. The husband brought suit against the primary care physician, including a request for punitive damages based on the financial incentives to the physician for delaying the referral. Although the jury returned a verdict in favor of the husband and against the primary care physician, the judge refused to allow the issue of financial incentives go to the jury, avoiding the potential for a large punitive damage award.[17] Risks leading to punitive damages are of added concern because, often, physician insurance policies exclude coverage of punitive damage awards, leaving the physician responsible for such damages.

The lesson, as in the *Fox* case, is that the physician must be careful when financial incentives are correlated with patient care, or lack thereof. Liability exposure may increase under such incentive plans. One way to lessen this exposure is to disclose financial incentives to the patient up front as part of the informed consent process. Some states are studying a statutory mandate that the consent process include disclosure of potential financial conflicts of interest. However, many physicians are reticent to disclose this information and may not even have such information readily available. A more general rule, is to ensure that the medical reasons for care, or a decision not to provide certain care, are carefully documented to show your focus on the patient's well being at the time care decisions are made.

In summary, in an era in which controlling the cost of medicine is central to the health care delivery system, it is critical that the physician be able to show that he/she exercised independent judgment. Should conflict arise between a physician and the managed care organization, the physician should advise the managed care organization of his/her medical judgment and document calls made to the company. The medical record should include a clear and succinct statement of why the requested care is necessary and the attempts to provide this information to the managed care organization. Appeal mechanisms of the managed care organization's utilization review decision should be exhausted when the physician believes the patient will suffer without the requested care. Documentation should include the name of the managed care personnel spoken to regarding approval of the requested care, with the dates of these contacts noted as well. The patient must be informed of the managed care organization's decision and the risks of not following the physician's recommended care. The physician's efforts to appeal the utilization review decision should also be noted to the patient. In cases in which the physician's provider contract with the managed care organization includes "gag rules" prohibiting adverse comments regarding the managed organization, it is critical such communications with the patient be simple, objective statements of fact.

If the patient decides to follow the decision of the managed care provider against the physician's advice, a request for assignment by the managed care organization of another physician should be considered. In the alternative, the physician should consider having the patient sign an informed refusal of care or an against medical

[17] *Ching v. Gaines, Ventura County Superior Court, November 1995.*

advice form. If the patient decides to follow the physician's recommendations for care, despite lack of approval from the managed care organization, the physician should, likewise, carefully document the basis for the care delivered, and consider obtaining a consultation to support the care decisions. The consultant should document his/her concurrence with the care recommendations also. The patient may wish to use this information to further contest coverage, or, perhaps, to provide a basis for the company's legal liability. In some instances, the patient may want to take the issue to the state insurance commission. Regardless, the physician's documentation will help protect him/her from liability should complications in care arise.

• CONSULTING OPINIONS AND LIABILITY RISKS

At the beginning of this chapter the significant liability risks of the surgeon were noted. Although the risk of lawsuits arising from surgery itself remains great, the perioperative period is a particularly risky time for a missed or delayed diagnosis. Claims for missed or delayed diagnosis have become more frequent than claims directly relating to surgery itself. Part of this increase is believed to be attributable to the managed care environment, where there are incentives to do fewer tests and keep patients in the hospital for fewer days. Patients often come to the hospital the day of the surgery with most of the preoperative assessment having taken place in the outpatient setting. The third-party payor is pushing to get the patient home after surgery and may be wary of approving payment for significant diagnostic procedures or additional lengths of stay. To support the request for more care, the primary physician turns to consultants for concurring opinions. The primary physician may also call a consultant to provide more specialized expertise for a particular medical problem. There are a variety of exposures that arise with the use of consultants. Defining the role of the consultant and the extent of his/her responsibility is sometimes difficult. These and other related issues are particularly important to perioperative medicine. When the consultant is called, the primary physician may decide to follow the advice of the consultant. If there is a resulting bad outcome, what is the liability of the primary physician versus that of the consultant? What is the liability when the consultant's advice is not followed, resulting in an adverse outcome?

The decision to request a consultation is one of personal judgment, but cases show that liability can result. One such case was a medical malpractice action in which the patient alleged she sustained an injury to her ulnar nerve during an operation to remove her right first rib and right cervical rib, resulting in a causalgia. The patient sustained her burden of proving malpractice on the part of the physicians for failing to secure a neurological consultation before making their decision to perform the operation, relying on testimony of a neurologist acting as the expert witness for the patient. This expert witness answered a hypothetical question, stating that he would have initially prescribed a regimen of physiotherapy rather than surgery, laying a foundation for the jury to find that had a neurology consult been requested, the patient would have been given an alternative to surgery. The patient successfully established that her ulnar nerve was negligently injured during the course of the operation. The jury returned a verdict in excess of $2 million in favor of the patient, which was upheld on appeal.[18]

The lesson in this case is that the informed consent discussion must include alternative care. This is especially the case if surgery carries significant risk. If a reasonable alternative to surgery is available, the physician should offer the patient a consult with a physician in that area of medicine: in this case, neurology.

In a second case, a 38-year-old mother of 4 children died as a result of a stroke following a hysterectomy when a blood clot traveled from the heart to a cerebral artery. The patient told the gynecologist that she was under the care of a cardiologist and had been given a thorough workup 12 days before the surgery. The patient stated her cardiologist had found her in good health and cleared her for an operation. However, the cardiologist never contacted the gynecologist, nor did the gynecologist contact the cardiologist or request an independent workup. Expert and fact witnesses (treating physician, pathologist) at the trial could not state whether the clot existed before surgery, nor whether it would, or could, have been detected before surgery. The patient's estate argued that the patient's gynecologist was negligent in not having obtained a consultation from a cardiologist to examine the patient within 24 hours before surgery. This time the jury did not find that the burden of proof had been met by the plaintiff, and instead, returned a verdict in favor of the physician.[19]

The central lesson is one of communication. In the first case, the missing link was a full and informed consent, which would have required a discussion of alternatives, including physiotherapy. In the second case, evidence showed that the patient was aware of potential cardiac problems and that they were discussed. However, as the treating physician one is responsible for assessing the patient's health and should not rely solely on a patient's own representation of health status. In this instance, the jury did not find the physician's negligence to be the proximate cause of the patient's death. If evidence of the presence of the clot before the surgery had existed, there would have been a basis for a jury to have connected the patient's death to the lack of a cardiac consultation, and, thus, a possibility of finding the physician negligent. The importance of doing an appropriate patient assessment with follow-up on particular risk factors before surgery cannot be overemphasized.

Likewise, after surgery, when a patient's health deteriorates for unexplained reasons or does not improve as anticipated, it is important to fully explore the reasons for the complications, including requesting reasonable consultations. However, once a consultation is requested, it is perilous to ignore the consultant's advice. The patient, or his/her legal surrogate decision-maker, must understand the opinions of the consultant as well as those of the primary physician, even if the primary physician does not recommend following the consultant's advice. Decision-making remains a patient right and the physician must ensure that the patient has information reasonably necessary to make fully informed decisions about his/her care.

....

[18] *Sternemann v. Langs, et. al., 460 NYS 2d 614 (1983).*

[19] *Bartley v. Pailet, MD, et. al., 527 So 2d 430 (LO. Ct. of App., 4th Cir., 1988).*

Although this is the general rule, it is sometimes difficult to establish the causal legal connection required allowing a plaintiff to recover from the primary physician. In one case, a 71-year-old patient had a history of a prior myocardial infarction (MI). He suffered from angina and debilitating rheumatoid arthritis. The patient was evaluated for elective left-knee replacement surgery. A preoperative electrocardiogram (ECG) was performed with two interpretations—one concluded the changes were "consistent with prior MI," the other concluded the changes were "more likely caused by an aneurysm." A decision was made to postpone surgery until a cardiac workup could be completed. This was done and the patient was admitted for surgery. A third cardiac consultant found no new changes in the latest ECG and stated that given the patient's history, the surgery posed a risk of another MI. Knee surgery was performed and 3 days later, the patient's left lower extremity was cold and without pulses. The defendant vascular surgeon determined the popliteal artery in the patient's left leg was occluded. The cardiologist saw the patient as he was complaining of shortness of breath and chest pain. After noting changes in the latest ECG, the cardiologist ordered the patient be transferred to the cardiac care unit. Instead, the vascular surgeon performed a thrombectomy to salvage the patient's leg. Two days later the patient suffered a cardiac arrest and died.

When this case went to trial, a summary disposition was granted in favor of the vascular surgeon; a directed verdict in favor of the cardiologist and hospital was granted after a jury trial. The patient's wife appealed, but the trial court's decision was upheld on appeal. The appellate court found that the evidence was insufficient to establish that the consulting cardiologist was negligent with respect to the care of a knee surgery patient where there was no evidence of standard of care or proximate cause. In this instance, the appellate court stated that it was the orthopedic surgeon's choice to follow or ignore the consulting physician's advice. The evidence was insufficient to prove the allegations of failure to diagnose an active MI, failure to consult with the patient's wife and advise her of the patient's status, and failure to place the diagnosis of peripheral vascular disease on the list of diagnoses, as reported by the consultant. On cross examination, the plaintiff's expert testified that he was not familiar with the standard of care for surgeons.[20]

The case represents the value of having excellent legal counsel. More importantly, the case is evidence of the parameters of a consultant's role and responsibility. It is not necessary that the primary physician follow the advice of the consultant, nor that the consultant communicate directly with the patient. What is required is that the primary physician take into account the opinions of the consultant and assure that the patient has information regarding all of the risks of care, including those identified by the consultant. In cases in which the patient is not informed by the primary physician of issues and/or recommendations of a consultant, a court may impose liability on the consultant for not ensuring that the patient was appropriately informed. As such, the consultant must inform the patient directly of his/her findings and/or recommendations, or follow-up with the primary attending to ensure the patient was told of the consultant's findings and/or recommendations.

[20] *Carlton v. St. John Hospital, et. al., 451 N.W.2d 543 (MI Ct. of App., 1990).*

LIABILITY FOR A BAD OUTCOME

Liability may also result directly from alleged injuries sustained during the preoperative or postoperative period. In the preoperative period, being able to show, through proper documentation, that an adequate work-up of the patient was done is essential. When this can be shown, a favorable outcome in the event of a lawsuit is likely. For example, a medical malpractice action was brought against a surgeon and an anesthesiologist on behalf of the children of a patient who died from complications caused by the anesthetic administered during a tonsillectomy. After striking claims against the surgeon, the District Court entered judgment in favor of the anesthesiologist. Subsequently, the court's decision was appealed and the Court of Appeals overturned the dismissal of claims against the surgeon, and the case was remanded for retrial. The Court of Appeals, however, upheld the decision of the lower court with respect to the anesthesiologist, finding evidence that supported the anesthesiologist did obtain an adequate history and medical evaluation, informed consent, and was not negligent in her choice of anesthetic.[21]

It is essential to perform and document a presurgical evaluation, reviewed in light of a full medical history. Clear evidence of this documentation is critical to proving a physician is not liable for a patient's bad outcome, which is a foreseeable risk of the surgery and use of anesthetics.

In a second case, a widow sued a cardiothoracic surgeon under the wrongful death and survival statute for improper treatment of her deceased husband. The patient had coronary bypass surgery performed and suffered a stroke postoperatively. He went into a coma and subsequently died. The plaintiff asserted that the physician was negligent in choosing a course of surgical treatment, rather than medical treatment. Again, the physician was successful in defending against malpractice allegations. The trial court entered a summary judgment for the physician and the case was upheld on appeal.[22]

The lesson is that documentation of the informed consent discussion with the patient, including a discussion of reasonable alternatives to surgery, is critical. Where such a discussion can be documented, together with an appropriate presurgical patient evaluation showing the patient's fitness for surgery, the ability to successfully defend a medical malpractice claim is increased significantly.

A third case exemplifies how a different result can occur. The children of a patient sued to recover for the death of their mother because of alleged medical malpractice on the part of the physician and hospital authority. The patient died following an elective gastroplasty. Both sides in the case agreed that the patient was not at high-risk for complications from this surgical procedure. According to the progress notes of the physician, the surgery was uneventful and the patient was taken to the recovery room. She responded normally during 3 hours of observation. Because the intensive care unit (ICU) was full and the patient was doing well, she was transferred to

[21] *Granado, et. al. V. Madsen, et. al., 720 S.W.2d 866 (TX. Ct. of App., 1987).*

[22] *Milkie v. Metni, M.D., 658 S.W. 2d 678 (TX. Ct. of App., 1983).*

her room rather than given an ICU bed. She subsequently suffered a cardiac arrest and lapsed into a coma. She was removed from life support and died.

The Superior Court entered summary judgment in the physician's favor, and the patient's children appealed. The Court of Appeals reversed, holding that an expert's opinion that the patient should have been kept in the ICU, rather than returned to her hospital room, raised material issues of fact as to negligence and proximate cause, precluding summary judgment.[23]

The lesson in this case can be viewed from several perspectives. As a general rule, if the physician changes his/her normal practice—i.e., sending the patient to his/her room rather than the ICU—the physician risks not being able to justify that the standard of care was met. This situation is complicated by hospital and reimbursement pressures to get the patient into the least costly environment. As discussed earlier in this chapter, defense of a physician becomes much more difficult when a bad outcome results. Instead, the physician should have explicit protocols for when a patient goes to his/her room versus when the patient is sent to the ICU. Isolated exceptions should be avoided, particularly if they come at a time when a hospital or physician is under obvious financial pressure.

Another example of liability risks in postoperative care can be seen in the case in which a patient suffered a fractured ankle in an automobile accident. The orthopedic surgeon had performed surgery without apparent complication. After visiting the patient one hour after the surgery, the surgeon left the hospital. The patient subsequently suffered a cardiac arrest, lapsed into a coma, and died within a few days. The plaintiff asserted that the physician failed to give proper postoperative orders, including failure to order monitoring of the patient's heart. According to the plaintiff's medical expert, this failure deviated from the accepted standards of medical practice and contributed to the decedent's demise. A jury decided in favor of the physician. However, on appeal, the Supreme Court held that the trial court erred in refusing to charge that the doctor's obligation included giving proper instructions to the hospital staff and seeing that his orders were carried out. The error was peculiarly prejudicial because the crux of the plaintiff's negligence theory was the *doctor's* failure to give proper instructions. The decision was reversed and remanded for a new trial.[24]

The lesson from this case is a fundamental one. The physician is generally considered responsible for patient care decisions. Assessment of the patient, and orders for appropriate monitoring and/or medications, are equally the responsibility of the physician. A physician cannot leave the patient in the care of nurses without giving a full assessment of the patient's condition and without ordering any special monitoring which may be required under the circumstances.

Finally, a third case involved a medical malpractice action brought against a nurse anesthetist and recovery-room nurse for the death of a 16-year-old girl. The patient was admitted for arthroscopic surgery of the left knee. The procedure was performed under general anesthesia administered by the nurse anesthetist. At the

[23] *Hooker v. Headley, 385 S.E.2d 732 (GA. Ct. of App., 1989).*
[24] *Lium v. Ploski, 449 N.Y.S. 2d 297 (S.Ct. N.Y., 1982).*

conclusion of the surgery, the patient was moved to the recovery room and was left in the care of the recovery room nurse. The patient went into cardiac arrest within 10 to 15 minutes after her arrival. She sustained severe brain damage, remained in a coma for 5 days and then died. The plaintiff's medical expert testified to the negligent behavior of the nurse anesthetist and recovery room staff. He stated that it was his opinion that the patient's death was caused by the negligent administration of anesthesia and by the failure on the part of the recovery room staff to adequately monitor the condition and initiate proper resuscitative measures. The trial judge granted the involuntary dismissal motion because he concluded that the plaintiff's cause of action was inadequately supported by expert testimony. He characterized the testimony as offering only a new opinion and excluded from evidence the report of an anesthesiologist consulted by the medical examiner in attempting to determine the cause of death. On appeal, the court found the physician's expert testimony established a *prima facie* case of negligence against the nurse anesthetist and the recovery room nurse, and also found that the anesthesiologist's report that was solicited and relied upon by the medical examiner to reach a final conclusion as to the cause of the patient's death, was admissible.[25]

The important lesson, again, is that the physician or nurse anesthetist is responsible not only for the administration of anesthesia, but for ensuring the patient's condition is stable after the surgery and that appropriate instructions have been given to the recovery room for monitoring. If the patient's condition is unstable, then the physician or nurse anesthetist has an obligation to remain with the patient or assure that someone equally trained is available to the patient. In many states, the physician may also be responsible for assessing the ability of the nurses and adequacy of the hospital facilities. In such cases, the physician's liability stems from his/her being found to be the "captain of the ship."

• ROLES AND RESPONSIBILITIES

Many of the cases examined depend on the role of the defendant physician and the responsibilities of that physician. The following example shows how difficult it can be to allocate responsibility when looking in hindsight, and the importance of clearly delineating roles at the outset of patient care.

In a hypothetical case, a 50-year-old female was admitted to the hospital in June 1994 for evaluation of progressive, bilateral lower extremity spasticity. A cervical myelogram on June 18th revealed spinal stenosis at C4-5 and C5-6. Cervical laminectomy was performed the same day with dural opening for disc exploration. The patient did well postoperatively, although she experienced tongue swelling, thought to be related to operative positioning. One day postoperatively, June 19th, the patient had significant bilateral upper extremity weakness. She complained of severe neck and head pain and earache and exhibited some mental status changes. Neurologic examination revealed bilateral positive Babinski's reflex. Laboratory studies

[25] *Pearson v. St. Paul, et.al., 531 A. 2nd 744 (N.J. Sup. Ct., 1987).*

revealed an increase in her white blood cell count (WBC) from 6,900 preoperatively to 26,500 by June 21st. Because of concern with her tongue swelling, she was transferred to the neurosurgical ICU for monitoring of her airway. On June 22nd, at roughly 6:30 am, the neurosurgery team made rounds and found the patient to have a good airway and an improved gait. The plan was to return the patient to the floor. The attending neurosurgeon then left town, and a second attending neurosurgeon was on call with a senior neurosurgery resident responsible for the patient. At approximately 8:30 am, the attending neurologist, acting as the ICU attending neurologist, was asked during morning rounds to examine the patient because the patient was agitated. The ICU attending neurologist and an ICU housestaff anesthesiologist found the patient attempting to get out of bed and pushing the nurses. The ICU attending neurologist asked the patient to stop this behavior and the patient responded by doing so. The ICU attending neurologist reviewed the patient chart and noted a history of alcohol use. The patient told the ICU attending neurologist that she had a history of alcohol abuse and stated that although she reported on admission that she had stopped drinking for 3 years, she had been drinking just before hospitalization. The ICU attending neurologist considered alcohol withdrawal to be the most likely explanation for the patient's agitation and recommended to the housestaff that Ativan be prescribed. The ICU attending neurologist did not see the patient again. However, during the afternoon of June 22nd, the patient became incoherent and ceased following commands. The ICU housestaff anesthesiologist made multiple calls to the senior neurosurgery resident to discuss performing a lumbar puncture (LP) to test for meningitis. The neurosurgery resident disagreed with the need for a lumbar puncture and declined the request for authority to perform it. At approximately 7:00 or 8:00 pm, the ICU housestaff neurologist called the ICU attending neurologist regarding the need for an LP. During this conversation, the ICU housestaff anesthesiologist was interrupted by a call from the chief neurosurgery resident who was responding to a page from the neurologist housestaff. After listening to the history presented by the housestaff anesthesiologist, the chief neurosurgery resident ordered a head computed tomography (CT) and, if not contraindicated, an LP. The LP was done some time after 11:00 pm on June 22 and was positive for pneumococcal meningitis. Antibiotics were started immediately. The patient required intubation on the morning of June 23rd, and following intubation, a head CT revealed cerebral edema. Intracranial pressure bolts were placed and mannitol administered. However, the patient died on June 23rd.

The question of who was ultimately responsible for the patient in the postoperative period is a central concern in determining liability. The on-call neurosurgeon had most likely not established a physician-patient relationship because he had never had any contact regarding the patient. As a result, he is not likely to have liability exposure, although he may have to struggle through a number of legal proceedings before being dismissed. The question of vicarious responsibility of the attending neurosurgeon for the acts or omissions of his residents and the responsibility of the ICU attending neurologist's responsibilities for ICU patients is not clear, and presents potential liability exposure. Overall, liability in the case is clear, and the matter may be best resolved through settlement. Most importantly, this hypothetic case stands as clear testament to the need to establish the roles and responsibilities of each member of the patient's health care provider team up front, before care is delivered. This helps minimize liability, but more importantly, helps ensure that the patient gets needed care in a timely manner.

In many respects, the liability aspects of medicine have become more complex. Determining responsibilities and ferreting out various incentives and disincentives to provide appropriate care is not always easy. Because medicine is able to perform more and technical miracles, the risks of complications during the perioperative period may lead to increases in claims. The need to carefully assess a patient before surgery and closely monitor a patient after surgery cannot be underestimated. The liability risks that follow for failure to do so have been evident in the wide variety of cases examined in this chapter. Documentation of patient care and good patient communication remain central to minimizing these risks. Lawsuits can sometimes result, regardless of the care provided, but most often, these claims can be successfully defended with support from qualified medical experts and excellent legal counsel.

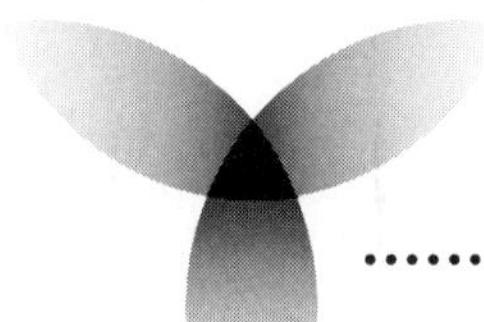

Chapter 48

General Management Issues

William T. Ross, Jr, MD, MBA

Central to the practice of perioperative medicine is the delivery of demanding phases of medical care; especially those involving the timely application of appropriate, often highly technical, aspects of care. Some examples of this are the accurate evaluation and planning for perioperative care of patients with complex medical and surgical disease; the coordination of elements of perioperative care provided by a variety of health care providers; and timely, effective communication with and education of perioperative patients so they can understand the progress of treatment and be able to work with health care providers throughout the perioperative encounter. Characteristically perioperative care involves the application of 'high-tech' tools, techniques, and personnel in circumstances requiring special vigilance. The tools available to perioperative physicians include the full range of pharmaceuticals, monitoring, and life-support techniques and, perhaps, most importantly, a broad understanding of normal and abnormal pathology, physiology, and pharmacology. Perioperative medicine can be characterized by the integration of the elements of highly sophisticated care into a system of care for individual patients.

Because of the highly specialized nature of perioperative medicine, its practitioners have tended to minimize or disregard its relationship to other elements in the health care arena. Increasingly, patients seeking medical care find it in a framework in which they or their employers have contracted, for example a managed care organization (MCO), to provide their care in return for prepaid fees. The MCO, in turn, may use or contract with health care providers to actually deliver care to patients in ways structured to reduce the MCO's costs of providing that care. Such schemes may have primary physicians function as "gatekeepers" to control referral of patients to sources of specialized care. Typically, practitioners of perioperative medicine work downstream from gatekeepers, and although they will be affected by MCO rules and practice patterns, the effects are indirect and somewhat remote in their minds. One must never lose sight of the fact that perioperative medicine is practiced in a larger environment. Perioperative medicine cannot exist in isolation from other branches of health care, but it does have its unique characteristics. It will have to clearly describe what its work is, what its results are, and what its costs are to effectively participate in the restructuring of health care now underway.

• MEDICINE AND THE MARKETPLACE

Those who practice perioperative medicine need to have a working understanding of the relationship of their practice to the overarching medical marketplace. In the 1980s and 1990s those paying for health care (increasingly these have been purchasers of care for large groups of patients) focused on reducing the costs of providing care to patients. Compared to reimbursement before the 1980s, this has had the effect of shifting the risk of higher costs from payers (largely insurers and an ever-decreasing fraction of patients paying for their own health care) to providers (practitioners and facilities). This shift has delivered alarming, even threatening, messages to providers, and particularly to practitioners who were never equipped by their education, training, or experience to deal with such issues. It is not surprising that such a threat to the general status quo and to their incomes, in particular, evokes expressions of anger and hostility.

Some of the current discord between providers and MCOs arises from a lack of mutually acceptable valuation of clinical activities because health care is not delivered under free-market circumstances. The discord becomes more understandable considering the effect of intermediaries and other competing interests involved in the care of patients. Intermediaries include insurers, employers, health maintenance organizations (HMOs) and MCO's. Other interests include patients, facilities, health care providers, MCOs payers, managers, accrediting organizations, regulators, legislators, and society at large (i.e., "The Public"). Each of these interests has its own priorities, terminology and jargon, and until recently, have tended to function relatively independently from one another. The ability of providers to make any possible care available to patients and to pass escalating costs back to insurers or employers is being severely limited by the advent of managed care.

Since the 1980s, payer reviews of the work of health care providers have demanded more and more documentation of the care rendered. Providers are being required to maintain and furnish documentary evidence of the charges they give for the services they have provided. The consequence of these trends has been a great effort to document various elements of care. The documentation required by third-party payers is tested by audits of patients' medical records and by reconciling items on patient bills with entries found in the medical record. Failure of the medical record to support billings to federal medical programs has resulted in threats of prosecution of health care providers for fraud. These have resulted in multimillion dollar settlements in the form of refunds from providers to the government. It is clear that absence of documentation will be taken as evidence that a service, or one of its components, was not provided. There is, seemingly, no way for health care providers to function in the evolving health care arena without making substantial investments in systems and personnel to assure compliance with the documentation requirements of MCOs and other payers. While such documentation of the work they perform is a change from the past business practices of health care organizations, it needs to be clearly recognized that business practices of traditional health care organizations have seriously lagged behind those of most other enterprises in the United States. As providers acquire such expertise, the possibility exists that opportunities will develop allowing providers to bring their own expertise into discussions with the payers, thereby, permitting more effective dialogues regarding the structure of systems of care for patients.

A polarizing concern in approaching the evaluation of health care outcome has been the contrasting of quality of care issues (how good is the product) with cost containment as a central goal of payers. A primer describing the present (1996) state of the debate about quality of care in medicine is contained in a series of six articles and an editorial recently published in the *New England Journal of Medicine.*

Over the last decade the realization that control of costs can work to conserve assets available to facilities and to providers has become generally understood to be a source of benefit to patients (e.g., better care at a lower price), providers (e.g., greater profit—or retained net income), and payers (e.g., lower expenditures to meet contractual obligations to their enrollees). Net income or profit for facilities, providers and organizations is the excess of revenue over expenses (expenses are generically referred to as "costs"). Profits are available to the owners (shareholders) of an entity, a portion of which may be distributed as dividends. In the case of "not for profit" organizations (e.g., some hospitals) owners traditionally do not share in profits. Such organizations have emphasized providing services, rather than maximizing income, and have used retained net income in greater measure to further the work of the organization. It is this shift of health care providers away from a "not for profit/service" position toward a "for profit" position, that has led to much of the present confusion, even hostility, in today's health-care delivery arena.

• MANAGING QUALITY: STRUCTURE, PROCESS, AND OUTCOME

The 1990s have seen a groundswell of interest in defining and measuring quality of care. Before this, the professional judgment of physicians was accepted as the standard by which quality was defined. Now, purchasers of health care are requiring providers to describe the quality of the health care services they will provide. The result of this has become apparent in several areas. For years, Medicare and most states have required accreditation of hospitals and ambulatory surgical centers by a nationally recognized accrediting organization as a prerequisite to reimbursement under the Medicare program. Much of the data formerly collected for such reviews has been based largely on administrative or billing data, and lacked clinical details. Currently, a number of sophisticated tools for measuring quality of care are available.

Health care facilities are increasingly required to be evaluated by one of several accrediting agencies, including the Joint Commission for the Accreditation of Hospital Organizations (JCAHO) and the Accreditation Association for Ambulatory Health Care (AAAHC). These are generally independent organizations developed to evaluate and report on the quality of health care facility organizations. Most have developed in response to a perceived need by the facilities to provide benchmarks, by which to assess their quality of care, and to provide data for broad quality comparisons between facilities. In most instances the accrediting organizations have, over time, moved toward a status, independent from the facilities they evaluate. They are now supported by fees they charge for evaluative site visits (2 days and $4000 for an accreditation visit to an ambulatory surgical facility, compared to $50,000 and 5 days for a visit to a large tertiary care hospital), sales of educational and "how to" materials, and by support from outside sources, including philanthropic grants.

The reviewing organizations examine structure and process of a facility undergoing an accreditation review during a site visit. Most of the data is obtained by reviewing the facility's bylaws, medical records, and by comparison of the facility's documentation of its actual process with its stated process as contained in its policy and procedure manuals. Historically, accreditation reviews have consisted of information review recorded in the course of caring for patients, and using that as a proxy for direct, continuing observation of process.

Those involved in providing for the care of patients, including perioperative care, should be acquainted with the way health care delivery organizations are being evaluated. In the aggregate, large health care organizations provide care for millions of people. Thus, the pressure and the effort expended to objectively describe the quality of the care they provide is enormous. Tools available to evaluate the performance of these organizations are relatively new and continue to be critiqued and undergo further development. The National Committee for Quality Assurance (NCQA), formed in 1979 by managed-care trade groups, was strengthened in 1995 when it appeared that the Department of Health and Human Services would move to monitor health plans at the federal level. The National Committee for Quality Assurance has developed the Health Plan Employer Data and Information Set (HEDIS), an instrument to collect, standardize, and measure the performance of MCOs. The present edition of HEDIS (version 2.5) contains 60 performance indicators, only two of which measure a health outcome. Version 3.0 of HEDIS has been released in draft form and includes additional performance measures and more outcome indicators. However, the draft fails to assess how plans will address serious illness.

Yet, HEDIS appears to be the major instrument available to evaluate MCOs and their requests for NCQA accreditation based on it, are rapidly increasing. It would appear that NCQA accreditation is directed mainly at an assessment of quality near the time plan participants (patients) approach the plan for an episode of care. The result is that to the extent that health care is being assessed, it will be assessed at the level of the primary physicians (gatekeepers). Thus, perioperative care will not be directly assessed by instruments such as HEDIS. This will leave patients with serious illness and who require a greater intensity of care (including, but not limited to perioperative care) to have their quality of care assessed by other mechanisms.

Perioperative physicians should view this as an opportunity to objectively assess their own work.

Recent reports indicate that managed care targets healthier, hence, less costly, patients to receive low-cost preventive interventions, leading to favorable responses to patient-satisfaction surveys. Some reports have documented disproportionate enrollments of healthy patients by managed-care health plans. Perioperative medicine should address such concerns. We should vigorously seek opportunities to study and report not only the direct results of care of the perioperative patient, but particularly longer-term ("downstream") outcomes. From a pragmatic position, we should seek opportunities to personally interact with patients in ways that are seen as helpful, friendly, supportive and lead to an increased public awareness of our roles and capabilities. We need to show that the care we provide is valuable and communicate that idea beyond the operating room.

• PROCESS AND OUTCOME

Elements of quality of care may be divided into widely accepted categories of structure, process, and outcome. Structural information describes the characteristics of facilities or practitioners (e.g., ownership of an ambulatory surgical center or a physician's specialty). Process data describe the characteristics of encounters between practitioners and patients (e.g., steps taken in the course of making a diagnosis). Outcome data describe the patient's subsequent health status (e.g., increased exercise tolerance following coronary bypass surgery). The relative contributions made individually by structure, process, and outcome to quality of care have no constant relation, but Brook, McGlynn, and Cleary have advanced the notion that both process and outcome measures can provide valid information concerning the quality of care. They view process measures as more sensitive measures of quality than outcome measures.

Consider an outcome study to examine the issue of requiring patients to be NPO before surgery. Since the incidence of aspiration in modern anesthetic practice is low (less than 1 in 10,000 pediatric anesthetics), a sample in excess of 100,000 anesthetics would be required to establish norms. Additional larger samples would be required to examine the effects of any interventions on this incidence. In circumstances in which the incidence of the condition being examined is greater than in the previous example (a few percent, for example), the utility of outcome studies becomes more practical.

Now consider a method that uses process criteria to evaluate quality of care. The specific process used to minimize the incidence of aspiration of gastric contents would have to have been previously validated using scientific evidence and/or clinical judgment. If the validation determined that patients who fasted in excess of 4 hours were at low risk of aspiration during anesthesia, a criterion could be established that defined excellent care if 98% of surgical patients were fasted for more than 4 hours, and average care if 94% of surgical patients were fasted for more than 4 hours. These explicit expectations could then be applied to clinical practice to test the level of preoperative care being provided. The evaluation of process is often easier to conduct and less costly in terms of size of samples, and of time to completion. Data from such process studies extended over time can be applied relatively easily to clinical settings.

A number of techniques to evaluate process and outcome have been described and additional instruments have been devised to assess the quality of care delivered by facilities and MCOs. An in-depth discussion is beyond the scope of this chapter, but discussions providing additional detail are listed in the bibliography.

STANDARDIZING DEFINITIONS

Progress toward the development of conceptual frameworks, within which perioperative patient care may be evaluated, requires that each term and circumstance surrounding perioperative care be unambiguously defined. The work of developing definitions of the elements of care is crucial to the development of databases recording events related to patient care. Only with clear, consistently defined data can information from different sources be merged or compared.

In describing the utilization of surgical facilities, Brown used eight primary times to record readily identified sentinel events occurring during the operative care of patients (e.g., time of day a patient entered the operating room, time of day anesthetic care began, time of day anesthetic induction was complete, time of day the incision was made, etc.). He then used differences between pairs of these sentinel events to determine various intervals during the care of surgical patients (e.g., anesthesia-preparation time is the difference between the time anesthetic induction was completed and the time anesthetic care began). Ratios (and other computations) using these time intervals and other time intervals, such as the time a given operating room is staffed and available for the care of patients, permits the calculation of derived values, such as the percent utilization, used in measuring the utilization of surgical facilities. In 1996, the Association of Anesthesia Clinical Directors published and widely distributed a glossary defining procedural times and terms useful in describing and managing the flow of patients through operating rooms.

The goal of outcome research is to fill gaps in medical knowledge and to direct practitioners to the best courses of action for their patients. The study of the outcome of a particular intervention offers an opportunity to define the range of results produced. The prospective definition of the question(s) to be answered is crucial to the power of outcome studies. Results of interventions may be clinical (e.g., a change in hemoglobin following treatment of pernicious anemia with vitamin B_{12}) or economic (e.g., wage and salary income of patients in the second year following different coronary revascularization procedures). Increasingly, these results are from perspectives extending beyond the strictly technical assessment of the success of a medical intervention (e.g., a surgical procedure removed a diseased organ). This is not intended to imply that physicians deliberately make decisions not in their patients' best interest, given the information currently at hand. It does emphasize a need for health care providers to seek, more broadly, the downstream effects of treatments they provide. Research into patient outcome is undergoing fundamental shifts in design, analysis, and importance with respect to validation of (or failure to validate) systems of health care.

CONCLUSION

Perioperative physicians have the task of deciding when to focus on outcome and when to focus on process issues. Clinical outcome studies have tended to be smaller and more narrowly focused than examination of process. Involvement in process change demands that perioperative physicians interact with other interests in the total system of health care. A systems approach to the organization of health care can provide opportunities for contributions from many disciplines to broadly applicable programs of perioperative care. Ultimately, systems of perioperative care will develop, having general applicability not limited to particular institutions or reimbursement schemes. To participate in and to contribute to these developments, perioperative physicians need to find a voice and reach beyond local, time-limited issues.

BIBLIOGRAPHY

Angell M, Kassirer JP: Quality and the medical marketplace—following elephants, *N Engl J Med* 335:883–885, 1996.

Bartling AC: Trends in managed care, *Healthcare Exec* 6-11, March/April 1995.

Berwick DM: Part 5: payment by capitation and the quality of care, *N Engl J Med* 335:1227–1231, 1996.

Blumenthal D: Part 1: quality of care—what Is it? *N Engl J Med* 335:891–893, 1996.

Blumenthal D: Part 4: the origins of the quality of care debate, *N Engl J Med* 335:1146–1149, 1996.

Blumenthal D, Epstein AM: Part 6: the role of physicians in the future of quality management, *N Engl J Med* 335:1328–1331, 1996.

Bodenheimer T: The HMO backlash—righteous or reactionary? *N Engl J Med* 335:1601–1604, 1996.

Brook RH, McGlynn EA, Cleary PD: Part 2: measuring quality of care, *N Engl J Med* 335:966–970, 1996.

Brown ACD: Computer management of operating room time information with proposed standard definitions for the measurement of utilization. In Blum BL, editor: *Proceedings of the Sixth Annual Symposium on Computer Applications in Medical Care*, Computer Society Press, Los Alamitos, CA, 1982.

Chassin MR: Part 3: improving the quality of care, *N Engl J Med* 335:1060–1063, 1996.

Davenport TH: Managing in the new world of process, *Public Productivity and Management Review* 18:133–147, 1994.

Donham RT, Mazzei WJ, Jones RL: Glossary of times used for scheduling and monitoring of diagnostic and therapeutic procedures, *Am J Anesthesiol* 23(suppl 5):2–12, 1996.

Fendrick AM, et al: Understanding the behavioral response to medical innovation, *Am J Man Care* 2:793–799, 1996.

Finkler S: The distinction between cost and charges, *Ann Inter Med* 96:102–109, 1992.

Iglehart JK: The national committee for quality assurance, *N Engl J Med* 335:995–999, 1996.

Johnson EA: The public's future perspective on managed care, *Health Care Manage Rev* 20(2):45–47, 1995.

Kassirer JP: The new health care game, *N Engl J Med* 335:433, 1996.

Klock PA, Roizen MF: More or better—educating the patient about the anesthesiologist's role as perioperative physician, *Anesth Analg* 83:671–672, 1996.

Macario A, et al: Where are the costs in perioperative care? analysis of hospital costs and charges for inpatient surgical care, *Anesthesiology* 83:1138–1144, 1995.

Moskowitz DB: Managed care: the third generation, *Chief Exec* 12–17, Jan/Feb 1996.

Orkin FK: Meaningful cost reduction—penny wise, pound foolish, *Anesthesiology* 83:1135–1137, 1995.

Pollard JB, Zboray AL, Mazze RI: Economic benefits attributed to opening a preoperative evaluation clinic for outpatients, *Anesth Analg* 83:407–410, 1996.

Ware JE, et al: Differences in 4-year health outcomes for elderly and poor, chronically ill patients treated in HMO and fee-for-service systems, *JAMA* 276:1039–1047, 1996.

Zvara DA, et al: The importance of the postoperative anesthetic visit: do repeated visits improve patient satisfaction or physician recognition? *Anesth Analg* 83:793–797, 1996.

Index

D

Q

R